Flow Cytometry in Neoplastic Hematology

This fourth edition presents an updated and expanded text and illustrations to reflect continued morphologic, immunophenotypic, and especially molecular advances in the field of neoplastic hematology, mostly due to the rapidly expanding application of next-generation sequencing. Those advances not only allow a more reliable diagnosis of the majority of tumors and identification of early changes such as monoclonal B-cell lymphocytosis or clonal hematopoiesis of indeterminate potential (CHIP), but also in many cases identify mutations or phenotypic changes in tumors that can be targeted by mutation-specific or antigen-specific drugs.

This edition incorporates the updated WHO classification of hematopoietic tumors and new immunophenotypic and molecular markers to provide a thorough pathologic overview of hematologic neoplasms while focusing on flow cytometric features. Special emphasis has been put on hematological neoplasms with crucial clinical significance such as acute promyelocytic leukemia, other acute leukemias, and difficult areas in flow cytometry. Flow cytometric features in AML, MDS, CMML, CLL, and measurable residual disease were significantly expanded. There are many new comparative tables, illustrations, and diagrams of algorithmic approaches.

Wojciech Gorczyca, MD, PhD, is Director of Flow Cytometry/Hematopathology at Bioreference Laboratories, OPKO Health Companies, Elmwood Park, New Jersey, USA. His many publications include *Atlas of Differential Diagnosis in Neoplastic Hematopathology, Fourth Edition,* and *Cytogenetics, FISH and Molecular Testing in Hematologic Malignancies.*

From the reviews of the previous edition: "The third edition of this book is a valuable addition... comprehensive... clearly written, well illustrated and supported by extensive references... Since there is a great deal of detailed information, it will serve as a useful reference for immunophenotyping laboratories as well as being an educational tool for others."

—Barbara J. Bain, *British Journal of Haematology*

Flow Cytometry in Neoplastic Hematology

Morphologic-Immunophenotypic-Genetic Correlation

Fourth Edition

Wojciech Gorczyca, MD, PhD
Director of Flow Cytometry/Hematopathology
Bioreference Laboratories, OPKO Health Companies
Elmwood Park, New Jersey, USA

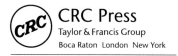

CRC Press
Taylor & Francis Group
Boca Raton London New York

CRC Press is an imprint of the
Taylor & Francis Group, an **informa** business

Fourth edition published 2023
by CRC Press
6000 Broken Sound Parkway NW, Suite 300, Boca Raton, FL 33487-2742
and by CRC Press

4 Park Square, Milton Park, Abingdon, Oxon, OX14 4RN

CRC Press is an imprint of Taylor & Francis Group, LLC

© 2023 Wojciech Gorczyca

Library of Congress Cataloging-in-Publication Data

Names: Gorczyca, Wojciech, 1959- author.
Title: Flow cytometry in neoplastic hematology : morphologic-immunophenotypic-genetic correlation / Wojciech Gorczyca.
Description: Fourth edition. | Boca Raton : CRC Press, 2023. | Includes bibliographical references and index.
Identifiers: LCCN 2022032059 (print) | LCCN 2022032060 (ebook) | ISBN 9781032055251 (hardback) | ISBN 9781032055268 (paperback) | ISBN 9781003197935 (ebook)
Subjects: MESH: Hematologic Neoplasms--diagnosis | Flow Cytometry | Leukemia, Lymphoid--diagnosis | Leukemia, Myeloid, Acute--diagnosis
Classification: LCC RC280.H47 (print) | LCC RC280.H47 (ebook) | NLM WH 525 | DDC 616.99/418--dc23/eng/20220817
LC record available at https://lccn.loc.gov/2022032059
LC ebook record available at https://lccn.loc.gov/2022032060

ISBN: 978-1-032-05525-1 (hbk)
ISBN: 978-1-032-05526-8 (pbk)
ISBN: 978-1-003-19793-5 (ebk)

DOI: 10.1201/9781003197935

Typeset in Warnock Pro
by KnowledgeWorks Global Ltd.

To my wife Elżbieta, my daughters, Marta, Ewa, and Małgorzata, and my grandchildren,
Emily and Kaiden, with love.

To my teachers in pathology, cytopathology, flow cytometry, and hematopathology,
Late Professor S. Woyke, Professor W. Olszewski, Late Dr. Z. Darzynkiewicz, and Dr. J. Weisberger.

CONTENTS

Contents

PREFACE

This fourth edition presents an updated and expanded text and illustrations to reflect continued morphologic, immunophenotypic, and especially molecular advances in the field of neoplastic hematology, mostly due to the rapidly expanding application of next-generation sequencing. Those advances not only allow a more reliable diagnosis of the majority of tumors and identification of early changes such as monoclonal B-cell lymphocytosis or clonal hematopoiesis of indeterminate potential (CHIP), but also in many cases identify mutations or phenotypic changes in tumors that can be targeted by mutation-specific or antigen-specific drugs.

This edition incorporates the updated WHO classification of hematopoietic tumors and new immunophenotypic and molecular markers to provide a thorough pathologic overview of hematologic neoplasms while focusing on flow cytometric features. Special emphasis has been put on hematological neoplasms with crucial clinical significance such as acute promyelocytic leukemia, other acute leukemias, and difficult areas in flow cytometry. Flow cytometric features in AML, MDS, CMML, CLL, and measurable residual disease were significantly expanded. There are many new comparative tables, illustrations, and diagrams of algorithmic approaches.

I would like to thank Robert Peden and the entire editorial office of CRC Press/Taylor & Francis Group for their help and support. I am also very grateful to my colleagues and co-workers at Bioreference Laboratories, especially all the hematopathologists (Drs. L. Alexa, D. Buzaid, S. Cote, L. Feldman, Y. Fan, P-S. Lee, Y. Pang, R. Persad, J. Talwar, and J. Weisensel), Maria Pawlik, former manager of Flow Cytometry Laboratory, and the whole flow cytometry department (D. Gusciora, H. Baybagan, R. Gurango, J. Rana, E. Gutowska, J, Hernandez, S. Salem and P. Patal).

Wojciech Gorczyca, MD, PhD
Director, Flow Cytometry/Hematopathology
Bioreference Laboratories, OPKO Health Companies
Elmwood Park, New Jersey, USA
November 2021

ABBREVIATIONS

AA	aplastic anemia
aCML	atypical chronic myeloid leukemia MDS/MPN with neutrophilia
AEL	acute erythroid leukemia
AITL	angioimmunoblastic T-cell lymphoma (nodal TFH cell lymphoma, angioimmunoblastic type)
ALCL	anaplastic large cell lymphoma
ALIP	abnormal localization of immature precursors
ALK	anaplastic lymphoma kinase
ALL	acute lymphoblastic leukemia
AML	acute myeloid leukemia
AMML	acute myelomonocytic leukemia
AML-MRC	acute myeloid leukemia with myelodysplasia-related changes
APL	acute promyelocytic leukemia
APL-v	acute promyelocytic leukemia, hypogranular variant
APMF	acute panmyelosis with myelofibrosis
ARCH	age-related clonal hematopoiesis
ATLL	adult T-cell lymphoma/leukemia
AUL	acute undifferentiated leukemia
B-ALL	B-cell acute lymphoblastic leukemia
BCL1	B-cell lymphoma 1 (cyclin D1) protein encoded by CCND1 gene
BCL2	B-cell lymphoma 2 apoptosis regulating protein encoded by BCL2 gene
BCR	breakpoint cluster region gene
BL	Burkitt lymphoma
BM	bone marrow
BP	blast phase
BPDCN	blastic plasmacytoid dendritic cell neoplasm
BRAF	v-raf murine sarcoma viral oncogene homolog B1
C-ALCL	cutaneous anaplastic large cell lymphoma
CBF	core binding factor
CBL-MZ	clonal B-cell lymphocytosis of marginal zone origin
CCUS	clonal cytopenia of unknown significance
CD	cluster designation
CEL	chronic eosinophilic leukemia
cFL	classic follicular lymphoma
cHL	classic Hodgkin lymphoma
CHIP	clonal hematopoiesis of indeterminate potential
CHOP	clonal hematopoiesis with oncogenic potential
CLL	chronic lymphocytic leukemia
CLPD-NK	chronic lymphoproliferative disorder of NK-cells
CML	chronic myeloid leukemia (BCR-ABL1+)
CMML	chronic myelomonocytic leukemia
CMR	complete molecular response
CNL	chronic neutrophilic leukemia
CP	chronic phase
DH	double hit
DLBCL	diffuse large B-cell lymphoma

EATL	enteropathy-associated T-cell lymphoma
EBV	Epstein-Barr virus
EBER	Epstein-Barr virus early RNA
EMT	extramedullary myeloid tumor
ENKTL	extranodal NK/T-cell lymphoma, nasal type
ET	essential thrombocythemia
ETP-ALL	early T-cell precursor ALL
FC	flow cytometry
FISH	fluorescence in situ hybridization
FITC	fluorescein isothiocyanate
FL	follicular lymphoma
FSC	forward scatter
FTCL	follicular T-cell lymphoma
GPI	glycosylphosphatidylinositol
HGBL, NOS	high grade B-cell lymphoma, not otherwise specific
HGBL-R	high grade B-cell lymphoma with rearrangement of MYC and BCL2 (and/or BCL6), double (or triple) hit lymphoma
H&E	hematoxylin and eosin
HCL	hairy cell leukemia
HCL-v	hairy cell leukemia variant
HL	Hodgkin lymphoma
HLH	hemophagocytic lymphohistiocytosis
HSTL	hepatosplenic T-cell lymphoma
IgG4-RD	immunoglobulin G4 related disease
IGVH	immunoglobulin heavy-chain variable gene
ISFN	In situ follicular neoplasia
iso	isochromosome
IVLBCL	intravascular large B-cell lymphoma
JAK2	Janus kinase 2
FLBL	follicular large B-cell lymphoma
LBL	lymphoblastic lymphoma
LGL	large granular lymphocyte
L-NN-MCL	leukemic non-nodal mantle cell lymphoma
LPL	lymphoplasmacytic lymphoma
LyG	lymphomatoid granulomatosis
LyP	lymphomatoid papulosis
MALT	mucosa associated lymphoid tissue
MBL	monoclonal B-cell lymphocytosis
MCL	mantle cell lymphoma
MDS	myelodysplastic neoplasm
MDS-IB	myelodysplastic neoplasm with increased blasts
MDS-LB	myelodysplastic neoplasm with low blasts
MDS-SF3B1	myelodysplastic neoplasm with SF3B1 mutation
MDS/MPN-N	MDS/MPN with neutrophilia (previously classified as aCML)
MF	mycosis fungoides
MGUS	monoclonal gammopathy of undetermined significance
MEITL	monomorphic epitheliotropic intestinal T-cell lymphoma
MPAL	mixed phenotype acute leukemia

MPL	myeloproliferative leukemia virus oncogene	**Post-PV-MF**	post polycythemia vera myelofibrosis
MPN	myeloproliferative neoplasm	**Pre-PMF**	prefibrotic primary myelofibrosis (early primary myelofibrosis)
MPO	myeloperoxidase	**PV**	polycythemia vera
MRD	measurable (minimal) residual disease	**PTCL**	peripheral T-cell lymphoma
MUM1	multiple myeloma 1 (oncogene)	**PTCL-TFH**	peripheral T-cell lymphoma with follicular T-helper phenotype
MZL	marginal zone B-cell lymphoma	**PTFL**	pediatric type follicular lymphoma
NHL	non-Hodgkin lymphoma	**RARA**	retinoic acid receptor a gene
NK	natural killer	**SBLPN**	splenic B-cell lymphoma/leukemia with prominent nucleoli
NLPHL	nodular lymphocyte predominant Hodgkin lymphoma	**SDRPL**	splenic diffuse red pulp small B-cell lymphoma
NMZL	nodal marginal zone lymphoma	**SLL**	small lymphocytic lymphoma
NPM	nucleophosmin gene	**SM**	systemic mastocytosis
NSE	nonspecific esterase	**SMZL**	splenic marginal zone lymphoma
PCFCL	primary cutaneous follicle center lymphoma	**SPCM**	smoldering plasma cell myeloma
PGD-TCL	primary cutaneous γδ T-cell lymphoma	**SPTCL**	subcutaneous panniculitis-like T-cell lymphoma
PCM	plasma cell myeloma	**SS**	Sézary's syndrome
PCR	polymerase chain reaction	**SSC**	side scatter
PD1	programmed death 1	**T-ALL**	T-cell acute lymphoblastic leukemia
PDC	plasmacytoid dendritic cell	**TFH**	T follicular helper (cell)
PDGFRA	alpha-type platelet-derived growth factor receptor gene	**THRLBL**	T-cell/histiocyte-rich large B-cell lymphoma
PDGFRB	beta-type platelet-derived growth factor receptor gene	**TCR**	T-cell receptor
PE	phycoerythrin	**TdT**	terminal deoxynucleotidyl transferase
PEL	primary effusion lymphoma	**TIA1**	T-cell-restricted intracellular antigen-1
PerCP	peridinium chlorophyll protein complex	**T-LGL**	T-cell large granular lymphocyte
Ph	Philadelphia chromosome	**T-LGLL**	T-cell large granular lymphocyte leukemia
PLL	prolymphocytic leukemia	**T-PLL**	T-cell prolymphocytic leukemia
PMBL	primary mediastinal large B-cell lymphoma	**WBC**	white blood cell (count)
PMF	primary myelofibrosis	**WM**	Waldenström macroglobulinemia
PML	promyelocytic leukemia gene		
Post-ET-MF	post essential thrombocythemia myelofibrosis		

1

INTRODUCTION TO FLOW CYTOMETRY

Flow cytometry (FC) has become an important test in clinical laboratory for the diagnosis, subclassification, and post-treatment monitoring of hematologic neoplasms [1–24]. FC results allow to choose in a timely manner most appropriate further genetic testing to establish the definite diagnosis and to further characterize the malignant process. Multiparameter FC measures simultaneously and rapidly numerous surface and/or intracytoplasmic markers on a single cell, allowing for accurate phenotypic characterization of analyzed population(s) in various, even complex samples (such as bone marrow [BM]). While no single marker permits a definite lineage assignment, analysis with panels of antibodies allows for separation of hematologic tumors into very precise subtypes with different prognosis and treatment requirements, as defined by current World Health Organization classification of hematopoietic and lymphoid tumors [25]. FC analysis can precisely differentiate between B- and T-cell malignancies, between mature (peripheral) and precursor tumors, and among the latter, determine the myeloid or lymphoid lineage. In acute leukemia, a highly heterogeneous disease divided into acute myeloid leukemia (AML), acute lymphoblastic leukemia (ALL), acute undifferentiated leukemia (AUL), and mixed phenotype acute leukemia (MPAL), FC helps in subclassification and prognosis, prompts additional genetic testing, and monitors the response after treatment (minimal residual disease, MRD).

FC analysis requires fresh (unfixed) material. Types of specimens suitable for FC include blood, BM aspirate, fresh tissue samples, fine needle aspirates, effusions (pleural, peritoneal), and other body fluids (e.g., cerebrospinal fluid; CSF). In FC protocol, the sample is incubated with antibodies, followed by red blood cell lysis, washing, fixation in paraformaldehyde, and FC analysis. Whole blood lysis represents the most used technique for sample preparation [26–28]. Routinely 5,000–10,000 cells are collected (in MRD protocols 500,000 events). Monoclonal antibodies used in FC are conjugated with fluorochromes, which are excited or stimulated by laser(s) in FC. FC is much faster than immunohistochemistry and can analyze thousands of cells within seconds. Another advantage of FC immunophenotyping is that it allows correlation of several markers on a single cell, and detects intensity of staining and aberrant expression of antigens. FC has high sensitivity for B-cell lymphoproliferative disorders and acute leukemia and high specificity for several categories of those neoplasms. All these properties are used in diagnostic hematopathology for subclassification of neoplasms. The major disadvantage of FC is a need for liquid cell suspension and therefore lack of correlation with histomorphologic features (tissue architecture). FC requires viable fresh (unfixed) material. In a subset of neoplasms, especially high-grade lymphomas, decreased viability often precludes accurate FC analysis.

The major roles of flow cytometry

Identification of acute promyelocytic leukemia (APL)

The classic (hypergranular) variant of acute promyelocytic leukemia (APL) is characterized by high side scatter (SSC), positive CD117, negative CD11c, CD34, and HLA-DR, and positive myeloid markers expression (myeloperoxidase, CD13, and CD33; Figure 1.1) [9, 11]. Less common, hypogranular variant of APL shows similar phenotype to classic APL, except for low SSC and often positive expression of CD2 and CD34.

Identification of acute leukemia and increased blasts

Myeloblasts. The first step in diagnosis and classification of acute leukemia by FC is to identify the presence of blasts and determine their lineage. Myeloblasts are usually characterized by expression of CD117 and/or CD34, HLA-DR, CD133, CD13, CD33, and CD38. The expression of CD45 is moderate and SSC is low (Figure 1.2). Subset of myeloblasts may be positive for TdT, CD123, CD71, CD7, and CD11c. Occasional cases may be HLA-DR-negative. AML is diagnosed with ≥20% blasts (or blasts equivalents) in the BM, except for AML with t(15;17), inv(16), or t(8;21), which do not require 20% threshold for the diagnosis.

Monoblasts. Monoblasts are characterized by positive CD64 (moderate or bright), bright CD45 (usually stronger than in myeloblasts), positive HLA-DR, positive CD11b, CD11c, CD4, CD36, and often positive CD2, CD56, CD71, and/or CD123 (Figure 1.3). The expression of CD14 varies from positive (bright), heterogeneous (variable), dim, or partial to completely negative, depending on the degree of maturation (immature monoblasts are usually CD14⁻). Expression of CD11b, although often positive, may be partial, dim, or variable ("smeary"). Rare cases may be positive for blastic markers (CD34 and/or CD117).

Erythroblasts. Erythroblasts are positive for CD71, glycophorin A (GPHA, CD235a), e-cadherin, and hemoglobin A. Less mature erythroid precursor are often positive for CD117.

Megakaryoblasts. Megakaryoblasts are positive for CD41 and CD61. Very immature forms may express CD34.

Blastic plasmacytoid dendritic cell neoplasm (BPDCN). BPDCB is positive for CD4, CD36, CD38, CD43, CD45, CD56 (bright), CD71, HLA-DR, CD303 (blood dendritic cell antigen-2; BDCA-2), CD123, and HLA-DR (Figure 1.4) [29]. CD45 is positive and may range from dim to moderate expression. Side scatter is low.

B-cell acute lymphoblastic leukemia/lymphoma (B-ALL/LBL). B-lymphoblasts are typically positive or CD34, TdT, HLA-DR, CD19, CD22, CD38, and CD10 with negative to dim CD45 and negative CD20 (Figure 1.5). Subset of B-ALL cases is negative for CD10 and subset of cases may be CD71⁺, CD123⁺,

DOI: 10.1201/9781003197935-1

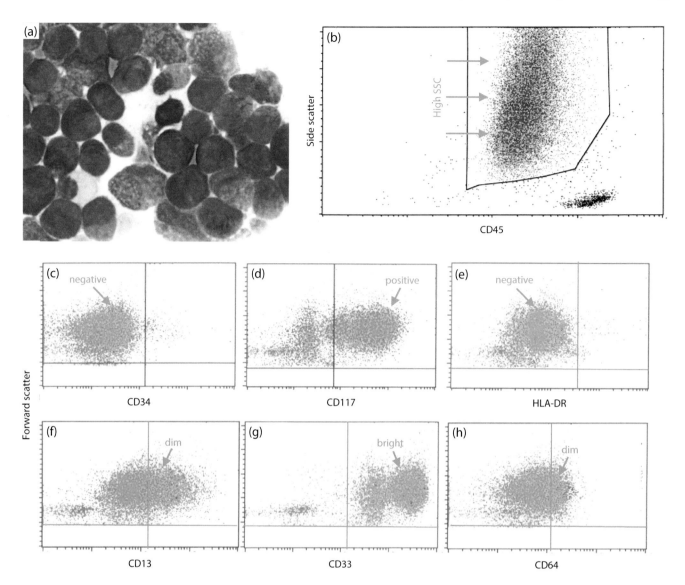

FIGURE 1.1   APL: typical flow cytometry pattern. Neoplastic promyelocytes are characterized by hypergranular cytoplasm with Auer rods (a). Flow cytometry features includes high side scatter (b, arrows), lack of CD34 (c), positive CD117 (d), lack of HLA-DR (e), positive CD13 (f), positive CD33 (g), and dimly positiveCD64 (h).

or partially CD20⁺. Blasts may express myeloid antigens (usually CD13 or CD33, rarely CD15).

T-cell acute lymphoblastic leukemia/lymphoma (T-ALL/LBL). T-lymphoblasts are positive for CD34 and/or TdT, do not express surface CD3 (cytoplasmic CD3 is positive), and are positive for one or more of the T-cell markers (CD2, CD5, and/or CD7; Figure 1.6). They are either dual CD4/CD8⁺ or dual CD4/CD8⁻. Subset of T-ALL is positive for CD1a and/or CD10. Early T-cell precursor T-ALL (ETP-ALL) shows often aberrant expression of CD13 and CD117, and lack of CD1a, surface CD3, and CD5 expression [30–34].

Acute undifferentiated leukemia (AUL). AUL is positive for some of the blastic markers (TdT, CD34), CD38 and HLA-DR, and does not express markers specific for myeloid or lymphoid lineages [35–38]. Dim and/or partial expression of CD10 or CD123 may be seen.

Mixed phenotype acute leukemia (MPAL). MPAL co-expresses myeloid (or monocytic) markers with B- or T-cell lineage specific marker (rarely B- and T-cell markers) [35, 37, 39–43]. MPALs are often positive for CD34, TdT, and HLA-DR. Lineage assignment criteria for myeloid lineage include (1) myeloperoxidase (MPO) or (2) monocytic differentiation (at least two of the following: CD11c, CD14, CD64, nonspecific esterase, and lysozyme) [44]. T-lineage is assigned with (1) strong cytoplasmic CD3 or (2) surface CD3 expression. B-lineage is assigned when there is (1) strong CD19 expression with at least one of the following strongly expressed: CD79a, cytoplasmic CD22, or CD10, or (2) weak CD19 with at least two of the following strongly expressed: CD79a, cytoplasmic CD22, or CD10.

Identification of clonal B-cells and clonal plasma cells

The major roles of FC in management of patients with lymphomas are assignment of lineage, differentiation between reactive and clonal B-cells, and subclassification of B-cell neoplasm based

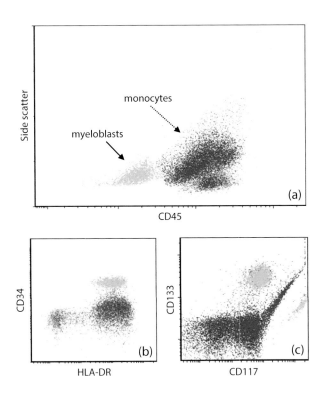

on aberrant phenotype of B-cells and their forward scatter. This is especially important in samples from blood, in which there is no tissue available for immunohistochemistry and molecular abnormalities are often not specific for a definite subclassification of neoplastic process (e.g., in CLL). The most commonly used markers in evaluation of B-cell neoplasms include CD5, CD10, CD11c, CD19, CD20, CD22, CD23, CD25, CD34, CD38, CD43, CD45, CD79, CD81, CD103, CD200, surface kappa, and surface lambda. The most commonly used markers in evaluation of plasma cell neoplasms include CD19, CD20, CD38, CD45, CD56, CD81, CD117, CD138, CD200, cytoplasmic kappa, and cytoplasmic lambda. B-cell lymphomas show prominent and cohesive population of light chain-restricted B-cells (Figure 1.7). Normal (mature) B-cells consist of two populations, one expressing kappa (κ) and the other lambda (λ) light chain immunoglobulins. Subset of mature B-cell proliferation may be surface light chain immunoglobulin negative. FC analysis of kappa and lambda expression, apart from evaluation of clonality, may also help in further classification of B-cell neoplasm. Dim or negative kappa and lambda expression is typical for chronic lymphocytic leukemia (CLL)/small lymphocytic lymphoma (CLL/SLL). Subset of DLBCL, FL, and BL may also be surface light chain negative. Lack of light chain expression is typical for hematogones and B-ALL. Germinal center cells from follicular hyperplasia may also show diminished expression of light chain with variable kappa and negative to dim lambda, which in rare cases may be confused with clonal CD10+ B-cell process. B-cells from pleural effusions are often completely surface light chain negative. Mature B lymphocytes exhibit allelic exclusion in which only a single class of light chain, either kappa or lambda, are expressed. However, very rare B-cell neoplasms, especially CLL, may show dual expression of both light chains.

FIGURE 1.2 Identification of myeloblasts (acute myelomonocytic leukemia, AMML). Myeloblasts (green dots) show moderate CD45 and low side scatter placing them is "blastic" gate on CD45 versus SSC display (a). They are usually positive for HLA-DR (b), CD34 (b), CD133 (c), and CD117 (c). Monocytes are represented by blue dots.

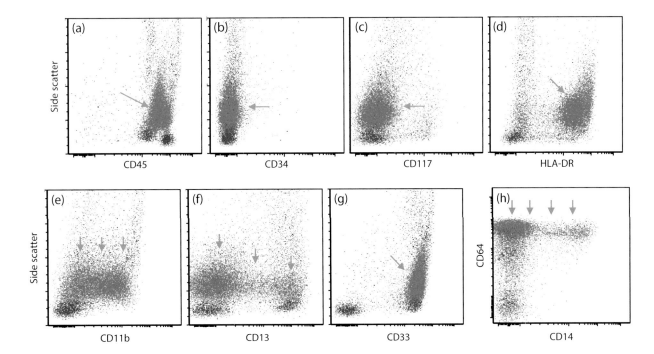

FIGURE 1.3 Acute monoblastic leukemia. Monoblasts (green dots, arrow) show bright expression of CD45 and slightly increased side scatter (a). CD34 and CD117 are not expressed (b–c), HLA-DR is positive (d), CD11b is variably expressed with subset of cells being negative and subset showing dim expression (e). There is aberrant, mostly negative CD13 expression (f) and both CD33 and CD64 are brightly expressed (g–h). CD14 is mostly negative (h).

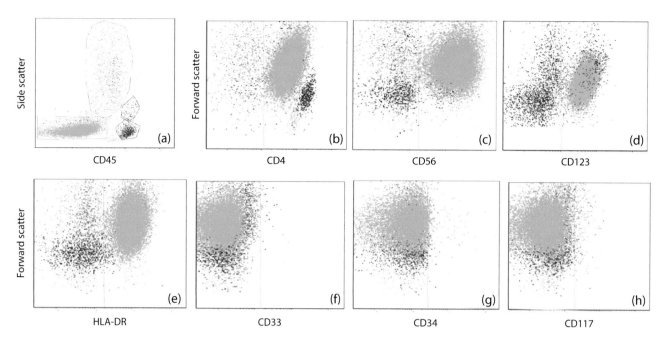

FIGURE 1.4 BPDCN shows low side scatter (a), negative to dim CD45 (a), positive CD4 (b), CD56 (c), CD123 (d), and HLA-DR (e), and does not express CD33 (f), CD34 (g), and CD117 (h).

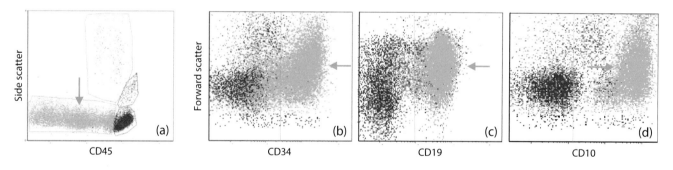

FIGURE 1.5 B-lymphoblasts (green dots, arrow) show negative to dim CD45 (a), low side scatter (a), and positive expression of CD34 (b), CD19 (c), and CD10 (d).

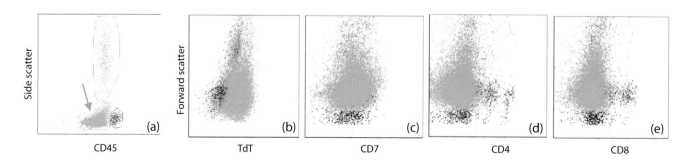

FIGURE 1.6 T-lymphoblasts (green dots; arrow) are CD45+ (a), have low side scatter (a), express TdT (b), CD7 (c) and are either dual CD4/CD8-negative (d–e) or dual CD4/CD8-positive (not shown).

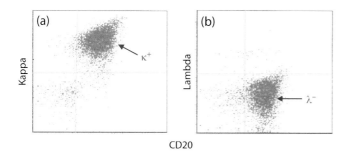

FIGURE 1.7 Identification of clonal B-cells: B-cells (red dots, arrow) show CD20 expression and κ restriction (a). There is no λ expression (b).

B-cell markers (CD19, CD20, CD22, CD79a) are positive. Subset of B-cell lymphoproliferations is positive for CD5 or CD10. Plasma cells are bright positive for CD38 and CD138. Benign plasma cells express CD19, CD27, CD45, CD81, and polytypic pattern of expression of cytoplasmic light chain immunoglobulins and are negative for CD28, CD56, CD117, and CD200. Malignant plasma cells have increased to variable forward scatter (FSC) and are often CD19$^-$, CD45$^-$, CD20$^-$, CD27$^-$, CD28$^+$, CD56$^+$, CD117$^+$, and CD200$^+$ and show restricted expression of either cytoplasmic kappa or cytoplasmic lambda. Clonal plasma cells accompanying low grade B-cell lymphomas with plasmacytic differentiation show low to medium FSC, may be CD19$^+$ and/or CD45$^+$, and are usually CD56$^-$ and CD117$^-$.

Identification of atypical T-cells
T-cell lymphomas can be suspected by FC based on loss or aberrant (dim or variable) expression of the T antigens (CD2, CD3, CD5, and/or CD7), aberrant expression of CD4 or CD8 (subset restriction, dual-positive CD4/CD8 expression or lack of both markers), increased forward scatter (FSC), lack of CD26 or CD45, or presence of additional markers such as CD10, CD25, CD30, CD56, CD57, or CD103 (Figure 1.8).

Diagnosis of paroxysmal nocturnal hemoglobinuria (PNH)
PNH FC evaluates the expression of GPI-anchored proteins on erythrocytes, granulocytes, and monocytes [45–53]. The demonstration of the absence of GPI-linked proteins in a significant fraction (large clone) of peripheral blood erythrocytes, neutrophils, and monocytes is diagnostic of PNH [45, 53]. Red blood cells are evaluated using CD235a (glycophorin A; GPHA) and CD59, white blood cells are evaluated using FLAER, CD24, CD15, and CD45 (for neutrophils), and FLAER, CD14, CD64, and CD45 (for monocytes).

Diagnosis and subclassification of lymphoproliferative neoplasms involving blood
FC analysis helps to identify and subclassify lymphoproliferations with predominant blood involvement such as CLL, B- and T-cell prolymphocytic leukemia (PLL), Sézary syndrome (SS), hairy cell leukemia (HCL) and its variant, leukemic non-nodal mantle cell lymphoma (L-NN-MCL), adult T-cell lymphoma/leukemia (ATLL), T-cell large granular leukemia (T-LGLL), and other lymphoproliferations presenting in leukemic phase including those in early stages or of undetermined clinical significance such as monoclonal B-cell lymphocytosis (MBL) [54–67].

Measurable (minimal) residual disease (MRD) analysis by flow cytometry
In many disorders, including (but not limited to) AML, B-ALL, CLL, and plasma cell myeloma (PCM), the level of MRD after therapy is an independent predictor of outcome [68–79].

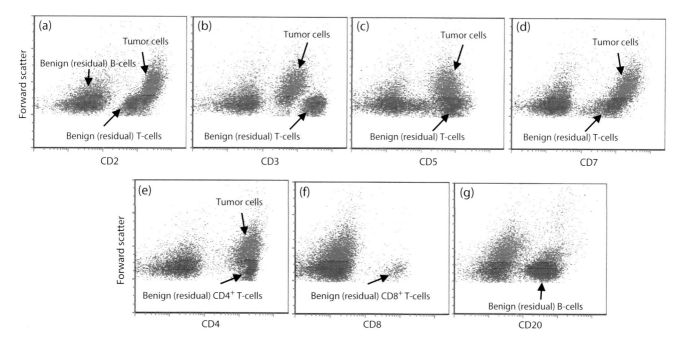

FIGURE 1.8 Identification of abnormal T-cells: increased forward scatter. PTCL with positive expression of all pan T-cell antigens (a–d). The neoplastic cells have increased forward scatter (compare with residual B-cells (g) and benign T-cells) and show dim CD3 (b). The expression of CD5 is slightly dimmer when compared to benign T-cells (c), and the expression of both CD2 and CD7 is slightly brighter (a and d). Neoplastic T-cells are CD4$^+$ (e–f). Residual B-cells have low forward scatter and positive CD20 (g).

Currently, the two most popular methods for MRD analysis are FC and real-time quantitative polymerase chain reaction (PCR). In acute leukemias, the basic principle of MRD analysis by FC is to identify aberrant phenotype of blasts (leukemia-associated immunophenotype, LAIP) that differ from the phenotype of normal hematopoietic cells, and to use LAIP to trace residual leukemia after treatment (see Chapter 25). In CLL, FC provides reliable detection of residual CLL cells down to the level of 0.0010% (10⁻⁵) with a single-tube assay which includes CD3, CD5, CD19, CD20, CD23, CD43, CD79b, CD81, and CD200 [80, 81].

Cell sorting by flow cytometry

The cell sorting by FC is used to purify and collect samples for additional testing. Heterogeneous mixtures of cells are placed in suspension and passed single file across one or more laser interrogation points. Separation of antibody conjugated cells generally exploits specific cell labeling with magnetic beads or with fluorescent tags. Light signals emitted from the particles are collected and correlated to entities such as cell morphology, surface and intracellular protein expression, gene expression, and cellular physiology. The cells can be separated based on conjugated fluorescent markers or beads, and without those, termed a label-free separation. The label-free separation methods can be divided into active (electrokinetic, acoustic, and magnetic cell separation) and passive [82] electrokinetic cell separation. Based on user-defined parameters, individual cells can then be diverted from the fluid stream and collected into viable, homogeneous fractions at exceptionally high speeds and a purity that approaches 100% [24, 83].

Flow cytometry in hematological emergencies

Circulating promyelocytes

Identification of even few promyelocytes in blood by FC or on blood smear (Figure 1.9) should prompt immediate BM analysis, as those cases are associated with either BM involvement by APL or imminent development of APL. Rapid molecular testing for *PML-RARA* by quantitative PCR and/or FISH should also be offered from blood sample to confirm the diagnosis of APL.

Aplastic anemia

Aplastic anemia (AA) is a rare, life-threatening disorder characterized by suppression of BM function (trilineage aplasia) resulting in progressive pancytopenia. AA is diagnosed when BM has <25% cellularity and blood analysis shows neutrophils <0.5 × 10⁹/L, platelets <20 × 10⁹/L, and reticulocyte count <20 × 10⁹/L. AA can be congenital or acquired. The inherited form is rare and includes Fanconi anemia, congenital keratosis, congenital pure red cell aplasia, and Shwachman-Diamond syndrome [84, 85]. Immune destruction of hemopoietic stem cells by T-lymphocytes plays an important role in pathogenesis, as shown by successful treatment with immunosuppressive agents, leading to transfusion independence or complete recovery of peripheral blood counts in a proportion of patients. BM analysis and FC help to exclude constitutional marrow failures, MDS, aleukemic leukemias, HCL, and APL (among others). Cases of AA complicating systemic lupus erythematosus or certain medications have been reported.

Acute leukemia

Presence of circulating blasts is discussed above.

Hyperleukocytosis

Hyperleukocytosis (WBC >100 × 10⁹/L) is a high-risk medical emergency associated with life-threatening complications, such as disseminated intravascular coagulation (DIC), leukostasis, and tumor lysis syndrome.

Diagnostic considerations of hyperleukocytosis include (Figure 1.10):

- B-cell and T-cell acute lymphoblastic leukemia (B-ALL; T-ALL)
- AML
- Chronic myeloid leukemia (CML, *BCR-ABL1⁺*)
- Primary myelofibrosis (PMF; rare cases)
- CLL and other B-cell lymphoproliferations
- Occasional T-cell lymphoproliferations, such as T-cell prolymphocytic leukemia (T-PLL) or adult T-cell leukemia/lymphoma (ATLL)

Severe pancytopenia/cytopenia

Pancytopenia is defined as a decrease in all three blood cell lines, which results in symptoms associated with anemia, leukopenia, and/or thrombocytopenia. FC plays important role in

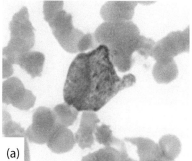
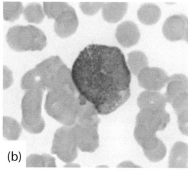
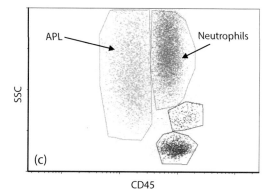

FIGURE 1.9 Circulating promyelocytes (APL). (a, b) Blood smear showing atypical promyelocytes. (c) FC showing promyelocytes (green dots) with high side scatter (SSC) and dimmer expression of CD45 when compared to neutrophils.

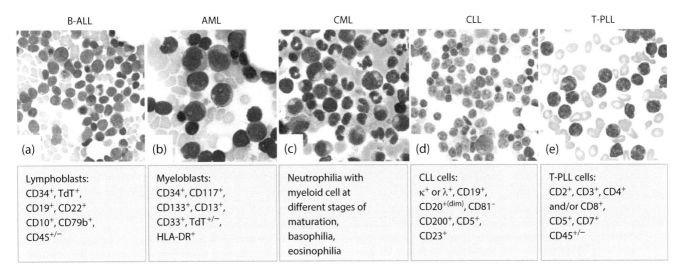

FIGURE 1.10 Etiology of hyperleukocytosis: B-ALL (a), AML (b), CML (c), CLL (d), and T-PLL (e).

establishing the diagnosis in many of conditions associated with severe cytopenia/pancytopenia.

Differential diagnosis of pancytopenia and/or severe cytopenia (anemia, leukopenia, or thrombocytopenia) includes:

- Myelodysplastic neoplasm (MDS)
- AML ("aleukemic")
- APL
- Acute erythroid leukemia (AEL, pure erythroid leukemia)
- PMF
- Post polycythemia vera (PV) myelofibrosis (post PV-MF)
- Post essential thrombocythemia (ET) myelofibrosis (post ET-MF)
- Systemic mastocytosis (SM)
- HCL
- T-LGL leukemia (TLLL)
- Paroxysmal nocturnal hemoglobinuria (PNH)
- Hemophagocytic lymphohistiocytosis (HLH; Figure 1.11)
- Metastatic tumor/other BM infiltrative process
- AA, congenital or acquired

- Gelatinous transformation of BM
- Hypersplenism
- Toxic marrow damage (therapy, toxins, radiation)
- Infections (sepsis, malaria, viruses, other)

10-color flow cytometry analysis

Within the past few years, instrument manufacturers have begun to produce benchtop instruments capable of the simultaneous detection of 10 or more fluorochromes, and with the advent of an increasing variety of fluorochromes suitable for immunophenotyping, the possibility of high-level multicolor FC is rapidly becoming a reality [20, 74, 86, 87]. The most common flow cytometers use two lasers but instruments with five or more lasers allowing for the detection of >30 parameters are being recently available.

Advantages of 10-color FC panels [17, 20, 88]:

- Increased accuracy to identify an abnormal population within complex samples. Given the large number of

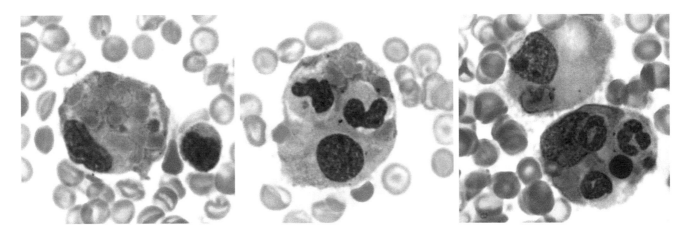

FIGURE 1.11 Hemophagocytic lymphohistiocytosis (HLH).

hematopoietic neoplasms, the 10-color approach is better suited to provide many disease-specific combinations of antibodies and therefore render more specific diagnoses. In addition, there it has better ability to identify small populations of abnormal cells before or after therapy.

- Better precision and specificity to identify and characterize rare events (cells) within predominant benign "background". These issues are of particular importance in the identification of small abnormal populations (e.g., MRD detection).
- Making better use of small specimens (limited, paucicellular samples). Clinical FC laboratories are increasingly asked to evaluate smaller amounts of material, such as fine-needle aspirates, CSF, and body fluids, in which the number of cells for evaluation is often the factor limiting analysis. Porwit and Rajab described one tube 14-antibody screening panel suitable for detection of major B- and T-cell abnormalities, enumeration of blasts and MDS-related abnormalities [88]. Figure 1.12 illustrates identification of Burkitt lymphoma (BL) in CSF by modified 1 tube 15-antibody panel.

- Saving the time needed to run and analyze samples (saving turnaround time and technologist' time). The use of increased numbers of antibodies in a single tube results in fewer tubes needing to be processed, with resultant savings not only in specimen volume (as mentioned earlier), but also in instrument time for acquisition, and technologist time to process, acquire and analyze ("gate") the specimen.
- Decreasing the number of additional flow tests ("add-ons"). The use of increased number of antibodies tested in the new 10-color panel allows to decrease significantly the number of add-on tests in the laboratory.
- Saving the volume of reagents. Through the use of more reagents per tube and using less tubes, redundancies of reagents within panels are reduced, resulting in savings in the volume of reagent consumed.
- Providing more efficient collection of larger numbers of events. The processing of fewer tubes and the use of smaller specimens would provide the ability to routinely collect larger numbers of events.
- Standardization. The use of larger panels that include many of the most popular combinations of antibodies enables a

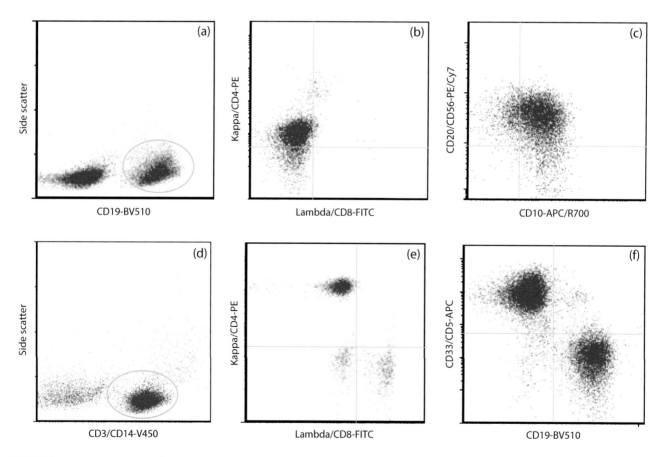

FIGURE 1.12 Burkitt lymphoma involving cerebrospinal fluid (CSF). FC analysis using 1 tube 10-color, 15-antibodies screening panel (CD3, CD4, CD5, CD8, CD10, CD14, CD19, CD20, CD33, CD34, CD45, CD56, CD117, kappa, and lambda). B-cells gated based on CD19 expression (a) show dim kappa expression (b) and co-expression of CD10 and CD20 (c). T-cells gated based on CD3 expression (d) show normal CD4:CD8 ratio (e). Ungated cells (f) show presence of CD5+ T-cells and CD19+ B-cells (f).

standardized approach to this type of analysis between different laboratories that is currently lacking.

The disadvantages of 10-color FC panels [20, 22–24]:

- Higher cost for instrumentation. The ability to perform 10-color FC relies on the use of multi-laser benchtop instruments with sophisticated collection optics. Such instruments are more expensive than prior 1- or 2-laser flow cytometers.
- The greater expertise is needed to understand a variety of technical issues. Analysis is more complex and time consuming when compared to 6-color panel. The 10-color panel needs highly trained personnel to analyze complex data.
- More complex data analysis (information overload) leading to increased time for the computer to acquire and display the data.
- Non-specific binding of antibodies. Each antibody and fluorochrome have the propensity for some degree of binding to cells via mechanisms unrelated to the epitope being detected (i.e., nonspecific binding). This disadvantage does not apply specifically to 10-color flow panel. Many cells (e.g., B-cells, natural killer [NK] cells, macrophages, promyelocytes, etc.) show non-specific staining (due to Fcγ receptors on their surface which can bind to the Fc region of the antibody used in the panel). High antibody concentration can also increase non-specific binding. Therefore, use of blocking reagents and proper titration of all antibodies are needed to maximize the signal to noise ratio. The correct isotypic control antibodies obtained from the same vendor and used at the same concentration as antibody of interest help to ensure that the observed staining is due to specific antibody binding rather than an artifacts. Presence of dead cells can also lead to false positives due to autofluorescence and increased non-specific antibody binding. Certain fluorochromes show increased binding to compromised or dying cells and debris, giving rise to significantly increased background on some samples. This is particularly true of reagents containing the cyanine dyes Cy5, Cy5.5, or Cy7, as well as Texas Red, and is less true of the fluorochromes Pacific Blue, fluorescein isothiocyanate (FITC), phycoerythrin (PE), Alexa 594, and allophycocyanin (APC).
- The spillover of one fluorochrome into the detection channel of the other fluorochrome. The spillover is more pronounced with several fluorochromes used in new 10-color panel when compared to old 6-color panels. The use of the spillover correction by a technique called "compensation" and by selecting the fluorochromes that have little or no overlap with each other. When tandem fluorochromes are used, it is important to separately compensate for each reagent containing a tandem fluorochrome, as the spectral emission properties commonly vary among lots, between manufacturers, and over time (e.g., if PE–Texas Red is attached to three different antibodies in a panel, compensation settings for each must be individually determined). This often results in the need for individual compensation settings for each separate reagent combination (i.e., tube-specific compensation), a process easily implemented using software compensation. One of the most common problems with the spillover includes PE and PE-Cy7 fluorochromes. For example, if the same tube of antigens includes kappa-PE and CD10-PE-Cy7, bright expression of kappa (conjugated with PE) in B-cell lymphomas may lead to false positive expression of CD10 (conjugated with PE-Cy7) leading to incorrect subclassification of lymphoma to germinal center cell origin. Or reversely, bright expression of CD10 conjugated with PE-Cy7 (e.g., in B-ALL) may lead to falsely positive expression of kappa (conjugated with PE).

- New tandem dyes may be more prone for degradation. Tandem dyes are less stable than single dye and can differ from a lot to lot in their energy transfer efficiency. It is necessary for the laboratory to take steps to avoid tandem dye degradation and consider its impact upon results. New tandems (e.g., APC-H7) are more stable than older ones (e.g., APC-Cy7).

Recommended combination of fluorochromes used in 10-color FC panels

The common lasers used are 488 nm (blue light), 405 nm (violet light), 532 nm (green light), 522 nm (green), 561 nm (green-yellow), 592 nm (yellow), 612 nm (orange), 633 nm (red), 640 nm (red), and 355 nm (ultraviolet). The design of the FC panel depends on planned role of the given panel (e.g., screening versus MRD analysis), clinical setting of the laboratory, the optical system used (instrument configuration: type and number of lasers and detectors, optical filters), cost, users' experience, available software to analyze data, and volume of cases in the lab. The best fluorochromes should be bright with a significant difference between the positive and negative (background) staining. The basic principle is that highly expressed antigens should be coupled with dim fluorochromes and dimly expressed antigens should be coupled with bright fluorochromes (e.g., bright CD8 with PacB; dimmer CD7 with PE). The background fluorescence is influenced by signal level, cell autofluorescence, non-specific staining, electronic noise, and optical background from other fluorochromes used in the panel (spectral overlap or spillover). Proper compensation allows decrease of the spillover, but choice of the reagents (fluorochromes) should be based on their potential spectral overlap with each other.

Common choices of fluorochromes for 10-color FC panel (Table 1.1):

- FITC or Alexa Fluor 488
- PE
- PerCP-Cy5.5 (peridinin chlorophyll protein-cyanin 5.5) or PE-Cy5.5
- PE-Cy7
- APC or Alexa Fluor 647
- APC-R700 or Alexa Fluor 680
- APC-H7 (allophycocyanin-hilite 7) or APC-Cy7
- BV 421 (Brilliant violet 421) or BD Horizon V450
- BV 510 or V500C
- BV 605

Antigen selection for FC panels

Table 1.2 presents most used markers for each cell lineage and Table 1.3 presents panels to be considered for specific hematopoietic neoplasm.

TABLE 1.1: Fluorochrome Characteristics

Laser Wavelength	Fluorochrome	Filter	Intensity of Fluorescence
Violet (407 nm)	Pacific Blue (PacB)	450/50	Moderate
	DAPI	450/50	
	Brilliant Violet 421	450/50	Very bright
	BD Horizon V450	450/50	Moderate
	Am-Cyan	525/50 or 550/20	
	BD Horizon V500	525/50 or 550/20	Dim
	BV 605		Very bright
Blue (488 nm)	FITC	530/30	Moderate
	Alexa Fluor 488	530/30	Moderate
	PE	575/26	Very bright
	PE-Texas Red (PE-TR; ECD)	610/20	
	BD Horizon PE-CF594	610/20	Very bright
	PE-Cy5	695/40 or 670/14	
	PE-Cy5.5	695/40	Very bright
	PerCP-Cy5.5	695/40	Bright
	PE-Cy7	780/60	Bright
	Krome Orange (KO)	550/40	
Yellow (594 nm)	Alexa Fluor 594 (AF594)	616/25	
Red (635 nm)	APC	670/30	Very bright
	Alexa Fluor 647	660/20	Bright
	Alexa Fluor 700 (AF 700)	730/40	
	APC-Alexa Fluor 700	730/40	
	APC-Cy7	780/60	Dim
	APC-H7	780/60	Dim
	APC-C750	780/60	

TABLE 1.2: Lineage Associated Markers Commonly Used by FC

Target	Antigens
B-cells	CD19, CD20, CD22, CD79a/b, s.kappa, s.lambda
T- and NK-cells	CD2, CD3, CD4, CD5, CD7, CD8, CD16, CD26, CD30, CD52, CD56, CD57, TCRαβ, TCRγδ
Pan-myeloid cells	CD13, CD15, CD33, MPO
Blasts	CD34, CD117, CD133, TdT
Granulocytes/neutrophils	CD10, CD11b, CD13, CD15, CD16, CD33
Monocytes/dendritic cells	CD4, CD11b, CD11c, CD13, CD14, CD36, CD64, CD123
Erythroid cells/precursors	GPHA (CD235a), CD71, CD117
Mast cells	CD2, CD25, CD117
Plasma cells	CD27, CD38, CD81, CD138, c.kappa, c.lambda, c.IgG, c.IgM, c.IgA, c.IgD
Megakaryocytes	CD41, CD61
Hematopoietic cells	CD45
Activation and other markers	HLA-DR, CD30, CD1a, CD38, CD25, CD103, CD200

Abbreviations: s, surface; c, cytoplasmic; GPHA, glycophorin A; TdT, terminal deoxynucleotidyl transferase.

TABLE 1.3: Antibodies Used to Identify Common Hematopoietic Neoplasms by FC

Neoplasm	Antigens
B-cell neoplasm	CD5, CD10, CD11c, CD19, CD20, CD22, CD25, CD38, CD43, CD45, CD52, CD71, CD79a/b, CD81, CD103, CD200, s.kappa, s.lambda
T- and NK-cell neoplasms	CD2, CD3, CD4, CD5, CD7, CD8, CD10, CD16, CD25, CD26, CD30, CD45, CD52, CD56, CD57, CD103, TCRαβ, TCRγδ
Acute myeloid leukemia, MDS/MPN	CD2, CD4, CD7, CD10, CD11b, CD11c, CD13, CD14, CD15, CD33, CD34, CD36, CD38, CD45, CD56, CD64, CD71, CD117, CD123, HLA-DR, MPO, TdT
B-cell ALL	CD10, CD13, CD19, CD20, CD22, CD45, CD79a/b, CD10, CD13, CD33, CD34, CD38, CD45, TdT
T-cell ALL	CD1a, CD2, s.CD3, c.CD3, CD4, CD5, CD7, CD8, CD10, CD13, CD33, CD38, CD45, CD34, TdT
Mast cell neoplasms	CD2, CD25, CD45, CD117
Plasma cell neoplasms	CD19, CD20, CD23, CD27, CD33, CD38, CD45, CD56, CD81, CD138, CD200, c.kappa, c.lambda, c.IgG, c.IgM, c.IgA, c.IgD
BPDCN	CD2, CD4, CD7, CD13, CD33, CD34, CD45, CD56, CD123, HLA-DR
MPAL and AUL	s.CD3, c.CD3, CD10, CD13, CD14, CD19, c.CD22, CD33, CD34, CD41, CD45, CD61, CD64, CD71, c.CD79a, CD117, HLA-DR, MPO, TdT

Abbreviations: s, surface; c, cytoplasmic; ALL, acute lymphoblastic leukemia; GPHA, glycophorin A; TdT, terminal deoxynucleotidyl transferase, MDS, myelodysplastic neoplasm; MPN, myeloproliferative neoplasm; BPDCN, blastic plasmacytoid dendritic cell neoplasm; MPAL, mixed phenotype acute leukemia; AUL, acute undifferentiated leukemia.

Automated flow cytometry data analysis

FC data are most often analyzed using a series of two-dimensional dot plots with manual "gating", as presented below in this chapter. The manual gating, which relies on the technologist's knowledge and experience, is one of the largest variables in the outcome of a FC-based analysis [89, 90]. In addition, the interpretation of data obtained from typical 10-color FC analysis, comparing 10 or more parameters with each other, is becoming very complex and difficult. Therefore, an automated FC data analysis (mass cytometry and more recently spectral flow cytometry, SFC) for identification and characterization of often complex cell populations and high dimensional cytometry data has been increasingly used, mostly in research and biotechnology or pharmaceutical laboratories [89–92]. Dimensionality reduction and/or cell clustering algorithms are commonly used to visualize and interpret high dimensional data. The t-distributed stochastic neighbor embedding (t-SNE) is one of the most often used software [93]. Its algorithm reduces data dimensionality by incorporating all parameters obtained during FC analysis, while maintaining the data structure. Cells with similar properties are plotted closer together that creates a two-dimensional map (t-SNE map) [91]. Other programs with graphical user interfaces include PhenoGraph, UMAP (uniform manifold approximation and projection), viSNE (visualization SNE), SPADE1 (spanning-tree progression analysis of density-normalized events), FlowSOM, and Citrus [91, 93, 94]. Software for automated FC analysis is available from Becton, Dickinson & Company (FACS Diva and Flow Jo), Beckman Coulter (Kaluza), De Novo Software (FCS Express), Verity Software House (Gemstone), and Applied Cytometry (VenturiOne). Figure 1.13 shows an example of t-SNE FC visualizations with cell populations color-coded according to clustering results displayed on classic biaxial dot plots. The computational cytometry with data-driven automated algorithms decreases technical variability in analysis of complex populations, reduce bias, and have better efficiency when compared to classic FC

approach [93, 95]. The automated FC software can be divided based on the algorithm learning methods into two categories, supervised and unsupervised. In supervised learning methods, the algorithms learn from training data with known outcomes in order to build a model to classify new inputs. In unsupervised learning, no training data set is needed, and the goal is to correctly identify and quantify cell populations [93]. Dimensionality reduction in t-SNE takes data with multiple parameters and reduces it to two dimensions which can be easily interpreted and presented in two-dimensional scatter plot, called t-SNE map [89]. In this map, different cell populations will visually appear as distinct clusters. The single cells can be then assigned to the t-SNE map by using automated clustering algorithms. SPADE (spanning-tree progression analysis of density-normalized events) consists of connected nodes that represent clusters of cells with similar properties, providing information about the main cellular lineages and relationship between different cell populations. SFC is expected to help in evaluation of samples with complex but subtle changes, such as dysmaturation of maturing myeloid cells in MDS, myeloproliferative neoplasm (MPN), or mixed MDS/MPN. It is also possible that t-SNE or similar automated approaches to data analysis may replace in the future scoring systems used currently in the diagnosis of certain hematopoietic neoplasms, such as CLL or MDS.

Flow cytometry parameters

Gating strategies

The gating strategies applied to samples from blood or BM are presented in Chapter 2. In samples other than blood or BM (e.g., lymph node and effusion) gating aims at elimination of non-viable elements. Figure 1.14 (a–b) illustrates gating strategy applied in the FC analysis of lymph node and other solid organs or effusions (spleen is most often analyzed using BM/blood strategy). The non-viable cells are excluded from analysis by gating on "viability" dye-negative population(s) [7-amino-actinomycin D (7-AAD), propidium iodide (PI), calcein blue, "aqua" viability dye, etc.]. High grade lymphomas are often characterized by increased number of non-viable cells or complete drop-out of neoplastic cells, leaving only benign (residual) lymphocytes for analysis. Non-viable cells have tendency for non-specific adsorption of antibodies leading to non-conclusive or non-interpretable results, and therefore FC results with increased number of non-viable cells must be interpreted with caution (preferably comparing analysis with and without poorly preserved populations). Some benign and malignant populations may show decreased expression of viability dyes mimicking non-viable cells due to non-specific adsorption of "viability" dyes, best exemplified by benign and neoplastic eosinophils (Figure 1.14, c–d) or neoplastic promyelocytes in APL. Low-grade (small cell) lymphomas tend to remain viable, even when the analysis by FC is delayed.

Pattern of antigen expression

FC immunophenotyping includes the evaluation of the expression of specific antigens (markers) along with light scatter properties of the cells. The analyzed parameters are compared to that expected in normal (benign) counterpart. Presence of any difference in the pattern of expression, e.g., lack of antigen expression, decreased or increased intensity of staining, variable (heterogeneous) expression or presence of a marker which is not typically seen in normal counterpart (e.g., lymphoid markers in myeloid cells or pan-myeloid markers in lymphoid cells) allows for identification of abnormal population. In many cases, and especially in tumors with predominance of neoplastic population (without benign cells which could be used as controls) correlation with staining of negative controls

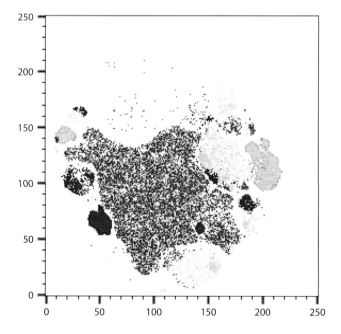

FIGURE 1.13 t-SNE map (color codes: purple, monocytes; red, T-cells; green, NK-cell; blue, B-cells; and gray, ungated cells). Blood sample stained with CD3, CD10, CD14, CD20, CD27, CD45, CD56, and CD57.

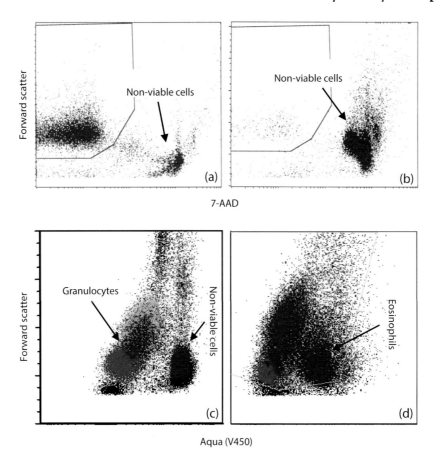

FIGURE 1.14 (a–b) Gating strategy of flow cytometric samples from lymph node (and other "solid" organs). Non-viable cells, which are labeled by 7-AAD (arrow) are excluded from analysis. Only 7-AAD-negative (viable) cells are further analyzed. Similar results may be achieved with other fluorochromes, e.g., propidium iodide. Both panels (a–b) represent lymph node with B-cell lymphoma: majority of cells in sample A are viable (7-AAD-negative) whereas majority of cell in sample B are non-viable (7-AAD-positive). Non-viable cells tend to scatter less light in forward direction and therefore are characterized by low forward scatter, when compared to viable cells. (c–d) Comparison of granulocytes and non-viable cells (c) with eosinophils (d) based on forward scatter versus aqua (viability) staining. Note much brighter aqua staining of non-viable cells.

maybe invaluable in excluding non-specific ("background") staining and thus deciding which results are truly positive. Although numeric evaluation of flow results (percent of cells positive for specific antigen) is crucial in rendering flow diagnosis (e.g., in analysis of number of CD34$^+$ blasts, percent of CD34$^+$ hematogones among all CD34$^+$ precursors, CD4:CD8 ratio or percentage of CD10$^-$ granulocytes, etc.), analysis of pattern of antigen expression is as important, because often only aberrant pattern of expression helps in establishing the correct diagnosis. Figure 1.15 shows a case of CLL with bi-clonal kappa and lambda expression. This case proves that focusing solely on numbers when analyzing FC results instead of considering also pattern of antigen expression may lead to erroneous interpretation of a case as benign (polytypic) instead of malignant (bi-clonal) composed of two separate kappa$^+$ and lambda$^+$ clones. In situation when FC abnormalities are more subtle such as abnormal pattern of expression of "maturation" pattern (e.g., by comparing the expression of CD11b versus CD16, or CD10 versus CD15, etc.) only careful comparison of FC results with patterns typically observed in benign (control) cases enables correct identification of features of dysgranulopoiesis (see Chapter 19).

Once the abnormal population is identified, evaluation of additional markers may be helpful for further characterization of the process and often allows for disease monitoring.

Based on the immunophenotypic features, possible entities or specific diagnoses (whenever possible) are suggested along with recommendation for additional testing (when applicable), such as morphology (e.g., blast enumeration; nodular or diffuse pattern of lymph node involvement), cytogenetics, FISH (e.g., *PML-RARA, IGH-BCL2, MYC*), PCR (e.g., *BCR-ABL1*, T- or B-cell clonality), next gene sequencing (NGS) for specific mutation(s) (e.g., *JAK2, CALR, MPL, NPM1, MYD88*, etc.), radiologic imaging studies (e.g., bone lesions in patients with plasma cell neoplasm), and specific laboratory data (e.g., serum M protein, serum erythropoietin level, viral studies for HTLV1, serum calcium levels, etc.).

Intensity of staining

The results of the staining are determined by the comparison between negative controls and the intensity of staining with each antibody (Figures 1.16–1.18). The negative staining can be defined by the fluorescence intensity similar to that of negative controls. The staining is positive when the expression (fluorescence intensity) of any given marker (antibody) is greater than that of a negative (isotypic) control. Even in heterogeneous (complex) samples such as blood or BM specimens, the use of "built-in" negative controls is limited and may lead to misinterpretation of the

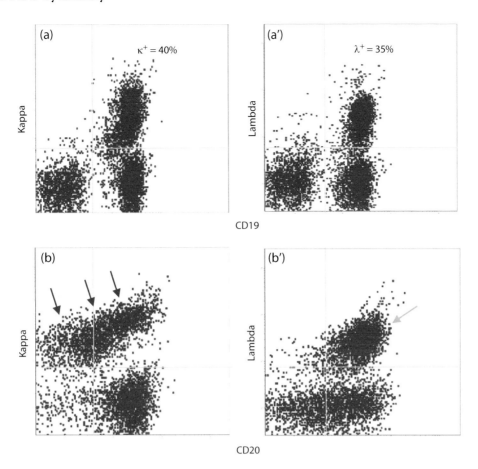

FIGURE 1.15 Analysis of percent of kappa⁺ and lambda⁺ B-cells in this CLL may suggest polytypic process (a, a′), but careful evaluation of pattern of antigen expression (CD20 versus kappa and lambda) indicate bi-clonal B-cell lymphoproliferative process: kappa⁺ B-cells show variable CD20 expression (b; red arrows) whereas lambda⁺ B-cells show more cohesive cluster of cells (b′; gray arrow).

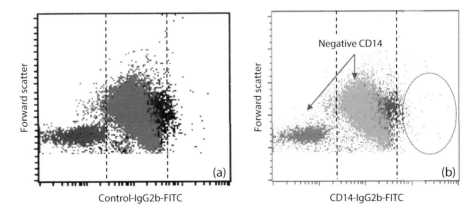

FIGURE 1.16 Assessing the staining results: the staining intensity for each antibody is compared with the negative control. Myelomonocytic population (green and blue dots) in panel b appears to express CD14, when compared to overtly negative lymphocytes (red dots). However, the intensity of the expression of CD14 is similar to non-specific staining with isotypic control (panel a), and therefore the result for CD14 have to be interpreted as negative. In this sample, only the cells located within the dotted circle (close to and beyond 10^3 on *x*-axis) would be considered positive. These panels show also that the "built-in" negative controls (in this case lymphocytes, which do not express CD14) cannot be used reliably as a negative control, since the population of interest may be characterized by a very high non-specific "background" staining (a).

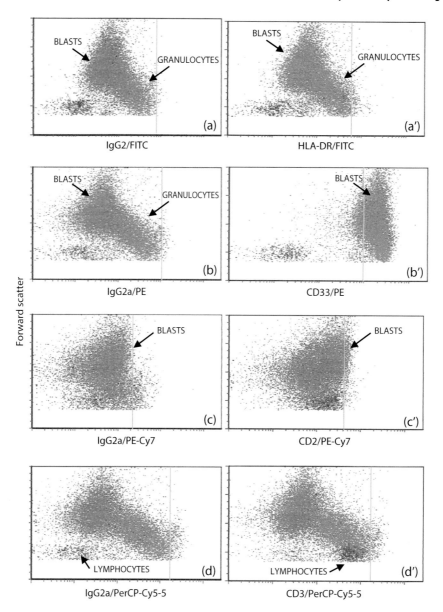

FIGURE 1.17 High non-specific (background) staining. Flow cytometry shows three distinct populations: blasts (green dots), granulocytes (gray dots) and lymphocytes (red dots). Based on control staining (left column; a–d) blasts are positive for CD33 (b′) and CD2 (c′), granulocytes are positive for CD33 (b′) and lymphocytes are positive for CD2 (c′) and CD3 (d′). All 3 populations do not express HLA-DR (a′).

results. Different cell populations often display variable intensity of "background" (non-specific) staining. Some cells (e.g., monocytic cells, atypical promyelocytes, and large lymphomatous cells with decreased viability) often display high non-specific staining (Figures 1.17 and 1.18). Therefore, the threshold between positive and negative expression should be established for each cell population based on the control (negative) sample and not by comparison with other population known to be negative for a specific marker. As illustrated in Figure 1.16, if only staining with CD14 was performed, each population with intensity greater than observed in lymphocytes (red dots), which do not express CD14 would be considered positive. However, as it is evident from the staining with negative (isotypic) control antibody (Figure 1.16a), the abnormal cells (green and blue dots) have extremely high nonspecific staining which is similar to that observed with CD14 (Figure 1.16b). Figure 1.17 illustrates the different level of

background (non-specific) staining among different populations (myeloblasts, granulocytes and benign T-lymphocytes) in the BM involved by AML. Only careful comparison of antigen expression for each population with that of non-specific staining (control) allows for the proper characterization of identified cells as positive or negative for a given marker.

The intensity of expression of any antigen can be categorized into dim, moderate, bright, and variable (Figure 1.18). The expression of an antigen may be homogeneous (e.g., all cells show dim pattern of expression), variable, or "smeary" (e.g., ranging from dim to moderate to bright) or partial (e.g., subset of cells is negative, and subset is positive for a given marker). The intensity of staining of any population is compared to that of benign counterpart and reported as either normal or abnormal. Each cell types have different pattern of antigen expression, for example, bright CD38 expression and negative CD45 expression is normal for

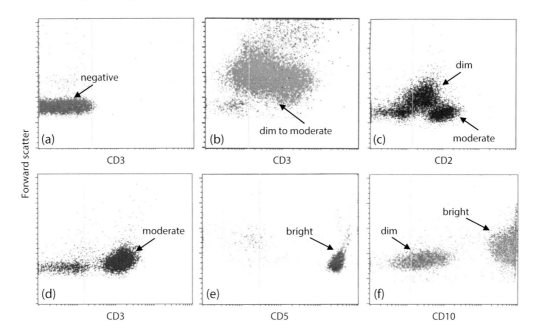

FIGURE 1.18 Intensity of antigen expression, see text for details.

benign plasma cells, whereas bright CD45 expression and moderate CD20 expression is normal for benign B-cells. In Figure 1.18a, red dots representing lymphocytes are negative for CD3. Dim staining is defined by the fluorescence intensity which is slightly increased when compared to negative control. The cells in Figure 1.18b have dim to moderate expression of CD3. Moderate staining is defined by at least one log decade brighter than negative control (Figure 1.18c–d). Figure 1.18c shows two populations of cells: one with dim and other with moderate expression of CD2. The abnormal population of lymphocytes (dim CD2) has increased forward scatter (FSC) suggesting larger cell size when compared to benign lymphocytes (moderate CD2). Bright staining is at least two log decades brighter than negative control. T-PLL cells (red; Figure 1.18e) and B-lymphoblasts (Figure 1.18f) display bright expression of CD5 and CD10, respectively. Based on the FC consensus meeting in Bethesda, the recommended descriptions of antibody distribution are "Negative", "Positive", or "Partially expressed" (relative to an appropriate negative control population) and the recommended descriptions of antibody fluorescence intensity are "Dim", "Bright", and "Heterogeneous", with the intensity relative to the closest normal hematolymphoid population [23].

The co-expression of antigens

The diagnosis and subclassification of hematopoietic tumors rely not only on the distinction between positive and negative expression of analyzed marker or the fluorescence intensity, but also on the proper identification of the co-expression of two or more markers by the same population of cells. The possibility to analyze the co-expression of several antigens on single cell is one of the biggest advantages of multicolor (multiparameter) FC analysis. Among B-cell lymphoproliferations, co-expression of B-cell markers with CD5 and CD23 is seen typically in CLL/SLL, CD25, and CD103 in HCL, CD10 and BCL2 in follicular lymphoma (FL), CD5 in mantle cell lymphoma (MCL), and CD10 and CD43 in BL. T-cell lymphomas may show co-expression of T-cell antigens with CD30 (e.g., anaplastic large cell lymphoma, ALCL), CD10 (nodal T-cell lymphomas with T-follicular helper (TFH) phenotype, including AITL,

and follicular T-cell lymphoma; FTCL), CD103 (enteropathy-associated T-cell lymphoma, EATL), and CD16/CD56/CD57 (T-cell large granular lymphocyte leukemia, T-LGLL; T/NK-cell lymphoproliferations). The majority of normal BM blasts co-express CD34 and CD117, while discordant CD34 and CD117 expression by blasts may indicate neoplastic processes. Figure 1.19 illustrates co-expression of different antigens by hematopoietic tumors.

Aberrant expression of antigens

Benign B-cells are positive for B-cell markers (e.g., CD19, CD20, CD22, CD79a, and CD79b) and negative for T-cell markers, and conversely, normal T-cells are positive for T-cell antigens (CD2, CD3, CD5, and CD7) and are negative for B-cell markers. Other cell lineages have also characteristic immunophenotypic profiles, e.g., benign monocytes display bright expression of CD11b, CD11c, CD14, and CD64 and are positive for HLA-DR, neutrophils are positive for pan-myeloid antigens (CD13, CD33), CD10, CD11b, and CD16, and benign plasma cells are positive for CD119, CD38, CD45, CD138, and are negative for CD56 and CD117. See Table 1.4.

TABLE 1.4: Frequency of Aberrant Antigen Expression in B-Cell Lymphomas

CD5⁻ MCL	11%
CD23⁻ CLL/SLL	4%
CD10⁺ HCL	12%
CD19⁺ PCM	2%
CD10⁻ FL	6%
CD5⁺ FL	1%
CD5⁺ MZL	10%–15%
CD56⁺ DLBCL	<1%
CD2⁺ CLL/SLL	<1%
CD200⁺ MCL	4%
CD5⁺ DLBCL	5%–20%
CD10⁺ LPL/WM	5%–10%

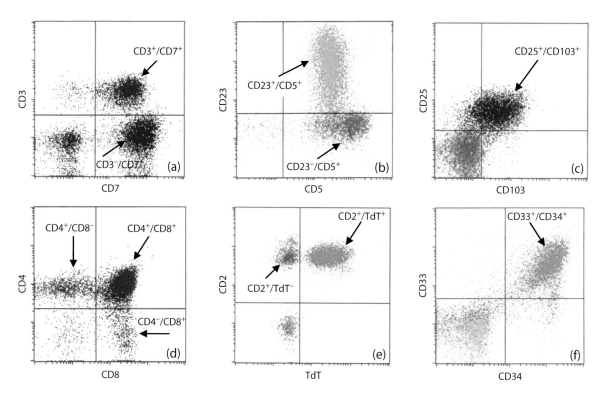

FIGURE 1.19   Co-expression of antigens. (a) Two populations of T-cells are identified by comparing the expression of CD3 and CD7. Normal (benign) T-cells (upper right quadrant) co-express CD3 and CD7, whereas neoplastic cells (lower right quadrant) lack CD3. (b) B-CLL/SLL is characterized by co-expression of CD5 and CD23 (upper right quadrant) in contrast to benign T-cells which have brighter expression of CD5 and do not express CD23 (lower right quadrant). (c) HCL is characterized by co-expression of CD25 and CD103. (d) Immature T-cell population (thymocytes from thymoma) display co-expression of CD4 and CD8 (upper right quadrant). Mature T-cells are either CD4+ (upper left quadrant) or CD8+ (lower right quadrant). (e) Immature T-cell population co-expressing CD2 and TdT (upper right quadrant); benign T-cells express CD2 but are TdT− (upper left quadrant). (f) Myeloblasts co-expressing CD34 and CD33 (arrow).

Identification of aberrant antigen expression helps to identify neoplastic process and allows for identification of MRD or early relapse in follow-up studies [13, 19, 96–113]. Types of aberrant antigen expression in FC studies include "lineage infidelity" (presence of markers associated with different cell lineage, such as B-cell makers on T-cells, T-cell markers on B-cells or myeloblasts, myeloid antigens in B-lymphoblasts or plasma cells, NK-cell marker CD56 on monoblasts), absence of an antigen which is normally positive (e.g., lack of HLA-DR or CD14 in monocytes, lack of surface CD3 in some T-cell neoplasms, lack of CD20 in B-cell lymphomas, and lack of CD45 in B- and T-cell lymphomas or leukemias), or unusually dim or bright expression of marker (e.g., bright CD10 in B-ALL, dim CD13 or CD33 in AML, bright CD11c expression in HCL, dim CD19 in FL, and dim or partial pan-T-cell markers in T-cell lymphomas). See Table 1.5.

Aberrant expression of T/NK cell-associated antigens (other than CD5 and CD43) on B-cell lymphomas is a known but

uncommonly observed phenomenon [114–116]. Neoplastic plasma cells often express CD56 and CD117 [117], CLL may show aberrant expression of CD2, CD4, or CD7, and rare cases of diffuse large B-cell lymphoma (DLBCL) may be CD56+. Aberrant expression of CD43 is often seen in CLL, MCL, BL, and subset of marginal zone lymphomas. Aberrant expression of CD200 is typical for CLL, HCL, and PCM. "Lineage infidelity" is also seen in acute leukemias, including positive expression of CD7 by myeloblasts and CD19 and CD56 in AML with t(8;21). T-cells in AITL are often positive for CD10 and other T-follicular helper markers [13, 118]. Maturing myeloid cells in MDS or MPN often display abnormal expression of CD56 [99]. Inaba et al. reported aberrant expression of T-cell antigens in 24.2% of B-cell lymphomas [116] and Quintanilla-Martinez et al. reported CD20+ T-cell lymphoma [119]. The co-expression of CD5 and CD23 is typical for CLL/SLL, but subset of cases may show aberrant lack of CD23. Similarly, co-expression of CD5 is typical for MCL but ~10% of cases show lack of CD5. Another example of aberrant loss of antigen expression includes CD10− FL or CD20− CLL (or less often other B-cell lymphoproliferations). See Table 1.6.

TABLE 1.5: Aberrant Expression of T-cell Antigens in Non-T-Cell Disorders

CD2	APL, BPDCN, mast cell disease, rare cases of CLL/SLL
CD3	PEL
CD5	SLL/CLL, MCL, some MZL, rare cases of FL, de novo DLBCL, thymoma/thymic carcinoma
CD7	AML, APL, BPDCN, monocytic leukemia
CD8	CLL (rare cases)

TABLE 1.6: Aberrant Expression of Pan-B Antigens in Non-B-Cell Disorders

CD19	Acute myeloid leukemia with t(8;21)
CD20	Peripheral T-cell lymphoma, NOS (rare cases)
CD79a	Megakaryocytes (non-specific staining)

Figure 1.20 presents several examples of aberrant antigen expression: DLBCL with aberrant expression of CD56 (Figure 1.20a); HCL with aberrant expression of CD2 on a subset of leukemic cells (Figure 1.20b; arrow); CLL/SLL with co-expression of CD8 (Figure 1.20c; arrow); and PTCL with aberrant expression of CD20 (arrow) on a subset of T-cells (Figure 1.20d) and MZL with MZL with aberrant expression of CD13 (Figure 1.20e). Similar to aberrant expression of an antigen, lack of a marker which is present help to identify and define abnormal cell population (Figure 1.21): acute monoblastic leukemia with aberrant loss of HLA-DR expression (Figure 1.21a); B-cell acute lymphoblastic leukemia (B-ALL) with loss of CD45 expression (Figure 1.21b); DLBCL with loss of CD20 (Figure 1.21c); and PTCL with aberrant loss of surface CD3 expression (Figure 1.21d).

Forward and side (orthogonal) light scatter

In FC analysis, cells are tagged with fluorochromes-conjugated monoclonal antibodies directed toward specific surface,

cytoplasmic, or nuclear antigens. Intrinsic physical properties of the cells, especially their size and cytoplasmic granularity, are measured simultaneously with fluorescence emission as the fluorochrome-tagged cells pass through laser light. The light scatter is measured in two different directions, forward (forward scatter or FSC) and at 90° (side scatter or SSC). The SSC (right angle/orthogonal light scatter) corresponds to the granularity of the cytoplasm and indicates the internal complexity of the cell (Figure 1.22; y axis). The cells with agranular cytoplasm (i.e., lymphocytes) have low SSC, whereas cells with granular cytoplasm (i.e., neutrophils, eosinophils, hypergranular promyelocytes) have high SSC. Forward angle light scatter (forward scatter; FSC) corresponds to cell size (Figures 1.23 and 1.24). Large cells have higher FSC when compared to smaller cells: note the difference between myeloblasts and monoblasts in Figure 1.23 and between small lymphocytes (red dots), large lymphocytes (blue dots), and cancer cells (orange dots) in Figure 1.24.

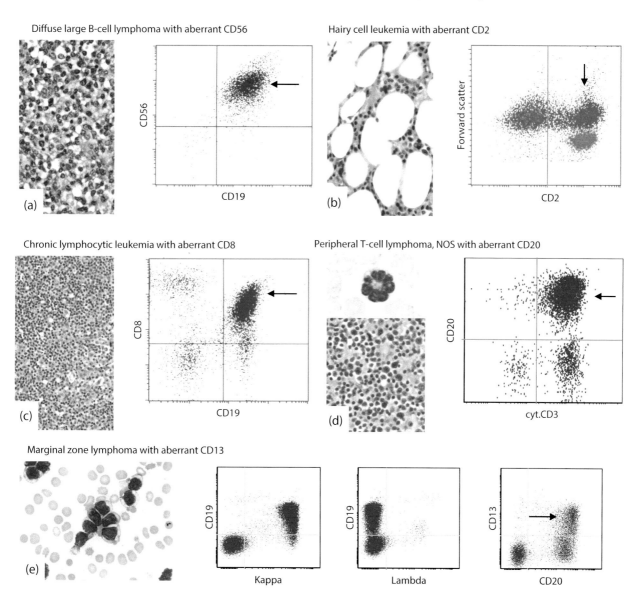

FIGURE 1.20   Aberrant antigen expression. (a) DLBCL with aberrant expression of CD56; (b) HCL with aberrant expression of CD2 on a subset of leukemic cells; (c) CLL/SLL with co-expression of CD8 (arrow); (d) PTCL with aberrant expression of CD20 (arrow) on a subset of T-cells; (e) MZL with aberrant expression of CD13 (arrow).

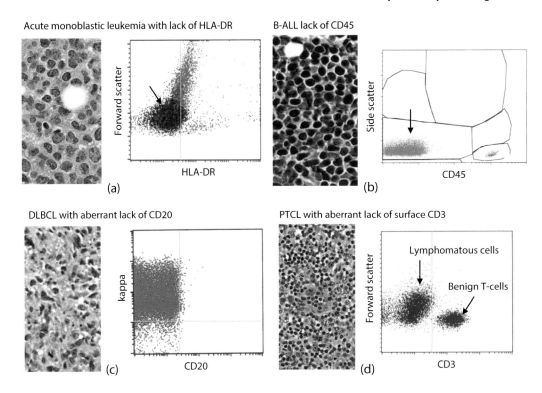

FIGURE 1.21 Aberrant lack of antigen expression. (a) Acute monoblastic leukemia with aberrant loss of HLA-DR expression; (b) B-ALL with loss of CD45 expression; (c) DLBCL with loss of CD20; (d) PTCL with aberrant loss of surface CD3 expression.

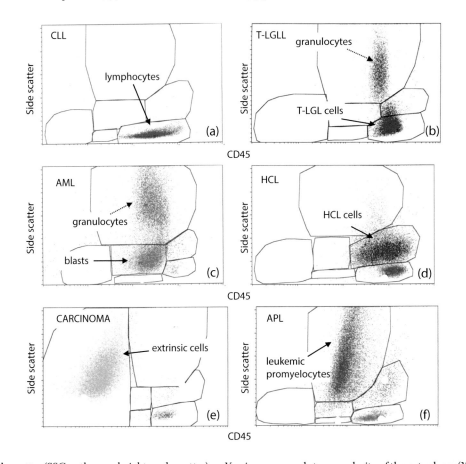

FIGURE 1.22 Side scatter (SSC; orthogonal, right angle scatter) on Y axis corresponds to granularity of the cytoplasm (X axis presents CD45 expression). Lymphocytes (a through f; red dots) have low SSC, whereas neutrophils (b–c), cancer cells (e) and atypical promyelocytes (f) have high SSC. Monocytes (b; blue dots), blasts (c; green dots) and HCL cells (d; blue dots) have higher SSC than lymphocytes (compare with red dots).

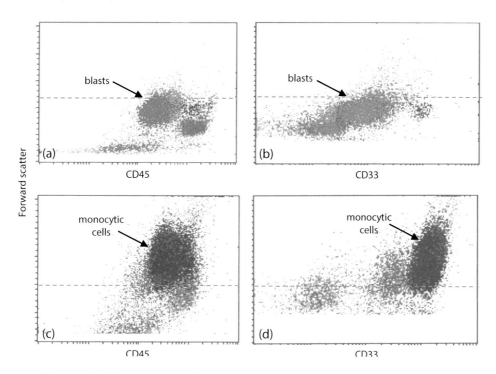

FIGURE 1.23 Forward scatter (FSC). Comparison of FSC (Y axis) between myeloblasts (a–b; green dots) and monoblasts (c–d; blue dots). Myeloblasts are smaller and therefore have lower FSC when compared to monocytic cells (compare with the location of dotted line in upper and lower panels or in relation to small lymphocytes marked with red dots).

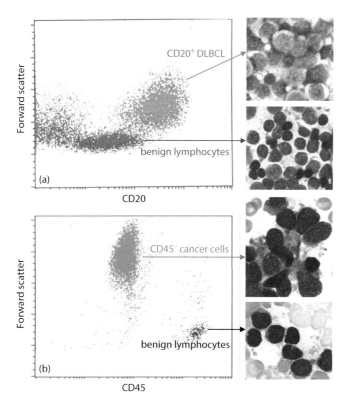

FIGURE 1.24 Forward scatter (FSC; Y axis): comparison between benign small lymphocytes (red dots, a), large lymphocytes of diffuse large B-cell lymphoma (blue dots; a) and metastatic cancer cells (orange dots; b).

Limitations of flow cytometry

Neoplasms with sparse neoplastic cells and/ or predominance of reactive elements
Hodgkin lymphoma

Hodgkin lymphoma (HL) is divided into classic Hodgkin lymphoma (cHL) and nodular lymphocyte predominant Hodgkin lymphoma (NLPHL; Figure 1.25) [25, 120–124]. Classic HL is a B-cell neoplasm characterized by the presence of Reed-Sternberg (R-S) cells and an accompanying polymorphic inflammatory infiltrate with eosinophils, histiocytes, small lymphocytes, and plasma cells. Based on the proportion of neoplastic cells (R-S cells and Hodgkin cells), the inflammatory background, and the amount of fibrosis, cHL is subdivided into four major subtypes: nodular sclerosis, lymphocyte-rich, mixed cellularity, and lymphocyte-depleted. NLPHL is a monoclonal B-cell neoplasm characterized by the presence of scattered large atypical CD20+ LP (lymphocyte predominant) cells also referred to as "popcorn cells", formerly known as L&H cells (lymphocyte and histiocyte cells) and a distinct nodular pattern on low magnification [25, 121, 124–129]. NLPHL involves most often peripheral lymph nodes (cervical, axillary, or inguinal lymph nodes), sparing usually mediastinal and axial lymph nodes. Mesenteric lymph node involvement can be seen but is rare. BM involvement is also rarely seen in NLPHL.

FC has limited role in the diagnosis of HL, where it serves mainly to exclude B- or T-cell disorders or in follow-up studies, to exclude secondary hematolymphoid tumors (e.g., post-therapy myeloid neoplasms or progression of HL into aggressive lymphomas). The neoplastic cells in classic HL (R-S and Hodgkin cells) and neoplastic cells in NLPHL (LP cells, lymphocyte predominant cells) are too large and too scarce to be harvested for routine

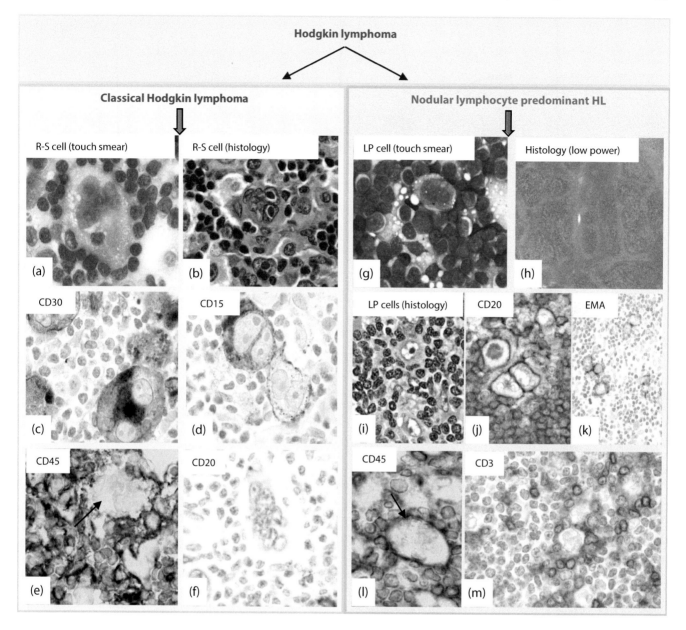

FIGURE 1.25 Classification of Hodgkin lymphomas. (a–f) classic HL: (a) touch imprint with Reed-Sternberg cells (R-S); (b) histologic section with typical multinucleated R-S cell; (c) positive CD30; (d) positive CD15; (e) negative CD45; and (f) negative CD20. (g–m) NLPHL: (g) touch imprint showing an atypical cell with large nucleus (LP cells, lymphocyte predominant); (h) low magnification of the lymph node showing nodular pattern; (i) high magnification showing typical LP cells (lymphocyte predominant, syn: "popcorn" or L&H cells); (j) positive CD20, (k) positive EMA; (l) positive CD45 (prominent membranous staining, compare with negative CD45 in R-S cells, e); (m) typical CD3+ T-cell rosettes around LP cells.

FC analysis (Figures 1.26 and 1.27), similarly to megakaryocytes in the analysis of the BM. In both classic HL and NLPHL, FC analysis often shows increased CD4:CD8 ratio (it may be normal or even reversed in occasional cases).

Despite difficulties in isolating neoplastic cells in cHL and NLPHL for FC analysis, several recent studies have tried to use FC in diagnosing HL and defining the phenotype of background T-cells [130–135]. Fromm et al. using 6-color FC approach characterized R-S cells by the increased side scatter and forward scatter, variably positive CD45 (in part due to bound T-cells), variable but mostly negative CD20 and CD64, and positive CD30, CD40, and CD95 [133, 134]. The immunophenotype of R-S cells depended on whether they were bound to T-cells (resetting) or represented pure

R-S cells after blocking the T-cells that surround Hodgkin cells in a preincubations step during sample preparation (CD58 and CD54 in R-S cells and CD2 and LFA-1 on T-cells). ALCL differs from cHL by strong CD45, variable CD30 and CD71, and lack of CD15, CD20, CD40, and CD64 expression, and DLBCL differs by bright CD20 and CD45 expression and lack of CD30, CD15, and CD64.

T-cell-rich/histiocytes-rich large B-cell lymphoma (THRLBL)

T-cell-rich/histiocytes-rich large B-cell lymphoma (THRLBL; Figure 1.28), characterized morphologically by predominance of reactive elements (small T-cells and histiocytes), and only rare neoplastic cells, most often yields negative results by FC for similar

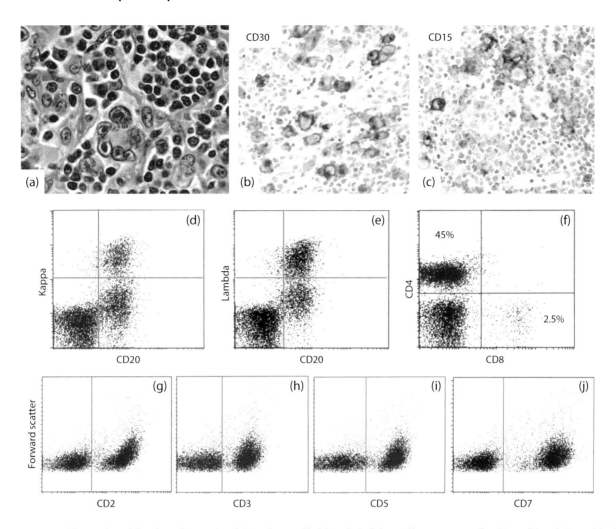

FIGURE 1.26 Classical Hodgkin lymphoma. Reed-Sternberg cells (a) and Hodgkin cells are positive for CD30 (b) and CD15 (c). Flow cytometry analysis (d–j) reveals only benign (polytypic) B-cells (d–f) and benign T-cells with increased CD4:CD8 ratio (f) and normal expression of pan-T-cell antigens (g–j).

reasons as in HL. Figure 1.29 shows the presence of rare neoplastic cells and predominance of reactive elements in THRLBL.

Nodal TFH cell lymphoma, angioimmunoblastic type (AITL)

AITL, especially early variant with preserved reactive, secondary follicles may show mostly reactive elements, may be difficult to identify by FC. The neoplastic T-cells are CD4+ and often show dim or negative expression of one or more of the pan-cell antigens, increased forward scatter and partial CD10 positivity. Subset of cells may be positive for CD71 (dim). Rare CD30+ cells are also often present. In some cases, the phenotypic atypia is easily identifiable (e.g., loss of CD3, CD5, and/or CD7), but immunophenotypic changes in the expression of pan-T-cell antigens may be subtle and abnormal population is identified through variable but increased forward scatter and CD4 restriction

Lymphoma in situ

FC plays very limited role in identifying lymphomas in situ. In situ follicular B-cell neoplasm (ISFN) is often discovered incidentally and comprise isolated scattered follicles colonized by monoclonal t(14;18)+ B-cells overexpressing BCL2 and CD10 within an otherwise uninvolved lymph node [25, 136, 137]. ISFNs are often

associated with prior or synchronous FL. Recently, BCL1+ (cyclin D1+) B cell infiltrate with MCL phenotype in the mantle zones of reactive-appearing lymphoid follicles or in colonic mucosa has been described and was termed in situ mantle cell neoplasm (IS-MCN). IS-MCN is an extremely rare phenomenon and represents either an early MCL (no overt lymphoma identified elsewhere) or an overt lymphoma (confirmed by morphologic and immunophenotypic analysis of concurrent tissues at different location) [138–143].

Neoplasms with prominent sclerosis (fibrosis)

Sclerotic tissue (e.g., lymph node with follicle center cell lymphoma or mediastinal large B-cell lymphoma) may be difficult to process for FC and yield enough cells for analysis (>10,000 cells are usually required).

Large cell and high-grade lymphomas

Even in cases of large B-cell lymphomas with numerous neoplastic cells, FC results may be negative or show only rare clonal cell, mostly due to selective drop-out of neoplastic cells (Figure 1.30), necrosis, or partial involvement. For similar reasons, other high-grade lymphomas, including anaplastic large cell lymphoma (Figure 1.31), may be missed by FC analysis.

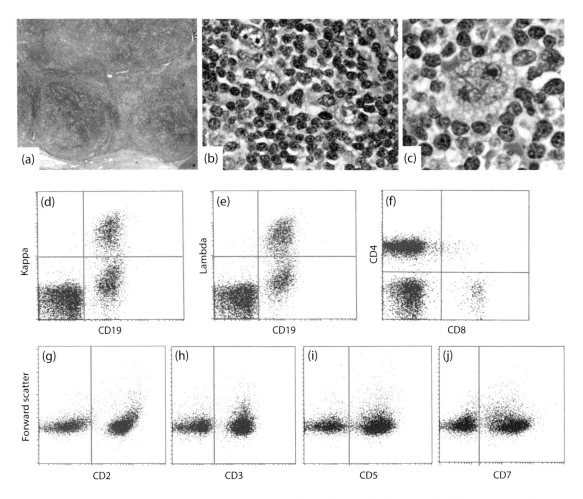

FIGURE 1.27 Nodular lymphocyte predominant Hodgkin lymphoma (NLPHL). The typical nodular patter on low power examination (a). Neoplastic cells (LP cells, also called "popcorn" cells or L&H cells) have large and multilobated or folded nuclei, prominent nucleoli and pale vesicular chromatin (b–c). Flow cytometry analysis shows polytypic B-cells (d–e) and T-cells with increased CD4:CD8 ratio (f) and normal pattern of expression of pan-T antigens (g–j).

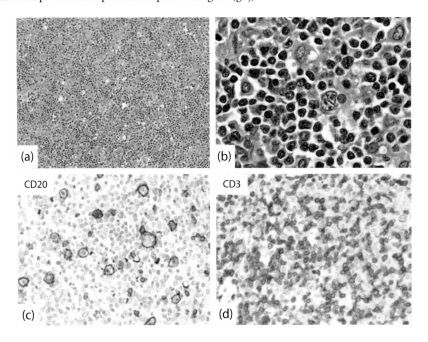

FIGURE 1.28 T-cell-rich large B-cell lymphoma. Atypical lymphoid infiltrate (a–b) with scattered large B-cell expressing CD20 (c) and predominance of small T-lymphocytes expressing CD3 (d).

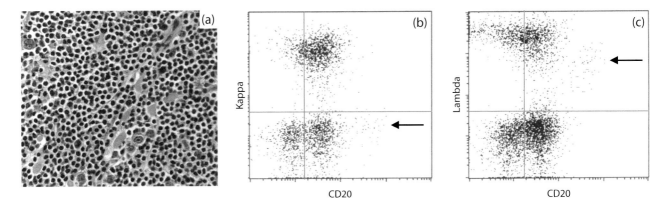

FIGURE 1.29 THRLBL. Tissue section (a) shows rare, atypical large lymphoid cells in the background of small lymphocytes. Flow cytometry (b–c) reveals minute clonal B-cell population (arrow) in the background of predominantly benign (polytypic) B-cells.

Lack of correlation with architectural (histologic) features

The other disadvantages of FC include loss of architectural relationship and correlation with histologic features, as specimen is disintegrated for staining and analysis. Architectural features are often crucial in subclassification of hematolymphoid tumors (e.g., FL versus diffuse lymphoma).

False negative FC results
Paratrabecular pattern of BM involvement

One of the major disadvantages of FC is discrepancies between FC and morphology. In the BM, lack of clonal B-cell population by FC analysis does not necessary excludes involvement by lymphoma. FC results may be falsely negative due to a paratrabecular distribution of neoplastic lymphoid aggregates (Figure 1.32).

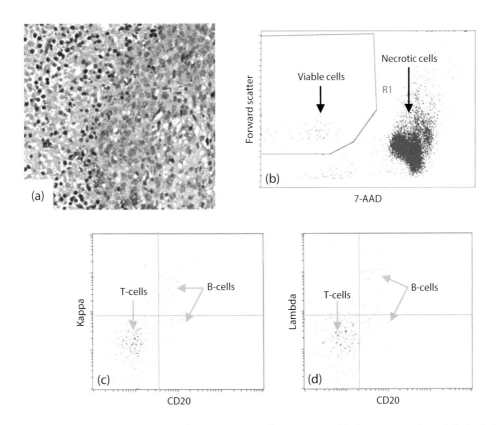

FIGURE 1.30 Diffuse large B-cell lymphoma with necrosis. Histologic section (a) shows necrosis and foci of viable tumor cells around blood vessels. Flow cytometry (b–d) results are negative due to predominance of necrotic cells in the sample (arrow). Rare T- and B-cells are identified (c–d).

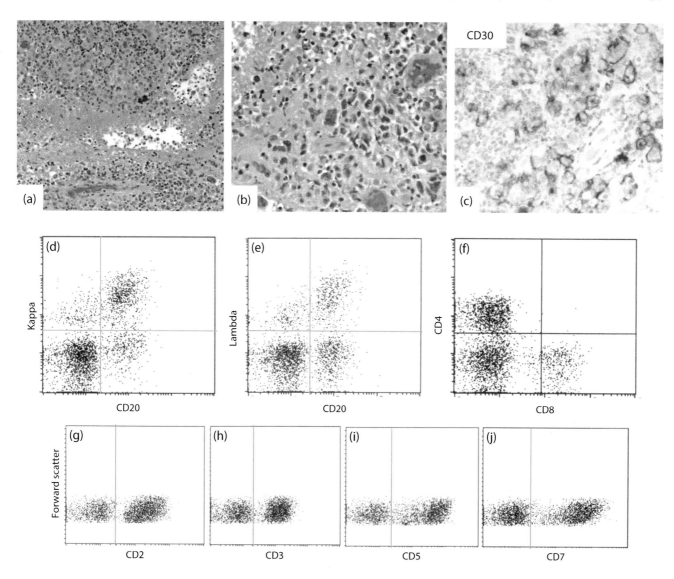

FIGURE 1.31 Anaplastic large cell lymphoma. Histologic sections (a–b) show numerous large neoplastic cells and areas of necrosis. Tumor cells are positive for CD30 (c). Flow cytometry shows only reactive B (d–e) and T-cells (f–j).

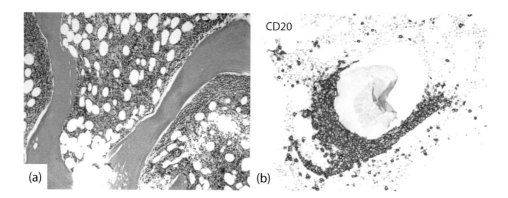

FIGURE 1.32 Bone marrow involved by follicular lymphoma (a, histology; b, immunostaining for CD20). Due to paratrabecular location of neoplastic lymphoid aggregates and/or due to reticulin fibrosis which often accompanies lymphoid infiltrate in the bone marrow, flow cytometry often does not reveal clonal B-cell population.

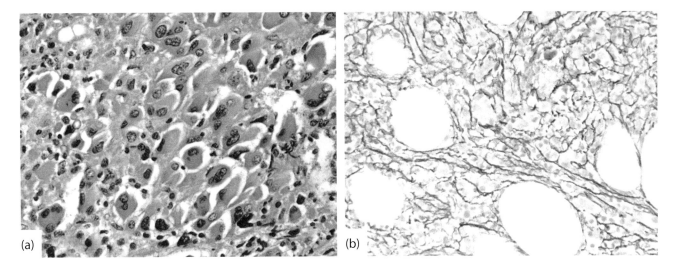

FIGURE 1.33   Acute megakaryoblastic leukemia (a) with prominent diffuse reticulin fibrosis (b). Fibrosis and predominance of large neoplastic cells (a) contribute to non-diagnostic FC results in many cases.

Increased reticulin fibrosis in BM
Due to tendency for some lymphomas (especially follicular lymphoma or lymphoplasmacytic lymphoma) for paratrabecular bone marrow involvement or increased reticulin fibrosis accompanying neoplastic infiltrate, clonal cells are not being aspirated into flow sample. In a series reported by Stacchini et al., FC and BM morphology agreed in 83.8% (both were positive or negative for lymphoma) and discrepant results were seen in 14.2% [144]. The latter group showed positive histology and negative FC (11.9%) or positive FC and histologically negative marrow (2.4%). Dunphy reported concordant results in 81.4% of cases; in 11.7% of cases, the morphology examination alone detected involvement, and in 4.7% of cases, FC detected involvement [145]. Perea et al. reported similar results (concordant results of FC and morphology in 79% and discordance in 21%) [146]. Prominent reticulin fibrosis often contributes to negative FC results (e.g., PMF or acute megakaryoblastic leukemia; Figure 1.33).

Focal BM or lymph node (or other tissue) involvement by neoplastic process
Focal (partial) involvement by neoplastic process, lymphoma in situ or uneven distribution of neoplastic cells (e.g., plasma cells or B-cells in BM), may lead to negative FC results.

Decreased viability of FC sample
Decreased viability of the sample may lead to false negative FC results. This is especially common in tumors with high proliferation rate (e.g., high grade lymphomas) or in when samples were mishandled (e.g., exposed to high temperatures, frozen or fixed).

Discrepant number of neoplastic cells
Bone marrow blasts
Since the FC analysis relies mostly on detection of membrane/cytoplasmic antigens, neoplastic cells with delicate and fragile cytoplasm are often underestimated or even absent, despite their abundance in the BM aspirate or core biopsy. Therefore, FC results cannot be used for specific diagnoses, which are based on numeric thresholds (e.g., 20% blasts for the diagnosis of AML or 10% plasma cells for the diagnosis of PCM).

Plasma cells
FC usually identifies fewer plasma cells than seen by immunohistochemistry in BM core biopsy or clot sections (Figure 1.34) or even aspirate smears. It is estimated that FC on average identifies 70% fewer plasma cells when compared to differential count of BM aspirate [147–149]. This poor recovery of plasma cells into FC samples is associated with susceptibility of plasma cells to destruction during sample preparation for FC, partial "hemodilution" of the sample and/or sampling error [117, 148]. The latter is caused by uneven distribution of plasma cells in the BM involved by PCM. Some patients with PCM may present with multiple lytic bone lesions but without intervening infiltration of BM (macrofocal PCM) [150]. The number of blasts may be underestimated by FC due to marrow fibrosis, uneven distribution of blasts in the BM, or abnormal phenotype of blasts, which lack typical markers of immaturity (CD34, CD117, and/or TdT).

Peripheral blood blasts
It is also not unusual to find much higher number of blasts by FC analysis of blood, when compared to actual number of blasts in the BM sample. This may be partially explained by abnormal "trafficking" of blasts in the BM with extensive fibrosis and/or presence of extramedullary hematopoiesis.

Dyserythropoiesis
The routine FC analysis does not evaluate red cell precursors, majority of which are eliminated from FC sample prior to the incubation with antibodies by using lysis procedure. Nucleated red cell precursors when present are underestimated and therefore the features of dyserythropoiesis are best evaluated on fresh BM aspirate smear (Figure 1.35). Recently, several FC methods have been used on non-lysed sample to evaluate dyserythropoiesis [151–153]. Della Porta et al. developed a quantitative FC approach to identify sideroblastic anemia by analyzing the expression of CD71, CD105, cytosolic H-ferritin, cytosolic L-ferritin, and mitochondrial ferritin in erythroblasts [153]. Compared with pathologic and healthy controls, MDS patients had higher expression of cytosolic H-ferritin and CD105, and lower expression of CD71 [153]. Mitochondrial ferritin was specifically detected in MDS with ring sideroblasts, and there was a close relationship between its expression and Prussian blue staining. The FC RED score

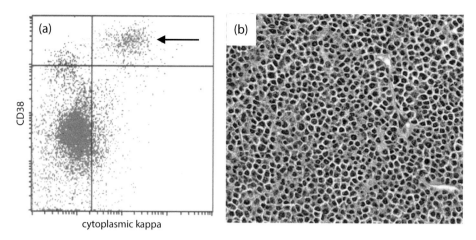

FIGURE 1.34 Multiple myeloma. The discrepancy between the number of clonal plasma cells detected by flow cytometry (a; arrow) and actual extent of bone marrow involvement (b) is due to drop-out of neoplastic cells during bone marrow aspiration and sample preparation. Plasma cells have delicate cytoplasm which often get destroyed during tissue processing leading to the under-representation of neoplastic cells on FC displays.

was developed as a whole BM FC protocol using the nuclear dye CyTRAK orange to gate nucleated cells without lysing red blood cells. The RED score is based on the evaluation of dyserythropoiesis with CD71 and CD36 coefficient of variation values and hemoglobin levels according to gender. It ranges from 0 to 7, with a RED score ≥3 predicting MDS with a sensitivity of 77.5% and a specificity of 90% [151, 152].

Dysgranulopoiesis

Many of the FC immunophenotypic abnormalities observed in patients with MDS are not specific and can be observed in reactive conditions, e.g., in post-chemotherapy marrow regeneration, viral infections, marrow involvement by lymphoma and treatment with growth factors (granulocyte colony-stimulating factor; G-CSF). MDS changes observed by FC may be similar to other myeloid disorders, especially MPNs or mixed MDS/MPN such as chronic myelomonocytic leukemia (CMML). Presence of prominent neutrophilia with eosinophilia, basophilia, and lymphopenia helps to differentiate CML from MDS. ET or MPNs in early stages of the disease often yield normal FC results, but differentiating MDS from some of the MPNs, especially early (pre-fibrotic) phase

of PMF is often not possible by FC analysis. Regenerating marrow may display marked myeloid shift, indicated by the predominance of granulocytes with low SSC and low-to-negative expression of CD10, CD11b, and CD16 and relatively bright CD33. CD56 may be aberrantly expressed on subset of granulocytes and/or monocytes in reactive conditions, including regenerating marrow, infections, and treatment with G-CSF. Maturing myeloid cells with prominent down-regulation of CD10 and CD16 need to be differentiated form neoplastic promyelocytes. Aberrant lack of expression of CD14 by monocytes is seen in PNH patients. Patients with viral infections, especially HIV often display aberrant pattern of myeloid maturation.

Differential diagnosis of CD10⁺ B-cell lymphomas

CD10⁺ B-cell lymphomas include FL, subset of DLBCL, BL, high grade B-cell lymphoma with rearrangement of *MYC* and *BCL2* (and/or *BCL6*) [HGBL-R], as well as rare cases of CD10⁺ mantle cell lymphoma (MCL), lymphoplasmacytic lymphoma (LPL), and HCL. Low grade FL is characterized by low forward scatter of clonal B-cells, dim CD19, negative or dim CD81 and CD200, lack of CD11c, and often positive CD38 expression. Co-expression

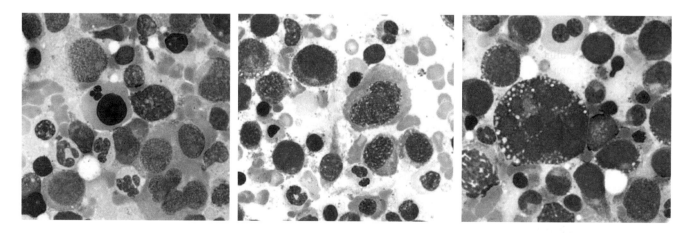

FIGURE 1.35 Bone marrow aspirate with prominent dyserythropoiesis representing MDS.

of CD5 with CD10 is most often associated with MCL. LPL is characterized by admixture of clonal IgM⁺ plasma cells in addition to clonal B-cell population and presence of *MYD88* mutation. HCL has typical bright expression of CD11c and co-expression of CD103 with CD25. The distinction between CD10⁺ B-cell lymphomas composed of medium to large cells (BL, high grade FL, HGBL-R, and DLBCL) is difficult, if not often possible by FC. Majority of high grade FLs show positive BCL2 expression, although subset of cases may be BCL2⁻. BL are BCL2⁻ and majority of HGBL-R are BCL2⁺. Common phenotypic features between HGBL-R and BL include positive CD71, bright expression of CD38 and CD81, and negative CD200. The final diagnosis is established based on histomorphology, Ki-67 index, and genetic profile including status of *BCL2*, *BCL6*, and *MYC* rearrangement (see Chapters 12 and 13 for details).

Phenotypic atypia of T-cells

The identification of neoplastic T-cell process based on aberrant phenotype revealed by FC is not always straightforward as various reactive processes may lead to activation and expansion of different T-cell subpopulations with or without subtle phenotypic changes. Diminished, partial, or negative expression of one or even two T-cell markers and/or increased FSC may be observed in reactive processes, including in viral infections (especially mononucleosis), treatment-associated changes, or in the sample involved by non-T-cell disorders. Memory T-cells show often decreased expression of CD7, NK cells are CD3 and CD5 negative, T-LGL cells are CD8⁺ and may show dimmer CD5. In normal and reactive conditions, the antigen most commonly showing aberrant expression is CD7, followed by CD5. In normal blood or BM samples, CD5 expression may be dim on a subset of benign T cells giving raise to two subtle T-cell populations, one with normal (moderate) CD5 and one with dim CD5. Minor population of CD7-negative T-cells can almost always be identified in benign samples from blood, BM or lymph nodes. Rare dual CD4/CD8⁺ T-cells or TCRγδ⁺ T-cells are also present in benign samples. In some reactive conditions, the CD7⁻ T-cell population may expand mimicking neoplastic process. This is especially common in patients with mononucleosis or in skin in patients with benign dermatoses. In a study by Weisberger et al., samples from all patients with infectious mononucleosis exhibited an activated (HLA-DR⁺, CD38⁺, CD8⁺) cytotoxic-suppressor T-cell population with aberrant down-regulation of CD7, and samples from 2 (8%) of 25 patients also showed down-regulation of CD5 [154]. Subset of normal NK cells may display dimmer expression of CD2 and CD7 [155].

T-LGL cell lymphocytosis and NK-cell lymphocytosis

It is often difficult to differentiate by FC analysis alone between reactive and malignant T-LGL or NK-cell proliferations. Two main variants of LGL proliferations can be recognized: T-cell T-LGLL and chronic lymphoproliferative disorder of NK cells (CLPD-NK), which account for more than 85% and 10% of cases, respectively. Another rare variant of LGL proliferation is called aggressive NK-cell leukemia, which is associated with Epstein-Barr virus (EBV) infection and poor prognosis. T-LGLL is usually an indolent and non-progressive disorder, and it has been suggested that it is at the end of a spectrum which ranges from a reactive/transient disorder, via a chronic lymphocytosis to clinically malignant disease requiring intensive therapy [156–159]. Chronic reactive proliferations of both TCRαβ⁺ and TCRγδ⁺ T-LGL- and NK cells are seen in various clinical conditions [160,

161]. In these cases, lymphocytosis is often <5 × 10⁹/L while in T-LGLL the lymphocytosis is often >5 × 10⁹/L. Differential diagnosis includes transient and chronic T-cell or NK-cell lymphocytosis in patients with viral infections, autoimmune disorders, patients with HCL or CLL, after chemotherapy or after organ transplantation (e.g., allogeneic BM transplant). Expansion of T-LGL cells is also observed in some patients with CML [162]. Differential diagnosis includes also T-cell clones of uncertain significance (T-CUS), which can be detected in patients with other malignancies and less often in healthy subjects [163] The T-CUS can be CD4⁻/CD8⁺ (78%), CD4⁻/CD8⁻ (12%), CD4⁺/CD8⁺ (9%), or CD4⁺/CD8⁻ (2%), with phenotypic features similar to T-LGLL, but with brighter CD2 and CD7 and dimmer CD3 expression [163]. In patients with LGL count in blood <0.5 × 10⁹/L without B-symptoms, cytopenias, infections, rheumatoid arthritis, and/or splenomegaly, and negative TCR gene rearrangement, diagnosis of T-LGLL is unlikely (they should be followed with FC analysis in 6 months). While the clonality of T-LGL process can be easily confirmed by TCR gene rearrangement, the confirmation of clonality in NK-cell neoplasms is difficult. Approximately one-third of CLPD-NK cases express restricted KIR (killer Ig-like receptor) antigens (CD158a, CD158b, and CD158c) while remaining third show absent KIR expression [66, 164, 165]. Since occasional reactive NK-cell proliferations can also have abnormal albeit transient expression of KIR, repeated studies are needed to definitively confirm NK-cell clonality [166].

APL with very dim or partial expression of CD117

Rare cases of APL may show very dim or partial expression of CD117, which may lead to false negative FC diagnosis. Careful attention to the pattern of CD45 versus side scatter showing dimmer CD45 expression and decreased side scatter (when compared to normal neutrophils), lack of CD10, CD11b, and CD16 expression by majority of myeloid cells, pattern of staining with viability dyes showing majority of cells in "non-viable" gate (positive staining for viability markers), as well as correlation with morphologic assessment of blood or BM aspirate smear help to make the correct diagnosis of APL and prompt rapid confirmatory testing by FISH and/or PCR for *PML-RARA* rearrangement.

APL with high, non-specific (auto)fluorescence

Some hematopoietic neoplasms may display non-specific autofluorescence leading to problems in determining between positive and negative antigen expressions. This is most commonly seen in APL, when majority of markers appears to be "positive" if analyzed without correlation with control (negative) staining. This high non-specific staining pattern in APL is one of the FC features helping in differential diagnosis between APL and HLA-DR-negative AML.

Classification of hematopoietic neoplasms

Hematopoietic neoplasms are subclassified broadly into lymphoid and myeloid neoplasms (Figure 1.36) [44, 167]. Both categories are further subdivided into immature tumors (acute leukemias, lymphoblastic lymphomas) and mature (chronic) tumors (B- and T-cell lymphomas, MDS, mastocytosis, and MPNs). Lymphoid neoplasms are categorized into either non-Hodgkin or HLs.

Non-Hodgkin lymphomas

Non-Hodgkin lymphomas (NHLs) are classified into B- or T-cell types and further subdivide into numerous histologic

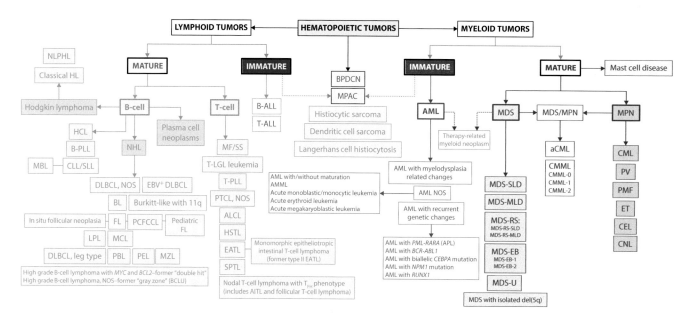

FIGURE 1.36 Classification of hematopoietic tumors.

Abbreviations: AITL, nodal TFH cell lymphoma angioimmunoblastic-type; aCML, atypical chronic myeloid leukemia; ALCL, anaplastic large cell lymphoma; ALL, acute lymphoblastic leukemia; AML, acute myeloid leukemia; AMML, acute myelomonocytic leukemia; BCLU, B-cell lymphoma, unclassifiable with features intermediate between BL and DLBCL; BL, Burkitt lymphoma; BPDCN, blastic plasmacytoid dendritic cell neoplasm; CEL, chronic eosinophilic leukemia; CML, chronic myeloid leukemia; CMML, chronic myelomonocytic leukemia; CNL, chronic neutrophilic leukemia; DLBCL, diffuse large B-cell lymphoma; EATL, enteropathy-associated T-cell lymphoma; EB, excess blasts; ET, essential thrombocythemia; HCL, hairy cell leukemia; HL, Hodgkin lymphoma; HSTL, hepatosplenic T-cell lymphoma; LPL, lymphoplasmacytic lymphoma; MBL, monoclonal B-cell lymphocytosis; MCL, mantle cell lymphoma; MLD, multilineage dysplasia; MPAL, mixed phenotype acute leukemia; MDS, myelodysplastic neoplasm; MDS-U, MDS unclassifiable; MF, mycosis fungoides; MPAL, mixed phenotype acute leukemia; MPN, myeloproliferative neoplasm; MZL, marginal zone lymphoma; NHL, non-Hodgkin lymphoma; NLPHL, nodular lymphocyte predominant Hodgkin lymphoma; NOS, not otherwise specified; PBL, plasmablastic lymphoma; PEL, primary effusion lymphoma; PCFCL, primary cutaneous follicle center lymphoma; PLL, prolymphocytic leukemia; PMF, primary myelofibrosis; PTCL, peripheral T-cell lymphoma; PV, polycythemia vera; RS, ring sideroblasts; SLD, single lineage dysplasia; SLL, small lymphocytic lymphoma; SPTL, subcutaneous panniculitis-like T-cell lymphoma; SS, Sézary syndrome; T$_{FH}$, T-follicular helper.

and phenotypic subtypes based on the stage of differentiation, histologic architecture, cell size, clinical data, and immunophenotype, and generally can be divided into indolent (low grade) and aggressive (high grade) [44, 168–192]. Mature B-cell neoplasms are the most common type of malignant lymphoma. The "low grade" category includes small lymphocytic lymphoma (SLL)/ CLL, low grade FL, primary cutaneous follicle center cell lymphoma (PCFCCL), marginal zone lymphoma (MZL) and lymphoplasmacytic lymphoma/ Waldenström macroglobulinemia (LPL/WM). Mantle cell lymphoma (MCL), although composed most often of small lymphocytes has a worse prognosis than most low-grade lymphomas. Subset of MCLs may have indolent clinical course (e.g., indolent leukemic non-nodal MCL or in situ mantle cell neoplasia). Leukemic non-nodal MCL display overlapping phenotypic and genetic features with CLL including lack of SOX11 expression, CD200 positivity, mutated *IGVH* and mostly less complex chromosomal changes [44, 167]. Subset of MCL may resemble morphologically and phenotypically MZL (MZL-like variant of MCL). Variants of FL include in situ follicular neoplasia, duodenal type FL, testicular FL and pediatric type FL. The large cell, "aggressive" group of B-cell lymphomas includes DLBCL and its variants, primary cutaneous DLBCL, leg type, EBV+ DLBCL, primary mediastinal large B-cell lymphoma (PMLBL), intravascular large B-cell

lymphoma (IVLBL), ALK+ large B-cell lymphoma, high grade lymphoma with rearrangement of MYC and BCL2 (and/or BCL6; HGBL-R), high grade lymphoma, not otherwise specified (HGBL, NOS), primary effusion lymphoma (PEL), blastoid and pleomorphic variants of MCL, BL, and plasmablastic lymphoma (PBL). Other disorders of B-cell origin include plasma cell neoplasms, HCL, and hairy cell leukemia variant (HCL-v).

T-cell lymphomas are diverse group of lymphoid neoplasms manifesting heterogeneous clinical, histologic, immunophenotypic, and cytogenetic features [64, 105, 193–213]. The classification of T-cell lymphoma is based largely on the histomorphologic features, phenotype, and clinical parameters. Predominantly nodal distribution is characteristic for T-cell lymphomas with T-follicular helper phenotype (T$_{FH}$) (which includes AITL and FTCL), peripheral T-cell lymphoma, not otherwise specified (PTCL, NOS), and anaplastic large cell lymphoma (ALCL). Extranodal location is seen in mycosis fungoides (MF), cutaneous ALCL, extranodal NK/T-cell lymphoma, nasal type, enteropathy-associated T-cell lymphoma (EATL), monomorphic epitheliotropic intestinal T-cell lymphoma (MEITL), hepatosplenic T-cell lymphoma (HSTL), and subcutaneous panniculitis-like T-cell lymphoma (SPTL). "Leukemic" presentation is typical for T-cell prolymphocytic leukemia (T-PLL), SS and T-LGL leukemia. ATLL may present as leukemic and nodal disease.

Hodgkin lymphomas

HL is divided into cHL and NLPHL. cHL is a B-cell neoplasm characterized by the presence of R-S cells and an accompanying polymorphic inflammatory infiltrate with eosinophils, histiocytes, small lymphocytes and plasma cells caused by cytokine production by the neoplastic cells. Based on the proportion of neoplastic cells (R-S cells and Hodgkin cells), the inflammatory background and the amount of fibrosis, HL is subdivided into four major subtypes: nodular sclerosis, lymphocyte-rich, mixed cellularity, and lymphocyte-depleted.

Immunodeficiency-associated lymphoproliferative disorders

These groups of disorders include post-transplant lymphoproliferative disorders and iatrogenic immunodeficiency-associated lymphoproliferative disorders.

Myeloproliferative neoplasms

MPNs represent a heterogeneous range of clonal hematopoietic stem cell diseases, which can be subdivided into classic and nonclassic myeloproliferative disorders [44, 214–226]. The first group includes chronic myeloid leukemia (CML, *BCR-ABL1*+) and three major non-CML categories: PV, ET, and PMF. Nonclassic myeloproliferative disorders include chronic neutrophilic leukemia (CNL), chronic eosinophilic leukemia, (CEL)/hypereosinophilic syndrome (HES), chronic basophilic leukemia, and MPNs, unclassifiable (MPN-U). Mastocytosis and myeloid/lymphoid neoplasms with eosinophilia and rearrangement of *PDGFA*, *PDGFRB*, or *FGFR1* constitute separate group of myeloid neoplasms.

Myelodysplastic neoplasms

MDS are divided into several categories: MDS with low blasts (MDS-LB), MDS, hypoplastic (MDS-h), MDS with increased blasts (MDS-IB), MDS with low blasts and SF3B1 mutation (MDS-SF3B1), and MDS with low blasts and isolated 5q deletion (MDS-5q). MDS-IB is further subdivided into type 1 (5%–9% blasts in the BM or 2%–4% blasts in blood) and type 2 (10%–19% blasts in the BM or 5%–19% blasts in blood) [44]. MDS (or AML) developing after exposure to chemo- or radiation therapy is classified as therapy-related myeloid neoplasm.

Myelodysplastic/myeloproliferative neoplasms

Myelodysplastic (MDS)/MPNs include CMML, atypical chronic myeloid leukemia (aCML; *BCR-ABL1*−), renamed in the updated WHO classification as myelodyplastic/myeloproliferative neoplasm with neutrophilia, MDS/MPN with SF3B1 mutation and thrombocytosis (MDS/MPN-SF3B1-T) and MDS/MPN, unclassifiable [44].

Acute myeloid leukemias

AML is divided into four major categories: (1) AML with recurrent genetic abnormalities; (2) AML with myelodysplasia-related changes; (3) therapy related myeloid neoplasms; and (4) AML, not otherwise specified (NOS). AML category includes also myeloid sarcoma (extramedullary myeloid tumor, EMT) and myeloid proliferations related to Down syndrome. The AML with recurrent genetic abnormalities include AML with t(8;21)/*RUNX1-RUNX1T1*, AML with inv(16)/*CBFB-MYH11*, APL with *PML-RARA*, AML with t(9;11)/*MLLT3-KMT2A*, AML with t(6;9)/*DEK-NUP214*, AML with inv(3), AML (megakaryoblastic) with t(1;22)/*RBM15-MKL1*,

AML with mutated *NPM1*, AML with biallelic mutations of *CEBPA*, and two provisional entities: AML with *BCR-ABL1* and AML with mutated *RUNX1*. The AML, NOS is further subdivided into AML with minimal differentiation, AML without maturation, AML with maturation, acute myelomonocytic leukemia (AMML), acute monoblastic (monocytic) leukemia, pure erythroid leukemia, acute basophilic leukemia, acute megakaryoblastic leukemia, and acute panmyelosis with myelofibrosis.

B-lymphoblastic leukemia/lymphoma

B-lymphoblastic leukemia/lymphoma (B-ALL) is subdivided into B-ALL, NOS, and B-ALL with recurrent genetic changes.

T-lymphoblastic leukemia/lymphoma

T-lymphoblastic leukemia/lymphoma (T-ALL) includes also two provisional entities: ETP-ALL and NK cell lymphoblastic leukemia/lymphoma.

Other hematopoietic tumors

Other tumors include mast cell disease (mastocytosis), myeloid/lymphoid neoplasms with eosinophilia and rearrangement of *PDGFRA*, *PDGFRB*, or *FGFR1*, AUL, MPAL, blastic plasmacytoid dendritic cell neoplasm (BPDCN), myeloid neoplasms with germline predisposition, gray zone lymphomas, histiocytic tumors, and Langerhans cell histiocytosis.

References

1. Borowitz, M.J., *Flow cytometry defended.* Am J Clin Pathol, 2000. **113**(4): p. 596–8.
2. Borowitz, M.J., et al., *U.S.-Canadian Consensus recommendations on the immunophenotypic analysis of hematologic neoplasia by flow cytometry: data analysis and interpretation.* Cytometry, 1997. **30**(5): p. 236–44.
3. Della Porta, M.G., et al., *Flow cytometry immunophenotyping for the evaluation of bone marrow dysplasia.* Cytometry B Clin Cytom, 2011. **80**(4): p. 201–11.
4. Baumgarth, N. and M. Roederer, *A practical approach to multicolor flow cytometry for immunophenotyping.* J Immunol Methods, 2000. **243**(1–2): p. 77–97.
5. Braylan, R.C., *Flow cytometry is becoming an indispensable tool in leukemia diagnosis and classification.* Cancer Invest, 1997. **15**(4): p. 382–3.
6. Braylan, R.C., et al., *U.S.-Canadian Consensus recommendations on the immunophenotypic analysis of hematologic neoplasia by flow cytometry: data reporting.* Cytometry, 1997. **30**(5): p. 245–8.
7. D'Archangelo, M., *Flow cytometry: new guidelines to support its clinical application.* Cytometry B Clin Cytom, 2007. **72**(3): p. 209–10.
8. Adachi, Y., et al., *A case of CD10-negative angioimmunoblastic T cell lymphoma with leukemic change and increased plasma cells mimicking plasma cell leukemia: a case report.* Oncol Lett, 2015. **10**(3): p. 1555–60.
9. Gorczyca, W., *Acute promyelocytic leukemia: four distinct patterns by flow cytometry immunophenotyping.* Pol J Pathol, 2012. **63**(1): p. 8–17.
10. Gorczyca, W., M.R. Melamed, and Z. Darzynkiewicz, *Analysis of apoptosis by flow cytometry.* Methods Mol Biol, 1998. **91**: p. 217–38.
11. Gorczyca, W., et al., *Immunophenotypic pattern of myeloid populations by flow cytometry analysis.* Methods Cell Biol, 2011. **103**: p. 221–66.
12. Gorczyca, W., et al., *Flow cytometry in the diagnosis of mediastinal tumors with emphasis on differentiating thymocytes from precursor T-lymphoblastic lymphoma/leukemia.* Leuk Lymphoma, 2004. **45**(3): p. 529–38.

13. Gorczyca, W., et al., *An approach to diagnosis of T-cell lympho-proliferative disorders by flow cytometry.* Cytometry, 2002. **50**(3): p. 177–90.

14. Kern, W., et al., *Clinical utility of multiparameter flow cytometry in the diagnosis of 1013 patients with suspected myelodysplastic syndrome: correlation to cytomorphology, cytogenetics, and clinical data.* Cancer, 2010. **116**(19): p. 4549–63.

15. Lee, D., G. Grigoriadis, and D. Westerman, *The role of multiparametric flow cytometry in the detection of minimal residual disease in acute leukaemia.* Pathology, 2015. **47**(7): p. 609–21.

16. Ossenkoppele, G.J., A.A. van de Loosdrecht, and G.J. Schuurhuis, *Review of the relevance of aberrant antigen expression by flow cytometry in myeloid neoplasms.* Br J Haematol, 2011. **153**(4): p. 421–36.

17. Porwit, A. and A. Rajab, *Flow cytometry immunophenotyping in integrated diagnostics of patients with newly diagnosed cytopenia: one tube 10-color 14-antibody screening panel and 3-tube extensive panel for detection of MDS-related features.* Int J Lab Hematol, 2015. **37** Suppl 1: p. 133–43.

18. Porwit, A., et al., *Revisiting guidelines for integration of flow cytometry results in the WHO classification of myelodysplastic syndromes-proposal from the International/European LeukemiaNet Working Group for Flow Cytometry in MDS.* Leukemia, 2014. **28**(9): p. 1793–8.

19. Weir, E.G. and M.J. Borowitz, *Flow cytometry in the diagnosis of acute leukemia.* Semin Hematol, 2001. **38**(2): p. 124–38.

20. Wood, B., *9-color and 10-color flow cytometry in the clinical laboratory.* Arch Pathol Lab Med, 2006. **130**(5): p. 680–90.

21. Wood, B.L., *Myeloid malignancies: myelodysplastic syndromes, myeloproliferative disorders, and acute myeloid leukemia.* Clin Lab Med, 2007. **27**(3): p. 551–75, vii.

22. Wood, B., *Multicolor immunophenotyping: human immune system hematopoiesis.* Methods Cell Biol, 2004. **75**: p. 559–76.

23. Wood, B.L., et al., *2006 Bethesda International Consensus recommendations on the immunophenotypic analysis of hematolymphoid neoplasia by flow cytometry: optimal reagents and reporting for the flow cytometric diagnosis of hematopoietic neoplasia.* Cytometry B Clin Cytom, 2007. **72 Suppl 1**: p. S14–S22.

24. McKinnon, K.M., *Flow cytometry: an overview.* Curr Protoc Immunol, 2018. **120**: p. 5.1.1–5.1.11.

25. Swerdlow, S.H., Campo, E., Harris, N. L., Jaffe, E. S., Pileri, S. A., Stein, H., Stein, H., Thiele, J., Arber, D.A., Le Beau M.M., Orazi, A., Siebert, R., eds. WHO classification of tumors of haematopoietic and lymphoid tissues. 2016, IARC: Lyon.

26. Borowitz, M.J., et al., *Immunophenotyping of acute leukemia by flow cytometric analysis. Use of CD45 and right-angle light scatter to gate on leukemic blasts in three-color analysis.* Am J Clin Pathol, 1993. **100**(5): p. 534–40.

27. Carter, P.H., et al., *Flow cytometric analysis of whole blood lysis, three anticoagulants, and five cell preparations.* Cytometry, 1992. **13**(1): p. 68–74.

28. Fleisher, T.A., C. Hagengruber, and G.E. Marti, *Immunophenotyping of normal lymphocytes.* Pathol Immunopathol Res, 1988. 7(5): p. 305–18.

29. Pagano, L., et al., *Blastic plasmacytoid dendritic cell neoplasm: diagnostic criteria and therapeutical approaches.* Br J Haematol, 2016. **174**(2): p. 188–202.

30. Coustan-Smith, E., et al., *Early T-cell precursor leukaemia: a subtype of very high-risk acute lymphoblastic leukaemia.* Lancet Oncol, 2009. **10**(2): p. 147–56.

31. Gutierrez, A. and A. Kentsis, *Acute myeloid/T-lymphoblastic leukaemia (AMTL): a distinct category of acute leukaemias with common pathogenesis in need of improved therapy.* Br J Haematol, 2018. **180**(6): p. 919–24.

32. Jain, N., et al., *Early T-cell precursor acute lymphoblastic leukemia/lymphoma (ETP-ALL/LBL) in adolescents and adults: a high-risk subtype.* Blood, 2016. **127**(15): p. 1863–9.

33. Khogeer, H., et al., *Early T precursor acute lymphoblastic leukaemia/lymphoma shows differential immunophenotypic characteristics including frequent CD33 expression and in vitro response to targeted CD33 therapy.* Br J Haematol, 2019. **186**(4): p. 538–48.

34. Noronha, E.P., et al., *T-lymphoid/myeloid mixed phenotype acute leukemia and early T-cell precursor lymphoblastic leukemia similarities with NOTCH1 mutation as a good prognostic factor.* Cancer Manag Res, 2019. **11**: p. 3933–43.

35. Bene, M.C. and A. Porwit, *Acute leukemias of ambiguous lineage.* Semin Diagn Pathol, 2012. **29**(1): p. 12–8.

36. Heesch, S., et al., *Acute leukemias of ambiguous lineage in adults: molecular and clinical characterization.* Ann Hematol, 2013. **92**(6): p. 747–58.

37. Porwit, A. and M.C. Bene, *Acute leukemias of ambiguous origin.* Am J Clin Pathol, 2015. **144**(3): p. 361–76.

38. Weinberg, O.K., et al., *Clinical, immunophenotypic, and genomic findings of acute undifferentiated leukemia and comparison to acute myeloid leukemia with minimal differentiation: a study from the bone marrow pathology group.* Mod Pathol, 2019. **32**(9): p. 1373–85.

39. Borowitz, M.J., *Mixed phenotype acute leukemia.* Cytometry B Clin Cytom, 2014. **86**(3): p. 152–3.

40. Charles, N.J. and D.F. Boyer, *Mixed-phenotype acute leukemia: diagnostic criteria and pitfalls.* Arch Pathol Lab Med, 2017. **141**(11): p. 1462–8.

41. Matutes, E., et al., *Mixed-phenotype acute leukemia: clinical and laboratory features and outcome in 100 patients defined according to the WHO 2008 classification.* Blood, 2011. **117**(11): p. 3163–71.

42. Porwit, A. and M.C. Bene, *Multiparameter flow cytometry applications in the diagnosis of mixed phenotype acute leukemia.* Cytometry B Clin Cytom, 2019. **96**(3): p. 183–94.

43. Wolach, O. and R.M. Stone, *How I treat mixed-phenotype acute leukemia.* Blood, 2015. **125**(16): p. 2477–85.

44. Arber, D.A., et al., *The 2016 revision to the World Health Organization classification of myeloid neoplasms and acute leukemia.* Blood, 2016. **127**(20): p. 2391–405.

45. Borowitz, M.J., et al., *Guidelines for the diagnosis and monitoring of paroxysmal nocturnal hemoglobinuria and related disorders by flow cytometry.* Cytometry B Clin Cytom, 2010. **78**(4): p. 211–30.

46. Brodsky, R.A., et al., *Improved detection and characterization of paroxysmal nocturnal hemoglobinuria using fluorescent aerolysin.* Am J Clin Pathol, 2000. **114**(3): p. 459–66.

47. Kwong, Y.L., et al., *Flow cytometric measurement of glycosylphosphatidyl-inositol-linked surface proteins on blood cells of patients with paroxysmal nocturnal hemoglobinuria.* Am J Clin Pathol, 1994. **102**(1): p. 30–5.

48. Richards, S.J. and D. Barnett, *The role of flow cytometry in the diagnosis of paroxysmal nocturnal hemoglobinuria in the clinical laboratory.* Clin Lab Med, 2007. **27**(3): p. 577–90, vii.

49. Richards, S.J., A.C. Rawstron, and P. Hillmen, *Application of flow cytometry to the diagnosis of paroxysmal nocturnal hemoglobinuria.* Cytometry, 2000. **42**(4): p. 223–33.

50. Seth, N., et al., *Utility of FLAER and CD157 in a five-color single-tube high sensitivity assay, for diagnosis of Paroxysmal Nocturnal Hemoglobinuria (PNH)-A standalone flow cytometry laboratory experience.* Int J Lab Hematol, 2021. **43**(2): p. 259–65.

51. Sutherland, D.R., et al., *Use of a FLAER-based WBC assay in the primary screening of PNH clones.* Am J Clin Pathol, 2009. **132**(4): p. 564–72.

52. van der Schoot, C.E., et al., *Deficiency of glycosyl-phosphatidylinositol-linked membrane glycoproteins of leukocytes in paroxysmal nocturnal hemoglobinuria, description of a new diagnostic cytofluorometric assay.* Blood, 1990. **76**(9): p. 1853–9.

53. Sutherland, D.R., et al., *ICCS/ESCCA consensus guidelines to detect GPI-deficient cells in paroxysmal nocturnal hemoglobinuria (PNH) and related disorders part 2 – reagent selection and assay optimization for high-sensitivity testing.* Cytometry B Clin Cytom, 2018. **94**(1): p. 23–48.

54. Delgado, J., et al., *Chronic lymphocytic leukemia: from molecular pathogenesis to novel therapeutic strategies.* Haematologica, 2020. **105**(9): p. 2205–17.

55. Nieto, W.G., et al., *Increased frequency (12%) of circulating chronic lymphocytic leukemia-like B-cell clones in healthy subjects using a highly sensitive multicolor flow cytometry approach.* Blood, 2009. **114**(1): p. 33–7.

56. Rawstron, A.C., *Monoclonal B-cell lymphocytosis: good news for patients and CLL investigators.* Leuk Lymphoma, 2007. **48**(6): p. 1057–8.

57. Shanafelt, T.D., et al., *Brief report: natural history of individuals with clinically recognized monoclonal B-cell lymphocytosis compared with patients with Rai 0 chronic lymphocytic leukemia.* J Clin Oncol, 2009. **27**(24): p. 3959–63.

58. Shao, H., et al., *Distinguishing hairy cell leukemia variant from hairy cell leukemia: development and validation of diagnostic criteria.* Leuk Res, 2013. **37**(4): p. 401–9.

59. Stetler-Stevenson, M. and P.R. Tembhare, *Diagnosis of hairy cell leukemia by flow cytometry.* Leuk Lymphoma, 2011. **52 Suppl 2**: p. 11–3.

60. Hu, Z., et al., *CD200 expression in mantle cell lymphoma identifies a unique subgroup of patients with frequent IGHV mutations, absence of SOX11 expression, and an indolent clinical course.* Mod Pathol, 2018. **31**(2): p. 327–36.

61. Ye, H., et al., *Smoldering mantle cell lymphoma.* J Exp Clin Cancer Res, 2017. **36**(1): p. 185.

62. Cook, L.B., et al., *Revised adult T-cell leukemia-lymphoma international consensus meeting report.* J Clin Oncol, 2019. **37**(8): p. 677–87.

63. Dearden, C.E., *T-cell prolymphocytic leukemia.* Med Oncol, 2006. **23**(1): p. 17–22.

64. Foucar, K., *Mature T-cell leukemias including T-prolymphocytic leukemia, adult T-cell leukemia/lymphoma, and Sezary syndrome.* Am J Clin Pathol, 2007. **127**(4): p. 496–510.

65. Scarisbrick, J.J., et al., *Blood classification and blood response criteria in mycosis fungoides and Sezary syndrome using flow cytometry: recommendations from the EORTC cutaneous lymphoma task force.* Eur J Cancer, 2018. **93**: p. 47–56.

66. de Mel, S., et al., *The utility of flow cytometry in differentiating NK/T cell lymphoma from indolent and reactive NK cell proliferations.* Cytometry B Clin Cytom, 2018. **94**(1): p. 159–68.

67. Lyapichev, K.A., et al., *Determination of immunophenotypic aberrancies provides better assessment of peripheral blood involvement by mycosis fungoides/Sezary syndrome than quantification of CD26- or CD7- CD4+ T-cells.* Cytometry B Clin Cytom, 2021. **100**(2): p. 183–91.

68. Al-Mawali, A., D. Gillis, and I. Lewis, *The role of multiparameter flow cytometry for detection of minimal residual disease in acute myeloid leukemia.* Am J Clin Pathol, 2009. **131**(1): p. 16–26.

69. Al-Mawali, A., A.D. Pinto, and S. Al-Zadjali, *CD34+CD38-CD123+ cells are present in virtually all acute myeloid leukaemia blasts: a promising single unique phenotype for minimal residual disease detection.* Acta Haematol, 2017. **138**(3): p. 175–81.

70. Arroz, M., et al., *Consensus guidelines on plasma cell myeloma minimal residual disease analysis and reporting.* Cytometry B Clin Cytom, 2015. **90**(1): p. 31–9.

71. Chen, X. and B.L. Wood, *Monitoring minimal residual disease in acute leukemia: technical challenges and interpretive complexities.* Blood Rev, 2017. **31**(2): p. 63–75.

72. Cherian, S., et al., *A novel flow cytometric assay for detection of residual disease in patients with B-lymphoblastic leukemia/lymphoma post anti-CD19 therapy.* Cytometry B Clin Cytom, 2018. **94**(1): p. 112–20.

73. de Tute, R.M., et al., *Minimal residual disease following autologous stem cell transplant in myeloma: impact on outcome is independent of induction regimen.* Haematologica, 2016. **101**(2): p. e69–e71.

74. Flores-Montero, J., et al., *Next generation flow for highly sensitive and standardized detection of minimal residual disease in multiple myeloma.* Leukemia, 2017. **31**(10): p. 2094–103.

75. Ossenkoppele, G. and G.J. Schuurhuis, *MRD in AML: does it already guide therapy decision-making?* Hematology Am Soc Hematol Educ Program, 2016. **2016**(1): p. 356–65.

76. Rawstron, A.C., et al., *Improving efficiency and sensitivity: European Research Initiative in CLL (ERIC) update on the international harmonised approach for flow cytometric residual disease monitoring in CLL.* Leukemia, 2013. **27**(1): p. 142–9.

77. Rawstron, A.C., et al., *Measuring disease levels in myeloma using flow cytometry in combination with other laboratory techniques: lessons from the past 20 years at the Leeds Haematological Malignancy Diagnostic Service.* Cytometry B Clin Cytom, 2016. **90**(1): p. 54–60.

78. Rawstron, A.C., B. Paiva, and M. Stetler-Stevenson, *Assessment of minimal residual disease in myeloma and the need for a consensus approach.* Cytometry B Clin Cytom, 2016. **90**(1): p. 21–5.

79. Schuurhuis, G.J., et al., *Minimal/measurable residual disease in AML: a consensus document from the European LeukemiaNet MRD Working Party.* Blood, 2018. **131**(12): p. 1275–91.

80. Rawstron, A.C., et al., *A complementary role of multiparameter flow cytometry and high-throughput sequencing for minimal residual disease detection in chronic lymphocytic leukemia: an European Research Initiative on CLL study.* Leukemia, 2016. **30**(4): p. 929–36.

81. Rawstron, A.C., et al., *Reproducible diagnosis of chronic lymphocytic leukemia by flow cytometry: an European Research Initiative on CLL (ERIC) & European Society for Clinical Cell Analysis (ESCCA) Harmonisation project.* Cytometry B Clin Cytom, 2018. **94**(1): p. 121–28.

82. Voronin, D.V., et al., *Detection of rare objects by flow cytometry: imaging, cell sorting, and deep learning approaches.* Int J Mol Sci, 2020. **21**(7): p. 2323.

83. Ibrahim, S.F. and G. van den Engh, *Flow cytometry and cell sorting.* Adv Biochem Eng Biotechnol, 2007. **106**: p. 19–39.

84. Bacigalupo, A., *Aplastic anemia: pathogenesis and treatment.* Hematology Am Soc Hematol Educ Program, 2007. 2007: p. 23–8.

85. Wang, L. and H. Liu, *Pathogenesis of aplastic anemia.* Hematology, 2019. **24**(1): p. 559–66.

86. Baumgarth, N. and M. Bigos, *Optimization of emission optics for multicolor flow cytometry.* Methods Cell Biol, 2004. **75**: p. 3–22.

87. Ommen, H.B., *Monitoring minimal residual disease in acute myeloid leukaemia: a review of the current evolving strategies.* Ther Adv Hematol, 2016. **7**(1): p. 3–16.

88. Rajab, A. and A. Porwit, *Screening bone marrow samples for abnormal lymphoid populations and myelodysplasia-related features with one 10-color 14-antibody screening tube.* Cytometry B Clin Cytom, 2015. **88**(4): p. 253–60.

89. Mair, F., et al., *The end of gating? An introduction to automated analysis of high dimensional cytometry data.* Eur J Immunol, 2016. **46**(1): p. 34–43.

90. Maecker, H.T., J.P. McCoy, and R. Nussenblatt, *Standardizing immunophenotyping for the Human Immunology Project.* Nat Rev Immunol, 2012. **12**(3): p. 191–200.

91. Ferrer-Font, L., et al., *High-dimensional data analysis algorithms yield comparable results for mass cytometry and spectral flow cytometry data.* Cytometry A, 2020. **97**(8): p. 824–31.

92. Finn, W.G., et al., *Analysis of clinical flow cytometric immunophenotyping data by clustering on statistical manifolds: treating flow cytometry data as high-dimensional objects.* Cytometry B Clin Cytom, 2008. **76B**(1): p. 1–7.

93. Cheung, M., et al., *Current trends in flow cytometry automated data analysis software.* Cytometry A, 2021. **99**(10): p. 1007–21.

94. Van Gassen, S., et al., *FlowSOM: using self-organizing maps for visualization and interpretation of cytometry data.* Cytometry A, 2015. **87**(7): p. 636–45.

95. Finak, G., et al., *Standardizing flow cytometry immunophenotyping analysis from the human immunophenotyping consortium.* Sci Rep, 2016. **6**: p. 20686.

96. Juco, J., J.T. Holden et al, *Immunophenotypic analysis of anaplastic large cell lymphoma by flow cytometry.* Am J Clin Pathol, 2003. **119**: p. 205–12.

97. Kampalath, B., M.P. Barcos, and C. Stewart, *Phenotypic heterogeneity of B cells in patients with chronic lymphocytic leukemia/small lymphocytic lymphoma.* Am J Clin Pathol, 2003. **119**(6): p. 824–32.

98. Bahia, D.M., et al., *Aberrant phenotypes in acute myeloid leukemia: a high frequency and its clinical significance.* Haematologica, 2001. **86**(8): p. 801–6.

99. Lanza, F., B.S. Castoldi, J.M. Goldman, *Abnormal expression of N-CAM (CD56) adhesion molecule on myeloid and progenitor cells from chronic myeloid leukemia.* Leukemia, 1993. **7**: p. 1570–75.

100. Tabernero, M.D., et al., *Adult precursor B-ALL with BCR/ABL gene rearrangements displays a unique immunophenotype based on the pattern of CD10, CD34, CD13 and CD38 expression.* Leukemia, 2001. **15**(3): p. 406–14.

101. Porwit, A., et al., *B-cell chronic lymphocytic leukaemia with aberrant expression of CD8 antigen.* Eur J Haematol, 1987. **39**(4): p. 311–7.

102. Schmidt, C.J., et al., *Aberrant antigen expression detected by multiparameter three color flow cytometry in intermediate and high grade B-cell lymphomas.* Leuk Lymphoma, 1999. **34**(5–6): p. 539–44.

103. Dong, H.Y., et al., *B-cell lymphomas with coexpression of CD5 and CD10.* Am J Clin Pathol, 2003. **119**(2): p. 218–30.

104. Gorczyca, W., *Flow cytometry immunophenotypic characteristics of monocytic population in acute monocytic leukemia (AML-M5), acute myelomonocytic leukemia (AML-M4), and chronic myelomonocytic leukemia (CMML).* Methods Cell Biol, 2004. **75**: p. 665–77.

105. Gorczyca, W., *Differential diagnosis of T-cell lymphoproliferative disorders by flow cytometry multicolor immunophenotyping. Correlation with morphology.* Methods Cell Biol, 2004. **75**: p. 595–621.

106. Jasionowski, T.M., et al., *Analysis of CD10+ hairy cell leukemia.* Am J Clin Pathol, 2003. **120**(2): p. 228–35.

107. Ludwig, W.D., et al., *Ambiguous phenotypes and genotypes in 16 children with acute leukemia as characterized by multiparameter analysis.* Blood, 1988. **71**(6): p. 1518–28.

108. Macedo, A., et al., *Phenotypic analysis of CD34 subpopulations in normal human bone marrow and its application for the detection of minimal residual disease.* Leukemia, 1995. **9**(11): p. 1896–901.

109. Macedo, A., et al., *Immunological detection of blast cell subpopulations in acute myeloblastic leukemia at diagnosis: implications for minimal residual disease studies.* Leukemia, 1995. **9**(6): p. 993–8.

110. Macedo, A., et al., *Characterization of aberrant phenotypes in acute myeloblastic leukemia.* Ann Hematol, 1995. **70**(4): p. 189–94.

111. Oelschlagel, U., et al., *Shift of aberrant antigen expression at relapse or at treatment failure in acute leukemia.* Cytometry, 2000. **42**(4): p. 247–53.

112. Ross, C.W., et al., *Immunophenotypic aberrancy in adult acute lymphoblastic leukemia.* Am J Clin Pathol, 1990. **94**(5): p. 590–9.

113. Terstappen, L.W., et al., *Flow cytometric characterization of acute myeloid leukemia. Part II. Phenotypic heterogeneity at diagnosis.* Leukemia, 1992. **6**(1): p. 70–80.

114. Kennedy, G.A., et al., *Identification of tumours with the CD43 only phenotype during the investigation of suspected lymphoma: a heterogeneous group not necessarily of T cell origin.* Pathology, 2002. **34**(1): p. 46–50.

115. Kaleem, Z., G. White, M.M. Zutter, *Aberrant expression of T-cell-associated antigens on B-cell non-Hodgkin lymphomas.* Am J Clin Pathol, 2001. **115**: p. 396–403.

116. Inaba, T., et al., *T-cell associated antigen-positive B-cell lymphoma.* Leuk Lymphoma, 2001. **42**(6): p. 1161–71.

117. Lin, P., et al., *Flow cytometric immunophenotypic analysis of 306 cases of multiple myeloma.* Am J Clin Pathol, 2004. **121**(4): p. 482–8.

118. Attygalle, A., et al., *Neoplastic T cells in angioimmunoblastic T-cell lymphoma express CD10.* Blood, 2002. **99**(2): p. 627–33.

119. Quintanilla-Martinez, L., et al., *CD20+ T-cell lymphoma. Neoplastic transformation of a normal T-cell subset.* Am J Clin Pathol, 1994. **102**(4): p. 483–9.

120. Egan, C. and S. Pittaluga, *Into the gray-zone: update on the diagnosis and classification of a rare lymphoma.* Expert Rev Hematol, 2020. **13**(1): p. 1–3.

121. Hartmann, S. and D.A. Eichenauer, *Nodular lymphocyte predominant Hodgkin lymphoma: pathology, clinical course and relation to T-cell/histiocyte rich large B-cell lymphoma.* Pathology, 2020. **52**(1): p. 142–53.

122. Pilichowska, M., et al., *Clinicopathologic consensus study of gray zone lymphoma with features intermediate between DLBCL and classical HL.* Blood Adv, 2017. **1**(26): p. 2600–9.

123. Sarkozy, C., et al., *Gray-zone lymphoma between cHL and large B-cell lymphoma: a histopathologic series from the LYSA.* Am J Surg Pathol, 2019. **43**(3): p. 341–51.

124. Wang, H.W., et al., *Diagnosis of Hodgkin lymphoma in the modern era.* Br J Haematol, 2019. **184**(1): p. 45–59.

125. Fan, Z., et al., *Characterization of variant patterns of nodular lymphocyte predominant Hodgkin lymphoma with immunohistologic and clinical correlation.* Am J Surg Pathol, 2003. **27**(10): p. 1346–56.

126. Agbay, R., et al., *Bone marrow involvement in patients with nodular lymphocyte predominant Hodgkin lymphoma.* Am J Surg Pathol, 2018. **42**(4): p. 492–99.

127. McKay, P., et al., *Guidelines for the investigation and management of nodular lymphocyte predominant Hodgkin lymphoma.* Br J Haematol, 2016. **172**(1): p. 32–43.

128. Hartmann, S., et al., *Nodular lymphocyte predominant Hodgkin lymphoma and T cell/histiocyte rich large B cell lymphoma-endpoints of a spectrum of one disease?* PLOS ONE, 2013. **8**(11): p. e78812.

129. Untanu, R.V., et al., *Variant histology, IgD and CD30 expression in low-risk pediatric nodular lymphocyte predominant Hodgkin lymphoma: a report from the Children's Oncology Group.* Pediatr Blood Cancer, 2018. **65**(1): p. 10.

130. Grewal, R.K., et al., *Use of flow cytometry in the phenotypic diagnosis of Hodgkin's lymphoma.* Cytometry B Clin Cytom, 2019. **96**(2): p. 116–27.

131. Fromm, J.R., S.J. Kussick, and B.L. Wood, *Identification and purification of classical Hodgkin cells from lymph nodes by flow cytometry and flow cytometric cell sorting.* Am J Clin Pathol, 2006. **126**(5): p. 764–80.

132. Fromm, J.R., A. Thomas, and B.L. Wood, *Flow cytometry can diagnose classical Hodgkin lymphoma in lymph nodes with high sensitivity and specificity.* Am J Clin Pathol, 2009. **131**(3): p. 322–32.

133. Fromm, J.R. and B.L. Wood, *A six-color flow cytometry assay for immunophenotyping classical Hodgkin lymphoma in lymph nodes.* Am J Clin Pathol, 2014. **141**(3): p. 388–96.

134. Wu, D., B.L. Wood, and J.R. Fromm, *Flow cytometry for non-Hodgkin and classical Hodgkin lymphoma.* Methods Mol Biol, 2013. **971**: p. 27–47.

135. Roshal, M., B.L. Wood, and J.R. Fromm, *Flow cytometric detection of the classical Hodgkin lymphoma: clinical and research applications.* Adv Hematol, 2011. **2011**: p. 387034.

136. Jegalian, A.G., et al., *Follicular lymphoma in situ: clinical implications and comparisons with partial involvement by follicular lymphoma.* Blood, 2011. **118**(11): p. 2976–84.

137. Oishi, N., S. Montes-Moreno, and A.L. Feldman, *In situ neoplasia in lymph node pathology.* Semin Diagn Pathol, 2018. **35**(1): p. 76–83.

138. Adam, P., et al., *Incidence of preclinical manifestations of mantle cell lymphoma and mantle cell lymphoma in situ in reactive lymphoid tissues.* Mod Pathol, 2012. **25**(12): p. 1629–36.

139. Aqel, N., et al., *In-situ mantle cell lymphoma–a report of two cases.* Histopathology, 2008. **52**(2): p. 256–60.

140. Carbone, A. and A. Santoro, *How I treat: diagnosing and managing "in situ" lymphoma.* Blood, 2011. **117**(15): p. 3954–60.

141. Edlefsen, K.L., et al., *Early lymph node involvement by mantle cell lymphoma limited to the germinal center: report of a case with a novel "follicular in situ" growth pattern.* Am J Clin Pathol, 2011. **136**(2): p. 276–81.

142. Neto, A.G., et al., *Colonic in situ mantle cell lymphoma.* Ann Diagn Pathol, 2012. **16**(6): p. 508–14.

143. Wilcox, R.A., *Cutaneous T-cell lymphoma: 2011 update on diagnosis, risk-stratification, and management.* Am J Hematol, 2011. **86**(11): p. 928–48.

144. Stacchini, A., et al., *Flow cytometry in the bone marrow staging of mature B-cell neoplasms.* Cytometry B Clin Cytom, 2003. **54**(1): p. 10–8.

145. Dunphy, C.H., *Combining morphology and flow cytometric immunophenotyping to evaluate bone marrow specimens for B-cell malignant neoplasms.* Am J Clin Pathol, 1998. **109**(5): p. 625–30.

146. Perea, G., et al., *Clinical utility of bone marrow flow cytometry in B-cell non-Hodgkin lymphomas (B-NHL).* Histopathology, 2004. **45**(3): p. 268–74.

147. Paiva, B., et al., *Multiparameter flow cytometry quantification of bone marrow plasma cells at diagnosis provides more prognostic information than morphological assessment in myeloma patients.* Haematologica, 2009. **94**(11): p. 1599–602.

148. Smock, K.J., S.L. Perkins, and D.W. Bahler, *Quantitation of plasma cells in bone marrow aspirates by flow cytometric analysis compared with morphologic assessment.* Arch Pathol Lab Med, 2007. **131**(6): p. 951–5.

149. Nadav, L., et al., *Diverse niches within multiple myeloma bone marrow aspirates affect plasma cell enumeration.* Br J Haematol, 2006. **133**(5): p. 530–2.

150. Dimopoulos, M.A., et al., *Macrofocal multiple myeloma in young patients: a distinct entity with favorable prognosis.* Leuk Lymphoma, 2006. **47**(8): p. 1553–6.

151. Park, S., et al., *Dyserythropoiesis evaluated by the RED score and hepcidin:ferritin ratio predicts response to erythropoietin in lower-risk myelodysplastic syndromes.* Haematologica, 2019. **104**(3): p. 497–504.

152. Mathis, S., et al., *Flow cytometric detection of dyserythropoiesis: a sensitive and powerful diagnostic tool for myelodysplastic syndromes.* Leukemia, 2013. **27**(10): p. 1981–7.

153. Della Porta, M.G., et al., *Flow cytometry evaluation of erythroid dysplasia in patients with myelodysplastic syndrome.* Leukemia, 2006. **20**(4): p. 549–55.

154. Weisberger, J., et al., *Down-regulation of pan-T-cell antigens, particularly CD7, in acute infectious mononucleosis.* Am J Clin Pathol, 2003. **120**(1): p. 49–55.

155. Morice, W.G., D. Jevremovic, and C.A. Hanson, *The expression of the novel cytotoxic protein granzyme M by large granular lymphocytic leukaemias of both T-cell and NK-cell lineage: an unexpected finding with implications regarding the pathobiology of these disorders.* Br J Haematol, 2007. **137**(3): p. 237–9.

156. Lamy, T. and T.P. Loughran, Jr., *Clinical features of large granular lymphocyte leukemia.* Semin Hematol, 2003. **40**(3): p. 185–95.

157. van Oostveen, J.W., et al., *Polyclonal expansion of T-cell receptor-gamma delta+ T lymphocytes associated with neutropenia and thrombocytopenia.* Leukemia, 1992. **6**(5): p. 410–8.

158. Langerak, A.W., Y. Sandberg, and J.J. van Dongen, *Spectrum of T-large granular lymphocyte lymphoproliferations: ranging from expanded activated effector T cells to T-cell leukaemia.* Br J Haematol, 2003. **123**(3): p. 561–2.

159. Dhodapkar, M.V., et al., *Clinical spectrum of clonal proliferations of T-large granular lymphocytes: a T-cell clonopathy of undetermined significance?* Blood, 1994. **84**(5): p. 1620–7.

160. Rose, M.G. and N. Berliner, *T-cell large granular lymphocyte leukemia and related disorders.* Oncologist, 2004. **9**(3): p. 247–58.

161. McClanahan, J., P.I. Fukushima, and M. Stetler-Stevenson, *Increased peripheral blood gamma delta T-cells in patients with lymphoid neoplasia: a diagnostic dilemma in flow cytometry.* Cytometry, 1999. **38**(6): p. 280–5.

162. Kreutzman, A., et al., *Mono/oligoclonal T and NK cells are common in chronic myeloid leukemia patients at diagnosis and expand during dasatinib therapy.* Blood, 2010. **116**(5): p. 772–82.

163. Shi, M., et al., *T-cell clones of uncertain significance are highly prevalent and show close resemblance to T-cell large granular lymphocytic leukemia. Implications for laboratory diagnostics.* Mod Pathol, 2020. **33**(10): p. 2046–57.

164. Morice, W.G., et al., *Demonstration of aberrant T-cell and natural killer-cell antigen expression in all cases of granular lymphocytic leukaemia.* Br J Haematol, 2003. **120**(6): p. 1026–36.

165. Morice, W.G., *The immunophenotypic attributes of NK cells and NK-cell lineage lymphoproliferative disorders.* Am J Clin Pathol, 2007. **127**(6): p. 881–6.

166. Morice, W.G., et al., *Chronic lymphoproliferative disorder of natural killer cells: a distinct entity with subtypes correlating with normal natural killer cell subsets.* Leukemia, 2010. **24**(4): p. 881–4.

167. Swerdlow, S.H., et al., *The 2016 revision of the World Health Organization classification of lymphoid neoplasms.* Blood, 2016. **127**(20): p. 2375–90.

168. Armitage, J.O. and D.D. Weisenburger, *New approach to classifying non-Hodgkin's lymphomas: clinical features of the major histologic subtypes. Non-Hodgkin's Lymphoma Classification Project.* J Clin Oncol, 1998. **16**(8): p. 2780–95.

169. Campo, E., *Genetic and molecular genetic studies in the diagnosis of B-cell lymphomas I: mantle cell lymphoma, follicular lymphoma, and Burkitt's lymphoma.* Hum Pathol, 2003. **34**(4): p. 330–5.

170. Frizzera, G., *Recent progress in lymphoma classification.* Curr Opin Oncol, 1997. **9**(5): p. 392–402.

171. Harris, N.L., *A practical approach to the pathology of lymphoid neoplasms: a revised European-American classification from the International Lymphoma Study Group.* Important Adv Oncol, 1995: p. 111–40.

172. Harris, E., et al., *Burkitt's lymphoma: single-centre experience with modified BFM protocol.* Clin Lab Haematol, 2002. **24**(2): p. 111–4.

173. Harris, N.L., J.A. Ferry, and S.H. Swerdlow, *Posttransplant lymphoproliferative disorders: summary of Society for Hematopathology Workshop.* Semin Diagn Pathol, 1997. **14**(1): p. 8–14.

174. Chadburn, A. and S. Narayanan, *Lymphoid malignancies: immunophenotypic analysis.* Adv Clin Chem, 2003. **37**: p. 293–353.

175. Jaffe, E.S., et al., *T-cell-rich B-cell lymphomas.* Am J Surg Pathol, 1991. **15**(5): p. 491–2.

176. Willemze, R., et al., *WHO-EORTC classification for cutaneous lymphomas.* Blood, 2005. **105**(10): p. 3768–85.

177. Willemze, R., et al., *Primary cutaneous large cell lymphomas of follicular center cell origin. A clinical follow-up study of nineteen patients.* J Am Acad Dermatol, 1987. **16**(3 Pt 1): p. 518–26.

178. Diebold, J., et al., *Diffuse large B-cell lymphoma: a clinicopathologic analysis of 444 cases classified according to the updated Kiel classification.* Leuk Lymphoma, 2002. **43**(1): p. 97–104.

179. Engelhard, M., et al., *Subclassification of diffuse large B-cell lymphomas according to the Kiel classification: distinction of centroblastic and immunoblastic lymphomas is a significant prognostic risk factor.* Blood, 1997. **89**(7): p. 2291–7.

180. Hans, C.P., et al., *Confirmation of the molecular classification of diffuse large B-cell lymphoma by immunohistochemistry using a tissue microarray.* Blood, 2004. **103**(1): p. 275–82.

181. Nakamura, N., et al., *The distinction between Burkitt lymphoma and diffuse large B-Cell lymphoma with c-myc rearrangement.* Mod Pathol, 2002. **15**(7): p. 771–6.

182. Weisberger, J., et al., *Differential diagnosis of malignant lymphomas and related disorders by specific pattern of expression of immunophenotypic markers revealed by multiparameter flow cytometry (review).* Int J Oncol, 2000. **17**(6): p. 1165–77.

183. Pileri, S.A., et al., *Diffuse large B-cell lymphoma: one or more entities? Present controversies and possible tools for its subclassification.* Histopathology, 2002. **41**(6): p. 482–509.

184. Falini, B., et al., *Lymphomas expressing ALK fusion protein(s) other than NPM-ALK.* Blood, 1999. **94**(10): p. 3509–15.

185. Isaacson, P.G., *Gastrointestinal lymphomas of T- and B-cell types.* Mod Pathol, 1999. **12**(2): p. 151–8.

186. Arcaini, L., et al., *Primary nodal marginal zone B-cell lymphoma: clinical features and prognostic assessment of a rare disease.* Br J Haematol, 2007. **136**(2): p. 301–4.

187. Boleti, E. and P.W. Johnson, *Primary mediastinal B-cell lymphoma.* Hematol Oncol, 2007. **25**(4): p. 157–63.

188. Davies, A.J., et al., *Transformation of follicular lymphoma to diffuse large B-cell lymphoma proceeds by distinct oncogenic mechanisms.* Br J Haematol, 2007. **136**(2): p. 286–93.

189. Ferreri, A.J. and C. Montalban, *Primary diffuse large B-cell lymphoma of the stomach.* Crit Rev Oncol Hematol, 2007. **63**(1): p. 65–71.

190. Goldaniga, M., et al., *A multicenter retrospective clinical study of CD5/CD10-negative chronic B cell leukemias.* Am J Hematol, 2008. **83**(5): p. 349–54.

191. Ponzoni, M., et al., *Definition, diagnosis, and management of intravascular large B-cell lymphoma: proposals and perspectives from an international consensus meeting.* J Clin Oncol, 2007. **25**(21): p. 3168–73.

192. Rawal, A., et al., *Site-specific morphologic differences in extranodal marginal zone B-cell lymphomas.* Arch Pathol Lab Med, 2007. **131**(11): p. 1673–8.

193. Savage, K.J., *Peripheral T-cell lymphomas.* Blood Rev, 2007. **21**(4): p. 201–16.

194. Savage, K.J., et al., *Characterization of peripheral T-cell lymphomas in a single North American institution by the WHO classification.* Ann Oncol, 2004. **15**(10): p. 1467–75.

195. Kluin, P.M., et al., *Peripheral T/NK-cell lymphoma: a report of the IXth Workshop of the European Association for Haematopathology.* Histopathology, 2001. **38**(3): p. 250–70.

196. Jaffe, E.S., *Nasal and nasal-type T/NK cell lymphoma: a unique form of lymphoma associated with the Epstein-Barr virus.* Histopathology, 1995. **27**(6): p. 581–3.

197. Jaffe, E.S., *Angioimmunoblastic T-cell lymphoma: new insights, but the clinical challenge remains.* Ann Oncol, 1995. **6**(7): p. 631–2.

198. Jaffe, E.S., *Classification of natural killer (NK) cell and NK-like T-cell malignancies.* Blood, 1996. **87**(4): p. 1207–10.

199. Jaffe, E.S., *Anaplastic large cell lymphoma: the shifting sands of diagnostic hematopathology.* Mod Pathol, 2001. **14**(3): p. 219–28.

200. Jaffe, E.S., *Pathobiology of peripheral T-cell lymphomas.* Hematology Am Soc Hematol Educ Program, 2006: p. 317–22.

201. Arrowsmith, E.R., et al., *Peripheral T-cell lymphomas: clinical features and prognostic factors of 92 cases defined by the revised European American lymphoma classification.* Leuk Lymphoma, 2003. **44**(2): p. 241–9.

202. Gallamini, A., et al., *Peripheral T-cell lymphoma unspecified (PTCL-U): a new prognostic model from a retrospective multicentric clinical study.* Blood, 2004. **103**(7): p. 2474–9.

203. Al-Hakeem, D.A., et al., *Extranodal NK/T-cell lymphoma, nasal type.* Oral Oncol, 2007. **43**(1): p. 4–14.

204. Attygalle, A.D., et al., *Distinguishing angioimmunoblastic T-cell lymphoma from peripheral T-cell lymphoma, unspecified, using morphology, immunophenotype and molecular genetics.* Histopathology, 2007. **50**(4): p. 498–508.

205. Dearden, C.E. and F.M. Foss, *Peripheral T-cell lymphomas: diagnosis and management.* Hematol Oncol Clin North Am, 2003. **17**(6): p. 1351–66.

206. Karube, K., et al., *Adult T-cell lymphoma/leukemia with angioimmunoblastic T-cell lymphomalike features: report of 11 cases.* Am J Surg Pathol, 2007. **31**(2): p. 216–23.

207. Kim, K., et al., *Clinical features of peripheral T-cell lymphomas in 78 patients diagnosed according to the Revised European-American lymphoma (REAL) classification.* Eur J Cancer, 2002. **38**(1): p. 75–81.

208. Loughran, T.P., Jr., *Chronic T-cell leukemia/lymphoma.* Cancer Control, 1998. **5**(1): p. 8–9.

209. Salhany, K.E., et al., *Subcutaneous panniculitis-like T-cell lymphoma: clinicopathologic, immunophenotypic, and genotypic analysis of alpha/beta and gamma/delta subtypes.* Am J Surg Pathol, 1998. **22**(7): p. 881–93.

210. Siegel, R.S., et al., *Primary cutaneous T-cell lymphoma: review and current concepts.* J Clin Oncol, 2000. **18**(15): p. 2908–25.

211. Tamaska, J., et al., *Hepatosplenic gamma delta T-cell lymphoma with ring chromosome 7, an isochromosome 7q equivalent clonal chromosomal aberration.* Virchows Arch, 2006. **449**(4): p. 479–83.

212. ten Berge, R.L., et al., *ALK-negative anaplastic large-cell lymphoma demonstrates similar poor prognosis to peripheral T-cell lymphoma, unspecified.* Histopathology, 2003. **43**(5): p. 462–9.

213. Willemze, R., et al., *Subcutaneous panniculitis-like T-cell lymphoma: definition, classification, and prognostic factors: an EORTC Cutaneous Lymphoma Group Study of 83 cases.* Blood, 2008. **111**(2): p. 838–45.

214. Michiels, J.J., et al., *Current diagnostic criteria for the chronic myeloproliferative disorders (MPD) essential thrombocythemia (ET), polycythemia vera (PV) and chronic idiopathic myelofibrosis (CIMF).* Pathol Biol (Paris), 2007. **55**(2): p. 92–104.

215. Moliterno, A.R., et al., *Molecular mimicry in the chronic myeloproliferative disorders: reciprocity between quantitative JAK2 V617F and Mpl expression.* Blood, 2006. **108**(12): p. 3913–5.

216. Spivak, J.L., *The chronic myeloproliferative disorders: clonality and clinical heterogeneity.* Semin Hematol, 2004. **41**(2 Suppl 3): p. 1–5.

217. Thiele, J. and H.M. Kvasnicka, *A critical reappraisal of the WHO classification of the chronic myeloproliferative disorders.* Leuk Lymphoma, 2006. **47**(3): p. 381–96.

218. Tefferi, A., et al., *Proposals and rationale for revision of the World Health Organization diagnostic criteria for polycythemia vera, essential thrombocythemia, and primary myelofibrosis: recommendations from an ad hoc international expert panel.* Blood, 2007. **110**(4): p. 1092–7.

219. Baxter, E.J., Scott, L. M., *Acquired mutation of the tyrosine kinase JAK2 in human myeloproliferative disorders.* Lancet, 2005. **365**: p. 1054–61.

220. Bousquet, M., et al., *Frequent detection of the JAK2 V617F mutation in bone marrow core biopsy specimens from chronic myeloproliferative disorders using the TaqMan polymerase chain reaction single nucleotide polymorphism genotyping assay. A retrospective study with pathologic correlations.* Hum Pathol, 2006. **37**(11): p. 1458–64.

221. Tefferi, A., et al., *Concomitant neutrophil JAK2 mutation screening and PRV-1 expression analysis in myeloproliferative disorders and secondary polycythaemia.* Br J Haematol, 2005. **131**(2): p. 166–71.

222. Cervantes, F. and G. Barosi, *Myelofibrosis with myeloid metaplasia: diagnosis, prognostic factors, and staging.* Semin Oncol, 2005. **32**(4): p. 395–402.

223. Gianelli, U., et al., *Essential thrombocythemia or chronic idiopathic myelofibrosis? A single-center study based on hematopoietic bone marrow histology.* Leuk Lymphoma, 2006. **47**(9): p. 1774–81.

224. Kreft, A., et al., *The incidence of myelofibrosis in essential thrombocythaemia, polycythaemia vera and chronic idiopathic myelofibrosis: a retrospective evaluation of sequential bone marrow biopsies.* Acta Haematol, 2005. **113**(2): p. 137–43.

225. Elliott, M.A., *Chronic neutrophilic leukemia and chronic myelomonocytic leukemia: WHO defined.* Best Pract Res Clin Haematol, 2006. **19**(3): p. 571–93.

226. Bench, A.J., et al., *Molecular diagnosis of the myeloproliferative neoplasms: UK guidelines for the detection of JAK2 V617F and other relevant mutations.* Br J Haematol, 2012. **160**(1): p. 25–34.

2

FLOW CYTOMETRY ANALYSIS OF BLOOD AND BONE MARROW

Bone marrow: Normal structure and hematopoiesis

Bone marrow (BM) in adult occupies the medullary spaces of large bones such as femur, hip, sternum, and humerus. The marrow cellularity changes with age and can be roughly estimated as *(100-age)%* (i.e., 100% at birth, 80% in childhood, 50% in a 50-year-old person, and 20% in an 80-year-old person). The primary function of the BM is the production of blood cells (hematopoiesis) in which early progenitor cells progressively differentiate into intermediate and mature elements. The BM (Figure 2.1) is composed of a matrix requisite for hematopoiesis and hemopoietic cells including rare pluripotent hemopoietic stem cells, myeloperoxidase (MPO) positive granulocytic precursors (CD34+ blasts, CD117+ blasts, and promyelocytes), glycophorin (GPHA, CD235a), and CD71 positive erythroid precursors, megakaryocytes (platelet precursors; CD61+), scattered monocytes (CD68+, CD163+), plasmacytoid dendritic cells (DCs) (CD123+), lymphocytes (positive for B- and T-cell markers), plasma cells (CD138+, MUM1+), mast cells (CD117+, mast cell tryptase+), adipocytes, blood vessels, and other stromal elements (e.g., osteoblasts, osteoclasts, fibroblasts, etc.). The area close to bone (paratrabecular zone) is composed mostly of myeloid precursors and intertrabecular area shows myeloid and erythroid precursors, sinusoids, and scattered megakaryocytes.

The BM contains progenitor cells called stem cells. Stem cells have the pluripotent capacity for both self-renewal and differentiation. The most undifferentiated cells (pluripotent stem cells) give rise to stem cells committed to a particular cell lineage (unipotent stem cells including common myeloid and common lymphoid progenitors). The stem cells express CD34, CD133, and CD59 and are usually negative for CD38, CD117, and CD33 (at least until they start to display lineage-specific potential). These cells give rise to all types of lymphocytes and myeloid cells. The myeloid lineage comprises all non-lymphoid white cells (neutrophils, monocytes, eosinophils, and basophils), mast cells, red cells, and megakaryocytes (platelets). Common myeloid progenitors differentiate into bi-potent cells, either megakaryocyte-erythroid progenitors or granulocytes-macrophage progenitors. The sequence of maturation stages on a BM aspirate smear stained with Wright-Giemsa for different cell types is presented in Figure 2.2. In healthy adults, the granulocytic series predominates over the erythroid series (the ratio is roughly 2:1 to 4:1). The recognized morphologic maturation stages in granulocytic lineage are myeloblasts, promyelocytes, myelocytes, metamyelocytes, bands, and polymorphonuclear leukocytes (neutrophils). Myeloblasts are round cells with high nuclear/cytoplasmic ratio, fine (immature) chromatin, scanty pale basophilic cytoplasm, and two or more prominent nucleoli. In a normal marrow core biopsy, blasts (CD34+) comprise up to 1%–2% of marrow cells. Promyelocytes are larger than blasts, have prominent nucleoli, and primary, azurophilic cytoplasmic granules. The chromatin features are coarser than in blasts. The neutrophil metamyelocytes are smaller than

promyelocytes, have coarser (more mature) chromatin, and its acidophilic cytoplasm shows azurophilic granules and many fine neutrophilic granules. They usually do not have nucleoli. Metamyelocytes are smaller than myelocytes and have more condensed chromatin, C-shaped nucleus, and neutrophilic granules in the cytoplasm. The nuclei of bands are elongated ("band-like") and narrow, and neutrophils show a segmented nucleus with two to five clumps joined by delicate strands of chromatin.

Megakaryocytic lineage includes megakaryoblasts, promegakaryocytes (granular), megakaryocytes, and "naked" nuclei. Megakaryoblasts have single nucleus (often irregular), few prominent nucleoli, and basophilic and agranular cytoplasm (early megakaryoblasts are indistinguishable morphologically from myeloblasts). Promegakaryocytes are larger than megakaryoblasts, have less basophilic cytoplasm, decreased nuclear/cytoplasmic ratio, and start to show nuclear lobes and cytoplasmic granules. Megakaryocytes are scattered individually, and usually do not exceed four to five per high power field (×400). They have irregular nuclei and pale, granular cytoplasm. Cytoplasmic fragments of megakaryocyte cells (platelets) are instrumental in primary hemostasis. Adults produce 10^{11} platelets daily (in normal conditions).

The erythroid lineage matures from stem cell to red cells (which carry oxygen to peripheral tissues) through proerythroblast (pronormoblast), basophilic normoblast (basophilic erythroblast), polychromatic normoblast (early polychromatic erythroblast), orthochromatic normoblast (late polychromatic erythroblasts), and reticulocyte. Pronormoblasts are large cells with prominent nucleolus, fine chromatin pattern, and deeply basophilic cytoplasm, which may be vacuolated. Basophilic normoblast is smaller, has more basophilic cytoplasm, coarse (granular) chromatin, and lacks nucleolus. Polychromatic normoblast is characterized by chromatin clumps and polychromatic cytoplasm, and orthochromatic normoblast is smaller, has eccentric nucleus with condensed chromatin, which becomes pyknotic at late stages of maturation.

The lymphoid lineage also matures from stem cell to mature lymphocyte. A lymphocyte will become either a B-cell (*b*ursal or *b*one marrow-derived) or a T-cell (*t*hymus-derived). T-cells are further subdivided into helper/inducer cells, suppressor/cytotoxic cells, and natural killer (NK) cells. T-cells regulate the B-cells, as well as kill infected cells in the body. The B-cells are programmed at birth to react against a specific glycoprotein sequence, or antigen. Each B-cell has surface immunoglobulin (antibody) which contains a specific kappa or lambda light chain configuration. If the B-cell encounters its antigen match, it undergoes clonal expansion, making millions of copies of itself and eventually differentiating into a plasma cell. Plasma cells pour out their immunoglobulin antibodies from their cytoplasm into the serum, thereby enabling the infection or intruder proteins to be eliminated. Programmed cell death (apoptosis) as well as suppressor T-cells prevents the clonal cells from becoming autonomous and hence neoplastic.

DOI: 10.1201/9781003197935-2

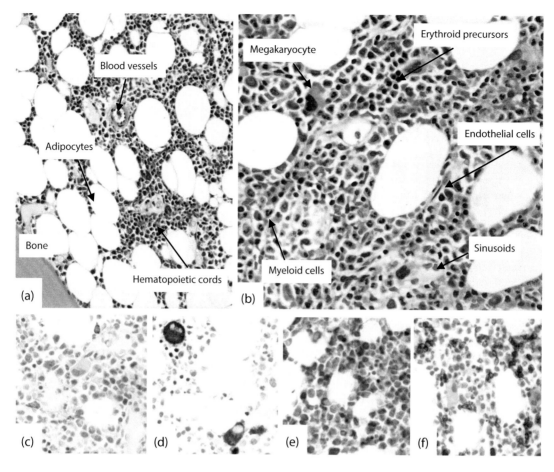

FIGURE 2.1   Bone marrow-normal histology: (a) low magnification; (b) higher magnification; (c) CD34 (blasts⁺); (d) CD61 (megakaryocytes⁺); (e) MPO (myeloid cells⁺); (f) GPHA (erythroid cells⁺).

Antigen expression during hematopoietic maturation

Hematopoietic cell differentiation starts from pluripotent stem cells and hematopoietic progenitor and precursor cells that become recruited and activated by cytokines and stromal cell signals to differentiate into lymphoid or myeloid cells. The myeloid series includes neutrophil, erythroid, monocytic, DCs, mast cell, basophil, eosinophil, and megakaryocytic lineages. Figure 2.3 presents antigenic profile of major cell types during normal hematopoiesis.

Granulocytic differentiation

Hematopoietic progenitors are positive for CD34, CD133, CD184, and HLA-DR. Neutrophilic maturation from blasts through promyelocytes, myelocytes, metamyelocytes, bands, and neutrophils is characterized by loss of CD34 and HLA-DR expression at promyelocytic stage and loss of CD117 expression at myelocyte stage, and acquisition of CD11b and CD11c expression at myelocytic stage and CD10 expression by neutrophils [1]. CD64 is expressed by promyelocytes through metamyelocytes. CD13 and CD33 are expressed at all stages of maturation with CD13 being brightly expressed by blasts and neutrophils, moderately by promyelocytes and dimly by metamyelocytes, and CD33 showing slight decrease in the intensity of CD33 expression as the cells become more mature. Granulocytic precursors display dim expression of CD45. The intensity of expression increases in the final stages of differentiation (based on the side scatter [SSC] and CD45 neutrophils can be often separated from

promyelocytes, myelocytes, metamyelocytes, and bands by having the strongest expression of CD45; Figure 2.4).

Myeloblasts are positive for CD34, CD38, HLA-DR, CD117, CD4, CD13 (dim), and CD33 (CD34 is expressed by all hematopoietic precursors, including early myeloblasts; CD117 expression appears after CD34). The expression of CD13 appears first, followed by acquisition of CD33 and increased expression of both CD13 and CD33. Promyelocytes lose CD34 and HLA-DR, retain CD117, and show positive expression of CD13 and CD33 (bright). They show dim expression of CD4 and start to acquire CD15. At the transition to myelocytes, the expression of CD117 is lost. The expression of CD13 diminishes at the transition from promyelocytes to myelocytes and then gradually increases. Myelocytes start to acquire the expression of CD11b, and its intensity increases as the cell matures to late myelocytes and metamyelocytes (at the same time, the expression of CD4 disappears). CD33 expression progressively decreases. Metamyelocytes start to express CD10 and CD16 which increases in intensity as the cells progress to mature neutrophils. Segmented forms display bright expression of CD11b, CD11c, CD10, CD16, and CD15. Other markers expressed at metamyelocytes/band/segmented stages include CD24, CD32, CD35, and CD65. Minute subset of normal granulocytes shows dim expression of CD64. CD14 and CD64 expressions are upregulated in infections and in patients on G-CSF therapy. Among glycosylphosphatidylinositol-anchored proteins (GPI-AP), CD55 and CD59 are constantly expressed along all the different stages of maturation; no significant differences are detected for CD59,

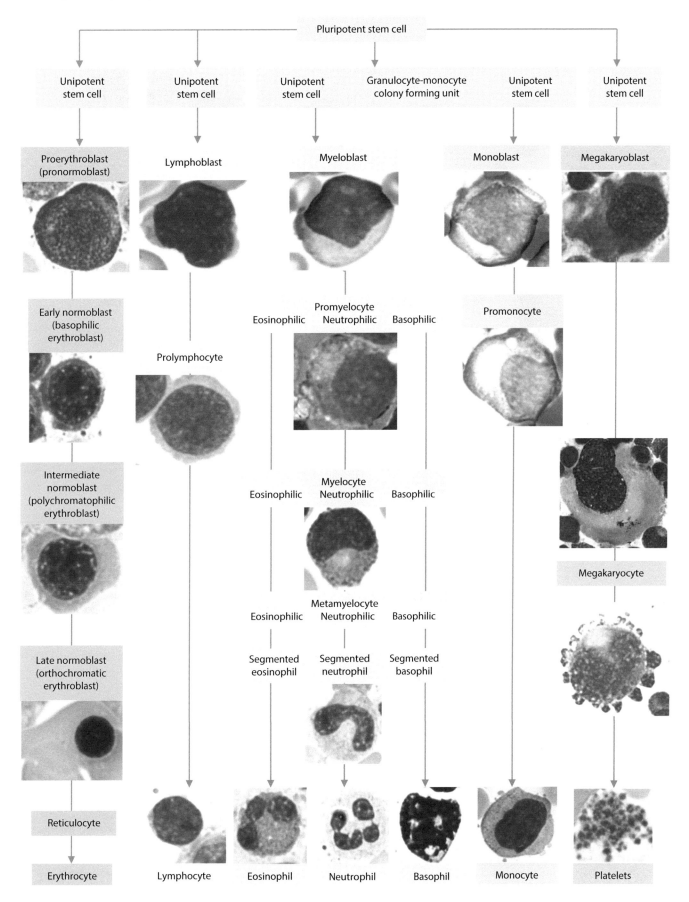

FIGURE 2.2 Hematopoiesis (see text for details).

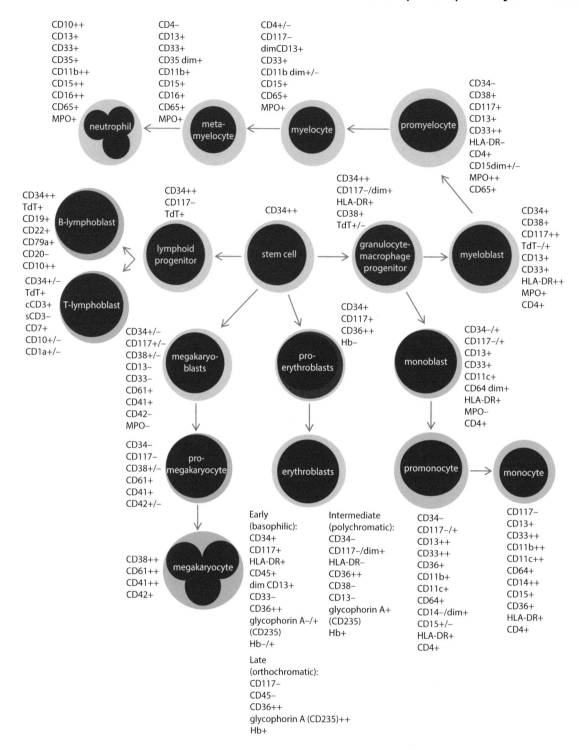

CD10++
CD13+
CD33+
CD35+
CD11b++
CD15++
CD16++
CD65+
MPO+

CD4−
CD13+
CD33+
CD35 dim+
CD11b+
CD15+
CD16+
CD65+
MPO+

CD4+/−
CD117−
dimCD13+
CD33+
CD11b dim+/−
CD15+
CD65+
MPO+

CD34−
CD38+
CD117+
CD13+
CD33++
HLA-DR−
CD4+
CD15dim+/−
MPO++
CD65+

neutrophil

meta-
myelocyte

myelocyte

promyelocyte

CD34++
TdT+
CD19+
CD22+
CD79a+
CD20−
CD10++

CD34++
CD117−
TdT+

CD34++

CD34++
CD117−/dim+
HLA-DR+
CD38+
TdT+/−

CD34+
CD38+
CD117++
TdT−/+
CD13+
CD33+
HLA-DR++
MPO+
CD4+

B-lymphoblast

lymphoid
progenitor

stem cell

granulocyte-
macrophage
progenitor

myeloblast

CD34+/−
TdT+
cCD3+
sCD3−
CD7+
CD10+/−
CD1a+/−

T-lymphoblast

CD34+/−
CD117+/−
CD38+/−
CD13−
CD33−
CD61+
CD41+
CD42−
MPO−

megakaryo-
blasts

CD34+
CD117+
CD36++
Hb−

pro-
erythroblasts

monoblast

CD34−/+
CD117−/+
CD13+
CD33+
CD11c+
CD64 dim+
HLA-DR+
MPO−
CD4+

CD34−
CD117−
CD38+/−
CD61+
CD41+
CD42+/−

pro-
megakaryocyte

erythroblasts

promonocyte

monocyte

CD38++
CD61++
CD41++
CD42+

megakaryocyte

Early
(basophilic):
CD34+
CD117+
HLA-DR+
CD45+
dim CD13+
CD33−
CD36++
glycophorin A−/+
(CD235)
Hb−/+

Late
(orthochromatic):
CD117−
CD45−
CD36++
glycophorin A (CD235)++
Hb+

Intermediate
(polychromatic):
CD34−
CD117−/dim+
HLA-DR−
CD36++
CD38−
CD13−
glycophorin A+
(CD235)
Hb+

CD34−
CD117−/+
CD13++
CD33++
CD36+
CD11b+
CD11c+
CD64+
CD14−/dim+
CD15+/−
HLA-DR+
CD4+

CD117−
CD13+
CD33++
CD11b++
CD11c++
CD64+
CD14++
CD15+
CD36+
HLA-DR+
CD4+

FIGURE 2.3   Antigen expression of major cell types during normal hematopoiesis.

but the expression of CD55 decreases from the early precursors to promyelocytes, and then increases along the maturation toward mature neutrophils. Figure 2.5 shows expression of CD10, CD11b, CD11c, CD16, and HLA-DR during normal myeloid maturation.

Any deviation from normal maturation pattern in myeloid lineage detected by FC can be fully integrated into the management of patients with an MDS suspicion (see Chapter 19). Apart from MDS, an abnormal maturation pattern can be seen in BM regeneration after immunosuppressive therapy or toxic marrow insult

(infections, nutritional deficiency, drugs), increased turnover of hematopoietic cells due to peripheral cell depletion (destruction), and uncontrolled expansion of neoplastic cells. False positive changes caused old sample (increased SSC of neutrophils or decreased number of monocytes) or presence of PNH clone, and false negative results (e.g., due to sample hemodilution) need to be excluded. In addition, EDTA (ethylenediaminetetraacetic acid) is known to influence marker expression (especially CD11b) and some authors recommend the use of heparin anticoagulants.

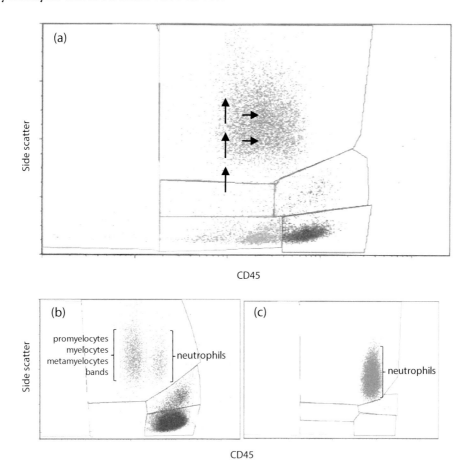

FIGURE 2.4 CD45 expression by granulocytes. The expression of CD45 increases as the cells reach final stages of differentiation into neutrophils (a). The direction of maturation is indicated in dot plot (b) by arrows (benign bone marrow sample from 11-month-old infant). Based on the CD45 versus side scatter (SSC), two populations of granulocytic cells can be identified: one with variable SSC and dimmer CD45 and the other with slightly lower SSC and brighter CD45. The first populations include promyelocytes, myelocytes, metamyelocytes, and bands, and the second population includes mostly mature neutrophils. The distinction between those two populations is more evident in plot (b) (benign bone marrow with relative T-cell lymphocytosis). Blood sample with reactive neutrophilia shows only one population of cells with very bright CD45.

Basophils show low SSC and dim to moderate CD45 (they often are located between blasts hematogones and lymphocytes on CD45 versus SSC display). Basophils are negative for CD15 and CD16 and have dimmer expression of CD13 when compared to neutrophils. Basophils are positive for CD9, CD13, CD22, CD25 (dim), CD33, CD36, CD38 (bright), CD45 (dimmer than lymphocytes and brighter than myeloblasts), and CD123 (bright), and are negative for CD19, CD34, CD64, CD117, and HLA-DR [2]. Eosinophils can be easily identified by flow cytometry by very low forward scatter, very high SSC, dimmer expression of CD13 and CD15 (compared to neutrophils), and lack of CD10 and CD16 (Figure 2.6).

Phenotypic profile of myeloid cells:

- *Myeloblasts*: SSC^{low}, variable FSC, CD4$^+$, CD10$^-$, CD11b$^-$, CD11c$^{+/-}$, CD13$^+$, CD33^{++}, CD34$^+$, CD38$^+$, CD117$^+$, HLA-DR$^+$, and CD123$^{+/-}$
- *Promyelocytes*: SSC^{high}, high FSC, CD4$^{+(dim)}$, CD11b$^-$, CD11c$^-$, CD13$^+$, CD15$^-$, CD16$^-$, CD33^{++}, CD34$^{-/+}$, CD38$^+$, CD64$^{+(dim)/-}$, CD117$^+$, and HLA-DR$^-$
- *Myelocytes*: high SSC, high FSC, CD4$^{+/-}$, CD11b$^{-/+}$, CD11c$^{-/+}$, CD10$^-$, CD16$^-$, CD33$^+$, CD34$^-$, CD38$^+$, CD117$^-$, and HLA-DR$^-$

- *Metamyelocytes*: SSC^{high}, high FSC, CD4$^-$, CD10$^{-/+}$, CD11b$^{+/-}$, CD11c$^{+/-}$, CD16$^{-/+}$, CD4$^-$, CD13$^+$, CD33$^+$, CD34$^-$, CD117$^-$, and HLA-DR$^-$
- *Neutrophils*: SSC^{high}, high FSC, CD4$^-$, CD10^{++}, CD11b^{++}, CD11c$^+$, CD13^{++}, CD15^{++}, CD16^{++}, CD33$^+$, CD34$^-$, CD38$^+$, CD117$^-$, and HLA-DR$^-$
- *Eosinophils*: SSC^{high}, very low FSC, CD4$^-$, CD10$^-$, CD11b$^+$, CD11c$^+$, CD13$^+$, CD15$^+$, CD16$^-$, CD33$^+$, CD34$^-$, CD38$^+$, CD117$^-$, and HLA-DR$^-$
- *Basophils*: SSC^{low}, moderate FSC, CD9$^+$, CD13$^+$, CD22$^+$, CD25$^+$, CD33$^+$, CD36$^+$, CD38^{++}, CD45^{++}, CD123$^+$, CD34$^-$, CD64$^-$, CD117$^-$, and HLA-DR$^-$
- *Early erythroid precursors*: CD45^{dim+}, SSC^{intermediate}, CD34$^+$, CD117$^+$, and CD235a$^-$
- *Proerythroblasts*: CD45$^{dim+/-}$, SSC^{intermediate}, CD34$^-$, CD36$^+$, CD117$^+$, CD71$^+$, and CD235a$^{+/-}$
- *Basophilic erythroblasts*: CD45$^{dim+/-}$, SSC^{intermediate}, CD34$^-$, CD36$^{+bright}$, CD117$^-$, CD71$^+$, and CD235a$^+$
- *Polychromatic erythroblasts*: CD45$^-$, SSC^{low}, CD34$^-$, CD36$^+$, CD117$^-$, CD71$^+$, and CD235a$^+$
- *Orthochromatic erythroblasts*: CD45$^-$, SSC^{low}, CD34$^-$, CD36$^{+/-}$, CD117$^-$, CD71$^+$, and CD235a$^+$

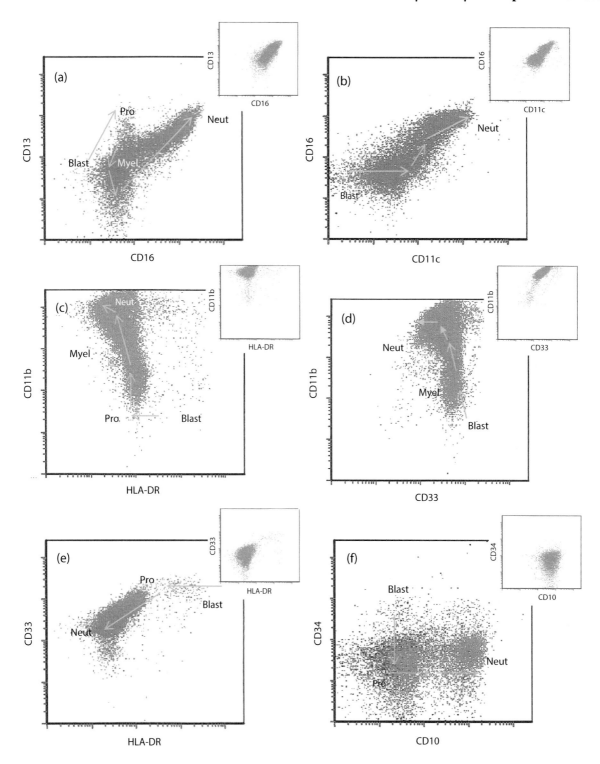

FIGURE 2.5 The expression of CD10, CD11b, CD16, CD11c, and HLA-DR during normal myeloid maturation (normal bone marrow samples; *insets show normal blood samples*). Myeloblasts gain CD13 as they mature to promyelocytes, and then lose its intensity as they become myelocytes; and then gain expression along the maturation toward mature neutrophils (a). CD16 expression starts to appear at metamyelocyte stage and is strongest in segmented forms (a–b). CD11b and CD11c expression gradually increases as the cells mature (b–c); neutrophils are brightly positive for both antigens. HLA-DR is positive in blasts and negative in promyelocytes and subsequent stages (c). CD33 is positive in all stages of granulocytic maturation, but the expression decreases as the cells mature (d–e). CD10 is positive in segmented forms (f). *Abbreviations*: Pro, promyelocytes; Myelo. Myelocytes; Neut, neutrophils.

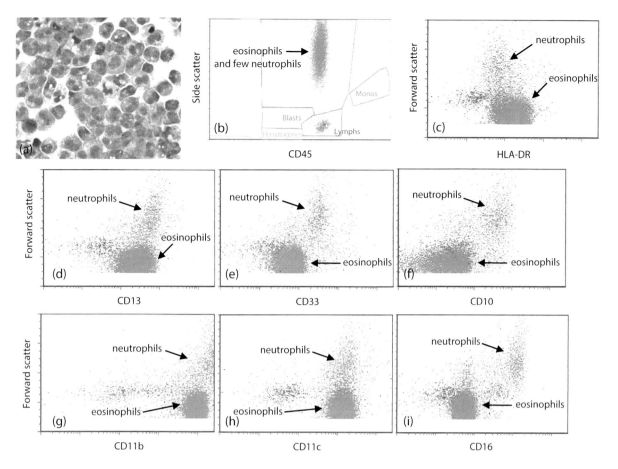

FIGURE 2.6 Flow cytometric features of eosinophils. Blood with marked eosinophilia (a; cytospin preparation from flow sample). Eosinophils, similarly to neutrophils, have high side scatter and moderate CD45 (b). Neutrophils are HLA-DR-negative, whereas eosinophils show dim HLA-DR (c). The expression of CD13 (d) and CD33 (e) is dimmer in eosinophils, when compared to neutrophils. Eosinophils are negative for CD10 (f), show bright expression of CD11b (g) and CD11c (h), and in contrast to neutrophils do not express CD16 (i).

Monocytic differentiation

Monocytic differentiation can be categorized into three stages: monoblasts, promonocytes, and monocytes. Early monoblasts express CD34, CD117, and HLA-DR. Late monoblasts start to lose CD34 and become CD4+. As the cells mature into promonocytes, expression of CD117 starts to diminish, CD34 is lost, and they start to acquire the expression of CD64, CD15, CD11b, and CD11c. Late promonocytes become positive for CD14. The expression of CD11b, CD11c, CD14, CD64, and HLA-DR becomes brighter as the monocytic cells become more mature. The expression of CD14 is strongest by mature cells (monocytes). In contrast to the neutrophils' differentiation, CD11b expression typically precedes CD15, and HLA-DR expression is retained. Mature monocytes in blood are positive for CD11b, CD11c, CD13, CD14, CD33, and CD64. Mature blood monocytes can be classified into three distinct populations (Figure 2.7): classical CD16−/CD14bright+ monocytes (classical monocytes, MO1), intermediate CD16+/CD14bright+ monocytes (MO2), and non-classical CD16+/CD14dim+ monocytes (MO3), with different gene expression profiles, chemokine receptor expression, and phagocytic activities [3, 4]. The MO1 constitutes the major monocyte population (85%) in healthy conditions. The proportion of CD16+/CD14dim+ non-classical monocytes increases in various inflammatory conditions, and in malignancies including plasma cell myeloma [5] and AML [6]. Monocytes give rise to tissue macrophages, osteoclasts (bone), Langerhans cells (skin, other), Kupffer cells (liver), and DCs (skin, other).

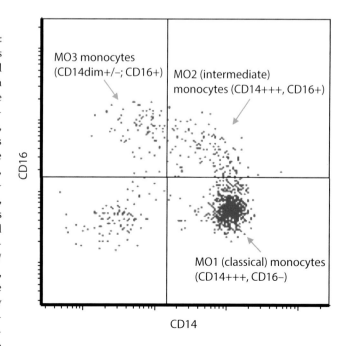

FIGURE 2.7 Classification of monocytes based on CD14 and CD16 expression (see text for details).

Erythroid differentiation

In the erythroid series, blasts are positive for CD34, CD38, CD45, CD117, and HLA-DR (moderate), proerythroblasts are positive for CD36, CD38, CD45, CD71, CD117, GPHA (CD235a; dim), and HLA-DR (moderate) and may express CD34, basophilic erythroblasts express CD36, CD71, glycophorin (CD235a; bright), and HLA-DR (dim) and polychromatophilic and orthochromatophilic erythroblasts express CD36, CD71, and glycophorin (CD235a; bright) [1]. Erythroid precursors progressively lose the expression of CD45.

Megakaryocytic differentiation

Megakaryoblasts are positive for CD45, CD34, CD38, HLA-DR (dim), and CD117. As they mature to megakaryocytes, they become positive for CD61 and lose the expression of HLA-DR, CD34, and CD117. Apart from CD61, megakaryocytes are positive for CD41, CD42, and CD29. Platelets lose the expression of CD38 and retain the expression of CD29, CD41, and CD61. They are CD45-negative.

B-cell differentiation

B-cells arise from BM precursors (progenitor B-cells; Figure 2.8). Progenitor B-cells (pro-B-lymphoblasts) undergo heavy chain rearrangement (*VDJ* gene segments in the H chain locus) to differentiate into precursor B-cells (pre-B) that express μ heavy chains. Pre-B-cells rearrange their immunoglobulin light chain genes (*VJ* gene segments) to become IgM+ immature B-cells and eventually mature to IgM+/IgD+ peripheral (mature) naïve B-cells, which circulate in blood and migrate to lymph nodes. The major stages of B-cell development in the BM include the hematopoietic stem cell (HSC), the multipotent progenitor (MPP), the common lymphoid progenitor (CLP), and then the progenitor B-cell (pro-B-cell), the precursor B-cell (pre-B- cell), and the immature B-cell [7]. The pro-B-cells can be further subdivided into

pre-pro-B, early pro-B, and late pro-B, and pre-B-cells into large pre-B and small pre-B. Pro-B-cells are positive for CD34, CD43, CD117 (C-Kit), B220 (CD45R), CD79a (Igα), CD79b (Igβ), CD10, and TdT, and gain CD19 expression (at early pro-B-cell stage). The pre-B-cells start expressing cytoplasmic μ heavy chains, express CD25, CD19, CD79a, CD79b, and B220 (CD45R), and lose CD117 and CD43 expressions at small pre-B stage. Immature B-cells are CD19+, CD43−, CD79a+, CD79b+, CD25−, CD117−, B220+, CD34+, and IgM+. Immature B-cells have a short half-life, and consists of T1 B-cells (IgM+high, IgD−, CD21−, CD23−, AA4.1+), which are located in the BM, and T2 B-cells which after entering spleen follicles acquire cell surface IgD, CD21, and CD23, and the ability to recirculate [7]. Once the B-cells mature, they start expressing CD22, CD24, and CD40. In the spleen, the B-cells can be subdivided into follicular B-cells (CD19+, B220+, IgMdim+, IgDbright+, CD21+moderate, and CD23+) and marginal zone B-cells (CD19+, B220+, IgMbright+, IgDdim+, CD21bright+, and CD23−). The expression of PAX5 and CD79a appears at the time of heavy chain gene rearrangements (transition from pro-B to pre-B), and the expression of CD20 appears at the time of immunoglobulin light chain rearrangement (immature B-cells). Naïve B-cells are negative for both CD34 and TdT, and often express CD5. Further differentiation of B-cells upon antigenic-induced stimulation occurs in secondary lymphoid tissues and gives rise to the germinal center reaction characterized by clonal expansion, class switch recombination at the *IGH* locus, somatic hypermutation of VH genes, and selection for increased affinity of a B-cell receptor for its unique antigenic epitope. Germinal centers contain large, highly proliferating centroblasts and smaller centrocytes. Final stages of B-cell maturation include transient generation of plasmablasts that secrete antibody while still dividing, short-lived extrafollicular plasma cells that secrete antigen-specific germ line-encoded antibodies

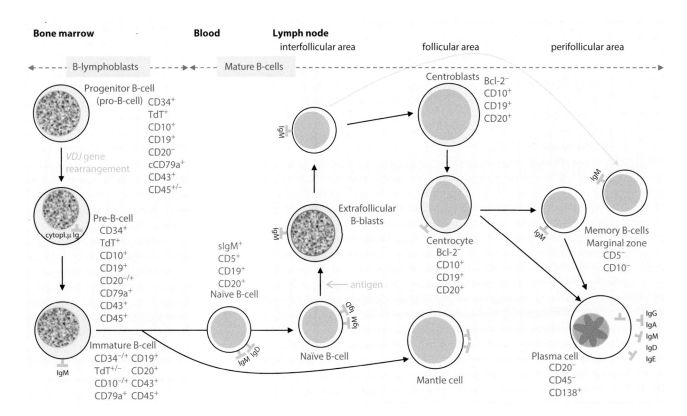

FIGURE 2.8 B-cell development.

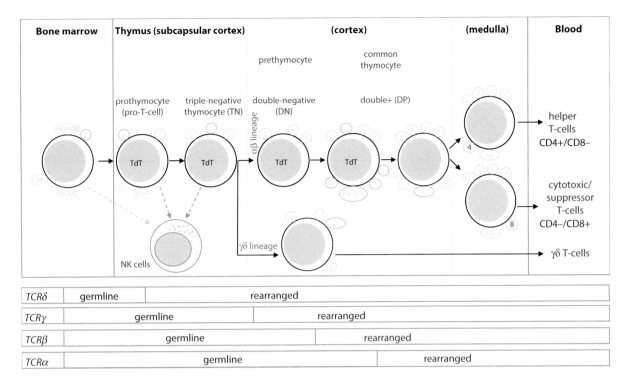

FIGURE 2.9 T-cell development.

and memory B-cells. Memory cells persist after antigen stimulation and expand during secondary responses and can terminally differentiate into antibody-secreting plasma cells.

T-cell differentiation

T-cells (Figure 2.9) arise from BM progenitor T-cells (prothymocytes, CD117+, CD44+, CD25−) that undergo maturation in the thymus and later in peripheral lymphoid tissues (e.g., blood, spleen, skin, mucosa). The earliest definite T-cells (early prothymocytes; pro-T-cells) evolve in the subcapsular region of the thymic cortex and are referred as triple-negative (TN) cells due to lack of expression of CD4, CD8, and surface CD3 (sCD3−/CD4−/CD8−). They are positive for CD2, CD7 (strong expression), CD34, CD44, TdT (nucleus), and cytoplasmic CD3 (c.CD3), and are characterized by a germ line configuration of TCRβ chain. In the process of differentiation, TN cells start to express CD1a and CD5, and progressively lose the expression of CD34 and intensity of CD7 expression. Further differentiation occurs in the thymic cortex, through several stages. Pre-T-cells are characterized by expression of TdT, CD7, CD2, CD5, and IL-7R.

Cortical thymocytes express TdT, CD1a, c.CD3, CD5, and CD7. They are initially negative for both CD4 and CD8 (double-negative T-cells; DN). In the thymic cortex, DN T-cells start to differentiate into double positive (DP) T-cells (CD4+/CD8+) through several stages. DN stage is characterized by continuous rearrangement of TCRB, TCRD, then TCRG, while TCRA rearrangement start occurring during the DP stage. During the transition from pro-T-cells to double-negative T-cells, cells rearrange TCRB gene, a process which is similar to IGH gene rearrangement (Dβ segment joins a Jβ segment, and then Vβ segment joins the DβJβ complex). At this point, cells start the commitment to either TCRγδ or TCRαβ lineages. If the TCRγδ rearrangement is successful, cells become Tγδ+. In subset of cells which undergo the rearrangements of β, α, and γ genes, β-chain forms a heterodimer with the pre-T-α-chain (surrogate α chain), termed pre-TCR complex and start differentiation

into αβ lineage, entering the DP phenotypic stage. The pre-TCR forms a complex with CD3 at the thymocyte surface; those cells are characterized by surface expression of pre-TCR and low CD3. The pre-TCR complex blocks further γδ differentiation (TCRG gene rearrangements are dysfunctional) and plays a major role in T-cell commitment to αβ lineage (with subsequent production of CD4+/CD8+ cells). T-cells committed to TCRαβ lineage mature into CD4+/CD8+ cells which express sCD3 and become negative for TdT. In the thymic medulla, DP cells finish the differentiation process, becoming either CD4+ or CD8+, and then enter the blood as mature T-helper (CD4+) or T-suppressor/cytotoxic (CD8+) cells. Medullary thymocytes have a phenotype of mature T-cells, which are either αβ or γδ, and demonstrate nongermline patterns of TCRG or TCRD genes. Mature T-cells are characterized by the membrane expression of TCR/CD3 complex.

Flow cytometry of blood and bone marrow: Gating strategies

The analysis of CD45 expression combined with side scatter (SSC; orthogonal light scatter) provides a simple and reproducible method for distinguishing major cell lineages in BM [8–17]. Figure 2.10 illustrates characteristic patterns seen in using this method and gating strategy applied in the flow cytometric (FC) analysis of blood and BM. Based on the intensity of CD45 staining (x-axis) and SSC (y-axis), one can distinguish several major cell populations in normal BM or blood: lymphocytes (bright CD45 and low SCC; red dots), monocytes (bright CD45 and increased SSC; blue dots), and granulocytes (moderate CD45 and high SSC; gray dots). In the normal BM samples, additional populations include blasts (moderate CD45 and low SSC), hematogones (moderate CD45, very low SSC), and plasma cells (negative CD45 and low or intermediate SSC). Majority of red blood cells and their precursors are eliminated from FC analysis by lysis. When present in the flow

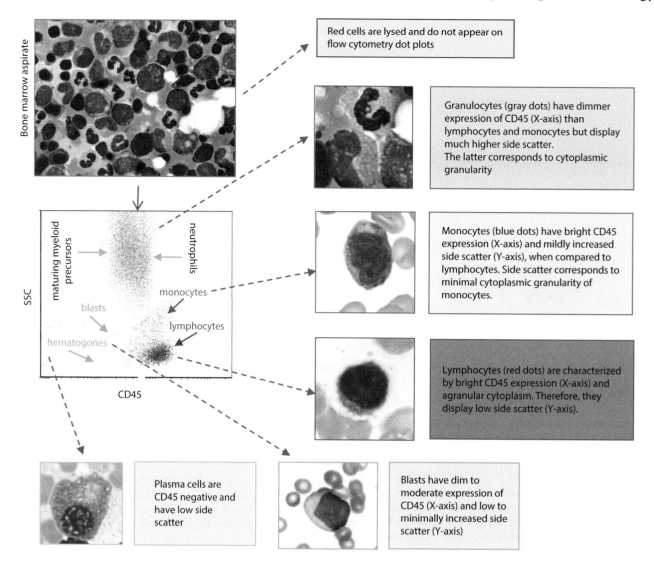

FIGURE 2.10 Gating strategy. Part of the sample from the bone marrow aspirate or blood (tube) is smeared on the microscope glass slide for morphologic correlation, while the rest is incubated with antibodies, lysed, fixed, and submitted for flow cytometry analysis; see text for details.

sample, red cell precursors are characterized by low SSC, negative CD45, positive GPHA (CD235a), and bright CD71. Figures 2.11–2.18 present distributions of some of the neoplastic populations in regard to the gates defined by CD45 *versus* SSC properties. Since malignant populations do not always display typical antigen expression or light scatter properties and do not fall into a specific gate, FC analysis should include also evaluation of antigens expression in open (ungated) mode (cluster analysis). For example, some myeloblasts display high SSC and dim or negative CD45, and might be underestimated if CD34 and/or CD117 analysis includes only cells with low SSC and moderate CD45. Based on antigen expression of ungated cells, the predefined gates can be modified (back-gating). After the data are acquired, each population is analyzed for specific markers (e.g., lymphocytes are analyzed for B-cell clonality and T-cell antigens expression, cells with dimmer CD45 expression and low SSC are analyzed for leukemic blasts, etc.). Flow data analysis should always include ungated display as well so that the abnormal population with different than typical CD45 *versus* SSC properties (see below) is not omitted.

Lymphocytic gate

Benign lymphocytes and the majority of mature (peripheral) lymphoproliferative disorders including CLL/SLL, T-LGL leukemia (T-LGLL), marginal zone lymphoma (MZL), follicular lymphoma (FL), and mature T-cell lymphomas have bright CD45 and low SSC (Figure 2.11; "lymphocytic" gate).

Monocytic gate

Benign and neoplastic monocytes (including chronic myelomonocytic leukemia and acute monoblastic leukemia) have bright CD45 expression, but SSC is higher than in lymphocytes (Figure 2.12; "monocytic" gate). A similar distribution is typical for hairy cell leukemia (HCL). Rare cases of large cell lymphomas and plasma cell myelomas may be placed in "monocytic" gate on CD45 versus SSC display. Also, maturing myeloid precursors with prominent features of dysgranulopoiesis (representing myelodysplastic syndrome; MDS) display markedly decreased SSC (due to degranulation) resulting in their location in "monocytic" gate.

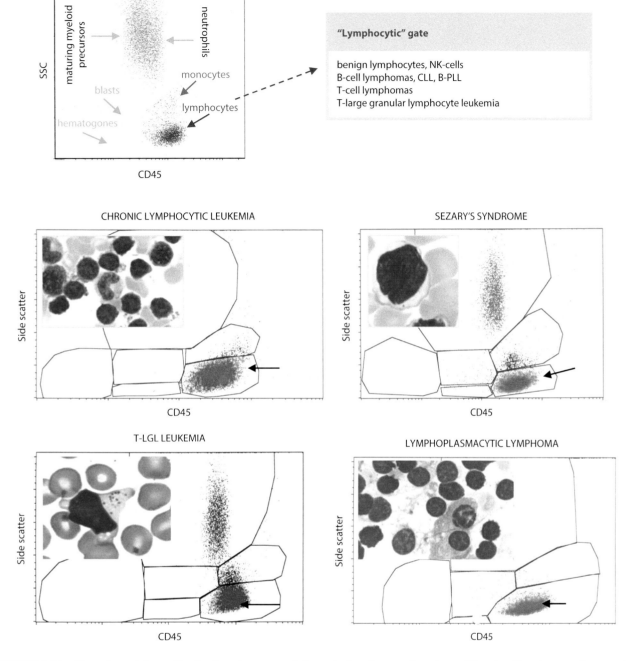

FIGURE 2.11 "Lymphocytic" gate. Benign lymphocytes and the majority of mature lymphoproliferative disorders are characterized by low side scatter (SSC) and bright expression of CD45 (red dots; arrow).

Hematogones gate

Normal B-cell precursors (hematogones; Figure 2.13) have very low SSC and dimmer expression of CD45 than displayed by normal lymphocytes. Lymphoblastic leukemias, occasional acute myeloid leukemias (AML), and mature B- and T-cell lymphoproliferations (e.g., CLL, T-PLL) may be located in hematogones gate.

Blast gate

Blasts usually have moderate CD45 expression and slightly increased SSC (Figure 2.14). B- and T-lymphoblastic leukemias, blastic plasmacytoid dendritic cell neoplasm (BPDCN), and occasional B- and T-cell lymphomas (most often large cell type) display similar location of neoplastic cells in the "blast" gate.

Plasmacytic gate

Neoplastic plasma cells usually are CD45⁻ and have high forward scatter (FSC) and low to slightly increased SSC (Figure 2.15). Similar properties are typical for nucleated red cell precursors. Many cases of B lymphoblastic leukemias (B-ALL) and occasional cases of acute myeloid leukemia (AML), BPDCN, chronic lymphocytic leukemia (CLL), or T-cell prolymphocytic leukemia (T-PLL) may be located in this gate.

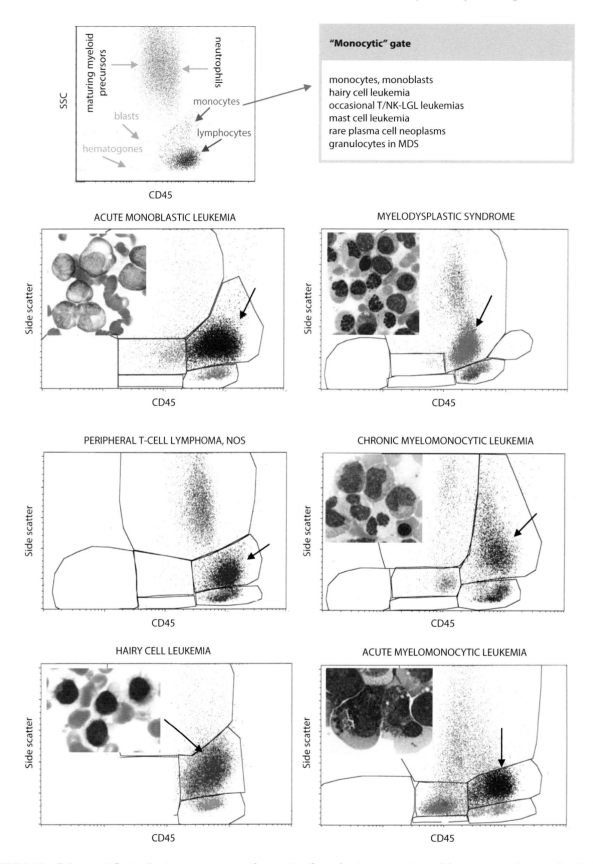

FIGURE 2.12 "Monocytic" gate. Benign monocytes and majority of neoplastic monocytic proliferations are characterized by bright CD45 expression and slightly increased side scatter (SSC). They appear above lymphocytic gate on CD45 versus SSC display (arrow). Apart from monocytic cells, similar SSC and CD45 properties are often seen in hairy cell leukemia and occasional lymphoproliferations, mast cell leukemia (unusual and rare form of mast cell disease), and markedly dysplastic granulocytes.

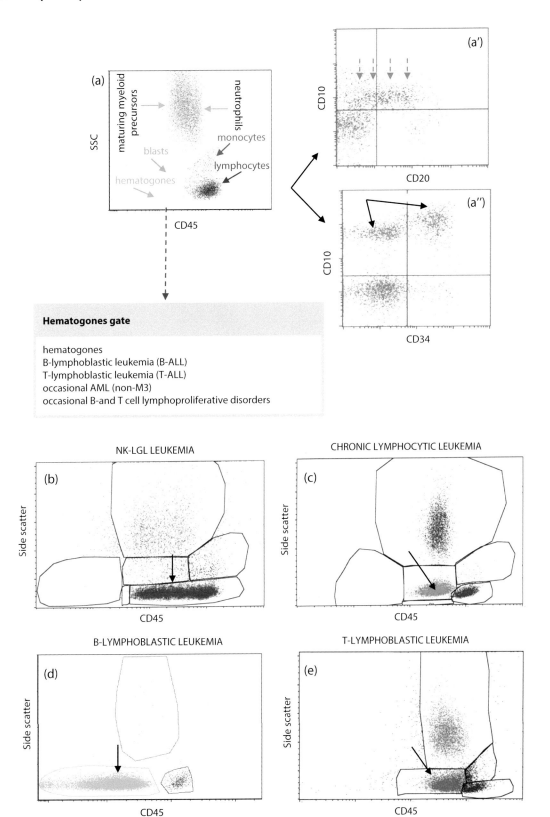

FIGURE 2.13 "Hematogones" gate (a). Hematogones are characterized by very low side scatter (SSC) and dimmer expression of CD45 when compared to lymphocytes (red dots); they have variable ("smeared") expression of CD20 (a'; broken arrows), and are positive for CD10 and partially for CD34 (a"). Occasional lymphoproliferative disorders and blasts may have similar to hematogones SSC and CD45 properties (b–e).

48

Flow Cytometry in Neoplastic Hematology

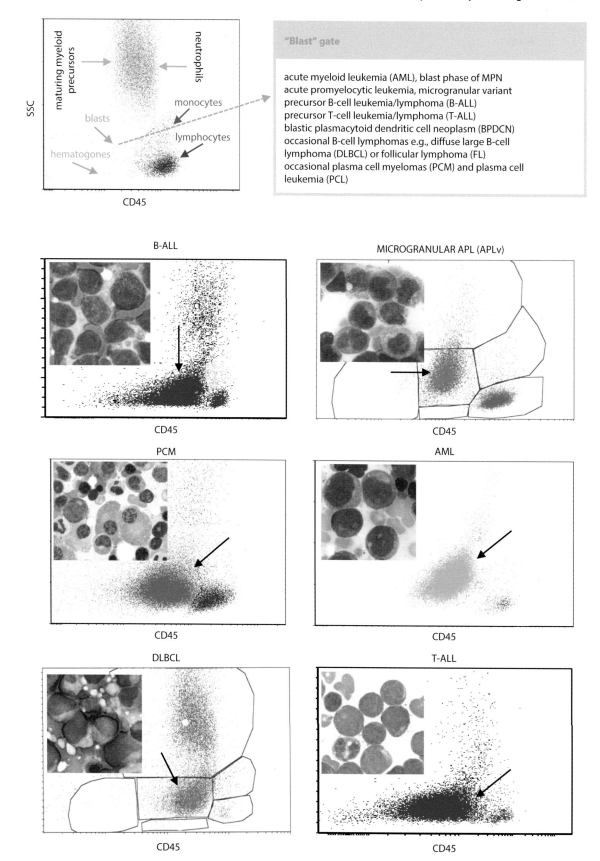

FIGURE 2.14 "Blast" gate. Myeloid precursors (blasts) have moderate CD45 and low side scatter (SSC). Occasional lymphoproliferative disorders, plasma cell tumors, as well as granulocytes with decreased granularity and microgranular APL have similar CD45 versus SSC characteristics.

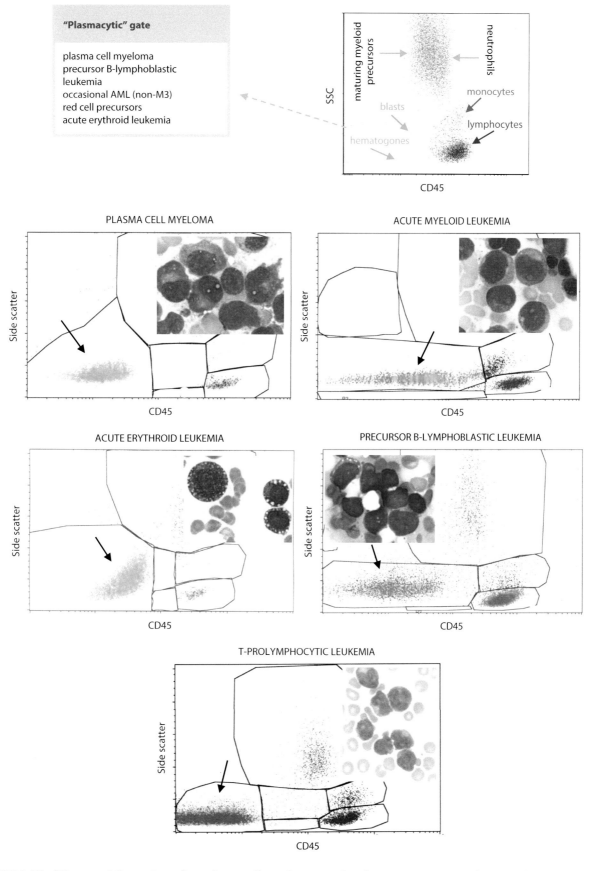

FIGURE 2.15 "Plasmacytic" gate. Apart from plasma cell neoplasms, erythroid precursors, occasional AML and B-ALL are characterized by negative CD45 and low side scatter. Rare T-PLL may be CD45-negative.

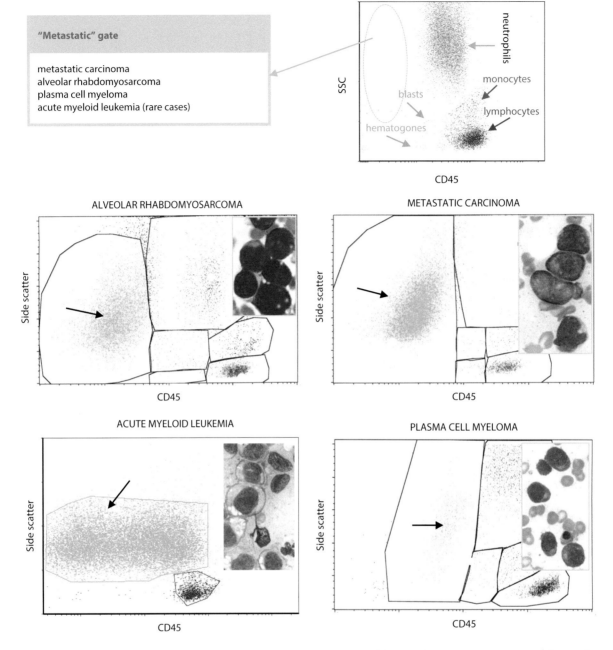

FIGURE 2.16   "Metastatic" gate. High side scatter and negative CD45 is typical for non-hematopoietic tumors and rare plasma cell neoplasms.

Metastatic gate

Extrinsic elements (e.g., small cell carcinoma) are CD45⁻ and usually display high SSC ("metastatic" gate; Figure 2.16). Erythroid precursors and occasional plasma cell tumors may be located in this gate.

Granulocytic gate

Granulocytes/maturing myeloid cells are characterized by moderate expression of CD45 and high SSC ("granulocytic" gate; Figure 2.17). Similar SSC properties are represented by classic (hypergranular) acute promyelocytic leukemia, mast cells, and occasional acute myeloid leukemias.

Blood: Normal flow cytometry pattern

Figure 2.18 presents the FC pattern of normal blood sample. The following reference ranges for normal peripheral blood cases were established on analysis of 120 cases (based on the expression of CD13 and CD33 for granulocytes/neutrophils, CD14 and CD64 for monocytes, CD19, CD20, and CD22 for B-cells, CD2, CD3, CD5, and CD7 for T-cells based, CD34 and CD117 for blasts). For age group 18–65 years (average ± SD): neutrophils 50.8% (±17.9), B-cells 4.5 (±2.6), T-cells 22.7 (±10.4), blasts 0.2 (±0.2), and monocytes 4.2 (±2.0). For age group >65 years (average ± SD): neutrophils 50.3% (±18.4),

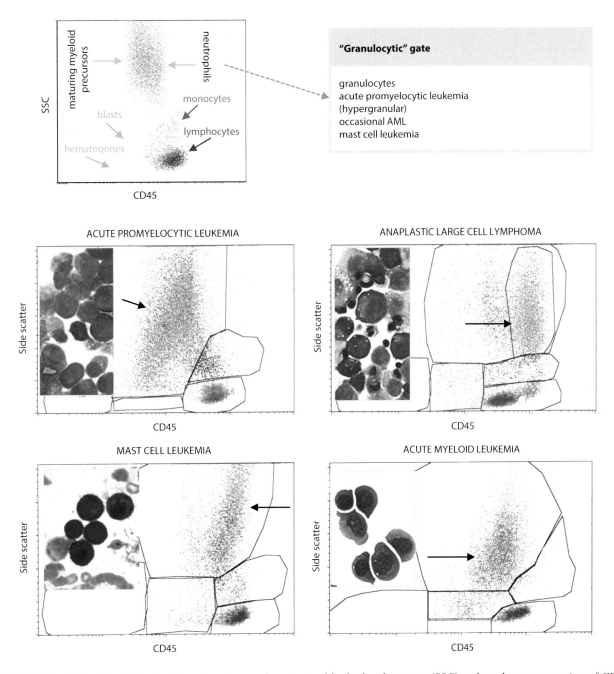

FIGURE 2.17 "Granulocytic" gate. Granulocytes are characterized by high side scatter (SSC) and moderate expression of CD45. Hematopoietic tumors with similar characteristics include mast cell proliferations, acute promyelocytic leukemia (hypergranular variant), and occasional large cell lymphomas and rare acute myeloid leukemias.

B-cells 3.5 (±2.4), T-cells 22.9 (±9.6), blasts 0.2 (±0.2), and monocytes 4.5 (±2.1). Table 2.1 presents the frequency of antigen expression in normal blood samples.

Bone marrow: Normal flow cytometry pattern

Figure 2.19 presents the FC pattern of normal BM sample. The following reference ranges for normal BM cases were established from the analysis of 120 cases (based on the expression of CD13 and CD33 for granulocytes/neutrophils, CD14 and CD64 for monocytes, CD19, CD20, and CD22 for B-cells, CD2, CD3, CD5, and CD7 for T-cells-based, CD34 and CD117 for blasts). For age group 18–65 years (average ± SD): granulocytes 60.3% (±20.1), B-cells 1.4 (±1.1), T-cells 9.8 (±6.1), blasts 1.2 (±0.9), and monocytes 3.4 (±3.3). For age group >65 years (average ± SD): granulocytes 60.6% (±20.0), B-cells 1.4 (±1.6), T-cells 8.2 (±6.1), blasts 1.1 (±0.7), and monocytes 4.0 (±4.4). Table 2.1 presents the frequency of antigen expression in normal BM samples.

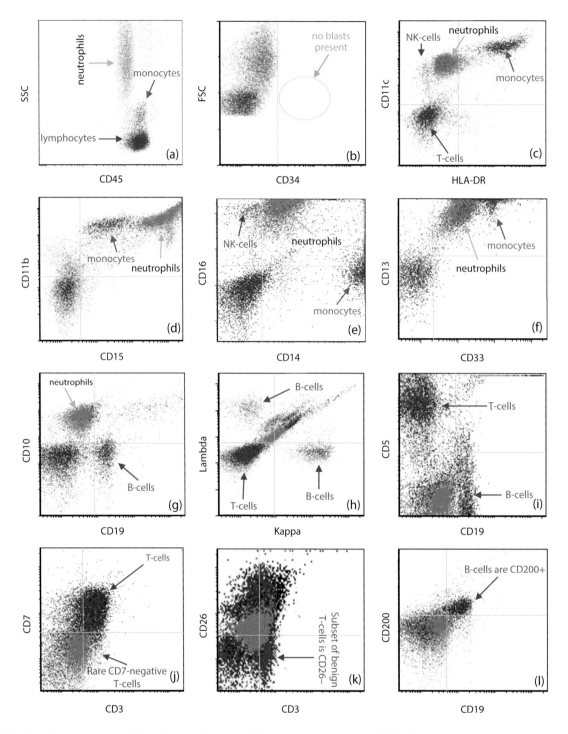

FIGURE 2.18 Flow cytometry of blood: normal pattern. CD45 versus side scatter (SSC) display (a) shows three major populations: neutrophils (gray dots), monocytes (blue dots), and lymphocytes (red dots). Neutrophils are characterized by high side scatter (SSC, a) and high forward scatter (FSC, b), while lymphocytes show low SSC and FSC. Normal blood sample shows either no blasts or only very few circulating blasts (b). Monocytes and neutrophils are CD11c+ (c), CD11b+ (d), and CD15+ (d). Monocytes show bright expression of CD14 (e) and CD33 (f), while neutrophils show dimmer CD33 when compared to monocytes (f) but are brightly positive for CD10 (g). NK-cells are CD11c+ (c) and CD16+ (e). Kappa versus lambda displays shows presence of polytypic B-cells (h) with kappa to lambda ratio ranging from 0.5:1 to 3:1 on average. B-cells are positive for CD19 (g, i) and T-cells are positive for CD5 (i); there are no or only very few CD5+ B-cells (the number of CD5+ B-cells is more pronounced in children and young adults). Majority of benign T-cells are positive for both CD3 and CD7 (j). Number of CD7-negative T-cells may increase in certain reactive conditions, such as viral infections. Majority of benign T-cells are positive for CD26, but most normal blood samples show minor fraction of CD26− T-cells (k). Number of benign T-cells with lack of CD26 may be higher when there is increased number of T-LGL cells. Benign B-cells are dimly positive for CD200 (l).

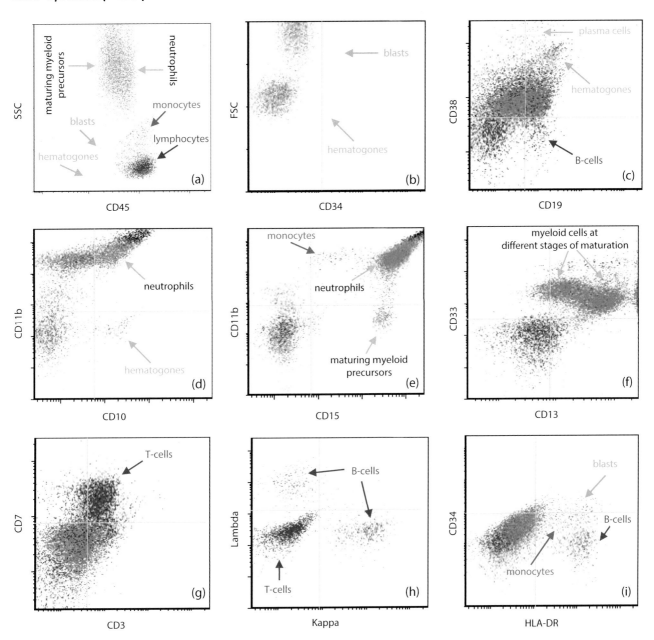

FIGURE 2.19 Flow cytometry of BM: normal pattern. CD45 versus side scatter (SSC) display (a) shows six major populations: myeloid cells at different stages of maturation (gray dots), monocytes (dark blue dots), lymphocytes (red dots), hematogones (light blue dots), and blasts (green dots). Myeloid cells (granulocytes) are characterized by high side scatter (SSC, a) and high forward scatter (FSC, b), while lymphocytes and hematogones show low SSC and FSC (a–b). Both hematogones and blasts are CD34⁺, but they differ in FSC (b). B-cells, hematogones and majority of benign plasma cells are CD19⁺ (c). The expression of CD38 is dim on myeloid cells, moderate to bright on blasts and hematogones, and very bright on plasma cells (c). Hematogones and most mature myeloid cells (neutrophils) are CD10⁺ (d). Monocytes and most mature myeloid cells (neutrophils, metamyelocytes, and myelocytes) show bright expression of CD11b (d–e) while less mature myeloid precursors are CD11b⁻. CD15 is positive on myeloid cells (granulocytes) and monocytes (e). Myeloid cells (neutrophils, maturing myeloid precursors, and monocytes) are positive for CD13 and CD33 (f); note variable pattern of expression of CD13 at different stages of maturation. Majority of benign T-cells are positive for both CD3 and CD7 (g). Benign B-cells show polytypic expression of surface light-chain immunoglobulins (kappa and lambda, (h), dot plots gated on lymphocytes only). The proportion of kappa to lambda (κ/λ ratio) is within the range of 0.5–3.0:1. HLA-DR is positive on blasts, B-cells, monocytes, and hematogones (i).

TABLE 2.1: Frequency of Antigens Expression in Benign Blood Samples (*n* = 100 Cases) and BM Samples (*n* = 100 Cases) in >18-Years-Old Patients (Numbers Represent the Percent of all Events Analyzed)

Antigen	Blood (Average % ± SD)	Bone Marrow (Average % ± SD)
CD2$^+$ cells	22.6 (±9.8)	9.8 (±6.8)
CD2$^+$ blasts	–	0.04 (±0.03)
CD3$^+$ cells	21.7 (±8.8)	8.7 (±5.9)
CD4$^+$ cells	13.9 (±7.5)	5.3 (±4.1)
CD5$^+$ cells	22.2 (±9.4)	8.9 (±5.8)
CD7$^+$ cells	19.5 (±7.8)	8.6 (±5.9)
CD7$^-$ T-cells	2.1 (±1.9)	–
CD7$^+$ blasts	–	0.01 (±0.02)
CD8$^+$ cells	8.6 (±14.1)	3.0 (±2.6)
CD10$^+$ lymphocytes	0.2 (±0.3)	0.2 (±0.7)
CD10$^+$ cells	58.8 (±12.7)	33.2 (±13.2)
CD11b$^+$ cells	61.3 (±13.4)	70.1 (±11.0)
CD11b$^+$ blasts	–	0.1 (±0.16)
CD11c$^+$ lymphocytes	3.5 (±2.1)	1.8 (±1.7)
CD11c$^+$ cells	56.2 (±13.3)	34.4 (±11.3)
CD13$^+$ cells	61.1 (±14.9)	56.6 (±15.3)
CD14$^+$ cells	4.7 (±2.0)	3.4 (±2.4)
CD14$^-$ monocytes	0.1 (±0.5)	0.03 (±0.04)
CD15$^+$ cells	57.2 (±16.8)	76.2 (±8.3)
CD15$^+$ blasts	–	0.15 (±0.2)
CD16$^+$ cells	61.6 (±13.7)	42.7 (±14.6)
CD19$^+$ cells	3.4 (±2.5)	1.3 (±1.2)
CD20$_+$ cells	3.3 (±2.6)	1.3 (±1.5)
CD22$_+$ cells	3.2 (±2.4)	1.5 (±1.3)
CD23$_+$ lymphocytes	1.5 (±1.6)	0.5 (±0.5)
CD26$_+$ lymphocytes	15.5 (±7.9)	–
CD26$^-$ T-cells	6.6 (±6.0)	–
CD33$_+$ cells	49.9 (±17.2)	60.1 (±27.0)
CD34$_+$ cells	0.2 (±0.3)	1.2 (±0.7)
CD38$_+$ cells	18.2 (±8.0)	7.7 (±4.6)
CD45$_+$ cells	97.7 (±3.3)	97.5 (±3.1)
CD56$^+$ lymphocytes	4.7 (±4.0)	–
CD56$^+$ granulocytes	1.7 (±1.1)	4.0 (±4.0)
CD56$^+$ blasts	–	0.05 (±0.03)
CD56$^+$ monocytes	1.1 (±0.9)	0.5 (±0.6)
CD57$^+$ T-cells	5.0 (±3.4)	2.3 (±2.2)
CD64$^+$ cells	22.0 (±12.4)	49.7 (±24.4)
CD64$^+$ monocytes	4.5 (±2.1)	4.0 (±3.9)
CD117$^+$ cells	0.2 (±0.6)	1.2 (±0.8)
HLA-DR$^+$ cells	16.9 (±3.8)	8.7 (±6.3)
HLA-DR$^-$ blasts	–	0.01 (±0.01)

References

1. Wood, B., *Multicolor immunophenotyping: human immune system hematopoiesis.* Methods Cell Biol, 2004. **75**: p. 559–76.
2. Pirruccello, S.J., K.H. Young, and P. Aoun, *Myeloblast phenotypic changes in myelodysplasia. CD34 and CD117 expression abnormalities are common.* Am J Clin Pathol, 2006. **125**(6): p. 884–94.
3. Ziegler-Heitbrock, L., et al., *Nomenclature of monocytes and dendritic cells in blood.* Blood, 2010. **116**(16): p. e74–e80.
4. Patnaik, M.M., et al., *Flow cytometry based monocyte subset analysis accurately distinguishes chronic myelomonocytic leukemia from myeloproliferative neoplasms with associated monocytosis.* Blood Cancer J, 2017. **7**(7): p. e584.
5. Sponaas, A.M., et al., *The proportion of CD16(+)CD14(dim) monocytes increases with tumor cell load in bone marrow of patients with multiple myeloma.* Immun Inflamm Dis, 2015. **3**(2): p. 94–102.
6. Ziegler-Heitbrock, L., *Blood monocytes and their subsets: established features and open questions.* Front Immunol, 2015. **6**: p. 423.
7. Ying Wang, J.L., P.D. Burrows, and J.-Y. Wang, *B cell development and maturation.* Adv Exp Med Biol, 2020. **1254**: p. 1–22.
8. Borowitz, M.J., et al., *Immunophenotyping of acute leukemia by flow cytometric analysis. Use of CD45 and right-angle light scatter to gate on leukemic blasts in three-color analysis.* Am J Clin Pathol, 1993. **100**(5): p. 534–40.
9. Craig, F.E. and K.A. Foon, *Flow cytometric immunophenotyping for hematologic neoplasms.* Blood, 2008. **111**(8): p. 3941–67.
10. Borowitz, M.J., et al., *U.S.-Canadian Consensus recommendations on the immunophenotypic analysis of hematologic neoplasia by flow cytometry: data analysis and interpretation.* Cytometry, 1997. **30**(5): p. 236–44.
11. Braylan, R.C., et al., *U.S.-Canadian Consensus recommendations on the immunophenotypic analysis of hematologic neoplasia by flow cytometry: data reporting.* Cytometry, 1997. **30**(5): p. 245–8.
12. D'Archangelo, M., *Flow cytometry: new guidelines to support its clinical application.* Cytometry B Clin Cytom, 2007. **72**(3): p. 209–10.
13. Davis, B.H., et al., *U.S.-Canadian Consensus recommendations on the immunophenotypic analysis of hematologic neoplasia by flow cytometry: medical indications.* Cytometry, 1997. **30**(5): p. 249–63.
14. Martinez, A., et al., *Routine use of immunophenotype by flow cytometry in tissues with suspected hematological malignances.* Cytometry, 2003. **56B**(1): p. 8–15.
15. Zeleznikova, T. and O. Babusikova, *The value of dot plot patterns and leukemia-associated phenotypes in AML diagnosis by multiparameter flow cytometry.* Neoplasma, 2005. **52**(6): p. 517–22.
16. Orfao, A., et al., *Clinically useful information provided by the flow cytometric immunophenotyping of hematological malignancies: current status and future directions.* Clin Chem, 1999. **45**(10): p. 1708–17.
17. Kussick, S.J. and B.L. Wood, *Using 4-color flow cytometry to identify abnormal myeloid populations.* Arch Pathol Lab Med, 2003. **127**(9): p. 1140–7.

3

IDENTIFICATION OF CLONAL B-CELL POPULATION

Polyclonal versus monoclonal B-cells

Polyclonal B-cells in blood and bone marrow

Lymphocytes composed approximately one-third of the total population of leukocytes in peripheral blood of newborns. Their relative and absolute number increases rapidly during the first 5 months of life, remains unchanged until 2 years of age, and gradually decreases to numbers observed in adults. Absolute numbers of B lymphocytes, which increase almost threefold during the first 5 months of life from the median value of 10.9%–27.3% remain almost unchanged until ~5 years of age, and gradually decrease thereafter to median 11.6% detected in young adults [1]. Non-memory population characterized by lack of CD27 expression composes the major subset of B lymphocytes. Gradual replacement of CD19$^+$CD27$^-$ non-memory B lymphocytes by CD27-positive B lymphocytes, considered to be memory cells, is completed in children of 10–16 years old [1]. Differential expression of IgD and CD27 allows to distinguish other subsets of B-cells, i.e., naive (CD19$^+$IgD$^+$CD27$^-$), non-switched memory/marginal zone (MZ)-like (CD19$^+$IgD$^+$CD27$^+$), and class-switched memory (CD19$^+$IgD$^-$CD27$^+$) B lymphocytes [1]. So-called transitional B cells with high expression of IgM and CD38 (CD19$^+$ IgM^{high}CD38^{high}) represent most recent B-cells released from bone marrow (BM). Their number is highest in children younger than 2 months, but their relative number decreases significantly during the first year of life and then remains almost invariable during the whole childhood. Their relative number in young adults is more than tenfold lower than in newborns, with the absolute counts being highest in children 2–5 months old [1] Normal mature B-cells consist of one population expressing kappa (κ) and the other lambda (λ) light chain immunoglobulins. The proportion of kappa to lambda (κ/λ ratio) is within the range of 0.5–3.0:1 in blood or BM.

Increased number of benign B-cells in blood is called polyclonal B-cell lymphocytosis (PPBL), first described by Gordon et al. [2]. The review of the literature shows that PPBL is diagnosed predominantly but not exclusively in women, usually smokers and is characterized by a moderate, chronic, and absolute lymphocytosis (>4 × 10^9/L) and atypical binucleated lymphocytes. Their immunophenotypic profile is most compatible with a memory MZ-like B-cell's population distinguished by the expression of CD27, IgM^{high}, CD21^{high}, CD5^{low}, and CD23^{low} [3, 4]. Rare cases of PBCL in newborns have also been described (Figure 3.1).

Benign (polytypic) B-cells from reactive process

Reactive lymph node (and other lymphoid tissues such as tonsils) shows polytypic expression of light chain immunoglobulins (kappa$^+$/lambda$^-$ and kappa$^-$/lambda$^+$ B-cells), occasional B-cells with CD10 expression and often partial CD23 expression on B-cells (Figure 3.2). The proportion of kappa to lambda (κ/λ ratio) is within the range of 1.2:1 to 2.7:1 in lymph nodes. In the florid reactive follicular hyperplasia (lymph nodes, tonsils, etc.), flow cytometry (FC) analysis shows increased number of B-cells with CD10 expression which often show variable ("smeary")

expression of light chain immunoglobulins with kappa being usually brighter than lambda (Figure 3.3) although in some patients, especially children and young adults the expression of lambda may be more pronounced (Figure 3.4).

Minor population of B-cells may be CD5$^+$ (more prominent in younger patients). FC analysis of lymph node (as well as from blood and BM) from patients with HIV often shows B-cells with strong kappa and lambda expression and poor resolution between kappa$^+$/kappa$^-$ and lambda$^+$/lambda$^-$ cells (Figure 3.5), giving the false impression of dual kappa and lambda positivity.

Clonal B-cell population

Kappa and lambda light-chain determination is of great importance in order to establish B-cell clonality. Mature B-cell neoplasms most often show a single clone of cells, expressing only one class of immunoglobulin light chains. Occasional B-cell lymphoproliferations show lack of detectable surface immunoglobulins when analyzed by FC. Identification of prominent and cohesive population of light chain-restricted B-cells by FC confirms B-cell lymphoma. Figure 3.6 shows clonal (κ$^+$) B-cell population. Identification of small B-cell clone or clonal population mixed with polytypic B-cells may be difficult. Separate analysis of cells with distinct immunophenotype (e.g., CD5, CD10, CD11c, CD38, CD43, or CD71 versus κ/λ), different intensity of expression of CD20 or CD19, and/or presence of cells with increased forward light scatter (FSC) is often helpful to identify neoplastic B-cells. Figure 3.7 shows partial involvement of the lymph node by marginal zone lymphoma (MZL). The identification of monoclonal B-cells was possible only by gating on B-cells with brighter CD20 expression and positive CD38. Figure 3.8 shows FC findings in a case of partial lymph node involvement by follicular lymphoma (FL). In some cases, gating on cells with high FSC (large cells) may be helpful in identifying clonal population (Figure 3.9).

Large cell lymphomas, especially those of high histological grade, often show selective drop-out of neoplastic cells and flow sample may display the predominance of reactive elements. Non-specific staining with certain antibodies (including kappa and lambda surface immunoglobulins), as a result of adherence of antibody to damaged (and therefore "sticky") cells, may result in erroneous FC interpretation. Exclusion of non-viable cells by proper gating and/or incubation of cells with a heating and blocking serum prior to the staining may improve the analysis.

Occasional B-cell lymphoproliferations show two clonal populations (one kappa$^+$ and one lambda$^+$), which represent either one process composed of two clones or a composite lymphoma. Different intensity of CD19, CD20, kappa or lambda expression, and/or presence of additional or different markers on one of the clones (e.g., CD5 or CD10) helps to identify process as malignant (instead of polytypic), as shown in Figure 3.10. Occasional cases of bi-clonal B-cell lymphoproliferations may be difficult to identify due to lack of heterogeneity in the expression of CD19, CD20,

DOI: 10.1201/9781003197935-3

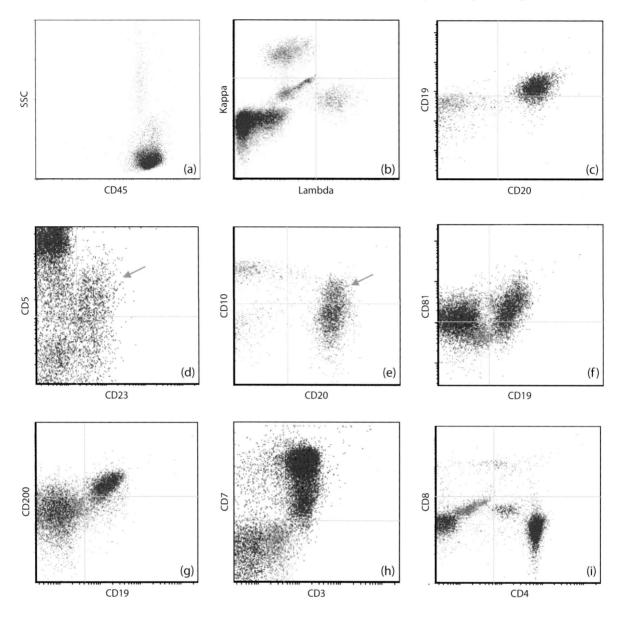

FIGURE 3.1 Benign polyclonal B-cell lymphocytosis in newborn. CD45 versus side scatter (SSC; a) shows predominance of lymphocytes (red dots). B-cells are polytypic (b) showing kappa+ and lambda+ populations. B-cells are positive for CD19 and CD20 (c) and show partial expression of CD5 and CD23 (d, arrow). Rare B-cells express also CD10 (e, arrow). B-cells show dim expression of CD81 (f) and moderate expression of CD200 (g). T-cells are positive for CD3 and CD7 (h) and show increased CD4:CD8 ratio (i).

kappa, and lambda (Figure 3.11) and correlation of those cases with molecular testing for B-cell clonality, morphologic evaluation, and review of clinical data are often crucial in establishing the definite diagnosis.

Clonal populations in reactive lymphoid hyperplasia

Although presence of clonal B-cell population is usually associated with malignancy, several studies demonstrated clonal B-cell populations in reactive conditions, especially in antigen-drive proliferation of mucosa-associated lymphoid tissue (MALT) in stomach, thyroid, orbit, and salivary gland [5–11]. Attygalle et al. reported six cases (four tonsils, two appendixes) of MZ hyperplasia with prominent intraepithelial B cells in children aged 3–11 years with clonal lambda+ cells (molecular

analysis did not confirm clonality) [11]. Lambda immunoglobulin light chain restriction has been also reported in multicentric Castleman's disease [12]. HHV8+ plasmablasts that show lambda light-chain restriction may localize in the mantle zone of B-cell follicles and coalesce to form microscopic lymphomas in some cases of multicentric Castleman's disease [13]. Kussick et al. described six cases of reactive follicular hyperplasia (five lymph nodes and one tonsil) without evidence of BCL2 overexpression or the t(14;18) in which FC identified prominent, clonal, follicle center B-cell populations [14]. The clonality in those six cases was confirmed by polymerase chain reaction (PCR). Of the six cases, five occurred in young males (8–28 years) with no known immunologic abnormality and one case in 32-year-old HIV+ woman. Some reactive lymph nodes, especially from patients

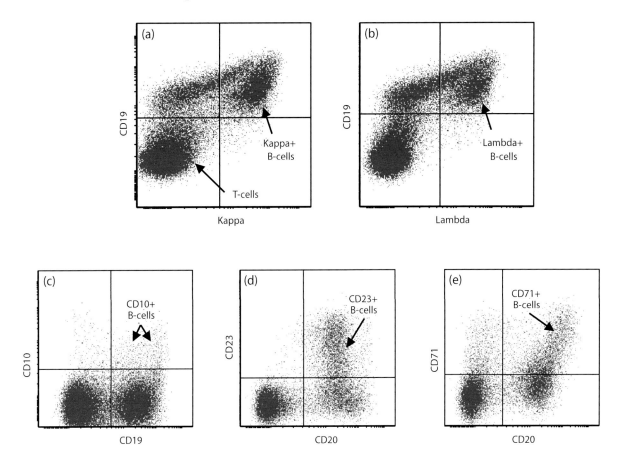

FIGURE 3.2 Benign (reactive) lymph node. B-cells show polytypic light chain immunoglobulins expression (a–b). Minor subset of B-cells is CD10+ (c; germinal center cells). Many of small B-cells are CD23+ (d; arrow), whereas activated B-cells are CD71+ (e; arrow).

with HIV infection, may show increased number of surface light chain-negative B-cells, expressing CD10. Lymph node with atypical MZ hyperplasia in children may show immunoglobulin lambda light-chain restriction by FC without clonal rearrangement of *IGH* gene by molecular (PCR) testing.

Clonal B-cells with non-detectable surface immunoglobulins

Plasma cells and primary mediastinal large B-cell lymphoma usually lack surface immunoglobulin expression by FC. Subset of other B-cell lymphoproliferations may also have non-detectable surface light chain immunoglobulins when analyzed by FC, most likely due to vary low density of antigens on the cells' surface. The most common type of lymphomas with lack of surface kappa (κ) and surface lambda (λ) expression by FC is FL (Figure 3.12), followed by diffuse large B-cell lymphoma (DLBCL; Figure 3.13), CLL/SLL, HCL, occasional Burkitt lymphomas (BLs, Figure 3.14), and rarely other B-cell lymphoproliferations. In the cases of FL, clonal B-cells are often accompanied by residual benign (polytypic) B-cells and numerous T-cells. The identification of neoplastic cells relies on the comparison of the number of cells with positive and negative immunoglobulin expression. In reactive processes, the number of κ+ cells should correspond to λ− cells, and *vice versa*, the number of λ+ cells should be similar to number of κ− cells. In FL with non-detectable surface immunoglobulins, there is a predominance of light chain immunoglobulin negative populations when compared to

cells expressing either kappa or lambda. Figure 3.15 shows variant of FL in which majority of lymphomatous cells are surface immunoglobulin negative, and only small subset shows kappa expression. B-cell lymphomas with non-detectable surface immunoglobulins need to be differentiated from B-cell lymphoblastic leukemia/lymphoma (B-ALL), hematogones, reactive conditions, and plasma cell neoplasms.

Reactive follicular hyperplasia versus follicular lymphoma

The distinction between FL and follicular hyperplasia may be occasionally difficult, especially when the latter shows significant number of CD10+ B-cells. Reactive lymph node with follicular hyperplasia shows typically two B-cell populations (Figure 3.16): CD10+ germinal center cells and CD10− B-cells. The latter are characterized by distinct kappa+ and lambda+ populations, moderate CD19 and CD20 expression, positive CD23, and negative CD71 expression. Germinal center cells show variable (heterogeneous) expression of both kappa and lambda (often with kappa slightly brighter than lambda), brighter CD20, slightly brighter CD19, negative CD23, and positive (dim or partial) CD71. The brighter expression of kappa by CD10+ B-cell population in follicular hyperplasia may be misinterpreted as clonal cells representing FL, especially in cases with predominance of CD10+ B-cells such as in florid follicular hyperplasia (Figure 3.17) or when FC sample such as fine needle aspirate represents predominantly reactive germinal center. Additionally, since the

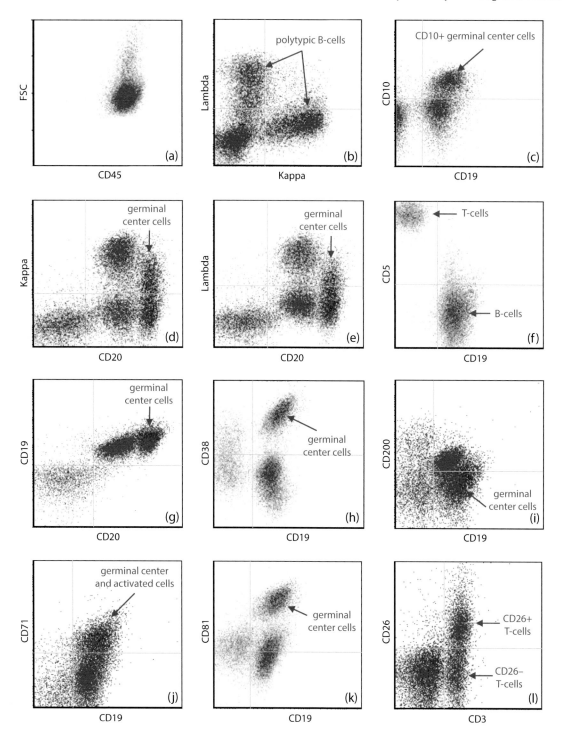

FIGURE 3.3   Florid reactive follicular hyperplasia (lymph node). In reactive lymph node with florid follicular hyperplasia, the majority of lymphocytes are small with low forward scatter (FSC, a). Only subset of germinal center cells and activated lymphocytes display
increased forward scatter (blue dots). B-cells show polytypic pattern of kappa and lambda expression (b). Benign germinal center
cells are CD10+ and show minimally brighter expression of CD19 than the rest of B-cells (c). The dot plots with CD20 versus light
chain immunoglobulin (d–e) show few distinct B-cell populations: germinal center B-cells with bright CD20 (arrows) and variable
("smeary") expression of surface light chain immunoglobulins with slight kappa predominance and non-germinal center B-cells with
dimmer CD20 and either kappa or lambda positivity. The predominance of kappa+ germinal centers cells is most typical, but some
cases with follicular hyperplasia (especially from children and young adults) may show lambda excess (see Figure 3.3). There are only
very few CD5+ B-cells (f); the number of B-cells expressing CD5 is more prominent in children. Dot plots g–k show difference in
expression of CD20 (g), CD38 (h), CD200 (i), CD71 (j), and CD81 (k) between germinal center cells and other B-cells. In reactive lymph
node minor subset of T-cells shows loss of CD26 expression (l).

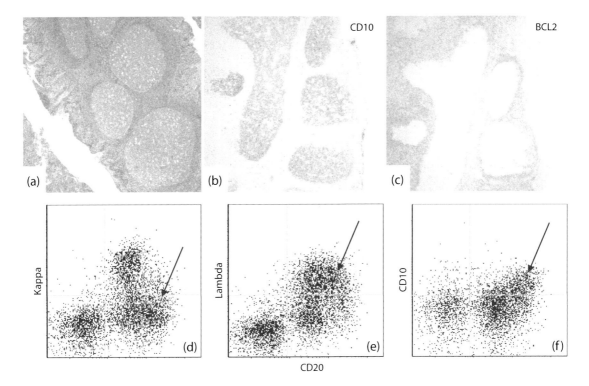

FIGURE 3.4 Follicular hyperplasia with germinal center cells showing lambda excess. Histologic section (H&E, a) shows follicular hyperplasia of tonsil from 4-year-old child. Immunostaining shows CD10⁺ (b) and BCL2⁻ (c) germinal centers. Flow cytometry (d–f) shows polytypic B-cells with distinct population of bright CD20⁺ germinal center cells (arrow) displaying variable expression of surface light chain immunoglobulins (d–e) with obvious lambda excess (compare d and e) and positive CD10 (f).

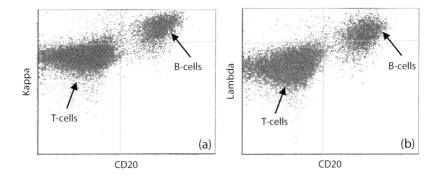

FIGURE 3.5 Polytypic B-cells in lymph node from HIV⁺ patient showing poor resolution between surface light chain positive and negative B-cells (a–b). B-cells appear as if they were dual kappa and lambda positive.

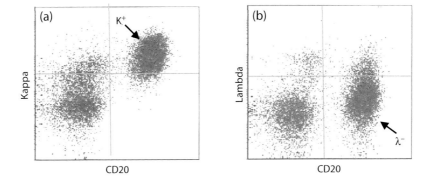

FIGURE 3.6 Clonal B-cells (kappa⁺; a). There is no lambda expression (b).

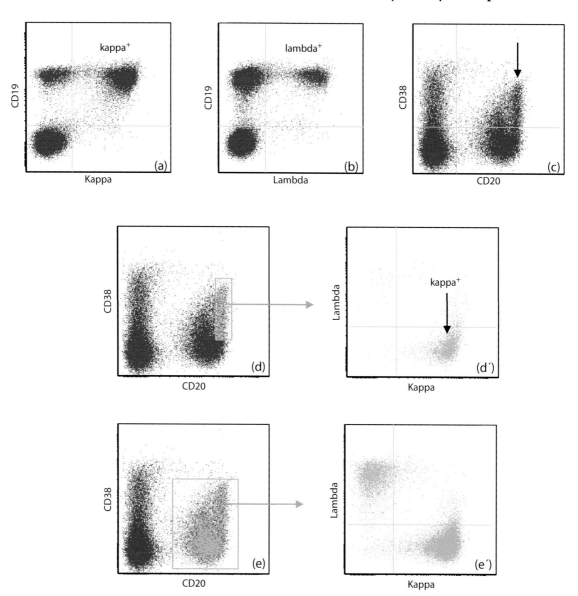

FIGURE 3.7 Partial lymph node involvement by MZL. FC analysis shows minute monoclonal B-cell population (kappa⁺) in the background of predominantly polytypic B-cells. Standard analysis of CD19 versus kappa and lambda (a–b) shows polytypic B-cells with slight kappa excess. A distinct, albeit minute population is noted on CD20 versus CD38 display (c, arrow). It shows brighter CD20 and positive CD38 expression. When analysis is confined to this population (d–d′), it shows kappa⁺ clone (compare with e–e′).

expression of both kappa and lambda by CD10⁺ reactive germinal center cells is dimmer than in CD10⁻ B-cells, the FC findings may be misinterpreted as surface negative cells, a feature often seen in FLs. Admixture of benign B-cells (sometimes predominant) in many cases of FL is yet another factor contributing to difficulties in differential diagnosis between FL and follicular hyperplasia by FC.

Several FC features help to distinguish reactive follicular hyperplasia from FL. In contrast to clonal B-cells, benign germinal center cells have heterogeneous ("smeary" or variable) expression of surface immunoglobulins (Figures 3.3 and 3.4). Lymphomatous cells from FL show distinct (cohesive) cluster of clonal B-cells without variable or "smeary" pattern or are surface immunoglobulin-negative. Occasional cases of FL may show dim expression of surface immunoglobulins, in which identification of clonal cells may be difficult. The expression of CD19 is often

dim in FL (Figure 3.18). In contrast, benign B-cells have moderate to bright expression of CD19. The expression of CD10 is often brighter in FL than in reactive germinal center cells and the expression of CD38 is often dimmer in FL when compared to reactive germinal center cells. Typical FL shows co-expression of CD10 and BCL2 (Figure 3.19) in contrast to reactive CD10⁺ germinal center cells which are BCL2⁻. However, subset of FL may be BCL2⁻ (more often in high grade FL). The morphologic and immunohistochemical evaluation of original sample should follow FC for final diagnosis. FISH studies for t(14;18)/*IGH-BCL2* and/or molecular test (PCR) for B-cell clonality may be needed in difficult cases. Increased forward scatter (FSC) of lymphomatous cells (another helpful diagnostic feature), suggests higher grade FL, which needs to be differentiated from DLBCL, BL, and high grade B-cell lymphoma with *MYC* and *BCL2* rearrangement (HGBL-R, double hit lymphoma).

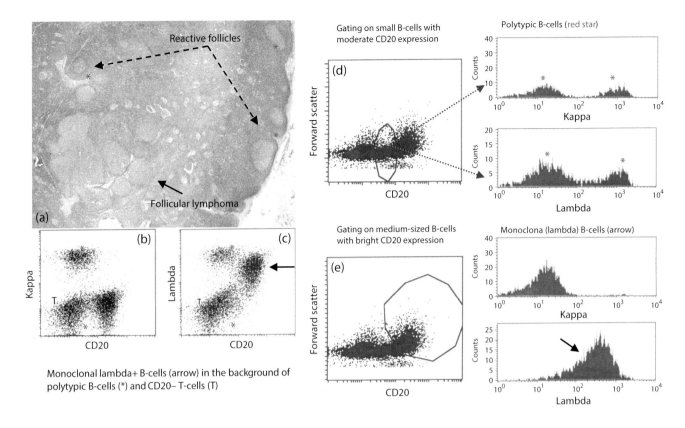

FIGURE 3.8   Partial involvement of the lymph node by follicular lymphoma. A histologic section (a) shows a lymph node with reactive follicles (*; dotted arrows) and a focus of FL (a; solid arrow). Flow cytometry (b–c) shows two populations of B-cells: those with moderate expression of CD20 (*) and those with bright expression of CD20 (c; arrow). The latter are monoclonal cells (λ⁺), representing FL. Residual benign B-cells with moderate CD20 expression are polytypic (*compare b and c*). The two populations differ not only in respect to the intensity of CD20 expression but also by forward scatter, which corresponds to cell size (d–e): gating on cells with moderate CD20 and low forward scatter (d) yields polytypic cells (*see histograms on the right*). Gating on cells with bright CD20 expression and slightly higher forward scatter (e) yields monoclonal λ+ population (arrow, *see histograms on the right*).

Monoclonal B-cell lymphocytosis

The presence of low numbers (<5×10^9/L) of circulating monoclonal B-cells (overall kappa to lambda ratio >3:1 or <0.3:1) in otherwise healthy subjects (no evidence of CLL/other lymphoproliferative disorders, adenopathy, or organomegaly) has been categorized as monoclonal B-cell lymphocytosis (MBL) [15–22]. Most MBLs (75%) have the phenotype of CLL with dim CD20 and dim surface immunoglobulins, and co-expression of CD5 and CD23 and are referred to as CLL-like MBL. The remaining two MBL types are classified as atypical CLL-like (CD5⁺/CD23⁻CD20⁺(dim or moderate) or CD5⁺/CD23⁺/CD20ᵇʳⁱᵍʰᵗ⁺) and CD5⁻ MBL (non-CLL-type or MZL-like, MZL-like). Non CLL-type MBL is also referred to as clonal B-cell lymphocytosis of marginal zone origin (CBL-MZ). The incidence of MBL increases with age, reaching a frequency >20% in persons >60 years and being more frequent among the relatives of patients with CLL. Based on a cutoff value of 0.5×10^9/L clonal B-cells, MBL is also subdivided into high-count MBL (≥0.5×10^9/L) and low-count MBL (<0.5×10^9/L).

MBL with CLL-like phenotype
MBL precedes CLL in most cases of CLL or small lymphocytic lymphoma. CLL-like MBL can be further subdivided into clinical MBL and population-screening MBL. The former is diagnosed in a clinical setting, is associated with lymphocytosis, and has a

concentration of clonal B-cells >1500/μL. Population-screening MBL is only detected during screening studies of healthy persons in the general population and is characterized by <50 clonal B-cells/μL ("low-count MBL"). The potential risk of progression of clinical MBL (previously termed MBL with lymphocytosis) into clinically overt CLL is ~1.1% per year. Rawstron et al. reported minute monoclonal B-cell populations (<3.5×10^9/L) with the phenotype of CLL in blood of 5% of healthy individuals (older than 60 years) [21, 23–25]. Nieto et al. analyzed the frequency of circulating monoclonal B-cells in 608 healthy subjects older than 40 years with normal blood count using a highly sensitive multicolor FC and found clonal CLL-like B-cells in 12% of patients (0.17±0.13 × 10^9/L) [19]. The clinical significance of monoclonal B-cell lymphocytosis is uncertain at the moment and long-term follow-up studies are needed to define its natural history (e.g., the risk of progression into CLL). Shanafelt et al. analyzed the relationship of absolute lymphocyte count (ALC) and B-cell count with clinical outcome in 459 patients with a clonal population with CLL phenotype to determine (1) whether the CLL diagnosis should be based on ALC or B-cell count, (2) what lymphocyte threshold should be used for diagnosis, and (3) whether any lymphocyte count has independent prognostic value after accounting for biologic/molecular prognostic markers [15, 26, 27]. B-cell count and ALC had similar value for predicting treatment-free survival and overall survival as continuous variables, but as binary factors, a B-cell threshold

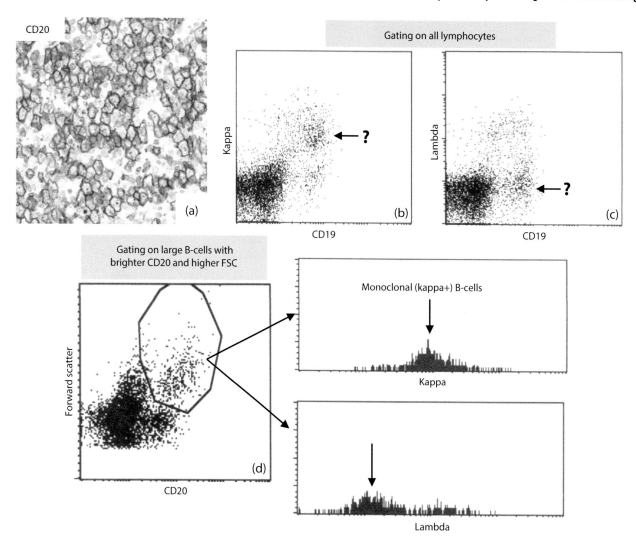

FIGURE 3.9 Diffuse large B-cell lymphoma: identification of clonal B-cells by gating on large cells (cells with high forward scatter). (a) Immunohistochemical staining for CD20 on tissue section from flow sample; (b–d) flow cytometry. Despite predominance of large B-cells in the tissue section (a), analysis of lymphocytic gate for kappa and lambda expression (b–c) shows only rare B-cells with suspicious cluster of kappa+ cells (arrow). Gating on large cell population with high forward scatter and brighter CD20 expression (d) shows obvious clonal population.

of 11×10^9/L best predicted survival. Fazi et al. evaluated 76 low-count MBLs with five-color FC: 90% of CLL-like MBL but only 44.4% atypical CLL and 66.7% CD5⁻ MBL persisted over time [18]. Population-screening CLL-like MBL had no relevant cell count change, and none developed an overt leukemia. In 50% of the cases, FISH showed CLL-related chromosomal abnormalities, including monoallelic or biallelic 13q deletions (43.8%), trisomy 12 (one case), and 17p deletions (two cases) [18, 28].

MBL with atypical CLL-like phenotype

MBLs with atypical CLL-like phenotype (e.g., with lack of CD23 or moderate to bright expression of CD20, negative CD200 or positive CD81) may present clinically similar to MBL with CLL-like phenotype or less often, MBL with t(11;14)/*CCND1* rearrangement (Figure 3.20). The latter most likely represents an indolent, non-nodal variant of mantle cell lymphoma (MCL) with mild lymphocytosis and leukemic blood involvement (with or without BM and spleen involvement). According to the 2016 WHO classification, there are two major known variants of MCL, classical which affects

the lymph nodes and extra nodal sites and have aggressive clinical course, and indolent leukemic non-nodal MCL (L-NN-MCL) [29]. L-NN-MCL is characterized by indolent clinical course, leukemic non-nodal presentation, and phenotype similar to CLL with positive CD200 and CD23 and often lack of SOX11 expression.

Clonal B-cell lymphocytosis of marginal zone origin (CBL-MZ)

Non-CLL MBL is characterized by immunophenotypic features suggestive of post germinal center derivation. Those cases have been recently termed clonal B-cell lymphocytosis of marginal zone origin (CBL-MZ) [22, 29–31]. CBL-MZ is characterized by the presence of clonal B cells in the blood and/or BM with morphologic and immunophenotypic features consistent with MZ derivation in otherwise healthy individuals. CBL-MZ is commonly associated with paraproteinemia (49%), usually immunoglobulin M (IgM), raising differential diagnosis with lymphoplasmacytic lymphoma/Waldenström macroglobulinemia (LPL/WM) [30]. Molecular testing for *MYD88* helps to identify LPL/WM (positive for *MYD88* mutation), although

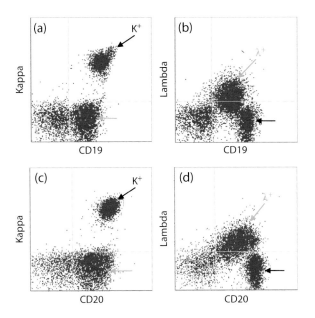

FIGURE 3.10 B-cell lymphoproliferative neoplasm composed of two distinct clonal populations, kappa⁺ (a) and lambda⁺ (b). Kappa positive clone (black arrow) is characterized by bright kappa expression, moderate CD19 (a, b) and moderate CD20 (c, d). Lambda positive clone (green arrow) shows dim CD19 (b) and dim CD20 (d).

further studies are needed to determine if presence of the mutation establishes LPL/WM diagnosis or that it can also be present in borderline CBL-MZ cases associated with paraproteinemia. Extended targeted next-generation sequencing revealed wide molecular heterogeneity with *MYD88* (14%), *PDE4DIP* (14%), *BIRC3* (11%), *CCND3* (11%), *NOTCH1* (11%), and *TNFAIP3* (11%) as the most mutated genes. Mutations of *MYD88* were "nonclassic" in most cases. Although some genetic lesions were overlapping with indolent lymphomas, mainly splenic B-cell lymphomas of MZ origin and splenic diffuse red pulp small B-cell lymphoma, the genetic profile of non-CLL CBL series seemed to suggest that various pathways could be involved in the pathogenesis of these disorders, not mirroring any specific lymphoma entity [31].

Aberrant expression of antigens in B-cell neoplasms

Benign B-cells are positive for B-cell markers (e.g., CD19, CD20, CD22, CD79a) and HLA-DR, and are negative for T-cell markers, CD4 and CD8, and conversely, normal T-cells are positive for T-antigens, CD4 or CD8, and are negative for B-cell markers (minor population of benign B-cells may be CD5⁺). Based on FC immunophenotyping, mature B-cell neoplasms can be broadly divided into several phenotypic categories: CD5⁺, CD10⁺, CD5⁻/CD10⁻, CD5⁺/CD10⁺, and CD103⁺ (detailed phenotypic classification of B-cell lymphoproliferations is presented in Chapter 12). CD5⁺ group includes chronic lymphocytic leukemia/small lymphocytic lymphoma (CLL/SLL), which typically is also CD23⁺ and CD200⁺, and MCL, which typically is CD200⁻ CD23⁻, and CD81⁺. Other CD5⁺ B-cell lymphomas include rare cases of MZL, DLBCL,

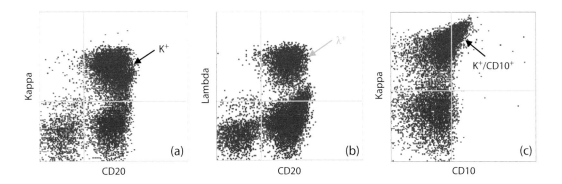

FIGURE 3.11 Blood with prominent B-cell lymphocytosis. Both kappa⁺ (a) and lambda⁺ (b) B-cells are noted mimicking polytypic process. The presence of marked B-cell lymphocytosis and dim CD10 expression (c) on minor subset of kappa⁺ B-cells should raise the possibility of a bi-clonal lymphoproliferative process. Molecular testing (PCR) showed clonal rearrangement of IGH.

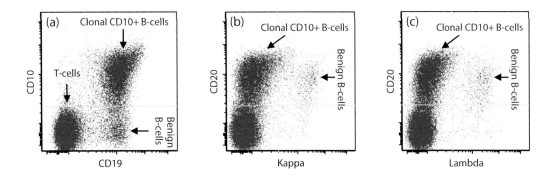

FIGURE 3.12 Follicular lymphoma with non-detectable surface immunoglobulins. Clonal B-cells are CD10⁺ (a) and do not express kappa (b) or lambda (c). Only benign (residual) B-cells show polytypic expression of kappa and lambda (b–c).

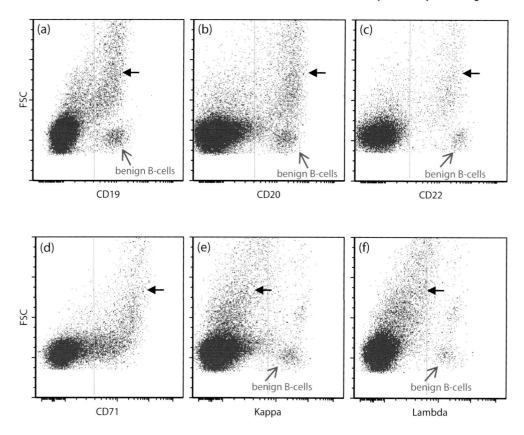

FIGURE 3.13 DLBCL with non-detectable surface immunoglobulins. When compared to normal (polytypic) B-cells, clonal B-cells (solid arrow) show very high forward scatter (FSC; a–f), slightly dimmer expression of CD19 (a), brighter CD20 (c), and dimmer CD22 (c). They are positive for CD71 (d) and appear both kappa and lambda negative (e–f), although very dim lambda expression cannot be excluded.

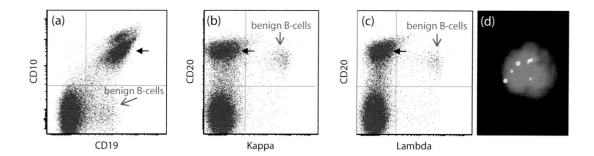

FIGURE 3.14 Burkitt lymphoma in a 4-year-old boy: clonal CD10⁺ B-cells (a; solid arrow) are negative for surface immunoglobulins (b–c). FISH studies confirmed *MYC* rearrangement (d).

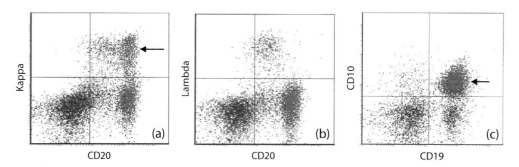

FIGURE 3.15 Follicular lymphoma. Majority of lymphomatous cells are surface immunoglobulin-negative (a–b; blue dots), but a minute subset shows kappa expression (a; arrow). All neoplastic cells express CD10 (c, arrow). Residual benign B-cells are polytypic (a–b; red dots) and do not express CD10 (c).

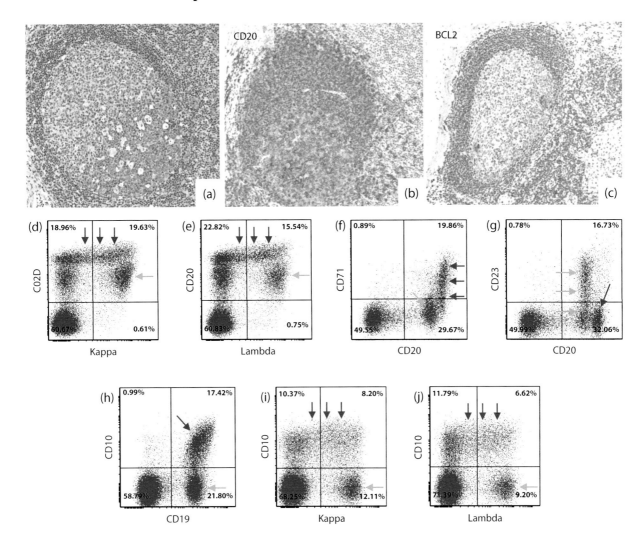

FIGURE 3.16 Benign lymph node with follicular hyperplasia. Reactive follicles (H&E section; a) express CD20 (b), and have BCL2⁻ germinal centers (c). Flow cytometry analysis (d–j) shows rather prominent polytypic B-cells composed of two distinct populations: B-cells with moderate CD20 (d–g; green arrows) and B-cells with bright CD20 (d–g; red arrows). B-cells with moderate CD20 represent non-germinal center B-cells, which are CD71⁻ (f; green arrow), CD23⁺ (g; green arrow), and CD10⁻ (h; green arrow). Germinal center cells are CD10⁺ (h; red arrow), CD71⁺ (f; red arrow), and CD23⁻ (g; red arrow). The expression of CD19 is similar to slightly brighter when compared to CD10⁻ B-cells (h). Germinal center cells are polytypic but show variable ("smeary") expression of surface light chain immunoglobulins (a–b; i–j; red arrows).

and LPL. CD10⁺ group includes FL, subset of DLBCL, Burkitt lymphoma, high grade lymphoma with rearrangement of MYC and BCL2 (HGBL-R, double hit lymphoma) and rare cases of MCL, hairy cell leukemia (HCL) and LPL. CD5⁻/CD10⁻ groups include MZL, LPL, subset of DLBCL, and rare cases of MCL. CD103⁺ group includes HCL and CD25⁻ hairy cell leukemia variant (HCL-v).

Typical mature B-cell lymphomas are characterized by bright expression of CD45, positive HLA-DR, and dim to moderate expression of B-cell markers (e.g., CD19, CD20, CD22, and CD79a); B lymphoblastic leukemia/lymphoma (B-ALL) usually displays negative or dim CD45, positive HLA-DR, and positive TdT and/or CD34, while majority of plasma cell neoplasms are characterized by bright expression of CD38 and CD138, negative CD45, CD19, and CD20, frequent expression of CD56 and/or CD117, and monotypic expression of cytoplasmic light and heavy chain immunoglobulins.

Examples of aberrant antigen expression in mature B-cell neoplasms include:

- CD5
  - positive CD5 expression in FL, MZL, and LPL (CD5 is typically positive in CLL and MCL)
  - lack of CD5 expression in MCL
- CD10
  - positive CD10 expression in HCL, LPL, MCL, or PCM (CD10 is typically positive in FL and BL, most often positive in HGBL-R and positive in subset of DLBCL)
  - lack of CD10 expression in FL
- CD11c
  - bright CD11c expression in HCL and less often other lymphoproliferations (HCL-v, MZL)
- CD13 and/or CD33 (pan-myeloid markers)
  - Positive expression in LPL, MZL (Figure 3.21), or CLL
- CD19
  - positive CD19 in PCM
  - dim CD19 in FL

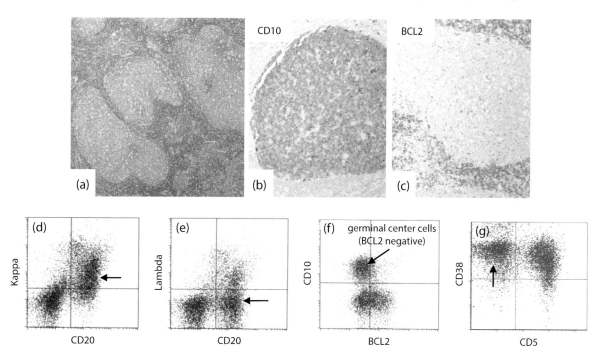

FIGURE 3.17 Florid follicular hyperplasia from HIV⁺ patient (H&E section; a); immunohistochemistry (b–c); and flow cytometry (d–e). Germinal center cells are positive for CD10 (b) and are negative for BCL2 (C). Flow cytometry reveals both T-cells (CD20⁻) and B-cells (CD20⁺). B-cells show strike predominance of CD10⁺ germinal center cells (d–g; arrow), which display variable ("smeared") expression of surface light chain immunoglobulins with brighter expression of kappa than lambda (compare d and e). CD10⁺ B-cells are BCL2⁻ (f). This pattern is characteristic for florid follicular hyperplasia and should not be confused with B-cell lymphoma of follicle center cell origin. Clonal B-cells from follicular lymphoma would not display "smeared" pattern of surface immunoglobulin (the cluster would be more cohesive) and in the majority of cases would be BCL2⁺. The expression of CD38 by CD10⁺ B-cells is often brighter in follicular hyperplasia (g; arrow) when compared to FL.

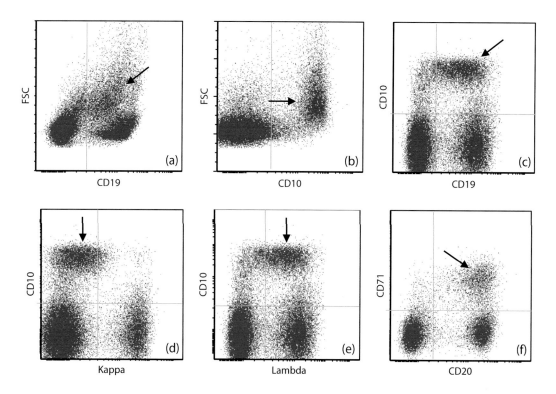

FIGURE 3.18 Follicular lymphoma composed of intermediate in size cells. Clonal B-cells display increased forward scatter (a–b; arrow), dim CD19 (a, c), positive CD10 (b–e), and lambda restriction (d–e). Subset of lymphomatous cells is CD71⁺ (e, arrow).

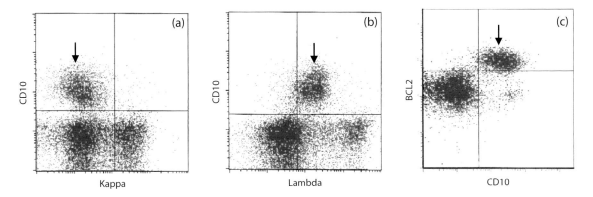

FIGURE 3.19 Follicular lymphoma: clonal B-cell (lambda⁺; a–b, arrow) are positive for BCL2 (c).

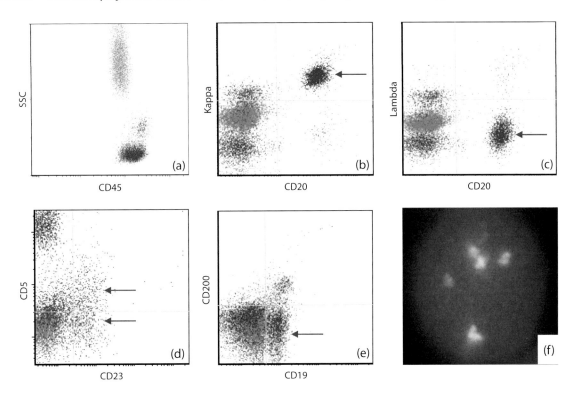

FIGURE 3.20 MBL with t(11;14) or I-NN-MCL. Flow cytometry (a–e) shows bright CD45 expression and low SSC (a), moderate kappa expression (a, compare with lambda, c), bright CD20 (b–c), co-expression of CD5 (partial) with CD23 (d), and negative CD200 (e; benign B-cells are CD200⁺). FISH analysis confirmed IGH/CCND1 rearrangement with one green (IGH), one orange (CCND1), and two yellow fusion signals (f).

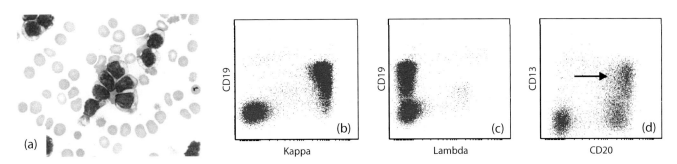

FIGURE 3.21 Aberrant expression of CD13 in MZL. Blood smear (a) shows atypical lymphoid cells. Flow cytometry (b–d) show positive CD19 (b–c), kappa restriction (b, compare with lambda, c), and aberrant albeit partial expression of CD13 (d; arrow; CD13 is positive only on subset of clonal CD20⁺ B-cells).

- CD20
  - lack of CD20 expression by mature B-cell lymphomas (excluding patients treated with Rituxan)
  - dim or very bright CD20 expression (different B-cell lymphomas)
- CD23
  - positive CD23 expression in MCL (CD23 is typically positive in CLL)
  - lack of CD23 expression in CLL/SLL
- CD43
  - positive CD43 expression in MZL, DLBCL, BL, other lymphomas (CD43 is typically positive in CLL and MCL)
- CD45
  - lack of CD45 expression in DLBCL or plasmablastic lymphoma (PBL)
  - positive CD45 in PCM
  - dim CD45 expression by mature B-cell lymphomas or CLL
- CD81
  - strong CD81 expression in MCL and BL, positive CD81 in HCL
- CD200
  - positive CD200 expression in PCM and rare cases of MCL (CD200 is typically positive in CLL)
  - lack of surface light chain immunoglobulins (except PCM)
- T-cell markers (other than CD5), including CD2, CD3, CD7, or CD8
  - positive expression in CLL, primary effusion lymphoma (PEL) or DLBCL (Figure 3.22)
- CD56
  - positive CD56 expression in PCM and in minor subset of DLBCL

- CD117
  - positive CD117 expression in PCM

B-cells versus plasma cells

Plasma cells are identified by FC using CD38 and CD138 antibodies. CD38 is a relatively broadly expressed marker, present in immature CD34+ precursors, including myeloblasts, lymphoblasts, B-cell progenitors (hematogones), monocytes, NK-cells, and in subset of activated B-cells and T-cells. During B-cell maturation, CD38 expression is remarkably high in B-lineage committed precursors and gradually decreases on immature B-lymphocytes in BM to become fully negative in naïve B-cells [32, 33]. Mature activated B-cells start expressing CD38 again, with high levels typically seen on germinal center B-cells and later further maturation to memory cells is associated with down-regulation of CD38 expression, while progression to plasma cells is associated with high level of expression. The intensity of expression of CD38 by plasma cells is much higher than that seen in all other hematopoietic cells and therefore CD38 is considered as one of the most reliable markers for the identification of plasma cells by FC [34]. CD138 is another marker with bright expression on plasma cells. Down-regulation of CD138 expression may be observed on aged sample as well as on samples exposed to heparin [35, 36].

Benign plasma cells have bright expression of CD38 and are most often positive for CD138, CD19, CD27, CD43, and CD81, dimly positive for CD45, and negative for CD20, CD22, surface immunoglobulins, CD56, CD117, CD200, and HLA-DR. Occasionally, subset of benign plasma cells may be CD56+ or CD45−. The expression of CD19 is usually heterogeneous with minor subset of plasma cells being negative (up to 30%). Similarly, small subset of benign plasma cells may be negative for CD45 and CD81, and positive for CD56. The pattern of expression of

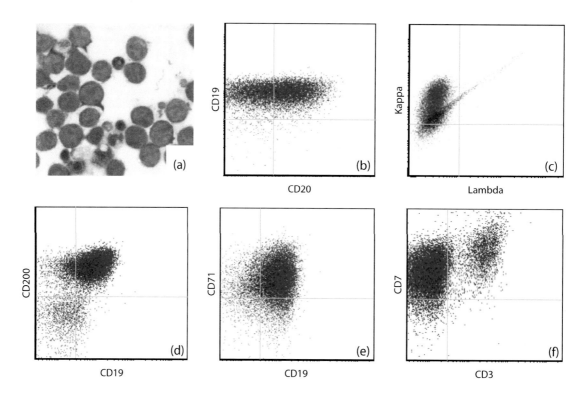

FIGURE 3.22 Testicular DLBCL with aberrant expression of CD7. Touch smear (a) shows atypical large lymphoid cells. Flow cytometry (b–f) shows clonal B-cells (blue dots) with dim CD19 (b), variable CD20 (b), kappa restriction (c), moderate CD200 (d), dim CD71 (e), and aberrant CD7 (f; red dots represent reactive T-cells which are positive for CD3 and CD7).

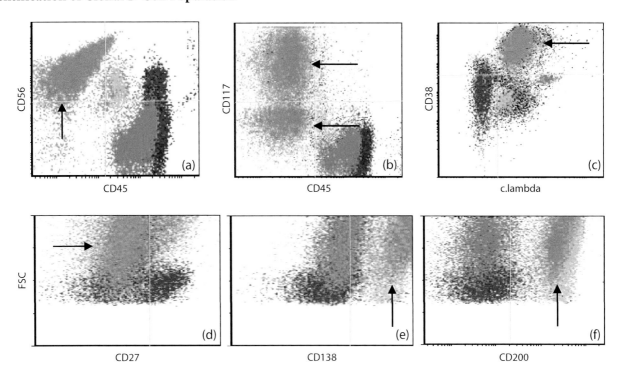

FIGURE 3.23 Plasma cell myeloma: typical phenotype of neoplastic plasma cells (orange dots, arrow) with lack of CD45 (a–b), positive CD56 (a) and CD117 (b, partial), bright expression of CD38 (c), cytoplasmic light chain restriction (c), negative CD27 (d), bright CD138 (e), and positive CD200 (f).

CD19, CD45, CD56, and CD81 reflects different stages of plasma cell maturation, with major subpopulation being CD19⁺, CD45⁺, CD81⁺, and CD56⁻ gradually progressing to minor CD19-/CD56⁻, and CD19⁻/CD56⁺ subpopulations [35, 37–40]. Expression of cytoplasmic immunoglobulins is polyclonal.

The clonal plasma cell component of B-cell lymphomas with plasmacytic differentiation (LPL/WM, subset of MZL, less often other B-cell lymphomas) has low to slightly increased FSC and often displays positive expression of CD19 and CD45 [41–43]. Plasma cell myelomas (PCMs) are usually negative for CD19, CD20, and CD45, show high or variable FSC, are brightly positive for CD38 and CD138, and often positive for CD56, CD200, and/or CD117 (Figure 3.23). When compared to benign plasma cells, plasma cell neoplasms show slightly dimmer expression of CD38 and slightly brighter expression of CD138. Rare cases of plasma cell neoplasms may show dim or even negative CD138. In most typical cases, distinction between B-cell lymphomas and plasma cell neoplasms is straightforward. Occasional cases of plasma cell neoplasms may show unusual phenotype with bright CD45, positive CD20, negative CD56 and CD117, or positive CD10, CD23, and HLA-DR, creating difficulties in differentiating them from B-cell lymphomas, especially those of high grade. Relatively bright expression of CD38 may be seen in DLBCL, anaplastic large cell lymphoma (ALCL), and other high-grade lymphoid neoplasms (BL, HGBL-R). Poorly differentiated PCM may be exceedingly difficult to differentiate morphologically and immunophenotypically from high grade B-cell lymphomas (e.g., PLB) or immature tumors (e.g., TdT⁺ high grade B-cell neoplasm). Table 3.1 compares the immunophenotypic profile of plasma cells and mature B-cells. Figure 3.24 shows PCM with aberrant phenotype including unusual expression of CD19 and HLA-DR and Figure 3.25 shows FL with unusual lack of CD45 mimicking malignant plasma cells.

TABLE 3.1: Comparison of Immunophenotypic Profile of B-Cells with Plasma Cells

	B-Cell Lymphomas	PCM
CD5	+/–	–
CD10	+/–	–/(+)
CD11c	+/–	–
CD13 or CD33	–	–/(+)
CD19	+	–/(+)
CD20	+bright a	–/(+)
CD22	+	–
CD23	+/–	–/(+)
CD38	+/–	+bright
CD43	–/+	+
CD45	+bright/(–)	–/(+)
CD56	–	+/(–)
CD79a	+	+/–
CD81	+/–	+/–
CD117	–	+/–
CD138	–	+bright
CD200	+/–b	+/(–)
Cyclin D1 (BCL1)	– (+ in MCL)	–/+
BCL6	–/+	–
HLA-DR	+	–/(+)
MUM1	–/+	+
PAX5	+	–/+
Surface κ or λ	+	–/(+)
Cytoplasmic κ or λ	–	+

Abbreviations: +, positive; (+), rarely positive; –, negative; (–), rarely negative.
ª CD20 maybe dim or negative (e.g., in CLL).
ᵇ CD200 is usually negative in MCL, FL, DLBCL.

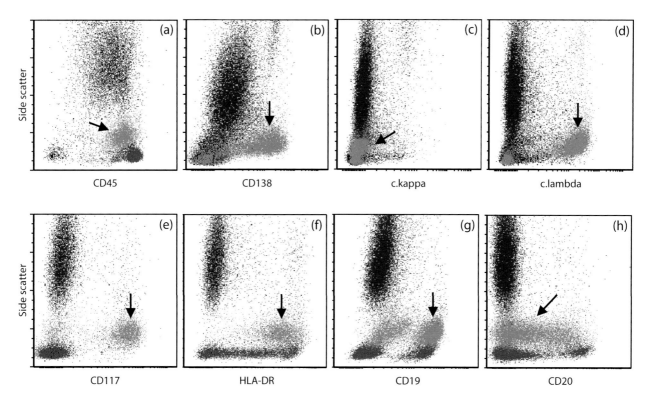

FIGURE 3.24 Plasma cell myeloma with aberrant expression of CD45 (a; orange dots, arrow), bright CD138 (b), monoclonal cytoplasmic lambda (c–d), aberrant CD117 (e), aberrant HLA-DR (f), aberrant CD19 (g), and partial CD20 expression (h).

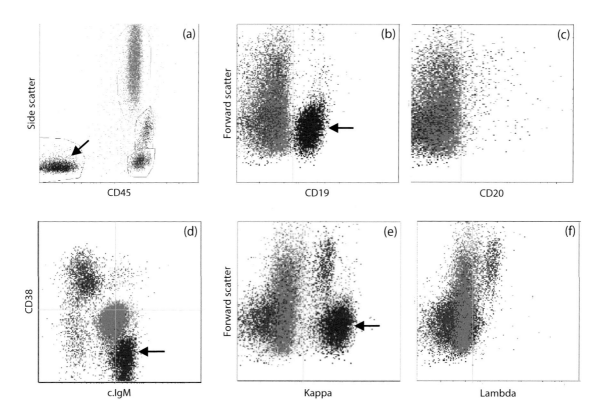

FIGURE 3.25 Follicular lymphoma with aberrant phenotype mimicking plasma cells. Patient had history of FL after treatment. Flow cytometry shows clonal B-cells with negative CD45 (a; arrow), positive CD19 (b), negative CD20 (c), negative CD38 (d), positive c.IgM (d), positive (surface) kappa (e), and negative (surface) lambda (f). Lack of CD20 (c) is associated with prior Rituxan treatment. Monocytes (e–f; blue dots) show non-specific staining with kappa and lambda. FISH studies confirmed t(14;18)/*BCL2-IGH* rearrangement (not shown).

Because of the bright expression of CD38 and/or CD138 by plasma cells, expression of the markers analyzed simultaneously in the same tube must be carefully evaluated after proper compensation for the potential "false-positive" expression due to fluorochrome spectral overlap.

Mature versus immature B-cells

B-cell population with lack of CD20 expression, bright CD10, lack of surface light chain immunoglobulins, and negative or dim CD45 raises the possibility of B-cell acute lymphoblastic leukemia/lymphoma (B-ALL/LBL) and requires additional testing for TdT and CD34. Table 3.2 compares the immunophenotypic features of mature and immature B-cell neoplasms. B-lymphoblasts are typically positive for TdT and/or CD34, positive for CD19, CD22, CD79a, and negative for CD20, show bright CD10 expression (subset of cases may be CD10−), show dim or negative CD45, positive CD43, and may be positive for myeloid markers (CD13 and/or CD33). Among mature B-cell proliferations only sporadic cases of CLL (and less often other B-cell lymphomas) may display positive CD13 (or CD33) expression. CD11c is often positive in mature B-cell lymphoproliferations (dim or partial in CLL, dim to moderate in MZL and bright in HCL), whereas majority of B-ALL are CD11c−. Hematogones, like B-ALL, are surface light chain immunoglobulin-negative (Figure 3.26) and are characterized by very low side scatter (SSC) and variable but mostly low FSC, variable expression of CD45 (from dim to moderate), partial positivity for CD34 and TdT, bright CD38, dim to moderate CD10, variable (heterogeneous) CD20 (with majority of cells negative and subset dimly positive with "smeary" expression) and lack of CD13/CD33 expression. Figure 3.27 shows typical FC pattern of B-ALL and Figure 3.28 shows typical FC pattern of hematogones.

TABLE 3.2: Comparison of Mature versus Immature B-Cell Neoplasms

	Mature B-Cell Lymphomas	B-ALL/LBL
CD5	−/+	−
CD10	−/+	+bright/(−)
CD11c	−/+	−
CD13	−	−/+
CD19	+ (dim in FL)	+
CD20	+	−/(+)
CD22	+	+
CD23	−/+	−
CD33	−	+/−
CD34	−	+/(−)
CD43	−/+	+
CD45	+bright	+/− (may be partial+)
CD56	−/(+)	−/(+)
CD79a	+	+
BCL6	−/+	−
HLA-DR	+	+
Surface κ/λ	+/(−)	−/(+)
TdT	−	+/(−)

Abbreviations: +, positive; (+), rarely positive; −, negative; (−), rarely negative.

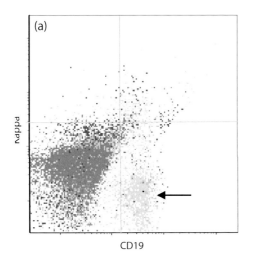
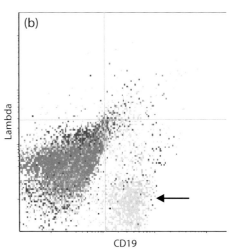

FIGURE 3.26 Hematogones (light blue dots; arrow) are negative for light chain surface immunoglobulins (a–b).

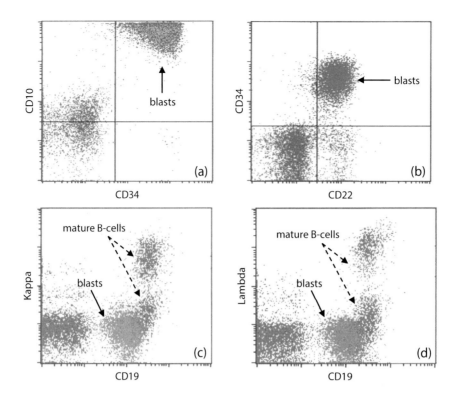

FIGURE 3.27 B-lymphoblasts (green dots; arrow) show bright CD10 (a), positive CD34 (a–b), and positive CD19 and CD22 (b–d). They are negative for surface light chain immunoglobulins (c–d). Note slightly dimmer expression of CD19 by lymphoblasts (c–d; solid arrow) when compared to residual (polytypic) benign B-cells (c–d; dashed arrows).

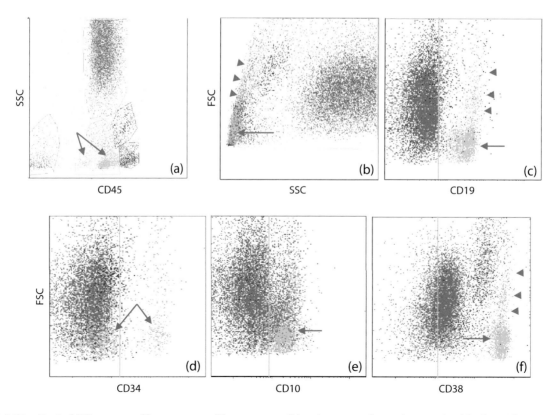

FIGURE 3.28 Typical FC pattern of hematogones. Hematogones (blue dots; arrow) are characterized by low side scatter (SSC; a), variable CD45 expression, often with distinct two populations (a), low forward scatter (FSC) on majority of cells (b–f) with only minor population of hematogones showing variably increased FSC (arrowheads), moderate CD19 (c), partial CD34 (d), moderate (not bright) CD10 (e), and bright CD38 (f).

References

1. Piatosa, B., et al., *B cell subsets in healthy children: reference values for evaluation of B cell maturation process in peripheral blood.* Cytometry B Clin Cytom, 2010. **78**(6): p. 372–81.

2. Gordon, D.S., et al., *Persistent polyclonal lymphocytosis of B lymphocytes.* N Engl J Med, 1982. **307**(4): p. 232–6.

3. Marcondes, N.A., et al., *Polyclonal B-cell lymphocytosis: report of three cases.* Cytometry B Clin Cytom, 2018. **94**(6): p. 953–5.

4. Salcedo, I., et al., *Persistent polyclonal B lymphocytosis: an expansion of cells showing IgVH gene mutations and phenotypic features of normal lymphocytes from the CD27+ marginal zone B-cell compartment.* Br J Haematol, 2002. **116**(3): p. 662–6.

5. Diss, T.C., et al., *B-cell monoclonality, Epstein Barr virus, and t(14;18) in myoepithelial sialadenitis and low-grade B-cell MALT lymphoma of the parotid gland.* Am J Surg Pathol, 1995. **19**(5): p. 531–6.

6. Quintana, P.G., et al., *Salivary gland lymphoid infiltrates associated with lymphoepithelial lesions: a clinicopathologic, immunophenotypic, and genotypic study.* Hum Pathol, 1997. **28**(7): p. 850–61.

7. Bahler, D.W. and S.H. Swerdlow, *Clonal salivary gland infiltrates associated with myoepithelial sialadenitis (Sjogren's syndrome) begin as nonmalignant antigen-selected expansions.* Blood, 1998. **91**(6): p. 1864–72.

8. Schulman, H., et al., *Gastric "pseudolymphoma" with restricted light chain expression in a patient with obscure gastrointestinal blood loss.* Dig Dis Sci, 1991. **36**(10): p. 1495–9.

9. Saxena, A., et al., *Distinct B-cell clonal bands in Helicobacter pylori gastritis with lymphoid hyperplasia.* J Pathol, 2000. **190**(1): p. 47–54.

10. Jakobiec, F.A., A. Neri, and D.M. Knowles, 2nd, *Genotypic monoclonality in immunophenotypically polyclonal orbital lymphoid tumors. A model of tumor progression in the lymphoid system. The 1986 Wendell Hughes lecture.* Ophthalmology, 1987. **94**(8): p. 980–94.

11. Attygalle, A.D., et al., *Atypical marginal zone hyperplasia of mucosa associated lymphoid tissue: a reactive condition of childhood showing immunoglobulin lambda light chain restriction.* Blood, 2004. **104**: p. 3343–8.

12. Du, M.Q., et al., *Kaposi sarcoma-associated herpes virus infects monotypic (IgM lambda) but polyclonal naive B cells in Castleman disease and associated lymphoproliferative disorders.* Blood, 2001. **97**(7): p. 2130–6.

13. Dupin, N., et al., *HHV-8 is associated with a plasmablastic variant of Castleman disease that is linked to HHV-8-positive plasmablastic lymphoma.* Blood, 2000. **95**(4): p. 1406–12.

14. Kussick, S.J., et al., *A distinctive nuclear morphology in acute myeloid leukemia is strongly associated with loss of HLA-DR expression and FLT3 internal tandem duplication.* Leukemia, 2004. **18**(10): p. 1591–8.

15. Shanafelt, T.D., et al., *B-cell count and survival: differentiating chronic lymphocytic leukemia from monoclonal B-cell lymphocytosis based on clinical outcome.* Blood, 2009. **113**(18): p. 4188–96.

16. Marti, G.E., et al., *B-cell monoclonal lymphocytosis and B-cell abnormalities in the setting of familial B-cell chronic lymphocytic leukemia.* Cytometry B Clin Cytom, 2003. **52**(1): p. 1–12.

17. Goldin, L.R., et al., *Common occurrence of monoclonal B-cell lymphocytosis among members of high-risk CLL families.* Br J Haematol, 2010. **151**(2): p. 152–8.

18. Fazi, C., et al., *General population low-count CLL-like MBL persists over time without clinical progression, although carrying the same cytogenetic abnormalities of CLL.* Blood, 2011. **118**(25): p. 6618–25.

19. Nieto, W.G., et al., *Increased frequency (12%) of circulating chronic lymphocytic leukemia-like B-cell clones in healthy subjects using a highly sensitive multicolor flow cytometry approach.* Blood, 2009. **114**(1): p. 33–7.

20. de Tute, R., et al., *Monoclonal B-cell lymphocytosis (MBL) in CLL families: substantial increase in relative risk for young adults.* Leukemia, 2006. **20**(4): p. 728–9.

21. Rawstron, A.C., et al., *Monoclonal B-cell lymphocytosis and chronic lymphocytic leukemia.* N Engl J Med, 2008. **359**(6): p. 575–83.

22. Xochelli, A., et al., *Clonal B-cell lymphocytosis exhibiting immunophenotypic features consistent with a marginal-zone origin: is this a distinct entity?* Blood, 2014. **123**(8): p. 1199–206.

23. Rawstron, A., P. Hillmen, and R. Houlston, *Clonal lymphocytes in persons without known chronic lymphocytic leukemia (CLL): implications of recent findings in family members of CLL patients.* Semin Hematol, 2004. **41**(3): p. 192–200.

24. Rawstron, A.C., et al., *Inherited predisposition to CLL is detectable as subclinical monoclonal B-lymphocyte expansion.* Blood, 2002. **100**(7): p. 2289–90.

25. Rawstron, A.C., et al., *Monoclonal B lymphocytes with the characteristics of "indolent" chronic lymphocytic leukemia are present in 3.5% of adults with normal blood counts.* Blood, 2002. **100**(2): p. 635–9.

26. Shanafelt, T.D., et al., *Brief report: natural history of individuals with clinically recognized monoclonal B-cell lymphocytosis compared with patients with Rai 0 chronic lymphocytic leukemia.* J Clin Oncol, 2009. **27**(24): p. 3959–63.

27. Shanafelt, T. and C.A. Hanson, *Monoclonal B-cell lymphocytosis: definitions and natural history.* Leuk Lymphoma, 2009. **50**(3): p. 493–7.

28. Fabris, S., et al., *Chromosome 2p gain in monoclonal B-cell lymphocytosis and in early stage chronic lymphocytic leukemia.* Am J Hematol, 2013. **88**(1): p. 24–31.

29. Swerdlow, S.H., Campo, E., Harris, N. L., Jaffe, E. S., Pileri, S. A., Stein, H., Stein, H., Thiele, J., Arber, D.A., Le Beau M.M., Orazi, A., Siebert, R., ed. *WHO classification of tumors of haematopoietic and lymphoid tissues.* 2016, IARC: Lyon.

30. Kalpadakis, C., et al., *Detection of L265P MYD-88 mutation in a series of clonal B-cell lymphocytosis of marginal zone origin (CBL-MZ).* Hematol Oncol, 2017. **35**(4): p. 542–7.

31. Defrancesco, I., et al., *Targeted next-generation sequencing reveals molecular heterogeneity in non-chronic lymphocytic leukemia clonal B-cell lymphocytosis.* Hematol Oncol, 2020. **38**(5): p. 689–97.

32. Quijano, S., et al., *Association between the proliferative rate of neoplastic B cells, their maturation stage, and underlying cytogenetic abnormalities in B-cell chronic lymphoproliferative disorders: analysis of a series of 432 patients.* Blood, 2008. **111**(10): p. 5130–41.

33. Perez-Andres, M., et al., *Human peripheral blood B-cell compartments: a crossroad in B-cell traffic.* Cytometry B Clin Cytom, 2010. **78 Suppl 1**: p. S47–S60.

34. Orfao, A., et al., *A new method for the analysis of plasma cell DNA content in multiple myeloma samples using a CD38/propidium iodide double staining technique.* Cytometry, 1994. **17**(4): p. 332–9.

35. Flores-Montero, J., et al., *Immunophenotype of normal vs. myeloma plasma cells: toward antibody panel specifications for MRD detection in multiple myeloma.* Cytometry B Clin Cytom, 2016. **90**(1): p. 61–72.

36. Jourdan, M., et al., *The myeloma cell antigen syndecan-1 is lost by apoptotic myeloma cells.* Br J Haematol, 1998. **100**(4): p. 637–46.

37. Robillard, N., et al., *Immunophenotype of normal and myelomatous plasma-cell subsets.* Front Immunol, 2014. **5**: p. 137.

38. Cannizzo, E., et al., *Multiparameter immunophenotyping by flow cytometry in multiple myeloma: the diagnostic utility of defining ranges of normal antigenic expression in comparison to histology.* Cytometry B Clin Cytom, 2010. **78**(4): p. 231–8.

39. Paiva, B., et al., *Clinical significance of CD81 expression by clonal plasma cells in high-risk smoldering and symptomatic multiple myeloma patients.* Leukemia, 2012. **26**(8): p. 1862–9.

40. Pojero, F., et al., *Old and new immunophenotypic markers in multiple myeloma for discrimination of responding and relapsing patients: the importance of "normal" residual plasma cell analysis.* Cytometry B Clin Cytom, 2015. **88**(3): p. 165–82.

41. Paiva, B., et al., *Multiparameter flow cytometry for the identification of the Waldenstrom's clone in IgM-MGUS and Waldenstrom's Macroglobulinemia: new criteria for differential diagnosis and risk stratification.* Leukemia, 2014. **28**(1): p. 166–73.

42. Morice, W.G., et al., *Novel immunophenotypic features of marrow lymphoplasmacytic lymphoma and correlation with Waldenstrom's macroglobulinemia.* Mod Pathol, 2009. **22**(6): p. 807–16.

43. Horna, P., et al., *Flow cytometric analysis of surface light chain expression patterns in B-cell lymphomas using monoclonal and polyclonal antibodies.* Am J Clin Pathol, 2011. **136**(6): p. 954–9.

4

IDENTIFICATION OF ABNORMAL T-CELL POPULATION

Introduction

Identification of abnormal T-cell population by flow cytometry (FC) is less straightforward than identification of clonal B-cells and requires the use of a broad panel of immunophenotypic markers and experience [1–11]. Additionally, final diagnosis and subclassification of T-cell lymphoproliferative disorders relies on multi-technology approach, which in addition to immunophenotyping by FC includes morphology, molecular testing for T-cell clonality (polymerase chain reaction [PCR]), cytogenetic/FISH studies [e.g., isochromosome 7; t(14;14)/inv(14), etc.], viral studies (e.g., HTLV-1), and detailed clinical and laboratory data.

Phenotype of benign T-cells
Benign T-cells are positive for T-cell markers (CD2, CD3, CD5, and CD7), CD4 or CD8, CD26, CD38, CD43, CD45, CD52, CD81, TCRαβ, and are negative for HLA-DR.

Blood and bone marrow
In normal blood samples (Table 4.1), the percentage of T-cells range from 2.5% to 45% (average 20.4%) with an average CD4:CD8 ratio of 2.3:1 (range 0.5:1 to 6.8:1). T-large granular lymphocytes (T-LGL cells) expressing CD2, CD3, CD5, CD7, CD8, and CD57 comprise between 0.1% and 14% of blood elements (average ~5%). Natural killer cells (NK-cells) which are positive for CD2, CD7, CD56, and often CD16 and negative for surface CD3 and CD5 comprise between 0.2% and 10% (average 3%). Dual CD4/CD8+ T-cells in blood comprise 0.2%–1% of total events. No significant population of CD10+ T-cells can be identified in blood samples. In normal bone marrow (BM) T-cells show similar FC features, with the main difference being smaller number of T-cells and lower CD4:CD8 ratio when compared to blood. Samples from patients recovering after chemotherapy for B-cell lymphomas/CLL or acute leukemia often show reversed CD4:CD8 ratio and increased number of NK-cells and/or T-LGL cells.

Reactive lymph nodes
In reactive lymph nodes (Table 4.2), T-cells comprise between 27% and 79% (average 54%). They do not display overtly aberrant phenotype, but subset of cells may show dimmer CD5 and/or CD7 expression. The CD4:CD8 ratio ranges from 2.1:1 to 8:1 (average 3.7:1). Lymph nodes from Hodgkin lymphoma cases show usually increased CD4:CD8 ratio (range 3.9:1 to 28:1; average 11.2:1), but there is no aberrant expression of pan-T-cell antigens. In benign samples the number of T-cells co-expressing CD4 and CD8 ranges from 0% to 1.5% (average 0.43%; SD 0.49), and dual CD4−/CD8− T-cells from 0% to 8% (average 0.9; SD 0.49) [3]. Peripheral blood from patients with confirmed infectious mononucleosis shows T-cells with expression of HLA-DR (42%–67%; average 51%), inverted CD4:CD8 ratio (0.12–0.6; average 0.33) and down-regulation of CD7 (dim expression) [3].

Activated T-cells in blood in viral infections
Activated T-cells in certain viral infections (human immunodeficiency virus, HIV; or Epstein-Barr virus, EBV) are characterized by decreased number of B-cells, increased percentages of total T-cells, cytotoxic-suppressor CD8+ T cells, CD4+/CD8+ T-cells,

activated HLA-DR+ T cells and T-follicular helper cells (CXCR5+/PD-1+/CD4+) compared to healthy controls. The CD4:CD8 ratio is often reversed and apart from aberrant expression of HLA-DR, T-cells show bright expression of CD38, increased forward scatter, down-regulation of CD5 expression and often diminished or completely absent expression of CD7 [12–14].

Aberrant T-cell phenotype by flow cytometry

Criteria used in identification of abnormal T-cell population by FC

- Loss or aberrant (dim, variable, partial) expression of the T-cell antigens (CD2, CD3, CD5, and/or CD7)
- Aberrant expression of CD4 or CD8 (subset restriction, dual-positive CD4/CD8 expression, or lack of both markers); aberrant (dim) expression of CD4 or CD8
- Loss or aberrant (dim, variable, partial) expression of CD45
- Increased forward light scatter (FSC)
- Aberrant expression of T-cell receptor (TCR), e.g., dim expression of TCRαβ, positive TCRγδ and lack of both TCRs
- Presence of blastic markers (TdT, CD34, CD1a, and/or CD117)
- Positive HLA-DR expression
- Expression of NK-cell associated markers (CD16, CD56, and/or CD57)
- Positive CD30
- Positive CD10
- Positive B-cell markers (CD19, CD20)
- Positive pan-myeloid markers (CD13, CD15, CD33)
- Positive CD103
- Loss of CD26
- Negative, very dim, or very bright CD38 expression
- Positive (strong) expression of CD25
- Presence of additional markers, such as CD11b, CD11c, or CD71

Increased forward scatter (FSC)
Normal T-cells have low FSC comparable to that of benign B-cells. Increased FSC may be observed in subset of T-cell lymphoproliferations characterized by predominance of intermediate to large lymphocytes. For example, many cases of T-cell prolymphocytic leukemia (T-PLL) are composed of medium-sized lymphocytes which are reflected by increased FSC (Figure 4.1). Anaplastic large cell lymphomas (ALCL) and subset of peripheral T-cell lymphomas (PTCL, NOS) display increased FSC reflecting large size of neoplastic cells (Figure 4.2). Majority of cases of T lymphoblastic leukemia/lymphoma (T-ALL) have cells of intermediate size with mildly increased FSC (Figure 4.3). Nodal TFH cell lymphoma, angioimmunoblastic-type (AITL) often shows admixture of benign (small) T-cells and neoplastic T-cells with variable FSC with subset of cells showing moderate to high FSC.

Complete loss or aberrant expression of T-cell antigen(s)
Loss of CD2, CD3, CD5, and/or CD7 or their aberrant expression (i.e., dim, partial, or variable expression) is present in majority of T-cell neoplasms (Table 4.3). Complete loss of the expression of at

DOI: 10.1201/9781003197935-4

TABLE 4.1: T-Cell Phenotype of Normal Blood Sample (n = 100 Cases)

	Average	Range	SD[c]
T-cells[a]	20.4%	2.5%–45%	10.8
CD4:CD8 ratio	2.3:1	0.5:1–6.8:1	1.3
CD4+/CD8+ T-cells[a]	0.19%	0%–2.3%	0.3
CD7– T-cells[b]	2.1%	1%–40%	1.9
NK-cells (CD3–/CD56+)[a]	3.5%	0.2%–10.3%	2.5
T-LGL cells (CD3+/CD57+)[a]	2.4%	0.1%–16%	2.7

[a] As percent of all events.
[b] As percent of all CD3+ T-cells.
[c] Standard deviation.

TABLE 4.2: T-Cell Phenotype in Reactive Lymph Nodes

	Average	Range	SD[c]
T-cells[a]	55.7%	22%–90%	14.7
CD4:CD8 ratio	3.9	0.2–14.5	3.4
CD4+/CD8+ T-cells[a]	0.4%	0%–2.6%	0.7
CD7– T-cells[b]	10.3%	1%–19%	5.3
B-cells[a]	32.6%	8%–74%	16.6
CD5+ B-cells[a]	0.8%	0.1%–2%	0.6

[a] As percent of all events.
[b] As percent of all CD3+ T-cells.
[c] Standard deviation.

least one T-cell antigens is seen in ~65% of cases (statistic based on phenotype of 567 tumors including 120 T-ALL and 457 mature T-cell disorders in author's series). T-cell neoplasms usually display loss of one T-cell marker (~41%), followed by loss of two antigens (~19%) and three antigens (6%), whereas complete loss of all four antigens is seen only in sporadic cases (1%), most often in null cell type of ALCL (Figure 4.4) and occasional T-ALL cases (Figure 4.3). T-ALL/LBLs more often show lack of at least one antigen when compared with mature (peripheral) tumors (~79% versus ~65%). Among mature (peripheral) T-cell neoplasms, lack of the expression of at least one T-cell antigen is observed most often in adult T-cell lymphoma/leukemia (ATLL; 100%) and NK-cell large granular lymphocyte leukemia (NK-LGLL; 100%), followed by ALCL (~91%), enteropathy-associated T-cell lymphoma/monomorphic epitheliotropic intestinal T-cell lymphoma (EATL/MEITL; ~86%), hepatosplenic T-cell lymphoma (HSTL; 83%), PTCL, not otherwise specified (PTCL; ~77%), AITL (~72%), and mycosis fungoides/Sézary's syndrome (MF/SS; ~71%). Aberrant loss of T-cell antigen(s) is seen least often in T-PLL (~27%) and T-LGL leukemia (T-LGLL; ~47%).

Among all T-cell neoplasms, CD2, CD3, CD5, and CD7 are negative in ~14%, ~37%, ~22%, and 32%, respectively. Mature (peripheral) tumors show most often loss of CD7 (~40%), followed by CD3 (~26%), CD5 (~25%), and CD2 (~9%), whereas T-ALL/LBL most often show loss of surface CD3 (~75%) followed by loss of 2 (~28%) and CD5 (~12%). In contrast to mature neoplasms, majority of T-ALL/LBL are strongly CD7+ (~98%) and only minor fraction of tumors is CD7– (~2%). LGL leukemia with NK-cell phenotype and NK-cell neoplasms are typically CD2+, surface CD3–, CD5–, and CD7+, whereas T-LGL leukemias (T-LGLL) are usually positive for surface CD3, show lack

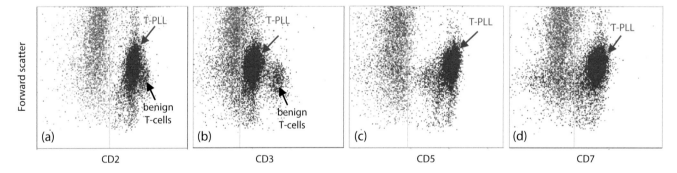

FIGURE 4.1 T-PLL (peripheral blood). Neoplastic T-cells (red arrow) show slightly increased forward scatter (FSC; a–d) when compared to residual benign T-cells (black arrow). In addition, T-PLL cells show slightly dimmer CD2 (a), dim CD3 (b), and moderate (normal) CD5 (c) and CD7 (d) expression.

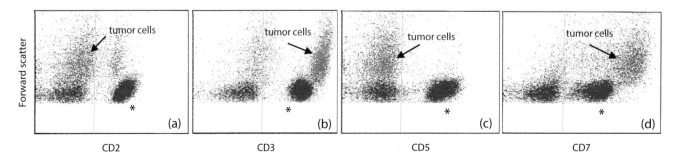

FIGURE 4.2 Identification of abnormal T-cells: aberrant expression of pan T-cell antigens and increased forward scatter. Benign (reactive) T-cells (a–d; red dots; *) have low FSC and display normal expression of CD2, CD3, CD5, and CD7. Neoplastic T-cells (a–d; blue dots; arrow) in addition to increased FSC (a–d) show aberrant loss of CD2 (a) and CD5 (c), and brighter expression of CD3 (b) and CD7 (d).

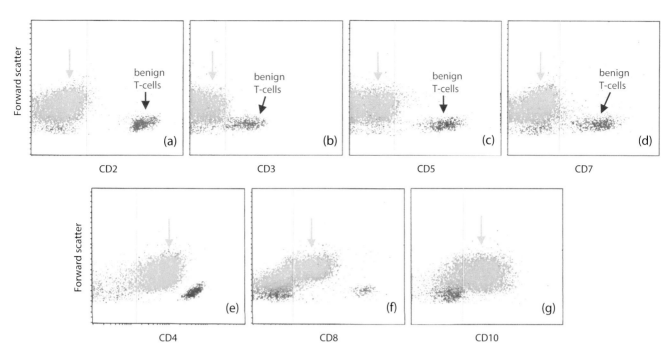

FIGURE 4.3 Identification of abnormal T-cells: mild increase in forward scatter and aberrant expression of pan T-cell antigens. T-ALL cells (a–g; green dots) show increased forward scatter (compare to residual small T-cells; red dots), negative expression of all T-cell antigens (CD2, CD3, CD5, and CD7; a–d; green arrow), dual CD4/CD8 positivity (e–f), and positive expression of CD10 (g). Rare residual, benign small T-cells (a–g; red dots) show normal phenotype and low forward scatter.

or dim expression of CD5 and/or CD7. T-PLL, AITL, and PTCL often show lack of CD7 and may be surface CD3⁻. ATLL, ALCL, MF/SS, and AITL often show lack CD7 expression (100%, ~73%, ~62%, and 52%, respectively). HSTL, EATL, and MEITL are usually CD5⁻.

Positive expression of all T antigens (CD2, CD3, CD5, and CD7) does not exclude T-cell neoplasm (Figures 4.5–4.7).

Positive expression of all four antigens (including expression on subset and dim/variable expression) can be identified in ~32% of cases (~35% in mature and ~22% in precursor T-cell neoplasms; Table 4.3). Lack of aberrant expression of T-cell markers (i.e., all markers have moderate to bright expression) is noted in ~13% of all tumors (~13% in mature and 8% in T-ALL), including ~8%

TABLE 4.3: Expression of T-Cell Antigens (CD2, CD3, CD5, and CD7) in T-Cell Neoplasms

Category	All Four Antigens Positive (%)				At Least One Antigen Negative (%)				
	All⁺	All Normal[a]	1 Aberrant[b]	>1 Aberrant[b]	≥1⁻	One⁻	Two⁻	Three⁻	Four⁻
All tumors[c]	32	(13)	(10)	(9)	67	(41)	(19)	(6)	(1)
T-ALL	**22**	**(8)**	**(9)**	**(5)**	**79**	**(52)**	**(20)**	**(7)**	**(1)**
Mature	**35**	**(13)**	**(10)**	**(12)**	**65**	**(38)**	**(20)**	**(6)**	**(1)**
PTCL	**23**	(8)	(8)	(7)	**77**	(48)	(23)	(6)	–
T-PLL	**73**	(52)	(11)	(10)	**27**	(23)	(4)	–	–
ALCL	**9**	(9)	–	–	**91**	(17)	(25)	(31)	(18)
ATLL	**0**	–	–	–	**100**	(76)	(18)	(6)	–
AITL	**28**	(12)	(5)	(11)	**72**	(54)	(13)	(5)	–
HSTL	**17**	–	(8.5)	(8.5)	**83**	(54)	(29)	–	–
T-LGLL	**53**	(~1)	(12)	(40)	**47**	(39)	(7)	(1)	–
NK-LGLL	**0**	–	–	–	**100**	–	(96)	(4)	–
EATL/MEITL	**14**	–	(14)	–	**86**	(58)	–	(14)	(14)
MF/SS	**31**	(12)	(11)	(8)	**71**	(52)	(15)	(4)	–

Abbreviations: T-ALL/LBL, T-cell acute lymphoblastic leukemia/lymphoma; T-PLL, T-cell prolymphocytic leukemia; PTCL, peripheral T-cell lymphoma; ALCL, anaplastic large cell lymphoma; AITL, nodal TFH cell lymphoma, angioimmunoblastic-type; ATLL, adult T-cell lymphoma/leukemia; MF/SS, mycosis fungoides/Sézary's syndrome; T-LGLL, T-cell large granular lymphocytes leukemia; NK-LGLL, NK-cell large granular lymphocyte leukemia; HSTL, hepatosplenic T-cell lymphoma; EATL, enteropathy-associated T-cell lymphoma; MEITL, monomorphic epitheliotropic intestinal T-cell lymphoma.

[a] Moderate or bright expression.

[b] Positive but either dim, partial, or variable expression.

[c] *n* = 567 cases (mature T-cell neoplasms, 447 cases; T-ALL, 120 cases).

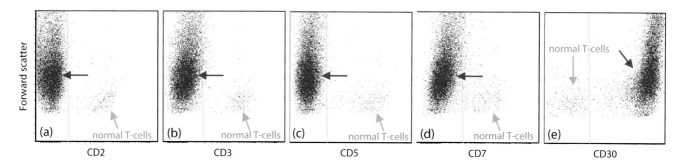

FIGURE 4.4 Identification of abnormal T-cells: aberrant expression of T-cell antigens. Tumor cells from ALCL ("null" cell type; a–d; red arrow) are negative for CD2 (a), CD3 (b), CD5 (c), and CD7 (d), have high forward scatter (a–d) and display bright expression of CD30 (e).

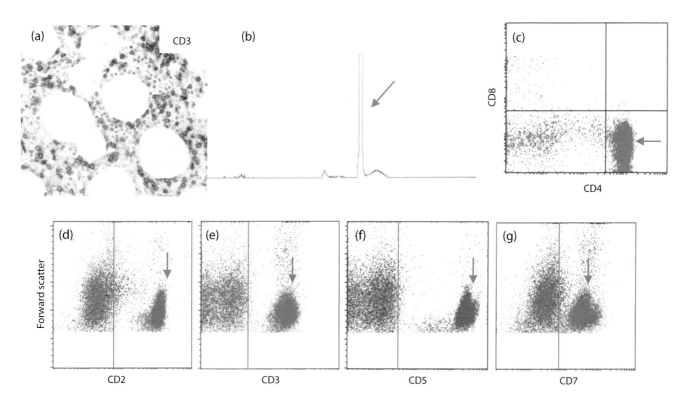

FIGURE 4.5 Identification of abnormal T-cells: positive expression of all pan T-cell antigens and CD4 restriction. T-PLL shows interstitial BM involvement (a, bone marrow staining for CD3) and clonal rearrangement of *TCR* gene (b). Flow cytometry immuno-phenotyping (c–g) shows normal expression of all pan-T antigens (d–g) and CD4 restriction (c).

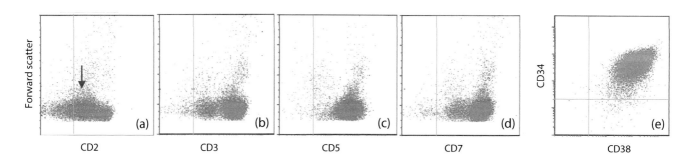

FIGURE 4.6 Identification of abnormal T-cells: positive expression of pan-T-cell antigens in T-ALL. The leukemic cells from T-ALL show positive expression of all pan T-cell antigens (a–d) with slightly dimmer CD2 (a; arrow). Positive surface CD3 (b) is rarely seen in T-ALL, as most of the T-leukemias are surface CD3 negative. CD5 shows moderate expression (c) and CD7 is brightly expression (d). Strong expression of both CD34 and CD38 (e) confirms the diagnosis of T-ALL.

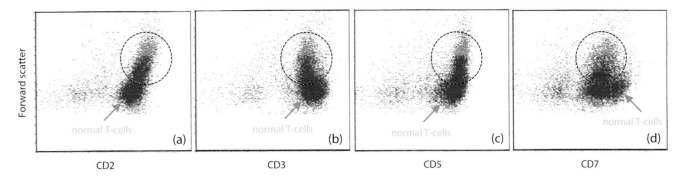

FIGURE 4.7 Identification of atypical T-cell population: positive expression of all pan-T-cell markers in nodal TFH cell lymphoma, angioimmunoblastic-type (AITL). Tumor cells from AITL (a–d; doted circle) show increased forward scatter and minimally brighter expression of CD2 (a) and CD5 (c), as well as minimally dimmer expression of CD3 (b) and CD7 (d), when compared to normal T-cells (arrow).

of PTCLs, ~1% of T-LGLL, ~9% of ALCL, ~12% of AITL, 12% of MF/SS, and ~52% of T-PLL. Figure 4.7 shows an example of AITL with positive expression of T-cell markers. Atypical T-cells in this case can be identified by increased FSC, slightly brighter CD2 and CD5 expression, and slightly dimmer CD3 and CD7 expression when compared to residual (normal) T-cells.

Aberrant T-cell phenotype is not specific for T-cell neoplasms. Various reactive processes may lead to activation and expansion of different T-cell subpopulations with or without subtle phenotypic changes. Diminished, partial or negative expression of one or even two T-cell markers and/or increased FSC may be observed in reactive processes, including in viral infections (especially mononucleosis), treatment-associated changes, or in the sample involved by non-T-cell disorders. Memory T-cells show often decreased expression of CD7, NK-cells are CD3 and CD5 negative, T-LGL cells are CD8+ and may show dimmer CD5. Lymph nodes involved by Hodgkin lymphoma usually show increased

CD4:CD8 ratio, increased number of CD4+/CD8+ T-cells and/or increased proportion of CD57+ T-cells. Occasional cases may show T-cells with aberrant phenotype requiring careful correlation of morphology with extensive immunophenotypic panel and molecular testing for T-cell clonality to differentiate between atypical yet reactive changes and PTCL with Reed-Sternberg-like cells. In normal and reactive conditions, the antigen most commonly showing aberrant expression is CD7, followed by CD5. In normal blood or BM samples, CD5 expression may be dim on a subset of benign T cells giving raise to two subtle T-cell populations, one with normal (moderate) CD5 and one with dim CD5. Minor population of CD7-negative T-cells can almost always be identified in benign samples from blood, BM or lymph nodes. Rare dual CD4/CD8+ T-cells or TCRγδ+ T-cells are also present in benign samples. In some reactive conditions, the CD7- T-cell population may expand mimicking neoplastic process. This is especially common in patients with mononucleosis (Figure 4.8) or in skin in patients

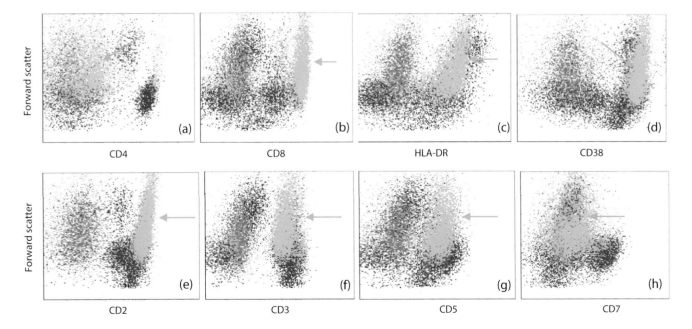

FIGURE 4.8 Aberrant expression of CD7 in patient with mononucleosis. The FC analysis of blood from 21 y/o patient with infectious mononucleosis shows significant population of atypical (activated) T-cells (green dots; arrow) with increased FSC (a–k), reversed CD4:CD8 ratio (a–b) due to predominance of CD8+ T-cells, positive activation markers, HLA-DR (c) and CD38 (d), positive CD2 (e), positive CD3 (f), positive CD5 (g), and aberrant loss of CD7 (h). PCR testing did not reveal clonal T-cell receptor (TCR) gene rearrangement (not shown).

with benign dermatoses. In a study by Weisberger et al., samples from all patients with infectious mononucleosis exhibited an activated (HLA-DR⁺, CD38⁺, CD8⁺) cytotoxic-suppressor T-cell population with aberrant down-regulation of CD7, and samples from 2 (8%) of 25 patients also showed down-regulation of CD5 [12]. Subset of normal NK-cells may display dimmer expression of CD2 and CD7 [15]. None of the non-T processes shows aberrant (dim) expression of more than two markers. Therefore, presence of dim expression for three or four T antigens is considered suggestive of T-cell lymphoma/leukemia. Diminished expression of one or more antigens is suggestive of malignancy, only if accompanied by other prominent abnormalities.

CD4/CD8 expression

Figure 4.9 shows examples of normal CD4:CD8 ratio. Restricted CD4 or CD8 expression (Figures 4.10 and 4.11), dual CD4/CD8 expression (Figure 4.12), or lack of both CD4 and CD8 (Figure 4.13), although not diagnostic of malignancy, raise the possibility of T-cell neoplasm and should be followed by evaluation of additional markers. Aberrant CD4:CD8 ratio may be seen in reactive conditions. Some non-T-cell disorders, such as Hodgkin lymphoma, may show marked predominance of CD4⁺ (or rarely CD8⁺) cells. Increased CD4:CD8 ratio may be also observed in granulomatous lymphadenitis (sarcoidosis) and reactive pleural effusions. In some viral infections, the CD4:CD8 ratio is reversed. Dual expression of CD4/CD8 is typical for thymocytes (*see below*) and therefore is not diagnostic for T-cell malignancy in the lesions obtained from mediastinum. T-cell lymphoproliferative disorders often contain significant component of residual benign (reactive) T-cells, which may obscure identification of CD4⁺ or CD8⁺ population of neoplastic T-cells (e.g., AITL). Careful evaluation of T-cell markers, FSC and additional markers (e.g., CD10)

is often helpful to identify abnormal population obscured by predominant benign elements. Table 4.4 shows the frequency of CD4 and CD8 expression in major types of mature T-cell neoplasms.

CD4⁺/CD8⁻

AITL, ATLL, and SS/MF are mostly CD4⁺. Majority of T-PLL (~61%), PTCL (~62%), and ALCL (~69%) express CD4, but they may be also CD8⁺, dual CD4/CD8⁺, or dual CD4/CD8⁻. Rare cases of T-ALL/LBL may be CD4⁺ (~10%). CD4 expression is not restricted to T-cell neoplasms. It is often present in acute myeloid leukemia, monocytes, and monocytic leukemias. Blastic plasmacytoid dendritic cell neoplasm (BPDCN) is CD4⁺/CD56⁺.

CD4⁻/CD8⁺

CD8⁺ T-cell neoplasms include the majority of T-LGLL, panniculitis-like T-cell lymphomas and EATL/MEITLs. Occasional cases of PTCL (~8%), T-PLL (~23%), ALCL (~18%), as well as rare cases of HSTL (17%) are CD8⁺; 3% of T-ALL cases are CD8⁺. Aberrant expression of CD8 may be seen in occasional B-cell lymphoproliferations (e.g., CLL).

CD4⁺/CD8⁺

Co-expression of CD4 and CD8 may be seen in very minute subset of benign T-cell in blood (average: 0.2%; range: 0%–2.3%; SD: 0.32) and/or bone marrow (average: 0.13%; range: 0%–2.7%; SD: 0.56). It is unusual in peripheral T-cell disorders, and most often indicate T-ALL/LBL. In the sample from mediastinum, dual CD4/CD8 expression is seen in thymocytes (either from thymic hyperplasia or thymoma). Among mature (peripheral) T-cell neoplasms, dual CD4/CD8 expression is observed in ~14% of T-PLL, ~4% of PTCL, ~3% of ALCL, and ~8% of T-LGLL. Dual positive CD4/CD8 expression comprises 36% of T-ALL/LBL cases.

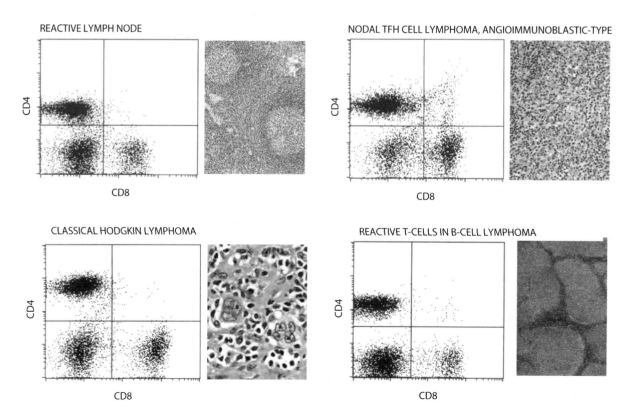

FIGURE 4.9 The CD4:CD8 ratio: normal pattern.

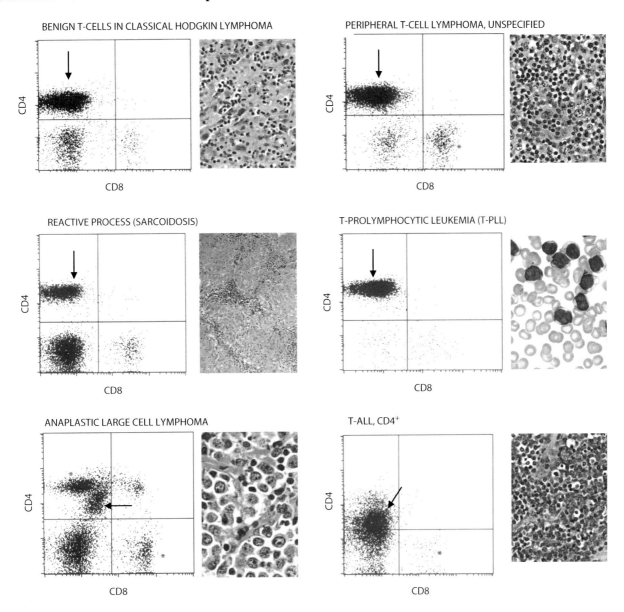

FIGURE 4.10 The CD4:CD8 ratio: predominance of CD4⁺ T-cells (arrow; red * represents residual benign T-cells).

CD4⁻/CD8⁻

Majority of T-ALL/LBLs are dual CD4/CD8-negative (~53%). CD4⁻/CD8⁻ phenotype is less common in mature T-cell lymphoproliferations. The latter are represented by EATL/MEITL (~14%), NK-cell LGLL (~69%), extranodal T/NK-cell lymphoma (nasal type), HSTL (~83%), non-hepatosplenic γδ T-cell lymphoma, followed by PTCL (~26%), T-PLL (~5%), ALCL (~9%), and T-LGLL (~8%).

Lack of CD45 or very dim CD45 expression

Lack of CD45 is rarely observed in peripheral T-cell disorders (~2%) or precursor T-cell neoplasms (~2%). Negative or dimly positive CD45 expression is highly suspicious for malignancy (Figure 4.14). Among mature (post-thymic) T-cell disorders, loss of CD45 is most often seen in T-PLL (~9%), followed by PTCL (~4%) and ALCL (~3%). Majority of mature T-cell disorders shows bright CD45 expression (~89%), whereas T-ALL/LBLs have most often moderate CD45 (~69%), followed by bright (~19%) and dim

(~12%) expression (Table 4.5). Benign (reactive) conditions do not show loss or aberrantly dim expression of CD45.

Presence of additional markers
HLA-DR

Benign T-cells and majority of T-cell neoplasms are negative for HLA-DR. Activated T-cells in reactive processes may show expression of HLA-DR, CD11c, and CD38 on subset. Figure 4.15 shows T-ALL case with unusual HLA-DR expression.

CD10

CD10 is positive in nodal lymphomas with T follicular helper cell (TFH) phenotype, which includes AITL, follicular T-cell lymphoma (FTCL), and nodal PTCL with T follicular helper phenotype (PTCL-TFH) [16, 17]. The WHO criteria specifically state that the expression of at least two TFH markers is required for the diagnosis of PTCL-TFH. TFH markers include CD10, BCL6,

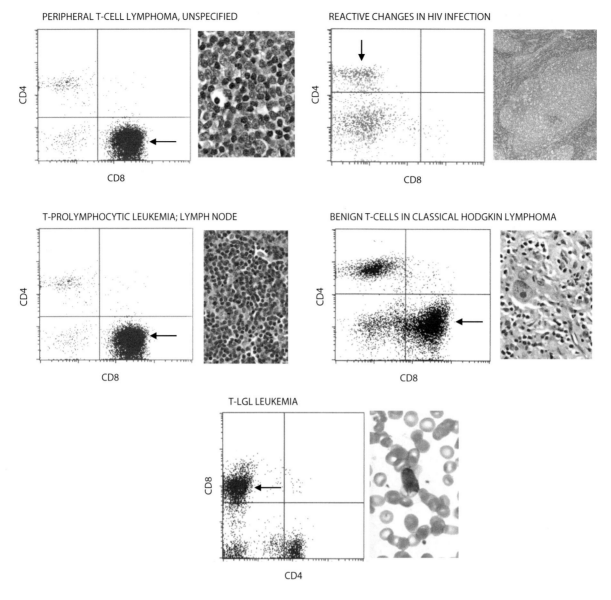

FIGURE 4.11 The CD4:CD8 ratio: CD8 predominance.

CXCL13, PD1 (CD279), ICOS, SAP (SLAM-associated protein), CXCR5, MAF (c-MAF), and CD200. T-cells in AITL often express CD10 (>60%; Figure 4.16). CD10 is positive on a subset of benign thymocytes (thymic tissue) and may be positive in occasional cases of PTCL and rare T-cell lymphomas from T-helper follicular cells. Approximately 30% of T-ALLs are CD10+ (Figure 4.17)

CD30
CD30 is expressed by ALCL (Figure 4.18) and a subset of other T-cell disorders, including PTCL, lymphomatoid papulosis (LyP), cutaneous ALCL, pagetoid reticulosis, and enteropathy-associated T-cell lymphoma (EATL). Subset of ATLL cases may show CD30 expression (most often seen in acute variant; Figure 15.4 in Chapter 15). Subset of cells in AITL is also CD30+.

CD25
CD25 is typically strongly positive in ATLL (Figure 4.19) but may be also positive in other T-cell disorders. CD25 is inconsistently

and variably expressed in other T-cell lymphomas (including Sézary's syndrome), in contrast to uniform and strong expression in ATLL.

CD103
CD103, a marker typical for hairy cell leukemia (HCL) and HCL variant (CD25− HCL), is often positive in EATL (Figure 4.20) and monomorphic epitheliotropic intestinal T-cell lymphoma (MEITL).

Other markers
Subset of T-cell lymphoblastic leukemia/lymphomas (T-ALL/LBL) may display aberrant expression of pan-myeloid markers, CD13 and/or CD33 (Figure 4.21). Very rare cases of PTCL co-express B-cell associated markers (CD19 and/or CD20). Dim expression of TCRαβ, lack of both TCR-associated antigens (αβ and γδ) or positive expression of TCRγδ on a significant proportion of T-cells usually indicates a malignant process.

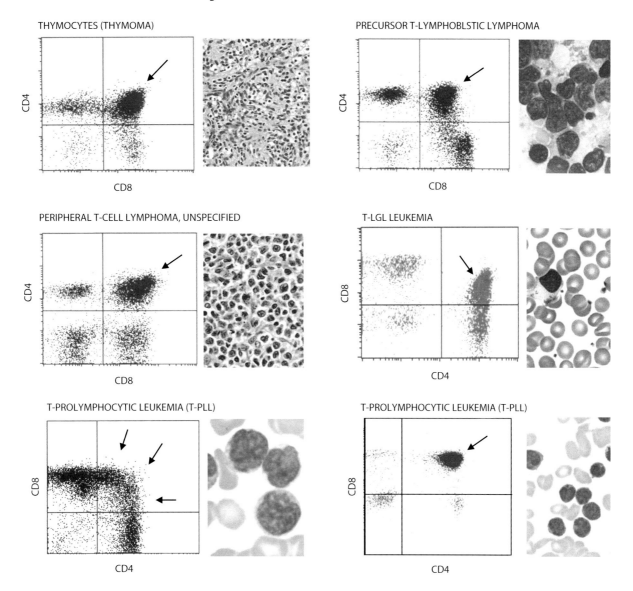

FIGURE 4.12   The CD4:CD8 ratio: dual CD4/CD8⁺ expression.

Loss of CD26 expression

Lack of CD26 expression is the most frequent phenotypic abnormality reported in mycosis fungoides (MF/Sézary syndrome), followed by loss of CD7 and CD2 [18–23]. The cutoff of 30% CD4⁺/CD26⁻ population has been reported as a reliable tool in differentiating MF/SS from inflammatory process [24]. Lack of CD26 is also typical for ATLL.

Loss of CD38 expression, aberrantly dim or bright CD38 expression

Negative or very dim CD38 expression is seen in T-cell neoplasms and was reported as a useful parameter in identifying atypical T-cell population in patient with MF/SS. Aberrantly bright CD38 may be seen in "high-grade" T-cell lymphomas (e.g., ALCL, subset of PTCL) or T-ALL/LBL.

Presence of blastic markers (TdT, CD34, CD1a, and/or CD117)

Presence of TdT, CD34, and/or CD1a indicates immature T-cell population, which represents either T-ALL or immature T-cells from thymic tissue (e.g., thymoma or thymic hyperplasia). CD117, marker associated with acute myeloid leukemia, systemic mastocytosis, and gastrointestinal stromal tumors can be rarely expressed in both peripheral (mature) and immature T-cell neoplasms (2.2% and 11.4%, respectively). Interestingly, among mature (peripheral) T-cell disorders CD117 expression is seen mostly in CD8⁺ T-PLL (Figure 4.22).

Expression of NK-cell associated markers (CD16, CD56, and/or CD57)

NK-cell markers (CD16, CD56, and CD57) are typically expressed by T-LGLL and T/NK-cell neoplasms. CD56 may be expressed in T-cell lymphomas including PTCL, ALCL, and hepatosplenic γδ

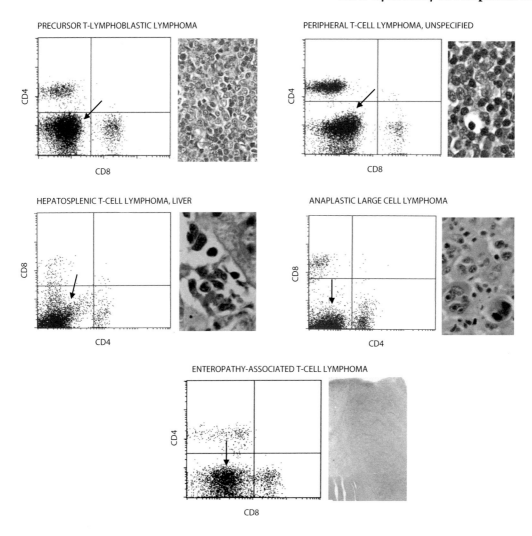

FIGURE 4.13   The CD4:CD8 ratio: dual CD4/CD8⁻ expression.

TABLE 4.4: CD4 and CD8 Expression in T-Cell Neoplasms[a]

Tumor	CD4⁺ (%)	CD8⁺ (%)	CD4⁺/CD8⁺ (%)	CD4⁻/CD8⁻ (%)
T-ALL/LBL	**8**	**3**	**36**	**53**
Mature	**51**	**27**	**4.5**	**17.5**
T-PLL	61	23	14	5
PTCL	61	9	4	26
ALCL	70	18	3	9
AITL	100	–	–	–
ATLL	100	–	–	–
MF/SS	94	6	–	4.2
T-LGLL	10	74	8	8
NK-LGLL	–	31	–	69
HSTL	–	17	–	83
EATL/MEITL	–	86	–	14

Abbreviations: T-ALL/LBL, T-cell acute lymphoblastic leukemia/lymphoma; T-PLL, T-cell prolymphocytic leukemia; PTCL, peripheral T-cell lymphoma; ALCL, anaplastic large cell lymphoma; AITL, angioimmunoblastic T-cell lymphoma; ATLL, adult T-cell lymphoma/leukemia; MF/SS, mycosis fungoides/Sézary's syndrome; T-LGLL, T-cell large granular lymphocytes leukemia; NK-LGLL, NK-cell large granular lymphocyte leukemia; HSTL, hepatosplenic T-cell lymphoma; EATL, enteropathy-associated T-cell lymphoma; MEITL, monomorphic epitheliotropic intestinal T-cell lymphoma.

[a]   *n* = 567 cases (mature T-cell neoplasms, 447 cases; T-ALL/LBL, 120 cases).

TABLE 4.5: CD45 Expression in T-Cell Neoplasms[a]

Tumor	CD45 Positive (%)			CD45 Negative (%)
	Bright	Moderate	Dim	
T-ALL/LBL	**19**	**69**	**12**	**2**
Mature	**89**	**8**	**1**	**2**
T-PLL	92	8	2	9
PTCL	87	7	2	4
ALCL	58	33	6	3
AITL	100	–	–	–
ATLL	92	8	–	–
MF/SS	88	12	–	–
T-LGLL	100	–	–	–
NK-LGLL	100	–	–	–
HSTL	100	–	–	–
EATL/MEITL	50	50	–	–

Abbreviations: T-ALL/LBL, T-cell acute lymphoblastic leukemia/lymphoma; T-PLL, T-cell prolymphocytic leukemia; PTCL, peripheral T-cell lymphoma; ALCL, anaplastic large cell lymphoma; AITL, angioimmunoblastic T-cell lymphoma; ATLL, adult T-cell lymphoma/leukemia; MF/SS, mycosis fungoides/Sézary's syndrome; T-LGLL, T-cell large granular lymphocytes leukemia; NK-LGLL, NK-cell large granular lymphocyte leukemia; HSTL, hepatosplenic T-cell lymphoma; EATL, enteropathy-associated T-cell lymphoma; MEITL, monomorphic epitheliotropic intestinal T-cell lymphoma.

[a]   *n* = 567 cases (mature T-cell neoplasms, 447 cases; T-ALL/LBL, 120 cases).

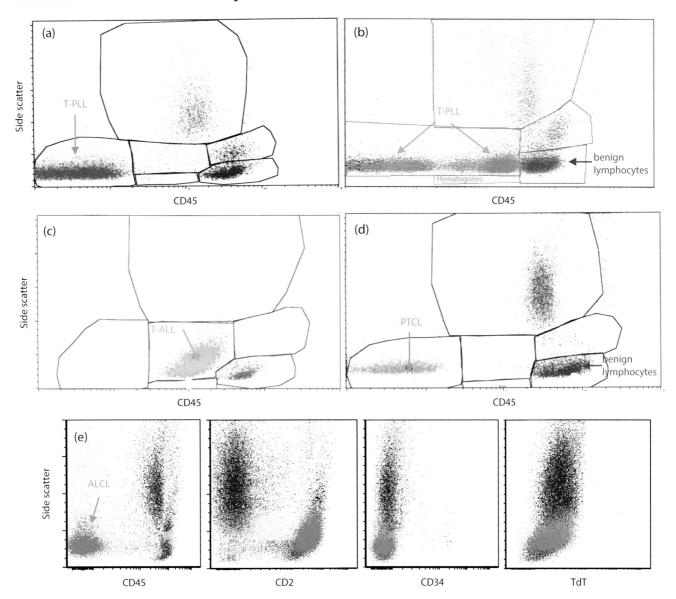

FIGURE 4.14 Aberrant expression of CD45: (a) T-PLL with negative CD45; (b) T-PLL with aberrant CD45 (subset of leukemic cells is negative and subset shows moderate CD45); (c) T-ALL with moderate CD45; (d) PTCL with negative CD45; and (e) ALCL with negative CD45 (T-cells are positive for CD2 and negative for CD34 and TdT).

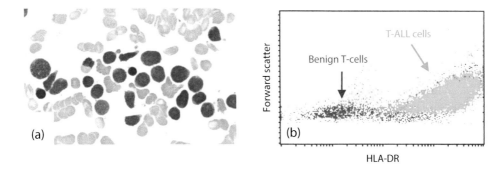

FIGURE 4.15 Additional markers in T-cell disorders: T-lymphoblasts (a) display aberrant expression of HLA-DR (b; green dots).

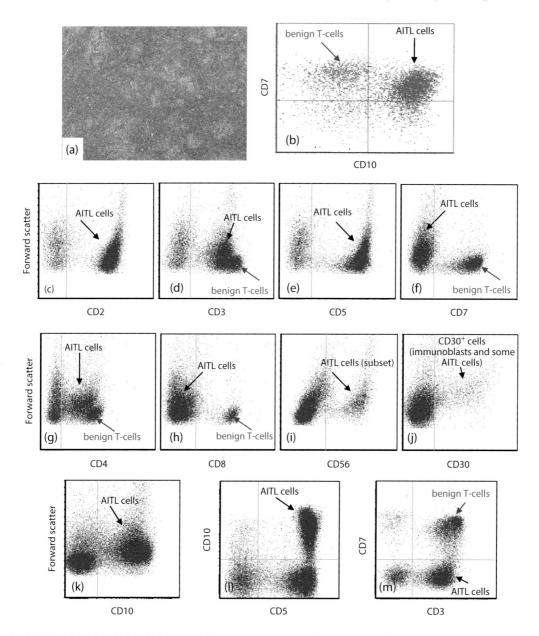

FIGURE 4.16 Additional markers in T-cell disorders: CD10 expression in nodal TFH cell lymphoma, angioimmunoblastic-type (AITL; two cases). (a–b) AITL (case #1) showing clusters of clear cells (a) with positive, but slightly dimmer expression of CD7 and positive CD10 (b). (c–m) AITL (case #2) with typical flow cytometry pattern. Tumor cells show partially increased forward scatter, positive CD2 (c), positive but dimmer CD3 (d), positive CD5 (e), negative CD7 (f), positive but dim CD4 (g), negative CD8 (h), partially positive CD56 (i), partially positive CD30 (j), and strongly positive CD10 (k–l). The CD3 versus CD7 display (m) shows loss of CD7 on neoplastic cells and slightly dimmer CD3 expression.

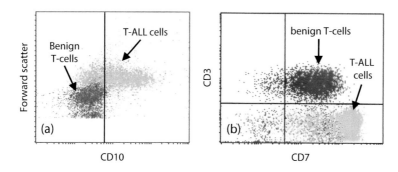

FIGURE 4.17 Additional markers in T-cell disorders: CD10 expression in T-ALL. Neoplastic cells express CD10 (a; green dots) and CD7 (b; green dots). Surface CD3 is negative (residual benign T-cells are positive for both CD3 and CD7 (red dots).

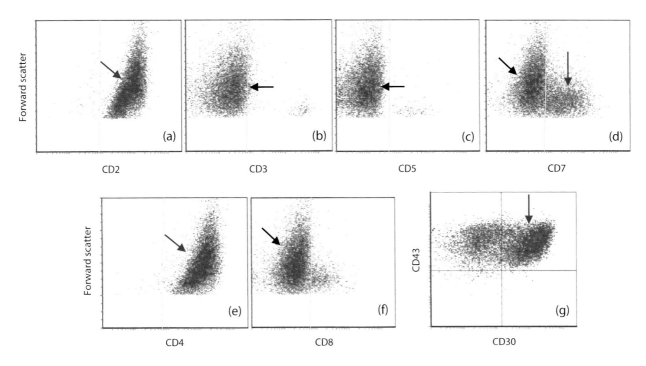

FIGURE 4.18 Additional markers in T-cell disorders: CD30 expression in ALCL. Tumor cells are positive for CD2 (a; red arrow), negative for CD3 (b; black arrow), negative for CD5 (c; black arrow), partially positive CD7 (d; red arrow shows $CD7^+$ cells and black arrow show major population of $CD7^-$ cells), positive for CD4 (e; red arrow), negative for CD8 (f; black arrow), positive for CD43 (g; upper quadrants), and mostly positive for CD30 (g; red arrow).

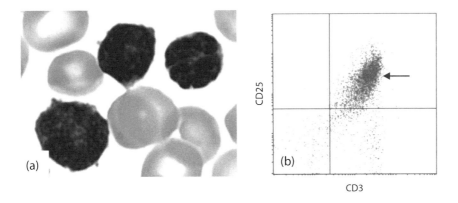

FIGURE 4.19 Additional markers in T-cell disorders: Neoplastic cells of adult T-cell leukemia/lymphoma (ATLL; a) are positive for CD25 (b; arrow).

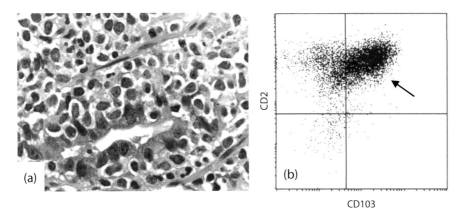

FIGURE 4.20 Additional markers in T-cell disorders: CD103 expression in enteropathy-type T-cell lymphoma.

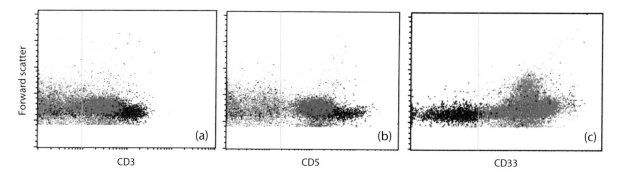

FIGURE 4.21 Additional markers in T-cell disorders: CD33 expression in T-ALL. Leukemic cells (green dots) are positive for CD3 (a; dim expression), CD5 (b; dim expression), and CD33 (c; heterogeneous expression). Residual (benign) T-cells have moderate CD3 (a) and CD5 (b) and are negative for CD33 (c; red dots). Granulocytes (gray dots) are CD33+ (c).

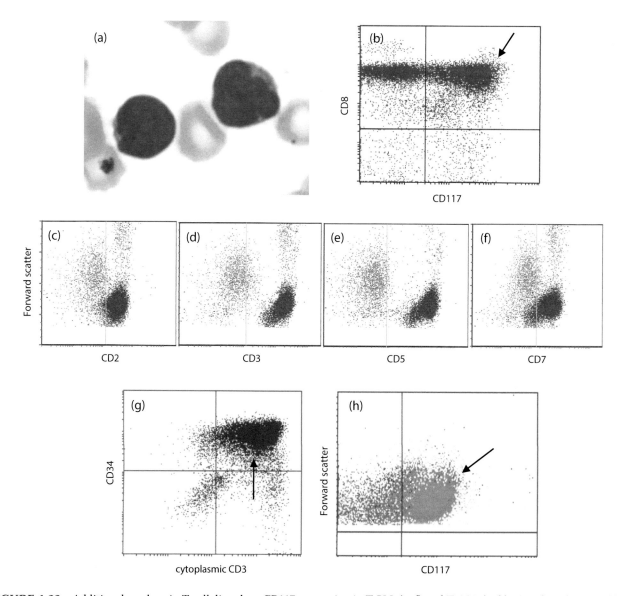

FIGURE 4.22 Additional markers in T-cell disorders: CD117 expression in T-PLL (a–f) and T-ALL (g–h). T prolymphocytes (a) co-express CD8 and CD117 (b; arrow). They do not display aberrant expression of pan-T-cell antigens (c–f). T-lymphoblastic are positive for CD34 (g), CCD3 (g), and CD117 (h).

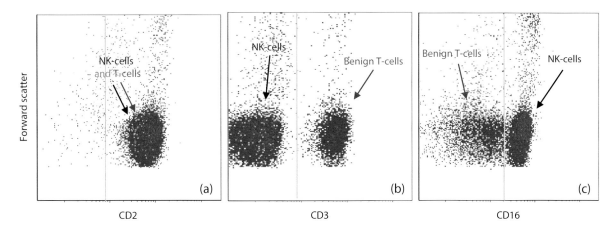

FIGURE 4.23 Additional markers in T-cell disorders: CD16 expression in NK-cells. NK-cells are typically positive for CD2 (a; arrow), negative for surface CD3 (b; solid arrow), and express CD16 (c; solid arrow) and/or CD56 (not shown).

T-cell lymphoma. Activated T-cells in reactive conditions may show dim CD56 expression on minute subset. Figure 4.23 shows CD16⁺ NK-cells.

Peripheral (mature) disorders versus T-ALL

Table 4.6 presents a comparison between the peripheral (mature) and precursor T-cell neoplasms. Presence of blastic markers (CD34, TdT) and CD1a indicates T-ALL/LBL (lack of both TdT

TABLE 4.6: Comparison Between the Phenotype of Mature and Precursor T-Cell Neoplasms

	Mature T-Cell Disorders (%)	T-ALL (%)
CD45		
Bright⁺	89	19
Moderate⁺	8	69
Dim⁺	1	12
Negative	2	2
T-cell antigens (surface)		
CD2⁺	91	71
CD3⁺	73	25
CD5⁺	75	87
CD7⁺	59	97
CD4/CD8 expression		
CD4⁺	51	8
CD8⁺	28	3
CD4/CD8⁺	5	36
CD4/CD8⁻	16	53
CD1a⁺	0	33
CD10⁺	7[a]	37
CD13⁺	0	7
CD33⁺	0	12
CD34⁺	0	36
CD117⁺	~2[b]	11
HLA-DR⁺	4	3
TdT⁺	0	86
TdT⁻/CD34⁻	100	3
TdT⁻/CD34⁻/CD1a⁻	100	1

[a] Angioimmunoblastic T-cell lymphoma.
[b] T-cell prolymphocytic leukemia.

and CD34 is observed in only 3% T-ALL cases). Aberrant expression of pan-myeloid antigens, CD13 and/or CD33 is seen in subset of T-ALL, but not in mature T-cell proliferations. T-ALLs usually have dim or moderate CD45 expression, whereas peripheral T-cell neoplasms typically display bright CD45. As far as T antigens are concerned, T-ALL are more often CD2⁻ and/or surface CD3⁻, and strongly CD7⁺, whereas peripheral tumors often show loss of CD7. The frequency of CD5 expression is comparable in both categories. Evaluation of CD4 and CD8 expression is very helpful in differential diagnosis: dual positive or dual negative CD4/CD8 expression is more often seen in T-ALL, whereas restricted CD4 or CD8 expression is more typical for mature neoplasms. Lack of TCR and positive CD10 or CD117 expression is seen more frequently in T-ALL.

T-cell markers expressed by non-T-cell processes

T antigens may be expressed by cells other than T-cells. CD2 is often expressed by monocytes and may be positive in acute promyelocytic leukemia (APL; hypogranular variant), BPDCN, mast cell tumors, and occasional cases of diffuse large B-cell lymphoma. CD3 is often expressed by B-cells of primary effusion lymphoma (PEL). Expression of CD3 (either surface or cytoplasmic) in conjunction with MPO or monocytic markers defines mixed phenotype acute leukemia (MPAL). CD5 is aberrantly expressed in B-CLL/SLL, mantle cell lymphoma, de novo CD5⁺ diffuse large B-cell lymphoma, and thymoma/thymic carcinoma. Rare cases of marginal zone lymphoma, lymphoplasmacytic lymphoma, and follicular lymphoma may also be CD5⁺. CD7 may be aberrantly expressed in AML, BPDCN, and acute monoblastic leukemia.

References

1. Ginaldi, L., et al., *Differential expression of CD3 and CD7 in T-cell malignancies: a quantitative study by flow cytometry.* Br J Haematol, 1996. **93**(4): p. 921–7.
2. Gorczyca, W., *Differential diagnosis of T-cell lymphoproliferative disorders by flow cytometry multicolor immunophenotyping. Correlation with morphology.* Methods Cell Biol, 2004. **75**: p. 595–621.

3. Gorczyca, W., et al., *An approach to diagnosis of T-cell lympho-proliferative disorders by flow cytometry.* Cytometry, 2002. **50**(3): p. 177–90.

4. Jennings, C.D. and K.A. Foon, *Recent advances in flow cytometry: application to the diagnosis of hematologic malignancy.* Blood, 1997. **90**(8): p. 2863–92.

5. Jiang, N.G., et al., *Flow cytometric immunophenotyping is of great value to diagnosis of natural killer cell neoplasms involving bone marrow and peripheral blood.* Ann Hematol, 2013. **92**(1): p. 89–96.

6. Juco, J., et al., *Immunophenotypic analysis of anaplastic large cell lymphoma by flow cytometry.* Am J Clin Pathol, 2003. **119**: p. 205–12.

7. Karube, K., et al., *Usefulness of flow cytometry for differential diagnosis of precursor and peripheral T-cell and NK-cell lymphomas: analysis of 490 cases.* Pathol Int, 2008. **58**(2): p. 89–97.

8. Klemke, C.D., et al., *The diagnosis of Sézary syndrome on peripheral blood by flow cytometry requires the use of multiple markers.* Br J Dermatol, 2008. **159**(4): p. 871–80.

9. Meyerson, H.J., *Flow cytometry for the diagnosis of mycosis fungoides.* G Ital Dermatol Venereol, 2008. **143**(1): p. 21–41.

10. Novelli, M., et al., *Flow cytometry immunophenotyping in mycosis fungoides.* J Am Acad Dermatol, 2008. **59**(3): p. 533–4.

11. Stacchini, A., et al., *The usefulness of flow cytometric CD10 detection in the differential diagnosis of peripheral T-cell lymphomas.* Am J Clin Pathol, 2007. **128**(5): p. 854–64.

12. Weisberger, J., et al., *Down-regulation of pan-T-cell antigens, particularly CD7, in acute infectious mononucleosis.* Am J Clin Pathol, 2003. **120**(1): p. 49–55.

13. Lima, M., et al., *Immunophenotype and TCR-Vbeta repertoire of peripheral blood T-cells in acute infectious mononucleosis.* Blood Cells Mol Dis, 2003. **30**(1): p. 1–12.

14. Qian, J., et al., *Altered ratio of circulating follicular regulatory T cells and follicular helper T cells during primary EBV infection.* Clin Exp Med, 2020. **20**(3): p. 373–80.

15. Morice, W.G., D. Jevremovic, and C.A. Hanson, *The expression of the novel cytotoxic protein granzyme M by large granular lymphocytic leukaemias of both T-cell and NK-cell lineage: an unexpected finding with implications regarding the pathobiology of these disorders.* Br J Haematol, 2007. **137**(3): p. 237–9.

16. Swerdlow, S.H., et al., ed. *WHO classification of tumors of haematopoietic and lymphoid tissues.* 2016, IARC: Lyon.

17. Swerdlow, S.H., et al., *The 2016 revision of the World Health Organization classification of lymphoid neoplasms.* Blood, 2016. **127**(20): p. 2375–90.

18. Novelli, M., et al., *Blood flow cytometry in Sézary syndrome: new insights on prognostic relevance and immunophenotypic changes during follow-up.* Am J Clin Pathol, 2015. **143**(1): p. 57–69.

19. Bernengo, M.G., et al., *The relevance of the CD4+ CD26- subset in the identification of circulating Sézary cells.* Br J Dermatol, 2001. **144**(1): p. 125–35.

20. Jones, D., et al., *Absence of CD26 expression is a useful marker for diagnosis of T-cell lymphoma in peripheral blood.* Am J Clin Pathol, 2001. **115**(6): p. 885–92.

21. Introcaso, C.E., et al., *Association of change in clinical status and change in the percentage of the CD4+CD26- lymphocyte population in patients with Sézary syndrome.* J Am Acad Dermatol, 2005. **53**(3): p. 428–34.

22. Kelemen, K., et al., *The usefulness of CD26 in flow cytometric analysis of peripheral blood in Sézary syndrome.* Am J Clin Pathol, 2008. **129**(1): p. 146–56.

23. Steinhoff, M., et al., *Prevalence of genetically defined tumor cells in CD7 as well as CD26 positive and negative circulating T-cell subsets in Sézary syndrome.* Leuk Res, 2009. **33**(1): p. 88–99.

24. Heid, J.B., et al., *FOXP3+CD25- tumor cells with regulatory function in Sézary syndrome.* J Invest Dermatol, 2009. **129**(12): p. 2875–85.

5

IDENTIFICATION OF MYELOBLASTS

Introduction

Identification of blasts (and blast equivalents) by flow cytometry (FC) is very important in the diagnosis and subclassification of acute leukemias, myelodysplastic neoplasms (MDS), myeloproliferative neoplasms (MPN), and in differential diagnosis of cells with "blastic" (immature) cytomorphologic features. FC analysis relies on the use of more than 300 markers (CD, cluster of differentiation), myeloperoxidase (MPO), terminal deoxynucleotidyl transferase (TdT), and orthogonal side scatter (SSC). It helps to differentiate between major types of acute leukemias, e.g., acute promyelocytic leukemia (APL) versus other HLA-DR⁻ (human leukemia antigen-DR) acute myeloid leukemias (AMLs), minimally differentiated AML versus acute lymphoblastic leukemia (ALL) and acute undifferentiated leukemia (AUL), acute monoblastic (monocytic) leukemia versus blastic plasmacytoid dendritic cell neoplasm (BPDCN), or B-cell acute lymphoblastic leukemia (B-ALL) versus T-cell acute lymphoblastic leukemia (T-ALL). Figure 5.1 presents an algorithm to the diagnosis and subclassification of acute leukemias. FC pattern often allows to raise the possibility of specific diagnoses such as APL and prompts additional confirmatory testing by fluorescence in-situ hybridization (FISH) and/or polymerase chain reaction (PCR). FC is also helpful in measurable (minimal) residual disease (MRD) evaluation after treatment. The FC panel should be broad since there is an overlap in the expression of some of the markers throughout acute leukemias of different lineages, e.g., CD33, a myeloid marker, may be positive in B-ALL and T-ALL, CD123 is positive in BPDCN and in subset of AMLs and ALLs, CD19, a B-cell marker, may be dimly positive in a subset of AML with maturation, and some of the T-cell antigens (CD2 and CD7) are often aberrantly expressed in AML. A rare variant of leukemia expressing CD34 and/or HLA-DR without an expression of lineage specific markers is classified as AUL. Another variant, termed mixed phenotype acute leukemia (MPAL) may show phenotypic features typical for both myeloid and lymphoid lineages (AML/B-ALL or AML/T-ALL).

Blasts and cells with blastic morphology

Blasts and atypical mononuclear cells with blast-like features include:

- AML: CD13⁺, CD33⁺, CD34⁺/rarely⁻, CD117⁺, CD133⁺/⁻, MPO⁺, CD81⁺/⁻, HLA-DR⁺/rarely⁻
- B-ALL: CD10⁺/⁻, CD19⁺, CD20⁻/rarely+(partial), CD22⁺, CD34⁺/rarely⁻, HLA-DR⁺, CD45⁻/+(dim), TdT⁺/rarely⁻
- T-ALL: CD1a⁻/⁺, CD2⁺, surface CD3⁻, cytoplasmic CD3⁺, CD5⁺/⁻, CD7⁺, CD4/CD8⁺ or CD4/CD8⁻, CD10⁻/⁺, CD34⁺, TdT⁺/⁻
- AUL: CD34⁺, HLA-DR⁺, CD3⁻, MPO⁻, TdT⁺/⁻, CD38⁺
- BPDCN: CD4⁺, CD13⁻, CD33⁻/⁺, CD56⁺(strong), CD123⁺(strong), CD11b⁻, CD11c⁻, HLA-DR⁺, CD45⁺, TdT⁻/⁺, MPO⁻, CD64⁻
- Blastoid variant of mantle cell lymphoma (MCL): CD19⁺, CD20⁺, CD5⁺, CD43⁺, CD81⁺, CD200⁻, positive for cyclin D1 (BCL1) and SOX11 by immunohistochemistry and *CCND1* rearrangement by FISH

- Blastic transformation of B- or T-cell lymphomas: history of B- or T-cell lymphoma
- Burkitt lymphoma (BL) and other high-grade B-cell lymphomas (HGBL): CD19⁺, CD20⁺, CD10⁺, CD71⁺, requires immunohistochemistry and FISH analysis to confirm the diagnosis
- Plasmablastic lymphoma (PBL): requires immunohistochemistry analysis to confirm the diagnosis
- Plasma cell myeloma (PCM) with plasmablastic features: positive for cytoplasmic light chain immunoglobulins, CD38, CD138 and often positive for CD56, CD200, and CD117, and negative for CD45, CD27, CD81, and CD20
- Immunoblastic variant of DLBCL: clonal B-cells with high forward scatter
- ALK⁺ DLBCL: requires immunohistochemistry analysis to confirm the diagnosis
- T-cell prolymphocytic leukemia (T-PLL): CD4 or CD8 positive (may be dual CD4/CD8 positive or negative), T-cell markers⁺
- Anaplastic large cell lymphoma (ALCL): T-cell markers⁺(rarely⁻), CD30⁺
- Metastatic tumors: require immunohistochemistry analysis to confirm the diagnosis
  - Metastatic carcinoma: CD45⁻, CD56⁺/⁻, CD117⁻/⁺, CD38⁻/⁺, keratin⁺
  - Rhabdomyosarcomas: CD45⁻, CD56⁺, CD90⁺, CD117⁺/⁻, myogenin⁺
  - Neuroblastoma: CD45⁻, CD56⁺, CD2⁺, CD81⁺
  - Primitive neuroectodermal tumors/Ewing sarcoma: CD45⁻, CD271⁺, CD99⁺
  - Wilms' tumor: CD45⁻, CD56⁺
  - Germ cell tumors: CD45⁻, CD56⁺, CD10⁺
  - Metastatic melanoma: CD45⁻, CD56⁺/⁻, CD10⁻/⁺, CD57⁺/⁻, CD117⁻/⁺

Leukemic stem cells (LSCs)

In 1994, Dick and colleagues showed that only the leukemic cells expressing the same markers as normal adult hematopoietic stem cells (HSCs; CD34⁺/CD38⁻) could initiate hematopoietic malignancy, and termed these cells as leukemia-initiating cells, leukemic stem cells (LSCs), or cancer stem cells (CSCs) [1–3]. Leukemias are now viewed as aberrant hematopoietic processes initiated by rare LSCs, which arise from the transformation of HSCs or committed progenitor cells [4]. Presence of LSCs, which are likely more therapy-resistant than majority of AML cells, have been shown to be responsible for the proliferation of disease and is implicated in relapse in patients with negative measurable residual disease (MRD) status. The occurrence of relapse in a proportion of patients achieving MRD⁻ status, roughly ranging between 20% and 25%, still represents a major drawback of all MRD studies [5, 6]. The surface markers of AML LSCs are considerably heterogeneous, including CD34⁺/CD38⁻, CD34⁺/CD38⁺, CD34⁺/CD38⁻/CD71⁻/HLA-DR⁻, and CD34⁻ subsets. Some of the surface antigens are negative in LSCs, such as CD19 and CD117,

DOI: 10.1201/9781003197935-5

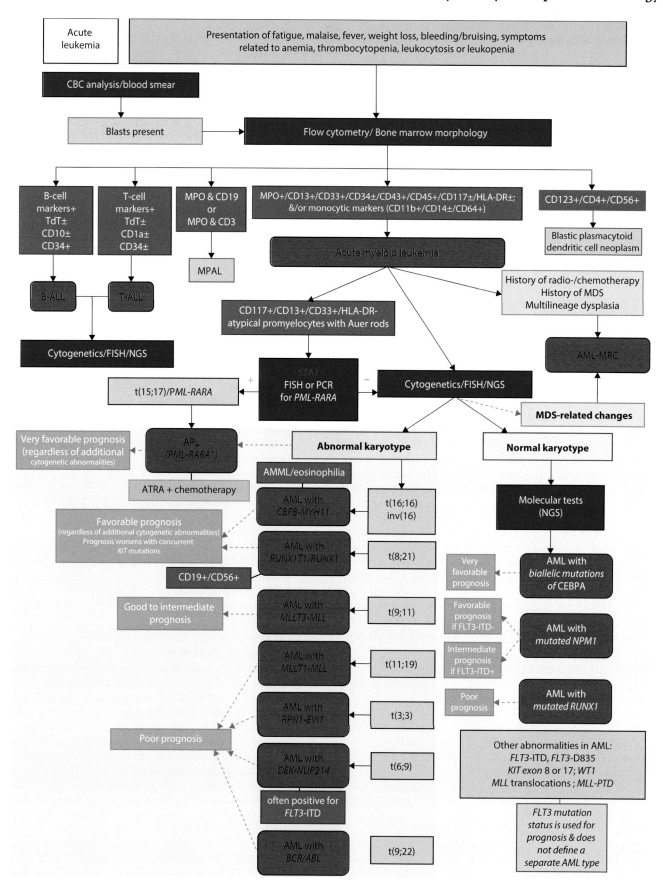

FIGURE 5.1   Algorithm to the diagnosis and subclassification of acute leukemias.

while other markers may be overexpressed in LSCs, including CD123, CD47, CD96, and TIM3.

AML definition and subclassification

AML is a clonal proliferation of immature hematopoietic precursors involving primarily the bone marrow (BM) and blood. AML represents a heterogeneous group of disorders with variable clinical presentation, cellular morphology, immunophenotype, chromosomal and molecular changes, therapeutic response, and overall prognosis [7–21]. Generally, AML can be defined as a clonal malignancy of transformed multipotent hematopoietic progenitor cell leading to accumulation of immature cells in the BM which replace normal elements causing cytopenias and their complications (e.g., fatigue due to anemia, infections due to granulocytopenia and bleeding due to thrombocytopenia). Leukemias may be associated with (hyper)leukocytosis or pancytopenia ("aleukemic" leukemia). Based on WHO criteria, ≥20% blasts (or blasts equivalents) are needed for the diagnosis of AML [except for AML with t(15;17), t(16;16/inv(16) and t(8;21) which can be diagnosed with <20% blasts]. AMLs with <20% blasts, which otherwise fulfill WHO criteria for the diagnosis are sometimes called "oligoblastic" AMLs.

The classification of myeloid neoplasm with increased blasts (<20%) and presence of *NPM1* mutations is somewhat controversial. *NPM1* mutations occurs most commonly in AML (classified as AML with *NPM1* mutation), but sporadic cases of other myeloid neoplasms, most commonly MDS (~2%) and chronic myelomonocytic leukemia (CMML; ~3%) may be *NPM1*+ [22]. Those cases can be classified as high-grade myeloid neoplasm with *NPM1* mutation representing either (1) "oligoblastic" AML (if the number of blasts is close to 20%), (2) MDS with *NPM1* mutation or (3) CMML with *NPM1* mutations. It is recommended that patients with either MDS or CMML with *NPM1* mutation should be treated aggressively with up-front chemotherapy rather than with MDS-directed protocols, as those neoplasms are associated with an aggressive clinical course, relatively rapid progression to overt AML and poor survival outcomes [22–27].

Therapy-related myeloid neoplasms include therapy-related acute myeloid leukemia (tAML), therapy-related myelodysplastic syndrome (tMDS), therapy-related myeloproliferative neoplasm (t(MPN), and therapy-related mixed myelodysplastic/myeloproliferative neoplasms (tMDS/MPN) occurring as late complications of cytotoxic chemotherapy and/or radiation therapy. Excluded from this category is transformation of MPN to AML, termed either blast phase or blast crisis, since it is often not possible to determine if this is a disease evolution or de novo therapy related neoplasm. Blast crisis is diagnosed with ≥20% blasts, while MPN with increased blasts not reaching 20% are termed MPN in accelerated phase. The current WHO classification replaced the French-American-British (FAB) classification.

The WHO classifies AML based on genetic, immunophenotypic, and clinical characteristics (Table 5.1):

- AML with defining genetic abnormalities
  - AML with t(15;17)/*PML-RARA* [acute promyelocytic leukemia, APL; FAB: AML-M3]
  - AML with t(8;21)/*RUNX1-RUNX1T1*
  - AML with *NPM1* mutation
  - AML with inv16(p13q22)/t(16;16)
  - AML with myelodysplasia-related changes
- Therapy related myeloid neoplasms

- AML, defined by differentiation
  - AML with minimal differentiation (FAB: AML-M0)
  - AML without maturation (FAB: AML-M1)
  - AML with maturation (FAB: AML-M2)
  - Acute myelomonocytic leukemia (AMML; FAB: AML-M4)
  - Acute monoblastic (monocytic) leukemia (FAB: AML-M5)
  - Acute (pure) erythroid leukemia (FAB: AML-M6)
  - Acute megakaryoblastic leukemia (FAB: AML-M7).

Morphology of AML

The requisite minimum of blasts for a diagnosis of acute leukemia is 20% in the BM or blood, as recommended in the WHO classification. AMLs associated with certain recurrent translocations such as t(15;17)(q22;q12), t(8;21)(q22;q22), and inv16(p13q22) is diagnosed even with <20% blasts/immature cells. For the purposes of diagnosing acute leukemia, abnormal promyelocytes (APL), monoblasts/promonocytes (acute monoblastic leukemia), and megakaryoblasts (acute megakaryoblastic leukemia) are considered blast equivalents. AML with *NPM1* mutation still requires 20% blasts for the diagnosis.

Three major types of myeloblasts are recognized based on nuclear and cytoplasmic characteristics (Figure 5.2). Type 1 myeloblasts have scanty, agranular cytoplasm, round or slightly irregular nuclei, fine chromatin, and a prominent nucleolus (usually more than one). A few granules in the cytoplasm may be occasionally seen. Type 2 myeloblasts are similar to type 1 except for the paucigranular cytoplasm (<15 primary azurophilic granules). Type 3 myeloblasts are characterized by numerous cytoplasmic granules (>20 granules). Abnormal promyelocytes from acute promyelocytic leukemia (hypergranular variant) are characterized by the presence of numerous small azurophilic cytoplasmic granules and Auer rods. In the microgranular variant of APL the atypical promyelocytes have a characteristic bilobed or dumb-bell shaped nuclei with delicate chromatin, bearing some resemblance to monoblasts. Monoblasts have large nuclei which are often folded or convoluted, finely dispersed chromatin and abundant pale cytoplasm. Occasional blasts may display erythrophagocytosis. This phenomenon is most commonly associated with monoblastic differentiation. Promonocytes are intermediate cells in maturation between monocytes and monoblasts; they are large with abundant, pale irregular cytoplasm, which may contain azurophilic granules. The nuclei are round or folded with finely dispersed chromatin and contain several inconspicuous nucleoli. Immature erythroid precursors have markedly basophilic cytoplasm with focally prominent vacuolation. Nuclei are large with coarse chromatin, irregular contours, and multinucleation. Dyserythropoietic features are prominent. Megakaryoblasts vary in morphologic appearance depending on the degree of differentiation. The most immature forms resemble myeloblasts, whereas cells with intermediate differentiation (promegakaryocytes) have more abundant cytoplasm with pseudopod formation. Occasional myeloblasts are small to intermediate and may resemble lymphoblasts or have "hand-mirror" appearance.

Evaluation of BM core biopsy reveals a hypercellular marrow with sheets of immature cells. Occasional acute leukemias presents with a hypocellular marrow or prominent fibrosis. Immunohistochemical staining of the core biopsy for CD34, TdT, and CD117 is very useful in establishing the diagnosis of AML in these situations. Subset of AML is associated with

TABLE 5.1: WHO Classification of Acute Myeloid Leukemias (AML)

1. AML with defining genetic abnormalities
1a. AML with balanced translocations/inversions

AML with t(8;21)/*RUNX1-RUNX1T1*	Large blasts with basophilic cytoplasm containing azurophilic granules; Auer rods; often aberrant expression of CD19 and CD56; expression of CD33 may be weak
AML with inv(16) or t(16;16)/*CBFB-MYH11*	Acute myelomonocytic leukemia features; increased eosinophils with atypical (immature) eosinophilic granules
Acute promyelocytic leukemia with t(15;17)*PML-RARA*	Atypical promyelocytes with Auer rods, lack of HLA-DR expression, sensitive to tretinoin (ATRA) and arsenic treatment, frequently complicated by disseminated intravascular coagulopathy (DIC)
AML with inv(3) or t(3;3)/*RPN1-MECOM*	Increased small hypolobated megakaryocytes; multilineage dysplasia, frequent CD7 expression in addition to blastic and myeloid markers
AML with t(6;9)/*DEK-NUP214*	Basophilia, multilineage dysplasia, affects younger patients
AML with t(9;11)/*KMT2A-MLLT3*	Monocytic features, more common in children, strong expression of CD33, CD64, CD4 and weak expression of CD13, CD34, and CD14
AML with t(1;22)/*RBM15-MKL1*	Megakaryoblastic features, positive for CD41, CD61, CD13, and CD33, often negative for CD34, CD45, and HLA-DR
AML with *BCR-ABL1* (provisional)	No history of CML, no evidence of biphenotypic phenotype

1b. AML with gene mutations

AML with mutated *NPM1*	Variable phenotype, but often with monocytic features, strong CD33 expression and often lack of HLA-DR and CD34, is associated with favorable prognosis (if normal karyotype and no accompanying *FLT3* mutations)
AML with biallelic mutation of *CEBPA*	Resembles morphologically and phenotypically AML, NOS, is associated with favorable prognosis
AML with mutated *RUNX1* (provisional)	Resembles morphologically and phenotypically AML, NOS

1c. AML with myelodysplasia-related changes (AML-MRC)

≥20% blasts; morphologic features of dysplasia in ≥50% of cells in at least two lineages; or AML arising from previous MDS or MDS/MPN; or AML with MDS-related cytogenetic abnormalities; absence of genetic changes typical for AML with recurrent genetic abnormalities, no prior history of toxic therapy

2. Therapy-related myeloid neoplasms

It includes therapy-related AML (tAML), MDS (tMDS), and MDS/MPN (t-MDS/MPN); often history of alkylating agents or radiotherapy; frequent genetic changes (usually chromosome 5 and 7 abnormalities or complex karyotype)

3. Acute myeloid leukemia, defined by differentiation

AML with minimal differentiation	No evidence of myeloid differentiation by morphology or cytochemistry (<3% blasts positive for MPO, SBB, and CAE); criteria for other types of acute leukemia are not fulfilled (e.g., prior therapy or specific genetic changes)
AML without maturation	Maturing cells in granulocytic lineage <10% of nucleated marrow cells; ≥3% blasts positive for MPO or SBB
AML with maturation	≥20% blasts; ≥10% maturing myeloid elements; <20% monocytes
Acute myelomonocytic leukemia	≥20% blasts (including promonocytes); ≥20% monocytes and their precursors
Acute monoblastic and monocytic leukemia	≥20% blasts (including promonocytes) in which ≥80% of leukemic cells are of monocytic lineage
Acute erythroid leukemia (AEL, pure erythroid leukemia)	>80% erythroid cells with ≥30% proerythroblasts, no evidence of significant myeloblastic component; erythroblasts usually are positive for GPHA, CD71, hemoglobin A, and E-cadherin (subset of cells may be CD117$^+$), lack CD34 and HLA-DR expression
Acute megakaryoblastic leukemia	≥20% blasts of which ≥50% are of megakaryocytic lineage, AML-MRC and tAML are excluded; blasts are positive for CD41, CD61, and CD42b, while CD45 and HLA-DR are often negative
Acute basophilic leukemia	Basophilic differentiation, blasts often positive for CD13, CD33, CD123, CD11b, and negative for CD34, CD117, and monocytic markers; does not fulfill criteria for any other specific AML category
Acute panmyelosis with myelofibrosis (APMF)	Increased blasts (≥20%) and marrow fibrosis; acute rapidly progressive clinical course of symptoms; does not fulfill criteria for any other specific AML category

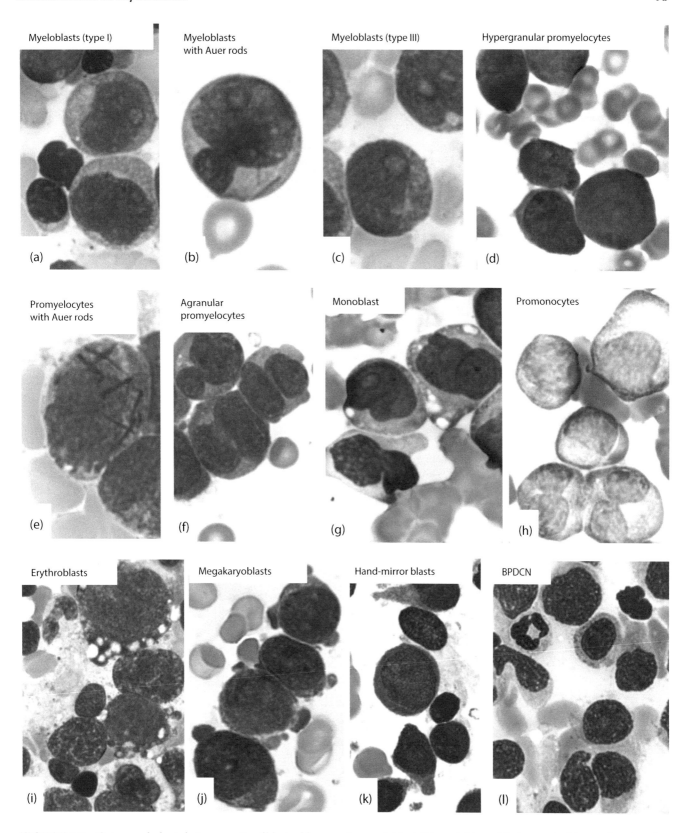

FIGURE 5.2 Cytomorphologic heterogeneity of blasts: (a) agranular myeloblast, (b) myeloblast with Auer rods, (c) granulated myeloblast, (d) hypergranular promyelocytes, (e) promyelocyte with numerous Auer rods, (f) agranular promyelocytes, (g) monoblasts, (h) promonocytes, (i) erythroblasts, (j) megakaryoblasts, (k) myeloblasts with hand-mirror features, and (l) BPDCN blasts.

eosinophilia. The majority of those cases belong to the category of acute myelomonocytic leukemia with eosinophilia (AML-M4Eo) and are associated with inv(16)/t(16;16) (variant of CBF+ AML). Occasional AML with eosinophilia, especially those preceded by chronic MPN associated with eosinophilia (e.g., chronic eosinophilic leukemia and mastocytosis with eosinophilia) may be associated with *FIP1L1/PDGFRA* fusion or show recurrent breakpoint clusters at chromosome bands 5q31-33, 8p11, and 9p24, which are linked to tyrosine kinase genes *PDGFRB*, *FGFR1*, and *JAK2*, respectively. As shown by Metzgeroth et al., patients with eosinophilia-associated hematological malignancies (including AML) with *FIP1L1/PDGFRA* fusion respond very well to treatment with tyrosine kinase inhibitors (e.g., imatinib) [28].

Identification of myeloblasts by flow cytometry

Introduction

Immunophenotyping plays an important role in the diagnosis and subclassification of acute leukemias (Tables 5.2 and 5.3). Myeloblasts, depending on specific subtype of AML are positive for CD34, CD117, CD133, CD138, MPO, HLA-DR, pan-myeloid antigens (CD13, CD33), CD4, monocytic markers (CD11b, CD11c, CD14, CD64), and TdT. In addition, there may be aberrant expression of B-cell associated markers (usually CD19), CD56 and some of the pan-T cell markers (most often CD7). TdT expression in AML has been proposed as a surrogate for *RUNX1* mutation [29, 30]. TdT expression in AML with minimal differentiation correlates with trisomy 13, inversely correlates with aberrations of chromosomes 5 and 7, and identifies a subset of patients with a better prognosis after stem cell transplant [31]. CD33 is a myeloid antigen expressed on blasts on most patients with AML. Evaluation of CD33 expression by FC in AML patients is clinically relevant due to CD33-targeted treatment strategies with

TABLE 5.2: Phenotypic Markers in Acute Myeloid Leukemia (AML) and Mixed Phenotype Acute Leukemia (MPAL)

AML

Precursor stage	CD34, CD38, CD117, CD133, HLA-DR, TdT
Granulocytic markers	CD10[a], CD13, CD15, CD16, CD33, CD65, cytoplasmic MPO, CD11b[a]
Monocytic markers	Nonspecific esterase (NSE), CD11c, CD14, CD64, lysozyme (muramidase), CD11b[a], CD36, NG2 homologue
Megakaryocytic markers	CD41, CD61, CD42
Erythroid markers	CD235a (glycophorin A), CD71, CD81, hemoglobin A, E-cadherin

MPAL

Myeloid lineage	MPO or evidence of monocytic differentiation (at least two of the following: NSE, CD11c, CD14, CD64, lysozyme)
B-lineage	1. CD19 (strong) with at least one of the following: CD79a, c.CD22, CD10, or 2. CD19 (weak) with at least 2 of the following: CD79a, c.CD22, CD10
T-lineage	CD3 (surface or cytoplasmic)

[a] CD10 is positive in neutrophils and CD11b is positive in neutrophils and monocytes.

toxin-conjugated humanized IgG4 anti-CD33 monoclonal antibody gemtuzumab ozogamicin (GO, Mylotarg), calicheamycin conjugates of anti-CD33 monoclonal antibody. In pediatric population, increased CD33 expression is directly associated with adverse disease features and inversely associated with low-risk disease [32]. Lower CD33 expression is associated with superior response to GO. In series reported by Pollard, there was a higher prevalence of low-risk disease features (e.g., CBF AML) in patients with low CD33 expression,

TABLE 5.3: Phenotype of Myeloblasts

	Myeloblasts	Neoplastic Promyelocytes	Monoblasts Promonocytes	Erythroblasts	Megakaryoblasts	BPDCN
CD4	−/+	−	+	−	−	+
CD7	−/+	−	−	−	−	−/+
CD11b	−	−	+/(−)	−	−	−
CD11c	+[dim]/−	−	+	−	−	−
CD13/CD33	+	+	+	−/(+)	−/+	−[1]
CD14	−	−	+/−[2]	−	−/+	−
CD34	+	−[3]	−/(+)	−/(+)	−/(+)	−
CD41/CD61	−	−	−	−	+	−
CD45	+	+	+	−/(+)	+	+
CD56	−/(+)	−/(+)	+/−	−	−	+
CD64	−/+[dim]	+[dim]	+	−	−	−
CD71	+[dim]/−	−/+[dim]	−/+[dim]	+[bright]	+/−	−
CD81	−/+	−		+[bright]	−	−
CD117	+	++	−/(+)	+[dim]	−/+	−/+
CD123	+/−	−	+/−	−/+	−/+	+
GPHA	−	−	−	−/(+)	−	−
HLA-DR	+/(−)	−	+/(−)	−/(+)	−/+	+
TdT	−/+	−	−	−	−	−/+
SSC	Low	High	Moderate	Variable	Variable	Low

Abbreviations: +, positive; (+), rarely positive; −, negative; (−), rarely negative; 1, CD33 rarely+; 2, if positive, expression often partial or variable (smeary); 3, hypogranular APL often CD34+; SSC, side scatter; BPDCN, blastic plasmacytoid dendritic cell neoplasm; GPHA, glycophorin (CD235a); TdT, terminal deoxynucleotidyl transferase.

whereas patients with high CD33 expression were more likely to have high risk disease (e.g., *FLT3-ITD*) [32]. In low-risk patients, high CD33 expression is associated with significantly inferior outcome. High blasts expression of CD33 may be a predictor of poor outcome.

Major antigens used in the diagnosis of AML
Immunophenotypic profile of major blast categories

- Myeloblasts: CD34+, CD117+, CD13+, CD33+. HLA-DR+(rarely−), CD45+, MPO+/−, CD45RA+, TdT+/−, CD7−/+, CD56−/+, CD71+/−, CD81+, CD133+
- Acute promyelocytic leukemia, hypergranular variant (APL): CD34−, CD117+(may be dim), CD13+, CD33+bright, CD11c−, HLA-DR−, MPO+, CD45+, TdT−, CD56−/+, CD64+(dim)/−, CD7−
- Monoblasts: CD34−/(rarely+), CD117−/rarely+, CD13+, CD33+, MPO−, HLA-DR+, CD45+, CD14+(may be partial or variable)/−, CD64+strong, CD11b+(may be partial or variable)/−, CD11c+, CD4+, CD56+/−, CD71+/−; CD123+/−
- Erythroblasts: CD34−, CD117+dim/−, CD13/CD33−, CD36+, HLA-DR−, MPO−, CD45−/dim+, TdT−, CD71bright+, CD81+, GPHA+/−
- Megakaryoblasts: CD34−/+, CD117+/rarely−, MPO−, CD13/CD33+/−, CD38+, HLA-DR−/+, CD45+/−, TdT−, CD41+/rarely−, CD42+, CD61+, CD71+
- BPDCN: CD4+, CD13−, CD33−/+, CD56+(strong), CD123+(strong), CD11b−, CD11c−, HLA-DR+, CD45+, TdT−/+, MPO−, CD64−
- AUL: CD34+, CD117−, MPO−, s.CD3−, c.CD3−, CD38+, HLA-DR+, CD45+, TdT+/−, CD7−/+, CD19−, CD14−, CD64−, CD11b−, CD11c−, CD56−, CD13−, CD33− (rare cases may show expression of one of myeloid markers: CD13, CD33, or CD117, but there is no co-expression of two or more of myeloid markers)

CD45 versus SSC (side scatter)
As can be expected from cytomorphologic and genotypic diversity of acute leukemias, FC features of AMLs are complex. Typical myeloblasts show moderate expression of CD45 and low SSC placing them in "blast gate" on CD45 versus SSC display (Figure 5.3a). Monoblasts have usually brighter CD45 and slightly higher SSC than myeloblasts (Figure 5.3b), whereas neoplastic promyelocytes from APL are characterized by moderate CD45 and high SSC (Figure 5.3c). Blasts in pure erythroid leukemia are usually CD45−, but some cases may show dim to moderate CD45 expression. The CD45 versus SSC pattern of megakaryoblasts is similar to blasts from AML with or without maturation. Some

AMLs may show negative, dim or partial CD45 expression (lack or CD45 is more typical for B-ALL). Rare cases of AML other than APL (AML with maturation or acute monoblastic leukemia) have high SSC mimicking either APL or granulocytes (maturing myeloid precursors) on CD45 versus SSC display.

Blastic versus maturation markers
Myeloblasts are usually identified by expression of "immature" (stem cell) markers such as TdT, CD34, CD117, and CD133 (Figure 5.4) and/or by lack of expression of markers typically present on mature cells (myelocytes, metamyelocytes, and neutrophils) such as CD10, CD11b, CD15, CD16, or CD65 (Figure 5.5). CD117 is positive in APL and majority of other AMLs, rare cases of ALL and rare cases of BPDCN. CD34 is positive in AUL and most AMLs, including minimally differentiated AML, AML without maturation, subset of AML with maturation, majority of hypogranular variant of APL and in poorly differentiated subtypes of monoblastic and megakaryoblastic leukemias. CD34 is negative in hypergranular (classic) APL, BPDCN, majority of acute monoblastic leukemias and in subset of AML with or without maturation. Lack of both CD34 and CD117 expression may be seen in acute monoblastic leukemia, subset of acute megakaryoblastic leukemias, pure erythroid leukemia, and rare cases of AML with/without maturation. In cases without CD34 and CD117, diagnosis of AML can be confirmed by additional markers, such as CD71 and GPHA for pure erythroid leukemia, CD11b, CD11c, CD14, CD64, and CD123 for acute monoblastic leukemia, and CD41 and CD61 for acute megakaryoblastic leukemia (Figure 5.6). Subset of AML, usually less differentiated, may express TdT. TdT expression in AML has been proposed as a surrogate for *RUNX1* mutation [29, 30]. TdT expression in AML with minimal differentiation correlates with trisomy 13, inversely correlates with aberrations of chromosomes 5 and 7, and identifies a subset of patients with a better prognosis after stem cell transplant [31].

MPO (myeloperoxidase)
Strong MPO expression by blasts indicates myeloid differentiation. FC interpretation of MPO expression may be difficult, especially in less differentiated AML, ALL, or MPAL. The discordant results of MPO expression in AML between FC and cytochemistry on BM aspirate smears (or immunohistochemistry on core biopsy or clot sections) have been well documented [33, 34]. 3% threshold has been used historically for MPO positivity by cytochemistry (on BM aspirate smears). In FC analysis 10% threshold has been recommended

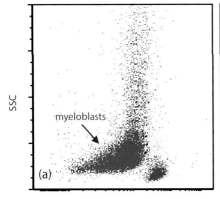
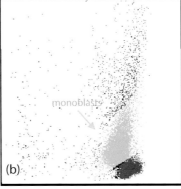
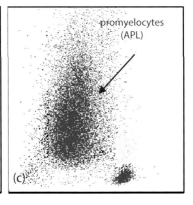

FIGURE 5.3 Identification of blasts: CD45 versus SSC. Myeloblasts typically show moderate CD45 and low SSC (a; blue dots). Monoblasts (b; green dots) in most cases have bright CD45 and slightly increased SSC when compared to myeloblasts. Neoplastic promyelocytes (c; blue dots) have high SSC and moderate CD45.

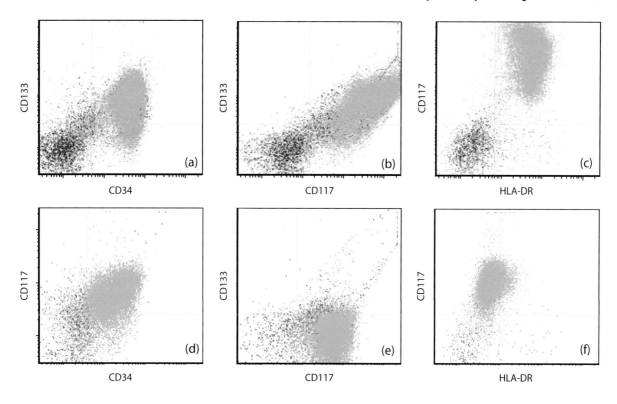

FIGURE 5.4   Case #1 (a–c). Myeloblasts (green dots) are positive for CD34 (a), CD133 (a–b), CD117 (b–c; bright expression), and HLA-DR (c). Case #2 (d–f). Myeloblasts (green dots) are positive for CD34 (d) and CD117 (d–f) and are negative for CD133 (e) and HLA-DR (f).

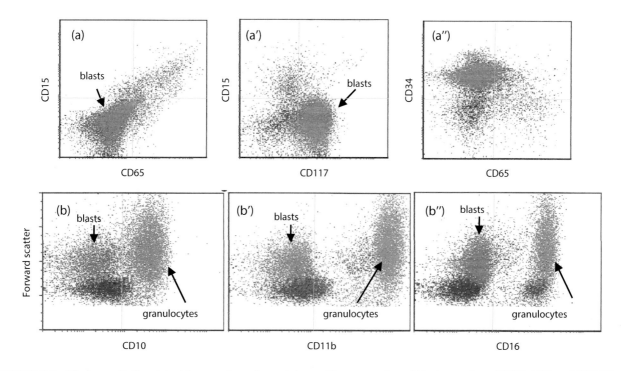

FIGURE 5.5   Blasts are distinguished from mature elements by positive expression of blastic markers (CD34, TdT, and CD117) and lack of expression of markers associated with maturation (CD10, CD11b, CD15, CD16, and CD65). Top panels (a) show myeloblasts negative for CD15 (a, a′) and CD65 (a, a″) and positive CD117 (a′) and CD34 (a″). Lower panels (b) display AML with maturation with blasts (green dots) negative for CD10 (b), CD11b (b′), and CD16 (b″). Note bright expression of those markers by maturing granulocytes (gray dots).

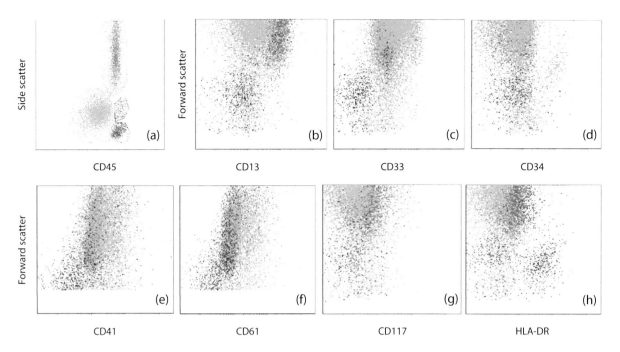

FIGURE 5.6 Acute megakaryoblastic leukemia without CD34 and CD117 expression. Megakaryoblasts (green dots) are characterized by positive CD45 (a), low SSC (a), high FSC (b–h), negative CD13 (b), positive CD33 (c), negative CD34 (d), positive CD41 (e), positive CD61 (f), negative CD117 (g), and negative HLA-DR (h).

[35–39], but in more recent study, Guy et al. proposed a threshold of 13% or 28% MPO positivity (using isotype control or normal lymphocytes as negative controls, respectively) [37]. The 13% MPO positivity threshold has sensitivity of 95.1% and specificity of 91.7%. As quantification of MPO expression by FC may be difficult, Borowitz suggested that MPO expression in B-ALL may not be sufficient for the diagnosis of MPAL if there is no expression of other myeloid markers (CD13 and CD33) [40]. Revised WHO classification (2016) recognized that some cases of otherwise typical B-ALL with homogeneous expression of lymphoid markers on a single blast population may express low level MPO using immunophenotypic methods without evidence of myeloid differentiation [21]. Figure 5.7 shows comparison of MPO expression by FC and cytochemistry.

CD13 and CD33

CD13 and CD33 are myeloid antigens expressed by blasts in most AMLs, CD13 being often dimmer than CD33 (Figure 5.8). The expression of CD13 or CD33 by blasts in AML may be aberrant,

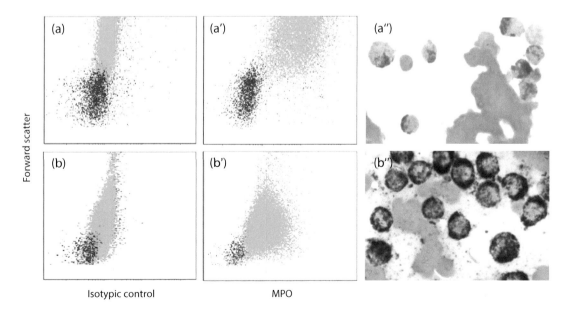

FIGURE 5.7 Comparison of MPO expression by FC and cytochemistry. Acute myeloid leukemia without maturation (a) shows strong MPO expression by FC (a, isotypic control; a′; MPO) and by cytochemistry (a″). Acute promyelocytic leukemia (b) shows dim expression of MPO by FC (isotypic control b; b′, MPO) but is strongly MPO positive by cytochemistry (b″).

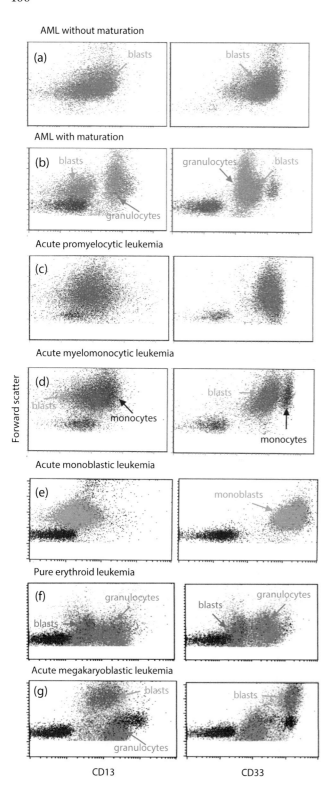

FIGURE 5.8 The expression of CD13 and CD33 in AML. Blasts from AML with or without maturation are most often positive for both CD13 and CD33 (a), the expression of CD13 often being dimmer than CD33. Subset of leukemias may show negative, dim or partial expression of either CD13 (b) or CD33. Neoplastic promyelocytes most often show dim CD13 and bright CD33 (c). Neoplastic monocytes have bright CD33 (d–e). Erythroblasts from pure erythroid leukemia are usually CD13/CD33-negative (f), whereas megakaryoblasts may be CD13 and/or CD33 positive (g).

either negative, dim, very bright, or partial. Acute monoblastic leukemia and APL usually show dim CD13 and bright CD33. Very bright expression of CD33 (much brighter than in maturing myeloid elements, neutrophils, or monocytes) is very useful parameter helpful in identifying APL by FC. Evaluation of CD33 expression by FC in AML patients is clinically relevant due to CD33-targeted treatment strategies with toxin-conjugated humanized IgG4 anti-CD33 monoclonal antibody gemtuzumab ozogamicin (GO, Mylotarg). In pediatric population, increased CD33 expression is directly associated with adverse disease features and inversely associated with low-risk disease [32]. Lower CD33 expression is associated with superior response to GO. In series reported by Pollard, there was a higher prevalence of low-risk disease features in patients with low CD33 expression, whereas patients with high CD33 expression were more likely to have high risk disease [32]. High blasts expression of CD33 may be a predictor of poor outcome.

CD14 and CD64
CD14 and CD64 are brightly positive in normal monocytes. Subset of AML, especially APL and acute megakaryoblastic leukemia may show dim CD64 expression. Acute monoblastic leukemias show bright expression of CD64 and positive CD11c but may be either negative, partially expressed or variably ("smeary") positive for CD14 as shown in Figure 5.9. BPDCN and AUL do not express CD14 and CD64.

CD11b and CD11c
Expression of CD11b and CD11c is most typical for acute monoblastic leukemia, in which CD11c is strongly positive, but the expression of CD11b maybe either negative, partial, dim, moderate or variable (Figure 5.10). Benign monocytes show bright expression of both CD11b and CD11c. Other AML subtypes (except for APL) often show dim, partial and less often moderate CD11c expression, but CD11b is usually negative or only dimly positive (most often on subset of blasts). CD11b may be seen in acute megakaryoblastic leukemia, especially in cases associated with Down syndrome (DS). Expression of CD11b in cytogenetically unfavorable AML was recently reported to be associated with monosomal karyotype and extremely poor prognosis [41].

CD45RA
CD45RA is expressed on leukemic cells in the majority of AML patients. It can be useful in evaluating the phenotype of LSCs (CD34+/CD38−) while monitoring patients on anti-LSC treatment [42].

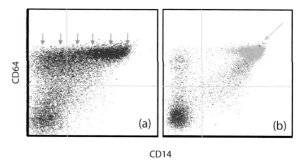

FIGURE 5.9 Identification of myeloblasts: expression of CD4 and CD64 in acute monoblastic leukemia. Monoblasts are positive for CD64 (a; bright expression) and often show variable ("smeary") pattern of CD14, ranging from negative to positive expression (a; arrows). In mature monocytes both CD14 and CD64 are brightly positive (b; arrow).

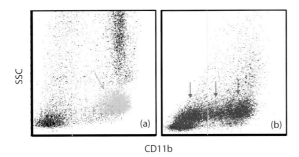

FIGURE 5.10 Identification of myeloblasts: expression of CD11b in acute monoblastic leukemia. Subset of acute monoblastic leukemias shows moderate to bright CD11b (a; green dots), but majority of cases have either variable ("smeary") CD11b (b, blue dots) with subset of cells negative and subset with variable positivity.

CD56

CD56 expression, often seen in acute monoblastic leukemia, may be also seen in other subtypes, including AML with t(8;21), APL, acute megakaryoblastic leukemia (especially in children) and acute leukemia with NK-cell differentiation. CD56, along with CD4 and CD123 expression is typical for BPDCN, which may also be positive for CD7 and/or CD117.

CD71

CD71 (transferrin receptor 1) is expressed at high levels on cells with high proliferation rate (similar to Ki-67) and on cells with high iron demand, such as maturing erythroid cells. Myeloblasts, promyelocytes and erythroblasts are CD71+, while more mature forms (myelocytes, metamyelocytes, neutrophils) are CD71-. Among acute leukemias, CD71 is strongly positive in acute (pure) erythroid leukemia and other AMLs, especially acute megakaryoblastic leukemia or poorly differentiated myeloid leukemias. APL and acute monoblastic leukemias are either CD71- or show only dim CD71 expression. Among lymphoblastic leukemias, CD71 expression is higher in T-ALL than in B-ALL [43]. CD71 is strongly positive in adult T-cell leukemia/lymphoma (ATLL), and majority of other high-grade lymphomas (e.g., Burkitt lymphoma, double hit lymphomas, ALCL or subset of diffuse large B-cell lymphoma).

CD123

CD123 (interleukin 3 receptor α) is a leukemia-associated antigen that is positive at high levels in blasts and is negative or expressed at low level in normal hematopoietic stem and progenitor cells. Immune-based therapies targeting CD123 are now being developed. The expression of CD123 is most typical for dendritic malignancies (e.g., BPDCN), but it can also be found in acute monoblastic leukemia and subset of AML, B-ALL, and T-ALL.

HLA-DR (human leukocyte antigen-DR)

Lack of HLA-DR is typical for APL (Figure 5.11). Occasional cases of non-APL AMLs may lack HLA-DR, but they differ from classic (hypergranular) APL by low SSC and often positive CD34 and CD11c. Hypogranular variant of APL, apart from CD117 and bright CD33 is often positive for CD34 and CD2, and lacks HLA-DR, CD11b, CD11c, and CD14. Approximately 8% of acute monoblastic leukemias are HLA-DR-. CD34-/HLA-DR- phenotype is often seen in AML with normal cytogenetics and FLT3-ITD [44]. Subset of AML with FLT3-ITD expresses CD7 and CD25. Lack of HLA-DR and CD34 is also often seen in AML with NPM1 mutations (Figure 5.12).

CD25

Gonen et al. identified CD25+ myeloblasts in 87 patients (13%), of which 92% had intermediate cytogenetic risk. CD25 expression was associated with expression of stem cell antigen, CD123 [45]. In multivariate analysis controlling for prognostic baseline characteristics and daunorubicin dose, CD25+ patients had inferior complete remission rate and overall survival compared to CD25- cases. CD25 was positively correlated with FLT3-ITD, DNMT3A- and NPM1-mutations. The adverse prognostic impact of FLT3-ITD+ AML was restricted to CD25+ patients. Importantly, CD25 expression improved AML prognostication independent of integrated, cytogenetic and mutational data, such that it re-allocated 11% of patients with integrated intermediate-risk disease based on cytogenetic/mutational profiling to the unfavorable-risk group improved the ability to identify patients at high risk of relapse. CD25+ status provides prognostic relevance in AML independent of known biomarkers and is correlated with stem-cell gene-expression signatures associated with adverse outcome in AML.

CD41 and CD61

CD41 and CD61 are positive in acute megakaryoblastic leukemia (AMKL; Figure 5.6). CD41 antigen is a transmembrane glycoprotein (IIb integrin, platelet GPIIb), essentially is restricted to megakaryocytes. CD41 is always non-covalently associated with CD61 (platelet GPIIIa, β3 integrin), to form the GPIIb-IIIa (CD41/CD61) complex.

Flow cytometric pattern in major AML subtypes

Minimally differentiated acute myeloid leukemia

FC phenotype of AML with minimal differentiation: s.CD3-, c.CD3-, CD4-, CD7+/-, CD11b-, CD11c-, CD13+, CD14-, CD15-, CD19-, c.CD22-, CD33+/-, CD34+, CD38+, CD36-, CD56-, CD64-, CD65-, c.CD79a-, CD117+, HLA-DR+, MPO-, TdT+/-

Blasts in AMLs with minimal differentiation are positive for CD34, CD117, CD13, and often CD33 and HLA-DR. TdT may be positive, and CD7 may be dimly positive or expressed by subset of blasts. Markers associated with myeloid or monocytic maturation (e.g., CD10, CD11b, CD14, CD15, CD64, or CD65), B-cell markers (CD22, cCD79a), and CD3 are negative. Similar phenotype to AML with minimal differentiation may be seen in subset of AML with myelodysplasia-related changes (AML-MRC).

AML with and without maturation

FC phenotype of AML without maturation: CD2-/rarely+, s.CD3-, c.CD3-, CD4-/+, CD7+/-, CD11b-/rarely+, CD13+, CD14-, CD15-, CD19-/rarely+, c.CD22-, CD33+/-, CD34+/rarely-, CD38+/rarely-, CD36-, CD64-, CD65-, c.CD79a-, CD117+, CD133+/-, HLA-DR+/rarely-, MPO rare blasts+, TdT+/-

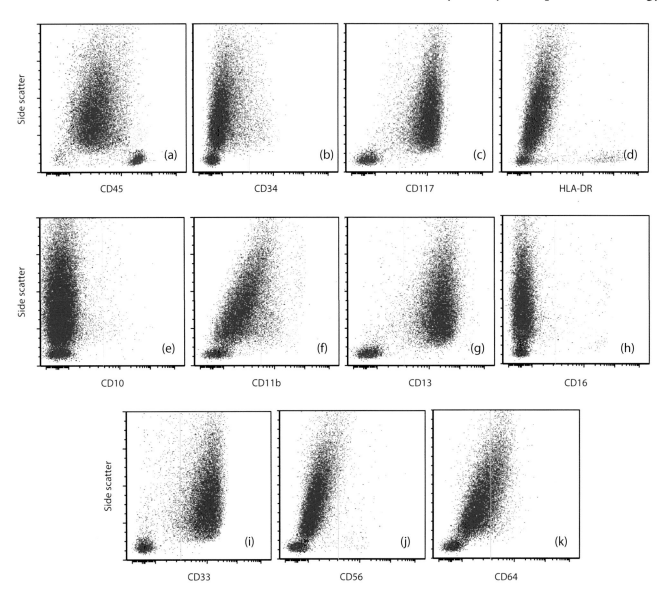

FIGURE 5.11 Acute promyelocytic leukemia (APL). Neoplastic promyelocytes (blue dots) are characterized by high side scatter (a–k; y axis), positive CD45 (a) negative CD34 (b), positive CD117 (c), negative HLA-DR (d), negative CD10 (e), negative CD11b (f), positive CD13 (g), negative CD16 (h), positive CD33 (i), negative CD56 (j), and negative to dimly positive CD64 (k). APL often show high non-specific "background" fluorescence and therefore the expression of specific markers need to be correlated with negative or "build-in" controls (e.g., with markers known to be negative such as CD3, CD8, CD19, CD20, etc.).

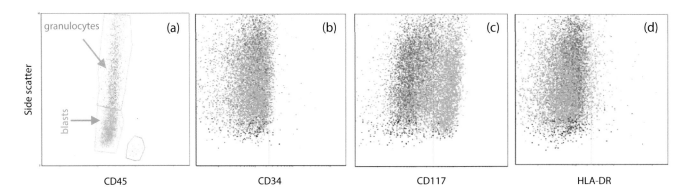

FIGURE 5.12 AML with *NPM1* mutations. Blasts (a–d; green dots) have low side scatter (a), moderate CD45 (a), negative CD34 (b), positive CD117 (c), and negative HLA-DR (d).

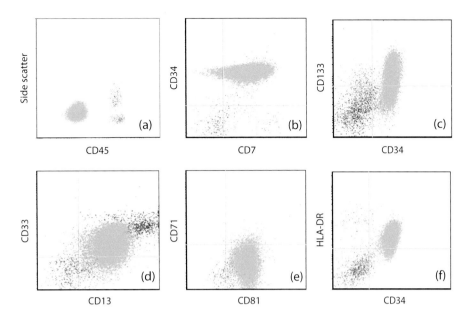

FIGURE 5.13 AML without maturation. Blasts (green dots) are characterized by low side scatter (a), dim CD45 expression (a), positive CD34 (b–c), aberrant expression of CD7 (b), positive CD133 (c), positive CD13 and CD33 (d), negative CD71 (e), dim expression of CD81 (e), and positive HLA-DR (f).

FC phenotype of AML with maturation: CD2$^{-/rarely+}$, s.CD3$^-$, c.CD3$^-$, CD4$^{-/+}$, CD7$^{+/-}$, CD11b$^{-/rarely+}$, CD11c$^{-/+}$, CD13$^+$, CD14$^-$, CD15$^{-/rarely+}$, CD19$^{-/rarely+}$, c.CD22$^-$, CD33$^{+/-}$, CD34$^{+/rarely-}$, CD38$^{+/rarely-}$, CD36$^-$, CD56$^{-/rarely+}$, CD64$^-$, CD65$^{-/rarely+}$, c.CD79a$^-$, CD117$^{+/rarely-}$, CD133$^{+/-}$, HLA-DR$^{+/rarely-}$, MPO$^+$, TdT$^{-/+}$

AML without maturation (Figure 5.13) and with maturation (Figure 5.14) are usually positive for CD4 (dim), CD11c (dim to moderate), CD13, CD33, CD34, CD117, and HLA-DR. In some cases, there is expression (often partial) of CD2, CD7, CD11b, CD19, CD56, and CD64. Subset of cases is CD34$^-$ and occasional cases are negative for HLA-DR. The correlation between genetic, morphologic, and phenotypic features in AMLs is presented in Table 5.4.

Acute promyelocytic leukemia (APL)

FC phenotype of APL
APL (hypergranular): CD2$^-$, s.CD3$^-$, c.CD3$^-$, CD4$^{-/+}$, CD7$^{+/-}$, CD11b$^-$, CD11c$^-$, CD13$^+$, CD14$^-$, CD15$^{-/rarely+(dim)}$, CD19$^-$, c.CD22$^-$, CD33$^{+bright}$, CD34$^-$, CD38$^+$, CD36$^-$, CD56$^{-/rarely+}$, CD64$^{-/dim+}$, CD65$^{-/rarely+}$, c.CD79a$^-$, CD117$^{+(may be dim)}$, CD133$^{-/rarely+}$, HLA-DR$^-$, MPO$^+$
APL-v (hypogranular): CD2$^{+/rarely-}$, s.CD3$^-$, c.CD3$^-$, CD4$^{-/+}$, CD7$^{+/-}$, CD11b$^-$, CD11c$^-$, CD13$^+$, CD14$^-$, CD15$^{-/rarely+(dim)}$, CD19$^-$, c.CD22$^-$, CD33$^{+bright}$, CD34$^{+/rarely-}$, CD38$^+$, CD36$^-$, CD56$^{-/rarely+}$, CD64$^{-/dim+}$, CD65$^{-/rarely+}$, c.CD79a$^-$, CD117$^{+(may be dim)}$, CD133$^{-/rarely+}$, HLA-DR$^-$, MPO$^+$

Classic (hypergranular) APL (Figure 5.11) has well recognized flow cytometric pattern with increased SSC, positive CD13 (often heterogeneous/variable expression), CD33 (very bright

expression), and CD117, lack of HLA-DR, CD11b, CD11c, and CD18, negative or weakly positive CD15 and CD65, negative CD34, and often positive CD64 (dim expression) [46, 47]. Lack of expression of HLA-DR is typical for APL but may be also seen in rare cases of other myeloid leukemias. Kussick et al. described HLA-DR$^-$/CD34$^-$ phenotype in AML with normal karyotype by conventional cytogenetics and association with *FLT3*-ITD [44]. AMLs with NPM1 mutation are often HLA-DR$^-$. Hypogranular APL (APL-v) is more difficult to diagnose by FC. Neoplastic promyelocytes in APL-v are usually positive for CD2, CD4, CD13, CD33, CD34, CD64, and CD117 (Figure 5.15). HLA-DR is negative, similarly to classic APL. Lack of HLA-DR, co-expression of CD2 and CD34, and lack of CD11b, CD11c, CD14, in conjunction with cytomorphology and cytochemistry (MPO, NSE) helps to differentiate APL-v from other types of AML, especially acute monoblastic leukemia. Occasional cases of APL may show very dim or partial expression of CD117, which in conjunction with lack of both CD34 and HLA-DR may lead to misdiagnosis as benign process. In those APL cases with very dim/partial CD117, careful correlation with cytomorphology, pattern of CD45 versus SSC, presence of high autofluorescence and characteristic bright expression of CD33 (much brighter than monocytes and normal neutrophils) help to identify APL. Figure 5.16 presents the summary of four flow cytometric patterns of APL: hypergranular (pattern 1), hypogranular (pattern 2), APL with partial involvement of blood or BM (pattern 3), and APL composed of hypergranular and hypogranular clones (pattern 4) [see details in Chapter 23].

AML with *NPM1* mutation

FC phenotype of AML with *NPM1* mutation: CD2$^{-/rarely+}$, s.CD3$^-$, c.CD3$^-$, CD4$^{-/+}$, CD5$^{+/-}$, CD7$^{+/-}$, CD11b$^{-/rarely+}$, CD11c$^+$, CD13$^{+/rarely-}$, CD14$^{-/rarely+}$, CD15$^{-/rarely+}$, CD19$^-$, c.CD22$^-$, CD33$^+$, CD34$^{-/rarely+}$, CD36$^-$, CD38$^+$, CD56$^{+/-}$, CD64$^{-/+}$, CD65$^{-/rarely+}$, CD79a$^-$, CD117$^+$, CD133$^{+/-}$, HLA-DR$^{-/+}$, MPO$^{+/-}$

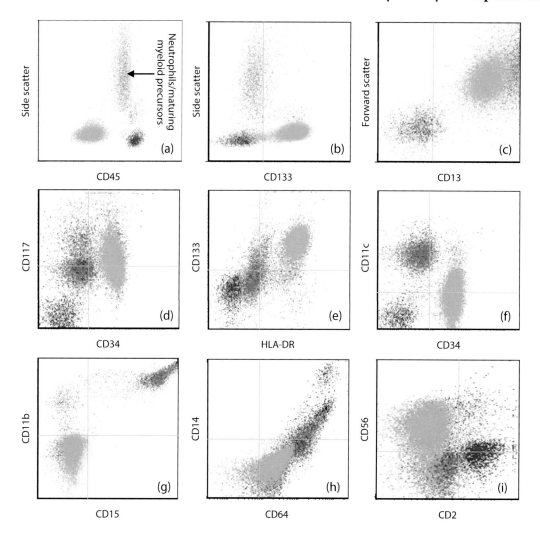

FIGURE 5.14   AML with maturation. Blasts (green dots) show dim expression of CD45 (a), low side scatter (a–b) and high forward scatter (c). Note the presence of maturing myeloid precursors and neutrophils (a, grey dots, arrow). Blasts display the following phenotype: CD133$^+$ (b), CD13$^+$ (c), CD34$^+$ (d), CD117^{dim+} (d), HLA-DR$^+$ (e), partially CD11c$^+$ (f), CD11b$^-$ (g), CD15$^-$ (g), CD14$^-$ (h), CD64$^-$ (h), and CD56$^+$ (i).

AML with NPM1 mutation shows variable phenotype, with significant subset of cases showing monocytic differentiation (AMML-like or acute monocytic leukemia-like) or features similar to APL-v. Blasts are often HLA-DR$^-$ and CD34$^-$.

Acute myelomonocytic leukemia (AMML)

FC phenotype of AMML
   Myeloblastic component: CD2$^{-/rarely+}$, s.CD3$^-$, c.CD3$^-$, CD4$^{-/+}$, CD7$^{+/-}$, CD11b$^{-/rarely+}$, CD11c$^{-/+}$, CD13$^+$, CD14$^-$, CD15$^{-/+}$, CD19$^{-/rarely+}$, c.CD22$^-$, CD33$^{+/-}$, CD34$^{+/rarely-}$, CD38$^{+/rarely-}$, CD36$^-$, CD56$^{-/rarely+}$, CD64$^-$, CD65$^{-/+}$, c.CD79a$^-$, CD117$^{+/rarely-}$, CD133$^{+/-}$, HLA-DR$^{+/rarely-}$, MPO$^+$, TdT$^{-/+}$
   Monocytic component: CD2$^{+/-}$, CD4$^+$, CD11b$^+$, CD11c$^+$, CD14$^+$, CD15$^+$, CD34$^-$, CD36$^+$, CD56$^{-/+}$, CD64$^+$, CD117$^-$, HLA-DR$^+$

AMML shows two distinct neoplastic populations: (1) myeloblasts and (2) monocytic cells (Figure 5.17). Myeloblasts usually show the phenotype similar to AML with/without maturation,

and monocytes are positive for CD4, CD11b, CD11c, CD14, CD64, and HLA-DR. In contrast to acute monoblastic leukemia or CMML, monocytes from acute myelomonocytic leukemia do not display in majority of cases overtly abnormal phenotype (such as loss or variable expression of CD14 or strongly positive CD56). Blasts with separate granulocytic and monocytic phenotypes are also typical for AML with inv(16)/t(16;16).

AML with t(8;21)/*RUNX1-RUNX1T1*

FC phenotype of AML with t(8;21): CD2$^{-/rarely+}$, s.CD3$^-$, c.CD3$^-$, CD4$^{-/+}$, CD7$^{+/rarely-}$, CD11b$^{-/rarely+}$, CD11c$^{-/+}$, CD13$^{+/rarely-}$, CD14$^-$, CD15$^{-/rarely+}$, CD19$^{+/rarely-}$, c.CD22$^-$, CD33$^{+/rarely-}$, CD34$^{+/rarely-}$, CD38$^{+/rarely-}$, CD36$^-$, CD56$^{+/rarely-}$, CD64$^-$, CD65$^{-/rarely+}$, CD79a$^{+/rarely-}$, CD117$^{+/rarely-}$, CD133$^{+/-}$, HLA-DR$^{+/rarely-}$, MPO$^+$, TdT$^{-/rarely+}$

Apart from blastic and myeloid markers, this variant of AML shows often positive expression of CD19 and CD56. HLA-DR is positive.

TABLE 5.4: Immunophenotypic-Morphologic-Genotypic Correlation in AML

Category	Phenotype	Morphology
AML with t(8;21)	Aberrant expression of B-cell antigens (CD19⁺, PAX5⁺, CD79a⁺) and CD56⁺	Blasts with perinuclear hofs and occasional Auer rods and/or pale pink colored granules
APL, hypergranular	HLA-DR⁻, CD34⁻, CD117⁺, MPO⁺	Numerous Auer rods ("fagot cells")
APL, hypogranular	HLA-DR⁻, CD34⁺, CD2⁺, CD117⁺, MPO⁺	Irregular nuclei
AML with *FLT3*-ITD	CD7⁺, CD34⁻, HLA-DR⁻, CD123⁺, CD133⁻, CD25⁺/⁻	"Cuplike nuclei" (nuclear invagination)
AML with *NPM1* mutation	CD34⁻, HLA-DR⁻, CD117⁺/⁻, CD64⁺	Nuclear invagination, myelomonocytic or monocytic features
AML with inv(16)/t(16;16)	Distinct populations of blasts (CD34⁺/CD117⁺) and monocytes (CD14⁺/CD64⁺); aberrant CD2 expression by blasts	Atypical immature eosinophils with purple or basophilic granules
AML with t(6;9)	Myeloid or monocytic phenotype	Blood with basophilia
AML with inv(3)/t(3;3)	Myeloid, monocytic or megakaryocytic phenotype, often CD7⁺	Monolobated or hypolobated megakaryocytes

Acute monoblastic leukemia

Phenotype of acute monoblastic (monocytic) leukemia: CD2⁻/⁺, s.CD3⁻, c.CD3⁻, CD4⁺, CD7⁺/⁻, CD11b⁺⁽ᵛᵃʳⁱᵃᵇˡᵉ⁾/ʳᵃʳᵉˡʸ⁻, CD11c⁺, CD13⁺, CD14⁻/⁺⁽ᵛᵃʳⁱᵃᵇˡᵉ/ᵖᵃʳᵗⁱᵃˡ⁾, CD15⁺, CD19⁻, c.CD22⁻, CD33⁺, CD34⁻/ʳᵃʳᵉˡʸ⁺, CD38⁺/ʳᵃʳᵉˡʸ⁻, CD36⁺, CD56⁺/ʳᵃʳᵉˡʸ⁻, CD64⁺, CD65⁺, c.CD79a⁻, CD117⁻/ʳᵃʳᵉˡʸ⁺, CD133⁻, HLA-DR⁺/ʳᵃʳᵉˡʸ⁻, MPO⁻/ʳᵃʳᵉˡʸ⁺

Monoblasts (promonocytes) from acute monoblastic (monocytic) leukemia usually have bright expression of CD45 and slightly increased SSC (Figures 5.18 and 5.19) placing them in a "monocytic" gate on CD45 versus SSC display. CD34 and CD117 are often negative but may be positive in less differentiated cases (CD117 more often than CD34). Monoblastic (monocytic) leukemias are positive for CD11b, CD11c, CD13 (dim), CD33 (bright), CD64, and HLA-DR and usually express also CD4 (dim), CD15,

CD56, and CD65. In contrast to benign monocytes, the expression of CD14 in monoblastic leukemia is either negative, partially positive, or heterogeneous ("smeary" with predominance of negative to dimly positive cells). CD123 may be positive. Apart from CD2 and CD56, monoblasts may also display aberrant expression of CD7, CD10, CD16, and CD23.

Acute erythroid leukemia (AEL, pure erythroid leukemia)

FC phenotype of AEL: CD45⁻/ʳᵃʳᵉˡʸ⁺, CD71⁺ᵇʳⁱᵍʰᵗ, GPHA⁻/⁺, CD117⁺⁽ᵒᶠᵗᵉⁿ ᵈⁱᵐ⁾/ʳᵃʳᵉˡʸ⁻, CD34⁻/ʳᵃʳᵉˡʸ⁺, CD36⁺, CD56⁻/ʳᵃʳᵉˡʸ⁺, HLA-DR⁻/ʳᵃʳᵉˡʸ⁺, TdT⁻

Blasts from AEL usually do not express CD45 and are positive for CD71 (strong expression; Figure 5.20). Other markers which are often positive include glycophorin A (GPHA; CD235a), CD117,

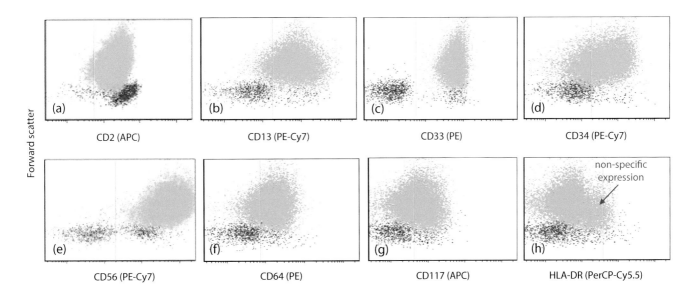

FIGURE 5.15 APL-v with typical phenotype and aberrant expression of CD56: CD2⁺ (a), CD13⁺ (b), CD33⁺ (c), CD34⁺ (d), CD56⁺ (e), CD64⁺ (f), CD117⁺ (g), and HLA-DR⁻ (h).

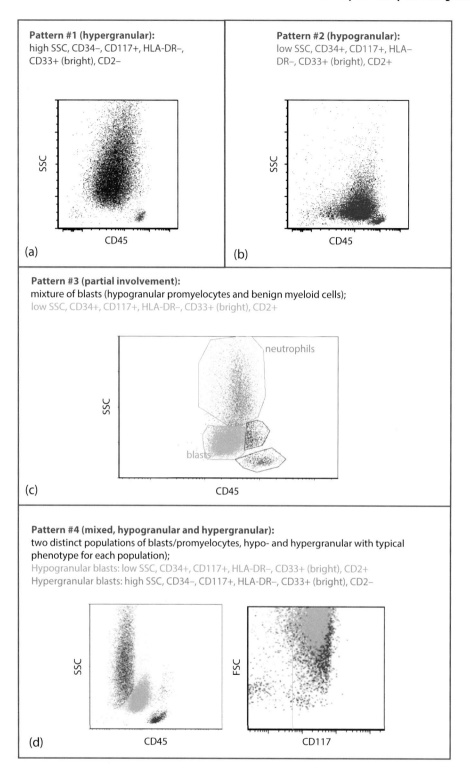

FIGURE 5.16 Four major patterns of APL in flow cytometry analysis. (a) The most common variant, hypergranular APL is characterized by high side scatter (SSC). (b) Hypogranular variant (pattern 2) is characterized by low side scatter (similar to majority of non-APL AMLs), positive CD117 and often positive expression of CD34 and CD2. (c) Pattern 3 shows partial involvement of blood or BM by APL with significant mixture of benign neutrophils and/or benign maturing myeloid precursors. (d) Pattern 4 shows presence of both hypergranular and hypogranular clones of APL. Both clones are positive for CD117, but only hypogranular blasts show positive expression of CD2 and CD34.

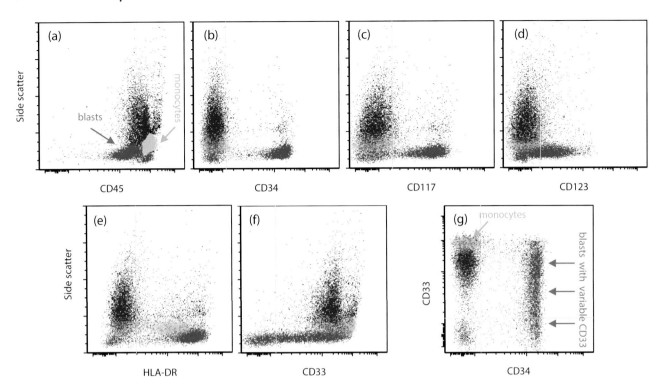

FIGURE 5.17 Acute myelomonocytic leukemia. Flow cytometry analysis shows blasts (≥20%; blue dots), monocytes (green dots), and granulocytes (purple dots). Blasts have low side scatter and dim to moderate CD45 (a), positive CD34 (b), CD117, (c), HLA-DR (d), and CD33 (e–f; aberrant variable expression). Monocytes have bright CD45 (a), positive HLA-DR (e), and bright CD33 (e–f).

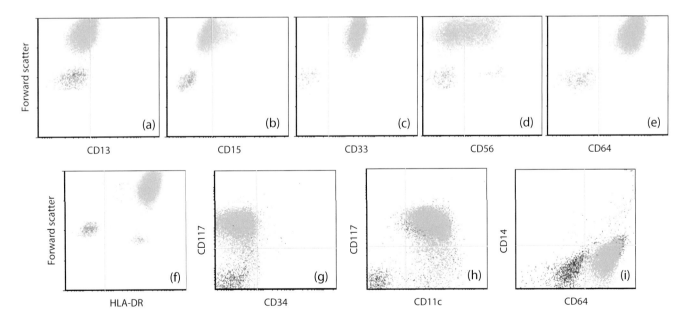

FIGURE 5.18 Acute monoblastic leukemia. Monoblasts (green dots) are characterized by high forward scatter (a–f), aberrant loss of CD13 (a), partially positive CD15 (b), bright expression of CD33 (c), partially positive CD56 (d), bright expression of CD64 (e), positive HLA-DR (f), negative CD34 (g), positive CD117 (g–h), positive CD11c (h), and aberrant loss of CD14 (i).

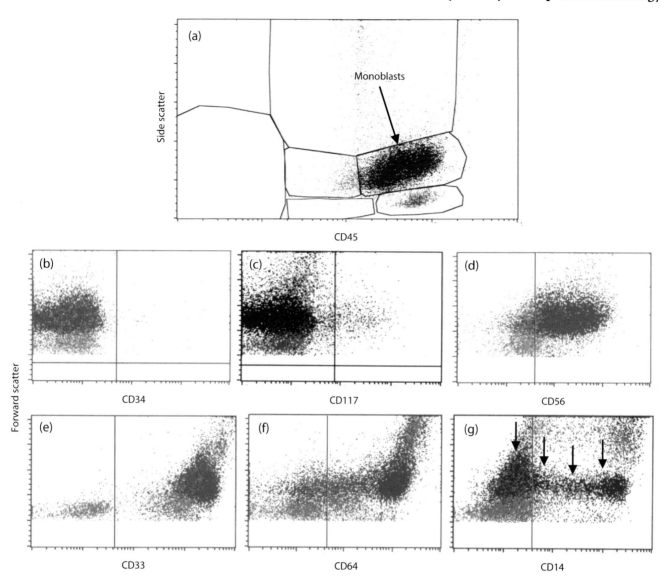

FIGURE 5.19 Acute monoblastic leukemia: monoblasts are CD45$^+$ (a), CD34$^-$ (b), CD117$^-$ (c), CD56$^+$ (d), CD33$^+$ (e), and CD64$^+$ (f). CD14 is variably expressed (g; arrows) with many blasts being negative.

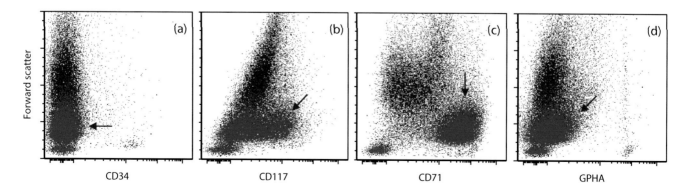

FIGURE 5.20 Acute erythroid leukemia (AEL, pure erythroid leukemia). Blasts (blue dots, arrow) are negative for CD34 (a), positive for CD117 (b), and strongly positive for CD71 (c). GPHA is negative (d).

CD43, E-cadherin, and hemoglobin A. CD34 and HLA-DR are most often negative. GPHA tends to stain more mature cells, whereas both CD71 and E-cadherin stain immature precursors.

Acute megakaryoblastic leukemia

FC phenotype of acute megakaryoblastic leukemia: CD7$^{-/rarely+}$, CD13$^{-/rarely+}$, CD15$^-$, CD33$^{+/-}$, CD34$^{+/rarely-}$, CD36$^+$, CD41$^+$, CD42b$^{+/rarely-}$, CD45$^{+/rarely-}$, CD61$^+$, CD64$^{+(dim/-)}$, CD71^{+dim}, CD117$^{+(often\ dim)/rarely-}$, CD56$^{-/rarely+}$, HLA-DR$^{-/rarely+(dim)}$, MPO$^-$, TdT$^-$

Blasts from acute megakaryoblastic leukemia express CD36, CD41, and CD61, may be positive for CD13, CD33, and CD117, and are negative for CD34 and TdT (Figure 5.6). CD45 and HLA-DR may be negative.

Leukemia-associated immunophenotype (LAIP)

Blasts often display aberrant immunophenotype (LAIP; leukemia-associated immunophenotype) which helps to differentiate MRD from normal marrow precursors:

- asynchronous antigen expression (e.g., expression of CD11b or CD15 by myeloblasts)
- lineage infidelity (expression of B- or T-cell markers, CD56, and/or CD10 by myeloblasts or monoblasts)
- antigen overexpression
- absence of lineage specific antigen (e.g., loss or partial expression of CD13 or CD33 by myeloblasts; loss of CD11b and/or CD14 by monoblasts)
- aberrant light-scatter properties (e.g., very high SSC)
- aberrant expression of CD45 (e.g., negative or partial expression)

Among antigens most commonly being aberrantly expressed by blasts in AML are CD7, and CD56, followed by CD2, CD5, CD11b, CD11c, CD10, CD15, CD19, CD45, CD65, and HLA-DR (Figures 5.21–5.23). The recognition of LAP can be used to monitor patients following chemotherapy or BM transplant and to help distinguish recovering BM form residual disease [48–59]. LAP can be identified in 60%–94% of patients with AML [54, 60, 61]. In series reported by Al-Mawali et al. the most common LAPs identified were CD117$^+$/CD15$^+$, CD117$^+$/CD65$^+$, CD34$^+$/CD15$^+$, and CD34$^+$/CD65$^+$ (these were present in 49%, 43%, 39%, and 29% of AML cases, respectively) [54]. Blasts in Down-syndrome-associated megakaryoblastic leukemia are more likely to express CD7 and CD11b than those in patients without DS [62].

Sensitivity of MRD detection by FC can approach 1 leukemic cell per 10^4–10^5 normal cells [54, 63, 64]. Based on the level of MRD (number of residual tumor cells determined by FC), San Miguel et al. suggested four risk categories for disease-free and overall survival in AML: very low-risk ($<10^{-4}$), low risk (10^{-3}–10^{-4}), intermediate risk (10^{-2}–10^{-3}), and high risk ($>10^{-2}$) [65]. The relapse-free survival rates at 3 years for these risk groups were 100%, 85%, 55%, and 25%, respectively. FC analysis enables the physicians to monitor treatment and modify it based of FC findings. Presence of blasts expressing CD34, CD123, CD25, and CD99 positively correlates with the internal tandem duplications (ITD) mutation in the *FLT3* gene in AML [66]. Detailed discussion of LAIP and MRD in AML is presented in Chapter 24.

Differential diagnosis of AML based on flow cytometry pattern

Myeloblasts versus lymphoblasts
AML is positive for CD117 and often also CD34 and usually express markers associated with granulocytic or monocytic differentiation, such CD11b, CD11c, CD13, CD14, CD15, CD33, CD64, CD65, and MPO. B-ALL is typically positive for TdT and CD34, negative for CD117 and displays B-antigens such as CD19, CD22, and CD79a (CD20 is most often absent). CD10 is often brightly positive in B-ALL and is negative in AML (rare monoblastic leukemias may be dimly CD10$^+$). T-ALL is positive for cytoplasmic CD3 (surface CD3 is most often negative), TdT, and CD7, and may be positive for CD34, CD1a, CD10, CD2, and CD5. It may show dual CD4/CD8 expression. TdT is more often positive in ALL, but may be positive in AML, especially less differentiated variants. Lymphoid markers, CD2, CD7, CD19, and CD56 may be aberrantly expressed by AML. The co-expression of CD19 and CD56 is seen in AML with t(8;21). CD2 is often expressed by acute monoblastic leukemia and hypogranular APL but may also be positive in AML with/without maturation. In AML with aberrant CD7, the expression of CD7 is often dim or partial, in contrast to usually bright expression of CD7 in T-ALL.

Both B- and T-ALL may display aberrant expression of CD13, CD33, and/or CD56. Presence of c.CD3 supports the diagnosis of T-ALL, whereas co-expression of CD19, CD22, and CD79a indicates B-ALL. Rare cases of T-ALL may show aberrant CD117 expression, most often indicating the specific subtype of T-ALL, early T-cell precursor ALL (ETP-ALL).

Myeloid lineage can be definitively confirmed by either positive MPO (FC, immunohistochemistry, or cytochemistry) or presence of at least two monocytic markers: non-specific esterase (NSE), CD11c, CD14, CD64, or lysozyme. T-lineage is defined by expression of c.CD3 or s.CD3, and B-lineage is defined by strong expression of CD19 and strong expression of at least **one** of the following antigens: CD10, CD79a, or c.CD22 (if the expression of CD19 is weak, strong expression of **two** of those additional markers is needed) [67]. Blasts expressing myeloid and lymphoid markers, as defined above, can be classified as MPAL (acute leukemia of ambiguous lineage; Figure 5.24). Acute leukemia (CD34$^{+/-}$, TdT$^{+/-}$, HLA-DR$^{+/-}$, CD38$^{+/-}$) without any specific myeloid or lymphoid markers, including c.CD3, GPHO, MPO, c.CD22, CD41, CD61, CD71, cCD79a, and strong CD19, is classified as AUL [67].

Monoblasts versus blastic plasmacytoid dendritic cells
Strong expression of CD4, CD56, and CD123 is typical for BPDCN, but those markers are by no means specific, as they are often positive in other leukemias, especially acute monoblastic leukemia. Therefore, differential diagnosis of BPDCN and acute monoblastic leukemia may be sometimes difficult by FC (Figure 5.25). In addition, blast phase of MPN or therapy-related myeloid neoplasm (post-therapy AML) often show unusual phenotype including strong expression of CD4 and CD56 requiring differential diagnosis from BPDCN. Presence of skin lesion, typical for BPDCN is often seen also in acute monoblastic leukemias (extramedullary myeloid tumor; monoblastic sarcoma). Apart from CD4, CD56, and CD123, both BPDCN and acute monoblastic leukemia are positive for HLA-DR and may be positive for

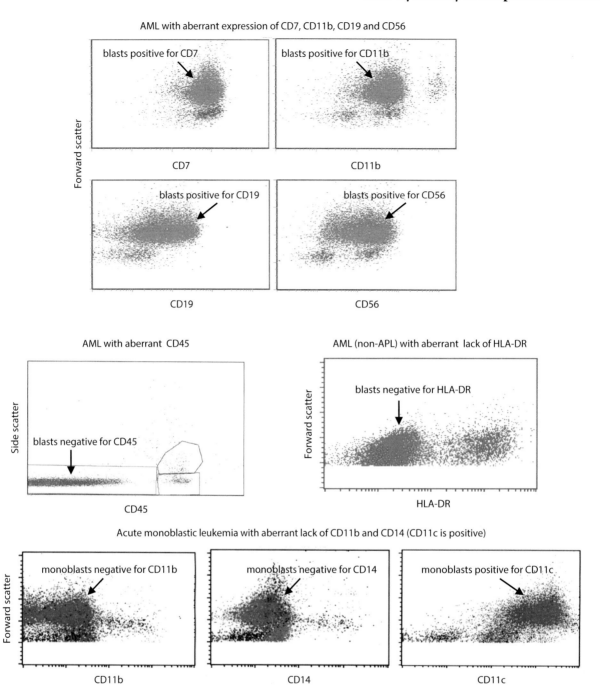

FIGURE 5.21 AML (4 cases) with aberrant immunophenotype (LAIP).

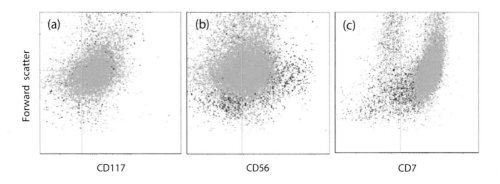

FIGURE 5.22 LAIP: blasts (green dots) are CD117 positive (a) and show aberrant expression of CD56 (b) and CD7 (c).

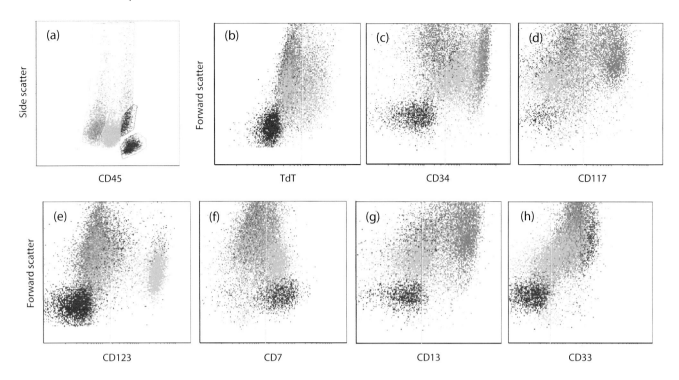

FIGURE 5.23 LAIP: two distinct populations of blasts are noted: one population (orange dots) shows dim CD45 (a), variable (mostly negative) TdT (b), bright CD34 (c), bright CD117 (d), negative CD123 (e), dim CD7 (f), bright CD13 (g), and moderate CD33 (h). The second population (green dots) shows moderate CD45 (a), partial TdT (b), dim to moderate CD34 (c), negative CD117 (d), bright CD123 (e), moderate CD7 (f), dim CD13 (g), and dim CD33 (h).

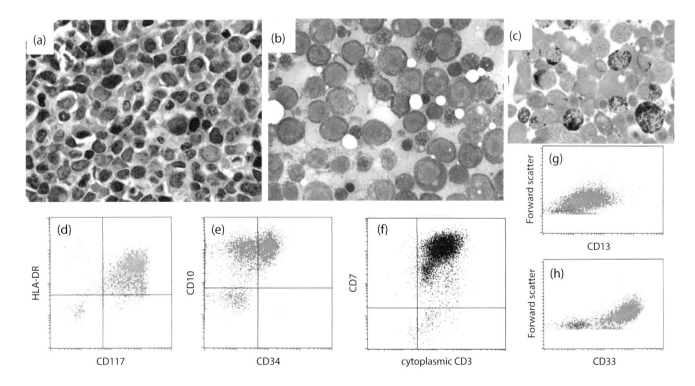

FIGURE 5.24 Mixed phenotype acute leukemia (MPAL; AML/T-ALL) – bone marrow. (a) Histologic section with H&E staining shows hypercellular bone marrow showing complete replacement by large blasts. (b) Aspirate smear shows blasts and rare erythroid precursors. (c) Blasts are positive for MPO (cytochemistry). (d–h) Flow cytometry analysis shows the following phenotype of blasts: HLA-DR+ (d), CD117+ (d), CD34+ (e), CD10+ (e), CD7+ (f), cytoplasmic CD3+ (f), CD13+ (g; dim expression), and CD33+ (h).

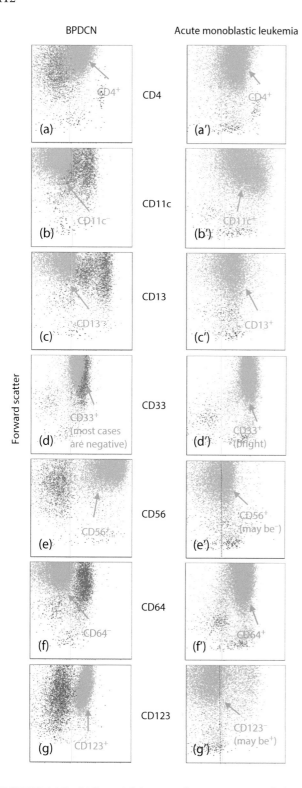

FIGURE 5.25 Differential diagnosis between BPDCN (left column) and acute monoblastic leukemia (right column). BPCDN is positive for CD4 (a), negative or CD11c (b), negative for CD13 (c) [rare cases may be CD13⁺], positive for CD33 (d) [majority of cases are CD33⁻], positive for CD56 (e), negative for CD64 (f), and positive for CD123 (g). Acute monoblastic leukemia is positive for CD4 (a′), positive for CD11c (b′), positive for CD13 (c′), positive for CD33 (d′), positive for CD56 (e′) [subset of cases is negative], positive or CD64 with bright expression (f′), and negative for CD123 (g′) [subset of cases may be positive].

CD2 and CD117. While some cases of BPDCN may show CD33, strong expression of both CD13 and CD33, or positive expression of CD13, CD33, and CD117 indicates acute monoblastic leukemia. Bright expression of CD64 and CD11c, positive CD11b and/or positive CD14 excludes BPDCN. In difficult cases, cytochemistry staining for NSE may help in differential diagnosis (positive NSE confirms acute monoblastic leukemia). FC pattern similar to BPDCN and acute monoblastic leukemia is seen in a subset of AML with *NPM1* mutation.

Monocytic versus granulocytic differentiation (monoblasts versus myeloblasts)

Acute monoblastic (monocytic) leukemia is positive for CD11c, CD13, CD15, CD33 (often bright), CD38, CD64, CD65, and HLA-DR. Many cases are also positive for CD4, CD11b, CD14, and CD56, and occasional cases express CD2, CD10, CD16, and/or CD23. Blastic markers, CD34, TdT, and CD117, are usually negative, but subset of cases (especially less differentiated) may be positive for CD117 or less often CD34. The expression of CD11b and CD14 varies from negative, partial, dim positive to variable ("smeary") but in more differentiated variants may be moderate or even bright (as in benign monocytes). The expression of CD45 is bright in most cases and SSC is slightly increased. Positive CD11b, CD11c, CD14, and HLA-DR in acute monoblastic leukemia differentiate it from APL (the latter is negative for these markers). Acute monoblastic leukemia often shows bright CD64, whereas the expression of CD64 in other types of AML, including APL is usually dim or negative. Positive CD11b, CD14, CD15, and CD65, and bright expression of CD11c and CD64 favor acute monoblastic leukemia over AML with/without maturation (the latter is most often negative for CD11b, CD14, CD15, CD65 and shows dim to moderate CD11c and CD64). CD56 is often positive in acute monoblastic leukemia, but it is not specific and may be expressed in other types of AML, plasma cell neoplasm, metastatic carcinoma with neuroendocrine features and BPDCN. Presence of ≥20% of monocytes and their precursors distinguishes AMML from cases of AML with/without maturation which may show minute population of monocytes. Strong expression of CD4, CD56, and CD123 by blasts without expression of myeloid markers should raise the possibility of BPDCN.

FC features which help to differentiate monoblasts from myeloblasts include:

- Moderate SSC (monoblasts) versus low SSC (myeloblasts)
- Bright CD45 (monoblasts) versus dim to moderate CD45 (myeloblasts)
- Bright CD64 expression (monoblasts) versus negative or dim CD64 (myeloblasts)
- Bright CD11c expression (monoblasts) versus negative or dim CD11c (myeloblasts)
- Positive CD11b (monoblasts)
- Positive CD14 (monoblasts)
- Bright CD34 expression (myeloblasts)
- Positive TdT (myeloblasts)
- Positive CD2, CD10, CD15, CD16, CD23, and/or CD65 favors monoblasts over myeloblasts
- CD56 expression is seen in monoblasts and myeloblasts but is more often present in acute monoblastic leukemia
- CD123 expression is seen in monoblasts and myeloblasts but is more often present in acute monoblastic leukemia

APL versus neutrophils/maturing myeloid precursors
Hypergranular (classic) APL has characteristic FC pattern (Figure 5.11):

- High SSC
- Moderate CD45
- Positive CD117 (may be dim)
- Negative HLA-DR
- Negative CD7, CD10, CD11b, CD11c, CD14, and CD34
- Dim (or negative) CD64
- Very bright CD33 (brighter than in normal neutrophils or monocytes)
- High (non-specific) background fluorescence, including non-specific staining with viability dyes mimicking non-viable cells

Granulocytes and maturing myeloid precursors (promyelocytes, myelocytes, metamyelocytes) have high SSC and moderate CD45 expression. APL shows similar SSC versus CD45 pattern, but the SSC in APL is slightly lower than in normal granulocytes and the expression of CD45 is rather homogenous, whereas maturing myeloid precursors show subset of cell with dimmer and subset of cells with brighter CD45 (reflecting different stages of myeloid maturation). In contrast to APL, granulocytes are positive for CD10, CD11b, CD11c, and CD16 and are negative for CD117 (Figure 5.26). Granulocytes/maturing myeloid precursors from MDS and MPN may display aberrant down-regulation of CD10, CD11b, CD16, and/or CD45 reflecting leftward shift and/or dysmaturation, as well as decreased SSC. Positive CD117 expression, negative CD11c and high SSC favor APL over abnormal (dyspoietic) granulocytes.

Hypogranular APL is characterized by:

- Low SSC
- Negative HLA-DR
- Positive CD117 (may be dim)
- Often positive CD2 and/or CD34
- Negative CD7, CD10, CD11b, CD11c, and CD14
- Dim (or negative) CD64
- Very bright CD33 (brighter than in normal neutrophils or monocytes)
- High (non-specific) background fluorescence, including non-specific staining with viability dyes mimicking non-viable cells

Benign granulocytes differ from hypogranular APL by higher SSC, negative CD117, negative CD34, and positive expression of CD10, CD11b, and CD16 (Figure 5.27).

APL versus HLA-DR-negative AML and AML with *NPM1* mutation
Blasts in non-APL AML usually have low SSC and are positive for HLA-DR and CD34, whereas neoplastic (hypergranular) promyelocytes have high SSC (they are located in the similar area as normal granulocytes on CD45 versus SSC dot plot display) and lack the expression of HLA-DR and CD34. In addition, hypergranular APL shows strong expression of CD33, negative CD4, negative CD11c, and dimly positive CD64. Rare cases of AML with/without maturation and acute monoblastic leukemia may be characterized by high SSC ("granulocytic" gate), similarly to classic APL (Figure 5.28).

HLA-DR-negative AML (Figure 5.29) may be difficult to differentiate by FC from hypogranular APL. Both leukemias are characterized by low SSC, positive CD117, positive or negative CD34, negative CD11b and positive myeloid markers (CD13 and CD33). Hypogranular APL often shows dim CD64 and positive for CD2 (usually dim or partial), whereas AML only rarely expresses CD2 and is most often CD64⁻. Positive CD4 and CD11c would favor AML (not APL). Correlation with cytologic features is often helpful, as even hypogranular APL shows occasional atypical promyelocytes with cytoplasmic granules or Auer rods. Final diagnosis should be based on FISH and PCR studies for *PML-RARA*.

AML with *NPM1* mutation is often HLA-DR⁻ and display low SSC and positive CD117, resembling hypogranular variant of APL.

The FC features that favor the diagnosis of NPM1⁺ AML over hypogranular APL include:

- Lack of CD2 expression in *NPM1⁺* AML (CD2 is often positive in hypogranular APL)
- Lack of CD4 expression in *NPM1⁺* AML (CD4 is positive in subset of hypogranular APL)
- Aberrant lack of CD13 (loss of CD13 is rarely seen in APL)
- Bright expression of CD33 (brighter than in normal neutrophils or monocytes) is typical for APL
- Lack of CD64 expression (APLs are often dim CD64⁺)
- Positive CD11c expression (APLs are CD11c⁻)
- Positive CD56 expression (CD56 may be positive in both entities, but is less common in APL)
- High (non-specific) background fluorescence, including non-specific staining with viability dyes mimicking non-viable cells is typical for APL

Hypogranular APL (APLv) versus acute monoblastic leukemia
Expression of HLA-DR, CD11b, and CD11c helps to differentiate acute monoblastic leukemia (HLA-DR⁺/CD11b⁺/⁻/CD11c⁺) from the hypogranular variant of APL (HLA-DR⁻/CD11b⁻/CD11c⁻). Moreover, monoblasts may show partial or variable ("smeary") expression of CD14, and may be positive for CD10, CD16, and/or CD23 (those markers are negative in APL). Acute monoblastic leukemia is typically HLA-DR⁺, with bright expression of this antigen, but occasional cases may be HLA-DR⁻. Both APL and acute monoblastic leukemia express CD64, but the expression is usually dim or partial in APL, and moderate or bright in acute monoblastic leukemia. Acute monoblastic leukemias often express CD56, whereas CD56 is only rarely positive in APL. Figure 5.30 compares FC features of acute monoblastic leukemia and hypogranular APL. In difficult cases, correlation with cytochemical staining for NSE and MPO on aspirate smears may help in differential diagnosis (APL is NSE⁻ and MPO⁺).

Blasts versus maturing myeloid precursors with leftward shift and/or dysmaturation
As mentioned above, myeloblasts differ from maturing myeloid precursors/neutrophils not only be expression of "blastic" markers (CD34, CD117, CD133, and TdT), but also by lack of markers associated with maturation, such as CD10, CD11b, CD15, CD16, or CD65. Occasional cases of AML show lack of expression of both CD34 and CD117. Additionally, subset of cases may show aberrant expression of markers typical for mature cells. On the other hand, mature elements from patients with MDS, MPN, regenerating marrow after chemotherapy or patients treated with

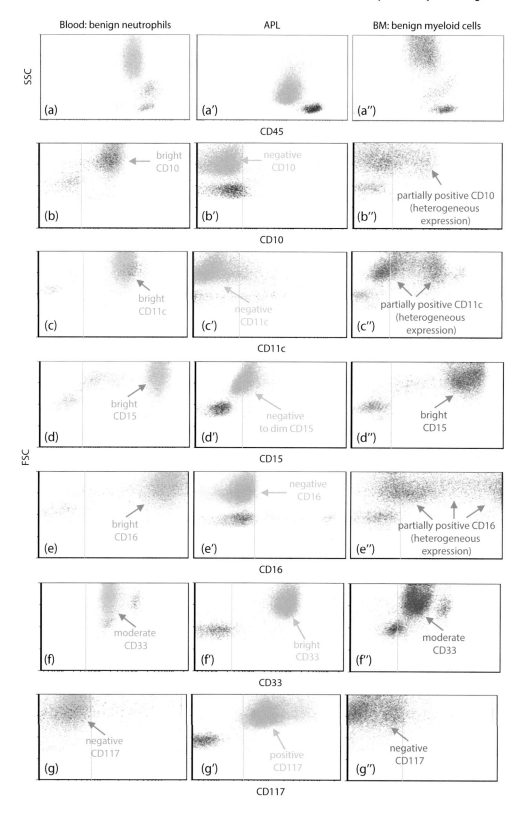

FIGURE 5.26 Comparison of the expression of CD45 (a–a″), CD10 (b–b″), CD11c (c–c″), CD15 (d–d″), CD16 (e–e″), CD33 (f–f″), and CD117 (g–g″) of benign neutrophils (left column; light blue dots), neoplastic promyelocytes from APL (middle column; green dots), and maturing myeloid precursors from benign BM (right column; dark blue dots). Neutrophils are characterized by moderate to birth CD45 (a), and bright expression of CD10 (b), CD11 (c), CD15 (d), and CD16 (e), moderate CD33 (f), and negative CD117 (g). APL is characterized by moderate CD45 (a′), negative CD10 (b′) and CD11c (c′), negative to partially dim CD15 (d′), negative CD16 (e′), bright CD33 (f′) and positive CD117 (g′). Benign maturing myeloid precursors show moderate CD45 (a″), variable CD10 (ranging from negative to positive; b″), variable CD11c (c″), bright CD15 (d″), variable CD16 (e″), moderate CD33 (f″), and negative CD117 (g″). *Abbreviation*: SSC, side scatter; FSC, forward scatter.

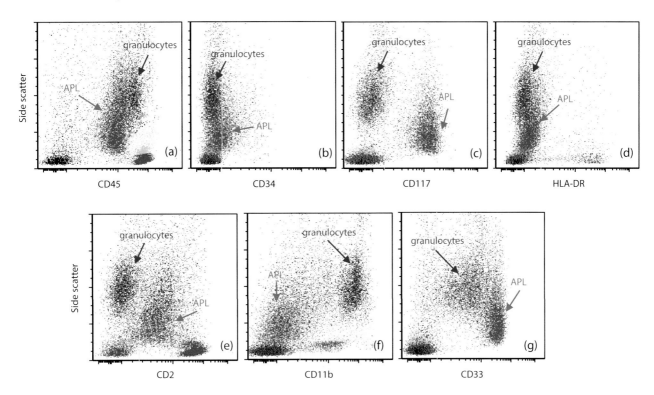

FIGURE 5.27 Phenotypic differences between hypogranular APL and granulocytes in the BM with partial involvement by APL. Hypogranular APL cells (blue dots) show low SSC (a–g), dim CD45 (a), negative to dim (partial) CD34 (b), positive CD117 (c), negative HLA-DR (d), positive CD2 (e), negative CD11b (f), and bright CD33 (g) whereas benign granulocytes (purple dots) show higher SSC (a), negative CD34 (b), negative CD117 (c), negative HLA-DR (d), negative CD2 (e), brightly positive CD11b (f), and dimmer CD33 (g).

granulocyte-colony stimulating factor (G-CSF, Neupogen) may show decreased SSC and often show prominent down-regulation of CD10, CD11b, CD15, and/or CD16 resulting in FC pattern similar to that seen in AML (Figure 5.31).

AML versus acute undifferentiated leukemia
AML versus MPAL (mixed phenotype acute leukemia)
MPAL, a variant of acute leukemia of ambiguous lineage) is a very rare disease with complex clinical, cytogenetic, immunophenotypic, and/or molecular genetic features and with adverse clinical outcome [21, 36, 68–71]. FC immunophenotyping using a broad phenotypic panel, immunohistochemical analysis and cytochemistry studies for myeloperoxidase and nonspecific esterase (NSE) are needed to establish the diagnosis of MPAL. Current WHO classification replaced previous scoring system proposed by the European Group for the immunological classification of Leukemias [21, 38, 68]. In the new WHO classification of leukemias, only markers considered most lineage-specific have been retained for lineage assignment [70]. The B-lineage is confirmed by strong expression of CD19 with at least one of the following strongly expressed: CD79a, cytoplasmic CD22 (c.CD22), or CD10 (if the expression of CD19 is dim, at least two of these markers need to be strongly positive). The T-lineage is confirmed by surface CD3 (s.CD3) positivity or strong cytoplasmic CD3 (c.CD3) expression. Myeloid lineage is confirmed by positive MPO staining (FC, cytochemistry, or immunohistochemistry) or presence of at least two monocytic markers: CD11c, CD14, CD64, lysosome, or NSE. Most cases of MPAL co-express myeloid markers with B- or T-cell lineage specific marker (Figure 5.13). Rare cases may co-express B- and T-cell markers. MPAL are often positive for CD34, TdT, and HLA-DR.

In MPAL cases with more than one blast population, different blast populations may display different phenotype, e.g., myeloblasts with MPO expression and B-lymphoblasts with CD19 and CD10 expression. The acute leukemia cases with two distinct blasts population, with one population showing the phenotype of AML with minimal differentiation (CD13+ and/or CD33+, CD117+/−, MPO−) and another with B- or T-lineage, can still be diagnosed as MPAL, but cases with one blast population showing B- or T-cell phenotype with some myeloid markers but without MPO (or monocytic markers) are diagnosed as ALL with aberrant expression of CD13 and/or CD33. Rare cases of otherwise typical B-ALL may display dim expression of MPO by FC [39, 40, 72–74], but in contrast to MPAL, there is no expression of other myeloid markers (CD13, CD33, CD117).

Subset of MPALs is positive for t(9;22)/*BCR-ABL1* or t(v;11q23)/*MLL*. MPAL co-expressing myeloid and T-lineage markers (myeloid/T MPAL) needs to be differentiated from early T-cell-precursor acute lymphoblastic leukemia (early T-cell precursor ALL). ETP-ALLs are usually dual CD4/CD8−, positive for CD2, CD7, TdT, c.CD3, negative for s.CD3, CD5, and CD1a (occasional cases may show dim CD5) and positive for myeloid/stem cell markers (CD117 and/or myeloid-associated antigens: CD11b, CD13, CD33, CD15, or CD65).

AML versus ETP-ALL
CD13, CD33, and CD117, markers usually associated with AML, may be present in ETP-ALL. ETP-ALL is a variant of T-ALL with distinct phenotype and unfavorable prognosis [75–80]. It differs from AML and MPAL by lack of myeloid or monocytic differentiation, as confirmed by negative staining for MPO and monocytic markers (CD64, CD14, and CD11c). ETP-ALL (Figure 5.32)

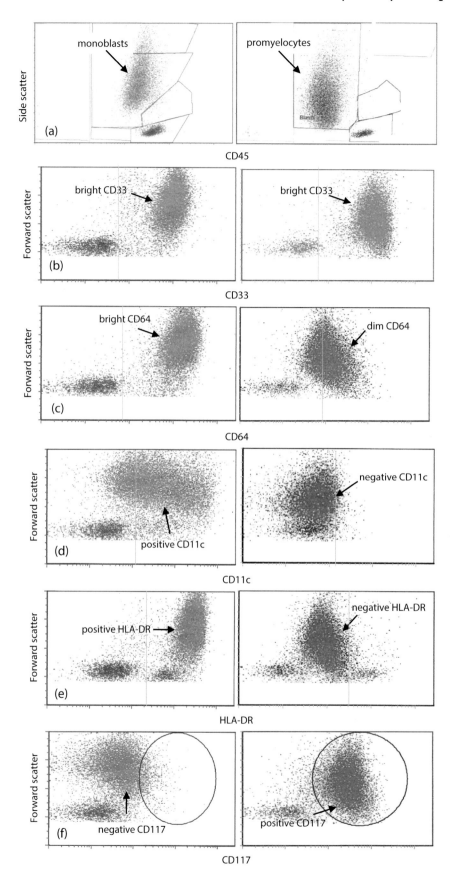

FIGURE 5.28 Comparison of acute monoblastic leukemia with high side scatter (left column) with APL (right column). Monoblasts with high side scatter show similar CD45 versus side scatter pattern to APL (a) and similar bright expression of CD33 (b). Acute monoblastic leukemia differs from APL by brighter expression of CD64 (c), positive CD11c (d), positive HLA-DR (e), and negative CD117 (f).

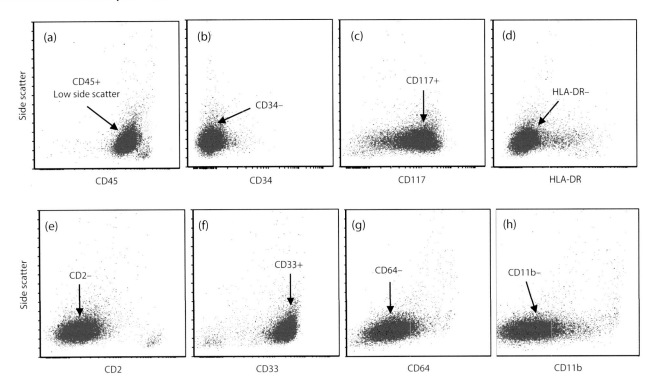

FIGURE 5.29 HLA-DR-negative AML without maturation. Blasts have low side scatter (a) and the following phenotype: CD45+ (a), CD34− (b), CD117+ (c), HLA-DR− (d), CD2− (e), CD33+ (f), CD64− (g), and CD11b− (h).

shows positive expression of CD2, c.CD3, CD7, TdT, CD11b, CD34, CD117, CD13, CD15, and HLA-DR, negative CD4, CD5, and CD1a and usually negative CD8.

AML versus plasma cell myeloma (PCM)

Neoplastic plasma cells are most often negative for CD45, HLA-DR, and myeloid markers, strongly positive for CD38 and CD138 with aberrant expression of CD56, CD117, and/or CD200, and therefore PCM rarely needs to be differentiated from AML when analyzed by FC. However, rare cases of PCM, especially relapsed or after treatment display poorly differentiated phenotype with dim to moderate CD45 and positive expression of CD117, CD33 and even HLA-DR, and may resemble myeloblasts on FC analysis, especially if there is loss of CD38 expression (e.g., after anti-CD38 treatment daratumumab). Figure 5.33 present a case of myeloma with such an unusual phenotype (CD38−, CD45+, CD56−, CD117+, and HLA-DR+). The morphologic features in conjunction with lack of myeloid markers expression, brightly positive CD138 and cytoplasmic light chain restriction help in making the correct diagnosis of PCM. In addition to occasional FC similarities between PCM and AML, also cytologic features of poorly differentiated (plasmablastic) PCM may mimic AML (Figure 5.34). Patients with HLA-DR+/CD117+ PCM have shorter overall survival and/or progression-free survival [81].

Transient abnormal myelopoiesis

In pediatric population, AML has to be differentiated from transient abnormal myelopoiesis (transient myeloproliferative disorder, TMD) associated with trisomy 21 [82–84]. About 10% of newborns with DS present with TMD, a pre-leukemia which resolves spontaneously in most cases [85]. Subset of DS patients with TMD progresses to true leukemia, usually with megakaryoblastic differentiation. The immunophenotype of blasts from children with TMD is characterized by the following phenotype: CD2−, CD4+(dim) (100%), CD7+ (100%), CD13+ (92%), CD14−, CD15−/+ (positive in 14%), CD33+ (100%), CD34+ (93%), CD38+ (100%), CD41/CD61+ (57%), CD56+ (93%), CD71+ (100%), CD117+ (100%), cytoplasmic MPO−, and HLA-DR+/− (positive in 30%) [86]. The phenotype of TMD is similar to DS-associated acute megakaryoblastic leukemia, except that the latter shows less often the expression of CD34 (50% versus 93%) [86].

Blastic markers in other disorders

CD34 is positive in vascular tumors, dermatofibrosarcoma protuberans and hematogones. CD117 is expressed by plasma cell neoplasms, mast cells, stromal tumors (e.g., GIST), small cell carcinoma, and subset of peripheral T-cell lymphoproliferative disorders (CD8+ T-PLL). TdT is positive in thymocytes and hematogones.

AML without expression of blastic markers

Rare AML cases are negative for CD34, CD117, and CD133 causing problems in differential diagnosis with neutrophils/maturing myeloid elements, especially with dysgranulopoiesis. As mentioned earlier, occasional cases of APL may show very dim or partial expression of CD117, which in conjunction with lack of both CD34 and HLA-DR may lead to misdiagnosis as benign process. In those APL cases with very dim/partial CD117, careful correlation with cytomorphology, pattern of CD45 versus SSC, presence of high autofluorescence, lack of CD11b and CD11c expression and characteristic bright expression of CD33 (much brighter than monocytes and normal neutrophils) help to identify APL. Cases with blastoid cytology and positive expression of CD56 and CD123 need to be differentiated from BPDCN, which typically shows the following phenotype: CD4+, CD7+/−, CD13−, CD33−, CD34−, CD45+, CD56+, CD117−/rare cases+, CD123+, and

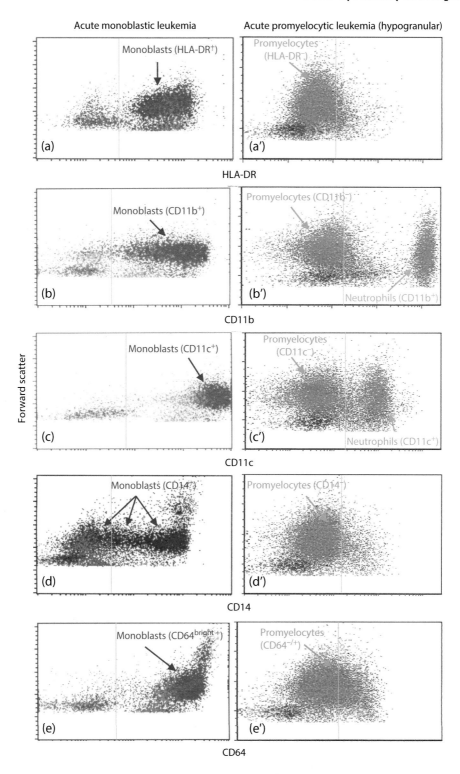

FIGURE 5.30 Comparison between acute monoblastic leukemia and hypogranular variant of acute promyelocytic leukemia. Monoblasts (left panels; blue dots) are positive for HLA-DR (a), CD11b (b), CD11c (c), CD14 (d, variable expression), and CD64 (e, bright expression), while promyelocytes (right panels; green dots) are negative for HLA-DR (a′), CD11b (b′), CD11c (c′), and CD14 (d′) and show dim/partial CD64 (e′). Residual neutrophils (gray dots) express both CD11b (b′) and CD11c (c′).

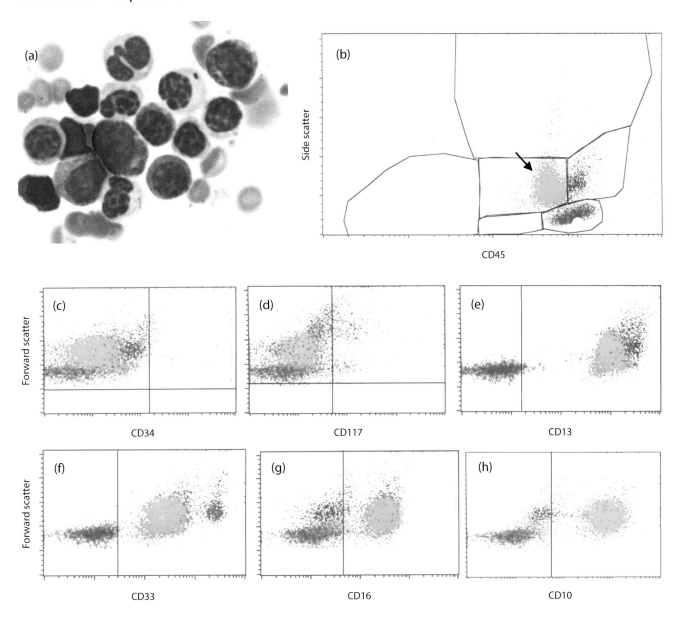

FIGURE 5.31 MDS: phenotypic features of dysmaturation (flow cytometry). Maturing myeloid precursors and neutrophils (green dots) display prominent features of dysgranulopoiesis in the form of hypogranular cytoplasm and nuclear abnormalities (a). Flow cytometry shows markedly decreased side scatter, placing myeloid cells in "blastic" gate (b; green dots). Blastic markers are negative (c–d) and there is normal expression of CD13 (e), CD33 (f), CD16 (g), and CD10 (h). Lack of CD34 and CD117 and normal expression of CD10 and CD16 help to differentiate dysplastic myeloid cells with low side scatter from myeloblasts.

HLA-DR⁺ (rare cases may show either CD13 or CD33 expression but in contrast to AML there is no expression of CD13, CD33, and CD117). In non-APL cases which lack blastic markers, correlation with cytomorphology and marrow studies is crucial to confirm acute leukemia. The very unusual phenotype of myeloblasts

(lack of blastic markers and presence of other phenotypic abnormalities) is often seen in therapy-related myeloid neoplasms and transformation (progression) to acute leukemia from either MDS or MPN, e.g., blast phase of CML. Figures 5.35 and 5.36 present examples of AMLs without expression of blastic markers.

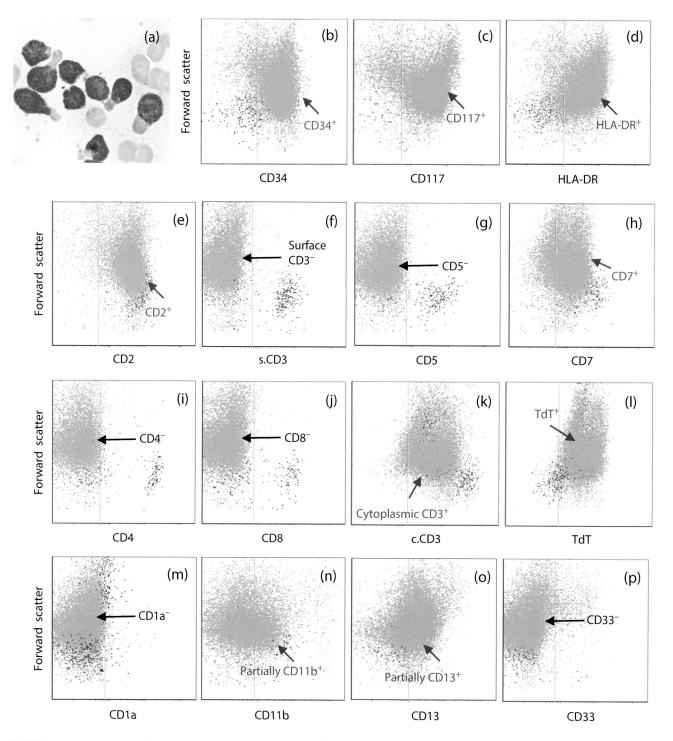

FIGURE 5.32 Early T-cell precursor acute lymphoblastic leukemia (ETP-ALL; bone marrow). T-lymphoblasts show hand-mirror appearance (a). They have the following phenotype: CD34+ (b), CD117+ (c), HLA-DR+ (d), CD2+ (e), surface CD3− (f), CD5− (g), CD7+ (h), CD4− (i), CD8− (j), cytoplasmic CD3+ (k), TdT+ (l) CD1a− (m), partially CD11b+ (n), CD13+ (o), and CD33− (p). Positive CD117, CD13, CD11b and negative CD5 and CD1a are typical for ETP-ALL.

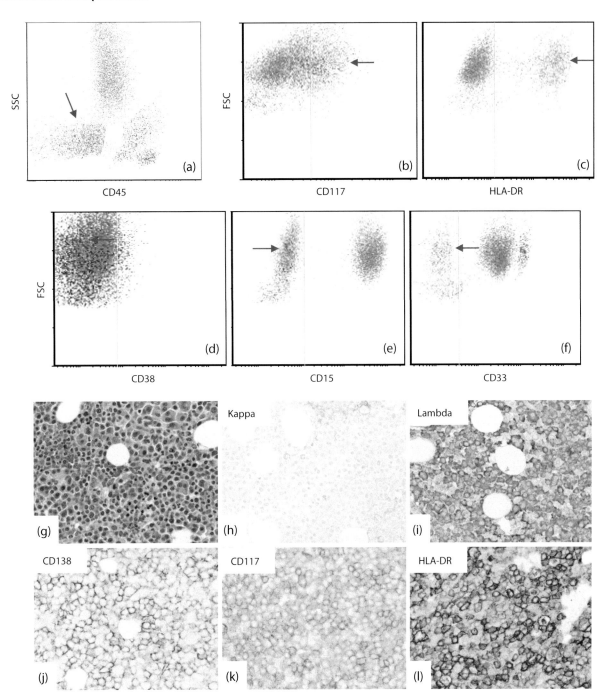

FIGURE 5.33 Recurrent PCM after therapy with unusual phenotype mimicking myeloblasts (CD45⁺, CD117⁺, and HLA-DR⁺). (a–f) Flow cytometry: plasma cells (magenta dots) show dim expression of CD45 (a), positive CD117 (b) and positive HLA-DR (c), negative CD38 (d), CD15 (e) and CD33 (f). Bright expression of CD138 and cytoplasmic lambda restriction (not shown) in conjunction with negative myeloid markers helped to confirm PCM and exclude myeloblasts. Subsequent BM morphologic analysis showed poorly differentiated PCM with plasmablastic features (g), negative kappa (h), and positive lambda (i), CD138 (j), CD117 (k), and HLA-DR (l).

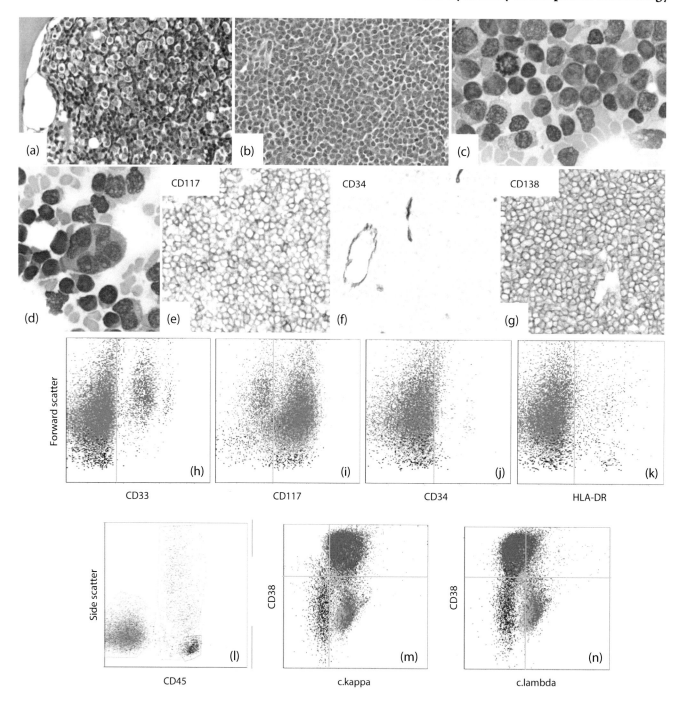

FIGURE 5.34 PCM with blastic morphology. Bone marrow core biopsy (a–b) shows total replacement of normal marrow elements by mononuclear cells with "blastic" morphology (a, original magnification ×200; b, original magnification ×400). Aspirate smear (c–d) shows neoplastic cells with prominent nucleoli, fine chromatin, and scanty basophilic cytoplasm. Occasional mitotic figures are also present. Some of the cells show multinucleation, a typical feature of plasma cell myeloma usually not observed in acute leukemias. Immunohistochemistry (e–g) shows positive CD117, negative CD34, and positive CD138. Flow cytometry (h–n) shows plasma cells (orange dots) with the following phenotype: CD33⁻ (h), CD117⁺ (i), CD34⁻ (j), HLA-DR⁻ (k), CD45⁻ (l), CD38⁺ (m–n), and cytoplasmic kappa restriction (m–n). Blastic morphology and positive CD117 expression mimic AML, but lack of CD45, CD34, HLA-DR, and CD33 in conjunction with presence of multinucleated cells and cytoplasmic light chain restriction help to diagnose myeloma rather than acute leukemia.

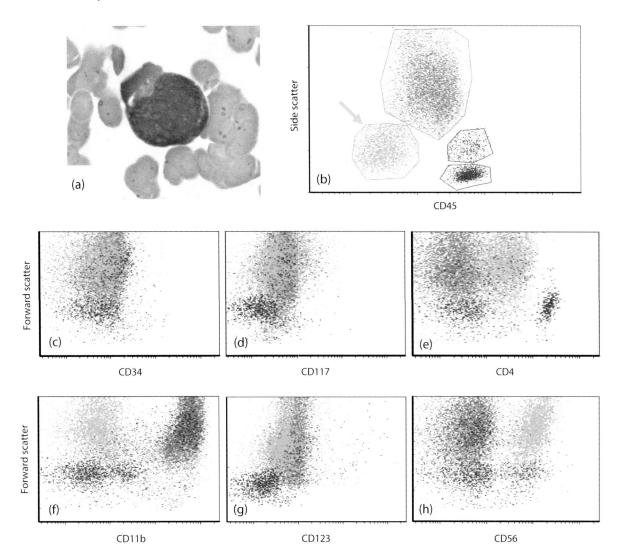

FIGURE 5.35 AML without expression of blastic markers (CD34 and CD117). (a) Aspirate smear showing large myeloblast. (b–h) Flow cytometry. Blasts (green dots) are dimly positive for CD45 (b), negative for CD34 (c) and CD117 (d), positive for CD4 (e), negative for CD11b (f) and CD123 (g), and positive for CD56 (h). Myeloid markers (CD13, CD33) were positive and monocytic markers (CD11c, CD14, and CD64) were negative. Lack of CD123 and presence of both CD13 and CD33 does not favor the diagnosis of blastic plasmacytoid dendritic cell neoplasm.

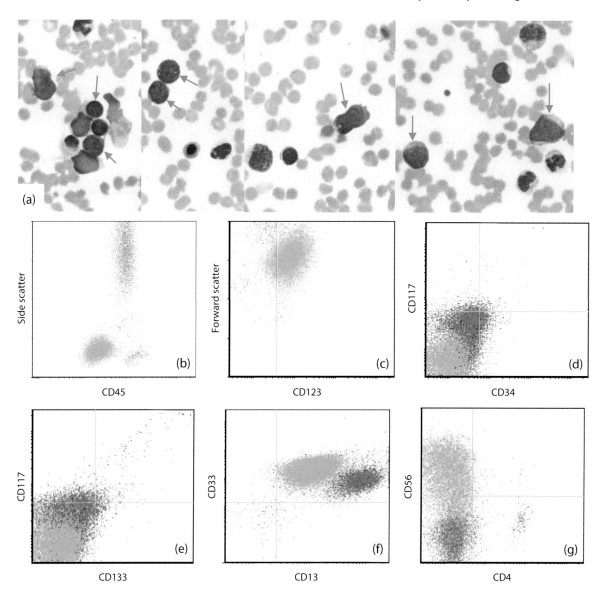

FIGURE 5.36 Blast phase of CML with unusual phenotype (lack of blastic markers). Blood smear (a, composite microphotograph) from patient with CML on targeted therapy with imatinib shows leukoerythroblastosis with numerous blasts (arrows). Flow cytometry (b–g) analysis shows blasts (green dots) with low side scatter (b), dim to moderate CD45 (b), high forward scatter (c), positive CD123 (c), lack of CD34, CD117, and CD133 (d–e), co-expression of CD13 and CD33 (f), positive CD56 (g), and negative CD4 (g).

References

1. Wang, X., S. Huang, and J.L. Chen, *Understanding of leukemic stem cells and their clinical implications.* Mol Cancer, 2017. **16**(1): p. 2.
2. Lapidot, T., et al., *A cell initiating human acute myeloid leukaemia after transplantation into SCID mice.* Nature, 1994. **367**(6464): p. 645–8.
3. Bonnet, D. and J.E. Dick, *Human acute myeloid leukemia is organized as a hierarchy that originates from a primitive hematopoietic cell.* Nat Med, 1997. **3**(7): p. 730–7.
4. Lane, S.W. and D.G. Gilliland, *Leukemia stem cells.* Semin Cancer Biol, 2010. **20**(2): p. 71–6.
5. Paietta, E., *Should minimal residual disease guide therapy in AML?* Best Pract Res Clin Haematol, 2015. **28**(2–3): p. 98–105.
6. Paietta, E., *Consensus on MRD in AML?* Blood, 2018. **131**(12): p. 1265–6.
7. Vardiman, J.W., et al., *The 2008 revision of the World Health Organization (WHO) classification of myeloid neoplasms and acute leukemia: rationale and important changes.* Blood, 2009. **114**(5): p. 937–51.
8. Grimwade, D. and F. Lo Coco, *Acute promyelocytic leukemia: a model for the role of molecular diagnosis and residual disease monitoring in directing treatment approach in acute myeloid leukemia.* Leukemia, 2002. **16**(10): p. 1959–73.
9. Appelbaum, F.R., et al., *Age and acute myeloid leukemia.* Blood, 2006. **107**(9): p. 3481–5.
10. Schnittger, S., et al., *Analysis of FLT3 length mutations in 1003 patients with acute myeloid leukemia: correlation to cytogenetics, FAB subtype, and prognosis in the AMLCG study and usefulness as a marker for the detection of minimal residual disease.* Blood, 2002. **100**(1): p. 59–66.
11. Stirewalt, D.L., et al., *FLT3, RAS, and TP53 mutations in elderly patients with acute myeloid leukemia.* Blood, 2001. **97**(11): p. 3589–95.
12. Mrozek, K., H. Dohner, and C.D. Bloomfield, *Influence of new molecular prognostic markers in patients with karyotypically*

normal acute myeloid leukemia: recent advances. Curr Opin Hematol, 2007. **14**(2): p. 106–14.

13. Grimwade, D., et al., *The predictive value of hierarchical cytogenetic classification in older adults with acute myeloid leukemia (AML): analysis of 1065 patients entered into the United Kingdom Medical Research Council AML11 trial.* Blood, 2001. **98**(5): p. 1312–20.

14. Byrd, J.C., et al., *Pretreatment cytogenetic abnormalities are predictive of induction success, cumulative incidence of relapse, and overall survival in adult patients with de novo acute myeloid leukemia: results from Cancer and Leukemia Group B (CALGB 8461).* Blood, 2002. **100**(13): p. 4325–36.

15. Dastugue, N., et al., *Prognostic significance of karyotype in de novo adult acute myeloid leukemia. The BGMT group.* Leukemia, 1995. **9**(9): p. 1491–8.

16. Bullinger, L., et al., *Use of gene-expression profiling to identify prognostic subclasses in adult acute myeloid leukemia.* N Engl J Med, 2004. **350**(16): p. 1605–16.

17. Dohner, H., et al., *Diagnosis and management of acute myeloid leukemia in adults: recommendations from an international expert panel, on behalf of the European LeukemiaNet.* Blood, 2010. **115**(3): p. 453–74.

18. Takahashi, S., *Current findings for recurring mutations in acute myeloid leukemia.* J Hematol Oncol, 2011. **4**: p. 36.

19. Patel, J.P., et al., *Prognostic relevance of integrated genetic profiling in acute myeloid leukemia.* N Engl J Med, 2012. **366**(12): p. 1079–89.

20. Grimwade, D., et al., *Refinement of cytogenetic classification in acute myeloid leukemia: determination of prognostic significance of rare recurring chromosomal abnormalities among 5876 younger adult patients treated in the United Kingdom Medical Research Council trials.* Blood, 2010. **116**(3): p. 354–65.

21. Arber, D.A., et al., *The 2016 revision to the World Health Organization classification of myeloid neoplasms and acute leukemia.* Blood, 2016. **127**(20): p. 2391–405.

22. Forghieri, F., et al., *NPM1-mutated myeloid neoplasms with <20% blasts: a really distinct clinico-pathologic entity?* Int J Mol Sci, 2020. **21**(23): p. 8975.

23. Matanes, F., et al., *Chronic myelomonocytic leukemia associated with myeloid sarcomas and NPM1 mutation: a case report and literature review.* Ther Adv Hematol, 2019. **10**: p. 2040620719854596.

24. Peng, J., et al., *Chronic myelomonocytic leukemia with nucleophosmin (NPM1) mutation.* Eur J Haematol, 2016. **96**(1): p. 65–71.

25. Zhang, Y., et al., *NPM1 mutations in myelodysplastic syndromes and acute myeloid leukemia with normal karyotype.* Leuk Res, 2007. **31**(1): p. 109–11.

26. Montalban-Bravo, G., et al., *NPM1 mutations define a specific subgroup of MDS and MDS/MPN patients with favorable outcomes with intensive chemotherapy.* Blood Adv, 2019. **3**(6): p. 922–33.

27. Bejar, R., *What biologic factors predict for transformation to AML?* Best Pract Res Clin Haematol, 2018. **31**(4): p. 341–5.

28. Metzgeroth, G., et al., *Recurrent finding of the FIP1L1-PDGFRA fusion gene in eosinophilia-associated acute myeloid leukemia and lymphoblastic T-cell lymphoma.* Leukemia, 2007. **21**(6): p. 1183–8.

29. Dobrea, C., et al., *"In situ" mantle cell lymphoma associated with hyaline-vascular Castleman disease.* Rom J Morphol Embryol, 2011. **52**(3 Suppl): p. 1147–51.

30. Neto, A.G., et al., *Colonic in situ mantle cell lymphoma.* Ann Diagn Pathol, 2012. **16**(6): p. 508–14.

31. Patel, K.P., et al., *TdT expression in acute myeloid leukemia with minimal differentiation is associated with distinctive clinicopathological features and better overall survival following stem cell transplantation.* Mod Pathol, 2013. **26**(2): p. 195–203.

32. Pollard, J.A., et al., *Correlation of CD33 expression level with disease characteristics and response to gemtuzamab ozogamicin containing chemotherapy in childhood AML.* Blood, 2012. **119**(16): p. 3705–11.

33. van den Ancker, W., et al., *A threshold of 10% for myeloperoxidase by flow cytometry is valid to classify acute leukemia of ambiguous and myeloid origin.* Cytometry B Clin Cytom, 2013. **84**(2): p. 114–8.

34. Peffault de Latour, R., et al., *Comparison of flow cytometry and enzyme cytochemistry for the detection of myeloperoxidase in acute myeloid leukaemia: interests of a new positivity threshold.* Br J Haematol, 2003. **122**(2): p. 211–6.

35. Craig, F.E. and K.A. Foon, *Flow cytometric immunophenotyping for hematologic neoplasms.* Blood, 2008. **111**(8): p. 3941–67.

36. Porwit, A. and M.C. Bene, *Acute leukemias of ambiguous origin.* Am J Clin Pathol, 2015. **144**(3): p. 361–76.

37. Guy, J., et al., *Flow cytometry thresholds of myeloperoxidase detection to discriminate between acute lymphoblastic or myeloblastic leukaemia.* Br J Haematol, 2013. **161**(4): p. 551–5.

38. Bene, M.C., et al., *Proposals for the immunological classification of acute leukemias. European Group for the Immunological Characterization of Leukemias (EGIL).* Leukemia, 1995. **9**(10): p. 1783–6.

39. Loghavi, S., J.L. Kutok, and J.L. Jorgensen, *B-acute lymphoblastic leukemia/lymphoblastic lymphoma.* Am J Clin Pathol, 2015. **144**(3): p. 393–410.

40. Borowitz, M.J., *Mixed phenotype acute leukemia.* Cytometry B Clin Cytom, 2014. **86**(3): p. 152–3.

41. Chen, M.H., et al., *CD11b expression correlates with monosomal karyotype and predicts an extremely poor prognosis in cytogenetically unfavorable acute myeloid leukemia.* Leuk Res, 2013. **37**(2): p. 122–8.

42. Kersten, B., et al., *CD45RA, a specific marker for leukaemia stem cell sub-populations in acute myeloid leukaemia.* Br J Haematol, 2016. **173**(2): p. 219–35.

43. Ploszynska, A., et al., *Cytometric evaluation of transferrin receptor 1 (CD71) in childhood acute lymphoblastic leukemia.* Folia Histochem Cytobiol, 2012. **50**(2): p. 304–11.

44. Kussick, S.J., et al., *A distinctive nuclear morphology in acute myeloid leukemia is strongly associated with loss of HLA-DR expression and FLT3 internal tandem duplication.* Leukemia, 2004. **18**(10): p. 1591–8.

45. Gonen, M., et al., *CD25 expression status improves prognostic risk classification in AML independent of established biomarkers: ECOG phase III trial, E1900.* Blood, 2012. **120**(11): p. 2297–306.

46. Swerdlow, S.H., Campo, E., Harris, N. L., Jaffe, E. S., Pileri, S. A., Stein, H., Stein, H., Thiele, J., Arber, D.A., Le Beau M.M., Orazi, A., Siebert, R., ed. WHO classification of tumors of haematopoietic and lymphoid tissues. 2016, IARC: Lyon.

47. Gorczyca, W., *Acute promyelocytic leukemia: four distinct patterns by flow cytometry immunophenotyping.* Pol J Pathol, 2012. **63**(1): p. 8–17.

48. Fleming, D.R., et al., *Diagnostic and clinical implications of lineage fidelity in acute leukemia patients undergoing allogeneic stem cell transplantation.* Leuk Lymphoma, 2000. **36**(3–4): p. 309–13.

49. Jennings, C.D. and K.A. Foon, *Flow cytometry: recent advances in diagnosis and monitoring of leukemia.* Cancer Invest, 1997. **15**(4): p. 384–99.

50. Campana, D. and E. Coustan-Smith, *Minimal residual disease studies by flow cytometry in acute leukemia.* Acta Haematol, 2004. **112**(1–2): p. 8–15.

51. Vidriales, M.B., et al., *Minimal residual disease monitoring by flow cytometry.* Best Pract Res Clin Haematol, 2003. **16**(4): p. 599–612.

52. San-Miguel, J.F., M.B. Vidriales, and A. Orfao, *Immunological evaluation of minimal residual disease (MRD) in acute myeloid leukaemia (AML).* Best Pract Res Clin Haematol, 2002. **15**(1): p. 105–18.

53. Coustan-Smith, E., et al., *Clinical significance of residual disease during treatment in childhood acute myeloid leukaemia.* Br J Haematol, 2003. **123**(2): p. 243–52.

54. Al-Mawali, A., et al., *Incidence, sensitivity, and specificity of leukemia-associated phenotypes in acute myeloid leukemia using specific five-color multiparameter flow cytometry.* Am J Clin Pathol, 2008. **129**(6): p. 934–45.

55. Al-Mawali, A., D. Gillis, and I. Lewis, *The role of multiparameter flow cytometry for detection of minimal residual disease in acute myeloid leukemia.* Am J Clin Pathol, 2009. **131**(1): p. 16–26.

56. Al-Mawali, A., et al., *The presence of leukaemia-associated phenotypes is an independent predictor of induction failure in acute myeloid leukaemia.* Int J Lab Hematol, 2009. **31**(1): p. 61–8.

57. Olaru, D., et al., *Multiparametric analysis of normal and post-chemotherapy bone marrow: implication for the detection of leukemia-associated immunophenotypes.* Cytometry B Clin Cytom, 2008. **74**(1): p. 17–24.

58. Voskova, D., et al., *Use of five-color staining improves the sensitivity of multiparameter flow cytomeric assessment of minimal residual disease in patients with acute myeloid leukemia.* Leuk Lymphoma, 2007. **48**(1): p. 80–8.

59. Voskova, D., et al., *Stability of leukemia-associated aberrant immunophenotypes in patients with acute myeloid leukemia between diagnosis and relapse: comparison with cytomorphologic, cytogenetic, and molecular genetic findings.* Cytometry B Clin Cytom, 2004. **62**(1): p. 25–38.

60. Reading, C.L., et al., *Expression of unusual immunophenotype combinations in acute myelogenous leukemia.* Blood, 1993. **81**(11): p. 3083–90.

61. Macedo, A., et al., *Characterization of aberrant phenotypes in acute myeloblastic leukemia.* Ann Hematol, 1995. **70**(4): p. 189–94.

62. Wang, L., et al., *Acute megakaryoblastic leukemia associated with trisomy 21 demonstrates a distinct immunophenotype.* Cytometry B Clin Cytom, 2015. **88**(4): p. 244–52.

63. Kern, W. and S. Schnittger, *Monitoring of acute myeloid leukemia by flow cytometry.* Curr Oncol Rep, 2003. **5**(5): p. 405–12.

64. Haferlach, T., et al., *Morphologic dysplasia in de novo acute myeloid leukemia (AML) is related to unfavorable cytogenetics but has no independent prognostic relevance under the conditions of intensive induction therapy: results of a multiparameter analysis from the German AML Cooperative Group studies.* J Clin Oncol, 2003. **21**(2): p. 256–65.

65. San Miguel, J.F., et al., *Early immunophenotypical evaluation of minimal residual disease in acute myeloid leukemia identifies different patient risk groups and may contribute to postinduction treatment stratification.* Blood, 2001. **98**(6): p. 1746–51.

66. Angelini, D.F., et al., *A leukemia-associated CD34/CD123/CD25/CD99+ immunophenotype identifies FLT3-mutated clones in acute myeloid leukemia.* Clin Cancer Res, 2015. **21**(17): p. 3977–85.

67. Valent, P. and R. Wieser, *Update on genetic and molecular markers associated with myelodysplastic syndromes.* Leuk Lymphoma, 2009. **50**(3): p. 341–8.

68. Matutes, E., et al., *Mixed-phenotype acute leukemia: clinical and laboratory features and outcome in 100 patients defined according to the WHO 2008 classification.* Blood, 2011. **117**(11): p. 3163–71.

69. Heesch, S., et al., *Acute leukemias of ambiguous lineage in adults: molecular and clinical characterization.* Ann Hematol, 2013. **92**(6): p. 747–58.

70. Bene, M.C. and A. Porwit, *Acute leukemias of ambiguous lineage.* Semin Diagn Pathol, 2012. **29**(1): p. 12–8.

71. Wolach, O. and R.M. Stone, *How I treat mixed-phenotype acute leukemia.* Blood, 2015. **125**(16): p. 2477–85.

72. Marcondes, N.A., F.B. Fernandes, and G.A. Faulhaber, *Lineage determination in acute leukemias.* Cytometry B Clin Cytom, 2014. **86**(3): p. 149.

73. Fuda, F. and W. Chen, *Lineage determination in mixed phenotype acute leukemia: response to Marcondes et al.* Cytometry B Clin Cytom, 2014. **86**(3): p. 150–1.

74. Zhou, Y., et al., *Advances in the molecular pathobiology of B-lymphoblastic leukemia.* Hum Pathol, 2012. **43**(9): p. 1347–62.

75. Coustan-Smith, E., et al., *Early T-cell precursor leukaemia: a subtype of very high-risk acute lymphoblastic leukaemia.* Lancet Oncol, 2009. **10**(2): p. 147–56.

76. Neumann, M., et al., *FLT3 mutations in early T-cell precursor ALL characterize a stem cell like leukemia and imply the clinical use of tyrosine kinase inhibitors.* PLoS One, 2013. **8**(1): p. e53190.

77. Neumann, M., et al., *Clinical and molecular characterization of early T-cell precursor leukemia: a high-risk subgroup in adult T-ALL with a high frequency of FLT3 mutations.* Blood Cancer J, 2012. **2**(1): p. e55.

78. You, M.J., L.J. Medeiros, and E.D. Hsi, *T-lymphoblastic leukemia/lymphoma.* Am J Clin Pathol, 2015. **144**(3): p. 411–22.

79. Zhang, J., et al., *The genetic basis of early T-cell precursor acute lymphoblastic leukaemia.* Nature, 2012. **481**(7380): p. 157–63.

80. Jain, N., et al., *Early T-cell precursor acute lymphoblastic leukemia/lymphoma (ETP-ALL/LBL) in adolescents and adults: a high-risk subtype.* Blood, 2016. **127**(15): p. 1863–9.

81. Wang, H., et al., *Association of CD117 and HLA-DR expression with shorter overall survival and/or progression-free survival in patients with multiple myeloma treated with bortezomib and thalidomide combination treatment without transplantation.* Oncol Lett, 2018. **16**(5): p. 5655–66.

82. Gamis, A.S., et al., *Natural history of transient myeloproliferative disorder clinically diagnosed in Down syndrome neonates: a report from the Children's Oncology Group Study A2971.* Blood, 2011. **118**(26): p. 6752–9.

83. Karandikar, N.J., et al., *Transient myeloproliferative disorder and acute myeloid leukemia in Down syndrome. An immunophenotypic analysis.* Am J Clin Pathol, 2001. **116**(2): p. 204–10.

84. Roy, A., et al., *Acute megakaryoblastic leukaemia (AMKL) and transient myeloproliferative disorder (TMD) in Down syndrome: a multi-step model of myeloid leukaemogenesis.* Br J Haematol, 2009. **147**(1): p. 3–12.

85. Zipursky, A., *Transient leukaemia–a benign form of leukaemia in newborn infants with trisomy 21.* Br J Haematol, 2003. **120**(6): p. 930–8.

86. Langebrake, C., U. Creutzig, and D. Reinhardt, *Immunophenotype of Down syndrome acute myeloid leukemia and transient myeloproliferative disease differs significantly from other diseases with morphologically identical or similar blasts.* Klin Padiatr, 2005. **217**(3): p. 126–34.

6

IDENTIFICATION OF LYMPHOBLASTS

Identification of B-lymphoblasts

B-cell maturation stages

B-cell differentiation is presented in Chapter 2. Generally, B-cell maturation stages can be divided into following categories [1–3]:

- Pro-B-cells [express CD34, CD43, CD117 (c-Kit), B220 (CD45R), CD10, TdT, and gain CD19 expression at early pro B-cell stage]
  - Pre-pro B-cells [CD19⁻]
  - Early pro B-cells [CD19⁺]
  - Late pro B-cells [CD19⁺]
- Pre-B-cells [start expressing cytoplasmic μ heavy chains, CD79a (Igα), CD79b (Igβ), and PAX5, express CD25, CD19, and B220 (CD45R), and lose CD117 and CD43 expression at small pre-B stage; the expression of CD20 appears at the time of immunoglobulin light chain rearrangement]
  - Large pre-B-cells
  - Small pre-B-cells [CD43⁻, CD117⁻]
- Immature B-cells [CD19⁺, CD43⁻, CD79a⁺, CD79b⁺, CD25⁻, CD117⁻, B220⁺, CD34⁺, and IgM⁺]
  - T1 B-cells [IgM⁺ʰⁱᵍʰ, IgD⁻, CD21⁻, CD23⁻, AA4.1⁺]
  - T2 B-cells [IgD⁺, CD21⁺, CD23⁺]
- Mature B-cells [CD5⁻/ʳᵃʳᵉˡʸ⁺, CD19⁺, CD20⁺⁽ᵐᵒᵈᵉʳᵃᵗᵉ ᵗᵒ ᵇʳⁱᵍʰᵗ⁾, TdT⁻, CD34⁻]
  - Follicular B-cells [CD10⁺, CD19⁺, B220⁺, IgMᵈⁱᵐ⁺, IgDᵇʳⁱᵍʰᵗ⁺. CD21ᵐᵒᵈᵉʳᵃᵗᵉ⁺, CD23⁻]
  - Marginal zone B-cells [CD10⁻, CD19⁺, B220⁺, IgMᵇʳⁱᵍʰᵗ⁺, IgDᵈⁱᵐ⁺. CD21ᵇʳⁱᵍʰᵗ⁺, CD23⁺]

Immunophenotype of B-lymphoblasts

B-ALL phenotype by flow cytometry: CD10⁺⁽ᵇʳⁱᵍʰᵗ⁾/ʳᵃʳᵉˡʸ⁻, CD13⁻/ʳᵃʳᵉˡʸ⁺, CD19⁺, CD20⁻/ʳᵃʳᵉˡʸ⁺, CD22⁺, CD33⁻/ʳᵃʳᵉˡʸ⁺, CD34⁺/ʳᵃʳᵉˡʸ⁻, CD38⁺⁽ᵇʳⁱᵍʰᵗ⁾, CD45⁻/⁺ᵈⁱᵐ, CD56⁻, CD71⁻/⁺ᵈⁱᵐ, CD79a⁺, CD81⁺ᵈⁱᵐ, CD123⁺/⁻, CD200⁺/⁻, HLA-DR⁺, MPO⁻, TdT⁺/ʳᵃʳᵉˡʸ⁻

Acute lymphoblastic leukemia (ALL) is the most common pediatric malignancy but occurs also in adults including elderly patients [4–8]. It can be divided into two major subtypes, B-cell ALL (B-ALL) and T-cell ALL (T-ALL), with B-ALL accounting for ~85% of cases [4, 5, 8]. B-ALL is a neoplasm of immature B-cell precursors usually involving blood and BM [4, 5, 9–12]. B-cell lymphoblasts can be identified by positive expression of CD19, CD22, CD79a, HLA-DR, CD38, CD10, CD81, TdT, and CD34, lack of surface light chain immunoglobulins expression (kappa and lambda), and negative or dim CD45 (Figures 6.1–6.4). Side scatter (SSC) is low to minimally increased and forward scatter (FSC) is variable (often moderate). Subset of B-ALLs is positive for CD13, CD15, CD20, CD33, CD71, CD123, and/or CD200 (Figures 6.1 and 6.5–6.7).

B-cell markers

B-lymphoblasts are positive for B-cell markers (CD19, CD22, CD79a, CD79b). Most cases show moderate CD19, but occasional cases have been reported with reduced level of CD19 expression. CD20 is most often negative (Figure 6.3), but occasional cases (~20%) show dim, partial, or variable (heterogeneous) CD20 expression (Figures 6.1, 6.5, and 6.6). When evaluating samples of patients with B-ALL for measurable (minimal) residual disease (MRD), non-specific expression of B-cell antigens (CD19, CD20) by natural killer (NK) cells must be excluded.

CD34 and TdT

CD34 is positive in 71% and TdT is positive in 85% of B-ALL. Lack of CD34 or its partial expression is especially common in B-ALL associated with Philadelphia chromosome [t(9;22)]. TdT is most often positive. Approximately 5% of B-ALL cases lack both TdT and CD34. The expression of CD34 is brighter and homogeneous in B-ALL when compared to hematogones.

CD71 and CD123

CD71 is positive on subset of B-ALL (10%–32%; Figure 6.7) but it is more often expressed by T-ALL [13, 14]. CD123 is often positive (Figure 6.7); stronger expression is usually noted in B-ALL with more mature phenotype.

CD45

CD45 may be completely negative, but most cases show variable (heterogeneous) CD45 expression ranging from negative to dim to partially moderate expression (Figure 6.4). Homogeneous, moderate CD45 expression can be seen in occasional cases, but bright CD45 (comparable to that of benign lymphocytes) is not typical for B-ALL.

CD10

Majority of B-ALL show bright CD10 expression (Figures 6.1 and 6.6), but some cases may be CD10⁻ (Figure 6.7). B-ALL associated with t(9;22)/*BCR-ABL1* often show bright CD10 expression, whereas B-ALL associated with *MLL* alteration are often CD10⁻. The expression of CD10 is brighter in B-ALL when compared to hematogones.

Myeloid markers (CD13, CD15, CD33, and CD65)

Subset of B-ALL/LBL may show aberrant expression of myeloid marker(s). CD33 is more often positive than CD13 or CD15 (co-expression of CD13 and CD33 antigens is rare). Aberrant expression of CD13 (Figure 6.1) or CD33 (Figure 6.7) is seen more frequently in B-ALL associated with Philadelphia chromosome. B-ALLs associated with *MLL* rearrangements show often aberrant expression of CD15 (Figure 6.6), CD33, and/or CD65 [15–17].

CD38

CD38 is positive in B-ALL. The expression of CD38 in B-ALL is usually dimmer when compared to hematogones. CD38 may be not expressed in hematogones (as well as in other cells that normally are CD38+) after targeted therapy with anti-CD38 antibody in patients with plasma cell myelomas.

DOI: 10.1201/9781003197935-6

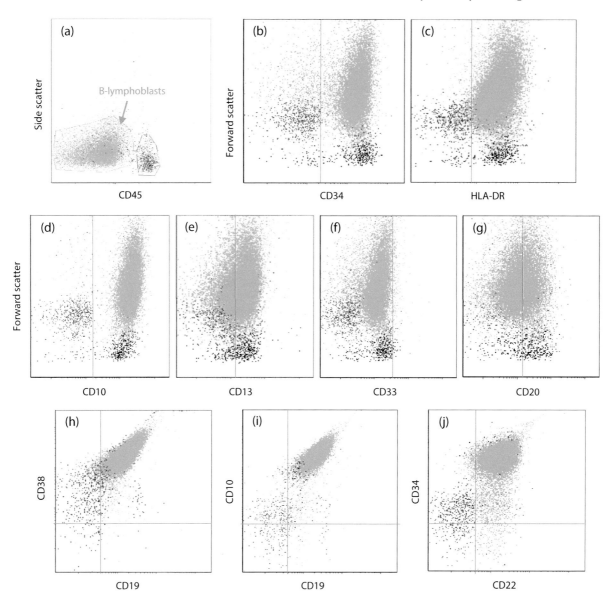

FIGURE 6.1 B-cell acute lymphoblastic leukemia (B-ALL): lymphoblasts (green dots) show low side scatter (SSC; a), negative to dim CD45 expression (a), increased, but variable forward scatter (b–g), positive CD34 (b), positive HLA-DR (c), bright expression of CD10 (d), dim expression of CD13 (e), negative CD33 (f), dim (partial) CD20 (g), moderate CD38 (h), and dim CD22 (j). The pattern of CD19 versus CD38 expression (h), CD19 versus CD10 expression (i) and CD22 versus CD34 expression (j), FSC and SSC properties of lymphoblasts, presence of aberrant CD13 or CD33 and lack of very dim CD45 expression often helps in differential diagnosis with hematogones.

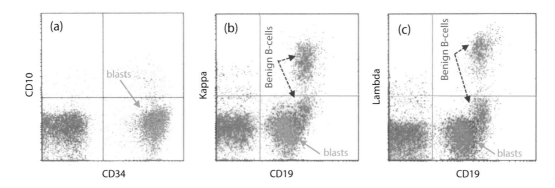

FIGURE 6.2 Identification of B-lymphoblasts – B-ALL/LBL. Lymphoblasts (green dots; arrow) are negative for CD10 (a), positive for CD34 (a), and positive for CD19 (b–c). There is no expression of surface light chain immunoglobulins (b–c). Note slightly dimmer expression of CD19 when compared to residual (polytypic) benign B-cells (b–c; dashed arrows).

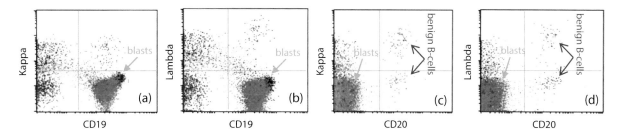

FIGURE 6.3 Identification of B-lymphoblasts. B-lymphoblasts are surface immunoglobulin-negative (a–d) and in majority of cases do not express CD20 (c–d).

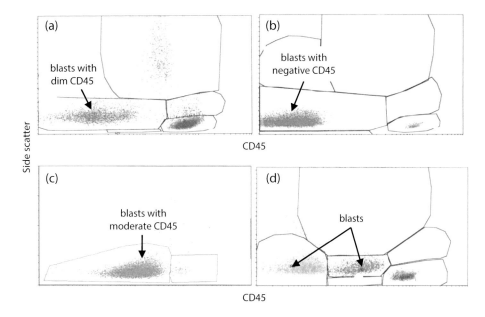

FIGURE 6.4 Identification of B-lymphoblasts: CD45 expression in B-ALL. Majority of B-ALL cases have dim CD45 (a), but the expression may be negative (b) or moderate (c). Rare cases show bimodal CD45 staining with one population of blasts positive and second population negative (d). The side scatter is typically low in B-ALL.

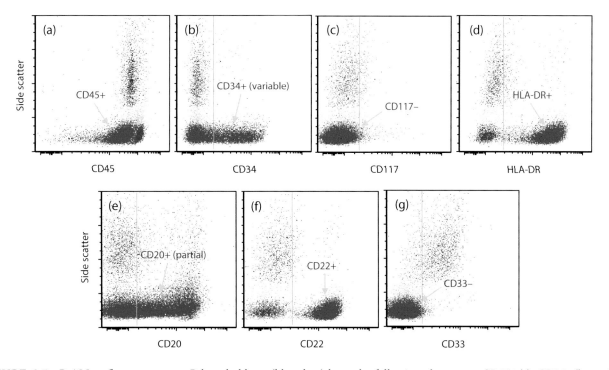

FIGURE 6.5 B-ALL – flow cytometry. B-lymphoblasts (blue dots) have the following phenotype: CD45+ (a), CD34+ (b; variable expression), CD117− (c), HLA-DR+ (d), CD20+ (e; variable and partial expression), CD22+ (f), and CD33− (g).

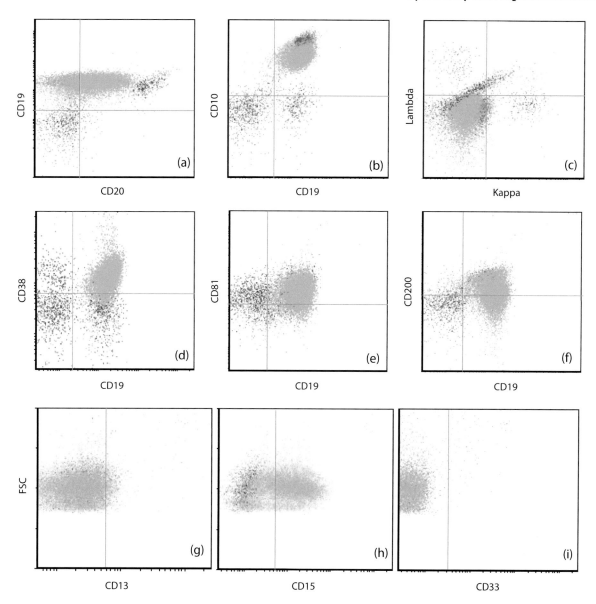

FIGURE 6.6 B-ALL with aberrant expression of CD15. B-lymphoblasts (green dots) show positive CD19 (a, b), partially dim CD20 (a), bright CD10 (b), negative surface light chain immunoglobulins (c), moderate CD38 (d), dim CD81 (e), and dim (partial) CD200 (f). Among myeloid antigens, CD13 is negative (g), CD15 is dimly positive (h), and CD33 is negative (i).

CD81 and CD200

CD81 is dimly positive (Figures 6.6–6.7) and CD200 is either dimly positive (Figure 6.6) or negative in B-ALL, but occasional cases may show moderate expression of CD200 (Figure 6.7). Similarly to CD38, CD81 is dimmer in blasts when compared to hematogones.

Surface light chain immunoglobulins (kappa and lambda)

The surface light-chain immunoglobulin restriction is rarely observed in B-ALL. It might be present in neoplasms arising from stages of precursor B-cell maturation. Surface light chain restriction is a feature of mature B-cell malignancies and can be seen in B-ALL cases associated with *MLL* gene rearrangements or BCR-ABL1 rearrangement (Figure 6.8). Negative or very dim expression of CD45, presence of myeloid antigens (CD13 or CD33), lack or dim and partial CD20 expression, and positive expression of

CD34 and/or TdT help to identify B-ALL with clonal surface kappa or lambda expression.

B-lymphoblasts versus hematogones

Maturing B-cell precursors (hematogones) can be identified by flow cytometry (FC) in majority of samples from BM (they comprise ~1% of marrow elements). Their number decreases with age but may be increased in regenerating BM from patients after chemotherapy or stem cell transplantation. Majority of patients with myelodysplastic syndromes (MDS) and myeloproliferative neoplasms (MPN) show lack of hematogones or significant decrease in their number (more pronounced in MPN than in MDS). The identification of hematogones is important in FC monitoring of B-ALL patients after treatment.

The phenotype of hematogones is variable depending on the stage of differentiation. Three distinct stages have been identified:

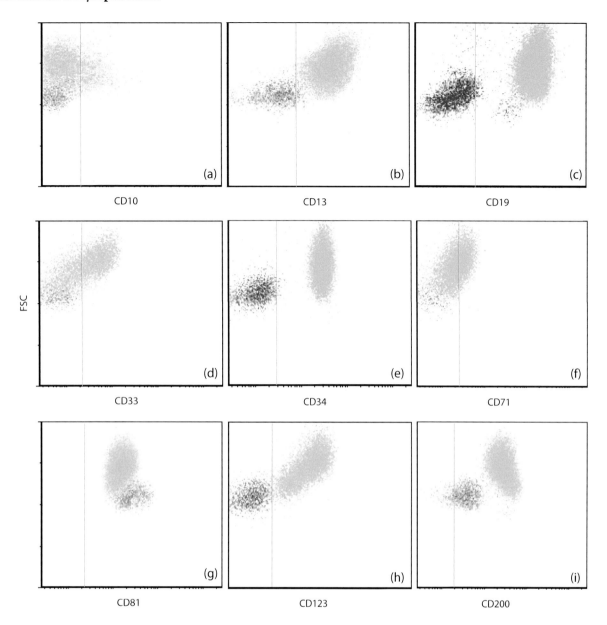

FIGURE 6.7 B-ALL with mostly negative CD10 (a), aberrant expression of CD13 (b), moderate CD19 (c), aberrant expression of CD33 (d), positive CD34 (e), negative to partially dim CD71 (f), dim CD81 (g), positive CD123 (h), and moderate CD200 (i).

stage I, II, and III hematogones [18, 19]. Stage I hematogones are positive for TdT, CD10, CD19, CD34, CD38, and CD58; stage II hematogones are positive for CD10, CD19, CD38, and cytoplasmic IgM and do not express CD34, CD58, and TdT; and stage III hematogones differ from stage II by acquiring dim (often variable) expression of CD20 and surface immunoglobulin light chains. At stage III hematogones, progressive acquisition of CD20 expression is associated with progressive loss of CD10 expression. The expression of CD45 varies with progressive increase in the intensity of CD45 expression as hematogones progress from stage I to stage III.

Generally, hematogones show exceptionally low SSC by FC and variable FSC, with majority of hematogones having low FSC and only minor subset showing increased (variable) FSC. Immunophenotyping shows variable (heterogeneous) expression of CD20 (ranging from negative to dim to moderate), partially positive

CD34 and variable expression of CD45 (Figures 6.9 and 6.10). A subset of hematogones with dim CD45 is usually CD34+ and a subset of hematogones with moderate CD45 is CD34−. The BM with increased number of hematogones shows spectrum of B-cell maturation with small proportion of very immature, CD19+/CD22+/CD20−/TdT+/CD34+ B-cells (I hematogones) and more mature CD10+/TdT−/sIg− cells (stage II hematogones) some of which express CD20 (stage III). Stage II hematogones usually predominate (~65%) [18, 20]. Hematogones are characteristically brightly positive for CD81 and dimly to moderately positive for CD200 (Figure 6.11).

B-lymphoblasts are characterized by higher SSC, slightly higher, but more cohesive FSC and presence of a cohesive cluster of cells on FC dot plot displays when compared to hematogones (Figures 6.12 and 6.13). Majority of hematogones have low forward scatter and only minor subset shows variably increased forward

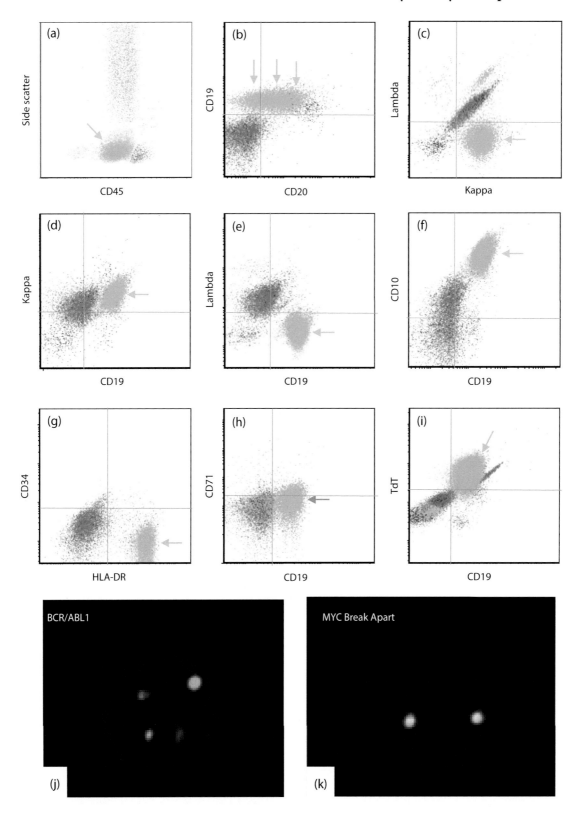

FIGURE 6.8 B-ALL with surface light chain immunoglobulin expression and BCR-ABL1 rearrangement (MYC negative). (a–i) Flow cytometry shows blasts (green dots, arrows) with moderate CD45 and low side scatter (a), positive CD19 (b), variably positive CD20 (b), kappa restriction (c–e), bright CD10 expression (f), negative CD34 (g), positive HLA-DR (g), negative CD71 (h), and positive TdT (i). FISH analysis showed BCR-ABL1 fusion (j: one green (BCR), one orange (ABL1), and two yellow fusion signals) and lack of MYC rearrangement (k: break apart probe with normal pattern, two orange/green fusion signals).

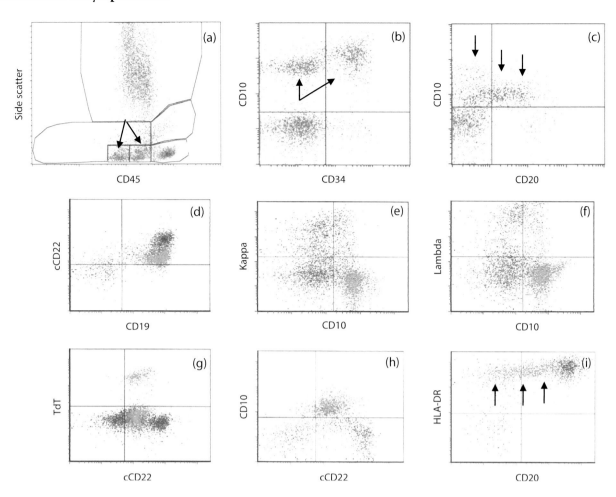

FIGURE 6.9 Hematogones (benign B-cell precursors). Two different bone marrow samples (a–c and d–i). Hematogones have very low side scatter and dim to moderate CD45. Based on CD45 and CD34 expression two distinct populations of hematogones can be identified. Less mature hematogones (a; green dots) show dim CD45 and positive CD34 (b). More mature hematogones have moderate CD45 expression (a, blue dots) and negative CD34 (b). Hematogones show bright expression of CD10 (b), but expression of CD10 becomes down-regulated as the cells mature (c). Typically for hematogones, the expression of CD20 is variable; earlier forms are CD20⁻, but as the cells mature, they become progressively CD20⁺ with characteristic heterogeneous ("smeary") pattern of CD20 expression (c). Hematogones are dim positive for cytoplasmic CD22 (d; blue dots) and CD19 (d; blue dots). Surface immunoglobulins are not expressed (e and f; blue dots). Similar to CD34, TdT shows bimodal staining: subset of cells is positive and more mature cells are negative (g). Parts h and I show typical dim expression of cytoplasmic CD22 and positive HLA-DR with smeary expression of CD20.

scatter. In contrast to B-lymphoblasts, hematogones show usually at least two distinct populations (stages I and II), and even for stage II hematogones, the expression of many markers is variable ("smeary"). This continuous fashion of antigen expression, most easily identifiable with CD10, CD20, and CD45 antigens, reflects changes in the level of antigen expression at different stages of B-cell maturation and is most helpful FC feature in differentiating hematogones from B-ALL. B-lymphoblasts show overexpression of CD58, CD22, CD34, CD10, and underexpression of CD81, CD45, and CD38 when compared to hematogones [21–23]. In contrast to hematogones, CD200 may be negative in B-ALL (~40%). B-ALL may be positive for CD123 (~30% of cases), whereas hematogones are CD123⁻. In contrast to B-ALL, hematogones do not display antigens from an inappropriate cell lineage (e.g., myeloid markers CD13, CD15, and/or CD33). The expression of CD10 is much brighter in B-ALL than in hematogones (subset of B-ALL may be CD10⁻) and the expression of CD38 is brighter in hematogones then in B-ALL. Similarly, the expression of CD81 is brighter in hematogones than in B-LL blasts. The expression of

TdT in hematogones is down-regulated (from negative to dim), as opposed to B-ALL blasts, which are strongly TdT⁺ (subset of B-ALL cases may be TdT⁻). Many B-ALL cases are either negative or dimly positive for CD45, whereas majority of hematogones (stage II) show moderate CD45. B-ALL are positive for CD58, whereas this antigen is only positive in early stages of B-cell maturation as the majority of hematogones are CD58⁻ [24]. Table 6.1 lists the major differences between hematogones and B-ALL.

Saumell et al. reported the distinct pattern of expression of LILRB1 (leukocyte immunoglobulin-like receptor B1; CD85j) in hematogones and neoplastic B-lymphoblasts, which might be useful in analysis of minimal residual disease (MRD) of B-ALL after treatment [25]. LILRB1 expression is higher on CD34⁺/CD10^bright⁺ stage I hematogones, which is downregulated to a dim level of expression on CD34⁻/CD10^moderate⁺ stage II hematogones and then upregulated to a moderate level of expression on CD10^dim⁺/CD20⁺ stage 3 hematogones [25]. In B-ALL, the expression of LILRB1 is homogeneous and brighter when compared to hematogones.

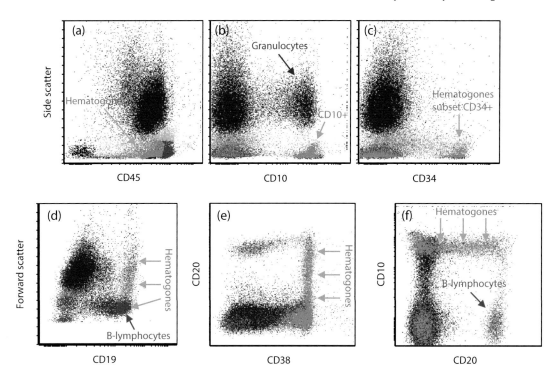

FIGURE 6.10 Hematogones (benign B-cell precursors). Hematogones (orange dots) are positive for CD45 and display very low side scatter (a). They are positive for CD10 (b), CD34 (c; partial), CD19 (d), and CD38 (e). One of the characteristic features of hematogones is increased, but variable forward scatter (d; arrows) and variable expression of CD20 (e–f; arrows).

B-ALL/LBL versus mature B-cell neoplasms

Burkitt lymphoma (BL) phenotype by flow cytometry: FSC^{increased}, sIg$^{+/rarely-}$, CD5$^{-/rarely+}$, CD10$^{+bright}$, BCL2$^-$, CD11c$^-$, CD19$^+$, CD20$^+$, CD22$^+$, CD23$^-$, CD25$^-$, CD34$^-$, CD38$^{+bright}$, CD43$^{+strong}$, CD45$^+$, CD71$^+$, CD79b^{+dim}, CD81$^{+moderate\ to\ bright}$, CD103$^-$, CD200$^{-/(may\ be\ dimly+)}$, and TdT$^-$

Plasmablastic lymphoma (PBL) phenotype by flow cytometry: FSC^{high}, sIg$^{+/rarely+}$, CD5$^{-/rarely+}$, CD10$^{-/rarely+}$, CD11c$^-$, CD19$^-$, CD20$^{-/+(dim)}$, CD23$^-$, CD25$^-$, CD30$^{-/+}$, CD34$^-$, CD38$^{+bright}$, CD43$^{-/rarely+}$, CD45$^{-/rarely+}$, CD56$^{+/-}$, CD71^{+dim}, CD79b$^{-/+dim}$, CD103$^-$, CD117$^{-/rarely+}$, CD200$^{+/-}$

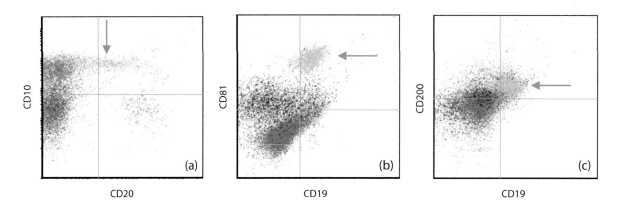

FIGURE 6.11 Hematogones (light blue dots; arrow) with typical pattern of expression of CD10 versus CD20 (a), CD19 versus CD81 (b), and CD19 versus CD200 (c). Note variable expression of CD20 (a), bright CD10 (a), bright CD81 (c), and dim CD200 (d).

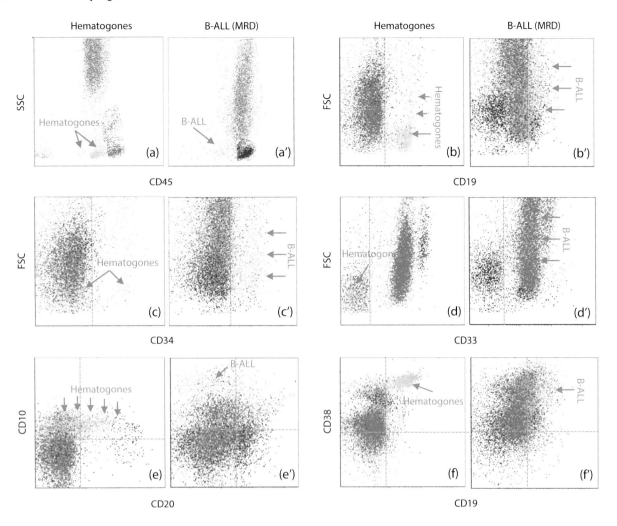

FIGURE 6.12 Comparison of FC features between hematogones and B-ALL (minimal residual disease). On CD45 versus SCC (a–a′) hematogones often show two distinct populations of cells with dim and moderate CD45, whereas B-ALL blasts usually form more cohesive population (a′). Hematogones have distinct forward scatter pattern (FSC, b–d) with major population showing very low FSC and minor population showing slightly increased, variable FSC ("comet"-like). B-ALL blasts are characterized by higher FSC (b′–d′). Hematogones show variable CD34 expression (c) with subset of less mature cells being CD34⁺ and subset of more mature hematogones being CD34⁻ (c); B-ALL blasts are uniformly CD34⁺ (c′). Hematogones do not display aberrant expression of CD33 (d) in contrast to B-ALL blasts which may be positive, as illustrated in d′. The pattern of staining with CD20 versus CD10 (e–e′) and CD19 versus CD38 (f–f′) is also helpful in differential diagnosis: hematogones show dimmer CD10 expression (e), partial CD20 expression (e), and brighter CD38 expression (f). The majority of B-ALL are CD20⁻.

High-grade B-cell lymphoma with *MYC* and *BCL2* rearrangement (HGBL-R) phenotype by flow cytometry: FSC^{increased}, sIg$^{+ (often dim)/rarely-}$, CD5⁻, CD10$^{+bright/rarely-}$, BCL2⁺, CD11c⁻, CD19⁺, CD20$^{+(may be dim)}$, CD22⁺, CD23⁻, CD25⁻, CD34⁻, CD38$^{+bright}$, CD43$^{+/-}$, CD45⁺, CD71⁺, CD81⁺, CD103⁻, CD123⁻, CD200⁻, and TdT⁻

Plasma cell myeloma (PCM) phenotype by flow cytometry: CD10$^{-/rarely+}$, CD19$^{-/rarely+}$, CD20$^{-/rarely dim+}$, cytoplasmic kappa⁺ or cytoplasmic lambda⁺, CD27⁻, CD33$^{-/rarely+}$, CD38$^{+bright}$, CD45⁻, CD56$^{+/less often-}$, CD81$^{-/dim+}$, CD117$^{+/less often-}$, CD138$^{+bright}$, CD200$^{+/less often-}$, HLA-DR$^{-/rarely+}$

Subset of mature B-cell lymphoproliferative disorders may show phenotypic or cytologic similarities with B-ALL. Some of the phenotypic characteristics of B-ALL, such as lack, partially dim or dim to moderate expression of CD45, negative, dim, or partial expression of CD20, positive CD10 and CD43 expression, or lack of surface light chain immunoglobulin expression may be seen in subset of mature B-cell lymphoproliferations. On the other hand, the presence of light-chain immunoglobulins restrictions revealed by FC does not necessarily exclude B-ALL, as it may be seen in minor subset of B-ALL cases (~5%–6%).

Dim to moderate CD45 expression is often seen in chronic lymphocytic leukemia (CLL) and lack of CD45 expression is typical for some B-cell lymphomas, generally high grade such as PBL or PCM. The phenotype of PBL is similar to plasma cell tumors with negative B-cell markers (CD19, CD20) except for CD79a being positive in 40% of cases, and negative CD45 (minor subset of cases may be dim CD45⁺).

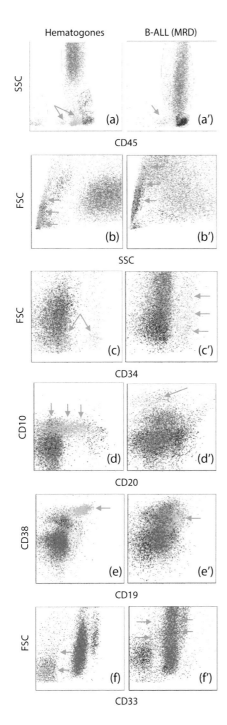

CD10 is expressed by follicular lymphoma (FL), subset of diffuse large B-cell lymphomas (DLBCL), high-grade B-cell lymphomas with *MYC* and *BCL2* (and/or *BCL6*) rearrangements (HGBL-R; double or triple hit lymphomas), and occasionally in other lymphoproliferations (e.g., mantle cell lymphoma, hairy cell leukemia, or lymphoplasmacytic lymphoma).

Negative, dim, or partial CD20 expression is seen in subset of CLL, and complete lack of CD20 is typical for PCM and PBL, as well as in mature B-cell lymphomas after therapy with Rituxan. Positive expression of surface light chain immunoglobulins (especially if strong), bright CD20 and CD45 expression, and lack of CD34 and TdT expression help to exclude B-ALL. Additional phenotypic features are also helpful in differential diagnosis, e.g., co-expression of CD5 and CD23 in CLL, positive CD5 in mantle cell lymphoma (MCL), strong expression of CD138 and positive EBV/EBER in PBL, or positive CD138, CD56, CD117 and cytoplasmic light and heavy chain immunoglobulins in PCM. Majority of mature B-cell lymphoproliferations show strong monotypic expression of either kappa or lambda. FL typically shows dim CD19, dim to moderate CD10, moderate CD20 and bright CD45. DLBCL may be CD10⁺ (or less often CD5⁺) and is characterized by increased forward scatter, light chain immunoglobulin restriction and moderate to bright CD20 and CD45.

The differentiation between BL and B-ALL may be difficult in some cases, as cytologic and phenotypic features between those two neoplasms overlap. Expression of surface μ heavy chain and one of the light chain immunoglobulins (kappa or lambda), bright CD20 and CD45 expression, and lack of TdT and CD34 favor the diagnosis of BL. CD58 expression is also much higher in BL than in B-ALL, as reported in a series of B-ALL and BL reported by Demina et al., with only CD58 expression being useful for differentiation between those two neoplasms [26, 27]. Expression of CD44 is lower in BL when compared to B-ALL, while expression of CD38 is often higher in BL than in B-ALL. *MYC* rearrangement typical for BL is only rarely reported in B-ALL. Figures 13.105–13.107 (Chapter 13) show FC features of BL. Figure 6.14 shows an unusual blastoid transformation of FL to B-cell neoplasm with two B-cell populations (mature and immature).

B-ALL versus acute myeloid leukemia (AML)

Phenotype of acute myeloid leukemia (AML) with minimal differentiation: s.CD3⁻, c.CD3⁻, CD4⁻, CD7⁺/⁻, CD11b⁻, CD11c⁻, CD13⁺, CD14⁻, CD15⁻, CD19⁻, c.CD22⁻, CD33⁺/⁻, CD34⁺, CD38⁺, CD36⁻, CD56⁻, CD64⁻, CD65⁻, c.CD79a⁻, CD117⁺, HLA-DR⁺, MPO⁻/few blasts⁺, TdT⁺/⁻

Phenotype of AML without maturation: CD2⁻/rarely⁺, s.CD3⁻, c.CD3⁻, CD4⁻/⁺, CD7⁺/⁻, CD11b⁻/rarely⁺, CD13⁺, CD14⁻, CD15⁻, CD19⁻/rarely⁺, c.CD22⁻, CD33⁺/⁻, CD34⁺/rarely⁻, CD38⁺/rarely⁻, CD36⁻, CD64⁻, CD65⁻, c.CD79a⁻, CD117⁺, CD133⁺/⁻, HLA-DR⁺/rarely⁻, MPOrare blasts⁺, TdT⁺/⁻

AML cases may be positive for B-cell antigens (especially CD19, less often CD79a), and B-ALL blasts may display aberrant

FIGURE 6.13 Hematogones versus B-ALL (MRD). Hematogones (blue dots; arrows) usually show two or event three distinct populations, which differ by intensity of CD45 expression (a). B-ALL blasts show homogenous population in regards to CD45 expression (a'). The forward scatter (FSC) of hematogones is variable but mostly low ad minor subset showing higher FSC (b). B-lymphoblasts most often show moderate to high FSC (b'). Only minor subset f hematogones is CD34⁺ (c), whereas B-lymphoblasts are most often positive for CD34 with rather homogeneous expression (c'). Hematogones show variable (heterogeneous) expression of CD20 (d), whereas B-lymphoblasts are usually CD20⁻ (d'). The expression of CD10 is brighter in B-ALL than in hematogones (d–d') and the expression of CD38 is brighter in hematogones (e–e'). In contrast to hematogones, B-lymphoblasts often display aberrant phenotype, including presence of CD33 (f–f').

TABLE 6.1: Comparison of B-ALL and Hematogones

	Hematogones	B-ALL
Overall pattern	More than one population (stages I and II) Variable ("smeary") pattern of antigen expression	Cohesive cluster of blasts
SSC	Low	Low to moderate
FSC	Low to variable on minor subset	Increased
CD2	Negative	Very rare cases positive
CD5	Negative	Very rare cases positive
CD10	Dim to moderate	Bright (rare cases CD10 negative)
CD13	Negative	May be positive
CD33	Negative	May be positive
CD19	Moderate	Moderate
CD20	Variable (negative to dim)	– (rare cases may be positive)
CD34	Positive and negative cells	Moderate (rarely negative)
CD38	Bright expression	Dim to moderate expression
CD45	Moderate (subset maybe dim)	Negative or dim
CD56	Negative	Very rare cases positive
CD58	Negative (stage I hematogones maybe positive)	Moderate
CD81	Bright	Dim
CD123	Mostly negative	Positive in subset
CD200	Dim to moderate	Negative or positive
TdT	Positive on subset	Moderate (subset of cases negative)

Abbreviations: SSC, side scatter; FSC, forward scatter; B-ALL, B-lymphoblastic leukemia.

expression of myeloid antigens, CD13, CD15, or CD33. Both types of leukemia are often positive for CD38 and HLA-DR and may be positive for TdT, CD71, and/or CD123. TdT is expressed more often in B-ALL, but it can also be positive in AML. AML can be differentiated from B-ALL by positive CD117, strong expression of both CD13, CD33, strongly positive MPO and lack of CD10 expression. In most cases of AML, expression of CD45 is dim to moderate while in B-ALL is negative, partially positive or dim. AML with monocytic differentiation can be distinguished by positive CD11b, CD11c, CD14, CD56, CD64, and CD123 expression. Acute erythroid leukemia (AEL) is positive for CD71 (bright expression) and often expresses glycophorin A (GPHA, CD235a) and/or hemoglobin A, lacks B-cell markers and CD10.

B-ALL versus mixed phenotype acute leukemia (MPAL)

Mixed phenotype acute leukemia (MPAL) is a rare and heterogeneous group of hematopoietic malignancies in which blasts show markers of multiple developmental lineages and cannot be clearly classified as acute myeloid or lymphoblastic leukemia [4, 28–31]. MPAL cases are often characterized by the presence of several subset of blasts, morphologically and/or immunophenotypically. Two patterns of antigen expression are associated with MPAL:

- co-expression of antigens classically associated with different lineages on the same cells (biphenotypic acute leukemia)
- co-occurrence in the same sample of two or more blast populations from different lineages (bilineal acute leukemia).

Current WHO classification replaced previous scoring system proposed by the European Group for the immunological classification of Leukemias [4]. In the new WHO classification of leukemias, only markers considered most lineage-specific have been retained for lineage assignment (Table 6.2). The B-lineage is

confirmed by strong expression of CD19 and positive at least one of the following markers: cytoplasmic CD22, cytoplasmic CD79a, or CD10. If the expression of CD19 is dim, those two additional markers are needed for B-lineage assignment. T-lineage is confirmed by either surface or cytoplasmic CD3 expression. Myeloid lineage is confirmed by positive myeloperoxidase (MPO) staining. If MPO is negative, MPAL can be diagnosed if blasts show strong expression of other myeloid markers such as CD117, CD33, and/or CD13. A clear differentiation toward the monocytic lineage (CD11c, CD14, CD64, or lysozyme) on a subpopulation of blasts may also define MPAL in the absence of MPO expression. MPAL co-expresses myeloid (or monocytic) markers with B- or T-cell lineage specific marker. It is often positive for CD34, TdT, and HLA-DR. MPAL is discussed in Chapter 26.

B-ALL versus TdT+ B-cell neoplasm with *BCL2* and/or *MYC* rearrangements

Rare B-cell neoplasms show blastic morphology, TdT expression, and *BCL2* rearrangement and occasionally *MYC* and *BCL6* rearrangement (double or triple hit lymphomas). These patients most often present with large abdominal and/or retroperitoneal masses and diffuse BM replacement by sheets of blasts. Blasts are medium to large in size and may show prominent cytoplasmic vacuoles especially in "double hit" cases. Tumor cells are positive for TdT, CD10, and CD19, negative or partially positive for CD34, negative or partially dimly positive for CD20, and negative for surface immunoglobulins [5]. Some of these neoplasms may represent transformation of prior low-grade lymphoma (e.g., FL; Figures 6.14 and 6.15). In some of these neoplasms, FC may show a mature B-cell lymphoma component and BM core biopsy may show peri- to paratrabecular infiltrate of small cells in addition to blasts [5].

De novo B-ALL with *BCL2* rearrangement [t(14;18)(q32;q21)] has also been reported [5, 32–37]. These tumors may be indistinguishable morphologically and immunophenotypically from FL with lymphoblastic transformation. It is suggested that the TdT+ B-cell lymphomas

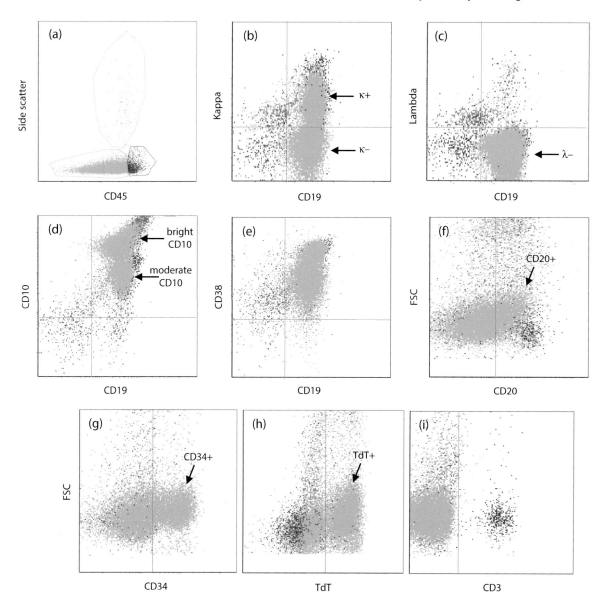

FIGURE 6.14 BM with mature and immature B-cell populations representing blastic transformation of follicular lymphoma. Blasts are dim CD45+ (a), lack surface light chain immunoglobulin expression (b–c), have bright CD10 (d), positive CD38 (e), negative CD20 (f), positive CD34 (g), and positive TdT (h). Mature B-cell component shows kappa restriction (b–c), moderate CD10 (d), positive CD20 (f), and negative both CD34 and TdT (g–h). Surface CD3 is negative (i).

TABLE 6.2: Phenotypic Criteria for MPAL

Myeloid lineage	1. MPO or
	2. evidence of monocytic differentiation (at least two of the following: NSE, CD11c, CD14, CD64, lysozyme)
B-lineage	1. CD19 (strong) with at least one of the following: CD79a, c.CD22, CD10, or
	2. CD19 (weak) with at least two of the following: CD79a, c.CD22, CD10
T-lineage	CD3 (surface or cytoplasmic)

Abbreviations: MPAL, mixed phenotype acute leukemia; NSE, non-specific esterase.
Source: Based on 2016 WHO classification (used with permission).

with *BCL2* and/or *MYC* rearrangement to be classified as "high-grade TdT+ blastic B-cell lymphoma/leukemia" [5]. They are aggressive with poor prognosis (reported survival duration of <1 year).

Identification of T-lymphoblasts

T-cell maturation stages

The phenotypic stages of T-cell development can be divided into [38]:

- pro-T: CD7+ (s.CD3−, c.CD3+, CD1a−, CD34+/−, CD2−, CD5−, and CD4−/CD8−)
- pre-T: CD2+ and/or CD5+ (s.CD3−, c.CD3+, CD7+, CD1a−, CD34+/− and CD4−/CD8− or CD4+/CD8+, TdT+)

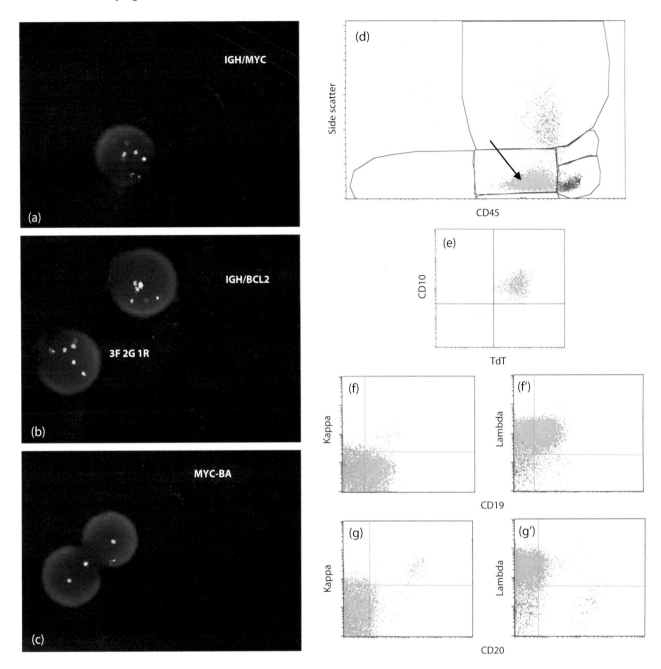

FIGURE 6.15 High grade B-cell lymphoma with TdT expression and rearrangements of *MYC* and *BCL2* representing blastic transformation of follicular lymphoma. (a–c) FISH analysis showing *MYC* rearrangement (a), *BCL2* rearrangement (b) and *MYC* break-apart dual color with split signals (c; red and green split signals; yellow, normal signal). (d–g) Flow cytometry analysis shows leukemic cells in blastic region (d; arrow) co-expressing CD10 and TdT (e) with clonal lambda expression (f, f′–g, g′), dim CD19 (f–f′), and negative CD20 (g–g′).

- cortical T: CD1a⁺ (s.CD3⁺/⁻, c.CD3⁺, CD2⁺, CD1a⁺, CD34⁻, CD4/CD8⁺)
- mature (medullary) T cells: either CD4⁺ or CD8⁺ (s.CD3⁺, CD1a⁻)

Based on the expression of CD1a and surface CD3 (s.CD3), WHO recognizes the following categories of T-ALL [4]:

- early T-ALL (CD1a⁻, s.CD3⁻)
- thymic T-ALL (CD1a⁺, s.CD3⁻)
- mature T-ALL (CD1a⁻, s.CD3⁺)

Immunophenotype of T-lymphoblasts

T-ALL phenotype by flow cytometry: CD1a⁻/⁺, CD2⁺, surface CD3⁻/rare cases⁺, cytoplasmic CD3⁺, CD4⁻/CD8⁻ or CD4⁺/CD8⁺, CD5⁺/⁻, CD7⁺, CD10⁻/⁺, CD13⁻/rarely⁺, CD15⁻/rarely⁺, CD33⁻/rarely⁺, CD34⁺/⁻, CD38⁺, CD56⁻/rare cases⁺, CD71⁻/⁺, CD79a⁻/rarely⁺, CD117⁻, CD123⁻, HLA-DR⁻, MPO⁻, TdT⁺/rarely⁻

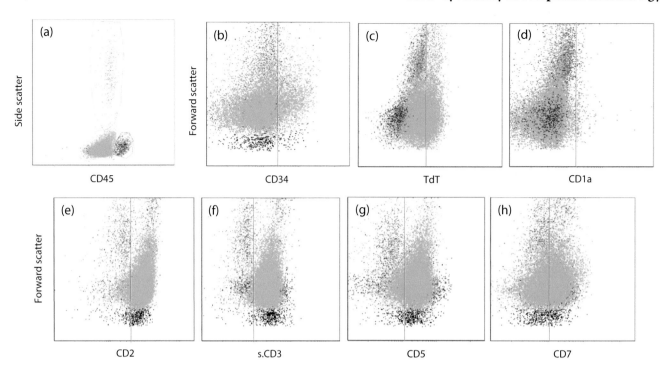

FIGURE 6.16 Identification of T-lymphoblasts. Blasts from T-ALL show moderate CD45 (a), partial CD34 (b), dim TdT (c), negative CD1a (d), and positive T-cell markers (CD2, CD3, CD5, and CD7; e–h). In contrast to the blasts in this case, majority of T-ALLs are surface CD3⁻ and have brighter CD7 expression.

T lymphoblastic leukemia/lymphoma (T-ALL/LBL) is an aggressive malignant neoplasm of immature T-cells [4, 39, 40]. T-lymphoblasts (Figures 6.16 and 6.17) are positive for T-cell markers [CD2, cytoplasmic CD3 (c.CD3), CD5, and CD7]. Surface CD3 (s.CD3) and HLA-DR are usually negative and CD7 expression is often bright. T-ALLs are either dual CD4/CD8⁻ or dual CD4/CD8⁺ (Figure 6.18). Only rare cases are positive for either CD4 or CD8. CD45 is most often positive (except for very early T-lymphoblasts) and majority of tumors are positive for TdT, CD34 and/or CD1a (Figures 6.18 and 6.19). Other markers, which may be positive in T-ALL, include CD10, CD43, CD71, and CD123. Subset of cases may be HLA-DR⁺ (Figure 6.20) and rare cases show aberrant expression of CD33. Recently, a variant of early T-ALL derived from early thymic cells (early T-cell precursors; ETP-ALL) has been recognized [9, 41–43]. The blasts of ETP-ALL are usually CD1a⁻, CD4⁻, CD5⁻, and CD8⁻ and are positive for CD117 and/or myeloid antigens.

Early T-cell precursor T-ALL (ETP-ALL)

ETP-ALL phenotype by flow cytometry: CD1a⁻, CD2⁺, surface CD3⁻, cytoplasmic CD3⁺, CD4⁻/CD8⁻ CD5⁻/dim+(<75%), CD7⁺, CD10⁻/⁺, CD13⁺, CD15⁻/rarely⁺, CD33⁺, CD34⁺/⁻, CD38⁺, CD56⁻/rare cases⁺, CD65⁺, CD71⁻/⁺, CD79a⁻/rarely⁺, CD117⁻/⁺, CD123⁻, HLA-DR⁻, MPO⁻, TdT⁺/rarely⁻

Subset of T-ALL shows the phenotype similar to early T-cell precursors of the thymus (ETP). ETP-ALL is a type of T-ALL that expresses a unique immunotype composed of early progenitor cell and myeloid markers [41, 42, 44, 45]. This leukemia comprises ~15% of T-ALL cases and is characterized by the absence

of CD1a, CD5, CD4, and CD8 expression and presence of one or more of myeloid or stem cell markers (CD11b, CD13, CD33, CD34, CD65, CD117, and/or HLA-DR) in at least 25% of the lymphoblasts [42, 43, 46]. Rare cases of ETP-ALL may be partially and dimly positive for CD5 (<75% of blasts) and/or CD4⁺. Early T-ALL differs from ETP-ALL by having ≥75% CD5 expression. The genetic alterations differ from non-ETP T-ALL and are more similar to myeloid leukemias or MPAL [43, 45, 47–49]. ETP-ALL is discussed in Chapter 18.

Mature (peripheral) T-cell neoplasms versus T-ALL

T-cell prolymphocytic leukemia (T-PLL) phenotype by flow cytometry: CD1a⁻, CD2⁺/⁻, CD3⁺/⁻, CD4⁺ (less often CD8⁺, CD4/CD8⁺ or CD4/CD8⁻), CD5⁺/⁻, CD7⁺/⁻, CD10⁻, CD25⁻, CD26⁺, CD34⁻, CD45⁺/rarely⁻, CD56⁻, CD57⁻, CD81⁺, CD117⁻/rarely⁺, CD200⁻, and TdT⁻

Angioimmunoblastic T-cell lymphoma (AITL) phenotype by flow cytometry: CD1a⁻, CD2⁺/⁻, CD3⁻/⁺, CD4⁺, CD5⁺/⁻, CD7⁺/⁻, CD8⁻, CD10⁺/rarely⁻, CD30⁻/rare cells⁺, CD34⁻, CD45⁺, CD56⁻, CD81⁺, CD200⁺/rarely⁻, and TdT⁻

Presence of blastic markers (CD34, TdT) and CD1a indicates T-ALL (lack of both TdT and CD34 is observed in only 5% T-ALL cases). Aberrant expression of myeloid antigens, CD13 and/or CD33 is seen in subset of T-ALL, but not in mature T-cell tumors. T-ALLs usually have dim or moderate CD45 expression,

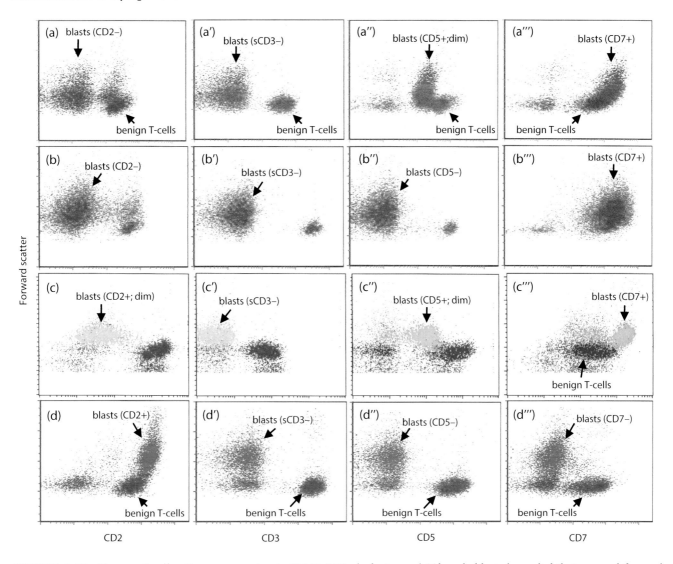

FIGURE 6.17 The pan-T-cell antigens expression in T-ALL/LBL. (a–b; 4 cases) T-lymphoblasts have slightly increased forward scatter when compared to benign T-cells (a–d). Blasts are most often negative for surface CD3 (a′, b′, c′, d′) and positive for CD7 (the expression of CD7 is usually brighter than in normal T-cells; a‴, b‴, c‴). CD2 and CD5 are positive in subset of cases, but are often aberrantly expressed (e.g. dim; a″, c, c″). Case d shows loss of all pan-T-cell markers except for CD2.

whereas peripheral T-cell tumors typically display bright CD45. T-PLL may show lack of CD45 expression and/or dual CD4/CD8 positivity, which in conjunction with cytologic features requires differential diagnosis from T-ALL (Figure 6.21). The immature T-cell neoplasms are more often CD2⁻ and/or surface CD3⁻, and bright CD7⁺, whereas peripheral (mature) tumors very often show positive surface CD3 and loss of CD7 expression. Enteropathy-associated T-cell lymphoma (EATL, formerly known as type I EATL), monomorphic epitheliotropic intestinal T-cell lymphoma (MEITL, formerly known as type II EATL) and hepatosplenic T-cell lymphoma (HSTL) are usually CD5⁻. HSTL is usually CD4/CD8⁻ (some cases may be CD8⁺) and EATL are often CD8⁺ but may be CD4⁻/CD8⁻. The frequency of CD5 expression is comparable with T-ALL and mature neoplasms. Evaluation of CD4 and CD8 expression is very helpful in differential diagnosis as dual positive or dual negative CD4/CD8 expression is more often seen in T-ALL, whereas presence of either CD4 or CD8 expression is more typical for mature neoplasms. Lack of TCR, positive CD10 or CD117 expression is seen more frequently in T-ALL. AITL and

nodal peripheral T-cell lymphoma with T-cell follicular helper (TFH) phenotype are often CD10⁺. Table 4.6 (Chapter 4) compares the phenotype of T-ALL with mature T-cell neoplasms.

Thymocytes versus T-lymphoblastic lymphoma

Flow cytometric characteristics of thymocytes (from thymoma or thymic hyperplasia):

Forward scatter shows two distinct populations (larger and smaller cells), CD1a⁺(subset), CD2⁺(variable), surface CD3⁺(subset; variable), cytoplasmic CD3⁺, CD4⁺/CD8⁺, CD5⁺(variable), CD7⁺(variable), CD10⁺(subset), CD13⁻, CD15⁻, CD33⁻, CD34⁺(subset), CD38⁺, CD56⁻, CD71⁺(subset), CD81⁺(variable), CD117⁻, CD123⁻, HLA-DR⁻, MPO⁻, TdT⁺(subset)

Dual positivity for CD4 and CD8 is rarely observed in peripheral (mature/post-thymic) T-cell lymphoproliferative disorders and,

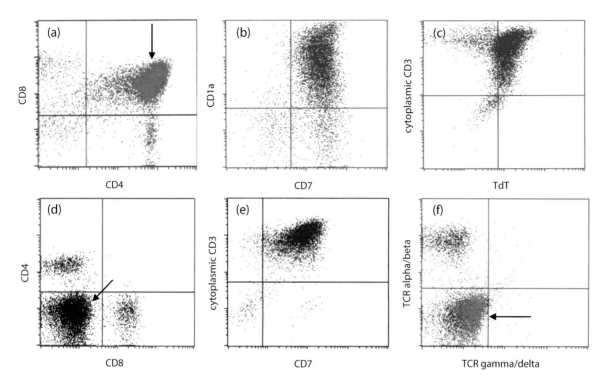

FIGURE 6.18 Identification of T-lymphoblasts by flow cytometry. The upper panels (a–c) present T-ALL with dual expression of CD4 and CD8 (a), positive CD1a (b), TdT and cytoplasmic CD3 (c). The lower panels (d–f) show T-ALL with dual CD4/CD8-negative phenotype (d) with positive staining for cytoplasmic CD3 (e) and negative TCR (f).

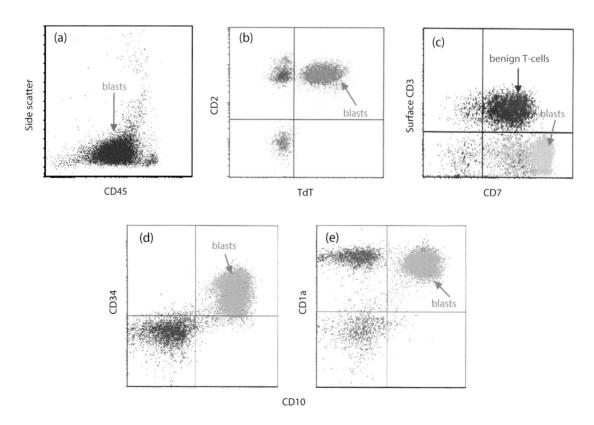

FIGURE 6.19 Identification of T-lymphoblasts by flow cytometry: T-lymphoblasts can be identified by moderate CD45 expression and low side scatter (a), positive TdT (b), lack of surface CD3 expression (c), positive CD34 (d), positive CD10 (d–e), and positive CD1a (e).

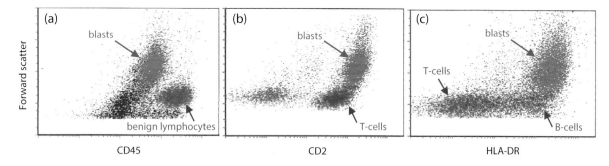

FIGURE 6.20 Identification of T-lymphoblasts. T-ALL/LBL blasts are positive for CD45 (a), CD2 (b) and show aberrant expression of HLA-DR (c).

therefore, when present is suspicious for an immature T-cell population (T-ALL shows co-expression of CD4 and CD8 in ~40% of cases). Thymocytes from either hyperplastic thymus or thymoma are always CD4/CD8⁺ and therefore the diagnosis of mediastinal T-ALL cannot be based on the presence of CD4/CD8 co-expression [50]. Regardless of whether from thymoma or benign thymic hyperplasia, immature T-cells (thymocytes) display characteristic variable expression of s.CD3 (Figures 6.22–6.24): majority of cells (small T-cells) show positive but variable ("smeary") CD3 expression, whereas larger T-cells are s.CD3 negative. This heterogeneous pattern of s.CD3 is never observed in surface CD3⁺ T-ALL. Small, more mature T-cells from thymoma/thymic hyperplasia are CD10⁻ and larger immature T-cells (surface CD3⁻) shows positive expression of CD10 (Figure 6.24), positive CD71 (Figure 6.25) and slightly brighter CD81 and dimmer CD200 (Figure 6.25). In a study by Ward et al., four distinct populations of T-cells, representing different stages of T-cell maturation could be identified in thymoma/thymic hyperplasia based on the expression of s.CD3 and BCL2: stage 1 with s.CD3⁻/BCL2⁺, stage 2 with s.CD3⁺dim/BCL2⁻, stage 3 with s.CD3⁺/BCL2⁻, and stage 4 with s.CD3⁺/BCL2⁺ [51]. In contrast to thymoma/thymic hyperplasia characterized by heterogeneous T-cell populations at different stages of maturation, T-ALL/LBL and reactive mediastinal lymph nodes had entirely homogeneous T-cell population [51].

Indolent T-lymphoblastic proliferation

Few cases of indolent T-lymphoblastic proliferations have been reported [39, 52–54]. It occurs in association with Castleman disease, HHV8⁺ multicentric Castleman disease, HHV8⁺

multicentric Castleman disease with associated polyclonal lambda-restricted "microlymphomas", various types of carcinoma, follicular dendritic tumors, marginal zone lymphoma, AITL or reactive (atypical) changes. It is characterized by focal collection of T-lymphoblasts with a cortical T-cell immunophenotype (CD4⁺, CD8⁺, CD1a⁺, and TdT⁺) [39], but subset of cases may also show population of CD4⁻/CD8⁻ T-cells [54]. It is negative for CD34 and most often show positive expression of surface CD3. There is no clonal rearrangement of *TCR* gene by PCR. Histologic sections show scattered immature T lymphoblasts without overt distortion of underlying architecture. There was no evidence of subsequent progression to T lymphoblastic leukemia.

Acute undifferentiated leukemia versus T-ALL

Acute undifferentiated leukemia (AUL) is a rare variant of acute leukemia which is positive for some of the blastic markers (TdT, CD34), CD38 and HLA-DR, and does not express markers specific for myeloid or lymphoid lineages. Negative surface and cytoplasmic CD3 excludes T-ALL.

T-ALL versus mixed phenotype acute leukemia (MPAL) and minimally differentiated AML with CD7 expression

MPAL co-expresses myeloid (or monocytic) markers with B- or T-cell lineage specific marker [28, 30, 47, 49]. MPALs are often positive for CD34, TdT, and HLA-DR. The T-lineage is confirmed by either surface or cytoplasmic CD3 expression. Myeloid lineage is confirmed by positive myeloperoxidase (MPO) staining (flow cytometry, cytochemistry, and/or immunohistochemistry) and

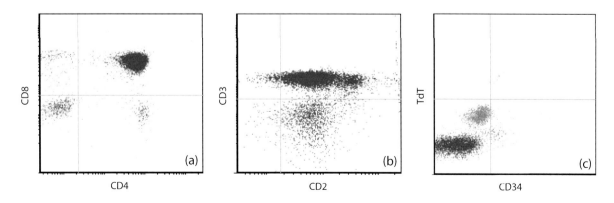

FIGURE 6.21 T-PLL with dual CD4/CD8 expression (a). In contrast to T-ALL, neoplastic T-cells in T-PLL are surface CD3⁺ (b) and lack CD34 and TdT expression (c).

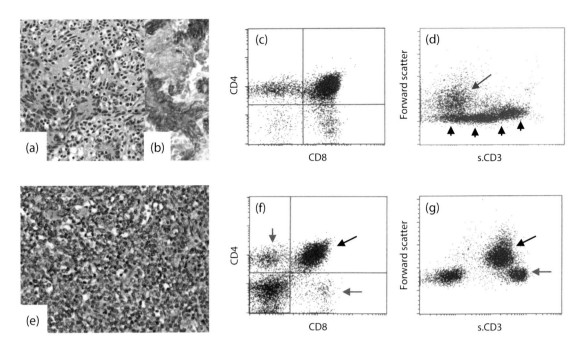

FIGURE 6.22 Comparison between flow cytometric features of thymocytes (a–d) and T-lymphoblasts (e–g). (a–b) Histologic section of thymoma. Tumor cells are positive for cytokeratin (AE1/AE3). Flow cytometric analysis reveals immature T-cells with dual expression of CD4/CD8 (c) and variable (smeared) expression of surface CD3 (d; black arrows). There is additional population of larger T-cells with negative expression of CD3 (red arrow). (e) T-lymphoblastic lymphoma (mediastinum). Lymphoblasts are dual positive for CD4/CD8 (f). There are distinct populations of benign T-cells expressing CD4 or CD8 (blue arrows). In contrast, thymocytes (c) shows gradual transition from CD4+/CD8 cells to CD4−/CD8+ cells with majority of cells positive for both antigens. T-lymphoblasts (black arrow) show moderate expression of surface CD3 (g) without typical for thymocytes smeared patter (compare with d). Normal (benign) T-cells (blue arrow, g) show brighter CD3 expression and lower forward scatter, when compared to lymphoblasts.

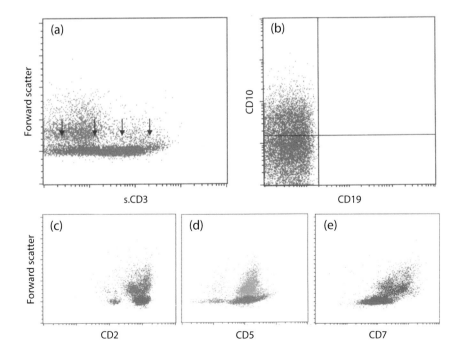

FIGURE 6.23 Thymocytes (thymoma/thymic hyperplasia) – flow cytometric characteristics. Thymocytes show characteristic smeared (variable) expression of surface CD3 on flow cytometric analysis (a; red arrows). Small cells (red dots, more mature cells) have variable expression of CD3, whereas larger cells (green dots; less mature cells) with increased forward scatter are CD3 negative (a). Those larger cells co-express CD10 (b). Both T-cell populations are positive for CD2 (c), CD5 (d), and CD7 (e).

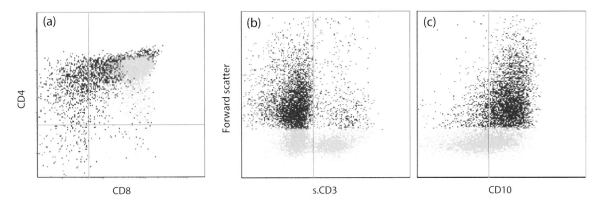

FIGURE 6.24 Thymocytes from thymoma are dual CD4/CD8 positive (a), show partial surface CD3 expression (b), and partial CD10 expression (c).

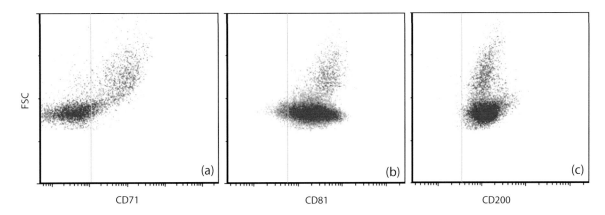

FIGURE 6.25 The expression of CD71, CD81, and CD200 by thymocytes. Small, more mature T-cells from thymoma/thymic hyperplasia (red dots) are CD71⁻ (a), and larger immature T-cells (blue dots) show positive expression of CD71 (a), slightly brighter CD81 (b), and dimmer CD200 (c).

monocytic lineage is confirmed by positive expression of at least two of the following markers: CD11c, CD14, CD64, lysosome, or nonspecific esterase (NSE). In the cases with negative MPO (e.g., minimally differentiated AML with aberrant CD7 expression), strong co-expression of CD13, CD33, and CD117 would indicate a myeloid differentiation. Subset of MPAL may show two distinct populations of blasts, one fulfilling the phenotypic criteria for AML and the other for either B-ALL or T-ALL (acute bi-lineal leukemia). A threshold 10% and more recently 13% MPO positive cells has been suggested for FC-based MPO analysis [38, 55].

Gutierrez et al. recently proposed to use the term of acute myeloid/T-lymphoblastic leukemia (AMTL) defined as acute leukemias that fit the diagnostic criteria of ETP-ALL or of T/myeloid MPALs, together with AMLs with clonal TCR gene rearrangements and evidence of T-lymphoid differentiation (CD3, CD7, CD2, or CD4 expression) [48]. Since aberrant expression of CD4 and CD7 is relatively common in acute megakaryoblastic leukemias, this subtype of AML should be excluded from the definition of AMTL [48]. Even with expression of myeloid markers, ETP-ALL is classified under T-ALL groups with the strong argument that the behavior of ETP-ALL is like other T-ALL in the most recent children's oncology group trials and in some adult studies. In their series, CD34, CD117, CD13/CD33, and CD11b had similar frequency distributions in both ETP-ALL and MPAL

(AML/T-ALL), whereas CD2 and HLA-DR were more frequent in the MPAL group (c.CD3 was present in more than 30% of blast cells, and MPO was found in more than 20% in MPAL) [48].

References

1. Ying Wang, J.L., P.D. Burrows, J.-Y. Wang, *B cell development and maturation*, in *B-cells in immunity and tolerance*. Adv Exp Med Biol, 2020. p. 1–22.
2. Brauninger, A., et al., *B-cell development in progressively transformed germinal centers: similarities and differences compared with classical germinal centers and lymphocyte-predominant Hodgkin disease*. Blood, 2001. **97**(3): p. 714–9.
3. Perez-Andres, M., et al., *Human peripheral blood B-cell compartments: a crossroad in B-cell traffic*. Cytometry B Clin Cytom, 2010. **78 Suppl 1**: p. S47–S60.
4. Swerdlow, S.H., Campo, E., Harris, N. L., Jaffe, E. S., Pileri, S. A., Stein, H., Stein, H., Thiele, J., Arber, D.A., Le Beau M.M., Orazi, A., Siebert, R., ed. *WHO classification of tumors of haematopoietic and lymphoid tissues*. 2016, IARC: Lyon.
5. Loghavi, S., J.L. Kutok, and J.L. Jorgensen, *B-acute lymphoblastic leukemia/lymphoblastic lymphoma*. Am J Clin Pathol, 2015. **144**(3): p. 393–410.
6. Ferrari, A., et al., *Acute lymphoblastic leukemia in the elderly: results of two different treatment approaches in 49 patients during a 25-year period*. Leukemia, 1995. **9**(10): p. 1643–7.

7. Pui, C.H., M.V. Relling, and J.R. Downing, *Acute lymphoblastic leukemia.* N Engl J Med, 2004. **350**(15): p. 1535–48.

8. Pagano, L., et al., *Acute lymphoblastic leukemia in the elderly. A twelve-year retrospective, single center study.* Haematologica, 2000. **85**(12): p. 1327–9.

9. Swerdlow, S.H., et al., *The 2016 revision of the World Health Organization classification of lymphoid neoplasms.* Blood, 2016. **127**(20): p. 2375–90.

10. Arber, D.A., et al., *The 2016 revision to the World Health Organization classification of myeloid neoplasms and acute leukemia.* Blood, 2016. **127**(20): p. 2391–405.

11. Borowitz, M.J., et al., *Immunophenotyping of acute leukemia by flow cytometric analysis. Use of CD45 and right-angle light scatter to gate on leukemic blasts in three-color analysis.* Am J Clin Pathol, 1993. **100**(5): p. 534–40.

12. Borowitz, M.J., et al., *Comparison of diagnostic and relapse flow cytometry phenotypes in childhood acute lymphoblastic leukemia: implications for residual disease detection: a report from the children's oncology group.* Cytometry B Clin Cytom, 2005. **68**(1): p. 18–24.

13. Koehler, M., et al., *Expression of activation antigens CD38 and CD71 is not clinically important in childhood acute lymphoblastic leukemia.* Leukemia, 1993. **7**(1): p. 41–5.

14. Das Gupta, A., J. Patil, and V.I. Shah, *Transferrin receptor expression by blast cells in acute lymphoblastic leukemia correlates with white cell count & immunophenotype.* Indian J Med Res, 1996. **104**: p. 226–33.

15. Seegmiller, A.C., et al., *Characterization of immunophenotypic aberrancies in 200 cases of B acute lymphoblastic leukemia.* Am J Clin Pathol, 2009. **132**(6): p. 940–9.

16. Pui, C.H., et al., *Reappraisal of the clinical and biologic significance of myeloid-associated antigen expression in childhood acute lymphoblastic leukemia.* J Clin Oncol, 1998. **16**(12): p. 3768–73.

17. Pui, C.H., et al., *Clinical characteristics and treatment outcome of childhood acute lymphoblastic leukemia with the t(4;11)(q21;q23): a collaborative study of 40 cases.* Blood, 1991. **77**(3): p. 440–7.

18. Carulli, G., et al., *Multiparameter flow cytometry to detect hematogones and to assess B-lymphocyte clonality in bone marrow samples from patients with non-Hodgkin lymphomas.* Hematol Rep, 2014. **6**(2): p. 5381.

19. Sedek, L., et al., *The immunophenotypes of blast cells in B-cell precursor acute lymphoblastic leukemia: how different are they from their normal counterparts?* Cytometry B Clin Cytom, 2014. **86**(5): p. 329–39.

20. Rimsza, L.M., et al., *Benign hematogone-rich lymphoid proliferations can be distinguished from B-lineage acute lymphoblastic leukemia by integration of morphology, immunophenotype, adhesion molecule expression, and architectural features.* Am J Clin Pathol, 2000. **114**(1): p. 66–75.

21. Nagant, C., et al., *Easy discrimination of hematogones from lymphoblasts in B-cell progenitor acute lymphoblastic leukemia patients using CD81/CD58 expression ratio.* Int J Lab Hematol, 2018. **40**(6): p. 734–9.

22. Muzzafar, T., et al., *Aberrant underexpression of CD81 in precursor B-cell acute lymphoblastic leukemia: utility in detection of minimal residual disease by flow cytometry.* Am J Clin Pathol, 2009. **132**(5): p. 692–8.

23. Tsitsikov, E., et al., *Role of CD81 and CD58 in minimal residual disease detection in pediatric B lymphoblastic leukemia.* Int J Lab Hematol, 2018. **40**(3): p. 343–51.

24. Lee, R.V., R.C. Braylan, and L.M. Rimsza, *CD58 expression decreases as nonmalignant B cells mature in bone marrow and is frequently overexpressed in adult and pediatric precursor B-cell acute lymphoblastic leukemia.* Am J Clin Pathol, 2005. **123**(1): p. 119–24.

25. Saumell Tutusaus, S., et al., *LILRB1: a novel diagnostic B-cell marker to distinguish neoplastic B lymphoblasts from hematogones.* Am J Clin Pathol, 2021. **156**(6): p. 941–9.

26. Demina, I., et al., *Additional flow cytometric studies for differential diagnosis between Burkitt lymphoma/leukemia and B-cell precursor acute lymphoblastic leukemia.* Leuk Res, 2021. **100**: p. 106491.

27. Demina, I., et al., *The use of additional immunophenotypic criteria for the differential diagnosis of Burkitt lymphoma/leukemia: An exemplary case report.* Leuk Res, 2021. **110**: p. 106662.

28. Matutes, E., et al., *Mixed-phenotype acute leukemia: clinical and laboratory features and outcome in 100 patients defined according to the WHO 2008 classification.* Blood, 2011. **117**(11): p. 3163–71.

29. Heesch, S., et al., *Acute leukemias of ambiguous lineage in adults: molecular and clinical characterization.* Ann Hematol, 2013. **92**(6): p. 747–58.

30. Bene, M.C. and A. Porwit, *Acute leukemias of ambiguous lineage.* Semin Diagn Pathol, 2012. **29**(1): p. 12–8.

31. Porwit, A. and M.C. Bene, *Multiparameter flow cytometry applications in the diagnosis of mixed phenotype acute leukemia.* Cytometry B Clin Cytom, 2019. **96**(3): p. 183–94.

32. Mufti, G.J., et al., *Common ALL with pre-B-cell features showing (8;14) and (14;18) chromosome translocations.* Blood, 1983. **62**(5): p. 1142–6.

33. Carli, M.G., et al., *Lymphoblastic lymphoma with primary splenic involvement and the classic 14;18 translocation.* Cancer Genet Cytogenet, 1991. **57**(1): p. 47–51.

34. Kramer, M.H., et al., *De novo acute B-cell leukemia with translocation t(14;18): an entity with a poor prognosis.* Leukemia, 1991. **5**(6): p. 473–8.

35. Nacheva, E., et al., *C-MYC translocations in de novo B-cell lineage acute leukemias with t(14;18)(cell lines Karpas 231 and 353).* Blood, 1993. **82**(1): p. 231–40.

36. Geyer, J.T., et al., *Lymphoblastic transformation of follicular lymphoma: a clinicopathologic and molecular analysis of 7 patients.* Hum Pathol, 2015. **46**(2): p. 260–71.

37. Subramaniyam, S., et al., *De novo B lymphoblastic leukemia/lymphoma in an adult with t(14;18)(q32;q21) and c-MYC gene rearrangement involving 10p13.* Leuk Lymphoma, 2011. **52**(11): p. 2195–9.

38. Bene, M.C., et al., *Proposals for the immunological classification of acute leukemias. European Group for the Immunological Characterization of Leukemias (EGIL).* Leukemia, 1995. **9**(10): p. 1783–6.

39. You, M.J., L.J. Medeiros, and E.D. Hsi, *T-lymphoblastic leukemia/lymphoma.* Am J Clin Pathol, 2015. **144**(3): p. 411–22.

40. Teachey, D.T. and D. O'Connor, *How I treat newly diagnosed T-cell acute lymphoblastic leukemia and T-cell lymphoblastic lymphoma in children.* Blood, 2020. **135**(3): p. 159–66.

41. Jain, N., et al., *Early T-cell precursor acute lymphoblastic leukemia/lymphoma (ETP-ALL/LBL) in adolescents and adults: a high-risk subtype.* Blood, 2016. **127**(15): p. 1863–9.

42. Coustan-Smith, E., et al., *Early T-cell precursor leukaemia: a subtype of very high-risk acute lymphoblastic leukaemia.* Lancet Oncol, 2009. **10**(2): p. 147–56.

43. Zhang, J., et al., *The genetic basis of early T-cell precursor acute lymphoblastic leukaemia.* Nature, 2012. **481**(7380): p. 157–63.

44. Khogeer, H., et al., *Early T precursor acute lymphoblastic leukaemia/lymphoma shows differential immunophenotypic characteristics including frequent CD33 expression and in vitro response to targeted CD33 therapy.* Br J Haematol, 2019. **186**(4): p. 538–48.

45. Noronha, E.P., et al., *T-lymphoid/myeloid mixed phenotype acute leukemia and early T-cell precursor lymphoblastic leukemia similarities with NOTCH1 mutation as a good prognostic factor.* Cancer Manag Res, 2019. **11**: p. 3933–43.

46. Patel, J.L., et al., *The immunophenotype of T-lymphoblastic lymphoma in children and adolescents: a Children's Oncology Group report.* Br J Haematol, 2012. **159**(4): p. 454–61.

47. Porwit, A. and M.C. Bene, *Acute leukemias of ambiguous origin.* Am J Clin Pathol, 2015. **144**(3): p. 361–76.

48. Gutierrez, A. and A. Kentsis, *Acute myeloid/T-lymphoblastic leukaemia (AMTL): a distinct category of acute leukaemias with common pathogenesis in need of improved therapy.* Br J Haematol, 2018. **180**(6): p. 919–24.

49. Wolach, O. and R.M. Stone, *How I treat mixed-phenotype acute leukemia.* Blood, 2015. **125**(16): p. 2477–85.

50. Gorczyca, W., et al., *Flow cytometry in the diagnosis of mediastinal tumors with emphasis on differentiating thymocytes from precursor T-lymphoblastic lymphoma/leukemia.* Leuk Lymphoma, 2004. **45**(3): p. 529–38.

51. Ward, N., et al., *Bcl-2 maturation pattern in T-cells distinguishes thymic neoplasm/hyperplasia, T-lymphoblastic lymphoma, and reactive lymph nodes.* Cytometry B Clin Cytom, 2018. **94**(3): p. 444–50.

52. Ohgami, R.S., et al., *Indolent T-lymphoblastic proliferation (iT-LBP): a review of clinical and pathologic features and distinction from malignant T-lymphoblastic lymphoma.* Adv Anat Pathol, 2013. **20**(3): p. 137–40.

53. Strauchen, J.A., *Indolent T-lymphoblastic proliferation: report of a case with an 11-year history and association with myasthenia gravis.* Am J Surg Pathol, 2001. **25**(3): p. 411–5.

54. Fromm, J.R., et al., *Flow cytometric features of incidental indolent T lymphoblastic proliferations.* Cytometry B Clin Cytom, 2020. **98**(3): p. 282–7.

55. van den Ancker, W., et al., *A threshold of 10% for myeloperoxidase by flow cytometry is valid to classify acute leukemia of ambiguous and myeloid origin.* Cytometry B Clin Cytom, 2013. **84**(2): p. 114–8.

7

IMMUNOPHENOTYPIC MARKERS IN FLOW CYTOMETRY

This chapter lists the most commonly used immunophenotypic markers in the diagnosis of hematological neoplasms applicable in flow cytometry (FC). Figure 7.1 shows algorithmic approach to immunophenotypic diagnosis of hematopoietic tumors, majority of which are CD45+. CD45− hematopoietic tumors include plasma cell myeloma (PCM), plasmablastic lymphoma (PBL), classic Hodgkin lymphoma (cHL), subset of B-cell acute lymphoblastic leukemia/lymphoma (B-ALL/LBL), subset of anaplastic large cell lymphomas (ALCLs), and occasionally in other T-cell lymphoproliferative disorders (subset of T-cell prolymphocytic leukemias [T-PLLs]), dendritic cell sarcoma, and occasional cases of DLBCL.

BCL2 (B-cell lymphoma/leukemia 2)

- **Benign:**
  - B-cells (CD10+ benign germinal center B-cells are negative)
  - T-cells
- **B-cell lymphoproliferations:**
  - Follicular lymphoma (FL) (majority)
  - Majority of B-cell lymphomas (Burkitt lymphoma (BL) is negative)
- **T-cell lymphoproliferations:**
  - Peripheral (mature) T-cell lymphoproliferations [anaplastic lymphoma kinase 1 (ALK1+) ALCL is negative]
- **Other tumors:**
  - Numerous other hematopoietic and non-hematopoietic tumors

The *BCL2* gene on chromosome 18q21 encodes a 26-kDa protein that inhibits apoptosis through the mitochondrial pathway. The *BCL2* gene was originally discovered in FLs with t(14;18)(q32;q21) translocation [1]. BCL2 protein can easily be detected by routine immunohistochemistry. BCL2 is widely expressed in normal lymphoid tissues but is absent in benign CD10+ germinal center B-cells. BCL2 positivity is helpful in differentiating FLs (BCL2+) from reactive follicular hyperplasia (BCL2−). Some FLs do not express BCL2 suggesting inhibition of apoptosis due to other factors (e.g., Bcl-X$_L$) rather than BCL2 overexpression [2]. Benign B-cells from mantle and marginal zones are BCL2+, and therefore immunostaining with BCL2 is not helpful in the diagnosis of MCL and MZL (including MALT lymphoma). DLBCL displays BCL2 expression in 30%–60% of cases, more frequently in nodal than in extranodal tumors [3–6]. BLs are BCL2−. BCL2 family proteins are expressed in subset of PTCLs and the level of expression correlates with some histological types, apoptotic rate, and proliferation [7]. In ALCL, BCL2 and ALK1 expressions are mutually exclusive [8]. BCL2 is expressed in ~60% of cases of HL, more often in nodular sclerosis type than in mixed cellularity type [9]. BCL2 is positive in subset of acute myeloid leukemia (AML) and acute lymphoblastic leukemia.

CD1a (cluster of differentiation 1a)

- **Benign:**
  - Cortical (common) thymocytes (thymic tissue, thymic hyperplasia)
  - Langerhans cells

- **Acute leukemias:**
  - T-cell acute lymphoblastic leukemia/lymphoma (T-ALL/LBL), subset
  - AML, minor subset of AMLs with monocytic differentiation
- **Myeloid neoplasms:**
  - Chronic myelomonocytic leukemia (CMML), cutaneous localization
- **Other tumors:**
  - Langerhans cell tumors (histiocytosis, sarcoma)
  - Thymoma
  - Indeterminate dendritic cell tumors/histiocytosis
  - Blastic indeterminate dendritic cell tumors

CD1 antigens consist of five different glycoproteins of which CD1a is most commonly used in FC. CD1a is a protein of 43–49 kDa expressed on dendritic cells and cortical thymocytes.

CD2

- **Benign:**
  - T-cells and NK cells
- **T/NK-cell lymphoproliferations:**
  - Peripheral (mature) T-cell lymphoproliferations
  - NK-cell proliferations including chronic lymphoproliferative disorders of NK cells
  - Aggressive NK-cell leukemia
- **B-cell lymphoproliferations:**
  - Chronic lymphocytic leukemia/small lymphocytic lymphoma (CLL/SLL), subset
  - B-cell lymphomas (rare cases)
- **Acute leukemias:**
  - T-ALL/LBL
  - AML, subset (often in acute monoblastic leukemia)
  - Hypogranular variant of APL-v
- **Myeloid tumors:**
  - CMML, subset
- **Other tumors:**
  - BPDCN, rare cases
  - Mast cell proliferations including systemic mastocytosis (SM)

CD2 is a pan T-cell antigen expressed by immature and mature T-cell disorders, including precursor T-ALL, PTCL, T-PLL, mycosis fungoides/Sézary's syndrome (MF/SS), adult T-cell leukemia/lymphoma (ATLL), T-large granular lymphocyte leukemia (T-LGL leukemia), NK-cell lymphoma/leukemia, extranodal NK/T-cell lymphoma, nasal type (ENKTL), aggressive NK-cell leukemia, AITL, ALCL, and cutaneous T-cell lymphomas (Figure 7.2). Subset of AML, especially acute monoblastic leukemia, mixed phenotype acute leukemia (MPAL), and BPDCN may show aberrant expression of CD2. Neoplastic mast cell proliferations show co-expression of CD2 and CD25. Hypogranular variant of APL often show aberrant CD2 expression (typical, hypergranular forms are most often CD2−). CD2 expression

DOI: 10.1201/9781003197935-7

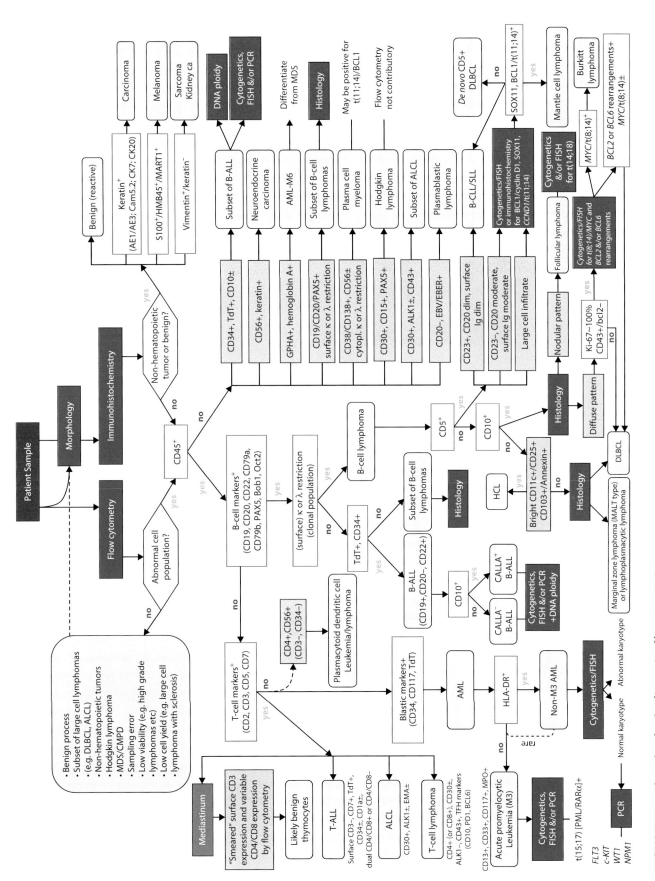

FIGURE 7.1 Algorithm for the diagnosis of hematopoietic tumors.

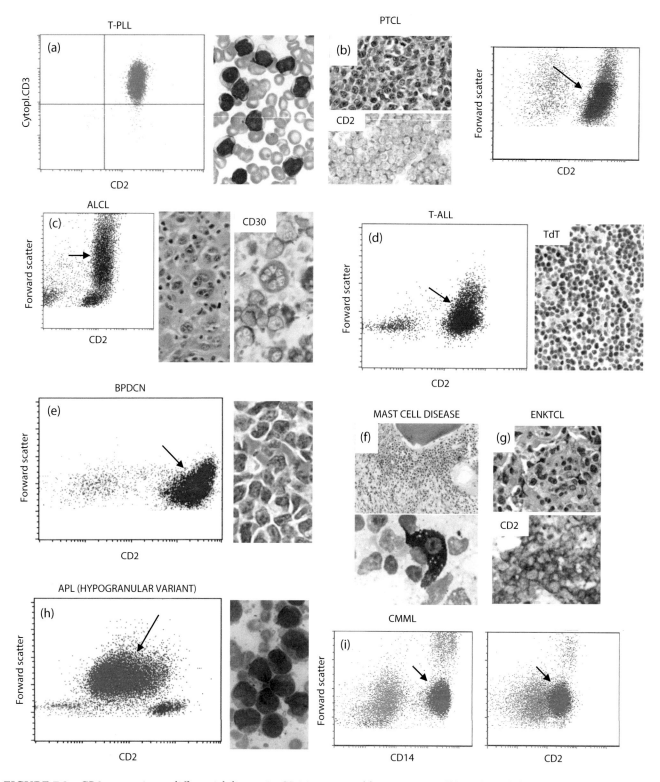

FIGURE 7.2 CD2 expression – differential diagnosis. CD2 is expressed by mature T-cell lymphoproliferative disorders including T-PLL (a), PTCL (b), and ALCL (c), precursor T-lymphoblastic leukemia/lymphoma (T-ALL, d), subset of blastic plasmacytoid dendritic cell neoplasm (BPDCN) (e), mast cell disease (f), extranodal NK/T-cell lymphoma, nasal type (ENKTL) (g), acute promyelocytic leukemia (APL), hypogranular variant (h), and monocytic proliferations, e.g., CMML (i).

(partial or complete) can be observed in 16% of CLL, and rarely in other B-cell lymphomas [10].

CD3

- *Benign:*
  - T-cells
- *B-cell lymphoproliferations:*
  - Isolated cases of primary effusion lymphoma (PEL), Epstein-Barr virus (EBV)+ B-cell lymphoma, PBL
- *T-cell lymphoproliferations:*
  - Peripheral (mature) T-cell lymphoproliferations
- *Acute leukemias:*
  - T-ALL/LBL
  - MPAL; AML/T-ALL
- *Other tumors:*
  - MPN with *FGFR1* rearrangement (8p11 myeloproliferative syndrome)

CD3 is the most specific marker for T-cell lymphoproliferations, being positive in both mature (peripheral) and subset of immature neoplasms. CD3 can be expressed on the membrane of the cells ("surface" antigen expression) and within the cytoplasm of the cell ("cytoplasmic" antigen expression). Surface CD3 expression is seen in T-cells, but the cytoplasmic expression is also present in NK cells. Immature T-cells that lack T-cell receptor gene rearrangements are negative for surface CD3. Precursor T-lymphoblastic neoplasms (T-ALL/LBL) usually do not express surface CD3 when analyzed by FC (cytoplasmic CD3 staining by FC and immunohistochemistry is often positive). Majority of mature (peripheral) T-cell lymphoproliferations are CD3+, but they may show either aberrant loss, dim or partial expression of CD3 especially in ALCL and other CD30+ T-cell lymphoproliferations, hepatosplenic T-cell lymphoma (HSTL) and enteropathy-associated T-cell lymphoma (EATL) [11–13]. In my series of cases, complete loss of surface CD3 expression is seen in 11% of T-PLL, 35% PTCL, not otherwise specified (PTCL, NOS), 33% of angioimmunoblastic T-cell lymphoma (AILT), 70% of ALCL, and 27% of ATLL, see Chapter 16 for details. Majority of EATLs are surface CD3−.

CD3 may be occasionally positive in PEL, a high-grade neoplasm of B-lineage associated with HHV8. CD3 expression has also been seen in non-HHV8-associated mature B-cell neoplasms, usually associated with EBV infection. MPN with *FGFR1* rearrangement (8p11 myeloproliferative syndrome) shows increased eosinophils and bilineal lymphoma/leukemia (often T-lymphoblastic and myeloid lineage), expressing CD3.

CD4 and CD8

CD4 expression:

- T-helper cells
- Dendritic cells
- Subset of peripheral T-cell lymphoproliferative disorders (PTCL, MF/SS, ATLL, ALCL)
- BPDCN
- Primary cutaneous CD4+ small/medium T-cell lymphoproliferative disorder
- Monocytes and monocytic neoplasms
- AML, subset
- ALK+ large B-cell lymphoma, rare cases
- Indolent T-cell lymphoproliferative disorder of the gastrointestinal (GI) tract, subset

CD8 expression:

- T-cell subset
- Subset of peripheral T-cell lymphoproliferative disorders (PTCL, ALCL, T-PLL)
- Monomorphic epitheliotropic intestinal T-cell lymphoma (MEITL)
- T-cell large granular lymphocyte leukemia (T-LGLL)
- Minor subset of chronic lymphoproliferative disorder of NK cells (dim and partial CD8 expression)
- CD8+ aggressive epidermotropic cutaneous T-cell lymphoma (CD8+ C-AECTCL)
- CD8+ cutaneous acral T-cell lymphoma (CD8+ C-ATCL)
- Subcutaneous panniculitis-like T-cell lymphoma (SPTCL)
- Very rare cases of MF
- Very rare cases of CLL and other mature B-cell neoplasms (PCM, LPL, MCL)
- Very rare cases of ENKTL
- Indolent T-cell lymphoproliferative disorder of the GI tract, subset

Dual CD4 and CD8 expression:

- T-prolymphocytic leukemia (T-PLL), subset
- T-cell acute lymphoblastic leukemia (T-ALL), subset
- ATLL, rare cases
- ALCL, rare cases
- PTCL, rare cases
- T-LGLL, rare cases

Dual CD4/CD8 negativity in T-cell lymphoproliferations:

- T-ALL, subset
- Chronic lymphoproliferative disorders of NK cells
- ENKTL
- Aggressive NK-cell leukemia
- HSTL
- PTCL, subset
- ALCL, subset
- T-PLL, subset

CD4 antigen is expressed by T-helper cells, monocytes, macrophages, and dendritic cells. The examples of hematolymphoid neoplasms expressing CD4 or CD8 are presented in Figure 7.3. CD4 is positive in peripheral T-cell lymphoproliferative neoplasms, BPDCN, and subset of myeloid proliferations including AML, CMML, acute monoblastic leukemia, and histiocytic tumors. Only rare cases of T-ALLs have restricted CD4 expression (majority of cases being either dual CD4/CD8+ or dual CD4/CD8−). Thymocytes from thymus or thymoma are dual CD4/CD8+. CD8 stains cytotoxic/suppressor T-cells and subset of NK-cells. CD8 is expressed by majority of T-LGL leukemias, SPTCL, and MEITL, rare cases of AETL, occasionally some other mature peripheral (mature) T-cell lymphoproliferations. In SPTCL CD8+ T-cells surround the adipocytes forming a characteristic low power rimming pattern. HSTL, T-LGL leukemia with NK-cell phenotype and aggressive NK-cell leukemia are dual CD4/CD8−. Very rare cases of mature B-cell lymphoproliferations may display aberrant expression of CD8 (most often CLL). Indolent T-cell lymphoproliferative disorder of the GI tract has been included as a provisional entity in the most recent WHO classification [14]. It is a

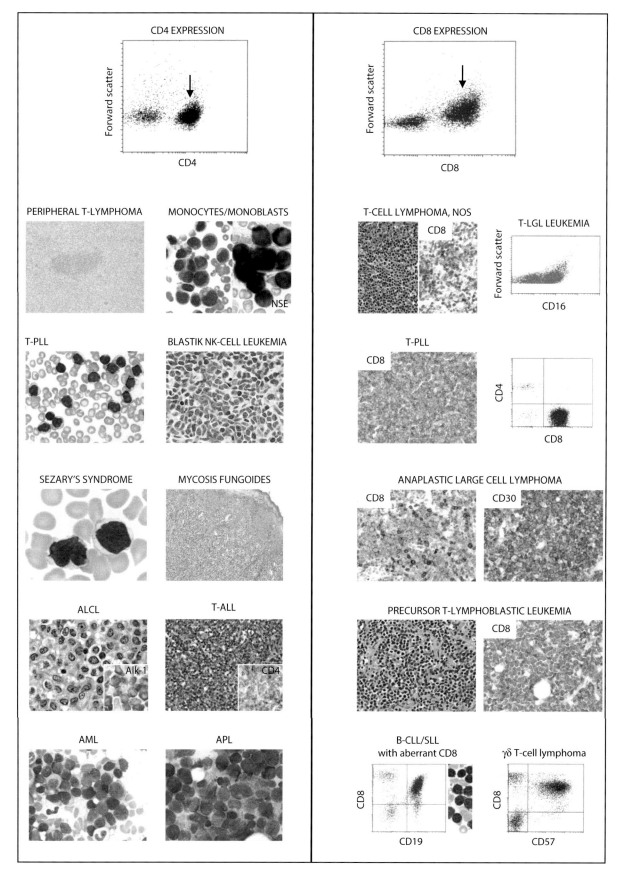

FIGURE 7.3   The expression of CD4 and CD8.

clonal T-cell lymphoproliferative disorder (CD4+ or CD8+) with an indolent clinical course [15–18].

CD5

- *Benign:*
  - T-cells
  - B-cells (subset) in children and young adults (number of CD5+ B-cells decreases with age)
- *B-cell lymphoproliferations:*
  - CLL/SLL
  - B-cell prolymphocytic leukemia (B-PLL), rare cases
  - Mantle cell lymphoma (MCL)
  - De novo CD5+ diffuse large B-cell lymphoma (DLBCL)
  - Marginal zone lymphoma (MZL), minor subset
  - Lymphoplasmacytic lymphoma (LPL), rare cases
  - FL, very rare cases
  - Intravascular large B-cell lymphoma (IVLBCL), subset
  - Hairy cell leukemia (HCL), very rare cases
- *T-cell lymphoproliferations:*
  - Peripheral (mature) T-cell lymphoproliferations with the exception of EATL, MEITL, and HSTL which are CD5−
- *Acute leukemias:*
  - T-ALL/LBL
  - MPAL; AML/T-ALL
- **Myeloid tumors:**
  - Aberrant CD5 expression by blasts in myelodysplastic syndrome (MDS)
- *Other tumors:*
  - BPDCN, rare cases

CD5, a 67-kDa pan-T-cell antigen is expressed by mature and immature T-cell lymphoproliferations. Aberrant loss of CD5 expression by benign T-cells may be seen in some reactive conditions (usually virus-associated infections) or after bone marrow (BM) transplant [19, 20]. The expression is often dimmer than in benign T-cells. Benign CD5+ B-cells may be present in blood and lymphoid tissues, more often in children and younger patients. The expression of CD5 is often aberrantly missing in neoplastic T-cell processes. HSTL and EATL are CD5−. NK cells and NK-cell tumors are CD5−. Myeloblasts from AML more often show aberrant expression of CD2 and CD7 than CD5, but MPAL may be CD5+.

Among B-cell disorders, CD5 is typically expressed in CLL/SLL and MCL. CLL/SLL differs from MCL by CD23 positivity, although some cases of CLL may be CD23− and rare MCL may be CD23+. Therefore, definite differentiation between MCL and CLL should be based on status of BCL1 (cyclin D1) by immunohistochemistry or *CCND1* rearrangement by FISH studies. Only a small proportion of DLBCL expresses CD5. Lack of BCL1 (cyclin D1) and SOX11 expression and lack of history of CLL/SLL distinguishes de novo CD5+ DLBCL from MCL and Richter's syndrome, respectively. The prognosis of de novo CD5+ DLBCL is worse than that for CD5− DLBCL. Subset of IVLBCLs, MZLs and rare cases of LPLs, FLs and HCLs may show CD5 expression. CD5+ splenic marginal zone lymphomas (SMZLs) do not differ clinically from typical CD5− cases, but more often show CD13 expression [21]. Phenotypic classification of mature B-cell lymphoproliferations is presented in Chapter 12.

CD7

- *Benign:*
  - T-cells
  - NK cells
- *B-cell lymphoproliferations:*
  - DLBCL, very rare cases
  - CLL/SLL, very rare cases
- *T/NK-cell lymphoproliferations:*
  - Peripheral (mature) T-cell lymphoproliferations
  - NK-cell proliferations including chronic lymphoproliferative disorders of NK cells
  - Aggressive NK-cell leukemia
- *Acute leukemias:*
  - T-ALL/LBL
  - AML, subset
  - MPAL; AML/T-ALL
- *Myeloid tumors:*
  - Aberrant CD7 expression by blasts in MDS
  - Aberrant CD7 expression by monocytes in CMML
- *Other tumors:*
  - BPDCN, subset

CD7 is a membrane-bound glycoprotein that is expressed very early in T-cell development. CD7 is a pan T-cell antigen expressed by peripheral (mature) T-cell lymphoproliferations and T-ALL. CD7 is very often aberrantly expressed (either negative or dim) in peripheral T-cell disorders. In precursor T-cell neoplasms CD7 is most often strongly positive (bright expression FC). Other hematopoietic tumors which may express CD7 include subset of BPDCN, MPAL, and AML (Figure 7.4). In AML, aberrant expression of CD7 represents one of the most common variants of leukemia-associated immunophenotype (LAIP). Acute promyelocytic leukemia (APL) and B-cell lymphoproliferations are typically CD7−. Among the latter, aberrant expression of non CD5 T-cell markers is very unusual and mostly represent expression of CD2 in CLL/SLL. Only sporadic cases of DLBCL and CLL/SLL show aberrant CD7. Blasts in MDS and monocytes in CMML often display aberrant CD7 expression (majority of juvenile myelomonocytic leukemias do not display aberrant expression of CD7, however).

CD10

- *Benign:*
  - Neutrophils (basophils and eosinophils are CD10−)
  - Germinal center B-cells
  - T follicular helper (TFH) cells
  - Thymocytes
  - Hematogones
- *B-cell lymphoproliferations:*
  - FL and its variants (e.g., pediatric type and duodenal type)
  - In situ follicular neoplasia (ISFN)
  - Primary cutaneous follicle center lymphoma (PCFCL), subset
  - BL
  - High grade B-cell lymphoma with *MYC* and *BCL2* rearrangements (HGBL-R, "double hit" lymphoma)
  - High grade B-cell lymphoma, not otherwise specified (HGBL, NOS), subset
  - DLBCL, subset
  - HCL, minor subset)
  - MCL, minor subset
  - LPL, rare cases
  - PBL, rare cases
  - Large B-cell lymphoma with *IRF4* rearrangement, subset
  - PCM, rare cases

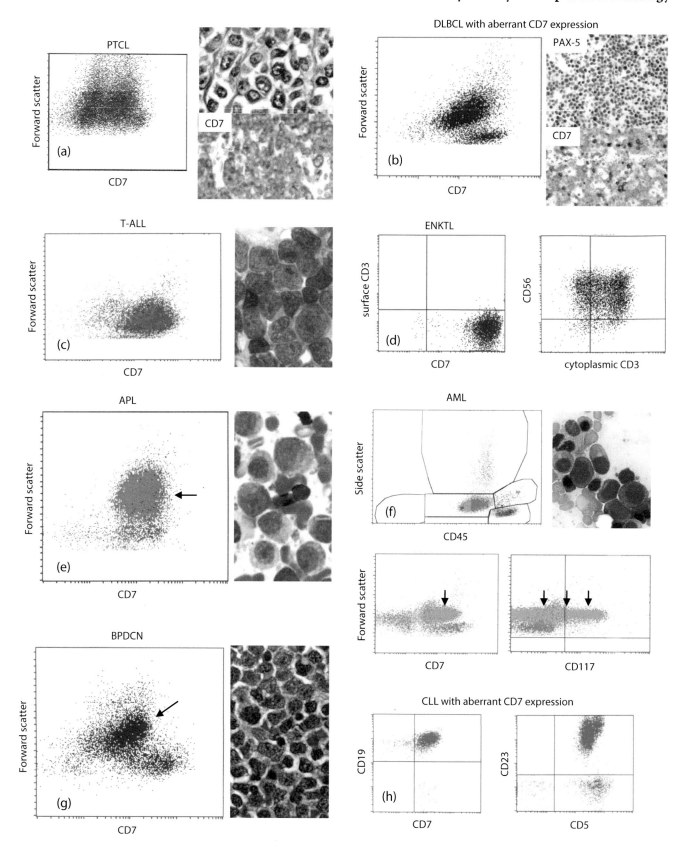

FIGURE 7.4 CD7 expression – differential diagnosis. CD7 is positive in significant subset of T-cell lymphoproliferative disorders, including PTCL (a), rare cases of DLBCL (b), rare cases of T-ALL (c), ENKTL (d), subset of APL (e), subset of AML (f), BPDCN (g), and rare cases of CLL (h).

- **T-cell lymphoproliferations:**
  - AITL, subset
  - Follicular T-cell lymphoma (FTCL)
  - Nodal PTCL with TFH phenotype
- **Acute leukemias:**
  - B-ALL/LBL
  - T-ALL/LBL, subset
  - MPAL; AML/B-ALL, subset
- **Myeloid tumors:**
  - Blasts in MDS may be CD10+
  - Lymphoid blast phase of chronic myeloid leukemia (CML)
- **Other tumors:**
  - Small cell carcinoma
  - Melanoma
  - Thymoma
  - Germ cell tumors

CD10 (Figure 7.5) is a 100-kDa cell surface metalloendopeptidase, known as a common acute lymphoblastic leukemia antigen (CALLA). Among hematopoietic cells, CD10 is expressed by immature B- and T-cells, germinal center B-cells, neutrophils, BL, majority of FLs, subset of DLBCL, high grade B-cell lymphoma with *MYC* and *BCL2* (and/or *BCL6*) rearrangements (HGBL-R; double or triple hit lymphoma), high grade B-cell lymphoma, not otherwise specified (HGBL, NOS), subset of MCL, subset of HCL and subset of LPL. Occasional FLs may be CD10⁻ (some cases may show discrepant FC and immunohistochemistry results with CD10 staining). Among precursor lymphoid neoplasms, CD10 is more often expressed by B-ALL than T-ALL. The expression of CD10 in B-ALL is very bright when analyzed by FC (immunohistochemistry shows strong membranous staining). Benign B-cell precursors (hematogones) are CD10+. CD10 is not expressed by erythroid and myeloid precursors. Rare cases of PCMs, malignant melanoma, and acute monoblastic leukemias may be CD10+.

Among T-cell lymphomas, CD10 is positive in nodal PTCL with T-follicular helper phenotype (PTCL-TFH), defined by expression of at least 2 or 3 TFH markers (CD10, BCL6, PD-1, CXCL13, and ICOS). In AITL, PD-1 and CXCL13 are positive in majority of cases (96% and 84%, respectively), whereas CD10 is noted only in subset of cases (66%) [22, 23]. Primary cutaneous CD4+ small/medium-sized pleomorphic T-cell lymphoproliferative disorder (CD4+ C-PTCLPD) similarly to AITL express BCL6, PD1 and CXCL13, but are CD10⁻ [24]. CD10 is expressed by rare cutaneous T-cell lymphomas with T$_{FH}$ phenotype [25].

Benign neutrophils display bright expression of CD10 (similar to CD16). Down-regulation of expression of both CD10 and CD16 by neutrophils may be seen in MDS. Aberrant CD10 expression may be seen in non-hematopoietic tumors especially small cell carcinoma (CD45⁻/CD10⁻/⁺/CD56⁺) or melanoma.

CD11b

- **Benign:**
  - Myeloid cells (neutrophils, eosinophils, basophils, subset of maturing myeloid precursors, monocytes)
  - Natural killer (NK) cells
  - CD8+ T-cells, subset
  - γδ+ T-cells, subset
  - Dendritic cells
- **T-cell lymphoproliferations:**
  - T-LGLL, subset
- **Acute leukemias:**
  - AML with/without maturation, minor subset
  - Acute monoblastic leukemia (often positive, but expression may be variable, dim, or partial)
- **Myeloid tumors:**
  - CMML
  - Juvenile myelomonocytic leukemia
  - Dysplastic neutrophils in MDS often show diminished expression of CD11b

CD11b is a type of cell surface receptor that is selectively expressed on leukocytes. This protein has several names such as integrin alpha M (ITGAM), complement component 3 receptor alpha chain (CR3a), and macrophage receptor 1 alpha subunit (MAC1a). CD11b is expressed by monocytes (macrophages), granulocytes, dendritic cells, and NK cells. It is negative on mature B- and T-cells, but activated CD8+ T-cells (e.g., in viral infections) and some T-LGL leukemia cells are often CD11b+ (at least partially). AMLs with monocytic differentiation are usually CD11b+, whereas myeloblasts from AML with or without maturation only sporadically display aberrant expression of CD11b. The CD11b+ AML is seen more often in cases with unfavorable cytogenetics and the expression of CD11b correlates with monosomal karyotype (defined as two or more autosomal monosomies, or one monosomy with other structural aberrations) and predicts an extremely poor prognosis [26]. APLs are CD11b⁻. Lack of CD11b and CD13 expression in transient myeloproliferative disorder helps to differentiate it from AML in infants with Down syndrome, which are usually CD11b+/CD13+ [27].

CD11c

- **Benign:**
  - Myeloid cells (neutrophils, eosinophils, basophils, subset of maturing myeloid precursors, monocytes)
  - CD8+ T-cells, subset
  - CD4+ T-cells, minor subset (upon activation)
  - NK cells, subset
  - Dendritic cells, subset
- **B-cell lymphoproliferations:**
  - CLL/SLL, often dim or partial expression
  - HCL, bright expression
  - Hairy cell leukemia variant (HCL-v), bright expression
  - MZL, subset (dim or partial expression)
  - Splenic diffuse red pulp B-cell lymphoma (SDRPL), moderate expression
  - DLBCL, subset
- **T-cell lymphoproliferations:**
  - T-LGLL, subset
  - HSTL
- **Acute leukemias:**
  - AML with/without maturation, subset (often partial or dim expression) [APL is CD11c⁻]
  - Acute monoblastic leukemia
- **Myeloid tumors:**
  - CMML
  - Juvenile myelomonocytic leukemia

CD11c is a member of the superfamily of glycoproteins that mediate cell–cell and cell–matrix interaction and is expressed strongly on monocytes and tissue macrophages, and less strongly on granulocytes and subsets of lymphocytes. Bright expression

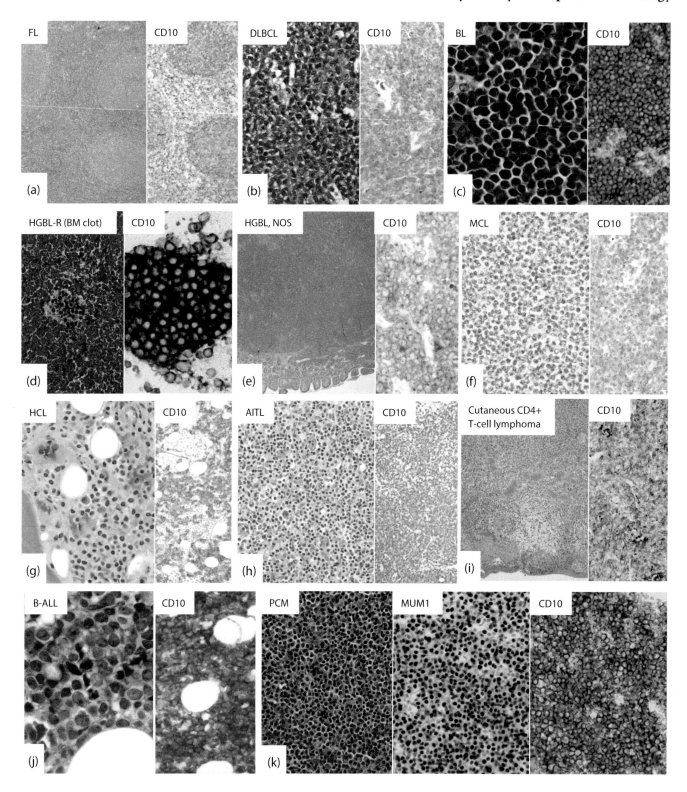

FIGURE 7.5 CD10 expression: differential diagnosis includes (a) follicular lymphoma (FL); (b) diffuse large B-cell lymphoma (DLBCL); (c) Burkitt lymphoma (BL); (d) "double-hit" lymphoma (HGBL-R); (e) HGBL, NOS; (f) mantle cell lymphoma (MCL); (g) hairy cell leukemia (HCL); (h) nodal TFH cell lymphoma, angioimmunoblastic-type (AITL); (i) cutaneous CD4+ small/intermediate T-cell lymphoma; (j) B-cell acute lymphoblastic leukemia/lymphoma (B-ALL/LBL); and (k) plasma cell myeloma (PCM).

of CD11c is typical for HCL and most cases of acute monoblastic leukemia. Other AMLs may express CD11c (dim, moderate, or partial), but APL both classic hypergranular and hypogranular variant (APL-v) are most often CD11c⁻. AML with *NPM1* mutation, which are often HLA-DR⁻ and CD34⁻ (like APL) are most often CD11c⁺. The CD11c may be dimly to moderately positive in other hematologic malignancies including CLL, MZL, and HCL-v. In contrast to CLL, MCLs are most often CD11c⁻ [28]. Expression of CD11c helps in differential diagnosis between SMZL with dim, partial, or negative expression, splenic diffuse red pulp B-cell lymphoma (SDRPL) with moderate expression and HCL which is brightly CD11c⁺. Among T-cell lymphoproliferations, CD11c may be seen in subset of CD8⁺ T-LGLL and HSTL.

CD13 and CD33

- *Benign:*
  - Neutrophils, maturing myeloid precursors
  - Eosinophils
  - Basophils
  - Myeloblasts
  - Monocytes and their precursors (promonocytes, monoblasts)
  - Mast cells, subset
- *B-cell lymphoproliferations:*
  - CLL, rare cases
  - PCM, rare cases
  - LPL, rare cases
  - MZL, rare cases
- *T-cell lymphoproliferations:*
  - ALCL, rare cases
- *Acute leukemias:*
  - AML (APL is characterized by variable CD13 and very bright CD33 expression)
  - B-cell acute lymphoblastic leukemia (B-ALL), subset
  - T-cell acute lymphoblastic leukemia (T-ALL), minor subset
  - Early T-cell precursor acute lymphoblastic leukemia (ETP-ALL)
- *Myeloid tumors:*
  - MDSs (the expression of CD13 and/or CD33 may be down- or up-regulated)
  - Myeloproliferative neoplasms (MPNs)
  - Mixed MDS/MPNs
- *Other tumors:*
  - BPDCN, subset

CD13 is positive in myeloid cells. During myeloid maturation, the expression of CD13 decreases from promyelocyte to metamyelocyte stage and later increases in final stages of neutrophilic maturation. The pan-myeloid antigens, CD13 and CD33 are expressed by AML and 10%–20% of ALL. CD13 is expressed by majority of AML. The CD33 molecule is a cell surface differentiation protein that is expressed on normal progenitor and myeloid cells, as well as on >80% of AML blasts. It belongs to the family of the sialic acid-binding immunoglobulin-like lectin (Siglec). With the availability of immunotherapy targeted for CD33, the analysis of CD33 expression is becoming very important for patients with acute leukemias. Among AML, the CD13 and/or CD33 are more often negative or dim in AML with t(8;21) when compared

to AML without this translocation. The discrepant CD13 and CD33 expression is seen in subset of AML (e.g., CD13⁺/CD33⁻ in minimally differentiated AML, CD13⁻/CD33⁺ in AML with maturation and *NPM1* mutation). APL typically shows variable expression of CD13 and very bright expression of CD33.

Subset of B-ALLs and T-ALLs may express CD13 and/or CD33. The aberrant expression of myeloid antigens (especially CD13 in conjunction with CD33, CD66c, and CD25) in B-ALL is often associated with t(9;22)/*BCR-ABL* rearrangement (Philadelphia chromosome and co-expression of CD13 and CD33 with t(12;17). Expression of CD13 by B-ALL has also been linked with chromosome 7 monosomy. In T-ALL, presence of CD13 and/or CD33 expression may be predictive of *ETV6* or *KMT2A* rearrangement. Myeloid antigen expression is characteristic for early T-cell precursor ALL (ETP-ALL).

Aberrant expression of CD13, CD33 and other myeloid antigens (CD11b, CD11c, CD15) may be seen in occasional cases of CLL and less often in other mature low-grade B-cell lymphomas (MZL, LPL/WM, B-PLL, SMZL) or minor subset of DLBCL. Rare cases of poorly differentiated PCMs may express CD13, CD15, or CD33. The expression of CD13 is seen more often in splenic MZL with positive CD5 expression [21]. CD13 expression by mature B-cell lymphomas more often show plasmacytic differentiation. FL and HCL do not express myeloid antigens. CD13 and/or CD33 may be aberrantly expressed in rare cases of ALCL [29–31].

CD14

- *Benign:*
  - Monocytes, bright expression (promonocytes and monoblasts show dimmer and/or partial expression)
- *Acute leukemias:*
  - Acute monoblastic leukemia, subset (often variable, partial, or dim expression)
  - Monocytic component in acute myelomonocytic leukemia (AMML)
- *Myeloid tumors:*
  - CMML
  - Juvenile myelomonocytic leukemia
  - MDSs may show aberrant expression of CD14 on neutrophils/maturing myeloid precursors

CD14 is 55 kDa glycoprotein which is brightly expressed by benign monocytes and majority of neoplastic monocytes from CMML and monocytic component of acute myelomonocytic leukemia (Figure 7.6). Monoblasts and promonocytes from acute monoblastic leukemia are either CD14⁻ or display partial or variable expression, ranging from negative to bright by FC analysis. Based on expression of CD14 and CD16, monocytes are subdivided into three categories: CD14^bright+/CD16⁻ classical monocytes (MO1), CD14^bright+/CD16⁺ intermediate monocytes (MO2), and CD14⁺/CD16^bright+ non-classical monocytes (MO3) [32–36]. In normal blood, classical monocytes predominate (~85%), followed by non-classical monocytes (~10%) and intermediate monocytes (~5%). CMML differs from reactive monocytosis by presence of predominantly classical (MO1) monocytes (CD14^bright+/CD16⁻) while presence of mixture of MO1, MO2, and MO3 monocytes is suggestive of reactive process. Benign neutrophils are CD14⁻ but neutrophils/maturing myeloid precursors from subset of MPN or MDS may be CD14⁺ (mild up-regulation of CD14 expression), especially in patients with monosomy 7 or del(5q). Similarly,

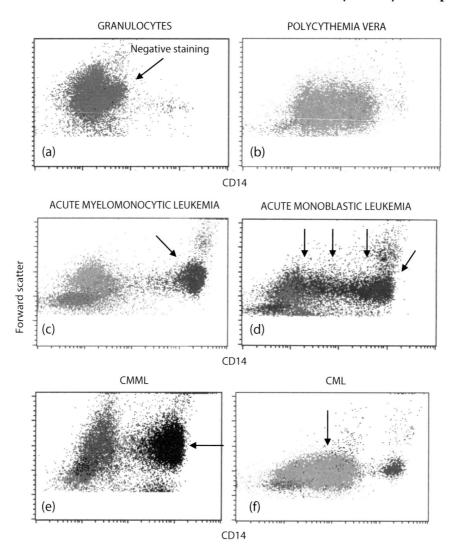

FIGURE 7.6 CD14 expression – differential diagnosis. Benign granulocytes (maturing myeloid cells) are negative for CD14 (a). Aberrant (dim) expression of CD14 (up-regulation) may be observed in subset of myeloproliferative disorders (e.g., PV, b; CML, f). Benign monocytes and neoplastic monocytes in majority of cases of CMML (e) and monocytic component of acute myelomonocytic leukemia (c) display bright expression of CD14. In contrast immature monocytic population from acute monoblastic leukemia is either CD14-negative or display variable expression (d, arrows).

aberrant expression of CD14 on neutrophils may be seen in transient myeloproliferative disorders in children with trisomy 21 or in patients with sepsis or after treatment with granulocyte-colony stimulating factors (G-CSF).

CD15

- *Benign:*
  - Neutrophils and maturing myeloid precursors
  - Monocytes
  - Eosinophils
  - Basophils, subset
  - Monocytes, classical (MO1, CD14⁺/CD16⁻)
- *B-cell lymphoproliferations:*
  - Rare cases of CLL, B-PLL, DLBCL, HCL, and PCM may show CD15 expression

- *T-cell lymphoproliferations:*
  - PTCL, NOS, rare cases
  - ALCL, rare cases
- *Acute leukemias:*
  - AML, subset
  - B-cell acute lymphoblastic leukemia (B-ALL), minor subset (most often pro-B-ALL)
- *Myeloid tumors:*
  - MDSs, blasts with aberrant CD15 expression
  - MPNs, blasts with aberrant CD15 expression
  - MDS/MPN
- *Other tumors:*
  - Hodgkin lymphoma, classic (cHL)

CD15 is expressed by granulocytes, classical monocytes, eosin-ophils, subset of basophils, neoplastic cells in CML, subset of

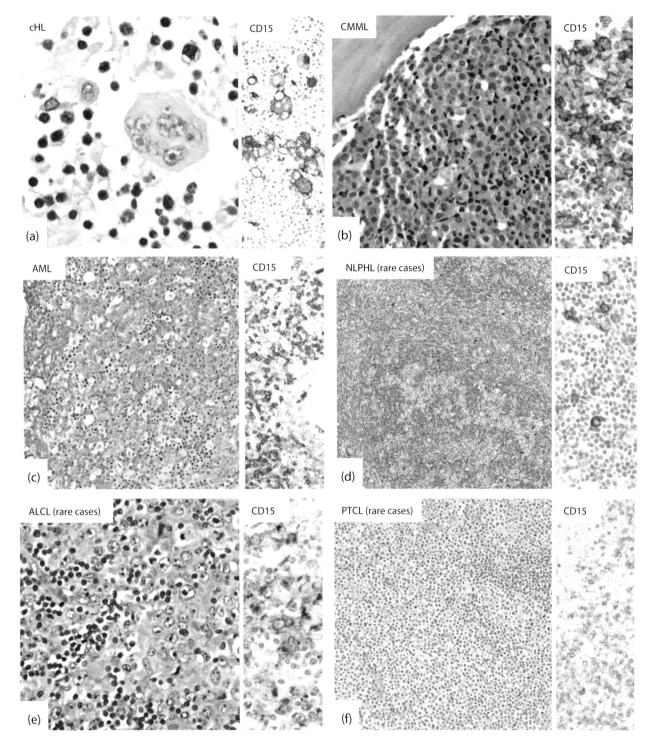

FIGURE 7.7 CD15 expression – differential diagnosis: (a) HL (classic); (b) CMML; (c) AML; (d) NLPHL (rare cases fixed in B5); (e) ALCL (rare cases); and (f) PTCL, not otherwise specified (rare cases).

AML and majority of neoplastic cells in cHL (Figure 7.7). Only very rare cases PTCLs (including ALCL and PTCL) display aberrant CD15 expression [37]. APL is either CD15⁻ or show dim (partial) CD15 expression. Mast cells and non-classical and intermediate monocytes are CD15⁻. CD15 is often present in non-hematopoietic malignancies. CD15 is also used routinely to identify neutrophils in paroxysmal nocturnal hemoglobinuria (PNH) FC panels.

CD16

- *Benign:*
  - Neutrophils
  - T-cells, subset (mostly γδT⁺ T-cells)
  - NK cells
  - Monocytes, minor subset (non-classical and intermediate monocytes)

- **T-cell lymphoproliferations:**
  - T-LGLL
  - Chronic lymphoproliferative disorder of NK cells
  - HSTL, subset
  - Aggressive NK-cell leukemia
- **Myeloid tumors:**
  - Dysplastic neutrophils in MDS often show diminished expression of CD16

CD16 has two different form, named CD16a (NK cells, majority of γδT+ T-cells and rare αβ+ T-cells) and CD16b (neutrophils, myelocytes, metamyelocytes). CD16 is expressed by neutrophils, T-LGL leukemia, chronic lymphoproliferations of NK cells, and HSTL. Benign monocytes usually display dim expression of CD16 on subset. Based on expression of CD14 and CD16, monocytes are classified into three categories: classical CD14$^{bright+}$/CD16$^-$ monocytes, intermediate CD14$^{bright+}$/CD16$^+$ monocytes, and nonclassical CD14^{dim+}/CD16$^+$ monocytes [32, 34, 36, 38]. Proportion of those three monocytes subsets is helpful in differential diagnosis between CMML (predominance of classical monocytes) and reactive monocytosis (admixture of classical, intermediate and non-classical monocytes). Myeloblasts and atypical promyelocytes of APL are CD16$^-$. Dysplastic granulocytes often display aberrant down-regulation of CD16 (lack of expression of CD16 suggests dysgranulopoiesis and leftward shift). Down regulation of CD16 expression by neutrophils is often seen in MDS and MPN (CML and primary myelofibrosis). Essential thrombocythemia (ET) and polycythemia vera (PV) most often show normal expression of both CD10 and CD16 by neutrophils. Comparing the pattern of expression of CD16 versus CD11b and CD16 versus CD13 is helpful in identifying abnormal pattern compatible with dysgranulopoiesis (see Chapter 19).

CD19

- **Benign:**
  - Hematogones
  - B-cells
  - Plasma cells (variable, often dim or partial expression)
- **B-cell lymphoproliferations:**
  - Majority of mature B-cell lymphoproliferative disorders (B-cell neoplasms which are often CD19$^-$ include PEL, ALK$^+$ large B-cell lymphoma, PBL and subset of post-transplant lymphoproliferative disorders)
  - PCM, rare cases
- **Acute leukemias:**
  - B-ALL/LBL
  - AML, subset (AML with t(8;21)/*RUNX1-RUNX1T1*)
  - MPAL; AML/B-ALL
- **Myeloid tumors:**
  - CML in lymphoid blast crisis
- **Other tumors:**
  - Nodular lymphocyte predominant Hodgkin lymphoma (NLPHL)

The CD19 molecule is a 95-kDa glycosylated type I integral membrane protein whose expression is limited to B-cells and follicular dendritic cells. CD19 is expressed by mature and immature B-cell neoplasms, NLPHL, benign plasma cells (variable expression), very rare plasma cell neoplasms, MPAL and subset of AML, usually associated with t(8;21)/*RUNX1-RUNX1T1* (which often co-expresses CD19 and CD56).

CD20

- **Benign:**
  - B-cells (germinal center cells show brighter expression than mantle cells)
- **B-cell lymphoproliferations:**
  - CLL, dim expression
  - HCL and HCL-v
  - Majority of B-cell lymphomas
  - PCM, minor subset
- **T-cell lymphoproliferations:**
  - Aberrant expression of CD20 may be seen in very rare cases (usually on subset of neoplastic cells) of PTCL, NOS, ALCL, T-PLL, follicular T-cell lymphoma (FTCL), and AITL
- **Acute leukemias:**
  - B-ALL/LBL, rare cases (usually dim and/or partial expression)
- **Other tumors:**
  - NLPHL
  - Hodgkin lymphoma, classic (cHL), minor subset
  - Thymoma, type A (spindle, medullary), subset

CD20 is present on late pre-B cells and mature B-cells, but not on precursor cells or terminally differentiated plasma cells (CD20 appears on the B-cell surface between immunoglobulin light chain gene rearrangement and the expression of surface Ig: it is expressed after CD19 and CD10 but before cytoplasmic μ chain expression). The function of CD20 remains poorly understood, although it has been implicated in B-cell activation, regulation of B-cell growth and regulation of transmembrane calcium flux. Apart from B-cell lymphoproliferations, CD20 is expressed on neoplastic cells (LP cells) in NLPHL, subset of classic HL and occasional plasma cell neoplasms. CD20$^+$ B-cell lymphomas often lose the CD20 positivity after anti-CD20 immunotherapy with rituximab (monoclonal antibody directed against CD20 antigen). Rituximab was shown to mediate antibody-dependent cellular cytotoxicity and complement-dependent cellular cytotoxicity and induce non-classic (caspase-independent) apoptosis of lymphoma cells in vitro.

CD20$^-$ B-cell lymphomas include the following (Figure 7.8):

- PBL
- PEL
- DLBCL associated with chronic inflammation
- ALK$^+$ large B-cell lymphoma
- DLBCL, rare cases

CD22

- **Benign:**
  - B-cells
  - Basophils, subset
- **B-cell lymphoproliferations:**
  - Majority of mature B-cell lymphoproliferative disorders (CLLs are CD22$^-$)
  - PCM, very rare cases
- **Acute leukemias:**
  - B-ALL/LBL, cytoplasmic expression of CD22

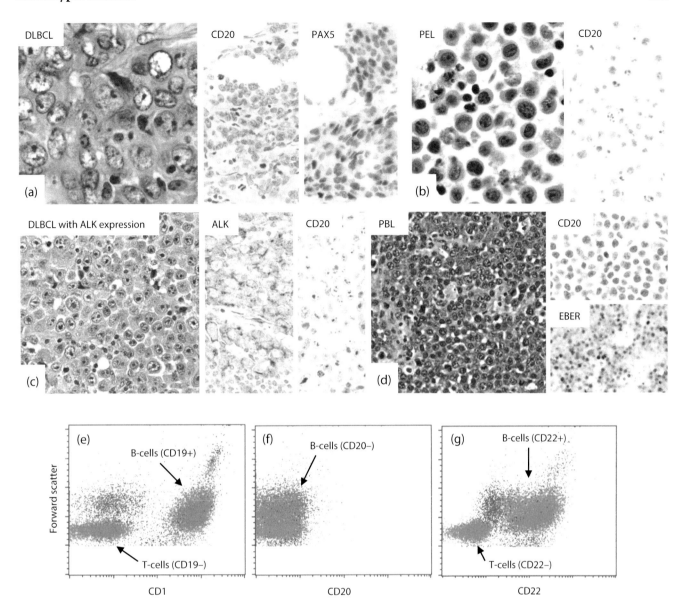

FIGURE 7.8 B-cell lymphomas with negative CD20 – differential diagnosis: (a) DLBCL (rare cases); (b) primary effusion lymphoma (PEL); (c) DLBCL with ALK-expression; (d) plasmablastic lymphoma (PBL); (e–g) after Rituxan treatment [lymphomatous cells are positive for CD19 (e) and CD22 (g) but display negative staining with CD20 (f; arrow)].

- • MPAL; AML/B-ALL
- • Acute basophilic leukemia, subset
- *Myeloid tumors:*
  - • Basophils in chronic and blast phase of CML are CD22+
- *Other tumors:*
  - • Mast cell neoplasms

CD22 is a B-cell specific marker (plasma cells are CD22−). CD22 is expressed by B-cell lymphoproliferations (both mature and precursor). CD22 expression is bright in HCL and splenic MZL and dim in other B-cell lymphoproliferations [39–42]. Plasma cell neoplasms and CLL are CD22−. Clonal plasma cell component of LPL may be CD22+. Basophils in CML and AMLs with basophilic differentiation may show CD22 expression (often together with CD13 and CD25 expression).

CD23

- *Benign:*
  - • B-cells, subset
  - • Plasma cells, subset
  - • Follicular dendritic cells (FDC)
  - • Activated T-cells, subset
  - • Activated monocytes, subset
- *B-cell lymphoproliferations:*
  - • CLL, strong expression
  - • FL, minor subset (diffuse variant is often CD23+)
  - • MZL, very rare cases
  - • B-PLL, rare cases
  - • LPL, rare cases
  - • HCL, rare cases

- • DLBCL, rare cases
- • Primary mediastinal large B-cell lymphoma (PMBL), subset
- • MCL, very rare cases
- • PCM, rare cases
- • *Acute leukemias:*
  - • Acute monoblastic leukemia, subset
- • *Myeloid tumors:*
  - • CMML, minor subset
- • *Other tumors:*
  - • Follicular dendritic cell tumors

CD23 is positive in benign B-cells in blood, mantle zone and germinal centers of lymph node and tonsil. CD23 is strongly expressed by majority of CLL/SLL. In contrast to CD5+/CD23+ CLL, most MCL cases are CD23– (only rare cases of MCL may be dimly CD23+). Subset of FL (especially diffuse variant) and DLBCL may be CD23+. B-cell lymphoproliferations which are usually CD23– include MCL, BL, HCL, majority of DLBCL, and majority of nodal and splenic MZL. Other hematopoietic tumors which may display aberrant CD23 expression include acute monoblastic leukemia and some CMML. Analysis of CD23 helps to assess FDC meshwork when evaluating nodal lymphomas (*see CD21, above*). Subset of benign plasma cells and plasma cell tumors express CD23.

CD24

CD24 is glycosylphosphatidylinositol (GPI)-linked protein also known as heat stable antigen (HSA). It is expressed on the surface of B cells (but not plasma cells), granulocytes, follicular dendritic cells, and epithelial cells. CD24 is used in FC panel for diagnosis of paroxysmal nocturnal hemoglobinuria (PNH). B-ALL and majority of mature B-cell lymphoproliferations are CD24+ (HCL, MZL and subset of DLBCL are usually negative or show dim expression).

CD25

- • *Benign:*
  - • T-cells, subset
  - • NK cells
  - • B-cells, minor subset (dim expression)
  - • Basophils
- • *B-cell lymphoproliferations:*
  - • HCL (HCL-v is CD25–)
  - • CLL, rare cases
  - • B-ALL, subset
  - • FL, rare cases
  - • Splenic marginal zone lymphoma (SMZL), subset
  - • B-cell lymphomas, subset (MCLs and splenic red pulp B-cell lymphoma are CD25–)
- • *T-cell lymphoproliferations:*
  - • ATLL, strong expression (100% of cases)
  - • ALCL, subset
  - • MF, subset
  - • PTCL, subset
  - • Follicular T-cell lymphoma (FTCL), subset
  - • ENKTL, majority of cases
- • *Acute leukemias:*
  - • AML, minor subset
  - • B-cell acute lymphoblastic leukemia (B-ALL), subset
  - • T-cell acute lymphoblastic leukemia (T-ALL), rare cases
- • *Myeloid tumors:*
  - • Chronic eosinophilic leukemia (CEL), subset
  - • CML in blast crisis, subset
- • *Other:*
  - • SM [benign mast cells are CD25–]
  - • Langerhans cell histiocytosis (LCH)

The CD25 (interleukin-2 receptor; IL-2R) is expressed by ATLL, HCL and subset of other T- and B-cell lymphoproliferative disorders (Figure 7.9). CD25 is often expressed by ALCL and is positive

HAIRY CELL LEUKEMIA

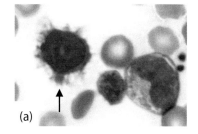
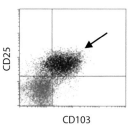

(a)

ADULT T-CELL LEUKEMIA/LYMPHOMA

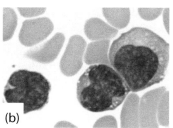
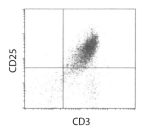

(b)

ANAPLASTIC LARGE CELL LYMPHOMA

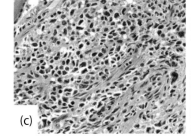
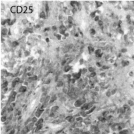

(c)

PERIPHERAL T-CELL LYMPHOMA, UNSPECIFIED

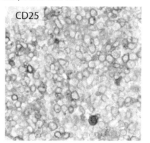

(d)

FIGURE 7.9 CD25 expression – differential diagnosis: (a) HCL; (b) ATLL; (c) ALCL (bone marrow); and (d) PTCL.

in subset of other T-cell lymphoproliferations, including PTCL, MF, FTCL, and ENKTL. AITL, HSTL, T-PLL, and T-LGLL are usually CD25⁻. CD25 is not expressed by HCL-v. Subset of AMLs may be positive for CD25. The expression of CD25 positively correlates with *FLT3*-ITD, *DNMT3A*, and *NPM1* mutations [43]. CD25 is expressed by neoplastic mast cell processes. Aberrant CD2 and/or CD25 expression on mast cells provides one minor criterion for a diagnosis of SM.

CD26

CD26 is a 110 kDa type II membrane protein expressed on the membrane of mature thymocytes, T lymphocytes (upregulated upon activation), B cells, NK cells, and macrophages. The analysis of CD26 is useful in evaluation patients with MF, which show loss of CD26 expression in 92% of cases of transformed MF [44]. Circulating neoplastic T-cells from patients with MF (Sézary's syndrome) and ATLL are negative for CD26 [45, 46].

CD27

- *Benign:*
  - T-cells, subset
  - NK cells
  - B-cells (memory cells)
  - Thymocytes
  - Plasma cells
- *B-cell lymphoproliferations:*
  - CLL
  - B-APLL
  - FL
  - LPL
  - SMZL
  - Nodal marginal zone lymphoma (NMZL)
  - DLBCL
  - BL
  - Monoclonal gammopathy of undetermined significance (MGUS) [CD27 is positive only in rare PCMs]
- *T-cell lymphoproliferations:*
  - Sézary's syndrome (SS), subset [MF is negative]
  - PTCL, minor subset
  - Follicular T-cell lymphoma (FTCL), subset
  - AITL, subset

CD30

- *Benign:*
  - Activated B- and T-cells (immunoblasts)
  - Atypical cell (immunoblasts) in EBV-lymphadenitis or Kikuchi lymphadenopathy
- *B-cell lymphoproliferations:*
  - DLBCL, subset
  - PEL
  - FL, rare cases
  - Primary mediastinal large B-cell lymphoma (PMBL)
  - Lymphomatoid granulomatosis (LyG)
  - PCM, rare cases
- *T-cell lymphoproliferations:*
  - ALCL, strong expression
  - PTCL, NOS, subset
  - Primary cutaneous anaplastic large cell lymphoma (C-ALCL)

- Pagetoid reticulosis (variant of MF)
- Lymphomatoid papulosis (LyP)
- Large cells in ATLL and subset of cells in acute form of ATLL
- Large cells in AITL
- Large cells in EATL
- Large cells in MF and transformed MF
- ENKTL, subset
- *Acute leukemias:*
  - AML, minor subset
- *Other tumors:*
  - Hodgkin lymphoma, classic (cHL)
  - Mediastinal grey zone lymphoma
  - Aggressive SM

CD30 (Figure 7.10) is a transmembrane glycoprotein and is a member of the tumor necrosis factor superfamily, that is expressed in activated B- and T-lymphocytes (with immunoblastic cytomorphology), cHL (100%), ALK⁺ ALCL (100%), ALK⁻ ALCL (100%), C-ALCL (100%), subset of DLBCL (subset), LyG, PEL (most cases), PMBL, large cells in EATL (>50%), LyP (60–100%), pagetoid reticulosis (a variant of MF, 100%), MF with large cell transformation, Sézary syndrome and occasional cases of FL and PCM. Both ALK⁺ and ALK⁻ ALCL have similar morphology with cohesive sheets of large cells often with characteristic intrasinusoidal distribution and presence of "hallmark" cells with indented, horseshoe, kidney-shaped nuclei. CD30 expression helps in subclassification of T-cell lymphomas. T-cell lymphomas with strong and uniform expression of CD30 include ALCL (both ALK⁺ and ALK⁻), ATLL, primary cutaneous C-ALCL, breast-implant-associated ALCL, MF with large cell transformation and rare cases of PTCL, NOS, and ENKTL. T-cell lymphomas with focal, variable, or weak expression of CD30 include AITL and subset of PTCL, EATL, ENKTL, and MEITL.

Benign mast cells are CD30⁻, but CD30 expression has been reported in aggressive SM and occasional mast cell leukemias. In classic HL and in ALCL, CD30 shows strong membranous staining and Golgi area staining. CD30 is expressed in 14%–21% of DLBCL and is associated with unique gene expression profiling, non-germinal-center origin and favorable prognosis [47, 48]. In AML, CD30 expression was reported to correlate with presence of *FLT3*-ITD mutation and leukocytosis [49] or high-risk disease [50]. Due to availability of targeted therapy for CD30⁺ lymphomas, it is recommended to include the intensity of CD30 staining (1+, 2+, 3+) and the percentage of tumor cells with membranous and/or Golgi pattern (presence of ≥1% or <1% staining in tumor cells).

CD34

- *Benign:*
  - Immature hematopoietic precursors including colony forming unit macrophage (CFU-M), CFU-G (granulocyte), burst-forming unit/erythroid (BFU-E)
  - Hematogones
  - Myeloblasts
  - Immature megakaryocytes
  - Mast cell progenitors
- *Acute leukemias:*
  - AML
  - B-cell acute lymphoblastic leukemia (B-ALL)
  - T-cell acute lymphoblastic leukemia (T-ALL), subset

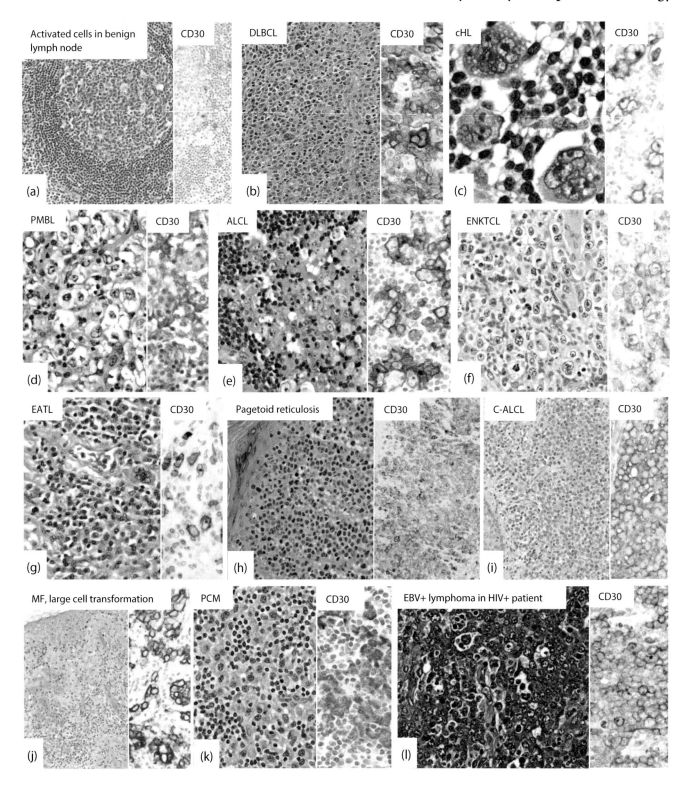

FIGURE 7.10 CD30 expression – differential diagnosis: (a) activated cells in reactive lymph node; (b) DLBCL; (c) classic HL; (d) primary mediastinal large B-cell lymphoma (PMBL); (e) ALCL; (f) extranodal NK/T-cell lymphoma, nasal type (ENKTL); (g) enteropathy-associated T-cell lymphoma (EATL); (h) Pagetoid reticulosis (variant of MF); (i) primary cutaneous ALCL (C-ALCL); (j) mycosis fungoides (MF) with large cell transformation; (k) plasma cell myeloma (PCM); (l) EBV-associated high grade lymphoma in HIV+ patient.

- Acute undifferentiated leukemia (AUL)
- Acute panmyelosis with myelofibrosis (APMF)
- Hypogranular variant of APL (APL-v) [classic, hypergranular APL is CD34⁻]
- MPAL
- *Myeloid tumors:*
  - Blasts and megakaryocytes in MDS
  - Circulating blasts in primary myelofibrosis (PMF)
  - CML in blast crisis
- *Other tumors:*
  - BPDCN, minor subset
  - Neuroblastoma

The CD34 is a small peptide attached to the cell membrane of a hematopoietic cell. It is a marker of myeloid immaturity expressed by developmentally early hematopoietic stem cells (erythroid, myeloid, and megakaryocytic precursors) and TdT⁺ immature lymphoid cells. Apart from blasts, CD34 stains also blood vessels and sinuses. The CD34 can be used by FC and by immunohistochemistry. CD34 is positive in both AML and acute lymphoblastic leukemia. Among AMLs, CD34 is not expressed by classic (hypergranular) APL and majority of acute monocytic leukemias. Hypogranular variant of APL (APL-v), on the other hand, is often CD34⁺. Apart from AML, CD34 is may be positive in B-ALL, T-ALL and in MPAL. BPDCNs are CD34⁻. AML with mutation of *NPM1* are often CD34⁻ and those without *NPM1* mutation but with *FLT3*-ITD are often CD34⁺ and TdT⁺ [51].

The immunophenotypic analysis of the CD34 staining in the BM by immunohistochemistry (number and distribution of blasts) and by FC (number of CD34⁺ blasts) is very useful in evaluation patients with MDS [52]. The number of CD34⁺ blasts in normal BM is usually <2% and blasts are scattered individually without forming significant clusters. In the MDS, not only CD34⁺ blasts are often increased but the distribution of blasts is abnormal with clustering in the intertrabecular areas (abnormal localization of immature precursors; ALIP). Presence of >2% blasts has prognostic significance for patients with MDS. By definition, presence of >5% blasts is diagnostic MDS with excess blasts (MDS-EB), and number of blasts >20% is indicative of AML Apart from increased number of blasts, identification of aberrant phenotype of CD34⁺ blasts by FC (e.g., CD117⁻, CD123⁺, down-regulation of CD13, CD33, or CD45 and aberrant expression of CD7 or CD56) often helps to diagnose indicate MDS. Increased number of CD34⁺ precursors is also observed in MPN, especially in accelerated phase or incipient blast crisis. the finding of 10%–19% of blasts in the blood and/or in BM, as well as the immunohistochemical detection of an increased number of CD34⁺ cells with cluster formation and/or an abnormal endosteal location in the BM, indicate an AP of the disease and presence of >20% blasts in blood or BM is diagnostic of blasts phase. In BM disorders with fibrosis (most often in primary myelofibrosis; PMF), the number of circulating blasts may be higher than in BM sample. Due to often suboptimal (hemodiluted) BM aspirate sample, there is also often discordance in the number of blasts seen in BM core biopsy and that reported by FC analysis of BM aspirate.

Correlation of the expression of CD34, CD117, PAX5, MUM1, CD71, and mast cell tryptase helps to differentiate between myeloblasts (CD34⁺/CD117⁺), hematogones (CD34⁺/PAX5⁺), mast cells (CD117⁺/tryptase⁺), immature basophils (tryptase⁺/CD34⁻/CD117⁻), immature erythroid cells (CD117⁺/⁻/CD71⁺/CD34⁻),

and plasma cells (CD117⁺/MUM1⁺). Among non-hematopoietic tumors, CD34 is expressed by vascular tumors, Kaposi's sarcoma, dermatofibrosarcoma protuberans, gastrointestinal stromal tumor (GIST), and some other soft tissue tumors.

Number of CD34⁺ circulating blasts is often increased in PMF and high grade MDS. In some PMF cases, number of CD34⁺ blasts in blood is higher than in BM, reflecting either abnormal cell trafficking due to marrow fibrosis and/or extramedullary hematopoiesis. Low grade MDS including MDS with reticulin fibrosis, essential thrombocythemia (ET) and polycythemia vera (PV) typically show lower number of circulating blasts when compared to PMF.

CD36

CD36 (glycoprotein IV) is monocytic marker (similar to CD14). CD36 is expressed by mature monocytes. CD36 may be expressed in subset of AML, usually with monocytic differentiation. In acute monoblastic (monocytic) leukemia, CD36 is more often positive that CD14. Only minor subsets of AML with/without maturation may show aberrant CD36 expression. APLs are CD36⁻, whereas acute megakaryoblastic leukemia are usually CD36⁺ (especially those associated with trisomy 21). CD36 was reported in 37% of patients in study by Perea [2-year leukemia-free survival (LFS) rate was 34% for CD36⁺ patients and 55% for CD36⁻ patients] [53]. CD36 is also reported in BPDCN.

CD38

- *Benign:*
  - Plasma cells
  - Activated (stimulated) B- and T-cells
  - Thymocytes
  - Hematogones
  - Neutrophils and maturing myeloid precursors
  - Eosinophils
  - Basophils
  - NK cells
  - Monocytes, classic (CD14^bright+/CD16⁻)
- *B-cell lymphoproliferations:*
  - PCM, bright expression
  - CLL, subset
  - MCL, major subset
  - DLBCL, subset
  - FL, subset
  - HCL, minor subset
  - PEL
  - DLBCL associated with chronic inflammation
  - PBL
  - ALK⁺ large B-cell lymphoma
  - BL
  - LPL
  - High grade B-cell lymphoma with *MYC* and *BCL2* rearrangement (HGBL-R)
  - MZL, subset
- *T-cell lymphoproliferations:*
  - ALCL, subset [ALK⁺ ALCL is often CD38⁻]
  - PTCL
  - ATLL, acute variant {chronic variant is negative]
  - T-PLL, subset
  - HTSL, majority

- T-LGLL, majority
- AITL, majority
- ENKTL, majority
- *Acute leukemias:*
  - AML, majority
  - B-cell acute lymphoblastic leukemia (B-ALL), majority
  - T-cell acute lymphoblastic leukemia (T-ALL), all cases
- *Myeloid tumors:*
  - Blasts and myeloid cells in MDS, MPN and mixed MDS/MPN
- *Other tumors:*
  - BPDCN, subset

CD38 is a transmembrane glycoprotein with a widespread cellular expression and functional activity. The CD38 expression is high in B-cell precursors and in terminally differentiated plasma cells, but low to absent in mature B-cells, where it can be induced by activatory signals. CD38 is often positive (dim to moderate) in AML. Among mature neoplasms, CD38 is often positive in MCL and may be positive in subset of CLL. CD38 is often positive in FL and may be positive in other B- and T-cell lymphoproliferations. T-cell neoplasms, especially ALCL or PTCL and high-grade B-cell lymphomas, such as high-grade B-cell lymphoma (HGBL) not otherwise specified, HGBL with rearrangement of *MYC* and *BCL2* (and/or *BCL6*) also called double or triple hit lymphoma and BL often show bright expression of CD38. Generally, bright expression of CD38 is typical for B-cell lymphomas with *MYC* rearrangement, being seen in 70% of B-cell lymphomas with *MYC* rearrangement (both DLBCL with *MYC* rearrangement and HGBL-R), and only in 17% of DLBCL without *MYC* rearrangement [54, 55]. CD38 is positive in subset of HCLs. HCL-v are CD38⁻.

Based on the percentage of clonal cells expressing CD38, CLL could be divided into two categories: one with <30% CD38⁺ leukemic cells and another with ≥30% cells. CLL with CD38 expression in more than 30% cells contained unmutated *IGVH* genes, whereas samples expressing less than 30% CD38⁺ contained mostly mutated cases indicating a strong inverse relationship between *IGVH* gene mutation and CD38 expression. The level of CD38⁺ cells correlates with clinical stage, response to treatment and overall survival: higher CD38 percentages correlates with more advanced stages, diffuse BM involvement, atypical morphology, deletion(11q), trisomy 12, poorer chemosensitivity and significantly shorter survival. In approximately 30% of patients with CLL the levels of CD38 expression and *IGVH* mutational status are discordant.

In patients with plasma cell myeloma treated with targeted therapy against CD38, the expression of CD38 may become negative in plasma cells and other cells normally positive for CD38 (e.g., hematogones).

CD43

- *Benign:*
  - T-cells
  - NK cells
  - Neutrophils
  - Eosinophils
  - Basophils
  - Mast cells
  - Monocytes
  - Hematogones
  - Erythroblasts/pronormoblasts
  - B-cells, minor subset (<10%)

- *B-cell lymphoproliferations:*
  - BL
  - MCL
  - CLL
  - MZL, subset
  - DLBCL, minor subset
  - Primary cutaneous DLBCL, leg type
  - ALK⁺ large B-cell lymphoma, rare cases
  - PCM
  - LPL, rare cases
  - HCL, subset [HCL-variant is CD43⁻]
- *T/NK-cell lymphoproliferations:*
  - Mature (peripheral) T-cell and NK-cell lymphomas
- *Acute leukemias:*
  - AML
  - B-cell acute lymphoblastic leukemia (B-ALL)
  - T-cell acute lymphoblastic leukemia (T-ALL)
- *Myeloid tumors:*
  - Blasts and myeloid cells in MDS, MPN and mixed MDS/MPN
- *Other tumors:*
  - BPDCN, subset
  - Langerhans cell sarcoma

CD43 is expressed by benign T-cells, mature T-cell lymphoproliferative disorders, CLL, MCL, BL, subset of DLBCL, subset of B-PLL, B-ALL, T-ALL, PCM, mast cell diseases, and histiocytes/histiocytic neoplasms. Benign B-cells are CD43-negative (except for terminal ileum [56]). Only small subset of FL may be CD43⁺. CD43 is not lineage specific since it is present on wide range of hematopoietic lesions, it is only rarely expressed on non-hematopoietic tumors and therefore is very useful in differentiating undifferentiated or anaplastic malignancies (hematopoietic versus non-hematopoietic). In subset of ALCL (null cell type), CD43 may be the only marker expressed apart from CD30 and ALK. CD43 expression is dimly positive in subset of HCL and predominantly negative in HCL-v.

CD45

CD45⁺ hematopoietic tumors
The leukocyte common antigen (LCA; CD45) is a complex family of high molecular weight glycoproteins expressed on majority of hematopoietic (white blood) cells and their progenitors, (maturing megakaryocytes and erythroid cells do not express CD45). CD45 is present on normal and malignant cells of myeloid, T-, and B-cell lineage. On white blood cells (WBCs), the level of CD45 is differentially expressed throughout maturation, being lower on blasts and immature forms and highest on mature myelomonocytic cells and lymphocytes.

CD45⁻ hematopoietic tumors (Figure 7.11)

- PCM
- Classic HL (Reed-Sternberg cells and Hodgkin cells)
- Acute erythroid leukemia (AEL)
- B-ALL/LBL, subset
- PBL
- Rare cases of ALCL and other mature T-cell lymphoproliferations
- AML, rare cases
- DLBCL, rare cases
- T-PLL, subset

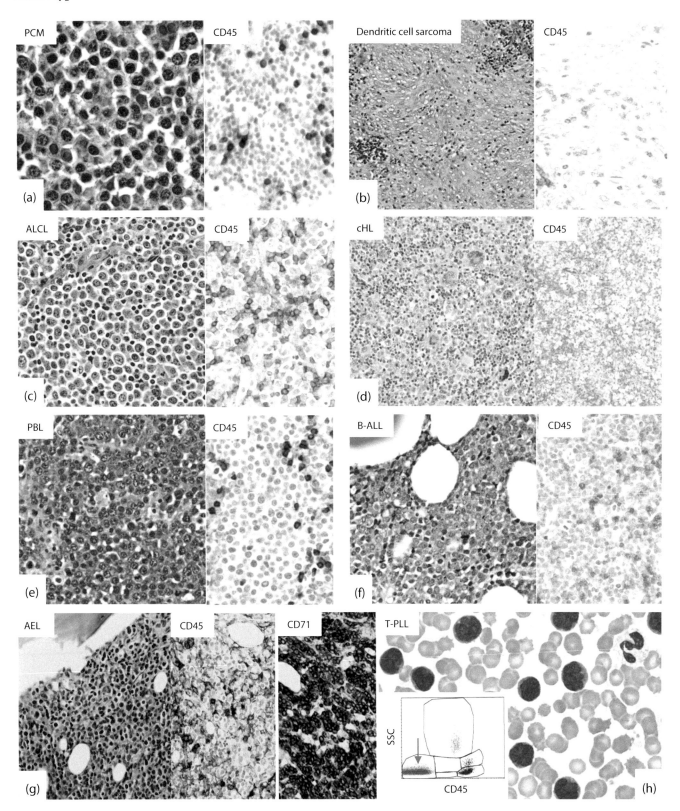

FIGURE 7.11 Hematopoietic tumors with negative CD45 expression – differential diagnosis: (a) plasma cell myeloma (PCM); (b) dendritic cell sarcoma; (c) anaplastic large cell lymphoma (ALCL); (d) classic HL; (e) plasmablastic lymphoma (PBL); (f) B-ALL (subset); (g) acute erythroid leukemia (AEL, negative CD45 and strongly positive CD71); (h) T-cell prolymphocytic leukemia (T-PLL) with negative CD45 expression by FC (orange dots. arrow), blood analysis.

CD49d

CD49d also known as integrin α4β1 (ITGB1; CD29) is a surface adhesion molecule which binds to the β-integrin CD29 to form very late antigen-4 (VLA-4). CD49d is emerging as one of the most valuable adverse prognostic markers in CLL/SLL [57–59]. CD49d is expressed by B- and T-lymphocytes, thymocytes, Langerhans cells, eosinophils, and monocytes. CD49d is considered positive if expressed by ≥30% of cells. CD49d is positive in approximately 40%–60% of CLL cases. Detection of CD49d is superior to CD38 and ZAP-70 in predicting overall and treatment-free survival in CLL [58]. High levels of CD49d protein and/or ITGB1 mRNA are significantly associated with shorter time form diagnosis to treatment and overall survival. This prognostic value of CD49d is independent of other prognostic parameters including FISH and *IGVH* status. Higher expression of CD49d is associated with unmutated IGVH and positive CD38 and ZAP70 expression. CD49d expression is lower among patients with deletion 11q and higher in patients with trisomy 12.

CD52

Monoclonal antibody therapy has emerged in the last decade as a promising approach in treating B- and T-cell malignancies. Alemtuzumab (Campath) is a humanized monoclonal antibody directed against the CD52 antigen. Similar to rituximab, Campath eliminates cells through antibody-dependent cell-mediated cellular toxicity, complement activation and apoptosis. CD52 is expressed on all normal and most malignant T-lymphocytes and majority of mature B-cell lymphoproliferations. Campath has been used in CLL, T-PLL, and low-grade non-Hodgkin lymphomas.

CD56

- *Benign:*
  - NK cells
- *B-cell lymphoproliferations:*
  - PCM, majority of cases
  - DLBCL, rare cases
- *T-cell lymphoproliferations:*
  - ENKTL
  - PTCL, subset
  - T-LGLL
  - Chronic lymphoproliferative disorder of NK cells
  - ALCL, subset
  - HTSL
  - MEITL
  - EATL, subset
  - Lymphomatoid papulosis (LyP), subset
  - Primary cutaneous γδ T-cell lymphoma (PCGD-TCL)
- *Acute leukemias:*
  - Acute monoblastic leukemia
  - AML, subset [most often AML with t(8;21)/*RUNX1-RUNX1T1*]
- *Myeloid tumors:*
  - Subset of neutrophils and maturing myeloid precursor in MDS, MPN, and mixed MDS/MPN
  - CMML, subset
- *Other tumors:*
  - BPDCN
  - Small cell carcinoma, carcinomas with neuroendocrine differentiation, malignant melanoma, neuroblastoma, Wilm's tumor, rhabdomyosarcoma

CD56 (Figure 7.12), a neural cell-adhesion molecule (N-CAM) is expressed by NK cells and a subset of T-cells and monocytes. Its expression is well recognized in hematolymphoid malignancies of NK-cell lineage, but also in PCM, AML, especially with monocytic differentiation, subset of APL, BPDCN, subset of PTCLs and ALCLs, and rare cases of DLBCL (especially extranodal). AML with t(8;21) is often displays co-expression of CD19 and CD56. Subset of LyP cases with cytotoxic phenotype expresses CD56. Among extranodal T-cell lymphomas, CD56 is positive in ENKTL, MEITL, EATL, HSTL, and PCGD-TCL. In contrast to PCM, majority of benign plasma cells are CD19+ and CD56−. CD56 expression is often upregulated in subset of granulocytes and monocytes from patients with MDS, MPNs, and mixed MDS/MPN (such as CMML).

CD57

- *Benign:*
  - Large granular lymphocytes (T-LGL)
  - CD8+ T-cells, subset
  - CD4+ T-cells, subset
  - NK cells, subset
- *T-cell lymphoproliferations:*
  - T-LGLL
  - Chronic lymphoproliferative disorder of NK cells, subset
  - T-PLL, rare cases (mostly dim and partial expression)
- *Acute leukemias:*
  - T-cell acute lymphoblastic leukemia (T-ALL), rare cases
- *Other tumors:*
  - Primitive neuroectodermal tumor (PNET)
  - Rhabdomyosarcoma
  - Small cell carcinoma

CD57 is expressed by NK cells and subset of T-cells. It is positive on T-LGL leukemia, subset of NK-cell neoplasms, and rare precursor T-cell lymphoblastic leukemias. In NLPHL there is often increased number of small benign CD57+ T-cells, which may form characteristic rosettes around large neoplastic cells (LP cells).

CD64

- *Benign:*
  - Monocytes (classical, CD14bright+/CD16−)
- *Acute leukemias:*
  - Acute monoblastic leukemia
  - AML, subset
  - APL, subset (dim or partial expression)
- *Myeloid tumors:*
  - CMML
  - Upregulation of CD64 on neutrophils may be seen in MDS

CD64 is expressed by monocytes, acute monoblastic leukemia, CMML, monocytic component of acute myelomonocytic leukemia, and blasts in subset of AML, including AML with or without maturation, APL (dim or partial expression), and acute megakaryoblastic leukemia. In contrast to acute leukemias with monocytic differentiation, the expression of CD64 in other types of AMLs is usually dim and/or partial.

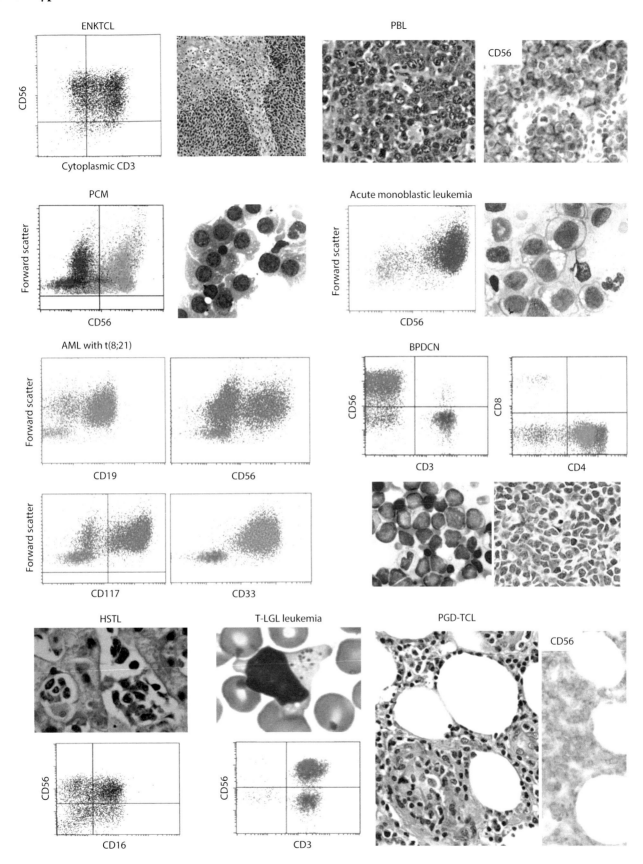

FIGURE 7.12(a) CD56 expression – differential diagnosis (see text for details, section: CD56).

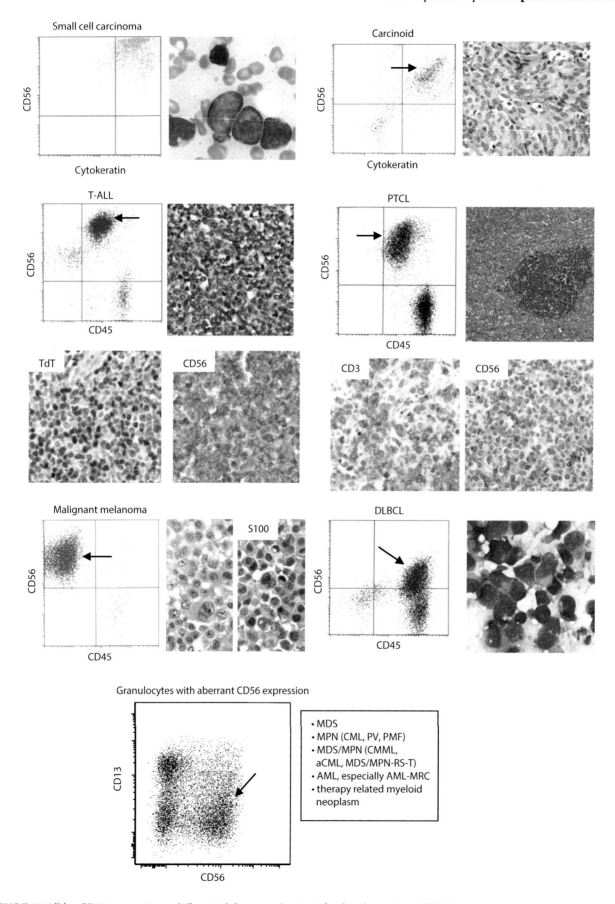

FIGURE 7.12(b)   CD56 expression – differential diagnosis (see text for details, section: CD56).

CD65

- *Benign:*
  - Neutrophils
  - Eosinophils
  - Basophils
  - Monocytes, subset
  - NK cells, minor subset
- *Acute leukemias:*
  - AML, subset
  - Early T-cell precursor acute lymphoblastic leukemia (ETP-ALL), subset

CD71 (transferrin receptor)

- *Benign:*
  - B- and T-cell precursors
  - Myeloblasts
  - Activated B- and T/NK cells
  - Erythroblasts/pronormoblasts
  - Germinal center B-cells (centroblasts)
  - Reactive follicular hyperplasia (CD10⁺ B-cells are CD71⁺)
- *B-cell lymphoproliferations:*
  - DLBCL, subset
  - BL
  - Primary mediastinal large B-cell lymphoma (PMBL)
  - Richter's transformation of CLL/SLL
  - Other high-grade lymphomas, especially high-grade B-cell lymphoma with *MYC* and *BCL2* rearrangements (HGBL-R) [low grade B-cell lymphomas are usually CD71⁻]
- *T-cell lymphoproliferations:*
  - PTCL, subset
  - ALCL, subset (expression may be bright)
  - ATLL, bright expression
- *Acute leukemias:*
  - AML, subset
  - AEL, bright expression
  - Acute megakaryoblastic leukemia
  - MPAL
  - B-cell acute lymphoblastic leukemia (B-ALL), minor subset (dim expression)
  - T-cell acute lymphoblastic leukemia (T-AL), subset
- *Myeloid tumors:*
  - Decreased expression of CD71 on erythroid precursors may be seen in MDS

CD71 is a transferrin receptor that mediates the uptake of transferrin-iron complexes. CD71 is strongly positive on erythroid precursors, myocytes, hepatocytes, endocrine pancreas cells, spermatocytes, basal keratinocytes, and placental syncytiotrophoblasts [60]. Among erythroid cells, CD71 is strongly positive in early precursors and the level of expression decreases gradually through the reticulocytes stage [61, 62]. In contrast to glycophorin A (GPHA; CD235a), CD71 is negative on red blood cells. In malignant tumors, CD71 is positive in AEL and high-grade lymphomas [62, 63]. By FC analysis, the expression of CD71 is often dimmer in BL than in aggressive DLBCLs. The expression of CD71 is decreased in dysplastic erythroid precursors [64, 65]. In BM biopsy specimens strong CD71 expression is restricted to erythroid lineage (myeloblasts, neoplastic plasma cells and metastatic carcinoma cells are usually negative) [62, 66]. Its expression is similar to e-cadherin, which stains early erythroid precursors. When analyzed by FC, CD71 positivity is seen in AML with or without maturation, acute monoblastic leukemia, acute myelomonocytic leukemia, MPAL, AEL, and acute megakaryoblastic leukemia. The expression of CD71 is either dim or negative in APL, acute monocytic leukemia or B-ALL. Similarly to CD34, progression from dysplasia to AML is associated with increased number of cells expressing CD71 [67].

CD79

- *Benign:*
  - B-cells
  - Hematogones
- *B-cell lymphoproliferations:*
  - Majority of mature B-cell lymphoproliferative disorders are CD79⁺ (CLL, PEL, and PBL are usually)
- *Acute leukemias:*
  - B-ALL/LBL
  - MPAL (AML, AML/B-ALL)
- *Other tumors:*
  - Non-hematopoietic tumors may be CD71⁺

CD79 is a heterodimer composed of two parts, α chain (CD79a) and β chain (CD79b). It is a B-cell marker which can be detected on B-cell surface or intracytoplasmic (most of the antibody epitopes are intracytoplasmic). All B-ALL are CD79a⁺ while CD79b is variably expressed with subset of cases being negative. Among benign cells, CD79 is expressed only by B-cells. CD79a and CD79b are positive in mature B-cell lymphoproliferative disorders and in subset of precursor B-cell neoplasms. CLL cases are CD79b⁻, while MCL are CD79b⁺. Immunohistochemical staining of the bone marrow with CD79a often shows non-specific labeling of megakaryocytes. Subset of PCMs is CD79a⁺.

CD81

- *Benign:*
  - Hematogones (bright expression)
  - Plasma cells
  - Myeloblasts
  - B-cells
  - T-cells
  - NK cells
  - Mast cells
  - Dendritic cells
- *B-cell lymphoproliferations:*
  - MCL, strong expression
  - HCL
  - FL, subset (dim expression)
  - DLBCL, subset (dim expression)
  - BL, strong expression
  - High grade B-cell lymphoma with *MYC* and *BCL2* rearrangement (HGBL-R), strong expression
  - HCL-v
  - PCM, minor subset
- *T-cell lymphoproliferations:*
  - Majority of T-cell lymphoproliferative disorders are CD81⁺
- *Acute leukemias:*
  - AML, major subset

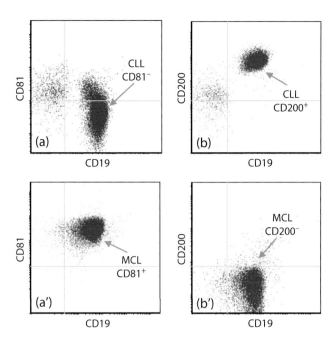

FIGURE 7.13 Comparison of CD81 and CD200 expression in CLL (a–b) and MCL (a′–b′). Note negative to partially dim CD81 expression in CLL (a) and strongly positive CD81 expression in MCL (a′). The expression of CD200 is strongly positive in CLL (b) and negative in MCL (b′).

- B-cell acute lymphoblastic leukemia (B-ALL) [dimmer expression than in hematogones]
- T-cell acute lymphoblastic leukemia (T-ALL)
- *Other tumors:*
  - Neuroblastoma
  - Rhabdomyosarcoma

CD81 is an integral surface membrane protein with 4 transmembrane domains (tetraspanin) that links with CD19 to form a multimolecular complex that is crucial for B-cell development and the humoral response. CD81 is positive in mature B-cell lymphoproliferative disorders. It is dimly expressed in B-ALL, which helps with differential diagnosis from hematogones (hematogones show bright expression of CD81). Benign plasma cells show a bright expression of CD81 while most malignant plasma cell neoplasm show either dim CD81 (~40%–45%) or are CD81− [68, 69]. Expression of CD81 by myeloma cells is associated with poor prognosis [68, 69]. BL is brightly positive and both FL and DLBCL show dimmer expression than in BL. CLL are CD81− and MCL are CD81+ (Figure 7.13). Both HCL and HCL-v are CD81+, but the expression of CD81 in HCL-v is much brighter than in HCL. PEL and CLL are CD81−.

CD103

- *Benign:*
  - Minor subset of T-cells in the GI tract and liver
  - Dendritic cells, subset
  - Rare circulating B-cells
- *B-cell lymphoproliferations:*
  - HCL
  - HCL-v
  - DLBCL, very rare cases

- Splenic diffuse red pulp B-cell lymphoma (SDRPL), very rare cases
- *T-cell lymphoproliferations:*
  - EATL
  - MEITL
  - PTCL, very rare cases
  - ATLL, very rare cases
  - T-PLL, rare cases
- *Other tumors:*
  - BPDCN, subset

CD103 is expressed by all cases of HCL and HCL-v (in rare cases the expression may be dim and/or partial). MEITL and EATL are also most often CD103+. Rare cases of other B-cell lymphoproliferative disorders, including large B-cell lymphoma may be (partially) CD103+.

CD117 (c-Kit)

- *Benign:*
  - Myeloblasts
  - Promyelocytes
  - Mast cells
- *B-cell lymphoproliferations:*
  - PCM, subset
- *T-cell lymphoproliferations:*
  - T-PLL, minor subset (most often CD8+ T-PLL)
- *Acute leukemias:*
  - AML
  - APL
  - Acute monoblastic leukemia, minor subset
  - MPAL, subset
  - T-cell acute lymphoblastic leukemia (T-ALL), rare cases
- *Myeloid tumors:*
  - Myeloid blasts in MDS, CMML, and MPN are CD117+. Abnormal expression of CD117 may be also seen in subset of maturing myeloid precursors
- *Other tumors:*
  - SM
  - BPDCN, minor subset
  - Malignant melanoma, subset
  - GIST
  - Small cell carcinoma, subset

CD117 (c-kit gene product) is positive in the majority of AMLs including AML with maturation and without maturation, acute myelomonocytic leukemia (myeloblastic component), AEL, and acute megakaryoblastic leukemia (Figure 7.14). The majority of acute monoblastic leukemias, however, are CD117−. Other hematopoietic tumors expressing CD117 include mast cell proliferations, plasma cell neoplasms, subset of T-cell acute lymphoblastic leukemia (T-ALL), and rare cases of CD8+ mature (peripheral) T-cell lymphoproliferations (e.g., T-PLL). Among non-hematopoietic lesions, CD117 is positive in GISTs and occasional malignant melanoma and poorly differentiated carcinomas/neuroendocrine tumors.

According to their CD34 and CD117 expressions, dendritic cells can be categorized into three maturational stages: (1) immature cell (CD34+), (2) intermediate cells (CD117+/CD34−), and (3) mature cells (CD34−/CD117−). These stages of maturation explain

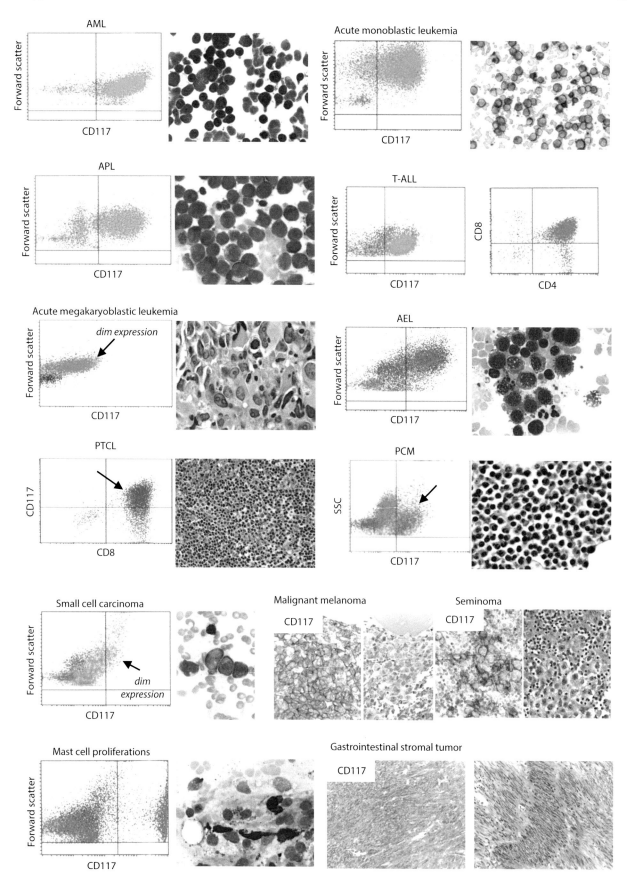

FIGURE 7.14   CD117 expression – differential diagnosis.

the variation in the clinical presentation of BPDCN, as well as its laboratory characteristics.

CD123

- *B-cell lymphoproliferations:*
  - HCL, bright expression
  - HCL-v, subset (lower intensity than in HCL)
- *Acute leukemias:*
  - AML, subset
  - B-cell acute lymphoblastic leukemia (B-ALL), subset
  - T-cell acute lymphoblastic leukemia (T-ALL), subset
  - AUL, minor subset
- *Myeloid tumors:*
  - CMML, subset
  - MDS, blasts may be CD123$^+$
- *Other tumors:*
  - SM
  - BPDCN
  - Dendritic cell neoplasms

CD123 antigen is an antibody that binds to the α-subunit of the interleukin-3 receptor. CD123 is expressed in AML, ALL, NK cell tumors, and dendritic cell neoplasms [70, 71]. CD123$^+$ AML often are positive for *FLT3*-ITD or *NPM1* mutations. It can be expressed also in mature B-cell disorders, such as HCL [70, 72]. The expression of CD123 in HCL is bright. HCL-v are mostly CD123$^-$, but subset of cases may show dim expression (~40%). Rare cases of other mature B-cell disorders (including SMLZ, CLL, MCL, and FL) may express CD123 but the expression is usually partial and/or dim [72]. BPDCN is characterized by co-expression of CD4, CD56, and CD123.

CD133

- *Benign:*
  - Myeloblasts
- *Acute leukemias:*
  - AML, subset
- *Myeloid tumors:*
  - Blasts in MDS and CMML may be CD133$^+$

CD133 is a primitive cell antigen that has been shown to be a more specific marker of hematopoietic stem cells than CD34. Although CD133 is expressed on CD34$^+$ cells in normal hematopoietic tissue, functional studies have revealed that an exceedingly rare population of CD133$^+$/CD34$^-$/CD38$^-$ cells has long-term in vitro and in vivo repopulating ability. In ALL, there is no correlation between CD133 expression and other markers but in AML group, there is a significant positive correlation between CD133 and HLA-DR, CD3, CD7 and TDT, CD13, and CD34.

CD138

- *Benign:*
  - Plasma cells
- *B-cell lymphoproliferations:*
  - PCM
  - ALK$^+$ large B-cell lymphoma
  - PBL
  - DLBCL, subset
  - PEL

CD138 and CD38 are most often expressed together. CD138 is expressed by majority of plasma cell neoplasms and subset of mature B-cell lymphoproliferations, predominantly PBL, ALK$^+$ large B-cell lymphoma and DLBCL with "activated" B-like phenotype or plasmablastic features. The expression of CD138 in plasma cell neoplasms is often dimmer than in benign plasma cells when analyzed by FC.

CD157

CD157 is a GPI-linked protein expressed on both neutrophils and monocytes. It is used in FC panels in analysis of PNH.

CD200

- *Benign:*
  - B-cells, subset
  - T-cells, subset (mostly TFH cells)
  - Thymocytes
  - Hematogones
- *B-cell lymphoproliferations:*
  - CLL
  - HCL
  - HCL-v, minor subset
  - MZL, minor subset (splenic marginal zone lymphomas are more often CD200$^+$)
  - Primary mediastinal large B-cell lymphoma (PMBL)
  - Splenic diffuse red pulp B-cell lymphoma (SDRPBL)
  - FL, minor subset
  - LPL, subset
  - PCM, subset
- *T-cell lymphoproliferations:*
  - AITL, subset
  - Primary cutaneous CD4$^+$ small/medium T-cell lymphoproliferative disorder
- *Acute leukemias:*
  - B-ALL/LBL
  - AML, subset
- *Myeloid tumors:*
  - Blasts in MDS may be CD200$^+$
- *Other tumors:*
  - Small cell carcinoma
  - Carcinoid

CD200 (OX-2) is an immunoglobulin superfamily membrane glycoprotein that is expressed by various cell types including B-cells, thymocytes, activated T-cells, and neuronal and endothelial cells. It is believed to exert an immunosuppressive effect via interaction with its receptor. It is not expressed by monocytes, NK cells, and granulocytes. CD200 demonstrates different expression patterns in a various B-cell lymphoproliferative disorders and B-cell lymphomas, with some tumors showing CD200 expression in majority of cases (CLL, HCL, SDRPBL), some being positive on subset (MZL, LPL, B-PLL) and some being mostly negative (HCL-v), MCL, BL, HGBL-R, DLBCL). CD200 expression improves the distinction between CLL (CD200$^+$) and MCL (CD200$^-$). Almost all of CLL cases (95%–100%), including atypical CLL (CD23$^-$) are CD200$^+$ while most of MCL cases (>92%) are CD200$^-$ (Figure 7.13). Apart from CLL, CD200 is positive in HCL (bright expression) and HCL-v (dim expression). Atypical CLL shows brighter expression when compared to typical CLL. DLBCL and FL are usually CD200$^-$, while MZLs are dimly positive only in minor subset of cases. High CD200 expression (≥50%) is associated with higher CD5, CD19, and CD23 expressions, older age, higher absolute lymphocytes count, hepatomegaly, splenomegaly, and a higher Rai stage. CD5$^+$ LPL/WM may show dim expression of CD200, which helps to differentiate from CLL, which show brighter expression of CD200. PCMs are often CD200$^+$ (50%–60%). Majority of T-cell lymphoproliferative disorders are CD200$^-$.

CD235a/GPHA (glycophorin A)

Glycophorin (GPHA, CD235a) is expressed on red blood cells and their precursors. The very early precursors are usually negative or only dimly positive (in contrast to CD71, which is most strongly expressed on early forms).

FLAER

FLAER or fluorescein-labeled proaerolysin, marketed as a liquid preparation (Cedarlane) is used in FC panel in evaluation of PNH.

HLA-DR (human leukocyte antigen-DR isotype)

- *Benign:*
  - B-cells
  - Hematogones
  - Myeloid, erythroid, and megakaryocytic precursors
  - Monocytes
  - Dendritic cells
- *B-cell lymphoproliferations:*
  - Mature B-cell lymphoproliferative disorders
  - PCM, very rare cases
- *T-cell lymphoproliferations:*
- *Acute leukemias:*
  - AML, majority of cases with few exceptions (e.g., *NPM1$^+$* AML). APL is HLA-DR$^-$
  - B-ALL/LBL
  - AUL
- *Other tumors:*
  - Blastic plasmacytoid dendritic cell tumor (BPDCN)

HLA-DR is expressed on B-cells at different stages of maturation, except for most mature plasma cells, hematopoietic progenitor cells, myeloid, erythroid, and megakaryocytic precursors, monocytes/macrophages, dendritic cells, and immature T-cells. HLA-DR is expressed on myeloblasts but is lost during maturation to the promyelocytic stage. Among malignant tumors, HLA-DR is positive on precursor and mature B-cell lymphoproliferations, majority of AML. Both hypergranular and hypogranular variants of APL are HLA-DR-negative. Plasma cell neoplasms and majority of T-cell lymphoma/leukemias (both mature and immature) do not express HLA-DR.

LILRB1 (leukocyte immunoglobulin-like receptor B1)

LILRB1 (CD85j) belongs to the type I transmembrane inhibitory leukocyte immunoglobulin-like receptor subfamily B member that can inhibit immune cell activation. It is expressed on lymphocytes and monocytes. Saumell et al. reported the distinct pattern of expression of LILRB1 in hematogones and neoplastic B-lymphoblasts, which might be useful in analysis of minimal residual disease (MRD) of B-ALL after treatment [73]. LILRB1 expression is higher on CD34$^+$/CD10$^{bright+}$ stage 1 hematogones, which is downregulated to a dim level of expression on CD34$^-$/CD10$^{moderate+}$ stage 2 hematogones and then upregulated to a moderate level of expression on CD10^{dim+}/CD20$^+$ stage 3 hematogones [73]. In B-ALL the expression of LILRB1 is homogeneous and brighter when compared to hematogones.

TCR beta F1 (T-cell receptor beta F1)

TCR Beta F1 antibody is directed against the beta chain of the alpha/beta T-cell receptor, thus staining most T lymphocytes and T-cell neoplasms with alpha/beta phenotype.

TCR gamma/delta

- *T-cell lymphoproliferations:*
  - PCGD-TCL
  - Aggressive cytotoxic T-cell lymphomas in the skin
  - T-LGLL, gamma/delta subtype
  - HSTL
  - PTCL, NOS, minor subset
- *Acute leukemias:*
  - T-ALL/LBL, minor subset

Majority of mature T-cell lymphoproliferations are positive for TCRαβ. Only small subset of tumors expresses TCRγδ, while subset of tumors is negative for both.

TdT (terminal deoxynucleotidyl transferase)

- *Benign:*
  - Thymocytes
  - Hematogones
- *B-cell lymphoproliferations:*
  - High grade B-cell lymphomas with TdT expression
- *Acute leukemias:*
  - B-ALL/LBL, subset
  - T-ALL/LBL, subset
  - AML, subset
  - AUL, subset
- *Other tumors:*
  - BPDCN, subset
  - Thymoma
  - Indolent T-lymphoblastic proliferations

TdT (Figure 7.15) is a unique intranuclear DNA polymerase. TdT is positive in acute lymphoblastic leukemia/lymphoma of both T- and B-cell lineage, subset of AMLs, most commonly in minimally differentiated AML, very rare cases of acute monoblastic leukemia and immature T-cells from thymic tissue (thymoma and thymic hyperplasia). In the series reported by Thalhammer-Scherrer et al., TdT was positive in 9.3% of AML (47% of AML with minimal differentiation), 86% of B-ALL and 69% of T-ALL [74].

Indolent T-lymphoblastic proliferations (IT-LBP) represent recently described extrathymic and extramedullary non-neoplastic lesions, often associated with hyaline vascular Castleman disease, low grade follicular dendritic cell sarcoma, MZL, or atypical reactive processes [75–78].

B-cell neoplasms with TdT expression but without other features of immaturity are rare and present a diagnostic challenge.

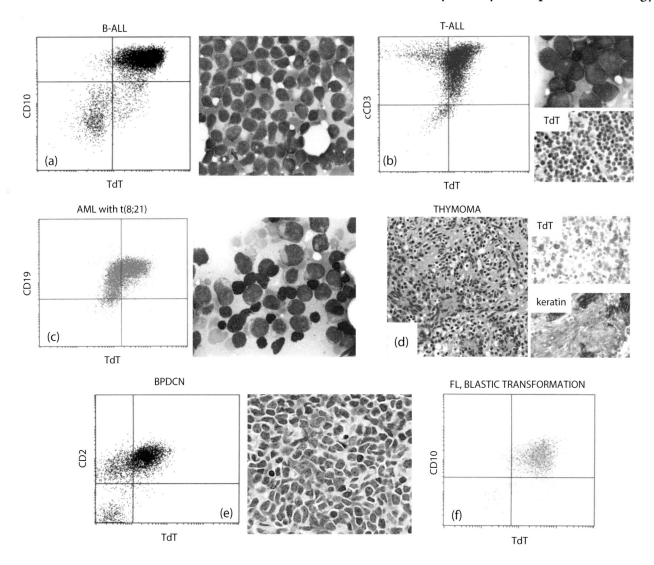

FIGURE 7.15   TdT expression: (a) B-ALL; (b) T-ALL; (c) AML; (d) thymoma; (e) BPDCN; (f) FL (blastic transformation).

Ok et al. described a group of high-grade lymphomas with TdT expression which represented [79]:

- De novo high grade B-cell lymphoma with *MYC*, *BCL2* and/or *BCL6* rearrangements double or triple hit lymphomas)
- TdT⁺ aggressive B-cell lymphoma arising in patients who had previously FL
- Initial relapse of TdT⁻ aggressive B-cell lymphoma in patients who previously had follicular lymphoma, followed by relapses in which the neoplasms acquired TdT expression
- Mature B-cell lymphoma that acquired TdT expression at relapse (this group included 1 case of EBV⁺ DLBCL and 1 cases of MCL)

References

1. Tsujimoto, Y., et al., *Involvement of the bcl-2 gene in human follicular lymphoma.* Science, 1985. **228**(4706): p. 1440–3.
2. Ghia, P., et al., *Unbalanced expression of bcl-2 family proteins in follicular lymphoma: contribution of CD40 signaling in promoting survival.* Blood, 1998. **91**(1): p. 244–51.
3. Mollejo, M., et al., *Monocytoid B cells. A comparative clinical pathological study of their distribution in different types of low-grade lymphomas.* Am J Surg Pathol, 1994. **18**(11): p. 1131–9.
4. Villuendas, R., et al., *Different bcl-2 protein expression in high-grade B-cell lymphomas derived from lymph node or mucosa-associated lymphoid tissue.* Am J Pathol, 1991. **139**(5): p. 989–93.
5. Skinnider, B.F., et al., *Bcl-6 and Bcl-2 protein expression in diffuse large B-cell lymphoma and follicular lymphoma: correlation with 3q27 and 18q21 chromosomal abnormalities.* Hum Pathol, 1999. **30**(7): p. 803–8.
6. Rantanen, S., et al., *Causes and consequences of BCL2 overexpression in diffuse large B-cell lymphoma.* Leuk Lymphoma, 2001. **42**(5): p. 1089–98.
7. Rassidakis, G.Z., et al., *BCL-2 family proteins in peripheral T-cell lymphomas: correlation with tumour apoptosis and proliferation.* J Pathol, 2003. **200**(2): p. 240–8.
8. Villalva, C., et al., *Bcl-2 expression in anaplastic large cell lymphoma.* Am J Pathol, 2001. **158**(5): p. 1889–90.
9. Rassidakis, G.Z., et al., *BCL-2 expression in Hodgkin and Reed-Sternberg cells of classical Hodgkin disease predicts a poorer prognosis in patients treated with ABVD or equivalent regimens.* Blood, 2002. **100**(12): p. 3935–41.
10. Kingma, D.W., et al., *CD2 is expressed by a subpopulation of normal B cells and is frequently present in mature B-cell neoplasms.* Cytometry, 2002. **50**(5): p. 243–8.

11. Geissinger, E., et al., *Disturbed expression of the T-cell receptor/ CD3 complex and associated signaling molecules in CD30⁺ T-cell lymphoproliferations.* Haematologica, 2010. **95**(10): p. 1697–704.

12. Bonzheim, I., et al., *Anaplastic large cell lymphomas lack the expression of T-cell receptor molecules or molecules of proximal T-cell receptor signaling.* Blood, 2004. **104**(10): p. 3358–60.

13. Tjon, J.M., et al., *Defective synthesis or association of T-cell receptor chains underlies loss of surface T-cell receptor-CD3 expression in enteropathy-associated T-cell lymphoma.* Blood, 2008. **112**(13): p. 5103–10.

14. Swerdlow, S.H., Campo, E., Harris, N. L., Jaffe, E. S., Pileri, S. A., Stein, H., Stein, H., Thiele, J., Arber, D.A., Le Beau M.M., Orazi, A., Siebert, R., ed. *WHO classification of tumors of haematopoietic and lymphoid tissues.* 2016, IARC: Lyon.

15. Soderquist, C.R. and G. Bhagat, *Gastrointestinal T- and NK-cell lymphomas and indolent lymphoproliferative disorders.* Semin Diagn Pathol, 2020. **37**(1): p. 11–23.

16. Matnani, R., et al., *Indolent T- and NK-cell lymphoproliferative disorders of the gastrointestinal tract: a review and update.* Hematol Oncol, 2017. **35**(1): p. 3–16.

17. Perry, A.M., et al., *Indolent T-cell lymphoproliferative disease of the gastrointestinal tract.* Blood, 2013. **122**(22): p. 3599–606.

18. van Vliet, C. and D.V. Spagnolo, *T- and NK-cell lymphoproliferative disorders of the gastrointestinal tract: review and update.* Pathology, 2020. **52**(1): p. 128–41.

19. Bierer, B.E., S.J. Burakoff, and B.R. Smith, *A large proportion of T lymphocytes lack CD5 expression after bone marrow transplantation.* Blood, 1989. **73**(5): p. 1359–66.

20. Indraccolo, S., et al., *A CD3⁺CD8⁺ T cell population lacking CD5 antigen expression is expanded in peripheral blood of human immunodeficiency virus-infected patients.* Clin Immunol Immunopathol, 1995. **77**(3): p. 253–61.

21. Kojima, M., et al., *Characteristics of CD5-positive splenic marginal zone lymphoma with leukemic manifestation ; clinical, flow cytometry, and histopathological findings of 11 cases.* J Clin Exp Hematop, 2010. **50**(2): p. 107–12.

22. Hsi, E.D., et al., *Analysis of Peripheral T-cell Lymphoma Diagnostic Workup in the United States.* Clin Lymphoma Myeloma Leuk, 2017. **17**(4): p. 193–200.

23. Fujisawa, M., S. Chiba, and M. Sakata-Yanagimoto, *Recent Progress in the Understanding of Angioimmunoblastic T-cell Lymphoma.* J Clin Exp Hematop, 2017. **57**(3): p. 109–19.

24. Cetinozman, F., P.M. Jansen, and R. Willemze, *Expression of programmed death-1 in primary cutaneous CD4-positive small/ medium-sized pleomorphic T-cell lymphoma, cutaneous pseudo-T-cell lymphoma, and other types of cutaneous T-cell lymphoma.* Am J Surg Pathol, 2012. **36**(1): p. 109–16.

25. Battistella, M., et al., *Primary cutaneous follicular helper T-cell lymphoma: a new subtype of cutaneous T-cell lymphoma reported in a series of 5 cases.* Arch Dermatol, 2012. **148**(7): p. 832–9.

26. Chen, M.H., et al., *CD11b expression correlates with monosomal karyotype and predicts an extremely poor prognosis in cytogenetically unfavorable acute myeloid leukemia.* Leuk Res, 2013. **37**(2): p. 122–8.

27. Karandikar, N.J., et al., *Transient myeloproliferative disorder and acute myeloid leukemia in Down syndrome. An immunophenotypic analysis.* Am J Clin Pathol, 2001. **116**(2): p. 204–10.

28. Kraus, T.S., et al., *The role of CD11c expression in the diagnosis of mantle cell lymphoma.* Am J Clin Pathol, 2010. **134**(2): p. 271–7.

29. Popnikolov, N.K., et al., *CD13-positive anaplastic large cell lymphoma of T-cell origin--a diagnostic and histogenetic problem.* Arch Pathol Lab Med, 2000. **124**(12): p. 1804–8.

30. Ries, S., et al., *CD13⁺ anaplastic large cell lymphoma with leukemic presentation and additional chromosomal abnormality.* Diagn Cytopathol, 2010. **38**(2): p. 141–6.

31. Dunphy, C.H., et al., *CD30⁺ anaplastic large-cell lymphoma with aberrant expression of CD13: case report and review of the literature.* J Clin Lab Anal, 2000. **14**(6): p. 299–304.

32. Ziegler-Heitbrock, L., *Blood monocytes and their subsets: established features and open questions.* Front Immunol, 2015. **6**: p. 423.

33. Patnaik, M.M., et al., *Flow cytometry based monocyte subset analysis accurately distinguishes chronic myelomonocytic leukemia from myeloproliferative neoplasms with associated monocytosis.* Blood Cancer J, 2017. **125**(23): p. 3618–26.

34. Kapellos, T.S., et al., *Human monocyte subsets and phenotypes in major chronic inflammatory diseases.* Front Immunol, 2019. **10**: p. 2035–40.

35. Talati, C., et al., *Monocyte subset analysis accurately distinguishes CMML from MDS and is associated with a favorable MDS prognosis.* Blood, 2017. **129**(13): p. 1881–3.

36. Hwang, S.M., et al., *Monocyte subsets to differentiate chronic myelomonocytic leukemia from reactive monocytosis.* J Clin Lab Anal, 2021. **35**(1): p. e23576.

37. Gorczyca, W., et al., *CD30-positive T-cell lymphomas co-expressing CD15: an immunohistochemical analysis.* Int J Oncol, 2003. **22**(2): p. 319–24.

38. Sponaas, A.M., et al., *The proportion of CD16(+)CD14(dim) monocytes increases with tumor cell load in bone marrow of patients with multiple myeloma.* Immun Inflamm Dis, 2015. **3**(2): p. 94–102.

39. Robbins, B.A., et al., *Diagnostic application of two-color flow cytometry in 161 cases of hairy cell leukemia.* Blood, 1993. **82**(4): p. 1277–87.

40. Sanchez, M.L., et al., *Incidence of phenotypic aberrations in a series of 467 patients with B chronic lymphoproliferative disorders: basis for the design of specific four-color stainings to be used for minimal residual disease investigation.* Leukemia, 2002. **16**(8): p. 1460–9.

41. Rossmann, E.D., et al., *Variability in B-cell antigen expression: implications for the treatment of B-cell lymphomas and leukemias with monoclonal antibodies.* Hematol J, 2001. **2**(5): p. 300–6.

42. Huang, J., et al., *Diagnostic usefulness of aberrant CD22 expression in differentiating neoplastic cells of B-cell chronic lymphoproliferative disorders from admixed benign B cells in four-color multiparameter flow cytometry.* Am J Clin Pathol, 2005. **123**(6): p. 826–32.

43. Gonen, M., et al., *CD25 expression status improves prognostic risk classification in AML independent of established biomarkers: ECOG phase III trial, E1900.* Blood, 2012. **120**(11): p. 2297–306.

44. Maitre, E., et al., *Usefulness of flow cytometry for the detection of cutaneous localization in malignant hematologic disorders.* Cytometry B Clin Cytom, 2019. **96**(4): p. 283–93.

45. Jones, D., et al., *Absence of CD26 expression is a useful marker for diagnosis of T-cell lymphoma in peripheral blood.* Am J Clin Pathol, 2001. **115**(6): p. 885–92.

46. Kelemen, K., et al., *The usefulness of CD26 in flow cytometric analysis of peripheral blood in Sézary syndrome.* Am J Clin Pathol, 2008. **129**(1): p. 146–56.

47. Hu, S., et al., *CD30 expression defines a novel subgroup of diffuse large B-cell lymphoma with favorable prognosis and distinct gene expression signature: a report from the International DLBCL Rituximab-CHOP Consortium Program Study.* Blood, 2013. **121**(14): p. 2715–24.

48. Campuzano-Zuluaga, G., et al., *Frequency and extent of CD30 expression in diffuse large B-cell lymphoma and its relation to clinical and biologic factors: a retrospective study of 167 cases.* Leuk Lymphoma, 2013. **54**(11): p. 2405–11.

49. Fathi, A.T., et al., *CD30 expression in acute myeloid leukemia is associated with FLT3-internal tandem duplication mutation and leukocytosis.* Leuk Lymphoma, 2013. **54**(4): p. 860–3.

50. Zheng, W., et al., *CD30 Expression in high-risk acute myeloid leukemia and myelodysplastic syndromes.* Clin Lymphoma Myeloma Leuk, 2013. **13**(3): p. 307–14.

51. Dalal, B.I., et al., *Detection of CD34, TdT, CD56, CD2, CD4, and CD14 by flow cytometry is associated with NPM1 and FLT3 mutation status in cytogenetically normal acute myeloid leukemia.* Clin Lymphoma Myeloma Leuk, 2012. **12**(4): p. 274–9.

52. De Smet, D., et al., *Diagnostic potential of CD34⁺ cell antigen expression in myelodysplastic syndromes.* Am J Clin Pathol, 2012. **138**(5): p. 732–43.

53. Perea, G., et al., *Adverse prognostic impact of CD36 and CD2 expression in adult de novo acute myeloid leukemia patients.* Leuk Res, 2005. **29**(10): p. 1109–16.

54. Alsuwaidan, A., et al., *Bright CD38 expression by flow cytometric analysis is a biomarker for double/triple hit lymphomas with a moderate sensitivity and high specificity.* Cytometry B Clin Cytom, 2019. **96**(5): p. 368–74.

55. Maleki, A., et al., *Bright CD38 expression is an indicator of MYC rearrangement.* Leuk Lymphoma, 2009. **50**(6): p. 1054–7.

56. Lee, P.S., et al., *Coexpression of CD43 by benign B cells in the terminal ileum.* Appl Immunohistochem Mol Morphol, 2005. **13**(2): p. 138–41.

57. Gooden, C.E., et al., *CD49d shows superior performance characteristics for flow cytometric prognostic testing in chronic lymphocytic leukemia/small lymphocytic lymphoma.* Cytometry B Clin Cytom, 2018. **94**(1): p. 129–35.

58. Bulian, P., et al., *CD49d is the strongest flow cytometry-based predictor of overall survival in chronic lymphocytic leukemia.* J Clin Oncol, 2014. **32**(9): p. 897–904.

59. Gattei, V., et al., *Relevance of CD49d protein expression as overall survival and progressive disease prognosticator in chronic lymphocytic leukemia.* Blood, 2008. **111**(2): p. 865–73.

60. Ponka, P. and C.N. Lok, *The transferrin receptor: role in health and disease.* Int J Biochem Cell Biol, 1999. **31**(10): p. 1111–37.

61. Nakahata, T. and N. Okumura, *Cell surface antigen expression in human erythroid progenitors: erythroid and megakaryocytic markers.* Leuk Lymphoma, 1994. **13**(5–6): p. 401–9.

62. Marsee, D.K., G.S. Pinkus, and H. Yu, *CD71 (transferrin receptor): an effective marker for erythroid precursors in bone marrow biopsy specimens.* Am J Clin Pathol, 2010. **134**(3): p. 429–35.

63. Davis, B.H., et al., *U.S.-Canadian Consensus recommendations on the immunophenotypic analysis of hematologic neoplasia by flow cytometry: medical indications.* Cytometry, 1997. **30**(5): p. 249–63.

64. Malcovati, L., et al., *Flow cytometry evaluation of erythroid and myeloid dysplasia in patients with myelodysplastic syndrome.* Leukemia, 2005. **19**(5): p. 776–83.

65. Della Porta, M.G., et al., *Flow cytometry evaluation of erythroid dysplasia in patients with myelodysplastic syndrome.* Leukemia, 2006. **20**(4): p. 549–55.

66. Dong, H.Y., S. Wilkes, and H. Yang, *CD71 is selectively and ubiquitously expressed at high levels in erythroid precursors of all maturation stages: a comparative immunochemical study with glycophorin A and hemoglobin A.* Am J Surg Pathol, 2011. **35**(5): p. 723–32.

67. Liu, Q., et al., *Significance of CD71 expression by flow cytometry in diagnosis of acute leukemia.* Leuk Lymphoma, 2014. **55**(4): p. 892–8.

68. Chen, F., et al., *Expression of CD81 and CD117 in plasma cell myeloma and the relationship to prognosis.* Cancer Med, 2018. 7(12): p. 5920–7.

69. Paiva, B., et al., *Clinical significance of CD81 expression by clonal plasma cells in high-risk smoldering and symptomatic multiple myeloma patients.* Leukemia, 2012. **26**(8): p. 1862–9.

70. Del Giudice, I., et al., *The diagnostic value of CD123 in B-cell disorders with hairy or villous lymphocytes.* Haematologica, 2004. **89**(3): p. 303–8.

71. Bain, B.J., *Bone marrow trephine biopsy.* J Clin Pathol, 2001. **54**(10): p. 737–42.

72. Bain, B.J., *Bone marrow aspiration.* J Clin Pathol, 2001. **54**(9): p. 657–63.

73. Saumell Tutusaus, S., et al., *LILRB1: a novel diagnostic B-cell marker to distinguish neoplastic B lymphoblasts from hematogones.* Am J Clin Pathol, 2021. **156**(6): p. 941–9.

74. Thalhammer-Scherrer, R., et al., *The immunophenotype of 325 adult acute leukemias: relationship to morphologic and molecular classification and proposal for a minimal screening program highly predictive for lineage discrimination.* Am J Clin Pathol, 2002. **117**(3): p. 380–9.

75. Ohgami, R.S., et al., *Indolent T-lymphoblastic proliferation (iT-LBP): a review of clinical and pathologic features and distinction from malignant T-lymphoblastic lymphoma.* Adv Anat Pathol, 2013. **20**(3): p. 137–40.

76. Strauchen, J.A., *Indolent T-lymphoblastic proliferation: report of a case with an 11-year history and association with myasthenia gravis.* Am J Surg Pathol, 2001. **25**(3): p. 411–5.

77. Ohgami, R.S., et al., *TdT⁺ T-lymphoblastic populations are increased in Castleman disease, in Castleman disease in association with follicular dendritic cell tumors, and in angioimmunoblastic T-cell lymphoma.* Am J Surg Pathol, 2012. **36**(11): p. 1619–28.

78. Fromm, J.R., et al., *Flow cytometric features of incidental indolent T lymphoblastic proliferations.* Cytometry B Clin Cytom, 2020. **98**(3): p. 282–7.

79. Ok, C.Y., et al., *High-grade B-cell lymphomas with TdT expression: a diagnostic and classification dilemma.* Mod Pathol, 2019. **32**(1): p. 48–58.

8

MORPHOLOGIC-FLOW CYTOMETRIC CORRELATION IN BLOOD

Normal blood

The flow cytometric features of normal blood are presented in Chapter 2.

Pancytopenia/cytopenia

Pancytopenia is defined as a decrease in all three blood cell lines which results in symptoms associated with anemia, leukopenia, and/or thrombocytopenia.

The differential diagnosis of pancytopenia and/or severe cytopenia (anemia, leukopenia, or thrombocytopenia) includes:

- Myelodysplastic neoplasm (MDS)
- AML ("aleukemic")
- Acute promyelocytic leukemia (APL)
- Acute erythroid leukemia (AEL, pure erythroid leukemia)
- Primary myelofibrosis (PMF)
- Post polycythemia vera (PV) myelofibrosis (post PV-MF)
- Post essential thrombocythemia (ET) myelofibrosis (post ET-MF)
- Systemic mastocytosis (SM)
- Hairy cell leukemia (HCL)
- T-LGL leukemia (T-LGLL)
- Paroxysmal nocturnal hemoglobinuria (PNH)
- Hemophagocytic lymphohistiocytosis (HLH)
- Metastatic tumor/other bone marrow (BM) infiltrative process
- Aplastic anemia (AA), congenital or acquired
- Gelatinous transformation of BM
- Hypersplenism
- Toxic marrow damage (therapy, toxins, radiation)
- Infections (sepsis, malaria, viruses, other)

There are numerous causes for pancytopenia, which can be divided into four main categories [1, 2]:

1. increased destruction of blood elements: autoimmune mechanisms, sepsis, other
2. sequestration (hypersplenism),
3. impaired production of blood elements: MDS, infiltrative marrow process such as PMF or systemic disease infiltrating BM such as leukemia, lymphoma, SM, carcinoma, granulomatous disease, AA, nutritional deficiencies (B12, other), toxic damage of BM due to drugs or radiation, infections, idiopathic, other.
4. combination of impaired production and peripheral destruction: PNH, HLH.

After clinical history and examination, complete blood count (CBC), blood smear analysis, and correlation with most relevant laboratory tests fail to determine the secondary etiology of pancytopenia, an evaluation of blood by flow cytometry (FC) and morphologic and genetic analysis of the BM would often follow. FC analysis would not only help identifying most series and urgent problems, such as APL or acute myeloid leukemia (AML), but

also helps to confirm or exclude many other disorders associated with pancytopenia (e.g., PNH, HCL, T-LGLL). In patients with MDS or PMF, FC analysis of blood may show circulating blasts, atypical phenotype of blasts, phenotypic atypia of monocytes and/or neutrophils, and decreased side scatter (SSC) of neutrophils. Both positive and negative FC results help in establishing the etiology of pancytopenia or refractory cytopenia. FC analysis of blood from patients with MDS may show circulating blasts, atypical phenotype of blasts, phenotypic atypia of monocytes and granulocytes, and/or SSC of neutrophils [3–11]. Occasional AML, especially APL, may present with pancytopenia. Figure 8.1 shows partial blood involvement by APL with scattered circulating promyelocytes. PMF may present as pancytopenia, anemia, leukoerythroblastosis, or prominent leukocytosis. Figure 8.2 compares FC findings in PMF with prominent leukocytosis with normal blood and normal BM. FC analysis of blood from patients with PMF shows circulating blasts and phenotypic atypia of granulocytes, especially aberrant expression of CD56. In some PMF cases, the number of blasts identified in blood may be higher than in BM (attributed to abnormal trafficking of blasts in fibrotic BM and/or extramedullary hematopoiesis). FC analysis of blood in patients with PMF showing increased circulating blasts helps in differential diagnosis of MDS with reticulin fibrosis, as those patients usually have lower number of blasts. HCL (Figure 8.3) often present with pancytopenia and lack of monocytes. T-LGLL (Figure 8.4) presents with severe neutropenia.

Neutrophilia

Algorithmic approach to neutrophilia is presented in Figure 21.3 in Chapter 21.

Differential diagnosis of neutrophilia includes:

- Leukemoid reaction
- Reactive neutrophilia due to inflammatory, infectious, acute hemorrhage/hemolysis, intoxication, burns, or metabolic diseases
- Paraneoplastic neutrophilia (associated with malignant diseases, such a carcinoma, Hodgkin lymphoma, or plasma cell myeloma [PCM])
- Neutrophilia associated with treatment (granulocyte colony stimulating factors, corticosteroids, lithium, other)
- Chronic myeloid leukemia (CML; *BCR-ABL1*+)
- Chronic neutrophilic leukemia (CNL)
- MDS/MPN with neutrophilia (formerly known as atypical CML)
- Myeloproliferative neoplasms (MPNs) other than CML
- Chronic myelomonocytic leukemia (CMML)

Leukemoid reaction may mimic leukemia, but its etiology is nonneoplastic. Leukemoid reaction is more common than myeloid malignancies. FC analysis of blood with reactive neutrophilia shows increased granulocytes to lymphocytes ratio with predominance of CD10+/CD11b+/CD16+/CD45^bright+ neutrophils. There is no aberrant expression of CD56 on significant subset of cells. In

DOI: 10.1201/9781003197935-8

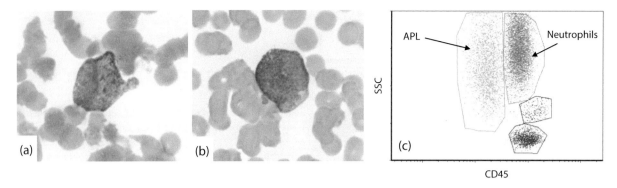

FIGURE 8.1 Circulating promyelocytes (APL). (a, b) Blood smear showing atypical promyelocytes; (c) FC showing promyelocytes (green dots) with high side scatter (SSC) and dimmer expression of CD45 when compared to neutrophils.

CML, blood smear shows myeloid leftward shift with rare blasts, eosinophilia and basophilia. FC analysis of blood resembles BM sample due to presence of blasts, decreased expression of CD10, CD11b, CD16, and CD45 by neutrophils (reflecting both leftward shift and dysmaturation) and often also aberrant expression of CD56 (Figure 8.5). Occasional cases of CML show circulating atypical immature B-cell population with hematogones-like FC features. The detailed description of morphology and FC findings in CML are presented in Chapter 21. CNL (Chapter 21) shows predominance of neutrophils without phenotypic features of leftward shift. Current WHO diagnostic criteria include leukocytosis of ≥25 × 10⁹/L (of which >80% are neutrophils) and with less than 10% of immature cells and less than 1% of blasts. Mutation of *CSF3R* T618I occurs frequently in CNL, although is not specific for this entity [12–18]. Rare cases of neutrophilia accompanying plasma cell neoplasms were reported to be positive for *SETBP1* mutations. Association between CNL and plasma cell neoplasms has also been reported. MDS/MPN with neutrophilia (known also as aCML, Chapter 20) is rare myeloid neoplasm characterized by overlap of myeloproliferative and myelodysplastic features, including leukocytosis with leftward-shifted granulocytic series, dysgranulopoiesis, dysmegakaryopoiesis, and dyserythropoiesis, but without basophilia and monocytosis [15, 19–22]. It usually affects older adults. In contrast to CML, there is no *BCR-ABL1* fusion or Philadelphia chromosome. Patients present with anemia and/or thrombocytopenia, high white blood cell count, splenomegaly and often hepatomegaly. Classic non-CML MPNs often present with neutrophilia. Hyperleukocytosis may complicate occasional cases of PMF. Presence of absolute monocytosis with differential count showing >10% monocytes suggests the diagnosis of CMML. Hyperleukocytosis may complicate occasional cases of PMF. Figure 8.2 compares FC analysis of blood from a patient with PMF and marked neutrophilia (WBC of 140,000/µL) with control samples from normal blood and normal BM.

Eosinophilia

The upper normal limit for the number of eosinophils in blood is 0.35–05 × 10⁹/L. Hypereosinophilia is defined as peripheral blood eosinophil counts >1.5 × 10⁹/L. Algorithmic approach to eosinophilia is presented in Figure 21.5 in Chapter 21.

Differential diagnosis of eosinophilia includes:

- Reactive eosinophilia
- Chronic eosinophilic leukemia (CEL)
- MPNs
- SM
- Eosinophilia accompanying hematologic neoplasms other than MPN

Eosinophils are negative for CD10 and CD16, positive for CD11b, CD13, CD15, CD33, and CD45 (bright), and have low forward scatter (FSC) and high SSC. They show typically non-specific staining with viability dyes, imitating non-viable elements. Eosinophils differ from neutrophils by very low FSC, slightly higher SSC, and negative expression of CD10 and CD16.

Reactive eosinophilia

Reactive eosinophilia is associated with parasitic infections (strongyloidiasis, hookworm infection, filariasis, scabies, isosporiasis), bacterial infections (chronic tuberculosis, resolving scarlet fever), HIV, allergic disorders (asthma, atopic dermatitis), drug hypersensitivity, Loeffler's syndrome, skin diseases (such as angiolymphoid hyperplasia), granulomatous disorders (sarcoidosis), certain non-hematologic neoplasms, abnormal T-cells with aberrant phenotype (may or may not be clonal), vasculitis, collagen vascular disorders, inflammatory bowel disease, hypoadrenalism, IL-2 therapy, radiation exposure, cholesterol embolization, and Kimura's disease.

Chronic eosinophilic leukemia (CEL) and other myeloproliferative neoplasms (MPNs) with eosinophilia

MPNs with eosinophilia include CEL (Figure 8.6), CML (*BCR-ABL1⁺*), hypereosinophilic syndrome (HES), and MPNs associated with rearrangement of *PDGFRA*, *PDGFRB*, or *FGFR1*. Diagnosis of CEL requires sustained eosinophilia >1.5 × 10⁹/L, lack of specific neoplasms which may be associated with eosinophilia (AML with inv16, *BCR-ABL⁺* CML, PV, ET, PMF, CNL, CMML, MDS/MPN with neutrophilia, MDS, and MPNs with *PDGFRA*, *PDGFRB*, or *FGFR1*), blasts <20% in blood and BM, and either evidence of clonality of eosinophils or an increased blasts (≥2% in blood and ≥5% in BM). Cases with no evidence of clonality or increased blasts are classified as idiopathic HES. HES is defined as eosinophilia (>1.5 × 10⁹/L) persisting for at least 6 months resulting in tissue damage, without underlying etiology (secondary eosinophilia) and no evidence of other malignancy associated with eosinophilia. Cases fulfilling the criteria for HES but without evidence of tissue damage are classified as idiopathic hypereosinophilia.

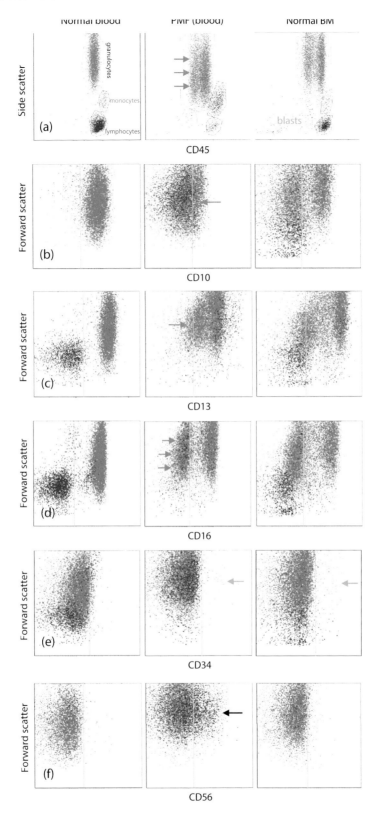

FIGURE 8.2 Flow cytometry of blood with marked leukocytosis (WBC = 140,000/μL) associated with primary myelofibrosis (PMF). The flow cytometry (FC) pattern of granulocytes in PMF (middle column) is compared with normal blood (left column) and normal BM (right column). Overall, the FC features of blood granulocytes in PMF resemble BM, indicating leftward shift. Subset of granulocytes show decreased expression of CD45 (a; arrows). The expression of CD10 in PMF is down-regulated (b; arrow), but does not show two distinct population seen in normal BM. The expression of CD13 (c) and CD16 (d) in PMF resemble pattern seen in BM and differs from uniformly bright expression of those antigens in normal blood. The staining with CD34 shows rare circulating blasts in PMF (e; arrow). In contrast to normal blood and BM, granulocytes (gray dots) and monocytes (blue dots) display aberrant expression of CD56 on subset of cells (f; arrow).

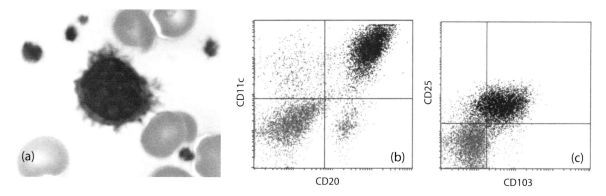

FIGURE 8.3   HCL. Smear from blood shows atypical lymphocytes with many cytoplasmic projections (a). Flow cytometry shows B-cells with bright CD11c and bright CD20 (b), and co-expression of CD25 with CD103 (c).

Eosinophilia accompanying other malignant disorders

Eosinophilia may be also seen in peripheral T-cell neoplasms, classic Hodgkin lymphoma (cHL), SM, and acute lymphoblastic leukemia (ALL).

Lymphocytic variant of hypereosinophilic syndrome

Lymphocytic variant of HES is a subset of HES with clonal T-cells. Flow cytometry analysis shows aberrant phenotype of T-cells in all cases (CD2+/CD3−/CD4+/CD5+/CD7−/+dim/CD8−/CD10rarely+) [23].

Lymphocytosis

Differential diagnosis of lymphocytosis includes:

- Reactive lymphocytosis
- Polyclonal T-cell lymphocytosis associated with thymoma
- Polyclonal B-cell lymphocytosis
- B- and T-cell lymphoproliferative neoplasms

Reactive lymphocytosis

Lymphocytosis is an increase in the number of lymphocytes in blood (>4 × 10⁹/L). Relative lymphocytosis is an increase in the percentage of lymphocytes in blood (usually >40%) and is mainly associated with severe neutropenia. Reactive lymphocytosis is transient and is associated most often with viral infections, post vaccination, and less often in some drug reactions/medication

or autoimmune disorders. Based on cytological features of lymphocytes in EBV or CMV infections reactive lymphocytes have been historically divided to Downy type 1 cells characterized by foamy basophilic cytoplasm and irregular, kidney-shaped nucleus, Downy type 2 cells with less basophilic cytoplasm, plasmacytoid features, and irregular cytoplasmic borders partially engulfing red blood cells, and Downey type 3 cells, which show features of reactive immunoblasts with fine chromatin and one or two more prominent nucleoli. Apart from viral infections, T-cell lymphocytosis of mature polytypic T-cells may be seen in patients with thymomas. Polyclonal B-cell lymphocytosis is a rare benign condition hematological disorder characterized by a selective expansion of circulating polyclonal marginal zone-like B cells (CD5−/CD10−). It is diagnosed predominantly in women, usually cigarette smokers and may have some familial (inherited?) occurrence.

Lymphoproliferative neoplasms

Lymphocytosis of mostly small lymphocytes can be seen in chronic lymphocytic leukemia (CLL), marginal zone lymphoma (MZL), occasional T-cell prolymphocytic leukemias (T-PLL) and reactive conditions. Small lymphocytes in CLL are round, have scant cytoplasm, and clumped chromatin. CLL composed of significant number of large cells with irregular nuclei and more dispersed chromatin are called atypical CLL. Prolymphocytes are medium-sized cells (twice the size of small lymphocytes) with round nucleus, prominent central nucleolus and more dispersed chromatin. Lymphocytosis of lymphocytes with predominance of prolymphocytes can be seen in splenic B-cell lymphoma/leukemia with prominent nucleoli and T-PLL. T-cell lymphoproliferations are generally characterized by more irregular nuclei when compared to most of B-cell lymphomas. T-cell prolymphocytes varies in size from small to medium, have pale basophilic and agranular cytoplasm and markedly irregular nuclei with prominent nucleoli (although variants reminiscent of CLL cytomorphology can also occur). Small to medium-sized lymphocytes with prominent cytoplasmic azurophilic granules are typical for T-large granular lymphocytes (T-LGL). Persistent lymphocytosis of T-LGL cells (>6 months) with >2 × 10⁹/L cells should raise the possibility of T-LGLL or chronic lymphoproliferative disorder of NK-cells (CLD-NK). Lymphocytosis with cytoplasmic projections (hairy cells or villous lymphocytes) is most often seen in HCL, hairy cell leukemia variant (HCL v), splenic lymphoma with villous lymphocytes (splenic marginal zone lymphoma; SMZL),

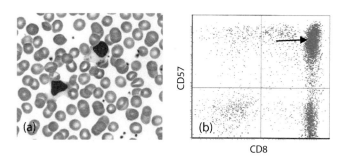

FIGURE 8.4   T-LGL leukemia. Atypical lymphoid cells with cytoplasmic granules (a) show co-expression of CD8 and CD57 (b; arrow).

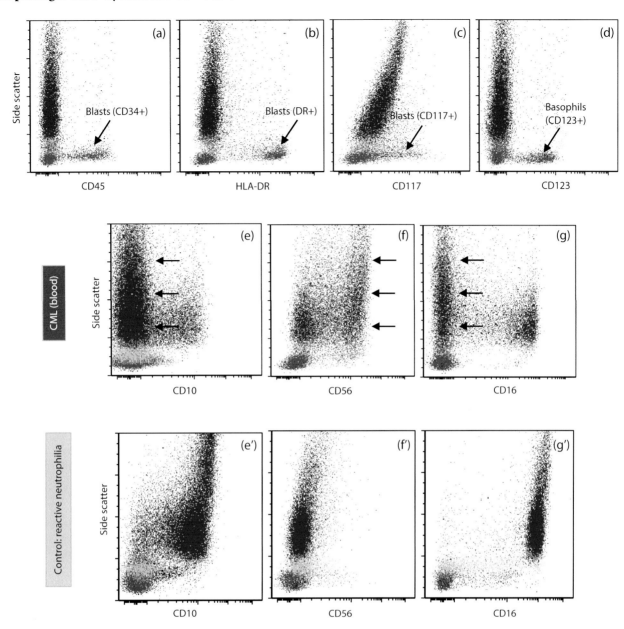

FIGURE 8.5 Flow cytometric features of CML in peripheral blood. The features differentiating CML from reactive neutrophilia include increased blasts expressing CD34, HLA-DR, and CD117 (a–c), increased basophils, expressing CD123 (d), decreased side scatter of granulocytes (e–g), down-regulation of CD10 (e; compare with control on e′), up-regulation of CD56 on granulocytes (f; compare with control on f′), and down-regulation of CD16 on granulocytes (g; compare with control on g′).

and splenic diffuse red pulp B-cell lymphoma (SDRPL). SDRPL characterized by circulating basophilic villous lymphocytes and diffuse infiltration of the splenic red pulp, is distinct from SMZL and HCL, but reminiscent of HCL-v. Lymphocytosis with nuclear outlines irregularities (indentations) can be seen in follicular lymphoma (FL) and mantle cell lymphoma (MCL). FL may be composed of predominantly small to medium-sized cell with elongated and indented (cleaved) nuclei (called centrocytes) and large cells with dispersed chromatin and 1–3 peripheral nucleoli (centroblasts). Large cells are at least three times larger than small lymphocytes. The lymphoid cells of MCL are usually small with clumped chromatin and prominent nuclear clefts, although

some cases are composed of more pleomorphic (or even blastoid) cells or small lymphocytes similar to CLL cells. Occasional cases of MCL present without adenopathy with indolent clinical course and blood involvement (leukemic non-nodal MCL; L-NN-MCL). Occasional cases of plasma cell leukemias (PCLs) may mimic HCL cytologically. Lymphocytosis with marked nuclear outlines irregularities, including "flower cells" is seen in adult T-cell leukemia/lymphoma (ATLL), and other T-cell lymphomas such as Sézary's syndrome (SS). Lymphocytosis of mostly large, highly atypical lymphocytes is seen most often in diffuse large B-cell lymphoma (DLBCL), anaplastic large cell lymphoma (ALCL), Burkitt lymphoma (BL), high grade B-cell lymphoma with *MYC*

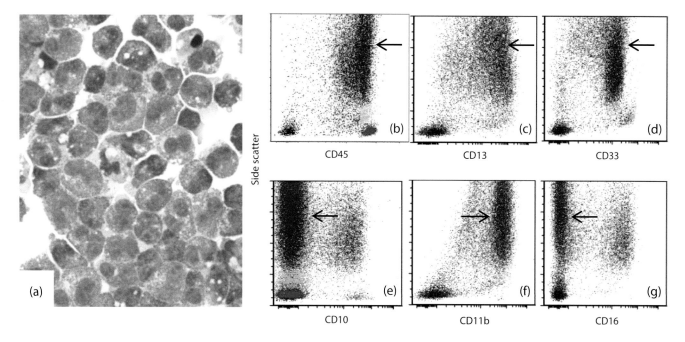

FIGURE 8.6 Chronic eosinophilic leukemia (CEL) – flow cytometry (FC) analysis. Eosinophils (a, cytospin preparation) have characteristic FC pattern (b–g) with high side scatter (b–g; arrow), positive CD45 (b), CD13 (c), and CD33 (d), negative CD10 (e), positive CD11b (f), and negative CD16 (g).

and *BCL2* (and/or *BCL6*) rearrangement (HGBL-R, "double hit" or "triple-hit" lymphoma), and peripheral T-cell lymphoma (PTCL). Lymphocytosis of medium-sized lymphocytes with blastoid features (fine chromatin, small nucleoli) can be seen lymphoblastic leukemia, and occasional mature lymphomas, e.g., BL or blastoid variant of MCL (see below). Figure 8.7 shows cytologic-flow cytometric correlation of lymphocytosis.

Summary of FC phenotypic profiles of most common causes of non-reactive lymphocytosis:

CLL: CD19$^+$, CD20$^{+(often\ dim)}$, surface light chain immunoglobulins$^{+(dim)/rarely-}$, CD5$^+$, CD23$^{+/rarely-}$, CD10$^-$, CD38$^{+(dim\ or\ partial)/-}$, CD43$^+$, CD71$^-$, CD81$^{-/+dim}$, CD200$^+$, CD11c$^{+/-}$, CD13$^{-/rarely+}$, CD2$^{-/rarely+}$

MCL: CD19$^+$, CD20$^+$, surface light chain immunoglobulin$^+$, CD5$^+$, CD10$^{-/rarely+}$, CD11c$^-$, CD23$^-$, CD38$^+$, CD43$^+$, CD71$^{-/+(dim\ or\ partial)}$, CD81$^{+strong}$, CD200$^-$

FL: CD19$^{+(often\ dim)}$, CD20$^+$, surface light chain immunoglobulin$^+$, CD5$^-$, CD10$^+$, CD11c$^-$, CD23$^-$, CD38$^{+/rarely-}$, CD43$^-$, CD71$^{-/+(dim\ or\ partial)}$, CD81$^{+(dim)/-}$, CD200$^{-/+(dim)}$

MZL: CD19$^+$, CD20$^+$, surface light chain immunoglobulin$^+$, CD5$^{-/rarely+}$, CD10$^-$, CD11c$^{+/-}$, CD23$^{-/+}$, CD38$^{+/-}$, CD43$^{-/+}$, CD81$^{+/-}$, CD200$^{-/rarely+}$

HCL-v: CD19$^+$, CD20$^+$, surface light chain immunoglobulin$^+$, CD5$^-$, CD10$^{-/rarely+}$, CD11c$^{+bright/rarely-}$, CD23$^{-/rarely+}$, CD25$^-$, CD38$^-$, CD43$^{-/+dim}$, CD71$^-$, CD81$^{+(often\ strong)}$, CD103$^+$, CD123$^{-/rarely+}$, CD200$^{-/+(dim)}$

SDRPL: sIg$^+$, CD5$^{-/rarely+}$, CD10$^-$, CD11c$^{-/+}$, CD19$^+$, CD20$^+$, CD22$^+$, CD23$^{-/rarely+}$, CD25$^-$, CD38$^-$, CD43$^{+(dim)/-}$, CD45$^+$, CD79b$^{+(moderate)}$, CD81$^{+/-}$, CD103$^{-/rarely+}$, CD123$^{-/rarely+}$, and CD200$^+$.

T-LGLL: CD2$^{+/rarely-}$, CD3$^{+/rarely-}$, CD8$^+$ (rarely CD4$^+$, CD4/CD8$^-$, or CD4/CD8$^+$), CD5$^{+/-}$, CD7$^{-/+}$, CD25$^-$, CD26$^{-/rarely+}$, CD16$^{-/rarely+}$, CD45$^+$, CD56$^{-/+}$, CD57$^{+/rarely-}$, CD81$^+$, CD200$^-$, TCRαβ$^+$ (rarely TCRγδ$^+$)

CLPD-NK: CD2$^+$, CD3$^-$, CD5$^-$, CD7$^{+/rarely-}$, CD4$^-$/CD8$^-$ (rarely CD8$^+$), CD25$^-$, CD26$^-$, CD16$^{+/rarely-}$, CD45$^+$, CD56$^{+/-}$, CD57$^{+/-}$, CD81$^+$, CD200$^-$, TCRαβ$^-$, TCRγδ$^-$

ALCL: high FSC, CD2$^{+/rarely-}$, CD3$^{+/-}$, CD4$^+$ or less often CD8$^+$ (rare tumors are either CD4/8$^-$ or CD4/CD8$^+$), CD5$^{+/-}$, CD7$^{-/rarely+}$, CD10$^-$, CD25$^{+/-}$, CD26$^{+/rarely-}$, CD30$^+$, CD43$^+$, CD45$^+$, CD56$^{-/rarely+}$

DLBCL: CD19$^+$, CD20$^+$, surface light chain immunoglobulin$^+$, CD5$^{-/rarely+}$, CD10$^{+/-}$, CD11c$^{-/rarely+}$, CD23$^-$, CD25$^{-/rarely+}$, CD38$^+$, CD43$^{-/+}$, CD71$^{+(dim\ or\ rarely\ strong)}$, CD81$^{+(dim)}$, CD200$^{-/rarely\ +(dim)}$

BL: CD19$^+$, CD20$^+$, surface light chain immunoglobulin$^+$, BCL2$^-$, CD5$^-$, CD10$^+$, CD11c$^-$, CD23$^-$, CD25$^-$, CD38$^+$, CD43$^{+(strong)}$, CD71$^{+(strong)}$, CD81$^{+(strong)}$, CD200$^{-/rarely\ +(dim)}$

T-PLL: CD2$^{+/-}$, CD3$^{+/-}$, CD4$^+$ (less often CD8$^+$, CD4/CD8$^+$ or CD4/CD8$^-$), CD5$^{+/-}$, CD7$^{+/-}$, CD25$^-$, CD26$^+$, CD45$^{+/rarely-}$, CD56$^-$, CD57$^-$, CD81$^+$, CD117$^{-/rarely+}$, CD200$^-$

ATLL: CD2$^{+/-}$, CD3$^{+/-}$, CD4$^+$ (rarely CD4/CD8$^+$), CD5$^+$, CD7$^-$, CD8$^-$, CD25$^+$, CD26$^-$, CD30$^{-/+}$, CD45$^+$, CD56$^-$, CD57$^-$, CCR4$^+$

MF/SS: CD2$^{+/-}$, CD3$^+$, CD4$^+$, CD5$^+$, CD7$^{-/rarely+}$, CD8$^-$, CD10$^-$, CD25$^{-/+}$, CD26$^-$, CD30$^{-/+}$

Erythrocytosis/polycythemia

The causes for erythrocytosis (increase in red blood cells relative to blood volume) or polycythemia (increase in both red blood cells and hemoglobin concentration) include:

- PV
- Reactive (secondary) erythrocytosis/polycythemia
- Inherited erythrocytosis (high oxygen-affinity hemoglobin, erythropoietin receptor mutation, 2,3-biphosphoglycerate mutase deficiency)

Algorithmic approach to erythrocytosis is presented in Figure 21.4 in Chapter 21. Secondary erythrocytosis is associated

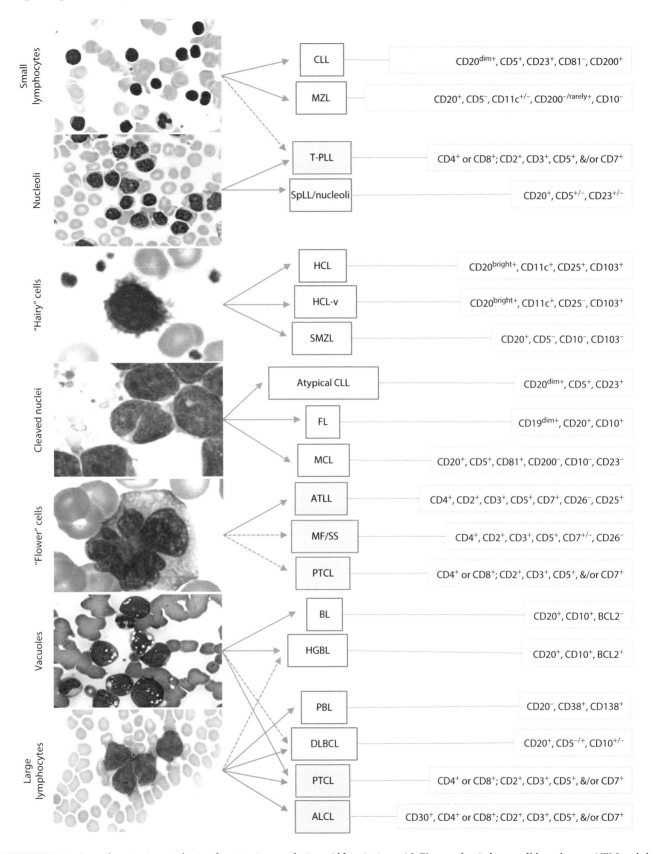

FIGURE 8.7 Lymphocytosis: cytologic-phenotypic correlation. *Abbreviations*: ALCL, anaplastic large cell lymphoma; ATLL, adult T-cell leukemia/lymphoma; BL, Burkitt lymphoma; CLL, chronic lymphocytic leukemia; DLBCL, diffuse large B-cell lymphoma; FL, follicular lymphoma; HCL, hairy cell leukemia; HCL-v, hairy cell leukemia variant; HGBL, high grade B-cell lymphoma; MCL, mantle cell lymphoma; MF/SS, mycosis fungoides/Sézary's syndrome; MZL, marginal zone lymphoma; PBL, plasmablastic lymphoma; PLL, prolymphocytic leukemia; SMZL, splenic marginal zone lymphoma; PTCL, peripheral T-cell lymphoma; SpLL/nucleoli, splenic B-cell lymphoma/leukemia with prominent nucleoli.

with hypoxia (lung disease, cardiac disease, high-altitude habitat, renal artery stenosis, intrinsic renal disease, obstructive sleep apnea), ectopic erythropoietin secretion (uterine leiomyoma, hepatocellular carcinoma, cerebellar hemangioblastoma), drug-associated (exogenous erythropoietin, androgen preparations) or relative due to dehydration. PV is the commonest MPN and the MPN most often complicated by arterial and venous thrombosis [24]. It is *JAK2*+ in all cases. Differential diagnosis of erythrocytosis is discussed in Chapter 21.

Basophilia

Differential diagnosis of basophilia includes:

- CML (*BCR-ABL1*+)
- ET
- PMF
- PV
- MDS (rare cases)
- Acute and chronic basophilic leukemia
- Acute megakaryoblastic leukemia
- Allergic reactions
- Chronic inflammation (inflammatory bowel disease, ulcerative colitis, rheumatoid arthritis)
- Infections

Basophils are characterized by intense azurophilic granules with dark blue segmented nuclei. By FC, they show moderate expression of CD45, positive myeloid markers (CD13 and CD33), positive CD11b, CD22, CD38, and bright CD123.

Thrombocytosis

Thrombocytosis can be seen in benign and malignant disorders, including:

- ET
- CML (*BCR-ABL1*+)
- PMF
- PV
- MDS with isolated deletion of 5q
- MDS/MPN with neutrophilia
- MDS/MPN with SF3B1 mutation and thrombocytosis (MDS/MPN-SF3B1-T)
- Unclassifiable MDS or MPN
- Acute megakaryoblastic leukemia
- Reactive (transient) thrombocytosis

Algorithmic approach to thrombocytosis is presented in Figure 21.2 in Chapter 21. Reactive thrombocytosis can be "acute" (transient) or sustained. The former is associated with acute blood loss, acute infection, or inflammation or after exercise. Sustained reactive thrombocytosis is associated with iron deficiency, chronic inflammations, drug effects, hemolysis, rebound following toxic therapy and in hyposplenism. ET is a relatively indolent and often asymptomatic clonal MPN that involves predominantly megakaryocytic lineage characterized primarily by a sustained elevation in platelets (≥450 × 10⁹/L), megakaryocytosis and minimal to absent BM fibrosis. Other MPNs, especially CML, PV and early PMF as well as some MDS (e.g., 5q⁻ syndrome) or mixed MDS/MPN disorders (e.g., MDS/MPN-RS-T) often present with thrombocytosis and therefore

comprehensive evaluation of the BM with cytogenetics, FC, fluorescence in situ hybridization (FISH), and molecular testing plays important role in establishing the final diagnosis. Thrombocytosis is rare in AML except for acute megakaryoblastic leukemia. It has also been reported in AML with i(17p), t(1;3), t(2;3) and other chromosome 3 abnormalities. Figure 8.8 shows increased number of atypical platelets in case of ET and acute megakaryoblastic leukemia.

Circulating blasts

Myeloblasts are variable is size (but generally larger than small lymphocytes), and mostly medium to large with scant or abundant gray or bluish cytoplasm, round, or oval nuclei with fine (delicate) chromatin and one or more large prominent nucleoli. Some myeloblasts contain azurophilic cytoplasmic granules or Auer rods. Lymphoblasts vary from small cells with scant cytoplasm to larger cells with more abundant cytoplasm. Cytoplasm may be vacuolated. Chromatin may be condensed (dark) in small blasts or dispersed, more delicate in larger blasts, which also may have several nucleoli. Some lymphoblasts show asymmetric location of nucleus and/or formation of cytoplasmic pseudopod giving so-called "hand-mirror" appearance. "Hand-mirror" cells are more typical for lymphoblastic leukemias, but they can also be seen in AMLs. Monoblasts are mostly large cells with abundant pale or blue cytoplasm with vacuoles and occasional pseudopod formation. The nuclei are round with delicate chromatin and prominent nucleoli. Promonocytes differ from monoblasts by irregular nuclear outlines, often with convoluted, folded, or grooved appearance and smaller, often inconspicuous nucleolus.

Blasts and atypical mononuclear cells with blast-like features include:

- AML
- B-cell and T-cell acute lymphoblastic leukemia (B-ALL/T-ALL)
- Blastic plasmacytoid dendritic cell neoplasm (BPDCN)
- Blastoid variant of MCL
- Blastic transformation of B- or T-cell lymphomas
- BL and other high-grade B-cell lymphomas (HGBLs)
- Plasmablastic lymphoma (PBL)
- PCM with plasmablastic features
- Immunoblastic variant of DLBCL
- ALK+ DLBCL
- ALCL
- Rhabdomyosarcoma and some other metastatic tumors

Figure 8.9 shows cytologic-flow cytometric correlation of blats and blast-like mononuclear cells. Apart from acute leukemias, blastic cytomorphology may be displayed by BPDCN, blastoid variant of MCL, variants of DLBCL (e.g., immunoblastic or ALK1+), BL, primary effusion lymphoma (PEL), high grade B-cell lymphoma with rearrangement of MYC and BCL2 (and/or BCL6; HGBL-R), PBL, PCM with plasmablastic features, some T-cell lymphomas, high grade transformation of mature B- or T-cell lymphomas, and some metastatic tumors.

Summary of FC phenotypic profiles of most common disorders with circulating blasts or "blast"-like cells:

AML: CD13+, CD33+, CD34+/rarely−, CD117+, CD133+/−, MPO+, CD81+/−, HLA-DR+/rarely−

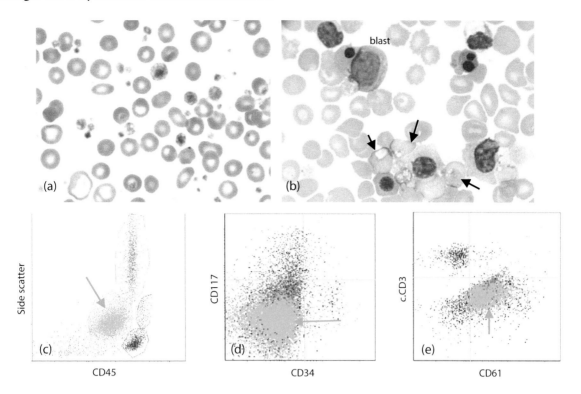

FIGURE 8.8   Thrombocytosis. Comparison between cytologic features of platelets in ET (a) and acute megakaryoblastic leukemia (b). Note strike cytologic atypia of platelets in the latter (arrow). By FC analysis, megakaryoblasts show moderate CD45 (c; green dots; arrow), negative CD34 and CD117 (d), and positive CD61 (e).

B-ALL: CD10$^{+/-}$, CD19^{+}, CD20$^{-/rarely+(partial)}$, CD22^{+}, CD34$^{+/rarely-}$, HLA-DR^{+}, CD45$^{-/+(dim)}$, TdT$^{+/rarely-}$

T-ALL: CD1a$^{-/+}$, CD2^{+}, surface CD3^{-}, cytoplasmic CD3^{+}, CD5$^{+/-}$, CD7^{+}, CD4/CD8^{+} or CD4/CD8^{-}, CD10$^{-/+}$, CD34^{+}, TdT$^{+/-}$

BPDCN: CD4^{+}, CD13^{-}, CD33$^{-/+}$, CD56$^{+(strong)}$, CD123$^{+(strong)}$, CD11b^{-}, CD11c^{-}, HLA-DR^{+}, CD45^{+}, TdT$^{-/+}$, MPO^{-}, CD64^{-}

DLBCL: CD19^{+}, CD20^{+}, surface light chain immunoglobulin^{+}, CD5$^{-/rarely+}$, CD10$^{+/-}$, CD11c$^{-/rarely+}$, CD23^{-}, CD25$^{-/rarely+}$, CD38^{+}, CD43$^{-/+}$, CD71$^{+(dim or rarely strong)}$, CD81$^{+(dim)}$, CD200$^{-/rarely+(dim)}$

BL: CD19^{+}, CD20^{+}, surface light chain immunoglobulin^{+}, BCL2^{-}, CD5^{-}, CD10^{+}, CD11c^{-}, CD23^{-}, CD25^{-}, CD38^{+}, CD43$^{+(strong)}$, CD71$^{+(strong)}$, CD81$^{+(strong)}$, CD200$^{-/rarely+(dim)}$

HGBL-R: CD19^{+}, CD20$^{+ (may be dim)}$, surface light chain immunoglobulin$^{+/rarely-}$, BCL2^{+}, CD5^{-}, CD10$^{+/rarely-}$, CD11c^{-}, CD23^{-}, CD25^{-}, CD38^{+}, CD43$^{+/-}$, CD71^{+}, CD81^{+}, CD200$^{-/+}$

Acute monoblastic leukemia: CD34$^{- (rarely+)}$, CD117$^{-/+}$, CD13^{+}, CD33^{++}, MPO^{-}, HLA-DR^{+}, CD45^{++}, CD14$^{+/-}$, CD64^{++}, CD11b$^{+/-}$, CD11c^{+}, CD4^{+}, CD56$^{+/-}$, CD71$^{+/-}$; CD123$^{+/-}$

B-PLL: CD19^{+}, CD20^{+}, surface light chain immunoglobulin^{+}, CD5$^{-/rare cases+}$, CD10^{-}, CD11c^{-}, CD23$^{-/+}$, CD38^{+}, CD43$^{-/+}$, CD71^{-}, CD81^{-}, CD200$^{+/rarely-}$

T-PLL: CD2$^{+/-}$, CD3$^{+/-}$, CD4^{+} (less often CD8^{+}, CD4/CD8^{+} or CD4/CD8^{-}), CD5$^{+/-}$, CD7$^{+/-}$, CD25^{-}, CD26^{+}, CD45$^{+/rarely-}$, CD56^{-}, CD57^{-}, CD81^{+}, CD117$^{-/rarely+}$, CD200^{-}

Monocytosis

Monocytes are large cells with abundant pale, clear or vacuolated cytoplasm and irregular (lobated) nuclei with rather dense chromatin and inconspicuous nucleoli. In neoplastic proliferations, mature monocytes show cytologic atypia in the form of abnormal nuclear lobation and/or cytoplasmic granulation. Immature monocytes (monoblasts and promonocytes) are characterized by more prominent nucleoli, finer chromatin and in the case of monoblasts, lack of nuclear convolutions and folds (see blasts, above). Algorithmic approach to monocytosis is presented in Figure 20.1 in Chapter 20.

Differential diagnosis of monocytosis include:

- Reactive monocytosis (infections, post-therapy, Hodgkin lymphoma, etc.)
- CMML
- CML (*BCR-ABL1*$^{+}$)
- MDS/MPN with neutrophilia (known as atypical CML)
- PMF and early (prefibrotic) stage of PMF (pre-PMF)
- PV
- ET
- Myeloid neoplasms with *PDGFRA*, *PDGFRB*, or *FGFR1* rearrangement
- MDS
- Juvenile myelomonocytic leukemia (JMML)
- CNL
- SM
- Acute myelomonocytic leukemia (AMML)
- Acute monocytic (monoblastic) leukemia
- AML with *NPM1* mutation
- BPDCN
- DLBCL with leukemic blood involvement

Reactive monocytosis

Reactive monocytosis occurs in patients with infections, autoimmune processes, after splenectomy and other stress-induced

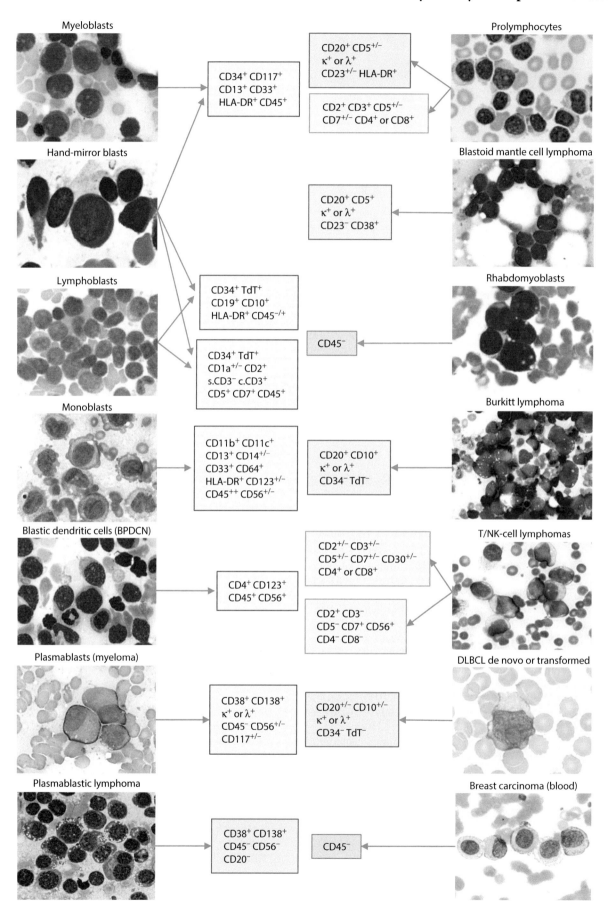

FIGURE 8.9 Blasts and blast-like cells: cytologic-immunophenotypic correlation.

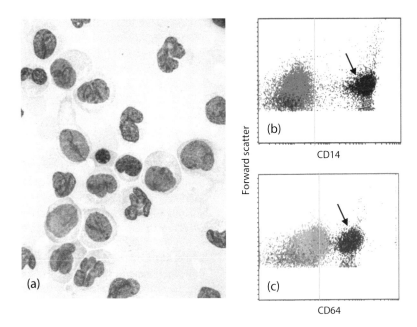

FIGURE 8.10 CMML. Neoplastic monocytes are mostly mature (a) and show bright expression of CD14 (b; arrow) and CD64 (c; arrow).

events (e.g., myocardial infarction) and in marrow regeneration after transplant or cytotoxic therapy. Infectious etiology includes tuberculosis and other bacterial infections (leptospirosis, listeriosis), fungal infections, infective endocarditis, viral infections (including SARS/COVID-19 associated disease), and in certain protozoal infections. Connective tissue disorders including systemic lupus erythematosus (SLE) and sarcoidosis, and lipid storage diseases may also lead to monocytosis in blood. Gastric carcinoma, PCM, lymphomas (Hodgkin and non-Hodgkin) can be also associated with monocytosis. Recovery from acute infections or the BM regeneration after cytotoxic therapy is often associated with transient monocytosis. Persistent etiology of monocytosis includes subacute or chronic infections (syphilis, brucellosis, malaria, tuberculosis, leishmaniosis, and rickettsial infections). Autoimmune disorders, such as sarcoidosis, ulcerative colitis, SLE, rheumatoid arthritis, and immune mediated thrombocytopenia (ITP may also be associated with persistent reactive monocytosis).

Benign (reactive) monocytes show bright expression CD11b, CD11c, CD13, CD14, CD15, CD33, CD36, and CD64, dim CD4, bright HLA-DR, and bright CD45. Minor subset of monocytes may be positive for CD2, CD16, and/or CDD56. Reactive monocytes usually do not display overtly aberrant phenotype [25]. Xu et al., showed alteration of one antigen on monocytes in 55% of the reactive monocytosis and abnormal expression of two or more antigens in only 15% of the cases [26]. The most common abnormalities in reactive monocytosis include decreased expression of CD13, CD15, CD36, and HLA-DR and aberrant expression of CD56.

CMML

CMML is a clonal hematopoietic malignancy with overlapping features of both MPN and an MDS [27–34]. CMML is defined by (1) persistent (at least 3 months) monocytosis (≥0.5 × 10⁹/L) with monocytes ≥10% of leukocytes in the blood; (2) <20% blasts

(blast count includes myeloblasts, monoblasts, and promonocytes); (3) lack of *BCR-ABL1* fusion (Philadelphia chromosome); (4) no rearrangement of *PDGFRA* or *PDGFRB*, and *PCM1-JAK2* fusion (should be specifically excluded in cases with eosinophilia); and (5) dysplastic features in one or more myeloid lineages [27]. Monocytes are mostly mature without significant cytologic atypia (Figure 8.10), but atypical monocytes with granulation, nuclear lobation or convolutions, grayish cytoplasm or even immature monocytes may be present. The mature monocytes are characterized by bright expression of CD11b, CD11c, CD13, CD14, CD15, CD33, CD36, CD45, CD64, and HLA-DR and positive CD4. Although reactive monocytosis may display subtle phenotypic atypia (most often aberrant expression of one of the antigens on subset of cells), prominent phenotypic atypia in the form of aberrant expression of at least two antigens or phenotypic atypia involving majority of monocytic population suggest CMML. The most commonly observed phenotypic changes in CMML include decreased or variable ("smeary") expression of CD11b, decreased CD13, CD15, CD36, CD33, and/or HLA-DR, decreased, variable or partial expression of CD14, and positive CD10, CD16, CD23, and/or CD56. Presence of aberrant phenotype of granulocytes (phenotypic features of dyspoiesis and/or leftward shift), presence of circulating blasts, increased number of blasts in the BM and lack of hematogones in the BM are additional FC features helpful in distinguishing CMML from reactive monocytosis. Based on the expression of CD14 and CD16, monocytes can be divided into CD14⁺/CD16⁻ (classical), CD14⁺/CD16⁺ (intermediate), and CD14^low/CD16⁺ (non-classical) monocytes [35]. Compared with healthy donors and patients with reactive monocytosis or another hematologic malignancy, CMML patients demonstrate a characteristic increase in the fraction of CD14⁺/CD16⁻ cells (cutoff value, 94.0%) and a decrease in the absolute number of CD14^low/CD16⁺ monocytes. [36]. Cases with absolute monocytes between 0.5 –1 × 10(9)/L, previously classified as oligomonocytic CMML [34] now belong to CMML category.

FC differential diagnosis between CMML and reactive monocytosis are discussed in Chapter 20.

CML and other MPNs

CML is characterized morphologically by prominent leukocytosis with blood smear showing predominance of granulocytes at different stages of maturation, basophilia, eosinophilia and scattered blasts, and nucleated erythroid precursors. CML shows also increased number of monocytes, which on occasional may be prominent, mimicking CMML. In most cases, however, granulocytes predominate. The diagnosis of CML is confirmed by presence of Philadelphia chromosome [t(9;22)] or the *BCR-ABL1* fusion. Presence of leukocytosis with eosinophilia in the absence of *BCR-ABL1* transcripts may indicate MPNs with *PDGFRA* or *PDGFRB* rearrangement, a rare neoplasm characterized by marked eosinophilia. Myeloid neoplasm with *PDGFRB* may often mimic CMML (it differs from CMML by prominent eosinophilia in addition to monocytosis). Monocytosis in PMF, ET, or PV patients can be seen at presentation, or appears later, especially during disease progression (often with appearance of dysplasia). Features overlapping in CMML and PMF include presence of leukocytosis, splenomegaly (in CMML, splenomegaly is usually associated with infiltration of spleen by leukemic CMML cells) and/or *JAK2* mutation. Presence of MPN-associated "driver" mutations (*JAK2*, *MPL*, or *CALR*) favors the diagnosis of PMF with monocytosis [27]. Those mutations, however, are not specific for PMF, as they may be present in CMML. PMF may also acquire secondary mutations, such as *TET2*, *DNMT3A*, *EZH2*, *ASXL1*, *SRSF2*, and *U2AF1*, which occur also commonly in CMML. In comparison to PMF with monocytosis, patients with CMML are older, have lower platelet count, higher BM blasts, presence of micromegakaryocytes or hypolobated forms and dysplasia in other lineages, higher frequency of *TET2* mutations and lower *JAK2* allelic burden. The neoplasms with overlapping features between PMF with monocytosis and CMML with marrow fibrosis may represent either "gray-zone" neoplasm (hybrid between PMF and CMML) or unusual PMF with monocytosis, dysplasia, and CMML-like mutations [27, 37–40].

MDS/MPN with neutrophilia (MDS/MPN-N)

In contrast to CMML, MDS/MPN-N, known as atypical CML (aCML) shows admixture of promyelocytes, myelocytes, and metamyelocytes which comprise at least 10% of leukocytes. All three BM lineages may display dyspoiesis. Staining of the BM aspirate with non-specific esterase (NSE) may be helpful to identify monocytes and differentiate CMML from MDS/MPN-N. Despite monocytosis in MDS/MPN-N, neutrophilia is still a predominant feature. Patients with significant neutrophilia but displaying monocytosis fulfilling the WHO criteria are diagnosed with CMML rather than MDS/MPN-N [41].

MDS

CMML shows dysplastic features which may involve all three lineages. Presence of dyspoiesis in conjunction with anemia and/or thrombocytopenia raises the possibility of MDS. In addition, subset of patients with MDS has monocytosis, but in contrast to CMML is not chronic or persistent. If dysplastic features are accompanied by absolute and persistent monocytosis, a diagnosis of CMML can be rendered, keeping in mind that there is a significant clinical, morphologic, and immunophenotypic overlap between MDS and CMML. MDS often is characterized by erythroid hyperplasia, whereas in CMML the myeloid to erythroid ratio is typically increased with normal or decreased erythropoiesis. Patients with MDS may progress into CMML [42–44]. Some MDS cases may show persistent nodular BM lesions composed of immature monocytes [45]. Monocytic leukemoid reaction in a patient with MDS has also been reported [46].

AMML

AMML has by definition at least 20% blasts (in CMML the number of blasts is <20%). Monocytes are usually mature but may display phenotypic atypia by FC analysis. AMML is discussed in Chapter 22. Presence of increased blasts, monocytes and atypical "eosinophilic" basophils should raise the suspicion of AML with *CBFB* rearrangement resulting from t(16;16) or inv(16).

Acute monoblastic (monocytic) leukemia

Acute monoblastic (monocytic) leukemia is characterized by presence of immature monocytes (promonocytes and monoblasts) with prominent cytologic and phenotypic atypia (Figure 8.11). Monoblasts are characterized by fine chromatin, round nuclei, nucleolus, and pale basophilic cytoplasm, whereas promonocytes have irregular, often folded nuclei, prominent nucleoli, and paler cytoplasm. Frequently immature monocytes display aberrant expression of CD14 (partial or complete loss; variable "smeary" expression) and positive CD56. In addition, poorly differentiated cases may be positive for CD34 and/or CD117. Aberrant expression of HLA-DR (negative or dim), CD10 (positive), CD33 (negative or dim), and CD11b (variable or dim) is also seen more often in acute monoblastic leukemia than in CMML. FC helps to differentiate acute monoblastic leukemia from hypogranular variant of APL and BPDCN, which often shows folded nuclei mimicking neoplastic monocytes (monoblasts).

BPDCN

Blasts of BPDCN shows variable cytomorphologic features ranging from those similar to lymphoblasts to those similar to myeloblasts or monoblasts. They are generally smaller than monoblasts and have less abundant cytoplasm, which is pale bluish, and only occasionally shows small vacuoles. Nuclei may be round or more pleomorphic with folds. Some blasts show eccentric location of nuclei with more bluish cytoplasm ("plasmacytoid" features). By FC, BPDCN shows characteristic co-expression of CD4, CD56, and CD123.

B-cell lymphoproliferations

DLBCL, BL, and HGBLs, as well as unusual "blastoid" variants of HCL or MCL may resemble cytologically immature monocytic cells. Flow cytometry immunophenotyping helps to distinguish between monoblasts and B-cell neoplasms (see Figure 22.28 in Chapter 22).

Leukoerythroblastosis

Leukoerythroblastosis called also myelophthisic anemia, is defined as presence of immature myeloid precursors and nucleated red cells in blood.

Differential diagnosis of leukoerythroblastosis include:

- PMF and other MPNs in fibrotic stage
- MDS/MPN-RS-T

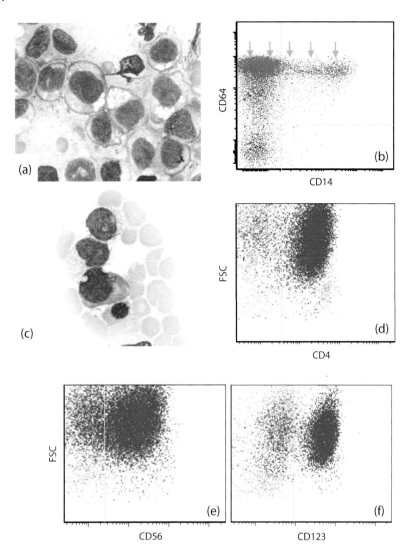

FIGURE 8.11 (a–b) Acute monoblastic leukemia. Monocytic cells are immature (a), represented mostly by monoblasts and pro-monocytes. FC analysis (b; green dots) shows bright CD64 expression and variable CD14 expression with majority of monocytic cells negative and minor subset showing variable expression (arrows). (c–f) Blastic plasmacytoid dendritic cell neoplasm (BPDCN). Blasts show slightly eccentric nuclei with irregular outlines, fine chromatin and nucleoli, and pale to vacuolated cytoplasm (c). FC analysis (d–f; magenta dots) shows co-expression of CD4 (d), CD56 (e), and CD123 (f).

- AML, especially AML with myelodysplasia-related changes (MDS-MRC) and reticulin fibrosis
- Infiltrative process in BM (metastatic carcinoma, lymphoma, Hodgkin lymphoma, PCM, CLL, mastocytosis, amyloidosis, granulomas, etc.)
- Infections

Circulating plasma cells

Circulating plasma cells can be identified in blood in the following processes:

- PCM
- PCL
- Reactive plasmacytosis in infections, drug reactions, and certain malignancies

- Reactive plasmacytosis in angioimmunoblastic T-cell lymphoma (AITL)

PCL is defined by circulating clonal plasma cells (>2 × 10⁹/L or ≥20% of leukocyte differential count) [27]. PCL (Figure 8.12) may be present at the time of diagnosis (primary PCL) or represent leukemic transformation of end-stage PCM (secondary PCL). Primary PCL is a high-risk feature for myeloma patients. Reactive plasma cells can be seen in blood in many conditions, including patients with viral infections (HIV, hepatitis), Staphylococcal sepsis, tuberculosis, treatment with intravenous immunoglobulins, drug reactions and autoimmune disorders, and in certain malignancies, especially AITL. In most cases of reactive plasmacytosis in blood the plasma cell count does not exceed 10%. Very prominent polytypic blood plasmacytosis mimicking PCL have been reported in AITL, parvovirus infections, mononucleosis-like reaction, and sickle cell disease [47–49].

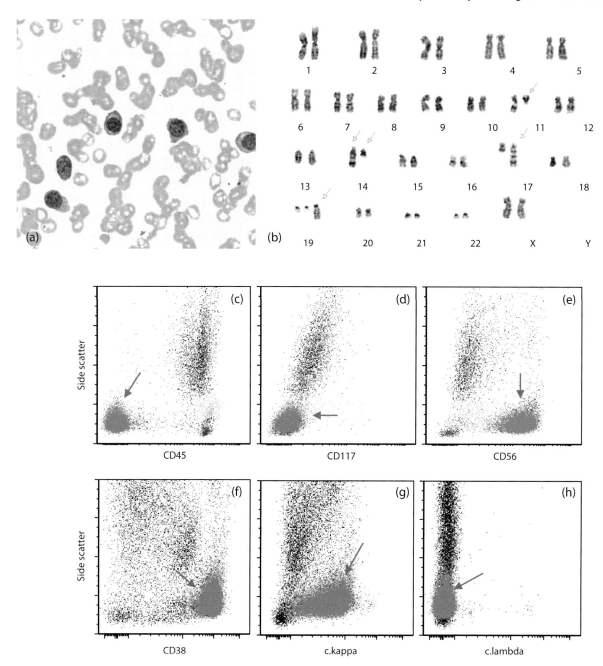

FIGURE 8.12 Plasma cell leukemia. (a) Blood smear with circulating plasma cells with mature cytologic features. (b) Complex chromosomal changes [including t(11;14)(q13;q32), add(14)(q11.2), add(17)(q25), +der(19)t(1;19)(q23;q12)]. (c–h) Flow cytometry shows negative CD45 (c), negative CD117 (d), positive CD56 (e), positive CD38 (f), and positive cytoplasmic kappa (g–h).

References

1. Gnanaraj, J., et al., *Approach to pancytopenia: diagnostic algorithm for clinical hematologists.* Blood Rev, 2018. **32**(5): p. 361–7.
2. Weinzierl, E.P. and D.A. Arber, *The differential diagnosis and bone marrow evaluation of new-onset pancytopenia.* Am J Clin Pathol, 2013. **139**(1): p. 9–29.
3. Bellos, F., et al., *Evaluation of flow cytometric assessment of myeloid nuclear differentiation antigen expression as a diagnostic marker for myelodysplastic syndromes in a series of 269 patients.* Cytometry B Clin Cytom, 2012. **82**(5): p. 295–304.
4. Cremers, E.M., et al., *Multiparameter flow cytometry is instrumental to distinguish myelodysplastic syndromes from non-neoplastic cytopenias.* Eur J Cancer, 2015. **54**: p. 49–56.
5. Della Porta, M.G., et al., *Flow cytometry immunophenotyping for the evaluation of bone marrow dysplasia.* Cytometry B Clin Cytom, 2011. **80**(4): p. 201–11.
6. Della Porta, M.G., et al., *Flow cytometry evaluation of erythroid dysplasia in patients with myelodysplastic syndrome.* Leukemia, 2006. **20**(4): p. 549–55.
7. Kern, W., et al., *Clinical utility of multiparameter flow cytometry in the diagnosis of 1013 patients with suspected myelodysplastic syndrome: correlation to cytomorphology, cytogenetics, and clinical data.* Cancer, 2010. **116**(19): p. 4549–63.
8. Ogata, K., *Diagnostic flow cytometry for low-grade myelodysplastic syndromes.* Hematol Oncol, 2008. **26**(4): p. 193–8.
9. Porwit, A. and A. Rajab, *Flow cytometry immunophenotyping in integrated diagnostics of patients with newly diagnosed cytopenia:*

one tube 10-color 14-antibody screening panel and 3-tube extensive panel for detection of MDS-related features. Int J Lab Hematol, 2015. **37 Suppl 1**: p. 133–43.

10. Reis-Alves, S.C., et al., *Improving the differential diagnosis between myelodysplastic syndromes and reactive peripheral cytopenias by multiparametric flow cytometry: the role of B-cell precursors.* Diagn Pathol, 2015. **10**: p. 44.

11. Stetler-Stevenson, M. and C.M. Yuan, *Myelodysplastic syndromes: the role of flow cytometry in diagnosis and prognosis.* Int J Lab Hematol, 2009. **31**(5): p. 479–83.

12. Elliott, M.A. and A. Tefferi, *Chronic neutrophilic leukemia 2014: update on diagnosis, molecular genetics, and management.* Am J Hematol, 2014. **89**(6): p. 651–8.

13. Elliott, M.A. and A. Tefferi, *Chronic neutrophilic leukemia 2016: update on diagnosis, molecular genetics, prognosis, and management.* Am J Hematol, 2016. **91**(3): p. 341–9.

14. Gotlib, J., et al., *The new genetics of chronic neutrophilic leukemia and atypical CML: implications for diagnosis and treatment.* Blood, 2013. **122**(10): p. 1707–11.

15. Haferlach, T., et al., *The diagnosis of BCR/ABL-negative chronic myeloproliferative diseases (CMPD): a comprehensive approach based on morphology, cytogenetics, and molecular markers.* Ann Hematol, 2008. **87**(1): p. 1–10.

16. Lasho, T.L., et al., *CALR mutation studies in chronic neutrophilic leukemia.* Am J Hematol, 2014. **89**(4): p. 450.

17. Lasho, T.L., et al., *Chronic neutrophilic leukemia with concurrent CSF3R and SETBP1 mutations: single colony clonality studies, in vitro sensitivity to JAK inhibitors and lack of treatment response to ruxolitinib.* Leukemia, 2014. **28**(6): p. 1363–5.

18. Tefferi, A., et al., *An overview on CALR and CSF3R mutations and a proposal for revision of WHO diagnostic criteria for myeloproliferative neoplasms.* Leukemia, 2014. **28**(7): p. 1407–13.

19. Wang, S.A., et al., *Atypical chronic myeloid leukemia is clinically distinct from unclassifiable myelodysplastic/myeloproliferative neoplasms.* Blood, 2014. **123**(17): p. 2645–51.

20. Schwartz, L.C. and J. Mascarenhas, *Current and evolving understanding of atypical chronic myeloid leukemia.* Blood Rev, 2019. **33**: p. 74–81.

21. Martiat, P., J.L. Michaux, and J. Rodhain, *Philadelphia-negative (Ph-) chronic myeloid leukemia (CML): comparison with Ph+ CML and chronic myelomonocytic leukemia. The Groupe Francais de Cytogenetique Hematologique.* Blood, 1991. **78**(1): p. 205–11.

22. Linder, K., C. Iragavarapu, and D. Liu, *SETBP1 mutations as a biomarker for myelodysplasia/myeloproliferative neoplasm overlap syndrome.* Biomark Res, 2017. **5**: p. 33.

23. Hu, Z., et al., *Lymphocytic variant of hypereosinophilic syndrome: a report of seven cases from a single institution.* Cytometry B Clin Cytom, 2021. **100**(3): p. 352–60.

24. Spivak, J.L., *How I treat polycythemia vera.* Blood, 2019. **134**(4): p. 341–52.

25. Gorczyca, W., *Flow cytometry immunophenotypic characteristics of monocytic population in acute monocytic leukemia (AML-M5), acute myelomonocytic leukemia (AML-M4), and chronic myelomonocytic leukemia (CMML).* Methods Cell Biol, 2004. **75**: p. 665–77.

26. Xu, Y., et al., *Flow cytometric analysis of monocytes as a tool for distinguishing chronic myelomonocytic leukemia from reactive monocytosis.* Am J Clin Pathol, 2005. **124**(5): p. 799–806.

27. Swerdlow, S.H., Campo, E., Harris, N. L., Jaffe, E. S., Pileri, S. A., Stein, H., Stein, H., Thiele, J., Arber, D.A., Le Beau M.M., Orazi, A., Siebert, R., ed. WHO classification of tumors of haematopoietic and lymphoid tissues. 2016, IARC: Lyon.

28. Patnaik, M.M., et al., *Chronic myelomonocytic leukaemia: a concise clinical and pathophysiological review.* Br J Haematol, 2014. **165**(3): p. 273–86.

29. Patnaik, M.M. and A. Tefferi, *Chronic myelomonocytic leukemia: 2018 update on diagnosis, risk stratification and management.* Am J Hematol, 2018. **93**(6): p. 824–40.

30. Itzykson, R., P. Fenaux, and E. Solary, *Chronic myelomonocytic leukemia: myelodysplastic or myeloproliferative?* Best Pract Res Clin Haematol, 2013. **26**(4): p. 387–400.

31. Itzykson, R. and E. Solary, *An evolutionary perspective on chronic myelomonocytic leukemia.* Leukemia, 2013. **27**(7): p. 1441–50.

32. Shen, Q., et al., *Flow cytometry immunophenotypic findings in chronic myelomonocytic leukemia and its utility in monitoring treatment response.* Eur J Haematol, 2015. **95**(2): p. 168–76.

33. Harrington, A.M., et al., *Immunophenotypes of chronic myelomonocytic leukemia (CMML) subtypes by flow cytometry. a comparison of CMML-1 vs CMML-2, myeloproliferative vs dysplastic, de novo vs therapy-related, and CMML-specific cytogenetic risk subtypes.* Am J Clin Pathol, 2016. **146**(2): p. 170–81.

34. Valent, P., et al., *Proposed diagnostic criteria for classical CMML, CMML variants and pre-CMML conditions.* Haematologica, 2019. **104**(10): p. 1935–49.

35. Ziegler-Heitbrock, L., et al., *Nomenclature of monocytes and dendritic cells in blood.* Blood, 2010. **116**(16): p. e74–e80.

36. Selimoglu-Buet, D., et al., *Characteristic repartition of monocyte subsets as a diagnostic signature of chronic myelomonocytic leukemia.* Blood, 2015. **125**(23): p. 3618–26.

37. Chapman, J., et al., *Myeloid neoplasms with features intermediate between primary myelofibrosis and chronic myelomonocytic leukemia.* Mod Pathol, 2018. **31**(3): p. 429–41.

38. Tefferi, A., et al., *CALR vs JAK2 vs MPL-mutated or triple-negative myelofibrosis: clinical, cytogenetic and molecular comparisons.* Leukemia, 2014. **28**(7): p. 1472–7.

39. Tefferi, A., et al., *One thousand patients with primary myelofibrosis: the mayo clinic experience.* Mayo Clin Proc, 2012. **87**(1): p. 25–33.

40. Tefferi, A., et al., *Monocytosis is a powerful and independent predictor of inferior survival in primary myelofibrosis.* Br J Haematol, 2018. **183**(5): p. 835–8.

41. Muramatsu, H., H. Makishima, and J.P. Maciejewski, *Chronic myelomonocytic leukemia and atypical chronic myeloid leukemia: novel pathogenetic lesions.* Semin Oncol, 2012. **39**(1): p. 67–73.

42. Rigolin, G.M., et al., *Myelodysplastic syndromes with monocytic component: hematologic and cytogenetic characterization.* Haematologica, 1997. **82**(1): p. 25–30.

43. Breccia, M., et al., *Chronic myelomonocytic leukemia with antecedent refractory anemia with excess blasts: further evidence for the arbitrary nature of current classification systems.* Leuk Lymphoma, 2008. **49**(7): p. 1292–6.

44. Wang, S.A., et al., *Chronic myelomonocytic leukemia evolving from preexisting myelodysplasia shares many features with de novo disease.* Am J Clin Pathol, 2006. **126**(5): p. 789–97.

45. Mongkonsritragoon, W., et al., *Nodular lesions of monocytic component in myelodysplastic syndrome.* Am J Clin Pathol, 1998. **110**(2): p. 154–62.

46. Moraes, M., J. Wilkes, and J.N. Lowder, *Monocytic leukemoid reaction, glucocorticoid therapy, and myelodysplastic syndrome.* Cleve Clin J Med, 1990. **57**(6): p. 571–4.

47. Nagoshi, H., et al., *Clinical manifestation of angioimmunoblastic T-cell lymphoma with exuberant plasmacytosis.* Int J Hematol, 2013. **98**(3): p. 366–74.

48. Ahsanuddin, A.N., R.K. Brynes, and S. Li, *Peripheral blood polyclonal plasmacytosis mimicking plasma cell leukemia in patients with angioimmunoblastic T-cell lymphoma: report of 3 cases and review of the literature.* Int J Clin Exp Pathol, 2011. **4**(4): p. 416–20.

49. Gawoski, J.M. and W.W. Ooi, *Dengue fever mimicking plasma cell leukemia.* Arch Pathol Lab Med, 2003. **127**(8): p. 1026–7.

9

MORPHOLOGIC-FLOW CYTOMETRIC CORRELATION IN BONE MARROW

Benign bone marrow

The flow cytometric features of normal bone marrow (BM) are presented in Chapter 2.

Increased blasts

Differential diagnosis of increased blasts in BM includes regenerating marrow after therapy or toxic insult, treatment with Neupogen, myelodysplastic neoplasm (MDS) with increased blasts (MDS-IB), chronic myelomonocytic leukemia (CMML), chronic myeloid leukemia (CML), and other myeloproliferative neoplasms (MPNs) in accelerated phase or blast crisis, acute promyelocytic leukemia (APL; Figure 9.1, see also Chapter 24), acute myeloid leukemia (AML) (Figure 9.2, see also Chapters 5, 22–24), blastic plasmacytoid dendritic cell neoplasm (BPDCN; see Chapter 27), B-cell acute lymphoblastic leukemia (B-ALL; see Chapters 6 and 17), and T-cell acute lymphoblastic leukemia (T-ALL; see Chapters 6 and 18). Normal BM shows less than 2%–3% of blasts. Based on the number of blasts in the BM, MDS is divided into MDS with increased blasts-1 (MDS-IB-1; 5%–9% of blasts) and MDS-IB-2 (10%–19% of blasts) [1]. CMML with <5% blasts in blood and <10% in BM is classified as CMML-1 and with 5–19% blasts in blood and 10-19% in BM as CMML-2. Current WHO classification of the hematopoietic tumors requires ≥20% of blasts for the diagnosis of AML (except for cases with certain recurrent genetic abnormalities) [1]. AMLs with t(15;17)/*PML-RARA*, t(8;21)/*RUNX1-RUNX1T1*, and t(16;16/inv(16)) can be diagnosed with <20% blasts [1]. Those leukemias are occasionally called "oligoblastic" AML. The classification of myeloid neoplasm with increased blasts (<20%) and presence of *NPM1* mutations is somewhat controversial. *NPM1* mutations occurs most commonly in AML (classified as AML with *NPM1* mutation), but sporadic cases of other myeloid neoplasms, most commonly MDS (~2%) and CMML (~3%) may be *NPM1*+ [2]. Those cases can be classified as high-grade myeloid neoplasm with *NPM1* mutation representing either (1) "oligoblastic" AML (if the number of blasts is close to 20%), (2) MDS with *NPM1* mutation, or (3) CMML with *NPM1* mutations. It is recommended that patients with either MDS or CMML with *NPM1* mutation should be treated aggressively with up-front chemotherapy rather than with MDS-directed protocols, as those neoplasms are associated with an aggressive clinical course, relatively rapid progression to overt AML and poor survival outcomes [2–7]. In WHO classification, blast phase (BP) of CML and other MPNs is defined by (1) ≥20% blasts; or (2) extramedullary blast proliferation. Current WHO classification does not recommend to diagnose ALL with <20% blasts in BM, and patients with <25% lymphoblasts in BM are usually classified as either B-cell lymphoblastic lymphoma (B-LBL) or T-cell lymphoblastic lymphoma (T-LBL), while patients with ≥25% blasts are diagnosed with B-ALL or T-ALL [1].

Summary of FC phenotypic profiles of blasts in BM:

AML: CD13+, CD33+, CD34+/rarely–, CD117+, CD133+/–, MPO+, CD81+/–, HLA-DR+/rarely–

Acute monoblastic (monocytic) leukemia: CD2–/+, s.CD3–, c.CD3–, CD4+, CD7+/–, CD11b+(variable)/rarely–, CD11c+, CD13+, CD14–/+(variable), CD15+, CD19–, c.CD22–, CD33+, CD34–/rarely+, CD38+/rarely–, CD36+, CD56+/rarely–, CD64+, CD65+, c.CD79a–, CD117–/rarely+, CD133–, HLA-DR+/rarely–, MPO–/rarely+

APL (hypergranular): CD2–, s.CD3–, c.CD3–, CD4–/+, CD7+/–, CD11b–, CD11c–, CD13+, CD14–, CD15–/rarely+(dim), CD19–, c.CD22–, CD33+bright, CD34–, CD38+, CD36–, CD56–/rarely+, CD64–/dim+, CD65–/rarely+, c.CD79a–, CD117+(may be dim), CD133–/rarely+, HLA-DR–, MPO+

APL-v (hypogranular): CD2+/rarely–, s.CD3–, c.CD3–, CD4–/+, CD7+/–, CD11b–, CD11c–, CD13+, CD14–, CD15–/rarely+(dim), CD19–, c.CD22–, CD33+bright, CD34+/rarely–, CD38+, CD36–, CD56–/rarely+, CD64–/dim+, CD65–/rarely+, c.CD79a–, CD117+(may be dim), CD133–/rarely+, HLA-DR–, MPO+

B-ALL: CD10+/–, CD19+, CD20–/rarely+(partial), CD22+, CD34+/rarely–, HLA-DR+, CD45–/+(dim), TdT+/rarely–

T-ALL: CD1a–/+, CD2+, surface CD3–, cytoplasmic CD3+, CD5+/–, CD7+, CD4/CD8+ or CD4/CD8–, CD10–/+, CD34+, TdT+/–

AUL: CD34+, HLA-DR+, TdT+/–, CD38+

BPDCN: CD4+, CD13–, CD33–/+, CD56+(strong), CD123+(strong), CD11b–, CD11c–, HLA-DR+, CD45+, TdT–/+, MPO–, CD64–

Diffuse small cell infiltrate

Lymphomas can display different histologic patterns of BM involvement, including diffuse, nodular, interstitial, paratrabecular, intrasinusoidal, and mixed. A diffuse infiltrate composed of small and occasionally intermediate lymphoid cells can be present in chronic lymphocytic leukemia (CLL; Figure 9.3), lymphoplasmacytic lymphoma (LPL), mantle cell lymphoma (MCL), marginal zone lymphoma (MZL), hairy cell leukemia (HCL, Figure 9.4), "lymphocytic" variant of plasma cell myeloma (PCM) composed of small to intermediate cells and in some T-cell lymphoproliferative disorders, including T-cell prolymphocytic leukemia (T-PLL), and T-cell large granular lymphocyte leukemia (T-LGLL). BM may be involved in acute variant of adult T-cell lymphoma/leukemia (ATLL): infiltrate is usually subtle (even in patients with prominent lymphocytosis), interstitial and patchy and may be accompanied by fibrosis. Rare cases of ATLL show mixed interstitial and focally paratrabecular infiltrate or diffuse BM involvement. Eosinophilia is often present. Differential diagnosis includes acute leukemias, especially lymphoblastic and reactive T-cell component in T-cell/histiocyte-rich large B-cell lymphoma (THRLBL), nodular lymphocyte predominant Hodgkin lymphoma (NLPHL), classic Hodgkin lymphoma (cHL), or some B-cell lymphomas after treatment (especially follicular lymphoma [FL]). In CLL diffuse infiltrate is seen mostly in advanced disease. Early stages of CLL show interstitial or nodular infiltrate composed mostly of small lymphocytes with admixture of prolymphocytes. Prolymphocytes form characteristic for CLL proliferation centers (well demarcated paler area on hematoxylin and eosin (H&E) section, composed of larger lymphocytes with

DOI: 10.1201/9781003197935-9

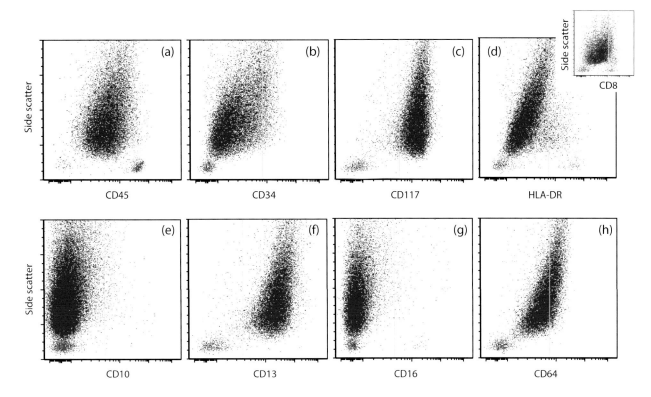

FIGURE 9.1 APL – flow cytometry of hypergranular variant. Neoplastic promyelocytes are characterized by high side scatter and moderate CD45 (a), negative CD34 (b), positive CD117 (c), negative HLA-DR (d; compare with negative staining for CD8, inset), negative CD10 (e), positive CD13 (f), negative CD16 (g), and dim CD64 (h).

more abundant cytoplasm). In HCL the infiltrate may be subtle, patchy, interstitial with residual hematopoiesis and increased reticulin fibrosis or diffuse replacing normal BM element. HCL cells have abundant clear cytoplasm with well demarcated borders, creating well known "fried-egg" appearance. Interstitial pattern in conjunction with intrasinusoidal infiltrate is seen in hairy cell leukemia variant (HCL-v) and some lymphomas (e.g., splenic marginal zone lymphoma, SMZL). Tables 9.1 and 9.2 summarize the most typical patterns of BM involvement in B- and T-cell lymphoproliferations.

Summary of FC phenotypic profiles in diffuse small cell infiltrate in BM:

CLL: $CD19^+$, $CD20^{+(often\ dim)}$, surface light chain immunoglobulins$^{+(dim)/rarely-}$, $CD5^+$, $CD23^{+/rarely-}$, $CD10^-$, $CD38^{+(dim\ or\ partial)/\ -}$, $CD43^+$, $CD71^-$, $CD81^{-/dim+}$, $CD200^+$, $CD11c^{+/-}$, $CD13^{-/rarely+}$, $CD2^{-/rarely+}$

MCL: $CD19^+$, $CD20^+$, surface light chain immunoglobulin$^+$, $CD5^+$, $CD10^{-/rarely+}$, $CD11c^-$, $CD23^-$, $CD38^+$, $CD43^+$, $CD71^{-/+(dim\ or\ partial)}$, $CD81^{+(strong)}$, $CD200^-$

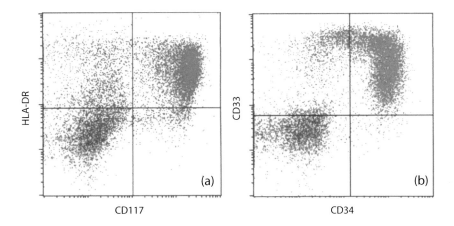

FIGURE 9.2 AML. Blasts (green dots) are positive for HLA-DR (a), CD117 (a), CD33 (b), and CD34 (b).

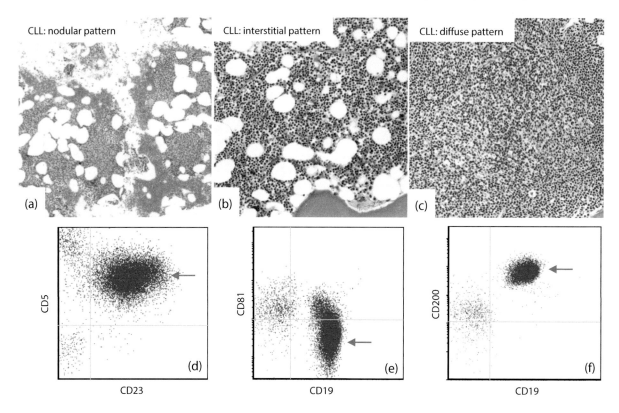

FIGURE 9.3 Chronic lymphocytic leukemia. Histomorphology (a–c) with three different patterns of involvement: nodular (a); interstitial (b); and diffuse lymphoid infiltrate with proliferation centers (c). Flow cytometry (d–f) shows typical immunophenotype of CLL (arrow) with co-expression of CD5 and CD23 (d), negative CD81 (e), and positive CD200 (f).

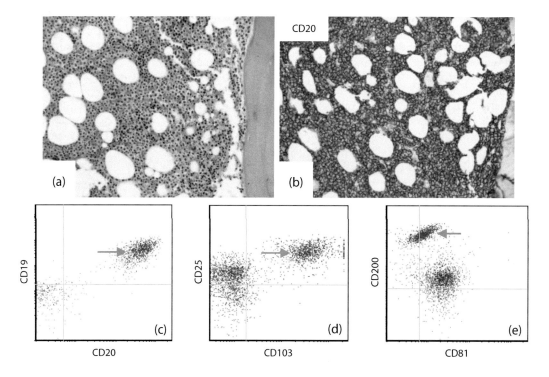

FIGURE 9.4 HCL with diffuse BM involvement. Histology (a) and immunohistochemical staining with CD20 (b) show total BM replacement by HCL. Flow cytometry (c–e) shows typical phenotypic profile of HCL (blue dots, arrow), bright expression of CD19 and CD20 (c), co-expression of CD25 and CD103 (d), bright CD200 (e), and negative to dim CD81 (e).

TABLE 9.1: Pattern of BM Involvement by Mature B-Cell Lymphoproliferative Neoplasms

	Pattern (Core Biopsy)	Phenotype (FC)
CLL	Interstitial, nodular, or diffuse	$\kappa^{+(dim)}$ or $\lambda^{+(dim)}$, CD20^{+dim}, CD5$^+$, CD10$^-$, CD11c$^{+/-}$, CD23$^{+/(-)}$, CD38$^{+/-}$, CD81$^{-/+dim}$, CD200$^+$
MCL	Interstitial, nodular and/or paratrabecular, rarely intrasinusoidal	κ^+ or λ^+, CD20$^+$, CD5$^+$, CD10$^-$, CD11c$^-$, CD23$^{-/(+)}$, CD38$^{+/(-)}$, CD81$^+$, CD200$^-$
LPL	Interstitial, diffuse, and/or paratrabecular	κ^+ or λ^+, CD20$^+$, CD5$^-$, CD10$^{-/(+)}$, CD11c$^-$, CD23$^-$, CD38$^{+/(-)}$, CD81$^{+dim/(-)}$, CD200$^-$
FL	Paratrabecular, nodular	κ^+ or λ^+, CD20$^+$, CD5$^-$, CD10$^{+/(-)}$, CD11c$^-$, CD23$^-$, CD38$^{+/(-)}$, CD81$^{-/+dim}$, CD200$^{-/+dim}$ with focal paratrabecular involvement, FC is often negative
SMZL	Intrasinusoidal, interstitial and/or nodular	κ^+ or λ^+, CD20$^+$, CD5$^{-/(+)}$, CD10$^-$, CD11c$^{+/-}$, CD23$^{-/(+)}$, CD38$^-$, CD81$^{-/+dim}$, CD200$^{-/(+dim)}$
HCL	Interstitial and/or diffuse, may be subtle or intrasinusoidal	κ^+ or λ^+, CD20$^+$, CD5$^-$, CD10$^{-/(+)}$, CD11c$^{+bright}$, CD23$^-$, CD25$^+$, CD81^{+dim}, CD103$^+$, CD200$^{+bright}$
DLBCL	Nodular, diffuse, rarely intrasinusoidal	κ^+ or λ^+, CD20$^+$, CD5$^{-/(+)}$, CD10$^{-/+}$, CD11c$^{-/(+)}$, CD23$^-$, CD38$^+$, CD81$^{+dim/-}$, CD200$^{-/(+)}$
THRLBL	Ill-defined nodular or diffuse	FC is usually negative
BL	Nodular or diffuse	κ^+ or λ^+, CD20$^+$, CD5$^{-/(+)}$, CD10$^{-/+}$, CD11c$^-$, CD23$^-$, CD38$^{-/+}$, CD81$^{+bright}$, CD200$^+$
IVLBCL	Intrasinusoidal or intravascular	FC is usually negative or show rare clonal B-cells

Abbreviations: +, positive; (+), rarely positive; −, negative; (−), rarely negative; κ, kappa; λ, lambda; FC, flow cytometry; CLL, chronic lymphocytic leukemia; MCL, mantle cell lymphoma; LPL, lymphoplasmacytic lymphoma; FL, follicular lymphoma; SMZL, splenic marginal zone lymphoma; HCL, hairy cell leukemia; DLBCL, diffuse large B-cell lymphoma; THRLBL, T-cell rich large B-cell lymphoma, BL, Burkitt lymphoma, IVLBCL, intravascular large B-cell lymphoma.

TABLE 9.2: Pattern of BM Involvement by Mature T-Cell Lymphoproliferative Disorders

	Pattern (Core Biopsy)	Comments
T-PLL	Interstitial and/or diffuse	Prolymphocytic cytology, often normal expression of all pan-T-cell antigens, present with prominent leukocytosis (lymphocytosis)
ATLL	Interstitial, focal (patchy) or diffuse (rarely paratrabecular), may be very subtle; often admixture of plasma cells and eosinophils	Medium to large cells with prominent ulcer irregularities, positive for HTLV1, co-expression of CD4 with CD25, and loss of CD7
T-LGL leukemia	Interstitial pattern, often subtle	Typical cytology on blood examination, co-expression of CD8 with CD57; Staining with CD57 in decalcified samples may be falsely negative. Patient may present with neutropenia and/or rheumatoid arthritis
AITL	Nodular, interstitial, paratrabecular, diffuse or mixed. Nodules are ill-defined and often progress into (focally) diffuse pattern. Infiltrate is very heterogeneous with lymphocytes, eosinophils, plasma cells, and histiocytes	Neoplastic T-cells are positive for CD4, pan-T-cell markers, and T follicular helper TFH) cell markers (PD1, CXCL13, BCL6, and/or CD10). The staining with CD10 in decalcified sample may be suboptimal
MF/SS	BM is negative or show subtle infiltrate, difficult to identify without immunostains	Many neoplastic cells have irregular and convoluted nuclear outlines; patients have history of skin lesion(s)
ALCL	Interstitial, nodular, focal, and/or rarely intrasinusoidal	Tumor cells are CD30$^+$ and may be ALK1$^+$
HSTL	Intrasinusoidal pattern, interstitial pattern, or both	Infiltrate may be accompanied by erythroid hyperplasia; tumor cells are positive for CD2, CD3, TIA1, granzyme B, and CD56; patients present with hepatosplenomegaly and/or spleen/liver tumors
PTCL, NOS	Focal, interstitial, nodular, diffuse, and/or rarely intrasinusoidal	History of nodal or extranodal PTCL, tumor cells positive for CD4 or CD8 and one or more pan-T-cell antigens
ENKTL	Random, interstitial, or diffuse and is often accompanied by macrophages and reticulin fibrosis	Tumor cells are positive for EBV/EBER, CD2, CD3, cytotoxic granule proteins (TIA1, granzyme B, perforin) and NK-cell markers (CD56, CD57). They lack CD5 expression

Abbreviations: T-PLL, T-cell prolymphocytic leukemia; ATLL, adult T-cell lymphoma/leukemia; T_LGL leukemia T-cell large granular lymphocytes leukemia; AITL, angioimmunoblastic T-cell lymphoma (currently termed nodal TFH cell lymphoma, angioimmunoblastic-type); MF/SS, mycosis fungoides/Sézary's syndrome; ALCL, anaplastic large cell lymphoma; HSTL, hepatosplenic T-cell lymphoma; PTCL, peripheral T-cell lymphoma, not otherwise specified; ENKTL, extranodal NK/T-cell lymphoma, nasal type.

FL: CD19$^{+(often\ dim)}$, CD20$^+$, surface light chain immunoglobulin$^+$, CD5$^-$, CD10$^+$, CD11c$^-$, CD23$^-$, CD38$^{+/rarely-}$, CD43$^-$, CD71$^{-/+(dim\ or\ partial)}$, CD81$^{+(dim)/-}$, CD200$^{-/+(dim)}$

MZL: CD19$^+$, CD20$^+$, surface light chain immunoglobulin$^+$, CD5$^{-/rare\ cases+}$, CD10$^-$, CD11c$^{+/-}$, CD23$^{-/+}$, CD38$^{+/-}$, CD43$^{-/+}$, CD81$^{+/-}$, CD200$^{-/rarely+}$

LPL: CD19$^+$, CD20$^+$, surface light chain immunoglobulin$^+$, CD5$^{-/rare\ cases+}$, CD10$^{-/rarely+}$, CD11c$^-$, CD13$^{-/rarely+}$, CD23$^{-/rarely+}$, CD25$^{+/rarely-}$, CD38$^{+/rarely-}$, CD43$^-$, CD71$^-$, CD81$^{+/-}$, CD200$^{(dim)/-}$

HCL: CD19$^+$, CD20$^+$, surface light chain immunoglobulin$^+$, CD5$^-$, CD10$^{-/rarely+}$, CD11c$^{+bright}$, CD23$^{-/rarely+}$, CD25$^+$, CD38$^-$, CD43$^{+(dim)/rarely-}$, CD71$^-$, CD81$^{+(dim)}$, CD103$^+$, CD123$^+$, CD200$^{+(bright)}$

T-PLL: CD2$^{+/-}$, CD3$^{+/-}$, CD4$^+$ (less often CD8$^+$, CD4/CD8$^+$ or CD4/CD8$^-$), CD5$^{+/-}$, CD7$^{+/-}$, CD25$^-$, CD26$^+$, CD45$^{+/rarely-}$, CD56$^-$, CD57$^-$, CD81$^+$, CD117$^{-/rarely+}$, CD200$^-$

HCL-v: CD19$^+$, CD20$^+$, surface light chain immunoglobulin$^+$, CD5$^-$, CD10$^{-/rarely+}$, CD11c$^{+bright/rarely-}$, CD23$^{-/rarely+}$, CD25$^-$, CD38$^-$, CD43$^{-/+dim}$, CD71$^-$, CD81$^{+(often\ strong)}$, CD103$^+$, CD123$^{-/rarely+}$, CD200$^{-/+(dim)}$

ATLL: CD2$^{+/-}$, CD3$^{+/-}$, CD4$^+$ (rarely CD4/CD8$^+$), CD5$^+$, CD7$^-$, CD8$^-$, CD25$^+$, CD26$^-$, CD45$^+$, CD56$^-$, CD57$^-$

T-LGLL: CD2$^{+/rarely-}$, CD3$^{+/rarely-}$, CD8$^+$ (rarely CD4$^+$, CD4/CD8$^-$, or CD4/CD8$^+$), CD5$^{+/-}$, CD7$^{-/+}$, CD25$^-$, CD26$^{-/rarely+}$, CD16$^{-/rarely+}$, CD45$^+$, CD56$^{-/+}$, CD57$^{+/rarely-}$, CD81$^+$, CD200$^-$, TCRαβ$^+$ (rarely TCRγδ$^+$)

THRLBL: predominance of small T-cells with normal phenotype

Diffuse intermediate/large cell infiltrate

Differential diagnosis of diffuse infiltrate of intermediate to large cells includes diffuse large B-cell lymphoma (DLBCL), anaplastic large cell lymphoma (ALCL; Figure 9.5), peripheral T-cell lymphoma (PTCL), B-ALL, T-ALL, PCM, AML, APL, acute monoblastic leukemia, acute erythroid leukemia (AEL), acute megakaryoblastic leukemia, Langerhans cell histiocytosis (LCH), BPDCN, and metastatic tumors. Two aggressive variants of MCL may show predominance of medium-sized blastoid cells (blastoid variant) and large pleomorphic cells (pleomorphic variant). Diffuse large or medium cell lymphoid infiltrate may represent Burkitt lymphoma (BL), DLCBL, high-grade B-cell lymphoma with *MYC* and *BCL2* rearrangement (HGBL-R), high grade B-cell lymphoma, not otherwise specified (HGBL, NOS), EBV$^+$ DLBCL, plasmablastic lymphoma (PBL), ALCL, PTCL, ATLL and occasional cases of cHL (see below). BL may present as leukemia with prominent blood and BM involvement (Figure 9.6). It is composed of medium cells with monomorphic appearance expressing CD20, BCL6, CD10, MYC, and Ki-67. Flow cytometry of BL shows clonal B-cells with increased (often variable) forward scatter, bright CD45, moderate expression of CD20 and surface light chain immunoglobulins, positive CD10, CD38, CD43, CD71, and CD81, and negative BCL2. FISH studies show rearrangement of *MYC* without concurrent *BCL2* or *BCL6* rearrangements. HGBL-R is defined by double (or triple) rearrangements involving *MYC* and *BCL2* (and/or *BCL6*), hence the name double-hit (DH) or triple-hit (TH) lymphoma. Morphologically and/or phenotypically HGBL-R may resemble BL or DLBCL. HGBL-R (DH or TH) often shows bright expression of CD10, CD38, and BCL2, dim CD20 and variably increased forward scatter. They may show flow cytometric features suggestive of immaturity, such as

negative or dim CD45 expression, lack or decreased (partial/dim) expression of CD20, lack of surface light chain immunoglobulins or rarely presence of TdT expression [8–10]. Among DH or TH lymphomas reported by Alsuwaidan et al., dim CD20 was noted in 32%, dim CD19 in 12%, bright CD38 in 56%, and lack of surface immunoglobulins in 23% [11]. Those cases need to be differentiated from transformed B-cell lymphomas (most often FLs). Based on cell of origin, major types of DLBCL includes germinal center B-cell like (GCB-like) and activated B-cell like (ABL-like) and based on cytomorphology DLBCL can be subdivided into centroblastic, immunoblastic or less common anaplastic. Some DLBCL may be accompanied by marked fibrosis mimicking primary myelofibrosis (PMF) or display cytologic features mimicking metastatic carcinoma. Presence of fibrosis, paratrabecular pattern of BM involvement or only focal marrow involvement may lead to false negative FC findings. In positive cases, DLBCL is characterized by high forward scatter, strong expression of CD20, often positive CD38 and surface light chain immunoglobulins, usually dim CD81 and usually negative CD200, and often positive CD71 (most cases show dim or partial CD71, but rare cases may be bright CD71$^+$). Subset of DLBCL cases may be positive for CD10 or less often CD5. CD5$^+$ DLBCL needs to be differentiated from Richter's syndrome. Comparison of the intensity of expression of CD39, CD43, CD81, and CD95 helps to differentiate between FL, DLBCL (GCB-like), DLBCL (ABC-like), and BL. Very strong expression of CD39 is typical for DLBCL, ABC-like, while DLBCL, GCB-like shows usually moderate CD39 and both FL and BL weak CD39 expression [12]. BL shows strong expression of CD43 while FL are often CD43$^-$ and DLBCL, GCB are weakly positive (CD43 is stronger in non-GCB DLBCL than in GCB DLBCL). CD81 expression is strong in BL, while is negative or week in FL or DLBCL and the expression of CD95 is negative o weak in BL and strong in DLBCL. Detection of DLBCL in BM by FC was reported to be associated with less favorable prognosis [13]. DLBCL needs to be differentiated from other large cell lymphomas, including CD20$^-$ plasmablastic lymphoma. DLBCL in BM without prior history of lymphoma (low grade or large cell type), without adenopathy or extranodal disease (including localized bone tumor) may represent rare case of primary BM large B-cell lymphoma [14, 15]. Scattered large neoplastic cells without forming sheets or aggregates can be seen in high grade myeloid neoplasms (e.g., MDS-IB), THRLBL, cHL, NLPHL, MZL with increased large cells, CLL with increased large cells and some T-cell lymphomas.

Summary of FC phenotypic profiles in diffuse intermediate to large cell infiltrate in BM:

DLBCL: CD19$^+$, CD20$^+$, surface light chain immunoglobulin$^+$, CD5$^{-/rarely+}$, CD10$^{+/-}$, CD11c$^{-/rarely+}$, CD23$^-$, CD25$^{-/rarely+}$, CD38$^+$, CD43$^{-/+}$, CD71$^{+(dim\ or\ rarely\ strong)}$, CD81$^{+(dim)}$, CD200$^{-/rarely\ +(dim)}$

HGBL-R: CD19$^+$, CD20$^{+(may\ be\ dim)}$, surface light chain immunoglobulin$^{+/rarely-}$, BCL2$^+$, CD5$^-$, CD10$^{+/rarely-}$, CD11c$^-$, CD23$^-$, CD25$^-$, CD38$^+$, CD43$^{+/-}$, CD71$^+$, CD81$^+$, CD200$^{-/+}$

MCL (pleomorphic variant): CD19$^+$, CD20$^+$, surface light chain immunoglobulin$^+$, sCD5$^+$, CD10$^{-/rarely+}$, CD11c$^-$, CD23$^-$, CD38$^+$, CD43$^+$, CD71$^{-/+(dim\ or\ partial)}$, CD81$^+$, CD200$^-$

BL: CD19$^+$, CD20$^+$, surface light chain immunoglobulin$^+$, BCL2$^-$, CD5$^-$, CD10$^+$, CD11c$^-$, CD23$^-$, CD25$^-$, CD38$^+$, CD43$^{+(strong)}$, CD71$^{+(strong)}$, CD81$^{+(strong)}$, CD200$^{-/rarely\ +(dim)}$

PTCL: CD2$^{+/-}$, CD3$^{+/-}$, CD4$^{+/-}$, CD5$^{+/-}$, CD7$^{-/+}$, CD8$^{-/+}$, CD10$^-$, CD30$^{-/rarely+}$, CD38$^+$, CD45$^+$, CD56$^{-/rarely+}$

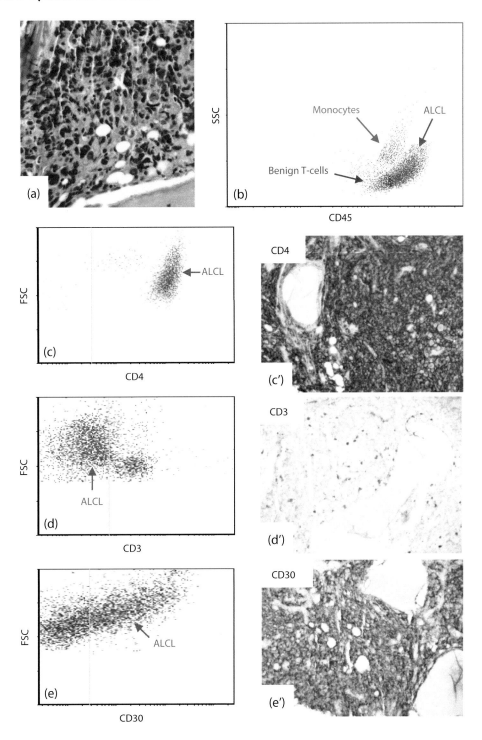

FIGURE 9.5 Anaplastic large cell lymphoma (ALCL) totally replacing BM. Histology section of BM core biopsy shows diffuse large cell lymphoid infiltrate (a). Flow cytometry (b–e) shows large cells with bright expression of CD45 (b, magenta dots), bright CD4 (c), negative CD3 (d), and positive CD30 (e). The forward scatter of ALCL cells is high (c–e). Immunohistochemical staining (c′–e′) confirmed flow cytometry findings with positive CD4 (c′), negative CD3 (d′), and positive CD30 (e′).

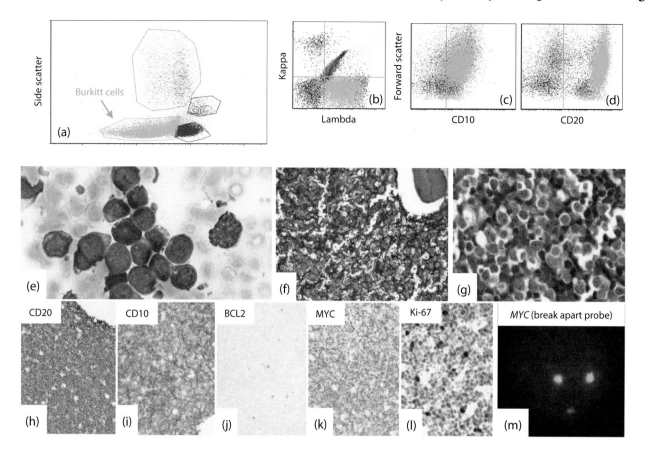

FIGURE 9.6 Burkitt leukemia (morphologic, immunophenotypic, and molecular analysis of blood and BM from 45-year-old patient). FC analysis showed 25% clonal B-cells in blood with low side scatter, dim to moderate expression of CD45 (a, green dots), monotypic lambda expression (b), positive CD10 (c), and bright CD20 (d). Aspirate smear (e) shows atypical cells with blastoid appearance. Histologic section from core biopsy (f–g, low and high power) shows diffuse infiltrate by monotonous medium-sized lymphoid cells. Immunohistochemistry analysis (h–l) shows positive CD20 (h) and CD10 (i), negative BCL2 (j), strong expression of MYC (>90%, k), and high Ki-67 index (l). FISH analysis (m) shows one green, one orange, and one yellow/green/orange fusion signal indicative of a chromosomal break in the *MYC* locus.

ALCL: high forward scatter, CD2$^{+/rarely-}$, CD3$^{+/-}$, CD4$^+$ or less often CD8$^+$ (rare tumors are either CD4/8$^-$ or CD4/CD8$^+$), CD5$^{+/-}$, CD7$^{-/rarely+}$, CD10$^-$, CD25$^{+/-}$, CD26$^{+/rarely-}$, CD30$^+$, CD43$^+$, CD45$^+$, CD56$^{-/rarely+}$

B-ALL: CD10$^{+(bright)/rarely-}$, CD13$^{-/rarely+}$, CD19$^+$, CD20$^{-/rarely+}$, CD22$^+$, CD33$^{-/rarely+}$, CD34$^{+/rarely-}$, CD38$^{+(bright)}$, CD45$^{-/+dim}$, CD56$^-$, CD71$^{-/+dim}$, CD79a$^+$, CD81^{+dim}, CD123$^{+/-}$, CD200$^{+/-}$, HLA-DR$^+$, MPO$^-$, TdT$^{+/rarely-}$

T-ALL: CD1a$^{-/+}$, CD2$^+$, surface CD3$^{-/rare cases+}$, cytoplasmic CD3$^+$, CD4$^-$/CD8$^-$ or CD4$^+$/CD8$^+$, CD5$^{+/-}$, CD7$^+$, CD10$^{-/+}$, CD13$^{-/rarely+}$, CD15$^{-/rarely+}$, CD33$^{-/rarely+}$, CD34$^{+/-}$, CD38$^+$, CD56$^{-/rare cases+}$, CD71$^{-/+}$, CD79a$^{-/rarely+}$, CD117$^-$, CD123$^-$, HLA-DR$^-$, MPO$^-$, TdT$^{+/rarely-}$

AML: CD13$^+$, CD33$^+$, CD34$^{+/rarely-}$, CD117$^+$, CD133$^{+/-}$, MPO$^+$, CD81$^{+/-}$, HLA-DR$^{+/rarely-}$

BPDCN: CD4$^+$, CD13$^-$, CD33$^{-/+}$, CD56$^{+(strong)}$, CD123$^{+(strong)}$, CD11b$^-$, CD11c$^-$, HLA-DR$^+$, CD45$^+$, TdT$^{-/+}$, MPO$^-$, CD64$^-$

APL: CD34$^-$, CD117$^+$, CD13$^+$, CD33$^{+bright}$, CD11c$^-$, HLA-DR$^-$, MPO$^+$, CD45$^+$, TdT$^-$, CD56$^{-/+}$, CD64$^{+(dim)/-}$, CD7$^-$

Acute monoblastic leukemia: CD34$^{-(rarely+)}$, CD117$^{-/+}$, CD13$^+$, CD33^{++}, MPO$^-$, HLA-DR$^+$, CD45^{++}, CD14$^{+/-}$, CD64^{++}, CD11b$^{+/-}$, CD11c$^+$, CD4$^+$, CD56$^{+/-}$, CD71$^{+/-}$; CD123$^{+/-}$

AEL: CD34$^-$, CD117$^{-/+}$, CD13/CD33$^-$, CD36$^+$, HLA-DR$^-$, MPO$^-$, CD45$^{-/dim+}$, TdT$^-$, CD71$^{bright+}$, CD81$^+$, GPHA$^{+/-}$

PCM: surface light chain immunoglobulins$^-$, cytoplasmic light chain immunoglobulins$^+$, cytoplasmic heavy chain immunoglobulins$^{+/-}$, CD38$^{+(bright)}$, CD138$^{+(bright)}$, CD56$^{+/rarely-}$, CD117$^{+/-}$, CD45$^{-/rarely+}$, CD20$^{-/rarely+}$, CD19$^-$, CD200$^{+/-}$

Metastatic carcinoma: CD45$^-$, CD56$^{+/-}$, CD117$^{-/+}$, CD38$^{-/+}$, keratin$^+$

Rhabdomyosarcomas: CD45$^-$, CD56$^+$, CD90$^+$, CD117$^{+/-}$, myogenin$^+$

Neuroblastoma: CD45$^-$, CD56$^+$, CD2$^+$, CD81$^+$

Primitive neuroectodermal tumors/Ewing sarcoma: CD45$^-$, CD271$^+$, CD99$^+$

Wilms' tumor: CD45$^-$, CD56$^+$

Germ cell tumors: CD45$^-$, CD56$^+$, CD10$^+$

Metastatic melanoma: CD45$^-$, CD56$^{+/-}$, CD10$^{-/+}$, CD57$^{+/-}$, CD117$^{-/+}$

Discrepancy between the size of lymphocytes in primary lymphoma and BM involvement

Occasional lymphomas may display differences in the phenotype and cytomorphologic features between primary site and BM. Comprehensive evaluation with immunophenotyping, cytogenetic/FISH and molecular studies for clonality may be necessary to exclude secondary tumors in those cases. DLBCL shows two variants of BM involvement: (1) involvement by large cells, which correspond to the size of the primary tumor, and (2) involvement by mostly small lymphocytes (as seen in low grade lymphomas) [16–18]. The former pattern is associated with poorer prognosis, whereas the discordant histologic pattern is associated with more frequent relapses, but similar 5-year survival to patient with DLBCL without BM involvement [16, 17].

Diffuse blastoid ("high-grade") infiltrate

Diffuse blastoid (or high-grade) infiltrate of BM may be seen blastoid variant of MCL, blastic transformation of low-grade lymphomas, BL, HGBL-R, ALCL, poorly differentiated PCM, variants of DLBCL (e.g., immunoblastic DLBCL or ALK$^+$ large B-cell lymphoma), T-PLL, PBL, and some metastatic tumors.

Summary of FC phenotypic profiles in blastoid ("high-grade") infiltrate in BM:

HGBL-R: CD19$^+$, CD20$^{+ \text{ (may be dim)}}$, surface light chain immunoglobulin$^{+/\text{rarely}-}$, BCL2$^+$, CD5$^-$, CD10$^{+/\text{rarely}-}$, CD11c$^-$, CD23$^-$, CD25$^-$, CD38$^+$, CD43$^{+/-}$, CD71$^+$, CD81$^+$, CD200$^{-/+}$

MCL (blastoid variant): CD19$^+$, CD20$^+$, surface light chain immunoglobulin$^+$, sCD5$^+$, CD10$^{-/\text{rarely}+}$, CD11c$^-$, CD23$^-$, CD38$^+$, CD43$^+$, CD71$^{-/+(\text{dim or partial})}$, CD81$^+$, CD200$^-$

BL: CD19$^+$, CD20$^+$, surface light chain immunoglobulin$^+$, BCL2$^-$, CD5$^-$, CD10$^+$, CD11c$^-$, CD23$^-$, CD25$^-$, CD38$^+$, CD43$^{+(\text{strong})}$, CD71$^{+(\text{strong})}$, CD81$^{+(\text{strong})}$, CD200$^{-/\text{rarely }+(\text{dim})}$

T-PLL: CD2$^{+/-}$, CD3$^{+/-}$, CD4$^+$ (less often CD8$^+$, CD4/CD8$^+$ or CD4/CD8$^-$), CD5$^{+/-}$, CD7$^{+/-}$, CD25$^-$, CD26$^+$, CD45$^{+/\text{rarely}-}$, CD56$^-$, CD57$^-$, CD81$^+$, CD117$^{-/\text{rarely}+}$, CD200$^-$

ALCL: high forward scatter, CD2$^{+/\text{rarely}-}$, CD3$^{+/-}$, CD4$^+$ or less often CD8$^+$ (rare tumors are either CD4/8$^-$ or CD4/CD8$^+$), CD5$^{+/-}$, CD7$^{-/\text{rarely}+}$, CD10$^-$, CD25$^{+/-}$, CD26$^{+/\text{rarely}-}$, CD30$^+$, CD43$^+$, CD45$^+$, CD56$^{-/\text{rarely}+}$

PCM (plasmablastic): surface light chain immunoglobulins$^-$, cytoplasmic light chain immunoglobulins$^+$, cytoplasmic heavy chain immunoglobulins$^{+/-}$, CD38$^{+(\text{bright})}$, CD138$^{+(\text{bright})}$, CD56$^{+/\text{rarely}-}$, CD117$^{+/-}$, CD45$^{-/\text{rarely}+}$, CD20$^{-/\text{rarely}+}$, CD19$^-$, CD200$^{+/-}$

Rhabdomyosarcomas: CD45$^-$, CD56$^+$, CD90$^+$, CD117$^{+/-}$, myogenin$^+$

Neuroblastoma: CD45$^-$, CD56$^+$, CD2$^+$, CD81$^+$

Primitive neuroectodermal tumors/Ewing sarcoma: CD45$^-$, CD271$^+$, CD99$^+$

Increased number of scattered large cells (other than megakaryocytes)

Scattered, highly atypical large cells can be seen in THRLBL, PTCL, cHL, NLPHL, cHL, and occasional cases of PCM with "anaplastic" features with large multinucleated and hyperchromatic cells mimicking atypical megakaryocytes. Flow cytometry analysis if often falsely negative in those neoplasm. Involvement of BM by NLPHL (advanced stage disease) is very rare, especially at presentation, and when present, raises the possibility of NLPHL progressing to large B-cell lymphoma or represents THRLBL, especially if T-cells do not express CD57 and there is minimal number of small B-cells in background of large, atypical cells. Patients with CLL may undergo large cell transformation into either DLBCL or cHL (Richter's transformation). BM biopsy may show in these cases scattered large cells with the phenotype of either DLBCL or cHL. In some cases, especially in patients treated with alemtuzumab large cells may be EBV/EBER$^+$.

Paratrabecular lymphoid infiltrate

Paratrabecular lymphoid aggregates most often indicate neoplastic process. Paratrabecular pattern is most typical for FL but may be also seen in other B-cell lymphomas, including LPL and MCL, and less often in DLBCL, PTCL, angioimmunoblastic T-cell lymphoma (AITL), ALCL, and rare cases of CLL. MZLs usually do not display paratrabecular pattern of BM involvement. If paratrabecular involvement of the BM is focal, flow cytometry is usually negative, but cases with prominent paratrabecular involvement are often positive as shown in the case of MCL in Figure 9.7.

Summary of FC phenotypic profiles in paratrabecular lymphoid infiltrate in BM:

FL: CD19$^{+(\text{often dim})}$, CD20$^+$, surface light chain immunoglobulin$^+$, CD5$^-$, CD10$^+$, CD11c$^-$, CD23$^-$, CD38$^{+/\text{rarely}-}$, CD43$^-$, CD71$^{-/+(\text{dim or partial})}$, CD81$^{+(\text{dim})/-}$, CD200$^{-/+(\text{dim})}$

LPL: CD19$^+$, CD20$^+$, surface light chain immunoglobulin$^+$, CD5$^{-/\text{rare cases}+}$, CD10$^{-/\text{rarely}+}$, CD11c$^-$, CD23$^{-/\text{rarely}+}$, CD25$^{+/\text{rarely}-}$, CD38$^{+/\text{rarely}-}$, CD43$^-$, CD71$^-$, CD81$^{+/-}$, CD200$^{+(\text{dim})/-}$

DLBCL: CD19$^+$, CD20$^+$, surface light chain immunoglobulin$^+$, CD5$^{-/\text{rarely}+}$, CD10$^{+/-}$, CD11c$^{-/\text{rarely}+}$, CD23$^-$, CD25$^{-/\text{rarely}+}$, CD38$^+$, CD43$^{-/+}$, CD71$^{+(\text{dim or rarely strong})}$, CD81$^{+(\text{dim})}$, CD200$^{-/\text{rarely }+(\text{dim})}$

MCL: CD19$^+$, CD20$^+$, surface light chain immunoglobulin$^+$, sCD5$^+$, CD10$^{-/\text{rarely}+}$, CD11c$^-$, CD23$^-$, CD38$^+$, CD43$^+$, CD71$^{-/+(\text{dim or partial})}$, CD81$^+$, CD200$^-$

PTCL: CD2$^{+/-}$, CD3$^{+/-}$, CD4$^{+/-}$, CD5$^{+/-}$, CD7$^{-/+}$, CD8$^{-/+}$, CD10$^-$, CD30$^{-/\text{rarely}+}$, CD38$^+$, CD45$^+$, CD56$^{-/\text{rarely}+}$

AITL: CD2$^{+/-}$, CD3$^{+/-}$, CD4$^+$, CD5$^{+/-}$, CD7$^{+/-}$, CD8$^-$, CD10$^{+/\text{rarely}-}$, CD30$^-$, CD45$^+$, CD56$^-$, CD81$^+$, CD200$^+$

CLL: CD19$^+$, CD20$^{+(\text{often dim})}$, surface light chain immunoglobulins$^{+(\text{dim})}$, CD5$^+$, CD23$^{+/\text{rarely}-}$, CD10$^-$, CD38$^{+(\text{dim or partial})/-}$, CD43$^+$, CD71$^-$, CD81$^{-/\text{dim}}$, CD200$^+$, CD11c$^{+/-}$,

Intrasinusoidal infiltrate

Intrasinusoidal infiltration is rarely found in the BM involved by lymphoma and is considered as a hallmark of SMZL. Apart from SMZL, an intrasinusoidal infiltrate (Figure 9.8) may be seen in T-cell lymphomas, e.g., hepatosplenic T-cell lymphoma (HSTL), ALCL, enteropathy associated T-cell lymphoma (EATL), and some B-cell lymphomas mainly, HCL variant (HCL-v), splenic diffuse red pulp small B-cell lymphoma (SDRPBL), MCL (rare), DLBCL, or intravascular large B-cell lymphoma (IVLBL). Whenever present, intrasinusoidal BM pattern by lymphoma should raise the possibility of splenic involvement [19]. Large cell lymphomas with intrasinusoidal distribution should also be differentiated for occasional cases of AEL (pure erythroid leukemia) and metastatic tumors, which may also display intrasinusoidal BM involvement.

Summary of FC phenotypic profiles in intrasinusoidal infiltrate in BM:

HSTL: CD2$^+$, CD3$^+$, CD4$^-$/CD8$^-$ (rare cases are CD4$^-$/CD8$^+$), CD5$^-$, CD7$^+$, CD16$^{-/\text{rarely}+}$, CD56$^+$, CD57$^-$, TCRγδ$^+$

HCL-v: CD19$^+$, CD20$^+$, surface light chain immunoglobulin$^+$, CD5$^-$, CD10$^{-/\text{rarely}+}$, CD11c$^{+\text{bright}/\text{rarely}-}$, CD23$^{-/\text{rarely}+}$, CD25$^-$, CD38$^-$, CD43$^{-/\text{dim}}$, CD71$^-$, CD81$^{+(\text{often strong})}$, CD103$^+$, CD123$^{-/\text{rarely}+}$, CD200$^{-/+(\text{dim})}$

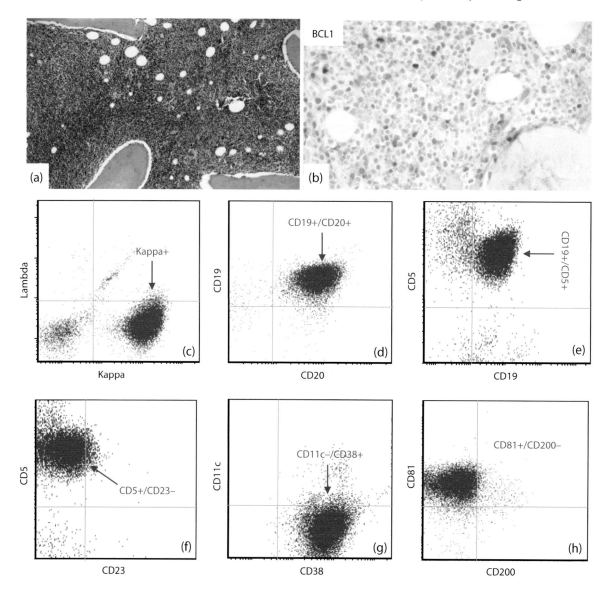

FIGURE 9.7 Mantle cell lymphoma (MCL) with paratrabecular BM involvement. Histology (a) shows atypical lymphoid infiltrate of mostly small lymphocytes with paratrabecular pattern. Lymphomatous cells are positive for BCL1 (cyclin D1; b). Flow cytometry (c–h) clonal B-cells with kappa restriction (c) and typical phenotypic features: moderate expression of both CD19 and CD20 (d), positive CD5 (e), negative CD23 (f), negative CD11c (g), positive CD38 (g), positive CD81 (h), and lack of CD200 (h).

SMZL: CD19$^+$, CD20$^+$, surface light chain immunoglobulin$^+$, CD5$^{-/\text{rare cases}+}$, CD10$^-$, CD11c$^{+/-}$, CD23$^{-/+}$, CD38$^{+/-}$, CD43$^{-/+}$, CD81$^{+/-}$, CD200$^{-/+}$

MCL: CD19$^+$, CD20$^+$, surface light chain immunoglobulin$^+$, sCD5$^+$, CD10$^{-/\text{rarely}+}$, CD11c$^-$, CD23$^-$, CD38$^+$, CD43$^+$, CD71$^{-/+(\text{dim or partial})}$, CD81$^+$, CD200$^-$

SDRPL: surface light chain immunoglobulin$^+$, CD5$^{-/\text{rarely}+}$, CD10$^-$, CD11c$^{-/+}$, CD19$^+$, CD20$^+$, CD22$^+$, CD23$^{-/\text{rarely}+}$, CD25$^-$, CD38$^-$, CD43$^{+(\text{dim})/-}$, CD45$^+$, CD79b$^{+(\text{moderate})}$, CD81$^{+/-}$, CD103$^{-/\text{rarely}+}$, CD123$^{-/\text{rarely}+}$, and CD200$^+$

AEL: CD34$^-$, CD117$^{-/+}$, CD13/CD33$^-$, CD36$^+$, HLA-DR$^-$, MPO$^-$, CD45$^{-/\text{dim}+}$, TdT$^-$, CD71$^{\text{bright}+}$, CD81$^+$, GPHA$^{+/-}$

Metastatic carcinoma: CD45$^-$, CD56$^{+/-}$, CD117$^{-/+}$, CD38$^{-/+}$, keratin$^+$

Lymphoid aggregates (nodular lymphoid infiltrate)

Reactive lymphoid aggregates are common findings, especially in patients with chronic immune stimulation, autoimmune disorders, infections and chronic MPNs, and their likelihood and number(s) increase with age. The differential diagnosis between reactive lymphoid aggregates and lymphoma (especially low grade) is often difficult, if not impossible, since many cytologic, histologic and immunophenotypic features overlap (especially between MZL and reactive lymphoid aggregates). Paratrabecular location, presence of prominent cytologic atypia or aberrant phenotype of lymphoid cells indicate lymphoma. On the other hand, small lymphoid aggregates composed of mixed population of small to intermediate lymphocytes, containing small blood vessels and rare histiocytes, located centrally between bone

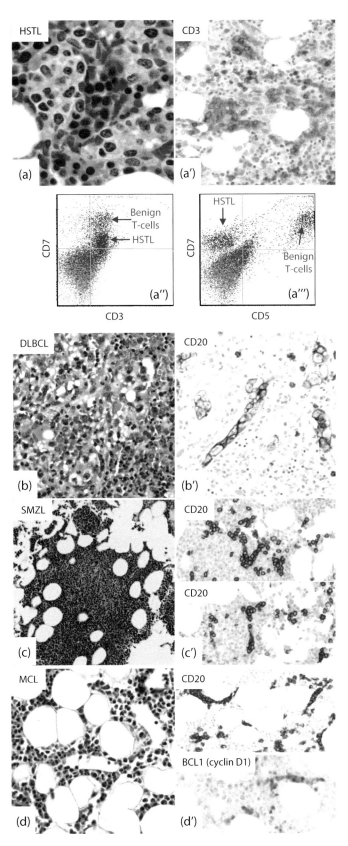

FIGURE 9.8 Bone marrow – intrasinusoidal infiltrate. (a) Hepatosplenic T-cell lymphoma (HSTL). Histology (a) shows clusters of large cells, which are CD3+ (a′) with intrasinusoidal distribution. Flow cytometry (a″–a‴) shows atypical T-cells (CD3+) with dim CD7 expression (a″) and negative CD5 (a‴). (b) DLBCL (b, histology; b′, CD20 immunostaining). (c) Splenic marginal zone lymphoma (SMZL). H&E section (c) shows mostly nodular infiltrate, and CD20 immunostaining (c′) shows intrasinusoidal lymphoma cells. (d) Mantle cell lymphoma (MCL) with prominent intrasinusoidal pattern (d, histology, d′, CD20 staining, and d″, BCL1 staining).

trabeculae suggest benign nature of the aggregates. The benign aggregates are usually well demarcated with intact follicular dendritic meshwork and without over reticulin fibrosis. They often show predominant population of small T-cells (CD4⁺>CD8⁺). Aggregates with germinal centers surrounded by a mantle zone show features similar to reactive follicles in the lymph node. The immunohistochemistry shows mixed B- and T-lymphocytes and CD10⁺/BCL2⁻/BCL6⁺ germinal center cells. B-cells in the mantle zone often express IgM and IgD. The presence of small T-cells per se, does not favor reactive aggregate over neoplastic process, since many lymphomas (especially FL or THRLBL) may have prominent admixture of benign small T-cells. In difficult cases, correlation with flow cytometry and/or molecular testing may be helpful in establishing definite diagnosis. Immunohistochemistry staining for kappa and lambda may be also helpful by showing monoclonal B-cells and/or plasma cells. The nodular lymphoid infiltrate in the BM can be seen in CLL, DLBCL, MZL, FL, MCL, PTCL, and rare cases of cHL, and ALCL. Nodular lymphoid infiltrate composed mostly of small mature lymphocytes with clusters of medium-sized cells with nucleoli (prolymphocytes) forming proliferation centers is typical for CLL and is not seen in other lymphomas. MZL, both nodal and extranodal may involve BM and usually shows nodular pattern (SMZL often displays intrasinusoidal component as well). MZL may show increased number of large cells, prompting the differential diagnosis of histologic transformation (HT) into DLBCL (see Chapter 11).

Summary of FC phenotypic profiles in nodular lymphoid infiltrate in BM:

CLL: CD19⁺, CD20⁺(often dim), surface light chain immunoglobulins⁺(dim), CD5⁺, CD23⁺/rarely⁻, CD10⁻, CD38⁺(dim or partial)/⁻, CD43⁺, CD71⁻, CD81⁻/dim, CD200⁺, CD11c⁺/⁻,

MCL: CD19⁺, CD20⁺, surface light chain immunoglobulin⁺, sCD5⁺, CD10⁻/rarely⁺, CD11c⁻, CD23⁻, CD38⁺, CD43⁺, CD71⁻/⁺(dim or partial), CD81⁺, CD200⁻

FL: CD19⁺(often dim), CD20⁺, surface light chain immunoglobulin⁺, CD5⁻, CD10⁺, CD11c⁻, CD23⁻, CD38⁺/rarely⁻, CD43⁻, CD71⁻/⁺(dim or partial), CD81⁺(dim)/⁻, CD200⁻/⁺(dim)

MZL: CD19⁺, CD20⁺, surface light chain immunoglobulin⁺, CD5⁻/rare cases⁺, CD10⁻, CD11c⁺/⁻, CD23⁻/⁺, CD38⁺/⁻, CD43⁻/⁺, CD81⁺/⁻, CD200⁻/rarely⁺

DLBCL: CD19⁺, CD20⁺, surface light chain immunoglobulin⁺, CD5⁻/rarely⁺, CD10⁺/⁻, CD11c⁻/rarely⁺, CD23⁻, CD25⁻/rarely⁺, CD38⁺, CD43⁻/⁺, CD71⁺(dim or rarely strong), CD81⁺(dim), CD200⁻/rarely ⁺(dim)

PTCL: CD2⁺/⁻, CD3⁺/⁻, CD4⁺/⁻, CD5⁺/⁻, CD7⁻/⁺, CD8⁻/⁺, CD10⁻, CD30⁻/rarely⁺, CD38⁺, CD45⁺, CD56⁻/rarely⁺

ALCL: high forward scatter, CD2⁺/rarely⁻, CD3⁺/⁻, CD4⁺ or less often CD8⁺ (rare tumors are either CD4/8⁻ or CD4/CD8⁺), CD5⁺/⁻, CD7⁻/rarely⁺, CD10⁻, CD25⁺/⁻, CD26⁺/rarely⁻, CD30⁺, CD43⁺, CD45⁺, CD56⁻/rarely⁺

Classic HL: predominance of small T-cells with normal phenotype

Pleomorphic lymphoid infiltrate

Pleomorphic lymphoid infiltrate with small lymphocytes mixed with larger lymphoid cells, scattered atypical large cells, histiocytes, eosinophils, with or without focal fibrosis is seen in classic HL (cHL), PTCL, AITL, and THRLBL. cHL shows pleomorphic

infiltrate with small lymphocytes, histiocytes, plasma cells, eosinophils, and rare, large, atypical cells (Hodgkin cells, Reed-Sternberg cells, and their variants), which is accompanied by fibrosis and pleomorphic inflammatory infiltrate with eosinophils, plasma cells, and histiocytes. Clusters of epithelioid cell granulomas may be present as well. cHL involving the BM needs to be differentiated from AITL, THRLBL, NLPHL, and PTCL. PTCL frequently involve BM, mostly with nodular or mixed patterns, and pleomorphic cellular composition with mixture of reactive and neoplastic cells. BM involvement by NLPHL is rare and usually is associated with advanced. BM involvement may be also seen after many relapses and most likely represents the disease progression into large B-cell lymphoma (THRLBL). BM involvement by lymphoma most often represent a systemic disease (secondary involvement by lymphoma arising elsewhere), but some lymphomas may arise primary in the BM or bone [14, 20–22]. Primary BM lymphoma is diagnosed only when there is no evidence of nodal or extranodal lymphoma and there is no mass in the bone. The primary BM lymphomas show heterogeneous histology (e.g., FL, DLBCL) and unfavorable outcome [14].

Summary of FC phenotypic profiles of pleomorphic lymphoid infiltrate in BM:

AITL: CD2⁺/⁻, CD3⁺/⁻, CD4⁺, CD5⁺/⁻, CD7⁺/⁻, CD8⁻, CD10⁺/rarely⁻, CD30⁻, CD45⁺, CD56⁻, CD81⁺, CD200⁺

PTCL: CD2⁺/⁻, CD3⁺/⁻, CD4⁺/⁻, CD5⁺/⁻, CD7⁻/⁺, CD8⁻/⁺, CD10⁻, CD30⁻/rarely⁺, CD38⁺, CD45⁺, CD56⁻/rarely⁺

THRLBL: predominance of small T-cells with normal phenotype

Classic HL: predominance of small T-cells with normal phenotype

Megakaryocytosis

The evaluation of megakaryocytes is an important part of comprehensive marrow analysis since the number of megakaryocytes and their cytomorphologic features often offer clues for the correct diagnosis in both benign and malignant conditions. Megakaryocytic hyperplasia without overt cytologic atypia is often seen in peripheral platelets destruction or sequestration. Reactive megakaryocytosis may be also seen in marrow involved by lymphoma. Among malignancies, prominent megakaryocytosis with cytologic atypia and often atypical megakaryocytic clustering is typical for MPNs, MDS, mixed MDS/MPN, AML with myelodysplasia-related changes and acute megakaryoblastic leukemia. Flow cytometry findings in MDS and MPN are described in Chapters 19 and 21.

Eosinophilia

The upper normal limit for the number of eosinophils in blood is $0.35–0.5 \times 10^9$/L. Hypereosinophilia is defined as peripheral blood eosinophil counts $>1.5 \times 10^9$/L ($>1{,}500$/μL). Increased eosinophils in the BM are often seen in both reactive and neoplastic processes. Differential diagnosis includes reactive eosinophilia in parasitic infections (strongyloidiasis, hookworm infection, filariasis, scabies, isosporiasis), bacterial infections (chronic tuberculosis, resolving scarlet fever), HIV, allergic disorders (asthma, atopic dermatitis), drug hypersensitivity, Loeffler's syndrome, skin diseases (such as angiolymphoid hyperplasia), granulomatous disorders (sarcoidosis), neoplasms (leukemia, lymphoma, adenocarcinoma), abnormal T-cells with aberrant phenotype (may or may not be clonal), vasculitis, collagen vascular disorders, inflammatory bowel disease, hypoadrenalism, IL-2 therapy, radiation exposure, cholesterol embolization, and Kimura's disease.

Chronic eosinophilic leukemia (CEL) is a MPN characterized by clonal proliferation of eosinophil precursors leading to persistent eosinophilia in blood, BM and peripheral tissues [1, 23–29]. Flow cytometric features of eosinophils in are shown in Figure 8.6 in Chapter 8. CEL, not otherwise specified (CEL, NOS) excludes patients with a Philadelphia chromosome (*BCR-ABL* fusion) or rearrangement of *PDGFRA*, *PDGFRB*, or *FGFR1*. Eosinophil count is >1.5 × 10⁹/L in the blood and blasts are <20% (blood or BM). Diagnosis of CEL requires an evidence for clonality of eosinophils and abnormal BM morphology (presence of dysplasia in one or more lineages). Those include peripheral T-cell disorders, cHL, systemic mastocytosis (SM), B-ALL [especially with t(5;14)], and classic MPNs (CML, PV, ET, PMF) [1, 24–26, 28–31]. Among T-cell neoplasm, the most associated with eosinophilia are CD4⁺ adult T-cell leukemia/lymphoma (ATLL), Sézary's syndrome (SS),

and AITL. In contrast to SS, eosinophilia is uncommon in T-PLL. Marked eosinophilia may be associated with B-ALL, leading to severe cardiac complications [32–34]. The eosinophilia in these patients can present before, concomitantly, or after the diagnosis of leukemia [32].

Cases with no evidence of clonality or increased blasts are classified as "idiopathic hypereosinophilic syndrome" (HES). HES is defined by eosinophilia (>1.5 × 10⁹/L) persisting for at least 6 months resulting in tissue damage, without underlying reactive etiology and malignancy associated with eosinophilia. Cases fulfilling the criteria for HES but without tissue damage are classified as idiopathic hypereosinophilia. Eosinophilia associated with rearrangement of *PDGFRA*, *PDGFRB*, or *FGFR1* is excluded from CEL and hypereosinophilic syndrome (HES) and constitutes separate myeloid neoplasms [1, 24, 30, 35]. Rearrangement of *PDGFRA* may lead to eosinophilia with either T-ALL, B-ALL, or myeloid leukemia [36]. Figure 9.9 shows an unusual case of metastatic carcinoma and concurrent MPN with eosinophilia and *PDGFRB/t(5;12)*.

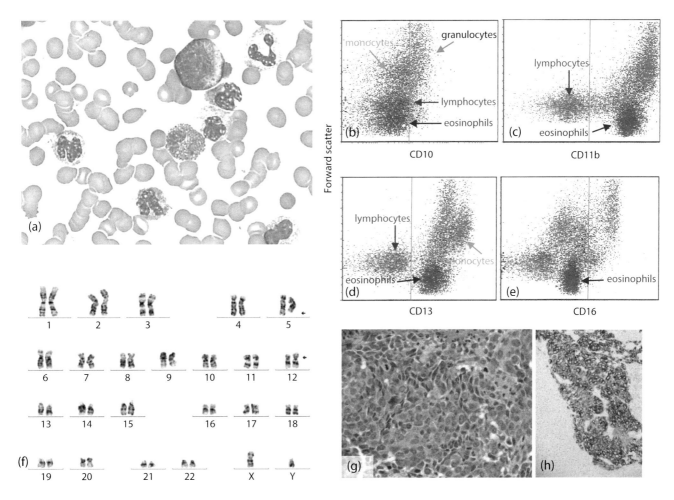

FIGURE 9.9 Unusual case of metastatic carcinoma to the bone marrow and myeloproliferative neoplasm with eosinophilia and *PDGFRB/t(5;12)*. CBC data revealed prominent leukocytosis. Blood smear (a) showed neutrophilia with eosinophilia. Flow cytometry analysis showed increased eosinophils (b–e; purple dots) with very low forward scatter (b–e), negative CD10 (b), positive CD11b (c) and CD13 (d), and negative CD16 (e). Both FISH and PCR tests were negative for *BCR-ABL1* rearrangement. Comprehensive bone marrow analysis showed t(5;12) by metaphase cytogenetics (f; small arrows) and core biopsy showed metastatic carcinoma (g; H&E section; objective ×400), confirmed by immunostaining with cytokeratin (h).

Erythroid hyperplasia with dyserythropoiesis

BM with erythroid hyperplasia is seen typically in patients with anemia (most pronounced in pernicious anemia). Erythroid hyperplasia can be seen in hemorrhagic and hemolytic states, thalassemia, secondary polycythemia, and after treatment with erythropoietin. Erythroid hyperplasia with cytomorphologic features of dyserythropoiesis is often seen in MDS, AML-MRD, and AEL (pure erythroid leukemia) [37–39].

The distinction between myeloid neoplasms with erythroid predominance, such as MDS with erythroid hyperplasia, AML-MRC, therapy-related myeloid neoplasm, and AEL can be difficult. Blasts <20% of all nucleated cells would favor MDS. Presence of ≥20% blasts and multilineage dysplasia in at least 50% of cells in two or more lineages indicates AML-MRC. The AML-MRC is also diagnosed when there is a prior history of MDS, or cytogenetic studies show typical MDS-related abnormalities. In patients with therapy-related myeloid neoplasm, regardless of the presence or absence of erythroid predominance (≥50% erythroid precursors) the prognosis is much worse than in AML with increased erythroid precursors (AEL or AML-MRC) [40]. Diagnostic considerations should include also prior erythropoietin therapy, which leads to erythroid hyperplasia with dyserythropoiesis. PV which most often shows panmyelosis, may be associated with decreased M:E ratio due to prominent erythropoiesis. Certain medications and congenital neutropenia lead to decreased M:E ratio due to reduced granulopoiesis. Figure 9.10 shows BM with bi-lineage

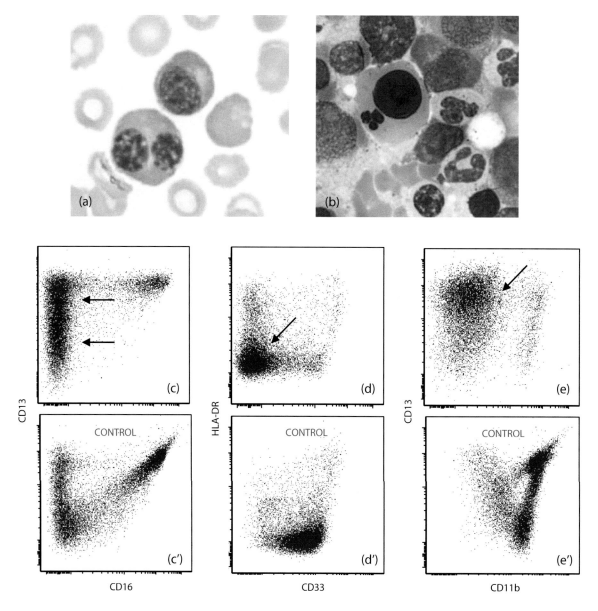

FIGURE 9.10 MDS. Dysgranulopoiesis in the form of Pelgeroid changes (a) and dyserythropoiesis with megaloblastoid changes and minute nuclear fragments in the cytoplasm (b). FC analysis shows decreased expression of CD16 (c; arrows), CD33 (d; arrow), and CD11b (e; arrow); compare with benign controls (c′–e′).

dysplasia (dyserythropoiesis and dyserythropoiesis) with typical flow cytometric features of dysgranulopoiesis.

Marrow infiltrate with fibrosis

Numerous reactive and malignant disorders are associated with BM fibrosis, including PMF, CML, PV, acute megakaryoblastic leukemia, SM, acute panmyelosis with myelofibrosis (APMF), infectious disease (granulomas), MDS with fibrosis, HCL, non-Hodgkin lymphoma, cHL, HIV infection, treatment with hematopoietic growth factors, following bone damage (necrosis, irradiation, fracture), some metabolic disorders, occasional PCM cases, autoimmune disorders (e.g. systemic lupus erythematosus, SLE), and metastatic tumors. The fibrosis is usually composed of reticulin fibers but may also include collagen. The latter may be accompanied by osteosclerosis. Special stains which are helpful in identifying fibrosis include Mallory's, van Gieson, Gomori's and Masson's. Both aspirate smears and flow cytometry are often not contributory in the cases with prominent BM fibrosis, as samples represents mostly blood elements.

Plasmacytosis

Increased number of plasma cells may be associated with reactive conditions (polyclonal plasmacytosis) and plasma cell neoplasms. Causes of reactive plasmacytosis include inflammatory conditions, chronic infections (mostly viral, but also certain bacterial), autoimmune disorders, hypersensitivity states, cHL, anemia (megaloblastic and iron deficiency), cirrhosis and occasional cases of CML, AML, and metastatic carcinoma. B-cell lymphomas may be accompanied by polyclonal or monoclonal plasmacytosis. Rarely, also some T-cell lymphoma, especially AITL may be associated with prominent

plasmacytosis mimicking plasma cell neoplasms (or plasma cell leukemia). PCM and monoclonal gammopathy of undetermined potential (MGUS) are defined by the presence of monoclonal plasma cell population. Presence of reactive, perivascular plasmacytosis is often seen in secondary polycythemia, and helps in differentiating it from PV. The reactive plasmacytosis, although sometimes very prominent, is usually composed of scattered, non-aggregated plasma cells, which are polytypic by immunohistochemistry and FC. Flow cytometric features of plasma cell neoplasms and differential diagnosis of BM plasmacytosis are presented in Chapter 14.

Metastatic tumors and other infiltrative processes

Extrinsic tumors are usually easily discernible by histomorphology and in some instances are also identified by flow cytometry (Figures 9.11 and 9.12). By flow cytometry, metastatic tumors are identified by lack of CD45 expression and frequent expression of CD56. Some metastatic tumors are also often positive for CD117 and may be positive for CD10. Rare cases of pancytopenia are caused by storage disorders, such as type 1 Gaucher disease, where abnormal accumulation and storage of glucocerebroside and related substances results in BM failure.

Summary of FC phenotypic profiles of metastatic tumors:

Metastatic carcinoma: CD45⁻, CD56⁺/⁻, CD117⁻/⁺, CD38⁻/⁺, keratin⁺
Rhabdomyosarcomas: CD45⁻, CD56⁺, CD90⁺, CD117⁺/⁻, myogenin⁺
Neuroblastoma: CD45⁻, CD56⁺, CD2⁺, CD81⁺
Primitive neuroectodermal tumors/Ewing sarcoma: CD45⁻, CD271⁺, CD99⁺

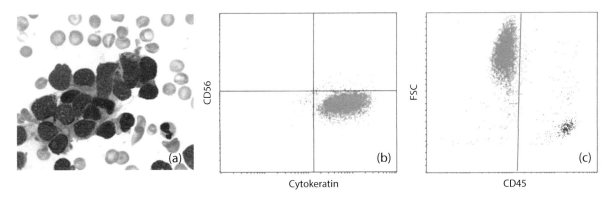

FIGURE 9.11 Metastatic carcinoma to the bone marrow: aspirate smear with cluster of cancer cells (a). Flow cytometry shows cytokeratin positive (b) and CD45 negative (c) population (orange dots).

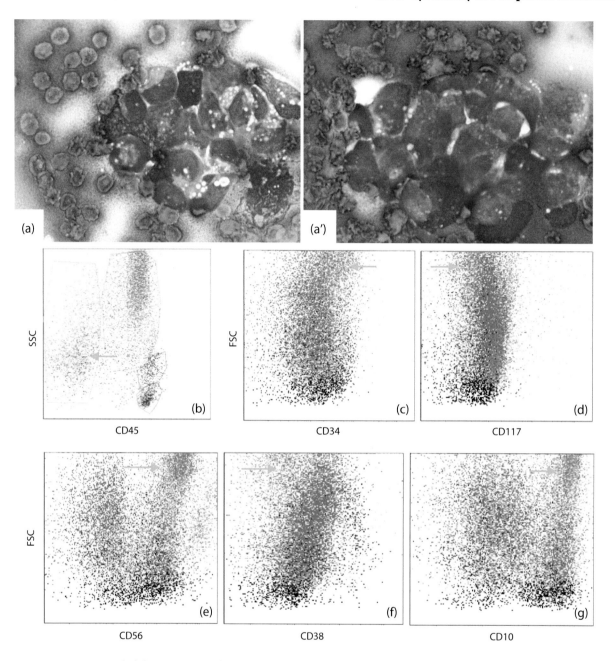

FIGURE 9.12 Metastatic rhabdomyosarcoma (24-year-old patient with history of rhabdomyosarcoma). Touch smears (a–a′) from BM shows clusters of large, highly atypical cells with cytoplasmic vacuoles and hyperchromatic, irregular nuclei. Flow cytometry analysis (b–g) shows cells with low side scatter (SSC, b) and high forward scatter (FSC, c–g). Tumor cells (subset of orange dots, arrow) show the following phenotype: CD45⁻ (b), CD34⁺ (c), CD117⁻ (d), CD56⁺ (e), CD38⁻ (f), and CD10⁺ (h).

References

1. Swerdlow, S.H., Campo, E., Harris, N.L., Jaffe, E.S., Pileri, S.A., Stein, H., et al., ed. *WHO classification of tumors of haematopoietic and lymphoid tissues.* 2016, IARC: Lyon.
2. Forghieri, F., et al., *NPM1-mutated myeloid neoplasms with <20% blasts: a really distinct clinico-pathologic entity?* Int J Mol Sci, 2020. **21**(23): p. 8975.
3. Matanes, F., et al., *Chronic myelomonocytic leukemia associated with myeloid sarcomas and NPM1 mutation: a case report and literature review.* Ther Adv Hematol, 2019. **10**: p. 2040620719854596.
4. Peng, J., et al., *Chronic myelomonocytic leukemia with nucleophosmin (NPM1) mutation.* Eur J Haematol, 2016. **96**(1): p. 65–71.
5. Zhang, Y., et al., *NPM1 mutations in myelodysplastic syndromes and acute myeloid leukemia with normal karyotype.* Leuk Res, 2007. **31**(1): p. 109–11.
6. Montalban-Bravo, G., et al., *NPM1 mutations define a specific subgroup of MDS and MDS/MPN patients with favorable outcomes with intensive chemotherapy.* Blood Adv, 2019. **3**(6): p. 922–33.
7. Bejar, R., *What biologic factors predict for transformation to AML?* Best Pract Res Clin Haematol, 2018. **31**(4): p. 341–5.
8. Moench, L., et al., *Double- and triple-hit lymphomas can present with features suggestive of immaturity, including TdT expression, and create diagnostic challenges.* Leuk Lymphoma, 2016. **57**(11): p. 2626–35.
9. Snuderl, M., et al., *B-cell lymphomas with concurrent IGH-BCL2 and MYC rearrangements are aggressive neoplasms with*

clinical and pathologic features distinct from Burkitt lymphoma and diffuse large B-cell lymphoma. Am J Surg Pathol, 2010. **34**(3): p. 327–40.

10. Wu, D., et al., *"Double-Hit" mature B-cell lymphomas show a common immunophenotype by flow cytometry that includes decreased CD20 expression.* Am J Clin Pathol, 2010. **134**(2): p. 258–65.

11. Alsuwaidan, A., et al., *Bright CD38 expression by flow cytometric analysis is a biomarker for double/triple hit lymphomas with a moderate sensitivity and high specificity.* Cytometry B Clin Cytom, 2019. **96**(5): p. 368–74.

12. Cardoso, C.C., et al., *The importance of CD39, CD43, CD81, and CD95 expression for differentiating B cell lymphoma by flow cytometry.* Cytometry B Clin Cytom, 2018. **94**(3): p. 451–8.

13. Martin-Moro, F., et al., *Bone marrow infiltration by flow cytometry at diffuse large B-cell lymphoma NOS diagnosis implies worse prognosis without considering bone marrow histology.* Cytometry B Clin Cytom, 2020. **98**(6): p. 525–8.

14. Martinez, A., et al., *Primary bone marrow lymphoma: an uncommon extranodal presentation of aggressive non-Hodgkin lymphomas.* Am J Surg Pathol, 2012. **36**(2): p. 296–304.

15. Yeh, Y.M., et al., *Large B cell lymphoma presenting initially in bone marrow, liver and spleen: an aggressive entity associated frequently with haemophagocytic syndrome.* Histopathology, 2010. **57**(6): p. 785–95.

16. Wannesson, L. and E. Chigrinova. *Concordant and discordant bone marrow involvement in diffuse large B-cell lymphoma: are they understudied phenomena?* J Clin Oncol, 2012. **30**(3): p. 336; author reply 336–7.

17. Chigrinova, E., et al., *Diffuse large B-cell lymphoma with concordant bone marrow involvement has peculiar genomic profile and poor clinical outcome.* Hematol Oncol, 2011. **29**(1): p. 38–41.

18. Said, J.W., *Aggressive B-cell lymphomas: how many categories do we need?* Mod Pathol, 2013. **26 Suppl 1**: p. S42–S56.

19. Pich, A., et al., *Intrasinusoidal bone marrow infiltration and splenic marginal zone lymphoma: a quantitative study.* Eur J Haematol, 2006. **76**(5): p. 392–8.

20. Bhagavathi, S., et al., *Primary bone diffuse large B-cell lymphoma: clinicopathologic study of 21 cases and review of literature.* Am J Surg Pathol, 2009. **33**(10): p. 1463–9.

21. Desai, S., et al., *Primary lymphoma of bone: a clinicopathologic study of 25 cases reported over 10 years.* J Surg Oncol, 1991. **46**(4): p. 265–9.

22. Dubey, P., et al., *Localized primary malignant lymphoma of bone.* Int J Radiat Oncol Biol Phys, 1997. **37**(5): p. 1087–93.

23. Tefferi, A., J. Thiele, and J.W. Vardiman, *The 2008 World Health Organization classification system for myeloproliferative neoplasms: order out of chaos.* Cancer, 2009. **115**(17): p. 3842–7.

24. Haferlach, T., et al., *The diagnosis of BCR/ABL-negative chronic myeloproliferative diseases (CMPD): a comprehensive approach based on morphology, cytogenetics, and molecular markers.* Ann Hematol, 2008. **87**(1): p. 1–10.

25. Wang, S.A., *The diagnostic work-up of hypereosinophilia.* Pathobiology, 2019. **86**(1): p. 39–52.

26. Noel, P., *Eosinophilic myeloid disorders.* Semin Hematol, 2012. **49**(2): p. 120–7.

27. Tefferi, A., R. Skoda, and J.W. Vardiman, *Myeloproliferative neoplasms: contemporary diagnosis using histology and genetics.* Nat Rev Clin Oncol, 2009. **6**(11): p. 627–37.

28. Valent, P., *Pathogenesis, classification, and therapy of eosinophilia and eosinophil disorders.* Blood Rev, 2009. **23**(4): p. 157–65.

29. Morsia, E., et al., *WHO defined chronic eosinophilic leukemia, not otherwise specified (CEL, NOS): A contemporary series from the Mayo Clinic.* Am J Hematol, 2020. **95**(7): p. E172–E174.

30. Gotlib, J., et al., *The FIP1L1-PDGFRalpha fusion tyrosine kinase in hypereosinophilic syndrome and chronic eosinophilic leukemia: implications for diagnosis, classification, and management.* Blood, 2004. **103**(8): p. 2879–91.

31. Gotlib, V., et al., *Eosinophilic variant of chronic myeloid leukemia with vascular complications.* Leuk Lymphoma, 2003. **44**(9): p. 1609–13.

32. Fishel, R.S., et al., *Acute lymphoblastic leukemia with eosinophilia.* Medicine (Baltimore), 1990. **69**(4): p. 232–43.

33. Invernizzi, R., et al., *Acute lymphoblastic leukemia and eosinophilia.* Haematologica, 1991. **76**(2): p. 167–8.

34. Roufosse, F., S. Garaud, and L. de Leval. *Lymphoproliferative disorders associated with hypereosinophilia.* Semin Hematol, 2012. **49**(2): p. 138–48.

35. Pardanani, A., et al., *FIP1L1-PDGFRA fusion: prevalence and clinicopathologic correlates in 89 consecutive patients with moderate to severe eosinophilia.* Blood, 2004. **104**(10): p. 3038–45.

36. Huang, Q., et al., *PDGFRA rearrangement leading to hypereosinophilia, T-lymphoblastic lymphoma, myeloproliferative neoplasm and precursor B-cell acute lymphoblastic leukemia.* Leukemia, 2011. **25**(2): p. 371–5.

37. Hasserjian, R.P., et al., *Acute erythroid leukemia: a reassessment using criteria refined in the 2008 WHO classification.* Blood, 2010. **115**(10): p. 1985–92.

38. Kasyan, A., et al., *Acute erythroid leukemia as defined in the World Health Organization classification is a rare and pathogenetically heterogeneous disease.* Mod Pathol, 2010. **23**(8): p. 1113–26.

39. Marsee, D.K., G.S. Pinkus, and H. Yu, *CD71 (transferrin receptor): an effective marker for erythroid precursors in bone marrow biopsy specimens.* Am J Clin Pathol, 2010. **134**(3): p. 429–35.

40. Zuo, Z., et al., *Acute myeloid leukemia (AML) with erythroid predominance exhibits clinical and molecular characteristics that differ from other types of AML.* PLoS One, 2012. 7(7): p. e41485.

10

MORPHOLOGIC-FLOW CYTOMETRIC CORRELATION IN LYMPH NODES

Reactive follicular hyperplasia

The lymph nodes act as a scaffolding system and are home for lymphocytes and monocytes/histiocytes in the lymphatic system. Lymph nodes are ovoid encapsulated structures composed of cortex (with primary and secondary follicles), paracortex (area between superficial cortex and medulla), and medulla (medullary cords with vessels and sinuses). The capsule and its extension within the lymph node parenchyma (trabeculae) together with reticular meshwork form supportive elements of the lymph node. The reticular meshwork is composed of reticular cells, dendritic cells, macrophages, and follicular dendritic cells (FDCs). Primary and secondary follicles are distributed within cortex (at the periphery of the lymph node). Primary follicles are composed of small and relatively monotonous B-cells, which are CD10$^-$ and BCL6$^-$ and positive for BCL2. Secondary (or reactive) follicles are composed of two zones: central, pale staining germinal centers and a darker staining mantle zone composed of mostly small lymphocytes. The mantle zone in the lymph nodes is usually homogenous without overt marginal zone, typical for follicles in the spleen. Certain reactive conditions in the lymph node may lead to the formation of easily identifiable marginal zone composed of so-called monocytoid B-cells. The germinal centers B-cells express CD10 and BCL6 and are negative for BCL2. They contain numerous larger lymphocytes with nucleoli (centroblasts), centrocytes (lymphocytes with irregular nuclei), small lymphocytes, tingible body macrophages, and dendritic reticulum cells. Few scattered T-cells expressing CD10 and PD1 are also present within reactive follicles. The secondary follicles often show polarization of their architecture with one pole composed of centrocytes (lighter zone) and the other with increased number of centroblasts and macrophages (darker zone). Polarization helps to differentiate reactive follicles from follicular lymphoma (FL). The polarization is easy to appreciate with Ki-67 or PD1 staining. Supporting the B-cells in the follicles are FDCs, best visualized by staining with CD21 and CD23. Intact (compact) distributions of FDC meshwork favor a reactive process, whereas an expanded or disrupted meshwork is seen in lymphomas.

The lymphoid cells between follicles (paracortex or interfollicular region) are composed predominantly of small T-cells with rare centroblasts (depending on the degree of activation), scattered interdigitating reticulum cells, and the high endothelial venules. Sinuses contain macrophages and patency is best evaluated by the examination of the subcapsular region. The immunohistochemical staining of the lymph node with selected antigens, including B-cell markers (CD19, CD20, CD22, CD79a, and PAX5), pan-T markers (CD2, CD3, CD5, and CD7), CD10, PD1, CD21, and BCL2, help to identify normal architecture and differentiate reactive process from lymphomas. Figure 10.1 shows typical flow cytometry (FC) pattern of reactive lymph node. In benign lymph nodes, the proportion of kappa to lambda (κ/λ ratio) is within the range of 1.2:1 to 2.7:1 in lymph nodes. In the florid reactive follicular hyperplasia (lymph nodes, tonsils, etc.), FC analysis shows increased number of B-cells with CD10 expression, which often show variable ("smeary") expression of light-chain immunoglobulins with kappa being usually brighter than lambda (Figure 10.2), although in some patients, especially children and young adults, the expression of lambda may be more pronounced (Figure 10.3).

Diffuse pattern with mostly small cells

Diffuse infiltrate of predominantly small lymphocytes is seen in small lymphocytic lymphoma/chronic lymphocytic leukemia (CLL/SLL), mantle cell lymphoma (MCL), nodal marginal zone lymphoma (NMZL), nodal involvement by hairy cell leukemia (HCL), FL with diffuse growth pattern (subset of FL with uncommon features), FL with prominent sclerosis, lymphoplasmacytic lymphoma (LPL), T-cell prolymphocytic leukemia (T-PLL), small cell variant of peripheral T-cell lymphoma (PTCL), small cell variant of anaplastic large cell lymphoma (ALCL), and lymphomatous or acute variants of adult T-cell lymphoma/leukemia (ATLL). Centrocytes are small to medium-size lymphocytes with irregular nuclear contours (cleaved cells), condensed chromatin, and scanty cytoplasm. Lymphocytes from MCL have indented nuclear outlines and small lymphocytes from SLL/CLL have round nucleic with condensed chromatin and scant cytoplasm. Lymph node with SLL/CLL show characteristic paler areas representing proliferation centers. FC shows dim expression of CD20 and surface light-chain immunoglobulins (subset of cases may be kappa and lambda negative), co-expression of CD5 and CD23, negative to dim CD81, negative CD71 and positive CD200 (Figure 10.4) [1–5]. In MCL, FC shows moderate expression of CD20 and light-chain immunoglobulins, positive CD5, CD38, and CD81, and negative CD11c, CD23, and CD200 [2, 6–11]. NMZL (Figure 10.5) shows clonal B-cells with non-specific phenotype (CD5$^-$, CD10$^-$) with moderate expression of CD20 (minor subset of cases may show aberrant expression of CD5) [1, 12–15]. Detailed FC patterns of low-grade B-cell lymphoproliferations are presented in Chapter 13.

Summary of FC phenotypic profiles in diffuse small cell infiltrate in LN:

CLL/SLL: CD19$^+$, CD20$^{+(often\ dim)}$, surface light-chain immunoglobulins$^{+(dim)}$, CD5$^+$, CD23$^{+/rarely-}$, CD10$^-$, CD38$^{+(dim\ or\ partial)/-}$, CD43$^+$, CD71$^-$, CD81$^{-/dim}$, CD200$^+$, CD11c$^{+/-}$,

MCL: CD19$^+$, CD20$^+$, surface light-chain immunoglobulin$^+$, CD5$^+$, CD10$^{-/rarely+}$, CD11c$^-$, CD23$^-$, CD38$^+$, CD43$^+$, CD71$^{-/+(dim\ or\ partial)}$, CD81$^+$, CD200$^-$

FL: CD19$^{+(often\ dim)}$, CD20$^+$, surface light-chain immunoglobulin$^+$, CD5$^-$, CD10$^+$, CD11c$^-$, CD23$^-$, CD38$^{+/rarely-}$, CD43$^-$, CD71$^{-/+(dim\ or\ partial)}$, CD81$^{+(dim)/-}$, CD200$^{-/+(dim)}$

MZL: CD19$^+$, CD20$^+$, surface light-chain immunoglobulin$^+$, CD5$^{-/rare\ cases+}$, CD10$^-$, CD11c$^{+/-}$, CD23$^{-/+}$, CD38$^{+/-}$, CD43$^{-/+}$, CD81$^{+/-}$, CD200$^{-/rarely+}$

LPL: CD19$^+$, CD20$^+$, surface light-chain immunoglobulin$^+$, CD5$^{-/rare\ cases+}$, CD10$^{-/rarely+}$, CD11c$^-$, CD23$^{-/rarely+}$, CD25$^{+/rarely-}$, CD38$^{+/rarely-}$, CD43$^-$, CD71$^-$, CD81$^{+/-}$, CD200$^{+(dim)/-}$

HCL: CD19$^+$, CD20$^+$, surface light-chain immunoglobulin$^+$, CD5$^-$, CD10$^{-/rarely+}$, CD11c$^{+bright}$, CD23$^{-/rarely+}$, CD25$^+$, CD38$^-$, CD43$^{+(dim)/rarely-}$, CD71$^-$, CD81$^{+(dim)}$, CD200$^{+(bright)}$

DOI: 10.1201/9781003197935-10

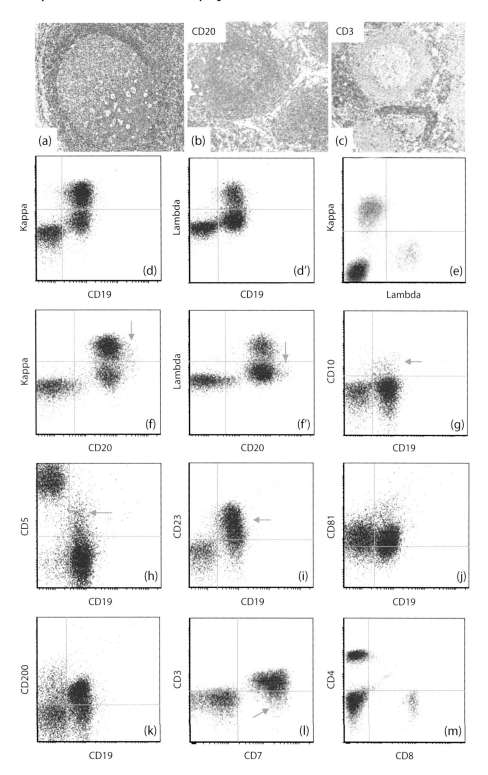

FIGURE 10.1 Flow cytometry pattern of benign (reactive) lymph node. (a–c) Benign lymph node – histology and immunohisto-chemistry. (a) Polarized germinal center with one pole composed of larger lymphocytes with macrophages and the other composed mostly of small lymphocytes (such polarization is typical for reactive follicles and helps to differentiate it from follicular lymphoma). (b) B-cells are visualized by staining with CD20. (c) T-cells are restricted to perifollicular area (CD3 staining). (d–m) Flow cytometry. B-cells are positive for CD19 (d–d′) with polytypic pattern of expression of kappa and lambda (d–f). The expression of CD20 is moderate (f–f′) with minor subset of cells (arrow) showing bright CD20. Rare B-cells express CD10 (g, arrow) and CD5 (h, arrow). Majority of benign B-cells are CD23+ (i, arrow). Both B- and T-cells are CD81+ (dim expression, j). Major subset of B-cells shows dim CD200 expression (k). T-cells are positive for CD3 and CD7 (l) with only few cells showing aberrant loss of CD7 (arrow). Major subset of T-cells is CD4+ and minor subset of T-cells is CD8+ (m).

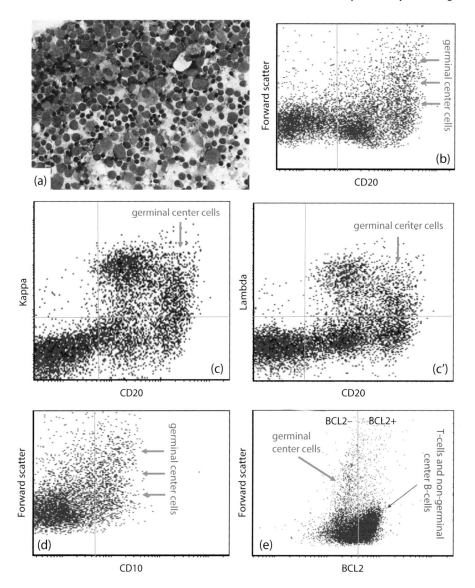

FIGURE 10.2 Flow cytometry pattern of florid follicular hyperplasia. (a) Touch smears from florid follicular hyperplasia often show increased number of large cells (centroblasts) mixed with small lymphocytes and tingible body macrophages. (b–e) Flow cytometry. Germinal center cells from benign follicular hyperplasia (blue dots, arrows) show bright CD20 expression (b), variable expression of surface light chain immunoglobulin (with kappa slightly stronger than lambda; c–c′) and increased forward scatter (b–e). Germinal center cells are CD10$^+$ (d) and BCL2$^-$ (e).

T-PLL: CD2$^{+/-}$, CD3$^{+/-}$, CD4$^+$ (less often CD8$^+$, CD4/CD8$^+$ or CD4/CD8$^-$), CD5$^{+/-}$, CD7$^{+/-}$, CD25$^-$, CD26$^+$, CD45$^{+/rarely-}$, CD56$^-$, CD57$^-$, CD81$^+$, CD117$^{-/rarely+}$, CD200$^-$

ATLL: CD2$^{+/-}$, CD3$^{+/-}$, CD4$^+$ (rarely CD4/CD8$^+$), CD5$^+$, CD7$^-$, CD8$^-$, CD25$^+$, CD26$^-$, CD45$^+$, CD56$^-$, CD57$^-$

Diffuse pattern with medium-sized and/or large cells

Diagnostic considerations of a diffuse infiltrate composed of large and/or intermediate in size cells include diffuse large B-cell lymphoma (DLBCL), PTCL, blastoid variant of MCL, extramedullary myeloid tumor (EMT; granulocytic sarcoma, monoblastic sarcoma), ALCL, plasmablastic lymphoma (PBL), Burkitt lymphoma (BL), high-grade B-cell lymphoma (HGBL) with *MYC*

and *BCL2* (HGBL-R, double or triple hit lymphoma), plasma cell neoplasm, B-cell and T-cell lymphoblastic lymphoma (B-LBL; T-LBL), histiocytic sarcoma, dendritic cell tumors, blastic plasmacytoid dendritic cell neoplasm (BPDCN), and non-hematopoietic tumors (e.g., carcinoma, melanoma, Ewing's sarcoma). Based on the expression of CD10, BCL6, and MUM1, DLBCL is subdivided into DLBCL, germinal center B-cell like (GCB-like; CD10$^+$, BCL6$^+$, MUM$^-$ or CD10$^-$, BCL6$^+$, MUM1$^-$), and non-germinal center type also called activated B-cell-like (ABC-like; CD10$^-$, BCL6$^{+/-}$, MUM1$^+$) [16–22]. In DLBCL, FC analysis shows clonal B-cells with high forward scatter, moderate expression of CD20, positive or negative CD10 expression, negative to dim/partial CD71, negative CD5 (minor subset of DLBCL may be CD5$^+$), often positive CD38, usually dim CD81 and usually negative CD200 (Figures 10.6 and 10.7) [23–29]. Comparison of the intensity of expression of CD39, CD43, CD81, and CD95

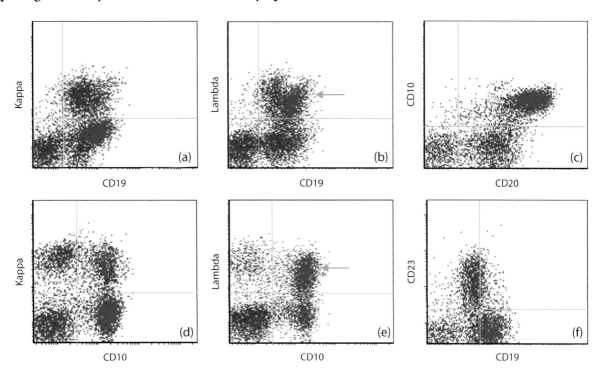

FIGURE 10.3 Flow cytometry pattern of florid follicular hyperplasia (11-year-old patient, lymph node). Based on CD19 expression, B-cells show two distinct populations: non-germinal center B-cells (red dots) with moderate CD19 expression (a–b) and polytypic pattern of kappa and lambda expression (a–b), and germinal center B-cells (blue dots) with bright CD19 and lambda excess (arrow). Germinal center B-cells show positive CD10 and bright CD20 expression (c). CD10⁺ B-cells are polytypic but show slight excess of lambda⁺ cells (d–e, arrow). Non-germinal center cells are CD23⁺ (f).

helps to differentiate between FL, DLBCL (GCB-like), DLBCL (ABC-like), and BL. Very strong expression of CD39 is typical for DLBCL, ABC-like, while DLBCL, GCB-like shows usually moderate CD39 and both FL and BL weak CD39 expressions [30]. Figure 10.8 compares FC features between low-grade FL and CD10⁺ DLBCL. BL shows strong expression of CD43 while FL is often CD43⁻ and DLBCL, GCB is weakly positive (CD43 is stronger in non-GCB DLBCL than in GCB DLBCL). CD81 expression is strong in BL, while is negative or weak in FL or DLBCL and the expression of CD95 is negative o weak in BL and strong in DLBCL. PTCL is positive for pan-T-cell antigens (often with aberrant expression of more than one marker), CD4 or CD8 restriction, increased forward scatter, bright CD45, and often positive CD38 [31–33]. Figure 10.9 shows correlation between immunohistochemistry and FC in the case of PTCL. Nodal TFH cell lymphoma, angioimmunoblastic-type (AITL) shows morphologically pleomorphic infiltrate and characteristic FC pattern with variably increased forward scatter. Detailed FC patterns of DLBCL and high-grade B-cell lymphoproliferations are presented in Chapter 13 and description of PTCL, AITL, and ALCL in Chapter 16.

Summary of FC phenotypic profiles in diffuse intermediate to large cell infiltrate in LN:

DLBCL: CD19⁺, CD20⁺, surface light-chain immunoglobulin⁺, CD5⁻/rarely+, CD10⁺/⁻, CD11c⁻/rarely+, CD23⁻, CD25⁻/rarely+, CD38⁺, CD43⁻/+, CD71⁺(dim or rarely strong), CD81⁺(dim), CD200⁻/rarely +(dim)

HGBL-R: CD19⁺, CD20⁺ (may be dim), surface light-chain immunoglobulin⁺/rarely−, BCL2⁺, CD5⁻, CD10⁺/rarely−, CD11c⁻, CD23⁻, CD25⁻, CD38⁺, CD43⁺/⁻, CD71⁺, CD81⁺, CD200⁻/+

MCL (pleomorphic variant): CD19⁺, CD20⁺, surface light-chain immunoglobulin⁺, sCD5⁺, CD10⁻/rarely+, CD11c⁻, CD23⁻, CD38⁺, CD43⁺, CD71⁻/+(dim or partial), CD81⁺, CD200⁻

BL: CD19⁺, CD20⁺, surface light-chain immunoglobulin⁺, BCL2⁻, CD5⁻, CD10⁺, CD11c⁻, CD23⁻, CD25⁻, CD38⁺, CD43⁺(strong), CD71⁺(strong), CD81⁺(strong), CD200⁻/rarely +(dim)

PTCL: CD2⁺/⁻, CD3⁺/⁻, CD4⁺/⁻, CD5⁺/⁻, CD7⁻/+, CD8⁻/+, CD10⁻, CD30⁻/rarely+, CD38⁺, CD45⁺, CD56⁻/rarely+

ALCL: high forward scatter, CD2⁺/rarely⁻, CD3⁺/⁻, CD4⁺ or less often CD8⁺ (rare tumors are either CD4/8⁻ or CD4/CD8⁺), CD5⁺/⁻, CD7⁻/rarely+, CD10⁻, CD25⁺/⁻, CD26⁺/rarely−, CD30⁺, CD43⁺, CD45⁺, CD56⁻/rarely+

B-ALL: CD10⁺(bright)/rarely−, CD13⁻/rarely+, CD19⁺, CD20⁻/rarely+, CD22⁺, CD33⁻/rarely+, CD34⁺/rarely−, CD38⁺(bright), CD45⁻/+dim, CD56⁻, CD71⁻/+dim, CD79a⁺, CD81⁺dim, CD123⁺/⁻, CD200⁺/⁻, HLA-DR⁺, MPO⁻, TdT⁺/rarely−

T-ALL: CD1a⁻/+, CD2⁺, surface CD3⁻/rare cases+, cytoplasmic CD3⁺, CD4⁻/CD8⁻ or CD4⁺/CD8⁺, CD5⁺/⁻, CD7⁺, CD10⁻/+, CD13⁻/rarely+, CD15⁻/rarely+, CD33⁻/rarely+, CD34⁺/⁻, CD38⁺, CD56⁻/rare cases+, CD71⁻/+, CD79a⁻/rarely+, CD117⁻, CD123⁻, HLA-DR⁻, MPO⁻, TdT⁺/rarely−

EMT: CD13⁺, CD33⁺, CD34⁺/rarely−, CD117⁺, CD133⁺/⁻, MPO⁺, CD81⁺/⁻, HLA-DR⁺/rarely−

BPDCN: CD4⁺, CD13⁻, CD33⁻/+, CD56⁺(strong), CD123⁺(strong), CD11b⁻, CD11c⁻, HLA-DR⁺, CD45⁺, TdT⁻/+, MPO⁻, CD64⁻

Metastatic carcinoma: CD45⁻, CD56⁺/⁻, CD117⁻/+, CD38⁻/+, keratin⁺

Rhabdomyosarcomas: CD45⁻, CD56⁺, CD90⁺, CD117⁺/⁻, myogenin⁺

Neuroblastoma: CD45⁻, CD56⁺, CD2⁺, CD81⁺

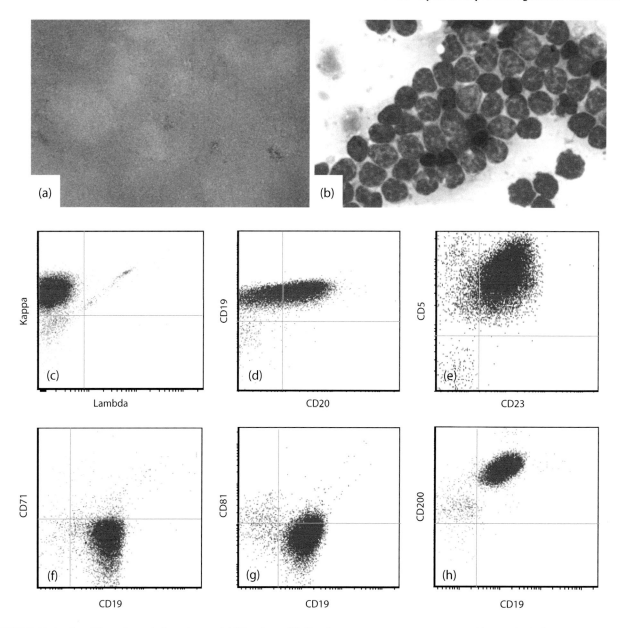

FIGURE 10.4 Small lymphocytic lymphoma. (a) Histology; (b) Cytology. Low power examination (a) reveals diffuse lymphoid infil-trate with typical paler areas (proliferation centers) giving rise to a pseudofollicular pattern. Touch smear (b) shows small round lym-phocytes with regular nuclear outlines and compact, darkly stained chromatin. (c–h) Flow cytometry. SLL/CLL cells are kappa$^+$ (c), CD19$^+$ (d), CD20$^+$ (dim expression, d), CD5$^+$ (e), CD23$^+$ (e), CD71$^-$ (f), CD81$^-$ (g), and CD200$^+$ (h).

Primitive neuroectodermal tumors/Ewing sarcoma: CD45$^-$, CD271$^+$, CD99$^+$

Metastatic melanoma: CD45$^-$, CD56$^{+/-}$, CD10$^{-/+}$, CD57$^{+/-}$, CD117$^{-/+}$

Mixed (pleomorphic) infiltrate

Diffuse pleomorphic infiltrate (Figure 10.10) with small, interme-diate, and large cells can be seen in Kikuchi lymphadenitis, EBV-associated atypical (reactive) hyperplasia, pleomorphic variant of MCL, nodal MZL with increased large cells, diffuse follicle cen-ter cell lymphoma (grade 2), AITL, PTCL, mixed cellularity clas-sic Hodgkin lymphoma (cHL), T-cell-rich/histiocyte-rich large B-cell lymphoma (TIIRLBL), EBV-associated DLBCL, HGBL;

Langerhans cell histiocytosis (LCH) and SLL/CLL with large cell transformation (Richter's syndrome). Pleomorphic infiltrate with increased vascularity is seen in late HIV infection and AITL.

Kikuchi lymphadenopathy (Kikuchi-Fujimoto disease/lymphadenitis) is a benign, self-limited disease often confused with B- and especially T-cell lymphomas due to effacement of lymph node architecture (at least partial) and scattered atypi-cal lymphocytes with immunoblastic features. The lymph node shows reactive germinal centers and focal areas of necrosis (necrosis may be subtle in early stages when only occasional apoptotic cells are present within histiocytic aggregates) [34–36]. The histiocytic cells with engulfed cellular debris have abun-dant cytoplasm and crescentic nuclei (C-shaped forms), a char-acteristic feature of Kikuchi disease. The infiltrate is composed

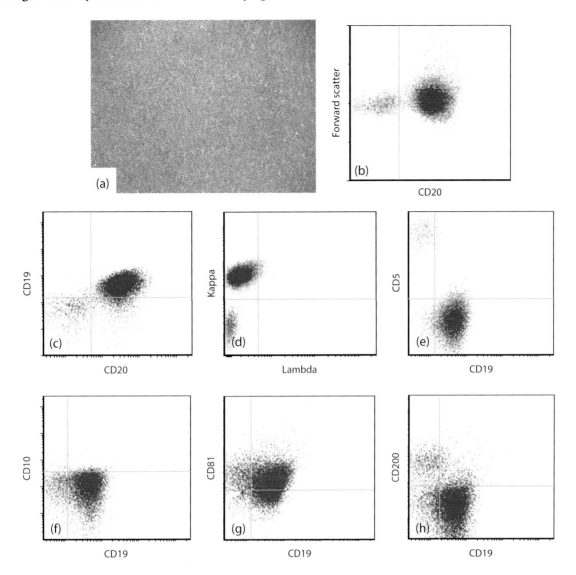

FIGURE 10.5 Flow cytometry pattern of nodal marginal zone lymphoma (NMZL). (a) Histology section shows diffuse lymphoid infiltrate of small cells. (b–h) Flow cytometry. B-cells show moderate CD20 expression and low forward scatter (b). They express CD20 and CD19 (c) and show moderate, expression of surface light chain immunoglobulin (d; presented case is kappa+). There is no CD5 (e) or CD10 (f) expression. Clonal B-cells in NMZL show dim CD81 expression (g), and negative CD200 (h).

of pleomorphic population of small, intermediate, to large lymphocytes (predominantly T-cells, especially in areas of necrosis; CD8+ T-cells are more abundant than CD4+), histiocytes (CD68+, CD163+, and CD4+), and plasmacytoid dendritic cells (CD123+, CD68+, and CD303+). Scattered weakly CD30+ immunoblasts may be present (they are of T-cell lineage, usually CD8+). Characteristically, there are no neutrophils and only rare plasma cells may be seen. Karyorrhectic debris are present in the necrotic areas and may be prominent. Based on the cellular composition, some authors distinguish several variants of Kikuchi lymphadenopathy: lymphohistiocytic, phagocytic, necrotic, and foamy cell type [37]. Lymphadenopathy in Kikuchi-Fujimoto disease may be accompanied by similar changes in the skin. Similar pattern to Kikuchi lymphadenopathy may be seen in systemic lupus erythematosus (SLE). SLE adenopathy differs by the presence of numerous plasma cells, hematoxylin bodies, and degenerated nuclear material in the blood walls (Azzopardi phenomenon). FC

analysis of Kikuchi disease shows reactive pattern with polytypic B-cells, minor subset of CD10+ B-cells, and many small T-cells with normal expression of pan T-cell antigens. The characteristic FC feature of Kikuchi lymphadenopathy is CD38 expression by the majority of CD19+ small B cells, expansion of mature T-cells (with CD8 predominance), lack of surface IgM on IgD+ B cells, and decreased expression of CD57 by both CD4+ and CD8+ T-cells [38].

Infiltrate with scattered large cells with irregular (binucleated, multilobed, or multinucleated) nuclei and prominent nucleoli is seen in cHL, PTCL, AITL, THRLBL, EBV+ DLBCL, NLPHL, EBV-associated lymphadenitis (infectious mononucleosis), Kimura disease, and CMV-associated lymphadenitis. Classical HL is characterized by the presence of Reed-Sternberg (R-S) cells, whereas typical form of NLPHL is characterized by scattered large cells with nucleoli (lymphocyte predominant cells; LP cells) within B-cell-rich nodules. R-S cells are large binucleated or

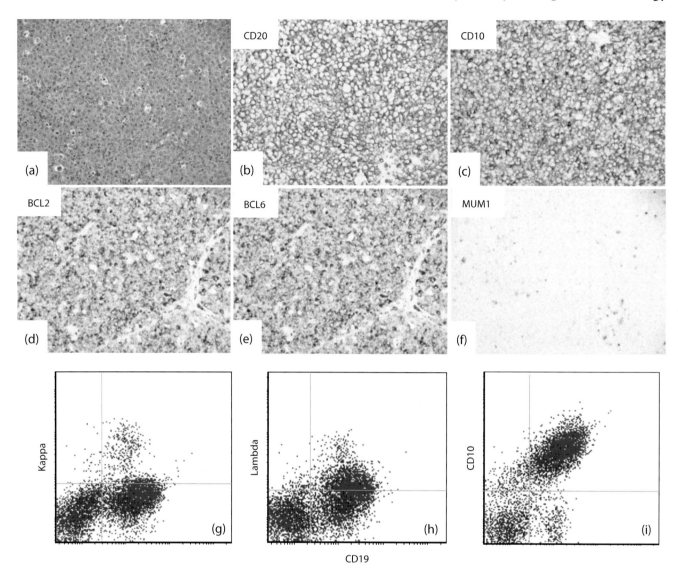

FIGURE 10.6 DLBCL, GCB-like. (a) Histology shows diffuse lymphoid infiltrate composed of large cells. (b–f) Immunohistochemistry. Lymphomatous cells are positive for CD20 (b), CD10 (c), BCL2 (d), and BCL6 (e). MUM1 is negative (f). (g–i) Flow cytometry shows clonal B-cells with negative kappa (g), dim lambda (h), and strong CD10 expression (i).

multinucleated (multilobated) cells with prominent eosinophilic nucleoli (often with clear halo around them), thick nuclear membrane, and amphophilic or eosinophilic cytoplasm. LP cells have multilobated nuclei, scanty cytoplasm, highly irregular nuclear contours, pale, vesicular chromatin, and prominent nucleoli. LP cells are surrounded by a rim of small T-cells (CD3⁺/CD57⁺ rosettes) and are most often located within nodules composed predominantly of small B-cells, in contrast to R-S cells, which are usually present within the T-cell-rich background with polymorphic inflammatory infiltrate with eosinophils, plasma cells, neutrophils, histiocytes, and small lymphocytes.

EBV-lymphadenitis (infectious mononucleosis) often shows cytologic atypia raising the possibility of malignancy (e.g., DLBCL, PTCL and especially, cHL). Lymph node is enlarged with mixed follicular and paracortical hyperplasia, small foci of necrosis, and very pleomorphic infiltrate composed of lymphocytes, histiocytes, and plasma cells. Interfollicular (paracortical) areas show increased number of larger atypical lymphocytes with immunoblastic, centroblastic, or plasmablastic cytomorphology,

which are either of B- or T-cell lineages. Those activated cells often express CD30. Scattered EBV-infected cells (either small- or medium-sized) are always present. Plasma cells are polytypic. T-cells often show increased number of CD8⁺ cells, some of which display cytologic atypia.

Summary of FC phenotypic profiles of pleomorphic lymphoid infiltrate in LN:

AITL: CD2$^{+/-}$, CD3$^{+/-}$, CD4$^+$, CD5$^{+/-}$, CD7$^{+/-}$, CD8$^-$, CD10$^{+/rarely-}$, CD30$^-$, CD45$^+$, CD56$^-$, CD81$^+$, CD200$^+$

DLBCL: CD19$^+$, CD20$^+$, surface light-chain immunoglobulin$^+$, CD5$^{-/rarely+}$, CD10$^{+/-}$, CD11c$^{-/rarely+}$, CD23$^-$, CD25$^{-/rarely+}$, CD38$^+$, CD43$^{-/+}$, CD71$^{+(dim or rarely strong)}$, CD81$^{+(dim)}$, CD200$^{-/rarely+(dim)}$

PTCL: CD2$^{+/-}$, CD3$^{+/-}$, CD4$^{+/-}$, CD5$^{+/-}$, CD7$^{-/+}$, CD8$^{-/+}$, CD10$^-$, CD30$^{-/rarely+}$, CD38$^+$, CD45$^+$, CD56$^{-/rarely+}$

THRLBL: predominance of small T-cells with normal phenotype

Classic HL: predominance of small T-cells with normal phenotype

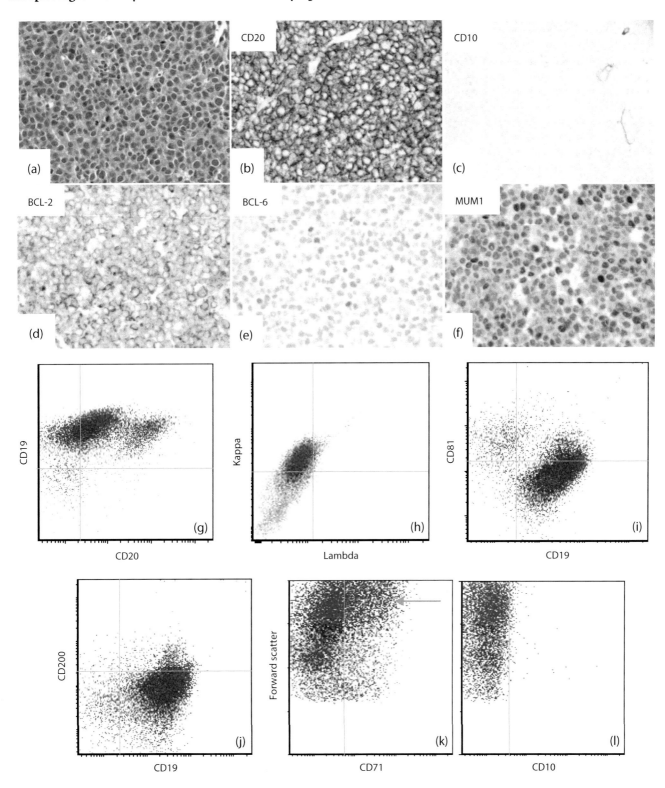

FIGURE 10.7 DLBCL, ABC-like. (a) Histology shows diffuse lymphoid infiltrate composed of large cells. (b–f) Immunohistochemistry. Lymphomatous cells are positive for CD20 (b), negative for CD10 (c), positive for BCL2 (d). BCL6 (e) and MUM1 (f). (g–l) Flow cytometry shows clonal B-cells with dim CD20 (g), moderate CD19 (g), kappa restriction (h), negative CD81 (i), and negative CD200 (j). The forward scatter of B-cells is high (k–l). There is partial dim expression of CD71 (k, arrow), and lack of CD10 (l).

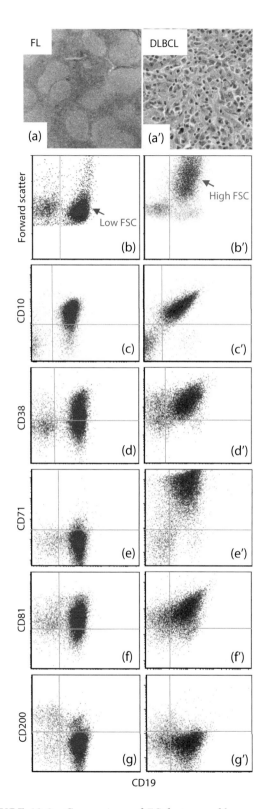

FIGURE 10.8 Comparison of FC features of low-grade FL (a, left column) and CD10⁺ DLBCL with GCB-like phenotype (a', right column). Low-grade FL display low forward scatter (b) and DLBCL shows high forward scatter (b'). Both lymphomas are positive for CD10 (c–c') and CD38 (d–d') with expression of CD38 being slightly dimmer in FL. In contrast to FL, DLBCL shows CD71 expression (e–e'). The expression of both CD81 and CD200 is often similar in those two lymphomas (f–f' and g–g').

Blastoid and/or "high-grade" infiltrate

Diffuse infiltrate of intermediate cells with blastic (blastoid) appearance is seen typically in precursor and high-grade neoplasms characterized by numerous mitotic figures, apoptotic cells, high Ki-67 index, starry-sky appearance and cells with prominent nucleoli, increased nuclear-cytoplasmic ratio, and often evenly distributed, fine chromatin. Some tumors may have hyperchromatic nuclei. Diagnostic considerations include B-cell lymphoblastic lymphoma (B-LBL), T-LBL, blastoid variant of MCL, immunoblastic variant of DLBCL, EMT (myeloid and monoblastic sarcoma), PBL, BPDCN, HGBL, not otherwise specified (HGBL, NOS) and HGBL with rearrangement of *MYC* and *BCL2* HGBL-R). HGBL-R is also termed double or triple hit (DH or TH) lymphoma. High-grade tumors with blastic features often show admixture of histiocytes, which engulf cellular debris (apoptotic bodies) giving raise to so-called starry-sky pattern when lymph node is examined on low power. This pattern is characteristic for BL, HGBL, NOS, HGBL-R, and precursor (lymphoblastic) tumors. Differential diagnosis of HGBLs is present in Chapters 12 and 13. BL in FC analysis (Figure 10.11) shows clonal B-cells with partially increased forward scatter, positive expression of B-cell markers, moderate expression of surface light-chain immunoglobulins, positive expression of CD10, moderate expression of CD19, strong expression of CD38 and CD43, dim or partial expression of CD71, positive CD81, and lack of BCL2 and CD20. BL shows stronger expression of CD43 when compared to FL or DLBCL (GCB-like). CD39 expression is negative or dim in BL (similar to FL) and strong in DLBCL (much stronger in non-germinal center type when compared to germinal center type) [30]. In contrast to BL, FLs often show dim expression of CD19 and dim or negative CD81. HGBL-R (DH or TH) often shows bright expression of CD10, CD38, and BCL2, dim CD20, and variably increased forward scatter. They may show flow cytometric features suggestive of immaturity, such as negative or dim CD45 expression, lack or decreased (partial/dim) expression of CD20, lack of surface light-chain immunoglobulins, or rarely presence of TdT expression [39–41]. Among DH or TH lymphomas reported by Alsuwaidan et al., dim CD20 was noted in 32%, dim CD19 in 12%, bright CD38 in 56%, and lack of surface immunoglobulins in 23% [42]. Those cases need to be differentiated from transformed B-cell lymphomas (most often FLs). Correlation with morphology, immunohistochemistry, and fluorescence in situ hybridization (FISH) studies is need for final subclassification of high-grade or "blastoid" lymphomas.

Summary of FC phenotypic profiles in blastoid ("high-grade) infiltrate in LN:

HGBL-R: CD19⁺, CD20⁺ (may be dim), surface light-chain immunoglobulin⁺/rarely⁻, BCL2⁺, CD5⁻, CD10⁺/rarely⁻, CD11c⁻, CD23⁻, CD25⁻, CD38⁺, CD43⁺/⁻, CD71⁺, CD81⁺, CD200⁻/⁺

MCL (blastoid variant): CD19⁺, CD20⁺, surface light-chain immunoglobulin⁺, sCD5⁺, CD10⁻/rarely⁺, CD11c⁻, CD23⁻, CD38⁺, CD43⁺, CD71⁻/⁺(dim or partial), CD81⁺, CD200⁻

BL: CD19⁺, CD20⁺, surface light-chain immunoglobulin⁺, BCL2⁻, CD5⁻, CD10⁺, CD11c⁻, CD23⁻, CD25⁻, CD38⁺, CD43⁺(strong), CD71⁺(strong), CD81⁺(strong), CD200⁻/rarely ⁺(dim)

T-PLL: CD2⁺/⁻, CD3⁺/⁻, CD4⁺ (less often CD8⁺, CD4/CD8⁺ or CD4/CD8⁻), CD5⁺/⁻, CD7⁺/⁻, CD25⁻, CD26⁺, CD45⁺/rarely⁻, CD56⁻, CD57⁻, CD81⁺, CD117⁻/rarely⁺, CD200⁻

ALCL: high forward scatter, CD2⁺/rarely⁻, CD3⁺/⁻, CD4⁺ or less often CD8⁺ (rare tumors are either CD4/8⁻ or CD4/CD8⁺),

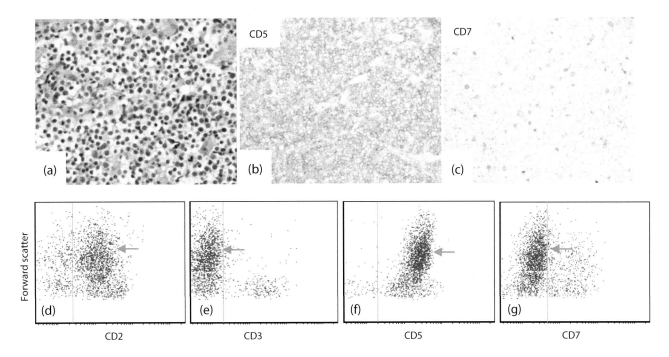

FIGURE 10.9 Peripheral T-cell lymphoma (PTCL). (a) Histology shows diffuse large cell lymphoid infiltrate with "clear" appearance. (b–c) Immunohistochemistry shows positive CD5 (b) and lack of CD7 expression (c). (d–g) Flow cytometry. Lymphomatous cells have increased forward scatter, positive CD2 (d), lack of surface CD3 expression (e), positive CD5 (f), and negative CD7 (g).

CD5$^{+/-}$, CD7$^{-/rarely+}$, CD10$^-$, CD25$^{+/-}$, CD26$^{+/rarely-}$, CD30$^+$, CD43$^+$, CD45$^+$, CD56$^{-/rarely+}$

B-ALL: CD10$^{+(bright)/rarely-}$, CD13$^{-/rarely+}$, CD19$^+$, CD20$^{-/rarely+}$, CD22$^+$, CD33$^{-/rarely+}$, CD34$^{+/rarely-}$, CD38$^{+(bright)}$, CD45$^{-/+dim}$, CD56$^-$, CD71$^{-/+dim}$, CD79a$^+$, CD81^{+dim}, CD123$^{+/-}$, CD200$^{+/-}$, HLA-DR$^+$, MPO$^-$, TdT$^{+/rarely-}$

T-ALL: CD1a$^{-/+}$, CD2$^+$, surface CD3$^{-/rare\ cases+}$, cytoplasmic CD3$^+$, CD4$^-$/CD8$^-$ or CD4$^+$/CD8$^+$, CD5$^{+/-}$, CD7$^+$, CD10$^{-/+}$, CD13$^{-/rarely+}$, CD15$^{-/rarely+}$, CD33$^{-/rarely+}$, CD34$^{+/-}$, CD38$^+$, CD56$^{-/rare\ cases+}$, CD71$^{-/+}$, CD79a$^{-/rarely+}$, CD117$^-$, CD123$^-$, HLA-DR$^-$, MPO$^-$, TdT$^{+/rarely-}$

EMT: CD13$^+$, CD33$^+$, CD34$^{+/rarely-}$, CD117$^+$, CD133$^{+/-}$, MPO$^+$, CD81$^{+/-}$, HLA-DR$^{+/rarely-}$

BPDCN: CD4$^+$, CD13$^-$, CD33$^{-/+}$, CD56$^{+(strong)}$, CD123$^{+(strong)}$, CD11b$^-$, CD11c$^-$, HLA-DR$^+$, CD45$^+$, TdT$^{-/+}$, MPO$^-$, CD64$^-$

Rhabdomyosarcomas: CD45$^-$, CD56$^+$, CD90$^+$, CD117$^{+/-}$, myogenin$^+$

Neuroblastoma: CD45$^-$, CD56$^+$, CD2$^+$, CD81$^+$

Primitive neuroectodermal tumors/Ewing sarcoma: CD45$^-$, CD271$^+$, CD99$^+$

Nodular pattern

The nodular ("follicular" pattern) is typical for several reactive conditions such as follicular hyperplasia, Toxoplasma lymphadenitis, Kimura disease, follicular hyperplasia with progressive transformation of germinal centers (PTGC), reactive process with mantle zone hyperplasia, Castleman's disease, rheumatoid lymphadenopathy, early HIV lymphadenopathy, and atypical follicular hyperplasia. The main differential diagnosis in the lymph node with nodular pattern includes follicular hyperplasia and FL (Figure 10.12). Nodularity (often vague) can be seen in SLL/

CLL with paler-staining proliferation centers composed of pro-lymphocytes ("pseudo-follicular" pattern), MCL, follicular T-cell lymphoma (FTCL), and nodal MZL. Fibrous bands dividing lymph node into prominent nodules with scattered large multi-lobated cells are characteristic for nodular sclerosis type of cHL, whereas a vague nodular pattern with scattered large cells in the background of small lymphocytes is typical for lymphocyte-rich cHL and nodular lymphocyte predominant Hodgkin lymphoma (NLPHL).

Summary of FC phenotypic profiles in nodular infiltrate in LN:

CLL: CD19$^+$, CD20$^{+(often\ dim)}$, surface light-chain immunoglobulins$^{+(dim)}$, CD5$^+$, CD23$^{+/rarely-}$, CD10$^-$, CD38$^{+(dim\ or\ partial)/-}$, CD43$^+$, CD71$^-$, CD81$^{-/dim}$, CD200$^+$, CD11c$^{+/-}$,

MCL: CD19$^+$, CD20$^+$, surface light-chain immunoglobulin$^+$, sCD5$^+$, CD10$^{-/rarely+}$, CD11c$^-$, CD23$^-$, CD38$^+$, CD43$^+$, CD71$^{-/+(dim\ or\ partial)}$, CD81$^+$, CD200$^-$

FL: CD19$^{+(often\ dim)}$, CD20$^+$, surface light-chain immunoglobulin$^+$, CD5$^-$, CD10$^+$, CD11c$^-$, CD23$^-$, CD38$^{+/rarely-}$, CD43$^-$, CD71$^{-/+(dim\ or\ partial)}$, CD81$^{+(dim)/-}$, CD200$^{-/+(dim)}$

FTCL: CD2$^{+/-}$, CD3$^{+/-}$, CD4$^+$, CD5$^{+/-}$, CD7$^{+/-}$, CD8$^-$, CD10$^+$, CD30$^-$, CD45$^+$, CD56$^-$, CD81$^+$, CD200$^+$

NMZL: CD19$^+$, CD20$^+$, surface light-chain immunoglobulin$^+$, CD5$^{-/rare\ cases+}$, CD10$^-$, CD11c$^{+/-}$, CD23$^{-/+}$, CD38$^{+/-}$, CD43$^{-/+}$, CD81$^{+/-}$, CD200$^{-/rarely+}$

Early AITL: CD2$^{+/-}$, CD3$^{+/-}$, CD4$^+$, CD5$^{+/-}$, CD7$^{+/-}$, CD8$^-$, CD10$^{+/rarely-}$, CD30$^-$, CD45$^+$, CD56$^-$, CD81$^+$, CD200$^+$

Classic HL: predominance of small T-cells with normal phenotype

NLPHL: predominance of small T-cells with normal phenotype

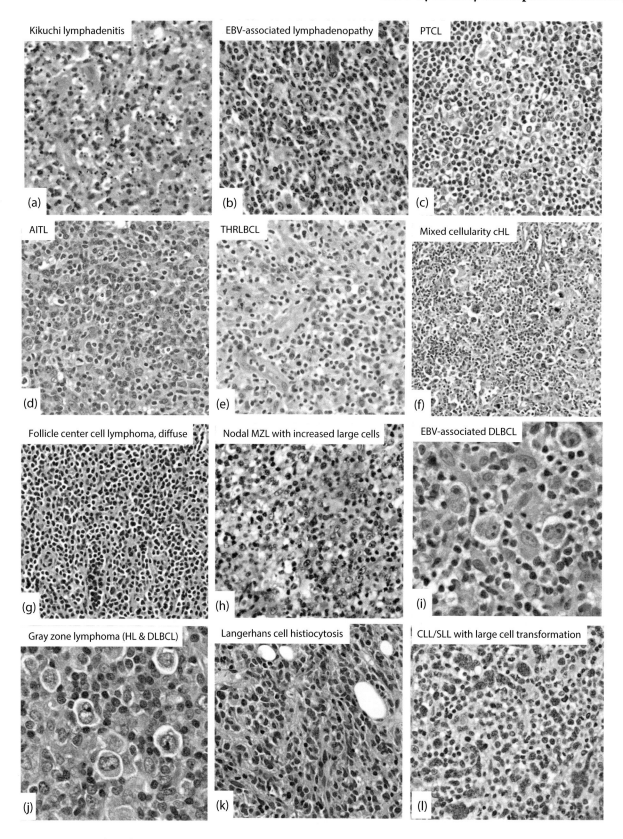

FIGURE 10.10 Lymph node with diffuse and pleomorphic infiltrate. Differential diagnosis includes (a) Kikuchi lymphadenitis; (b) EBV-associated atypical (reactive) hyperplasia; (c) peripheral T-cell lymphoma, unspecified (PTCL); (d) angioimmunoblastic T-cell lymphoma (AITL); (e) T-/histiocyte-rich large B-cell lymphoma (THRLBCL); (f) Hodgkin lymphoma, classic (mixed cellularity); (g) diffuse follicle center cell lymphoma (grade 2); (h) nodal marginal zone lymphoma with increased large cells; (i) EBV+ DLBCL; (j) mediastinal grey zone lymphoma; (k) Langerhans cell histiocytosis; and (l) small lymphocytic lymphoma (SLL/CLL) with large cell transformation (Richter's syndrome).

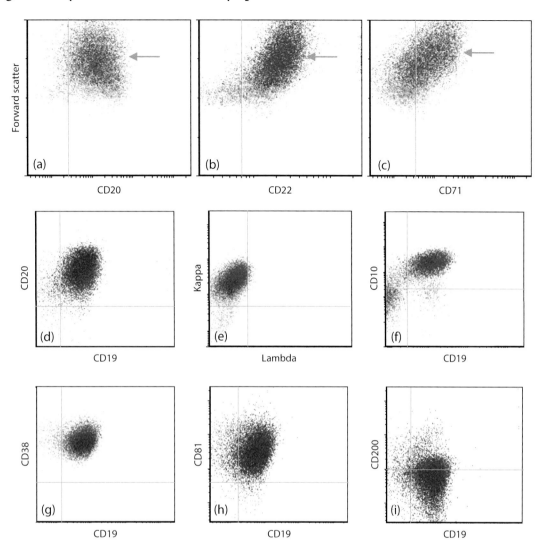

FIGURE 10.11 Flow cytometry of BL. Lymphomatous cells (blue dots, arrow) show increased forward scatter (a–c) and positive expression of CD20 (a), CD22 (b), CD71 (c), and CD19 (d). Kappa versus lambda scattergram (e) shows kappa restriction. The lymphoma cells are positive for CD10 (f), CD38 (g), and CD81 (h). CD200 is negative (i).

Paracortical (interfollicular; T-zone) pattern

A paracortical (interfollicular) infiltrate can be seen in AITL, especially early subtypes with preserved follicles (Figure 10.13), and occasionally in PTCL (so-called T-zone variant). It is also often seen in ALCL. Other lesions with prominent paracortical pattern include DLBCL (variant with interfollicular lymph node involvement), EMT, BPDCN, Castleman's disease, plasma cell neoplasms involving lymph nodes, cHL, metastatic tumors, HCL, mast cell disease, and LCH. Occasional cases of T-lymphoblastic lymphoma (T-LBL) show interfollicular pattern of involvement (Figure 18.4 in Chapter 18).

Summary of FC phenotypic profiles in paracortical infiltrate in LN:

DLBCL: CD19$^+$, CD20$^+$, surface light-chain immunoglobulin$^+$, CD5$^{-/rarely+}$, CD10$^{+/-}$, CD11c$^{-/rarely+}$, CD23$^-$, CD25$^{-/rarely+}$, CD38$^+$, CD43$^{-/+}$, CD71$^{+(dim\ or\ rarely\ strong)}$, CD81$^{+(dim)}$, CD200$^{-/rarely\ +(dim)}$

Early AITL: CD2$^{+/-}$, CD3$^{+/-}$, CD4$^+$, CD5$^{+/-}$, CD7$^{+/-}$, CD8$^-$, CD10$^{+/rarely-}$, CD30$^-$, CD45$^+$, CD56$^-$, CD81$^+$, CD200$^+$

Classic HL: predominance of small T-cells with normal phenotype

ALCL: high forward scatter, CD2$^{+/rarely-}$, CD3$^{+/-}$, CD4$^+$ or less often CD8$^+$ (rare tumors are either CD4/8$^-$ or CD4/CD8$^+$), CD5$^{+/-}$, CD7$^{-/rarely+}$, CD10$^-$, CD25$^{+/-}$, CD26$^{+/rarely-}$, CD30$^+$, CD43$^+$, CD45$^+$, CD56$^{-/rarely+}$

EMT: CD13$^+$, CD33$^+$, CD34$^{+/rarely-}$, CD117$^+$, CD133$^{+/-}$, MPO$^+$, CD81$^{+/-}$, HLA-DR$^{+/rarely-}$

BPDCN: CD4$^+$, CD13$^-$, CD33$^{-/+}$, CD56$^{+(strong)}$, CD123$^{+(strong)}$, CD11b$^-$, CD11c$^-$, HLA-DR$^+$, CD45$^+$, TdT$^{-/+}$, MPO$^-$, CD64$^-$

PTCL: CD2$^{+/-}$, CD3$^{+/-}$, CD4$^{+/-}$, CD5$^{+/-}$, CD7$^{-/+}$, CD8$^{-/+}$, CD10$^-$, CD30$^{-/rarely+}$, CD38$^+$, CD45$^+$, CD56$^{-/rarely+}$

Metastatic carcinoma: CD45$^-$, CD56$^{+/-}$, CD117$^{-/+}$, CD38$^{-/+}$, keratin$^+$

PCM: surface light-chain immunoglobulins$^-$, cytoplasmic light-chain immunoglobulins$^+$, cytoplasmic heavy chain immunoglobulins$^{+/-}$, CD38$^{+(bright)}$, CD138$^{+(bright)}$, CD56$^{+/rarely-}$, CD117$^{+/-}$, CD45$^{-/rarely+}$, CD20$^{-/rarely+}$, CD19$^-$, CD200$^{+/-}$

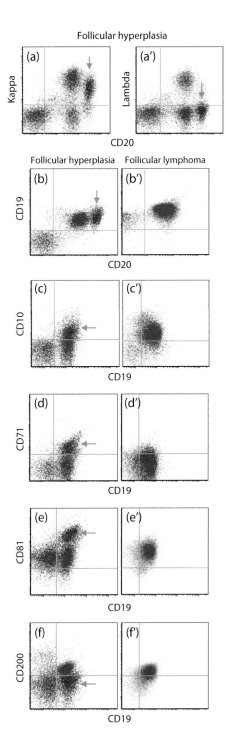

FIGURE 10.12 Comparison of flow cytometry pattern in follicular hyperplasia and follicular lymphoma (FL). Occasional cases of follicular hyperplasia show prominent population of CD10+ germinal center cells which show excess of kappa expression (a, a′; blue dots, arrow), and less often lambda excess. Follicular hyperplasia differs from FL by presence of population of B-cells with brighter CD20 expression (b, arrow), expression of CD10 on minor subset of B-cells (c, arrow), positive expression of CD71 on majority of germinal center cells (d, arrow), strong expression of CD81 (e, arrow), and lack of expression of CD200 by germinal center cells (f, arrow). Follicular lymphomas usually show homogenous expression of CD20 (b′) and CD10 (c′), lack of CD71 (d′), dim expression of CD81 (e′), and negative or dim expression of CD200 (f′).

T-ALL: CD1a[-/+], CD2+, surface CD3[-/rare cases+], cytoplasmic CD3+, CD4-/CD8- or CD4+/CD8+, CD5[+/-], CD7+, CD10[-/+], CD13[-/rarely+], CD15[-/rarely+], CD33[-/rarely+], CD34[+/-], CD38+, CD56[-/rare cases+], CD71[-/+], CD79a[-/rarely+], CD117-, CD123-, HLA-DR-, MPO-, TdT[+/rarely-]

Intrasinusoidal pattern

An intrasinusoidal pattern is typical for ALCL, metastatic non-hematopoietic tumors, occasional cases of DLBCL, intravascular large B-cell lymphoma (IVLBL), hepatosplenic T-cell lymphoma (HSTL), some cases of HC and variants of PTCL. In IVLBL tumor cells display mature B-cell phenotype expressing CD45, CD20 and other B-cell markers. The expression of CD20 is strong but rare CD20- cases have been reported. Majority of cases show a non-germinal center phenotype with MUM1 expression (75%–80%) [43]. Rare cases may be positive for CD30, display germinal center B-cell-like phenotype with CD10/BCL6 immunoreactivity (CD10 and BCL6 expression was noted in 13%–22% and 22%–26%, respectively) [43, 44]. Recent series by Matsue et al. did not report CD10 expression in IVLBL [45]. There is aberrant CD5 expression in significant proportion of cases (38%–47%) [43, 45, 46], more often than DLBCL, NOS. Ki-67 usually ranges from 60% to 100%. PD-L1 positivity is appreciated in 44%–50% of cases. Rare cases of cHL may show intrasinusoidal. Cutaneous CD30+ T-cell lymphoproliferations, such as lymphomatoid papulosis (LyP) and primary cutaneous ALCL (C-ALCL) can involve local lymph nodes with sinusoidal infiltration mimicking cHL or systemic ALCL.

Summary of FC phenotypic profiles in intrasinusoidal infiltrate in LN:

HTCL: CD2+, CD3+, CD4-/CD8- (rare cases are CD4-/CD8+), CD5-, CD7+, CD16[-/rarely+], CD56+, CD57-, TCRγδ+

DLBCL: CD19+, CD20[+/rarely-], surface light-chain immunoglobulin+, CD5[+/-], CD10[+/-], CD11c[-/rarely+], CD23-, CD25[-/rarely+], CD38+, CD43[-/+], CD71[+(dim or rarely strong)], CD81[+(dim)], CD200[-/rarely +(dim)]

IVLBL: CD19+, CD20+, surface light-chain immunoglobulin+, CD5[-/rarely+], CD10[+/-], CD30[-/rarely+],

ALCL and C-ALCL: high forward scatter, CD2[+/rarely-], CD3[+/-], CD4+ or less often CD8+ (rare tumors are either CD4/8- or CD4/CD8+), CD5[+/-], CD7[-/rarely+], CD10-, CD25[+/-], CD26[+/rarely-], CD30+, CD43+, CD45+, CD56[-/rarely+]

Metastatic carcinoma: CD45-, CD56[+/-], CD117[-/+], CD38[-/+], keratin+

Anaplastic infiltrate

Anaplastic infiltrate is characterized by highly atypical, pleomorphic, often bizarre cells with hyperchromatic nuclei and prominent nucleoli. Anaplastic features can be seen in anaplastic variant of DLBCL, anaplastic lymphoma kinase (ALK)+ DLBCL, ALK+ ALCL, ALK- ALCL, anaplastic (poorly differentiated) plasma cell myeloma (PCM), cHL, nodular sclerosis (syncytial variant), cHL, lymphocyte-depleted type), Langerhans cell sarcoma, anaplastic carcinoma and rare cases of EMT (myeloid sarcoma). ALCL is characterized by positive CD30 expression and aberrant expression of T-cell markers. Many cases show positive CD38 and CD71. DLBCL is positive for B-cell markers, CD38, HLA-DR and surface light-chain immunoglobulins. CD71 expression in DLBCL is usually partially dim, but occasional cases (especially with anaplastic or "high-grade" features) may show bright CD71 (Figure 10.8).

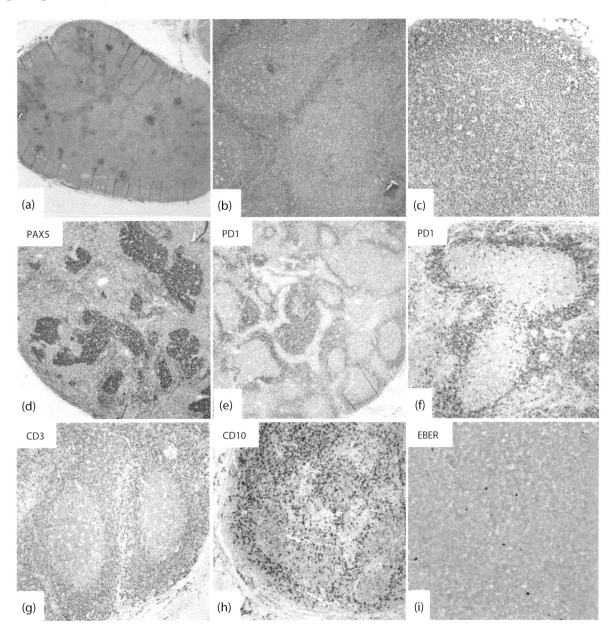

FIGURE 10.13 Perifollicular AITL with reactive germinal centers. The histologic section shows lymph node with numerous reactive germinal centers (a–c). The reactive B-cell follicles are positive for PAX5 (d). Neoplastic T-cell population is identified by immunostaining with PD1 (e–f, low and intermediate magnification), CD3 (g), and CD10 (h). Note dimmer expression of CD3 by neoplastic T-cells (immediately around the follicles) when compared to reactive T-cells in the background (g). The expression of CD10 is stronger among AITL cells than in germinal center cells (h). Scattered EBV-infected cells are noted by EBER (ISH) staining (i).

Anaplastic lymphoid infiltrate may be also seen in subset of ATLL and transformed mycosis fungoides.

Summary of FC phenotypic profiles in anaplastic infiltrate in LN:

DLBCL ("anaplastic" variant): CD19$^+$, CD20$^{+/rarely-}$, surface light-chain immunoglobulin$^+$, CD5$^{+/-}$, CD10$^{+/-}$, CD11c$^{-/rarely+}$, CD23$^-$, CD25$^{-/rarely+}$, CD38$^+$, CD43$^{-/+}$, CD71$^{+(dim\ or\ rarely\ strong)}$, CD81$^{+(dim)}$, CD200$^{-/rarely\ +(dim)}$

ALCL: high forward scatter, CD2$^{+/rarely-}$, CD3$^{+/-}$, CD4$^+$ or less often CD8$^+$ (rare tumors are either CD4/8$^-$ or CD4/CD8$^+$), CD5$^{+/-}$, CD7$^{-/rarely+}$, CD10$^-$, CD25$^{+/-}$, CD26$^{+/rarely-}$, CD30$^+$, CD43$^+$, CD45$^+$, CD56$^{-/rarely+}$

PCM ("anaplastic" variant): surface light-chain immunoglobulins$^-$, cytoplasmic light-chain immunoglobulins$^+$, cytoplasmic heavy chain immunoglobulins$^{+/-}$, CD38$^{+(bright)}$, CD138$^{+(bright)}$, CD56$^{+/rarely-}$, CD117$^{+/-}$, CD45$^{-/rarely+}$, CD20$^{-/rarely+}$, CD19$^-$, CD200$^{+/-}$

ATLL: CD2$^{+/-}$, CD3$^{+/-}$, CD4$^+$ (rarely CD4/CD8$^+$), CD5$^+$, CD7$^-$, CD8$^-$, CD25$^+$, CD26$^-$, CD30$^{+/-}$, CD45$^+$, CD56$^-$, CD57$^-$

Histiocyte-rich infiltrate

Numerous histiocytes are typically seen in reactive conditions, including sinus histiocytosis, infections, cat-scratch disease, tuberculosis, fungal lymphadenitis, toxoplasma lymphadenitis, sarcoidosis, dermatopathic lymphadenitis, Kikuchi lymphadenitis, and Rosai-Dorfman disease. Toxoplasmosis is characterized by prominent follicular hyperplasia with increased large cells and macrophages with tingible bodies, aggregates of monocytoid B-cells, plasma cells, and activated lymphocytes (immunoblasts) in medullary cords, and small granulomas, which are present in interfollicular and paracortical areas and often infiltrate reactive follicles. Sarcoidosis is characterized by granulomas in which some epithelioid cells contain crystalloid structures forming so-called asteroid body. Histiocytes with large vesicular nuclei, prominent nucleoli, abundant pale "wispy" or frothy cytoplasm, and engulfed lymphoid cells (emperipolesis or lymphocytophagocytosis) are typical for Rosai-Dorfman disease (sinus histiocytosis with massive lymphadenopathy [47]. Histiocytes in Rosai-Dorfman disease are positive for S100, CD4, CD11c, CD68, and CD163 and do not express CD1a or Langerin. Differential diagnosis of Rosai-Dorfman disease includes LCH, which is characterized by positive S100, CD1, and Langerin (CD207). Occasional hematolymphoid neoplasms have histiocyte-rich background or numerous histiocytic aggregates (granuloma-like). Those include histiocyte-rich large B-cell lymphoma (also called T-cell rich/histiocyte-rich large B-cell lymphoma; THRLBL), Lennert's lymphoma (a variant of PTCL), DLBCL with granulomas, NLPHL, and cHL. In lymph nodes involved by THRLBL, FC is most often negative, which is associated with paucity of neoplastic B-cells and predominance of reactive elements (T-cells and histiocytes), similar to cHL or NLPHL. By using FC sorting, Glynn and Fromm characterized immunophenotypic features of neoplastic B-cells in THRLBL: lack of surface immunoglobulins and overexpression of CD40, CD50, and CD54 when compared to DLBCL [48].

HS is a malignant tumor of the macrophage lineage. It occurs in lymph nodes and extranodal locations including skin, abdominal organs (intestinal tract), soft tissue, bone, and spleen. Morphologically, HS consists of large cell with diffuse, non-cohesive growth pattern or intrasinusoidal pattern. HSs are positive for CD4, CD11c, CD14, CD43, CD45, CD68, CD163, HAM56, lysozyme, and HLA-DR. Neoplastic cells lack the immunoreactivity with B- and T-cell markers. LCH is an "inflammatory" heterogeneous myeloid neoplasm of CD1a+/CD207+/S100+ dendritic cells (Langerhans cells) involving various organs in both children and adults. Langerhans cells express CD1a, S100, CD207, vimentin, HLA-DR, Langerin, and CD45. The expression of CD68 is weak and focal.

References

1. Jevremovic, D., et al., *CD5+ B-cell lymphoproliferative disorders: Beyond chronic lymphocytic leukemia and mantle cell lymphoma.* Leuk Res, 2010. **34**(9): p. 1235–8.
2. Sandes, A.F., et al., *CD200 has an important role in the differential diagnosis of mature B-cell neoplasms by multiparameter flow cytometry.* Cytometry B Clin Cytom, 2014. **86**(2): p. 98–105.
3. D'Arena, G., et al., *CD200 included in a 4-marker modified Matutes score provides optimal sensitivity and specificity for the diagnosis of chronic lymphocytic leukaemia.* Hematol Oncol, 2018. **36**(3): p. 543–6.
4. Mora, A., et al., *CD200 is a useful marker in the diagnosis of chronic lymphocytic leukemia.* Cytometry B Clin Cytom, 2019. **96**(2): p. 143–8.
5. Kohnke, T., et al., *Diagnosis of CLL revisited: increased specificity by a modified five-marker scoring system including CD200.* Br J Haematol, 2017. **179**(3): p. 480–7.
6. Kelemen, K., et al., *CD23+ mantle cell lymphoma: a clinical pathologic entity associated with superior outcome compared with CD23- disease.* Am J Clin Pathol, 2008. **130**(2): p. 166–77.
7. Hu, Z., et al., *CD200 expression in mantle cell lymphoma identifies a unique subgroup of patients with frequent IGHV mutations, absence of SOX11 expression, and an indolent clinical course.* Mod Pathol, 2018. **31**(2): p. 327–36.
8. Sorigue, M., et al., *Positive predictive value of CD200 positivity in the differential diagnosis of chronic lymphocytic leukemia.* Cytometry B Clin Cytom, 2019. **98**(5): p. 441–8.
9. Kraus, T.S., et al., *The role of CD11c expression in the diagnosis of mantle cell lymphoma.* Am J Clin Pathol, 2010. **134**(2): p. 271–7.
10. Falay, M., et al., *The role of CD200 and CD43 expression in differential diagnosis between chronic lymphocytic leukemia and mantle cell lymphoma.* Turk J Haematol, 2018. **35**(2): p. 94–98.
11. Kilo, M.N. and D.M. Dorfman, *The utility of flow cytometric immunophenotypic analysis in the distinction of small lymphocytic lymphoma/chronic lymphocytic leukemia from mantle cell lymphoma.* Am J Clin Pathol, 1996. **105**(4): p. 451–7.
12. Baseggio, L., et al., *CD5 expression identifies a subset of splenic marginal zone lymphomas with higher lymphocytosis: a clinico-pathological, cytogenetic and molecular study of 24 cases.* Haematologica, 2010. **95**(4): p. 604–12.
13. Jaso, J., et al., *CD5-positive mucosa-associated lymphoid tissue (MALT) lymphoma: a clinicopathologic study of 14 cases.* Hum Pathol, 2012. **43**(9): p. 1436–43.
14. Kojima, M., et al., *Characteristics of CD5-positive splenic marginal zone lymphoma with leukemic manifestation; clinical, flow cytometry, and histopathological findings of 11 cases.* J Clin Exp Hematop, 2010. **50**(2): p. 107–12.
15. Xochelli, A., et al., *Clonal B-cell lymphocytosis exhibiting immunophenotypic features consistent with a marginal-zone origin: is this a distinct entity?* Blood, 2014. **123**(8): p. 1199–206.
16. Campuzano-Zuluaga, G., et al., *Frequency and extent of CD30 expression in diffuse large B-cell lymphoma and its relation to clinical and biologic factors: a retrospective study of 167 cases.* Leuk Lymphoma, 2013. **54**(11): p. 2405–11.
17. Schmitz, R., et al., *Genetics and pathogenesis of diffuse large B-cell lymphoma.* N Engl J Med, 2018. **378**(15): p. 1396–407.
18. Gutierrez-Garcia, G., et al., *Gene-expression profiling and not immunophenotypic algorithms predicts prognosis in patients with diffuse large B-cell lymphoma treated with immunochemotherapy.* Blood, 2011. **117**(18): p. 4836–43.
19. Thieblemont, C., et al., *The germinal center/activated B-cell sub-classification has a prognostic impact for response to salvage therapy in relapsed/refractory diffuse large B-cell lymphoma: a bio-CORAL study.* J Clin Oncol, 2011. **29**(31): p. 4079–87.
20. Hwang, H.S., et al., *High concordance of gene expression profiling-correlated immunohistochemistry algorithms in diffuse large B-cell lymphoma, not otherwise specified.* Am J Surg Pathol, 2014. **38**(8): p. 1046–57.
21. Choi, W.W., et al., *A new immunostain algorithm classifies diffuse large B-cell lymphoma into molecular subtypes with high accuracy.* Clin Cancer Res, 2009. **15**(17): p. 5494–502.
22. Alizadeh, A.A., et al., *Distinct types of diffuse large B-cell lymphoma identified by gene expression profiling.* Nature, 2000. **403**(6769): p. 503–11.
23. Talaulikar, D., et al., *Clinical role of flow cytometry in redefining bone marrow involvement in diffuse large B-cell lymphoma (DLBCL) – a new perspective.* Histopathology, 2008. **52**(3): p. 340–7.
24. Xu, Y., R.W. McKenna, and S.H. Kroft, *Comparison of multiparameter flow cytometry with cluster analysis and immunohistochemistry for the detection of CD10 in diffuse large B-cell lymphomas.* Mod Pathol, 2002. **15**(4): p. 413–9.
25. Tsagarakis, N.J., et al., *Contribution of immunophenotype to the investigation and differential diagnosis of Burkitt lymphoma, double-hit high grade B-cell lymphoma, and single-hit MYC-rearranged diffuse large B-cell lymphoma.* Cytometry B Clin Cytom, 2020. **98**(5): p. 412–20.

26. McGowan, P., et al., *Differentiating between Burkitt lymphoma and CD10+ diffuse large B-cell lymphoma: the role of commonly used flow cytometry cell markers and the application of a multiparameter scoring system.* Am J Clin Pathol, 2012. **137**(4): p. 665–70.

27. Tomita, N., et al., *Diffuse large B cell lymphoma without immunoglobulin light chain restriction by flow cytometry.* Acta Haematol, 2009. **121**(4): p. 196–201.

28. Johnson, N.A., et al., *Diffuse large B-cell lymphoma: reduced CD20 expression is associated with an inferior survival.* Blood, 2009. **113**(16): p. 3773–80.

29. Schniederjan, S.D., et al., *A novel flow cytometric antibody panel for distinguishing Burkitt lymphoma from CD10+ diffuse large B-cell lymphoma.* Am J Clin Pathol, 2010. **133**(5): p. 718–26.

30. Cardoso, C.C., et al., *The importance of CD39, CD43, CD81, and CD95 expression for differentiating B cell lymphoma by flow cytometry.* Cytometry B Clin Cytom, 2018. **94**(3): p. 451–8.

31. Alikhan, M., et al., *Peripheral T-cell lymphomas of follicular helper T-cell type frequently display an aberrant CD3(–/dim)CD4(+) population by flow cytometry: an important clue to the diagnosis of a Hodgkin lymphoma mimic.* Mod Pathol, 2016. **29**(10): p. 1173–82.

32. Stacchini, A., et al., *The usefulness of flow cytometric CD10 detection in the differential diagnosis of peripheral T-cell lymphomas.* Am J Clin Pathol, 2007. **128**(5): p. 854–64.

33. Karube, K., et al., *Usefulness of flow cytometry for differential diagnosis of precursor and peripheral T-cell and NK-cell lymphomas: analysis of 490 cases.* Pathol Int, 2008. **58**(2): p. 89–97.

34. Pileri, S., et al., *Histiocytic necrotizing lymphadenitis without granulocytic infiltration.* Virchows Arch A Pathol Anat Histol, 1982. **395**(3): p. 257–71.

35. Felgar, R.E., et al., *Histiocytic necrotizing lymphadenitis (Kikuchi's disease): in situ end-labeling, immunohistochemical, and serologic evidence supporting cytotoxic lymphocyte-mediated apoptotic cell death.* Mod Pathol, 1997. **10**(3): p. 231–41.

36. Menasce, L.P., et al., *Histiocytic necrotizing lymphadenitis (Kikuchi-Fujimoto disease): continuing diagnostic difficulties.* Histopathology, 1998. **33**(3): p. 248–54.

37. Tsang, W.Y., J.K. Chan, and C.S. Ng, *Kikuchi's lymphadenitis. A morphologic analysis of 75 cases with special reference to unusual features.* Am J Surg Pathol, 1994. **18**(3): p. 219–31.

38. Scott, G.D., et al., *Histology-independent signature distinguishes Kikuchi-Fujimoto disease/systemic lupus erythematosus-associated lymphadenitis from benign and malignant lymphadenopathies.* Am J Clin Pathol, 2020. **154**(2): p. 215–24.

39. Moench, L., et al., *Double- and triple-hit lymphomas can present with features suggestive of immaturity, including TdT expression, and create diagnostic challenges.* Leuk Lymphoma, 2016. **57**(11): p. 2626–35.

40. Snuderl, M., et al., *B-cell lymphomas with concurrent IGH-BCL2 and MYC rearrangements are aggressive neoplasms with clinical and pathologic features distinct from Burkitt lymphoma and diffuse large B-cell lymphoma.* Am J Surg Pathol, 2010. **34**(3): p. 327–40.

41. Wu, D., et al., *"Double-Hit" mature B-cell lymphomas show a common immunophenotype by flow cytometry that includes decreased CD20 expression.* Am J Clin Pathol, 2010. **134**(2): p. 258–65.

42. Alsuwaidan, A., et al., *Bright CD38 expression by flow cytometric analysis is a biomarker for double/triple hit lymphomas with a moderate sensitivity and high specificity.* Cytometry B Clin Cytom, 2019. **96**(5): p. 368–74.

43. Murase, T., et al., *Intravascular large B-cell lymphoma (IVLBCL): a clinicopathologic study of 96 cases with special reference to the immunophenotypic heterogeneity of CD5.* Blood, 2007. **109**(2): p. 478–85.

44. Yegappan, S., et al., *Angiotropic lymphoma: an immunophenotypically and clinically heterogeneous lymphoma.* Mod Pathol, 2001. **14**(11): p. 1147–56.

45. Matsue, K., et al., *Diagnosis of intravascular large B cell lymphoma: novel insights into clinicopathological features from 42 patients at a single institution over 20 years.* Br J Haematol, 2019. **187**(3): p. 328–36.

46. Masaki, Y., et al., *Intravascular large B cell lymphoma: proposed of the strategy for early diagnosis and treatment of patients with rapid deteriorating condition.* Int J Hematol, 2009. **89**(5): p. 600–10.

47. Rosai, J. and R.F. Dorfman, *Sinus histiocytosis with massive lymphadenopathy. A newly recognized benign clinicopathological entity.* Arch Pathol, 1969. **87**(1): p. 63–70.

48. Glynn, E. and J.R. Fromm, *Immunophenotypic characterization and purification of neoplastic cells from lymph nodes involved by T-cell/histiocyte-rich large B-cell lymphoma by flow cytometry and flow cytometric cell sorting.* Cytometry B Clin Cytom, 2020. **98**(1): p. 88–98.

11

MOLECULAR-FLOW CYTOMETRIC CORRELATION

Introduction – Overview of genetic testing

Conventional cytogenetics, fluorescence in situ hybridization (FISH), and molecular testing by polymerase chain reaction (PCR) play an important and ever-expanding role in the diagnosis, prognostication, and monitoring patients with hematopoietic neoplasms (Tables 11.1 and 11.2). Flow cytometry (FC) pattern in some cases may be characteristic enough to suggest a neoplasm with specific molecular (genetic) changes (Table 11.3). Final diagnosis, nevertheless, should always be based on a combination of morphology, phenotype, and genetic testing.

Fluorescence in situ hybridization (FISH)

FISH uses test probes against target DNA in the nucleus of interphase cells or metaphase chromosomes. FISH allows the analysis of specific DNA changes in tissues (cells) or intact chromosomes and does not require metaphase chromosomes. Many of the clinical applications of FISH include chromosome enumeration using a-satellite probes (e.g., gain or loss of a chromosome), marker identification, genes mapping, deletion, amplification, or translocation as well as whole chromosome "painting". In hematologic malignancies, the most common chromosomal abnormalities targeted by FISH include t(9;22)/*BCR-ABL1* in chronic myeloid leukemia (CML) (and subset of acute myeloid leukemia [AML] and acute lymphoblastic leukemia [ALL]), t(15;17)/*PML-RARA* in acute promyelocytic leukemia (APL), t(14;18)/*IGH-BCL2* in follicular lymphoma (FL), t(11;14)/*CCND1-IGH* in mantle cell lymphoma (MCL), del(13q), del(11q), and del(17p)/*TP53* in chronic lymphocytic leukemia (CLL), del(5q) in myelodysplastic neoplasm (MDS) and AML, del(13q)*RB1*, t(11;14)/*CCND1-IGH*, and del(17p)*TP53* in plasma cell myeloma (PCM), t(8;14)/*MYC-IGH* in Burkitt lymphoma (BL), *MYC-IGH*, *BCL2* and *BCL6* rearrangements in high grade double or triple hit B-cell lymphomas, t(11;18)/*API2-MALT1* and t(14;18)/*IGH-MALT1* in marginal zone lymphoma (MALT lymphoma), t(8;21)/*RUNX1-RUNX1T1* in AML, inv16 in AML, and t(12;21)/*ETV6-RUNX1* in ALL.

The FISH probes can be generally subclassified into following categories: centromere-specific probes; whole chromosome ("painting") probes; single-copy (locus specific) genomic probes; and spectral karyotyping (SKY; multiplex metaphase FISH; multicolor FISH). Figure 11.1 presents introduction to analysis of FISH probes. FISH probes for chromosomal translocations are most widely used in evaluation of hematopoietic tumors. In the detection of translocation, two probes are labeled with different fluorochrome: normal cell will display four signals (two of each color), while cell with translocation will show two adjacent signals leading to different color of fluorescence signal. Dual-fusion probe consists of pair of probes labeled with two different colors (fluorochromes), green (e.g., FITC) and red (e.g., rhodamine) directed against translocations breakpoint regions in the two different genes involved in a reciprocal translocation. In normal cell there are two green and two red signals corresponding to two separate loci that are not in immediate proximity (no translocation). In cells with translocation between the targeted loci, there is one green and one red signal (normal chromosome) and one yellow signal indicating the fusion between two loci (yellow fluorescence being the result of overlap between green and red signals). Variant and complex pattern may be also identified and provide additional clinical information on the underlying chromosomal changes. Third color may be used to label specific chromosome (for example chromosome 9 in *BCR-ABL1* analysis; Figure 11.2). In the case of break-apart (BA) probe, the target DNA is labeled with two different probes directed at two opposite areas of the gene (3′ and 5′). The interpretation of results is opposite to that with fusion probes: fusion (yellow) signal is normal, and separate green and red signals indicate translocation (BA). The fusion of the signal seen as different colors (e.g., yellow) would indicate the normal allele, whereas the two different signals (e.g., red and green) would indicate the presence of translocation. The counterstain using either propidium iodide (PI) or DAPI can be used to identify chromosomes. Commonly used BA probes in hematologic tumors include *MLL*-BA (AML/ALL), *CBFB*-BA (AML), *RARA*-BA (APL), *MYC*-BA (BL and BCLU), *MALT1*-BA (MALT lymphoma), *ALK*-BA (ALCL), and *IGH*-BA (NHL/PCM).

Polymerase chain reaction (PCR)

PCR developed by Mullis and Faloona is a core technique for most tests used in molecular diagnostics [1–3]. It targets a segment of DNA (or RNA in reverse-transcriptase PCR) and produces multiple copies (usually between 10^7 and 10^{11}) of a DNA region of interest. PCR enables the detection of malignant cells below the threshold of karyotyping or morphology, even when combined with immunophenotyping. Fresh tissue is the best source of tissue for PCR analysis, but fixed tissue (formalin, ethanol) may also be used. Carnoy's, Zanker's, B5, and Bouin's fixatives are suboptimal for PCR. Tissues exposed to decalcifying solutions (e.g., bone marrow [BM] trephine core biopsy) are not suitable for PCR analysis. Three major steps in PCR include denaturation of double-stranded DNA into single-stranded DNA (ssDNA), hybridization (annealing) of oligonucleotide primers to both ends of a target sequence, and a synthesis achieved by addition of four nucleotide bases and a *Taq* polymerase. A PCR reaction usually involves 30–40 cycles. The denaturation is achieved by high temperature (95°C), which, by breaking the hydrogen bonds between complementary bases, creates single-stranded DNA. In the next step, the two primers join (hybridize) the single-stranded template DNA. In the final step (synthesis), *Taq* polymerase synthesizes new DNA strands, using the oligonucleotide primers as starting points.

Diagnosis of B-cell lymphomas is based most often on histomorphology and immunophenotyping (FC and/or immunohistochemistry), but many cases require also genetic testing for either more definite diagnosis and/or for subclassification. Assessment of clonality by immunoglobulin gene rearrangement is crucial in establishing the definite diagnosis in cases with atypical (ambiguous) histology and phenotype, very early (incipient) lymphoproliferations, pleomorphic infiltrate with paucity of neoplastic cells, low-grade B-cell lymphoproliferations, which may be difficult to diagnose based on morphology or cases with insufficient amount of tissue for morphologic/phenotypic analysis.

DOI: 10.1201/9781003197935-11

TABLE 11.1: Most Common Chromosomal and Molecular Changes in the Diagnosis of Hematopoietic Malignancies

Marker	Neoplasm
*ALK1-NPM/*t(2;5)	Anaplastic large cell lymphoma (ALCL), ALK1+
BCR-ABL1 /t(9;22)	Chronic myeloid leukemia (CML) in blast crisis
	Acute myeloid leukemia (AML)
	Acute lymphoblastic leukemia (ALL)
*BCL2-IGH/*t(14;18)	Follicular lymphoma (FL)
	Diffuse large B-cell lymphoma (DLBCL), subset
BRAF mutation	Hairy cell leukemia
CALR mutations	Essential thrombocythemia (ET)
	Primary myelofibrosis (PMF)
CSF3R mutations	Chronic neutrophilic leukemia (CNL)
	Occasional atypical CML (*BCR-ABL1*−)
del(5q)/del(5)	Myelodysplastic syndrome (MDS)
	5(q)-syndrome (MDS with isolated 5q deletion)
	AML, therapy related myeloid neoplasm
del(7q)/del(7)	AML, MDS, therapy-related myeloid neoplasm
del(13)	Chronic lymphocytic leukemia (CLL)
	Plasma cell myeloma (PCM)
del(17p)	Various neoplasms (poor prognosis)
i(7q)	Hepatosplenic T-cell lymphoma (HSTL)
inv(14) [*TCL1*]	T-cell prolymphocytic leukemia (T-PLL)
inv(16)/t(16;16)	AML with *CBFB-MYH11* (AMML with eosinophilia)
JAK2 mutation	Polycythemia vera (PV), ET, PMF
KTM2A (MLL) translocation	AML, ALL, mixed phenotype acute leukemia (MPAL)
	Specific *KMT2A* fusion partners are associated with the disease phenotype (lymphoblastic versus myeloid)
*MYC-IGH/*t(8;14)	Burkitt lymphoma
	Subset of DLBCL
NPM1 mutations	AML with *NPM1*
*PML-RARA/*t(15;17)	Acute promyelocytic leukemia (APL)
t(8;21)/*RUNX1-RUNX1T1*	AML with *RUNX1-RUNX1T1*
t(9;14)/*PAX5-IGH*	Lymphoplasmacytic lymphoma (LPL)
t(11;14)	Mantle cell lymphoma (MCL)
	PCM, subset
t(11;18)/*API2-MALT1*	Extranodal marginal zone B-cell lymphoma (MALT type)

T-cell lymphoproliferative disorders may display rearrangements of one, two, three, or four *TCR* genes. PCR analysis of *TCRB* and *TCRG* genes is most often used to confirm clonality, whereas *TCRD* is rarely used. *TCRA* gene is usually not targeted. The results of molecular tests for T-cell clonality have to be correlated with relevant clinical and laboratory information, including morphology and phenotype. Detection of clonality is not an equivalent of malignancy, since clonal T-cell population can be identified in nonmalignant conditions, including large granular lymphocytosis, immunodeficiency-associated disorders, autoimmune disorders,

TABLE 11.2: Mutations in Myeloid Neoplasms

	AML	MPN (not-CML)	MDS	MDS/MPN	CNL
FLT3	+		Rare cases (1%)	Rare cases (4%)	
NPM1	+		Rare cases (2%)	Rare cases (3%)	
CEBPA	+				
TET2		Rare cases	+	+	
SETBP1	+ (secondary)		+ (secondary)	+ (aCML)	
SRSF2			+	+	
SF3B1			+ (RARS)	+	
ASHL1		Rare cases	+	+	
DNMT3A	+	+	+	+	
JAK2		+	rare cases	+/−	
CALR		+ (ET, PMF)	rare cases (8%)		
CSF3R	aCML (subset)				+

Abbreviations: AML, acute myeloid leukemia; MPN, myeloproliferative neoplasm; MDS, myelodysplastic syndrome; CNL, chronic neutrophilic leukemia.

TABLE 11.3: Molecular (Genetic) Flow Cytometric Correlation

Molecular (Genetic Changes)	Flow Cytometry Features	Diagnosis
BCR-ABL1 [t(9;22)]	Blood: Increased myeloid to lymphoid ratio, eosinophilia (low forward scatter, high side scatter, CD10$^-$, CD16$^-$, CD13$^+$, CD11b$^+$, CD33$^+$); rare myeloblasts; rare immature B-cells; basophilia (CD11b$^+$, CD13$^+$, CD33$^+$, CD22$^+$); decreased expression of CD10, Cd11b and/or CD16 on granulocytes; partial CD56 expression on granulocytes	CML (*BCR-ABL1*$^+$)
IgH-CCND1 [t(11;14)]	Clonal B-cells with moderate CD20, moderate kappa or lambda expression, positive CD5, negative CD23, positive CD81, negative CD200 and positive CD38.	MCL
IgH-MYC [t(8;14)]	Clonal B-cells with positive CD10, positive CD71, negative BCL2 and moderate to bright CD20	BL
KTM2A (MLL) rearrangement	Depending on fusion partner, leukemia may show myeloid, lymphoid or mixed phenotype features. B-ALL blasts population may be accompanied by blasts with monocytic differentiation[a]	B-ALL, AML, T-ALL. Mixed phenotype acute leukemia (MPAL), often B-ALL/myeloid (monoblastic)
NPM1 mutations	Myeloblasts are often HLA-DR-negative, CD34-neagative, CD117$^+$ and may show monocytic differentiation	AML with *NPM1* mutation
PML-RARA [t(15;17)]	Atypical promyelocytes with high side scatter, moderate CD45, positive CD117, negative CD34, negative HLA-DR, negative CD4 and CD7, and negative CD11c	APL
RUNX1-RUNX1T1 [t(8;21)]	Myeloblasts (CD34$^+$, CD117$^+$, HLA-DR$^+$) are often positive for CD19 and CD56	AML with *RUNX1-RUNX1T1*
TCL1 translocations [t(14;14)]	Increased T-cells with CD4 or CD8 restriction (rarely CD4/CD8$^-$ or CD/CD8$^+$) and often normal expression of T-cell antigens	T-PLL

[a] Differential diagnosis between normal (mature) monocytes and neoplastic monocytes in cases of B-ALL versus MPAL may be difficult. Acute leukemia with KTM2A fusion often display "lineage plasticity" with phenotypic switch between myeloid and lymphoid lineages during the course of the disease.

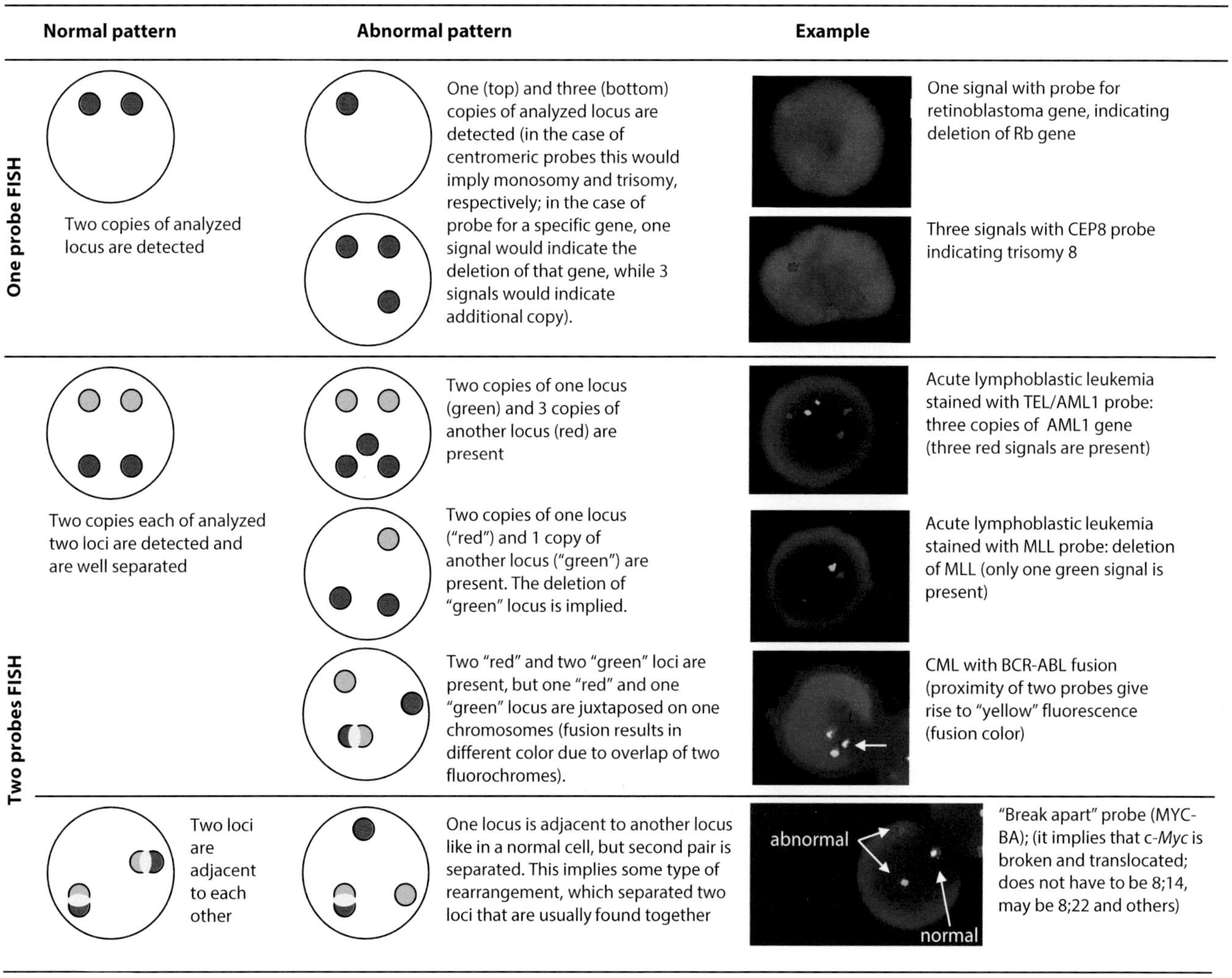

	Normal pattern	Abnormal pattern	Example

One probe FISH

Two copies of analyzed locus are detected

One (top) and three (bottom) copies of analyzed locus are detected (in the case of centromeric probes this would imply monosomy and trisomy, respectively; in the case of probe for a specific gene, one signal would indicate the deletion of that gene, while 3 signals would indicate additional copy).

One signal with probe for retinoblastoma gene, indicating deletion of Rb gene

Three signals with CEP8 probe indicating trisomy 8

Two probes FISH

Two copies each of analyzed two loci are detected and are well separated

Two copies of one locus (green) and 3 copies of another locus (red) are present

Acute lymphoblastic leukemia stained with TEL/AML1 probe: three copies of AML1 gene (three red signals are present)

Two copies of one locus ("red") and 1 copy of another locus ("green") are present. The deletion of "green" locus is implied.

Acute lymphoblastic leukemia stained with MLL probe: deletion of MLL (only one green signal is present)

Two "red" and two "green" loci are present, but one "red" and one "green" locus are juxtaposed on one chromosomes (fusion results in different color due to overlap of two fluorochromes).

CML with BCR-ABL fusion (proximity of two probes give rise to "yellow" fluorescence (fusion color)

Two loci are adjacent to each other

One locus is adjacent to another locus like in a normal cell, but second pair is separated. This implies some type of rearrangement, which separated two loci that are usually found together

"Break apart" probe (MYC-BA); (it implies that c-*Myc* is broken and translocated; does not have to be 8;14, may be 8;22 and others)

FIGURE 11.1 Interpretation of FISH results.

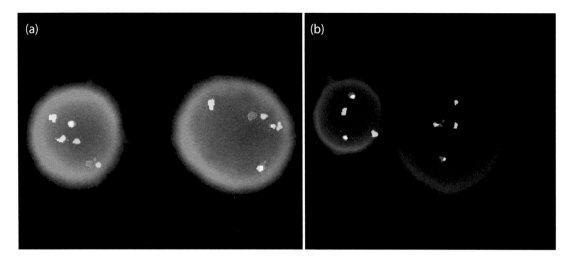

FIGURE 11.2 FISH analysis for *BCR-ABL* using three-color probes: aqua for argininosuccinate synthetase 1 (*ASS1*) gene on chromosome 9q34, green for *BCR* gene on chromosome 22, and red for *ABL* gene on chromosome 22. Several positive signals (yellow) are seen in case of CML (a); control sample (b) shows two green signals for normal chromosome 22 and two red and blue signals close to each other for normal chromosome 9.

viral infections and in healthy (elderly) individuals [4–14]. With advancing age, healthy individuals frequently demonstrate large clonal expansions of CD8+ T cells in the blood, which persist for long periods of time and appear to be maintained as a population of memory cells [12, 14]. Clonal expansion of CD4+ T-cells is less common [11]. Rheumatoid arthritis patients exhibited a significantly increased frequency of T cell expansions both in the CD8+ and CD8− subsets [9]. The clonal activation of peripheral T cells was found to correlate with disease activity in patient with systemic lupus erythematosus [8]. Monoclonal T-cell population is frequently detected in patients with celiac disease-associated ulcerative jejunitis (both in ulcer and intervening mucosa) with the same clone being detected in subsequent enteropathy-associated T-cell lymphoma [5]. Benign cutaneous infiltrates, including pseudolymphomas, have been reported with clonal T-cell populations. For example, Ponti et al. reported clonality in 2.3% of benign inflammatory disease in the skin [15]. Clonal expansion of T-LGL cells is often seen in solid organ transplant recipients [16].

Next-generation sequencing (NGS)

Next-generation sequencing (NGS) helps to identify genomic, transcriptional, and epigenetic changes in patients with hematologic neoplasms, that play crucial role in diagnostic process, helps in prognostication and guides the treatment decisions [17–24].

On the basis of literature review and Working Group consensus, Li et al. proposed to group clinical and experimental evidence of molecular changes into four levels [18]:

1. **Level A,** biomarkers that predict response or resistance to US FDA-approved therapies for a specific type of tumor or have been included in professional guidelines as therapeutic, diagnostic, and/or prognostic biomarkers for specific types of tumors
2. **Level B,** biomarkers that predict response or resistance to a therapy based on well-powered studies with consensus from experts in the field, or have diagnostic and/or prognostic significance of certain diseases based on well powered studies with expert consensus

3. **Level C,** biomarkers that predict response or resistance to therapies approved by FDA or professional associates for different tumor type (i.e., off-label use of a drug), serve as inclusion criteria for clinical trials, or have diagnostic and/or prognostic significance based on the results of multiple small studies
4. **Level D,** biomarkers that show plausible therapeutic significance based on preclinical studies or may assist disease diagnosis and/or prognosis themselves or along with other biomarkers based on small studies or multiple case reports with no consensus.

Somatic variants can be further subclassified into 4 tiers, based on their level of clinical significance in diagnosis, prognosis, and treatment in malignant neoplasms [18]:

- **Tier I** variants with strong clinical significance (includes level A and level B biomarkers).
  Examples of tier I mutations include the following:
  - *ASXL1* mutations are independently associated with an increased risk of leukemic transformation and decreased overall survival in myeloid malignancies (MDS, MDS/MPN, MPN); in AML *ASXL1* mutation is associated with decreased overall survival,
  - *BRAF* predicting response to vemurafenib in melanoma or HCL,
  - *CALR* helps determine the diagnosis of primary myelofibrosis (PMF) or essential thrombocythemia (ET); CALR mutations are associated with lower risk of thrombosis when compared to *JAK2-* or *MPL-*mutated ET; *CALR* type 1 mutations are associated with improved survival when compared to type 2,
  - *CBL* mutations may be associated with inferior prognosis in MDS/MPN,
  - *FLT3*-ITD predict poor prognosis in AML,
  - *JAK2* mutated PMF has been associated with intermediate prognosis and higher risk of leukemic transformation and thrombosis compared to *CALR*-mutated cases,
  - *KIT* is used to diagnose systemic mastocytosis (SM). *KIT* D816V mutation confers resistance to imatinib

mesylate and sunitinib, while response to other tyrosine kinase inhibitors remains under investigation,

- *NRAS* in AML and MDS indicate worse prognosis and possible progression from lower grade disease,
- *PML-RARA* predicts response to therapy with differentiation inducers (all-trans retinoic acid or arsenic),
- *RUNX1* p.Gln390Alafs*210 mutations are associated with increased risk of leukemic transformation, poor prognosis, and decreased overall survival in MDS,
- *SF3B1* is associated with MDS with ring sideroblasts and with mixed MDS/myeloproliferative neoplasm with ring sideroblasts and thrombocytosis (MDS/MPN-RS-T),
- *TET2* p.Glu1323 mutations may be predictive of improved responses to hypomethylating agents (e.g., Azacytidine),
- *TP53* predicts poor prognosis (decreased overall survival) in hematologic neoplasms,
- *U2AF1* mutations in MDS are associated with decreased overall survival and increased risk of leukemic transformation,
- **Tier II** variants of potential clinical significance (includes level C and level D biomarkers).

    Examples of type II mutations include:
    - *DNMT3* in AML and MDS is associated with rose prognosis,
    - *FLT3*-ITD predicts response to therapy with *FLT3* inhibitors in AML,
    - *JAK2* predicts response to ruxolitinib in PMF, *JAK2* inhibitors in ALL,
    - *NRAS* predicts poor prognosis in MDS,
    - *PHF6* mutations have been associated with reduced overall survival in AML in one study],
    - *SF3B1* predicts good prognosis in AML developing in patients with MDS,
    - *TET2* mutations help in the diagnosis of MDS and chronic myelomonocytic leukemia (CMML) (they often are seen in CHIP); they are associated with worse prognosis in AML,
    - *ZRSR2* is associated with poor prognosis in MDS.
- **Tier III** variants of unknown clinical significance [example: *RUNX1* p.Ser389Pro]
- **Tier IV** variants (benign or likely benign) (observed at significant allele frequency in general or specific subpopulation databases).

Molecular-flow cytometric correlation

Acute myeloid leukemia with *NPM1* mutations

> **Phenotype of AML with *NPM1* mutation:** CD2$^{-/rarely+}$, s.CD3$^-$, c.CD3$^-$, CD4$^{-/+}$, CD5$^{+/-}$, CD7$^{+/-}$, CD11b$^{-/rarely+}$, CD11c$^+$, CD13$^{+/rarely-}$, CD14$^{-/rarely+}$, CD15$^{-/rarely+}$, CD19$^-$, c.CD22$^-$, CD33$^+$, CD34$^{-/rarely+}$, CD36$^-$, CD38$^+$, CD56$^{+/-}$, CD64$^{-/+}$, CD65$^{-/rarely+}$, CD79a$^-$, CD117$^+$, CD133$^{+/-}$, HLA-DR$^{-/+}$, MPO$^{+/-}$

NPM1 mutations occur in:

- AML; subset
- Rare cases of MDS and mixed MDS/MPN neoplasms

AML carrying nucleophosmin (*NPM1*) mutations displays distinct molecular and clinical-pathological features that led to its inclusion as provisional entity in 2008 WHO classification [25–32]. *NPM1* is nucleocytoplasmic shuttling protein mainly localized in the nucleolus that has multiple functions, including interaction with *TP53* in controlling cell proliferation and apoptosis and controlling DNA repair and centrosome duplication during mitosis. *NPM1* mutations are now recognized as the most common genetic lesion in AML, present in 25%–35% of adult AML and in 45%–64% of patients with cytogenetically normal AML.

NPM1 mutations are rare in MDS or myelodysplastic/myeloproliferative neoplasm (MDS/MPN) ranging from 0% to 9%, with an overall frequency of 2% in MDS and 3% in CMML. Mutation burden does not correlate with number of blasts in BM, but *NPM1*-mutated MDS or MDS/MPN patients have an aggressive clinical course and higher rate of relatively rapid transformation to AML.

NPM1$^+$ AML often shows monocytic differentiation, a female preponderance, and lack of HLA-DR and CD34 expression. *NPM1* mutations are prognostically favorable in the absence of *FLT3*-ITD [30]. *NPM1* mutations also have favorable prognostic impact in older patients with cytogenetically normal AML, especially those age ≥70 years. In AML, *NPM1* mutations are usually secondary events, often occurring after *DNMT3A*, *IDH1*, and *NRAS* mutations. AML with *NPM1* mutations show wide immunophenotypic spectrum when analyzed by FC, but blasts tend to be CD34$^-$, CD117$^+$, CD33$^+$, CD38$^+$, HLA-DR$^-$, and CD11c$^+$ (Figure 11.3). Blasts display low side scatter (SSC). Many cases show monocytic differentiation, resembling acute myelomonocytic leukemia or acute monoblastic (monocytic) leukemia, and some cases resemble hypogranular variant of APL. Occasional cases resemble phenotypically

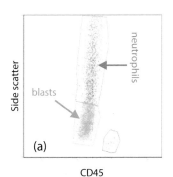
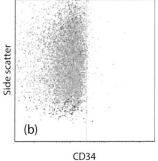
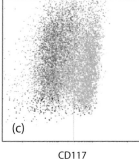
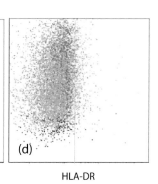

(a) CD45	(b) CD34	(c) CD117	(d) HLA-DR

FIGURE 11.3   AML with *NPM1* mutations: blasts (green dots) show low side scatter (a), negative CD34 (b), positive CD117 (c), and negative HLA-DR (d), resembling hypogranular variant of APL.

blastic plasmacytoid dendritic cell neoplasm (BPDCN) with positive CD56 expression and negative HLA-DR, CD11b, CD14, CD34, and CD64. Detailed description of AML with *NPM1* mutation and its differential diagnosis are described in Chapter 24.

Acute myeloid leukemia with t(8;21)/*RUNX1-RUNX1T1*

Phenotype of AML with t(8;21): CD2$^{-/rarely+}$, s.CD3$^-$, c.CD3$^-$, CD4$^{-/+}$, CD7$^{+/rarely-}$, CD11b$^{-/rarely+}$, CD11c$^{+/-+}$, CD13$^{+/rarely-}$, CD14$^-$, CD15$^{-/rarely+}$, CD19$^{+/rarely-}$, c.CD22$^-$, CD33$^{+/rarely-}$, CD34$^{+/rarely-}$, CD38$^{+/rarely-}$, CD36$^-$, CD56$^{+/rarely-}$, CD64$^-$, CD65$^{-/rarely+}$, CD79a$^{+/rarely-}$, CD117$^{+/rarely-}$, CD133$^{+/-}$, HLA-DR$^{+/rarely-}$, MPO$^+$, TdT$^{-/rarely+}$

Phenotypically, AML with t(8;21)/*RUNX1-RUNX1T1* is positive for myeloid antigens (CD13, CD33), HLA-DR, blastic markers (CD34, CD117, and CD133) and characteristically CD19 and CD56 (Figure 11.4). There is often aberrant expression of CD7, but CD10 is negative. Presence of t(8;21)/*RUNX1-RUNX1T1* puts this leukemia in the category of AML with recurrent genetic changes and not mixed phenotype acute leukemia (MPAL), despite co-expression of CD19 and myeloid markers. For the diagnosis of MPAL (B-ALL/AML), the B-lineage must be confirmed by strong expression of CD19 and positive expression of at least one (two, if CD19 is dimly positive) of the following markers: cytoplasmic CD22, cytoplasmic CD79a or CD10. Detailed description of AML with t(8;21) mutation and its differential diagnosis are described in Chapter 24.

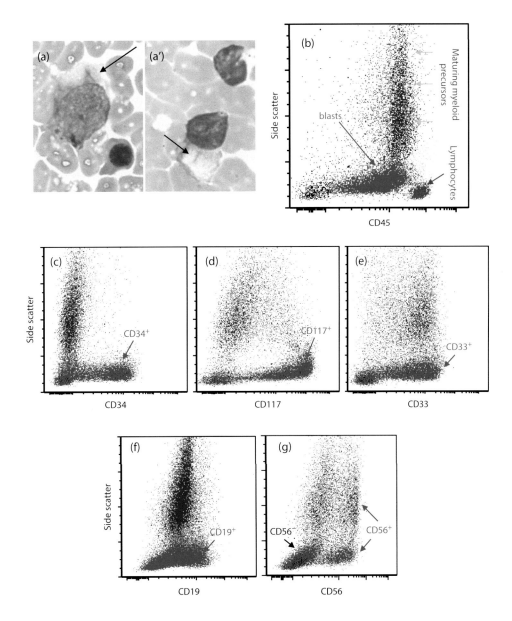

FIGURE 11.4 AML with *RUNX1-RUNX1T1* – flow cytometry. Blasts are large with nucleoli and occasional Auer rods (a; smear from flow sample). Flow cytometry (b–g) reveals phenotypic features of AML with maturation (b; blasts are represented by blue dots, and maturing myeloid precursors by purple dots). Blasts are positive for CD45 (b), CD34 (c), CD117 (d), CD33 (e), CD19 (f; partial), and CD56 (g; partial). Granulocytes show aberrant CD56 expression on subset (g).

Acute promyelocytic leukemia (APL) with t(15;17)/*PML-RARA*

PHENOTYPE OF APL

APL (hypergranular): CD2⁻, s.CD3⁻, c.CD3⁻, CD4⁻/⁺, CD7⁺/⁻, CD11b⁻, CD11c⁻, CD13⁺, CD14⁻, CD15⁻/rarely+(dim), CD19⁻, c.CD22⁻, CD33⁺bright, CD34⁻, CD38⁺, CD36⁻, CD56⁻/rarely+, CD64⁻/dim+, CD65⁻/rarely+, c.CD79a⁻, CD117⁺(may be dim), CD133⁻/rarely+, HLA-DR⁻, MPO⁺

APL-v (hypogranular): CD2⁺/rarely⁻, s.CD3⁻, c.CD3⁻, CD4⁻/⁺, CD7⁺/⁻, CD11b⁻, CD11c⁻, CD13⁺, CD14⁻, CD15⁻/rarely+(dim), CD19⁻, c.CD22⁻, CD33⁺bright, CD34⁺/rarely⁻, CD38⁺, CD36⁻, CD56⁻/rarely+, CD64⁻/dim+, CD65⁻/rarely+, c.CD79a⁻, CD117⁺(may be dim), CD133⁻/rarely+, HLA-DR⁻, MPO⁺

The t(15;17)(q24;q21) disrupts *PML* gene on chromosome 15q24 (15q22-24) and the gene encoding the retinoic acid receptor α (*RARA*) on chromosome 17q21 (17q12-21). The t(15;17) leads to the formation of two reciprocal fusion genes, *PML-RARA* on chromosome 15 and *RARA-PML* on chromosome 17. Seven different chromosomal translocations have been identified in APL, all involving *RARA* gene. Small subset of APL (less than 1%) carry *PLZF-RARA* fusion [t(11;17)], which is associated with lack of response to retinoic acid. Other *RARA* partners include *STAT5b* (17q11), *NPM1* (nucleophosmin, a gene mutated in substantial number of AML cases; 5q35), *NUMA1* nuclear matrix gene (11q13), *PRKAR1A* (17q23), and *FIP1L1* (4q12) [33–37].

Hypergranular (classic) APL has characteristic FC pattern with high SSC, moderate CD45, positive CD117, negative CD34, negative HLA-DR, negative CD11c, and often dim CD64 (Figure 11.5) [38]. Hypogranular APL in addition to markers positive in classic APL, is often positive for CD2 and CD34. Detailed description of APL and its differential diagnosis are described in Chapter 24.

Acute myeloid leukemia with inv(16)(p13.1q22)/t(16;16) (p13.1;q22), and del(16)(q22) [*CBFB-MYH11*]

PHENOTYPE OF AML WITH *CBFB-MYH11*

Blasts: CD2⁻/rarely+, s.CD3⁻, c.CD3⁻, CD4⁻/⁺, CD7⁺/rarely⁻, CD11b⁻/rarely+, CD11c⁻/⁺, CD13⁺/rarely⁻, CD14⁻, CD15⁻/rarely+, CD19⁻, c.CD22⁻, CD33⁺/rarely⁻, CD34⁺/rarely⁻, CD38⁺/rarely⁻, CD36⁻, CD56⁺/⁻, CD64⁻, CD65⁻/rarely+, CD79a⁻, CD117⁺/rarely⁻, CD133⁺/⁻, HLA-DR⁺/rarely⁻, MPO⁺, TdT⁻/rarely+
Monocytes: CD4⁺, CD11b⁺, CD11c⁺, CD13⁺, CD14⁺, CD33⁺, CD45⁺, CD56⁻/⁺, CD64⁺(bright)
Eosinophils: FSClow, SSChigh, CD10⁻, CD13⁺, CD16⁻, CD33⁺, CD123⁺/rarely⁻

AML with inv(16)/t(16;16) displays increased blasts and monocyted and is characterized by increased atypical (often immature) eosinophils with large basophilic granules intermixed with more typical eosinophilic granules (Figure 23.32; Chapter 23). In some cases, blasts are large with irregular nuclei and prominent cytoplasmic granules and occasional Auer rods (mimicking cytologically APL). FC shows mixed populations of blasts, monocytes, maturing myeloid cells, and atypical and immature (CD123⁺) eosinophils. Blasts are positive for CD13, CD33, CD34, and CD117, and often also HLA-DR and CD2. They may display aberrant expression of CD7, CD15, CD56, and CD65 and/or lack of HLA-DR. Monocytic cells are most often positive for CD11b, CD11c, CD13, CD14, CD64, and HLA-DR. Eosinophils are characterized by high SSC, low forward scatter (FSC), negative CD10 and CD16 and positive CD13, CD33, and often CD123.

Acute myeloid leukemia with *CEBPA* mutation
CEBPA mutation occurs in:

- AML
- Myeloid neoplasms with germline predisposition

CEBPA mutations are found in approximately 15% of AML patients and its presence is associated with a favorable response to standard treatment and better prognosis (survival) [39, 40]. The prognosis of AML with *CEBPA* is independent of other prognostic factors, including age and *FLT3* status, but appears to be more pronounced in patients with biallelic (double) mutation [41, 42]. AML with double-mutated *CEBPA* have other mutations, including *TET2* (34%), *GATA2* (21%), *WT1* (13.7%), *DNMT3A* (9.6%), *ASXL1* (9.5%), *NRAS* (8.4%), *KRAS* (3.2%), *IDH1/2* (6.3%), *FLT3*-internal tandem duplication (6.3%), *FLT3*-tyrosine kinase domain (2.1%), *NPM1* (2.1%), and *RUNX1* (1 of 94 cases) [43]. AML with *CEBPA* mutation is closely associated with CD7, CD15, CD34, and HLA-DR expression by blasts [44].

Mastocytosis with *KIT* mutation
KIT mutations occur in:

- AML; subset
- SM
- Chronic eosinophilic leukemia (CEL), very few cases reported
- BPDCN, rare cases

Presence of *KIT* mutations is associated with adverse outcome in core binding factor (CBF) positive AML, especially in the subgroup with *RUNX1-RUNX1T1* rearrangement. *KIT* mutations are detected in ~25% of CBF⁺ AML [45–50]. Few cases of CEL with KIT mutations have been reported; patients responded to imatinib [17]. The *KIT* D816V mutations is present in the majority of SM (>90%) with or without associated hematological neoplasm (AHN) [17]. Depending on the type of AHN additional mutations may be also present (*TET2, SRSF2, ASXL1, CBL, RUNX1,* and *RAS*). Unlike SM, mast cell

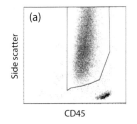
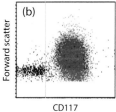
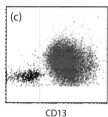
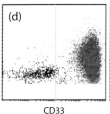
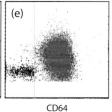

FIGURE 11.5 Acute promyelocytic leukemia (APL) – flow cytometry. Neoplastic promyelocytes (green dots) show high side scatter (a), positive CD117 (b), positive CD13 (c), positive CD33 (d), and positive CD64 (e).

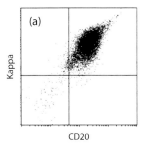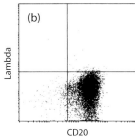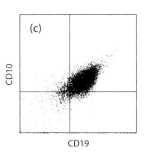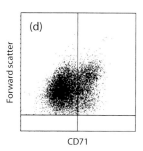

FIGURE 11.6 Burkitt lymphoma – flow cytometry. B-cells are CD20$^+$ (a–b), kappa positive (a), lambda negative (c), and show partial CD71 expression (d).

leukemia may harbor atypical *KIT* mutations, such as non-D816V mutations. *KIT* mutations have been seen in 9% of BPDCNs.

Burkitt lymphoma with t(8;14)/*MYC* rearrangement

BL phenotype by FC: FSC^{increased}, sIg$^{+/rarely-}$, CD5$^{-/rarely+}$, CD10$^{+bright}$, BCL2$^-$, CD11c$^-$, CD19$^+$, CD20$^+$, CD22$^+$, CD23$^-$, CD25$^-$, CD34$^-$, CD38$^{+bright}$, CD43$^{+strong}$, CD45$^+$, CD71$^+$, CD79b^{+dim}, CD81$^{+moderate\ to\ bright}$, CD103$^-$, CD200$^{-/(may\ be\ dimly+)}$, and TdT$^-$

MYC rearrangement occurs in:

- BL
- High grade B-cell lymphoma (HGBL) with *MYC* and *BCL2* (and/or *BCL6*) rearrangement (HGBL-R; double hit lymphoma)
- Diffuse large B-cell lymphoma (DLBCL), subset
- Plasmablastic lymphoma (PBL)
- PCM, rare cases
- Other B-cell lymphomas (sporadically)

FC analysis of BL shows clonal B-cell population with moderate to bright expression of CD20 and surface immunoglobulins, positive CD10, CD38, CD43, CD71, and CD81, increased FSC and negative BCL2 and CD200 (Figure 11.6). Differential diagnosis of BL includes other CD10$^+$ B-cell lymphoproliferations: DLBCL, HGBL with *MYC* a *BCL2* (and/or *BCL6*) rearrangements (HGBL-R), CD10$^+$ MCL, CD10$^+$ hairy cell leukemia (HCK), and B-lymphoblastic leukemia (B-ALL). Differential diagnosis requires correlation with histomorphology, Ki-67 immunostaining, and FISH studies (*MYC*, *BCL2*, and *BCL6*). HGBL-R with *MYC* and *BCL2* or *MYC* and *BCL6* rearrangements are also called double hit, and with *MYC*, *BCL2* and *BCL6* rearrangement, triple hit. Subset of DLBCL, which shows only *MYC* rearrangement (without concurrent *BCL2* and *BCL6*) may be also referred to as a single hit lymphoma.

High grade B-cell lymphoma with rearrangement of *MYC* and *BCL2* (and/or BCL6) [HGBL-R, double or triple hit lymphoma]

HGBL-R phenotype by FC: FSC^{increased}, sIg$^{+\ (often\ dim)/rarely-}$, CD5$^-$, CD10$^{+bright/rarely-}$, BCL2$^+$, CD11c$^-$, CD19$^+$, CD20$^{+(may\ be\ dim)}$, CD22$^+$, CD23$^-$, CD25$^-$, CD34$^-$, CD38$^{+bright}$, CD43$^{+/-}$, CD45$^+$, CD71$^+$, CD81$^+$, CD103$^-$, CD123$^-$, CD200$^-$, and TdT$^-$

B-cell markers (CD19, CD20, CD22, CD79a) are positive and majority of cases show monoclonal expression of surface immunoglobulins, but some cases (double-hit lymphomas) may be surface immunoglobulin negative. Most HGBL-R have germinal center phenotype with expression of CD10 (90%–100%). BCL2 protein is detected in up to 95% [51]. Majority of cases have strong expression of CD71 and co-expression of CD10 and BCL2 by FC. Surface light chain immunoglobulin expression by FC is often decreased and can be absent in 20% of cases [52]. Figures 13.110–13.112 (Chapter 13) show examples of FC findings in HGBL-R.

Chronic myeloid leukemia (CML) with t(9;22)/*BCR-ABL1*

BCR-ABL1 rearrangement occurs in:

- CML
- AML; subset
- B-cell acute lymphoblastic leukemia/lymphoma (B-ALL/LBL; subset)
- T-cell acute lymphoblastic leukemia/lymphoma (T-ALL/LBL; minor subset)

FC analysis of blood from patients with CML shows increased granulocytes to lymphocytes ratio due to myeloid hyperplasia and lymphopenia, a small population of blasts, eosinophilia, and basophilia and aberrant phenotype of granulocytes and monocytes. The phenotypic abnormalities of granulocytes include partially negative to dim expression CD10, CD11b, CD13, and CD16, and partially positive expression of CD56 (Figure 11.7). The SSC of granulocytes is deceased. In addition to an aberrant phenotype of granulocytes, the majority of CML cases also display an aberrant expression of CD56 by monocytes. Occasional cases of CML show a minor population of circulating immature B-cells resembling phenotypically hematogones in the BM. These atypical B-cells are positive for CD22, CD19, and CD10, and likely represent partially mature B-lymphoid precursors derived from Philadelphia$^+$ stem cells. In contrast to blood, FC features of CML in the BM are subtle and include lack of hematogones, increased myeloid to lymphoid ratio, increased myeloblasts, decreased SSC of granulocytes, subtle phenotypic atypia of granulocytes (increased population of CD10$^-$, CD11b$^-$, and/or CD16$^-$ cells, and/or increased population of CD56$^+$ cells), phenotypic atypia of monocytes (CD56 expression) and increased number of eosinophils and basophils. Eosinophils are characterized by high SSC, very low FSC, positive CD11b, CD13, CD33, and negative CD10 and CD16, and basophils are characterized by moderate to bright CD45 and slightly increased SSC, positive myeloid markers and often positive CD22 expression. CML is discussed in Chapter 21.

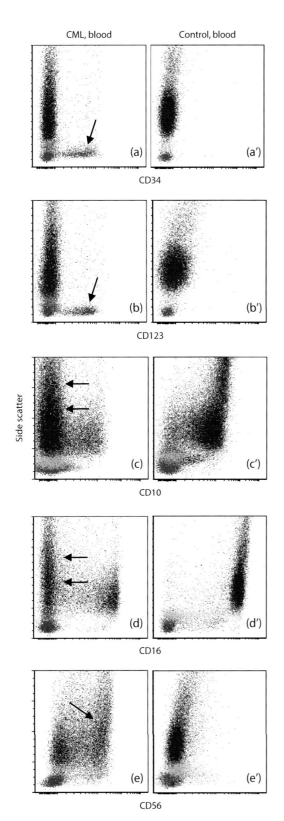

FIGURE 11.7 Flow cytometric pattern of CML in peripheral blood (CML, left column; control, right column). CML differs from healthy controls (normal blood and reactive neutrophilia) by presence of circulating blasts (a, arrow), basophilia (b, arrow), significant number of CD10-negative (c, arrows) and CD16-negative (D, arrows) granulocytes and up-regulation of CD56 (e, arrow).

Mantle cell lymphoma (MCL) with t(11;14)/*CCND1* rearrangement

MCL phenotype by FC: sIg^+(moderate), CD2^−, CD5^+/rarely−, CD10^−/rarely+, CD11c^−, CD19^+, CD20^+(moderate/bright), CD22^+, CD23^−/(rare cases +), CD25^−, CD38^+/rarely−, CD43^+/rarely−, CD45^+(bright), CD49d^−/+, CD79a^+, CD79b^+(bright), CD81^+strong, CD103^−, CD123^−/rarely+, and CD200^−.

CCND1 rearrangement occurs in:

• MCL
• PCM, subset

MCL is characterized by t(11;14) involving the rearrangement of *CCND1* gene. FC analysis shows clonal B-cells with moderate CD20, moderate kappa or lambda expression, positive CD5 and CD81, negative CD23 and CD200, and often positive CD38 expression. Rare cases may be CD10^+. CD11c is usually negative. FC features of MCL are presented in Figures 13.76–13.79 in Chapter 13.

T-cell prolymphocytic leukemia (T-PLL) with chromosome 14 abnormalities

T-PLL phenotype by FC: CD2^+/−, CD3^+/−, CD4^+ (less often CD8^+, CD4/CD8^+ or CD4/CD8^−), CD5^+/−, CD7^+/−, CD25^−, CD26^+, CD45^+/rarely−, CD56^−, CD57^−, CD81^+, CD117^−/rarely+, CD200^−

T-PLL is characterized by prominent lymphocytosis. In contrast to other T-cell lymphoproliferations, many T-PLL cases show normal expression of T-cell antigens (CD2, CD3, CD5, and CD7). Majority of cases are either CD4^+ or CD8^+, but occasional cases may be dual CD4/CD8^+ or dual CD4/CD8^−. Subset of CD8^+ cases may display dim or partial expression of CD117. The chromosomal translocations involving the T-cell receptor (TCR) gene and one of two protooncogenes (*TCL1* and *MTCP-1*) are seen in the majority of cases. Figure 11.8 presents T-PLL with typical chromosomal and phenotypic changes. Figures 16.4–16.8 in Chapter 16 show FC features of T-PLL.

Chronic neutrophilic leukemia (CNL) with *CSFR3* mutation
CSF3R mutation occurs in:

• Chronic neutrophilic leukemia (CNL)
• Atypical CML, rare cases atypical CML (aCML; *BCR-ABL1*-)
• Chronic myelomonocytic leukemia (CMML), rare cases
• AML (pediatric)

CSF3R mutations occur in majority of patients with CNL often together with mutation of SETBP1 or ASXL1 [17, 53–61]. *CSF3R* mutations have also been reported in <10% of aCML, AML (especially pediatric cases) as well as in 3% of CMML cases [17, 54, 56]. The most common *CSF3R* mutations are the membrane proximal mutation, T618I, and truncation mutations.

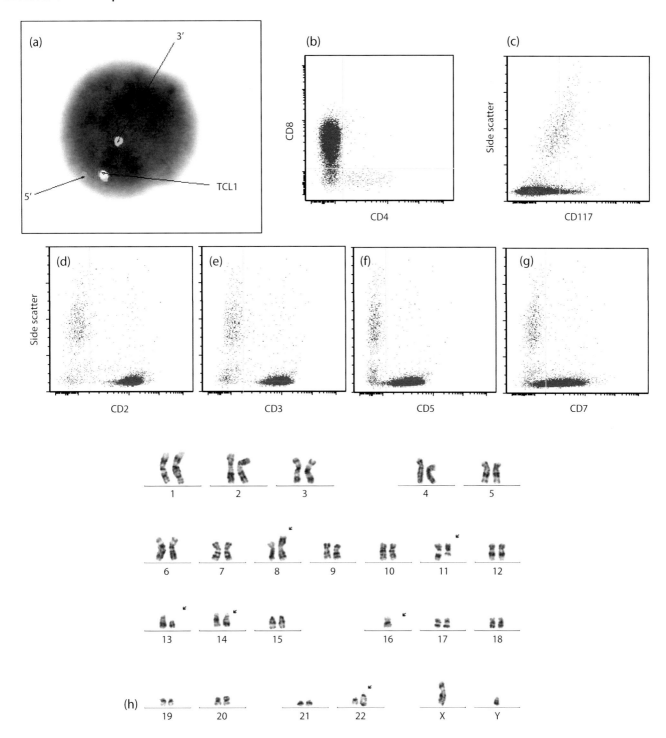

FIGURE 11.8 T-cell prolymphocytic leukemia. FISH analysis shows the rearrangement of *TCL1* gene (a). Flow cytometry shows CD8 restriction (b), dim CD17 on minute subset (c), and positive expression of all pan-T-cell antigens (d–g) with CD7 being slightly dimmer. Cytogenetic (h) shows inversion of chromosome 14 and isochromosome 8q typical for T-PLL, as well as other changes (11q/ATM deletion and 13q deletion).

Co-existence of *CSF3R* and *ASXL1* is associated with worse prognosis in CNL [62].

CNL is a rare and distinct *BCR-ABL1*-negative chronic myeloproliferative neoplasm defined by sustained (mature) neutrophilia defined by persistent mature neutrophilic leukocytosis, BM granulocyte hyperplasia, and frequent hepatosplenomegaly [17, 25, 56, 63–66]. It affects mostly elderly patients and is characterized by splenomegaly, hepatomegaly, persistent neutrophilic leukocytosis without significant leftward shift, toxic granulation and Döhle bodies, elevated leukocyte alkaline phosphatase and vitamin B12 levels. Blood smear shows marked neutrophilia with minimal left shift, predominance of segmented forms and bands (≥80%), prominent toxic granules. BM is hypercellular with increased M:E ratio due to expansion of neutrophilic granulopoiesis with granulocytic maturation pattern and without excess of myeloblasts or promyelocytes (<5% blasts in BM and <1% in blood). FC shows predominance of mature neutrophils.

Hepatosplenic T-cell lymphoma (HSTL) with isochromosome 7q

HTCL phenotype by FC: CD2$^+$, CD3$^+$, CD4$^-$/CD8$^-$ (rare cases are CD4$^-$/CD8$^+$), CD5$^-$, CD7$^+$, CD16$^{-/rarely+}$, CD56$^+$, CD57$^-$, TCRγδ$^+$

Hepatosplenic T-cell lymphoma (HSTL) is a rare form of extranodal lymphoma derived from cytotoxic γδ$^+$ T-cells, which occurs predominantly in young adults and shows male predominance [67–73]. Spleen shows prominent red pulp with sinuses and cords infiltrated by neoplastic T-cells and white pulp reduced or completely absent. The infiltrate is composed of atypical but monotonous population of medium-sized cells with characteristic intrasinusoidal distribution (the marked sinusoidal pattern is seen also in liver and BM). On FC analysis, the tumor cells are positive for CD2, CD3, CD45, and TCRγδ$^+$ [68–72, 74, 75]. Rare cases of HSTL TCRαβ$^+$ have been reported [76–79]. Majority of cases are CD7$^+$, TIA1$^+$, dual CD4/CD8$^-$, and CD5$^-$ (rare cases display dim expression of CD5). Only rare tumors may be CD4$^-$/CD8$^+$.

Anaplastic large cell lymphoma (ALCL) with t(2;5)/ALK rearrangement

ALCL phenotype by FC: high FSC, CD2$^{+/rarely-}$, CD3$^{+/-}$, CD4$^+$ or less often CD8$^+$ (rare tumors are either CD4/8$^-$ or CD4/CD8$^+$), CD5$^{+/-}$, CD7$^{-/rarely+}$, CD10$^-$, CD25$^{+/-}$, CD26$^{+/rarely-}$, CD30$^+$, CD43$^+$, CD45$^+$, CD56$^{-/rarely+}$

Anaplastic large cell lymphoma, anaplastic lymphoma kinase (ALK)-positive is a T-cell lymphoma composed of usually large cells with abundant cytoplasm and pleomorphic, often horseshoe-shaped nuclei, with a translocation involving the ALK gene and expression of ALK protein [17]. ALK$^+$ ALCL occurs in children and young adults (median age 34 years) and has male to female ratio of 3:2. ALK$^+$ ALCL frequently involves both lymph nodes and extranodal sites, including skin, bone, soft tissues, lung, and liver. BM is involved in 10%–30%. ALK$^+$ ALCL shows a wide range of morphological spectrum including common, lymphohistiocytic, small cell, giant cell, monomorphic and Hodgkin-like variants [25, 80–90]. FC may show cluster of cells with high FSC as well as increased SSC, which put tumor cells in "monocytic" or "granulocytic" regions on CD45 versus SSC display (as with other high grade lymphomas, FC often underestimate the number of tumor cells due to selective loss of tumor cells). The neoplastic cells often display aberrant T-cell phenotype, easily identifiable by FC data. Most cases show aberrant expression of T-cell markers with loss of surface CD3, CD5, or TCR. ALK$^+$ and ALK$^-$ ALCL differ in terms of genomic profiles [91]. The most common losses affect 17p13.3-p12 (25%), in which TP53 gene is

located, 6q21 (17%), the region containing PRDM1 and ATG5, 13q32.3-q33.3 and 16q23.2 (16%) [91]. More than 20% of ALCL show gains of different regions of the long arm of chromosome 1 and 16% cases show gains of 8q24.22. In ALK$^-$ ALCL, 52% show PRDM1 inactivation and/or loss of 17p (52%), and remaining 48% are negative for those changes, and in ALK$^+$ ALCL, 45% show genetic aberrations (in addition to ALK) and the remaining 55% are without additional genetic changes [91].

Hairy cell leukemia (HCL) with BRAF mutation

HCL phenotype by FC: sIg$^+$, CD5$^-$, CD10$^{-/rarely+}$, CD11c$^{+(bright)}$, CD19$^+$, CD20$^+$, CD22$^{+bright}$, CD23$^{-/rarely+}$, CD25$^+$, CD38$^-$, CD43$^{+(dim)/-}$, CD45$^+$, CD79b$^{+(moderate)}$, CD81$^{+(dim)}$, CD123$^{+(bright)}$, and CD200$^{+bright}$.

BRAF mutation occurs in:

- HCL
- AML, rare cases
- BPDCN, rare cases

BRAF mutations, reported typically in thyroid cancer and melanoma, have been also associated with HCL. Unlike that observed in other BRAF-mutated tumors that may carry mutations other than V600E (V600K and V600R in melanoma), HCL patients are V600E$^+$. Presence of BRAF mutations helps to distinguish HCL (BRAF$^+$) from hairy cell leukemia variant (HCL-v) and other B-cell lymphomas including splenic marginal zone lymphoma and splenic diffuse red pulp small B-cell lymphoma (BRAF$^-$) [39–43, 92–94]. BRAF V600E mutations are very specific for HCL occurring in 80%–90% of patients [43, 95]. BRAF mutations have been reported only in sporadic cases of other B-cell lymphoproliferations, including ~3% of B-CLL/CLL [96], B-cell prolymphocytic leukemia [97], Hodgkin lymphoma [98], splenic marginal zone lymphoma [99,100], and marginal zone lymphomas [101]. In MZL cases, BRAF mutations occur most commonly in nodal variant (16% of nodal MZL were reported to be BRAF$^+$) [101]. HCL with BRAF mutations was reported to respond to vemurafenib [102]. In AML, BRAF mutations are independently associated with a worse prognosis. BRAF inhibitors might be a useful therapeutic option for patients in this subgroup. BRAF mutations have been seen in 3% of BPDCNs.

HCL cells express B-cell markers, HLA-DR, CD25, CD103, CD11c, CD123, and CD200. The expression of CD11c is very bright. Rare cases may be CD10$^+$. Genetically, HCL is characterized by BRAF V600E mutation [39, 40, 42, 43, 103]. The detailed description of HCL is presented in Chapter 13.

Lymphoplasmacytic lymphoma/Waldenström macroglobulinemia (LPL/WM) with MYD88 mutation

LPL phenotype by FC: sIg$^+$, CD5$^{-/rarely+}$, CD10$^{-/rarely+}$, CD11c$^-$, CD19$^+$, CD20$^+$, CD22$^+$, CD23$^{-/rarely+}$, CD25$^{+/-}$, CD38$^{+/rarely-}$, CD43$^-$, CD45$^+$, CD79b$^-$, CD81$^{+(dim)/rarely-}$, CD103$^-$, CD123$^-$, and CD200$^{+dim/-}$. Clonal B-cells are often accompanied by clonal CD19$^+$/CD45$^+$/CD56$^-$/IgM$^+$ plasma cells.

MYD88 mutation occurs in:

- Lymphoplasmacytic lymphoma/Waldenström macroglobulinemia (LPL/WM)
- DLBCL (activated B-cell-like);
- Primary DLBCL of central nervous system
- Primary testicular DLBCL
- Cutaneous DLBCL, leg type (C-DLBCL-LT)
- IgM MGUS
- CLL/SLL, rare cases
- MZL, rare cases

MYD88 L265P mutation was identified in 79%–93% of patients with LPL/WM [104–108]. Poulain et al. identified alteration of the *MYD88* locus in 91% of WM patients, including 12% with gain on chromosome 3 at the 3p22 locus that included the *MYD88* gene [104, 105]. Ngo et al. identified *MYD88* L265P mutation in 29% of ABC DLBCL [107]. MZD88 mutations are rare in GCB subtype of DLBCL. 54% of patients with IgM type of MGUS also have *MYD88* mutations [108]. NGS has revealed recurring somatic mutations in LPL/WM, including *MYD88* (95%–97%), *CXCR4* (30%–40%), *ARID1A* (17%), and *CD79B* (8%–15%). Majority of LPL/WM are characterized by presence of *MYD88* L265P mutations [104, 106, 108–110]. MYD88 is detected less frequently in non-IgM LPL type (40%) [111]. The *MYD88* gene is located at chromosome 3q22.2 and encodes an adaptor protein in the interleukin-1 (IL-1) and toll-like receptor pathways. The primary consequence of *MYD88* mutation is NF-κB activation via Bruton tyrosine kinase and other molecules. Although highly prevalent in LPL/WM, *MYD88* has been described in other lymphomas, including 70% of primary DLBCL of central nervous system and testicular DLBCL, 50% of cutaneous DLBCL, leg type and 24% of ABC type of DLBCL, NOS [112]. Occasional CLL/SLL and splenic MZL cases also carry *MYD88* mutations [113–117].

LPL is defined as a low-grade B-cell neoplasm composed of a mixture of small lymphocytes, lymphocytes with plasmacytoid features and plasma cells, which does not fulfill the criteria for any of the other small B-cell lymphoid neoplasm [17, 105, 109, 118–122]. Monoclonal paraprotein (usually IgM) is often present but is not required for the diagnosis of LPL. B-cells have moderate to bright expression of surface immunoglobulin and dim to moderate expression of cytoplasmic IgM. They most often do not express CD5, CD10, or CD23, but CD25 and especially CD38 may be positive (CD38 dimmer than in plasma cells). The plasma cell population is usually smaller and is negative for surface immunoglobulins, brightly positive for cytoplasmic immunoglobulins (of the same isotype as B-cells), brightly positive for CD38/CD138, most often positive for cytoplasmic IgM, and often positive for CD19 and CD45. The identification of *MYD88* L265P gene mutation has been a major advance in the diagnosis of patients with LPL/WM [104, 108,109]. *MYD88* can be mutated also in subset of cases of non-IgM LPL.

Splenic marginal zone lymphoma (SMZL) with deletion 7q

MZL phenotype by FC: low FSC, sIg+, CD5−/rarely+, CD10−, CD11c+(dim)/rarely−, CD13−/rarely+, CD19+, CD20+moderate, CD22+, CD23−/rarely+, CD25−, CD38−/rarely+, CD43+/−, CD45+, CD81+, CD103−/rarely+, CD123−/rarely+, and CD200+/rarely−

Splenic marginal zone lymphoma (SMZL) (Figure 11.9) is positive for B-cell markers (CD19, CD20, CD22, CD79a), BCL2, surface IgM (or less often IgD), and light chain immunoglobulins, and in most cases is negative for CD5, CD10, CD23, CD43, CD103, and CD123. The expression of CD11c is variable (usually dim or partial), expression of CD81 is either negative or dimly positive, and expression of CD200 is often positive (usually moderate). Subset of SMZL (~30%) is positive for deletion 7q. BM biopsy often shows intrasinusoidal pattern of involvement or mixed pattern (intrasinusoidal, nodular, and occasionally paratrabecular). Deletion of 7q may be also seen in subset of splenic diffuse red pulp small B-cell lymphomas (SDRPL).

Follicular lymphoma with t(14;18)/*BCL2-IGH*

FL phenotype by FC: sIg+/rarely−, CD5−/rarely+, CD10+/rarely−, BCL2+/rarely−, CD11c−, CD19+(often dim), CD20+, CD22+, CD23−/rarely+, CD25−, CD38+/rarely−, CD43−/rarely+, CD45+, CD81+dim, CD103−, CD123−/rarely+, and CD200variable (+/−).

BCL2 rearrangement occurs in:

- FL
- DLBCL; subset
- HGBL with *MYC* and *BCL2* (and/or *BCL6*) rearrangement (HGBL-R, double or triple hit lymphoma)

FC analysis of FL (Figure 11.10) shows monotypic expression of surface light chain immunoglobulins (κ or λ), moderate to bright expression of CD20, dim expression of CD19 and positive expression of CD10 and BCL2 (subset of FL may be BCL2−). In many cases FC reveals two B-cell populations: a neoplastic population with monotypic expression of surface immunoglobulins and a subpopulation of residual benign (polytypic) B-cells, as well as increased number of reactive T-cells. Dim expression of CD19 and co-expression of CD10 and BCL2 usually confirm malignant process in these cases. A subset of FL may be negative for surface light chain immunoglobulins. Flow cytometric differential diagnosis includes other CD10+ B-cell lymphoproliferative disorders (DLBCL, subset of MCL, HGBL-R, subset of HCL and BL) and florid follicular hyperplasia (see Chapters 3, 12, and 13). Lymph node shows complete effacement of the architecture with prominent nodular (follicular) pattern. BM is often involved with a majority of cases showing paratrabecular pattern.

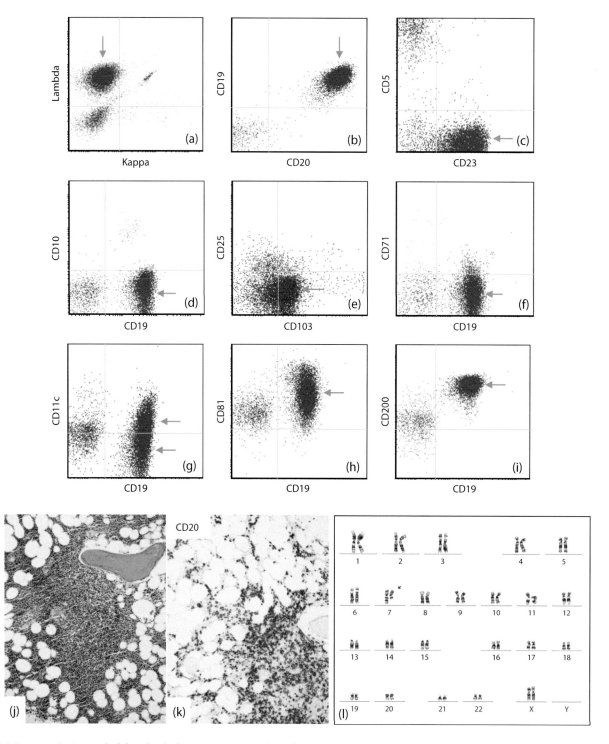

FIGURE 11.9 SMZL with del7q. (a–i) Flow cytometry analysis (bone marrow sample) shows clonal lambda+ B-cells (a, arrow) with bright expression of CD20 (b), negative CD5 (c), positive CD23 (c), negative CD10 (d; hematogones seen as light blue dots are CD10+), negative CD25 (e), partial dim CD103 (e), negative CD71 (f), partially dim CD11c (g), dim to moderate CD81 (h), and moderate CD200 (i). Histologic examination of BM core biopsy shows atypical lymphoid infiltrate with paratrabecular and intrasinusoidal components (j). Intrasinusoidal infiltrate is best visualized by CD20 staining (k). Cytogenetic studies show deletion 7q (l, arrow).

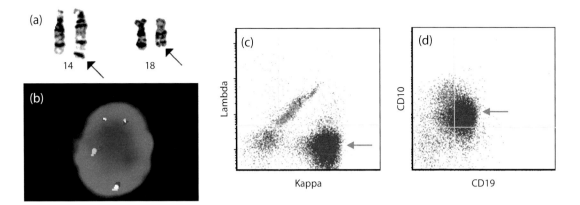

FIGURE 11.10 Follicular lymphoma with t(14;18) [*IGH-BCL2*]: (a) cytogenetics (partial karyotype); (b) FISH. (c–d) Flow cytometry shows clonal B-cells (kappa⁺; c) with CD10 expression (d).

References

1. Mullis, K., et al., *Specific enzymatic amplification of DNA in vitro: the polymerase chain reaction.* Cold Spring Harb Symp Quant Biol, 1986. **51 Pt 1**: p. 263–73.

2. Mullis, K., et al., *Specific enzymatic amplification of DNA in vitro: the polymerase chain reaction. 1986.* Biotechnology, 1992. **24**: p. 17–27.

3. Mullis, K.B. and F.A. Faloona, *Specific synthesis of DNA in vitro via a polymerase-catalyzed chain reaction.* Methods Enzymol, 1987. **155**: p. 335–50.

4. Holm, N., et al., *The value of molecular analysis by PCR in the diagnosis of cutaneous lymphocytic infiltrates.* J Cutan Pathol, 2002. **29**(8): p. 447–52.

5. Ashton-Key, M., et al., *Molecular analysis of T-cell clonality in ulcerative jejunitis and enteropathy-associated T-cell lymphoma.* Am J Pathol, 1997. **151**(2): p. 493–8.

6. Delfau-Larue, M.H., et al., *Prognostic significance of a polymerase chain reaction-detectable dominant T-lymphocyte clone in cutaneous lesions of patients with mycosis fungoides.* Blood, 1998. **92**(9): p. 3376–80.

7. Delfau-Larue, M.H., et al., *Diagnostic value of dominant T-cell clones in peripheral blood in 363 patients presenting consecutively with a clinical suspicion of cutaneous lymphoma.* Blood, 2000. **96**(9): p. 2987–92.

8. Kolowos, W., et al., *Detection of restricted junctional diversity of peripheral T cells in SLE patients by spectratyping.* Lupus, 1997. **6**(9): p. 701–7.

9. Hall, F.C., et al., *TCR beta spectratyping in RA: evidence of clonal expansions in peripheral blood lymphocytes.* Ann Rheum Dis, 1998. **57**(5): p. 319–22.

10. Wack, A., et al., *Age-related modifications of the human alphabeta T cell repertoire due to different clonal expansions in the CD4⁺ and CD8⁺ subsets.* Int Immunol, 1998. **10**(9): p. 1281–8.

11. Schwab, R., et al., *Expanded CD4⁺ and CD8⁺ T cell clones in elderly humans.* J Immunol, 1997. **158**(9): p. 4493–9.

12. Posnett, D.N., et al., *Clonal populations of T cells in normal elderly humans: the T cell equivalent to "benign monoclonal gammapathy".* J Exp Med, 1994. **179**(2): p. 609–18.

13. Lantelme, E., et al., *Clonal predominance, but preservation of a polyclonal reservoir, in the normal alpha beta T-cell repertoire.* Hum Immunol, 1997. **53**(1): p. 49–56.

14. Chamberlain, W.D., M.T. Falta, and B.L. Kotzin, *Functional subsets within clonally expanded CD8(+) memory T cells in elderly humans.* Clin Immunol, 2000. **94**(3): p. 160–72.

15. Ponti, R., et al., *T-cell receptor gamma gene rearrangement by multiplex polymerase chain reaction/heteroduplex analysis in patients with cutaneous T-cell lymphoma (mycosis fungoides/Sézary syndrome) and benign inflammatory disease: correlation with clinical, histological and immunophenotypical findings.* Br J Dermatol, 2005. **153**(3): p. 565–73.

16. Sabnani, I., et al., *Clonal T-large granular lymphocyte proliferation in solid organ transplant recipients.* Transplant Proc, 2006. **38**(10): p. 3437–40.

17. Swerdlow, S.H., Campo, E., Harris, N. L., Jaffe, E. S., Pileri, S. A., Stein, H., et al., ed. *WHO classification of tumors of haematopoietic and lymphoid tissues.* 2016, IARC: Lyon.

18. Li, M.M., et al., *Standards and guidelines for the interpretation and reporting of sequence variants in cancer: a joint consensus recommendation of the Association for Molecular Pathology, American Society of Clinical Oncology, and College of American Pathologists.* J Mol Diagn, 2017. **19**(1): p. 4–23.

19. Yohe, S. and B. Thyagarajan, *Review of clinical next-generation sequencing.* Arch Pathol Lab Med, 2017. **141**(11): p. 1544–57.

20. Alvarez-Larran, A., et al., *Genomic characterization in triple-negative primary myelofibrosis and other myeloid neoplasms with bone marrow fibrosis.* Ann Hematol, 2019. **98**(10): p. 2319–28.

21. Defrancesco, I., et al., *Targeted next-generation sequencing reveals molecular heterogeneity in non-chronic lymphocytic leukemia clonal B-cell lymphocytosis.* Hematol Oncol, 2020. **38**(5): p. 689–97.

22. Shabani Azim, F., et al., *Next generation sequencing in clinical oncology: applications, challenges and promises: a review article.* Iran J Public Health, 2018. **47**(10): p. 1453–7.

23. Skov, V., *Next generation sequencing in MPNs. Lessons from the past and prospects for use as predictors of prognosis and treatment responses.* Cancers (Basel), 2020. **12**(8): p. 2194.

24. Zhang, W., et al., *Novel bioinformatic classification system for genetic signatures identification in diffuse large B-cell lymphoma.* BMC Cancer, 2020. **20**(1): p. 714.

25. Swerdlow, S.H., Campo, E., Harris, N. L., Jaffe, E. S., Pileri, S. A., Stein, H., et al., ed. *WHO classification of tumors of haematopoietic and lymphoid tissues.* 2008, IARC: Lyon.

26. Falini, B., et al., *Cytoplasmic nucleophosmin in acute myelogenous leukemia with a normal karyotype.* N Engl J Med, 2005. **352**(3): p. 254–66.

27. Falini, B., et al., *Acute myeloid leukemia carrying cytoplasmic/mutated nucleophosmin (NPMc⁺ AML): biologic and clinical features.* Blood, 2007. **109**(3): p. 874–85.

28. Dohner, K., et al., *Mutant nucleophosmin (NPM1) predicts favorable prognosis in younger adults with acute myeloid leukemia and normal cytogenetics: interaction with other gene mutations.* Blood, 2005. **106**(12): p. 3740–6.

29. Patel, J.P., et al., *Prognostic relevance of integrated genetic profiling in acute myeloid leukemia.* N Engl J Med, 2012. **366**(12): p. 1079–89.

30. Schlenk, R.F., et al., *Mutations and treatment outcome in cytogenetically normal acute myeloid leukemia.* N Engl J Med, 2008. **358**(18): p. 1909–18.

31. Takahashi, S., *Current findings for recurring mutations in acute myeloid leukemia.* J Hematol Oncol, 2011. **4**: p. 36.

32. Verhaak, R.G., et al., *Mutations in nucleophosmin (NPM1) in acute myeloid leukemia (AML): association with other gene abnormalities and previously established gene expression signatures and their favorable prognostic significance.* Blood, 2005. **106**(12): p. 3747–54.

33. Brunel, V., et al., *Variant and masked translocations in acute promyelocytic leukemia.* Leuk Lymphoma, 1996. **22**(3–4): p. 221–8.

34. Chen, S.J., et al., *Rearrangements of the retinoic acid receptor alpha and promyelocytic leukemia zinc finger genes resulting from t(11;17) (q23;q21) in a patient with acute promyelocytic leukemia.* J Clin Invest, 1993. **91**(5): p. 2260–7.

35. Corey, S.J., et al., *A non-classical translocation involving 17q12 (retinoic acid receptor alpha) in acute promyelocytic leukemia (APML) with atypical features.* Leukemia, 1994. **8**(8): p. 1350–3.

36. Fenaux, P., C. Chomienne, and L. Degos, *Acute promyelocytic leukemia: biology and treatment.* Semin Oncol, 1997. **24**(1): p. 92–102.

37. Redner, R.L., et al., *The t(5;17) variant of acute promyelocytic leukemia expresses a nucleophosmin-retinoic acid receptor fusion.* Blood, 1996. **87**(3): p. 882–6.

38. Gorczyca, W., *Acute promyelocytic leukemia: four distinct patterns by flow cytometry immunophenotyping.* Pol J Pathol, 2012. **63**(1): p. 8–17.

39. Andrulis, M., et al., *Application of a BRAF V600E mutation-specific antibody for the diagnosis of hairy cell leukemia.* Am J Surg Pathol, 2012. **36**(12): p. 1796–800.

40. Arcaini, L., et al., *The BRAF V600E mutation in hairy cell leukemia and other mature B-cell neoplasms.* Blood, 2012. **119**(1): p. 188–91.

41. Shao, H., et al., *Distinguishing hairy cell leukemia variant from hairy cell leukemia: development and validation of diagnostic criteria.* Leuk Res, 2013. **37**(4): p. 401–9.

42. Tadmor, T., et al., *The BRAF-V600E mutation in hematological malignancies: a new player in hairy cell leukemia and Langerhans cell histiocytosis.* Leuk Lymphoma, 2012. **53**(12): p. 2339–40.

43. Tiacci, E., et al., *BRAF mutations in hairy-cell leukemia.* N Engl J Med, 2011. **364**(24): p. 2305–15.

44. Iriyama, N., et al., *Normal karyotype acute myeloid leukemia with the CD7+ CD15+ CD34+ HLA-DR+ immunophenotype is a clinically distinct entity with a favorable outcome.* Ann Hematol, 2014. **93**(6): p. 957–63.

45. Boissel, N., et al., *Incidence and prognostic impact of c-Kit, FLT3, and Ras gene mutations in core binding factor acute myeloid leukemia (CBF-AML).* Leukemia, 2006. **20**(6): p. 965–70.

46. Cairoli, R., et al., *Prognostic impact of c-KIT mutations in core binding factor leukemias: an Italian retrospective study.* Blood, 2006. **107**(9): p. 3463–8.

47. Paschka, P., et al., *Adverse prognostic significance of KIT mutations in adult acute myeloid leukemia with inv(16) and t(8;21): a Cancer and Leukemia Group B Study.* J Clin Oncol, 2006. **24**(24): p. 3904–11.

48. Schnittger, S., et al., *KIT-D816 mutations in AML1-ETO-positive AML are associated with impaired event-free and overall survival.* Blood, 2006. **107**(5): p. 1791–9.

49. Schwind, S., et al., *inv(16)/t(16;16) acute myeloid leukemia with non-type A CBFB-MYH11 fusions associate with distinct clinical and genetic features and lack KIT mutations.* Blood, 2013. **121**(2): p. 385–91.

50. Wakita, S., et al., *Importance of c-kit mutation detection method sensitivity in prognostic analyses of t(8;21)(q22;q22) acute myeloid leukemia.* Leukemia, 2011. **25**(9): p. 1423–32.

51. Aukema, S.M., et al., *Double-hit B-cell lymphomas.* Blood, 2011. **117**(8): p. 2319–31.

52. Alsuwaidan, A., et al., *Bright CD38 expression by flow cytometric analysis is a biomarker for double/triple hit lymphomas with a*

moderate sensitivity and high specificity. Cytometry B Clin Cytom, 2019. **96**(5): p. 368–74.

53. Menezes, J., et al., *CSF3R T618I co-occurs with mutations of splicing and epigenetic genes and with a new PIM3 truncated fusion gene in chronic neutrophilic leukemia.* Blood Cancer J, 2013. **3**: p. e158.

54. Maxson, J.E., et al., *Oncogenic CSF3R mutations in chronic neutrophilic leukemia and atypical CML.* N Engl J Med, 2013. **368**(19): p. 1781–90.

55. Elliott, M.A. and A. Tefferi, *Chronic neutrophilic leukemia 2016: update on diagnosis, molecular genetics, prognosis, and management.* Am J Hematol, 2016. **91**(3): p. 341–9.

56. Gotlib, J., et al., *The new genetics of chronic neutrophilic leukemia and atypical CML: implications for diagnosis and treatment.* Blood, 2013. **122**(10): p. 1707–11.

57. Lasho, T.L., et al., *Chronic neutrophilic leukemia with concurrent CSF3R and SETBP1 mutations: single colony clonality studies, in vitro sensitivity to JAK inhibitors and lack of treatment response to ruxolitinib.* Leukemia, 2014. **28**(6): p. 1363–5.

58. Luo, Q., et al., *CSF3R T618I, ASXL1 G942 fs and STAT5B N642H trimutation co-contribute to a rare chronic neutrophilic leukaemia manifested by rapidly progressive leucocytosis, severe infections, persistent fever and deep venous thrombosis.* Br J Haematol, 2018. **180**(6): p. 892–4.

59. Ouyang, Y., et al., *Clinical significance of CSF3R, SRSF2 and SETBP1 mutations in chronic neutrophilic leukemia and chronic myelomonocytic leukemia.* Oncotarget, 2017. **8**(13): p. 20834–41.

60. Szuber, N., et al., *CSF3R-mutated chronic neutrophilic leukemia: long-term outcome in 19 consecutive patients and risk model for survival.* Blood Cancer J, 2018. **8**(2): p. 21.

61. Zhang, H., et al., *Gain-of-function mutations in granulocyte colony-stimulating factor receptor (CSF3R) reveal distinct mechanisms of CSF3R activation.* J Biol Chem, 2018. **293**(19): p. 7387–96.

62. Elliott, M.A., et al., *ASXL1 mutations are frequent and prognostically detrimental in CSF3R-mutated chronic neutrophilic leukemia.* Am J Hematol, 2015. **90**(7): p. 653–6.

63. Elliott, M.A., *Chronic neutrophilic leukemia: a contemporary review.* Curr Hematol Rep, 2004. **3**(3): p. 210–7.

64. Elliott, M.A., *Chronic neutrophilic leukemia and chronic myelomonocytic leukemia: WHO defined.* Best Pract Res Clin Haematol, 2006. **19**(3): p. 571–93.

65. Haferlach, T., et al., *The diagnosis of BCR/ABL-negative chronic myeloproliferative diseases (CMPD): a comprehensive approach based on morphology, cytogenetics, and molecular markers.* Ann Hematol, 2008. **87**(1): p. 1–10.

66. Tefferi, A., R. Skoda, and J.W. Vardiman, *Myeloproliferative neoplasms: contemporary diagnosis using histology and genetics.* Nat Rev Clin Oncol, 2009. **6**(11): p. 627–37.

67. Ferreri, A.J., S. Govi, and S.A. Pileri, *Hepatosplenic gamma-delta T-cell lymphoma.* Crit Rev Oncol Hematol, 2012. **83**(2): p. 283–92.

68. Belhadj, K., et al., *Hepatosplenic gammadelta T-cell lymphoma is a rare clinicopathologic entity with poor outcome: report on a series of 21 patients.* Blood, 2003. **102**(13): p. 4261–9.

69. Cooke, C.B., et al., *Hepatosplenic T-cell lymphoma: a distinct clinicopathologic entity of cytotoxic gamma delta T-cell origin.* Blood, 1996. **88**(11): p. 4265–74.

70. Farcet, J.P., et al., *Hepatosplenic T-cell lymphoma: sinusal/sinusoidal localization of malignant cells expressing the T-cell receptor gamma delta.* Blood, 1990. **75**(11): p. 2213–9.

71. Vega, F., L.J. Medeiros, and P. Gaulard, *Hepatosplenic and other gammadelta T-cell lymphomas.* Am J Clin Pathol, 2007. **127**(6): p. 869–80.

72. Wong, K.F., et al., *Hepatosplenic gamma delta T-cell lymphoma. A distinctive aggressive lymphoma type.* Am J Surg Pathol, 1995. **19**(6): p. 718–26.

73. Yamaguchi, M., *Hepatosplenic gammadelta T-cell lymphoma: difficulty in diagnosis.* Intern Med, 2004. **43**(2): p. 83–4.

74. Gorczyca, W., et al., *An approach to diagnosis of T-cell lymphoproliferative disorders by flow cytometry.* Cytometry, 2002. **50**(3): p. 177–90.

75. Gorczyca, W., *Flow cytometry in neoplastic hematopathology.* 2006, Taylor and Francis: London, New York.

76. Kumar, S., C. Lawlor, and E.S. Jaffe, *Hepatosplenic T-cell lymphoma of alphabeta lineage.* Am J Surg Pathol, 2001. **25**(7): p. 970–1.

77. Lai, R., et al., *Hepatosplenic T-cell lymphoma of alphabeta lineage in a 16-year-old boy presenting with hemolytic anemia and thrombocytopenia.* Am J Surg Pathol, 2000. **24**(3): p. 459–63.

78. Macon, W.R., et al., *Hepatosplenic alphabeta T-cell lymphomas: a report of 14 cases and comparison with hepatosplenic gammadelta T-cell lymphomas.* Am J Surg Pathol, 2001. **25**(3): p. 285–96.

79. Suarez, F., et al., *Hepatosplenic alphabeta T-cell lymphoma: an unusual case with clinical, histologic, and cytogenetic features of gammadelta hepatosplenic T-cell lymphoma.* Am J Surg Pathol, 2000. **24**(7): p. 1027–32.

80. Falini, B., et al., *ALK expression defines a distinct group of T/null lymphomas ("ALK lymphomas") with a wide morphological spectrum.* Am J Pathol, 1998. **153**(3): p. 875–86.

81. Pileri, S.A., et al., *Anaplastic large cell lymphoma: a concept reviewed.* Adv Clin Path, 1998. **2**(4): p. 285–96.

82. Pileri, S.A., et al., *Anaplastic large cell lymphoma: update of findings.* Leuk Lymphoma, 1995. **18**(1–2): p. 17–25.

83. Ott, G., et al., *A lymphohistiocytic variant of anaplastic large cell lymphoma with demonstration of the t(2;5)(p23;q35) chromosome translocation.* Br J Haematol, 1998. **100**(1): p. 187–90.

84. Stein, H., et al., *CD30(+) anaplastic large cell lymphoma: a review of its histopathologic, genetic, and clinical features.* Blood, 2000. **96**(12): p. 3681–95.

85. Bayle, C., et al., *Leukaemic presentation of small cell variant anaplastic large cell lymphoma: report of four cases.* Br J Haematol, 1999. **104**(4): p. 680–8.

86. Kinney, M.C., et al., *A small-cell-predominant variant of primary Ki-1 (CD30)+ T-cell lymphoma.* Am J Surg Pathol, 1993. **17**(9): p. 859–68.

87. Chan, J.K., R. Buchanan, and C.D. Fletcher, *Sarcomatoid variant of anaplastic large-cell Ki-1 lymphoma.* Am J Surg Pathol, 1990. **14**(10): p. 983–8.

88. Lamant, L., et al., *Gene-expression profiling of systemic anaplastic large-cell lymphoma reveals differences based on ALK status and two distinct morphologic ALK+ subtypes.* Blood, 2007. **109**(5): p. 2156–64.

89. Zinzani, P.L., et al., *Anaplastic large cell lymphoma Hodgkin's-like: a randomized trial of ABVD versus MACOP-B with and without radiation therapy.* Blood, 1998. **92**(3): p. 790–4.

90. Ferreri, A.J., et al., *Anaplastic large cell lymphoma, ALK-positive.* Crit Rev Oncol Hematol, 2012. **83**(2): p. 293–302.

91. Boi, M., et al., *PRDM1/BLIMP1 is commonly inactivated in anaplastic large T-cell lymphoma.* Blood, 2013. **122**(15): p. 2683–93.

92. Traverse-Glehen, A., et al., *Splenic diffuse red pulp small-B cell lymphoma: toward the emergence of a new lymphoma entity.* Discov Med, 2012. **13**(71): p. 253–65.

93. Verma, S., et al., *Rapid detection and quantitation of BRAF mutations in hairy cell leukemia using a sensitive pyrosequencing assay.* Am J Clin Pathol, 2012. **138**(1): p. 153–6.

94. Xi, L., et al., *Both variant and IGHV4-34-expressing hairy cell leukemia lack the BRAF V600E mutation.* Blood, 2012. **119**(14): p. 3330–2.

95. Ewalt, M., et al., *Real-time PCR-based analysis of BRAF V600E mutation in low and intermediate grade lymphomas confirms frequent occurrence in hairy cell leukaemia.* Hematol Oncol, 2012. **30**(4): p. 190–3.

96. Jebaraj, B.M., et al., *BRAF mutations in chronic lymphocytic leukemia.* Leuk Lymphoma, 2012. **54**(6): p. 1177–82.

97. Langabeer, S.E., et al., *Incidence of the BRAF V600E mutation in chronic lymphocytic leukaemia and prolymphocytic leukaemia.* Leuk Res, 2012. **36**(4): p. 483–4.

98. Haefliger, S., et al., *PET-positive bone lesion due to Langerhans cell histiocytosis after BEACOPP therapy for Hodgkin lymphoma: how anamnesis, histopathological accuracy, and molecular analysis could resolve a clinical dilemma.* Ann Hematol, 2018. **97**(2): p. 355–7.

99. Raess, P.W., et al., *BRAF V600E is also seen in unclassifiable splenic B-cell lymphoma/leukemia, a potential mimic of hairy cell leukemia.* Blood, 2013. **122**(17): p. 3084–5.

100. Turakhia, S., et al., *Immunohistochemistry for BRAF V600E in the differential diagnosis of hairy cell leukemia vs other splenic B-cell lymphomas.* Am J Clin Pathol, 2015. **144**(1): p. 87–93.

101. Pillonel, V., et al., *High-throughput sequencing of nodal marginal zone lymphomas identifies recurrent BRAF mutations.* Leukemia, 2018. **32**(11): p. 2412–26.

102. Follows, G.A., et al., *Rapid response of biallelic BRAF V600E mutated hairy cell leukaemia to low dose vemurafenib.* Br J Haematol, 2013. **161**(1): p. 150–3.

103. Tiacci, E., et al., *Simple genetic diagnosis of hairy cell leukemia by sensitive detection of the BRAF-V600E mutation.* Blood, 2012. **119**(1): p. 192–5.

104. Poulain, S., et al., *MYD88 L265P mutation in Waldenstrom macroglobulinemia.* Blood, 2013. **121**(22): p. 4504–11.

105. Treon, S.P. and Z.R. Hunter, *A new era for Waldenstrom macroglobulinemia: MYD88 L265P.* Blood, 2013. **121**(22): p. 4434–6.

106. Hunter, Z.R., et al., *The genomic landscape of Waldenstrom macroglobulinemia is characterized by highly recurring MYD88 and WHIM-like CXCR4 mutations, and small somatic deletions associated with B-cell lymphomagenesis.* Blood, 2014. **123**(11): p. 1637–46.

107. Ngo, V.N., et al., *Oncogenically active MYD88 mutations in human lymphoma.* Nature, 2011. **470**(7332): p. 115–9.

108. Xu, L., et al., *MYD88 L265P in Waldenstrom macroglobulinemia, immunoglobulin M monoclonal gammopathy, and other B-cell lymphoproliferative disorders using conventional and quantitative allele-specific polymerase chain reaction.* Blood, 2013. **121**(11): p. 2051–8.

109. Treon, S.P., et al., *Genomic landscape of Waldenstrom macroglobulinemia.* Hematol Oncol Clin North Am, 2018. **32**(5): p. 745–52.

110. Hunter, Z.R., et al., *Insights into the genomic landscape of MYD88 wild-type Waldenstrom macroglobulinemia.* Blood Adv, 2018. **2**(21): p. 2937–46.

111. King, R.L., et al., *Lymphoplasmacytic lymphoma with a non-IgM paraprotein shows clinical and pathologic heterogeneity and may harbor MYD88 L265P mutations.* Am J Clin Pathol, 2016. **145**(6): p. 843–51.

112. Yu, X., et al., *MYD88 L265P mutation in lymphoid malignancies.* Cancer Res, 2018. **78**(10): p. 2457–62.

113. Martinez-Trillos, A., et al., *Mutations in TLR/MYD88 pathway identify a subset of young chronic lymphocytic leukemia patients with favorable outcome.* Blood, 2014. **123**(24): p. 3790–6.

114. Baliakas, P., et al., *Recurrent mutations refine prognosis in chronic lymphocytic leukemia.* Leukemia, 2015. **29**(2): p. 329–36.

115. Baliakas, P., et al., *Prognostic relevance of MYD88 mutations in CLL: the jury is still out.* Blood, 2015. **126**(8): p. 1043–4.

116. Martinez-Trillos, A., et al., *Clinical impact of MYD88 mutations in chronic lymphocytic leukemia.* Blood, 2016. **127**(12): p. 1611–3.

117. Martinez-Lopez, A., et al., *MYD88 (L265P) somatic mutation in marginal zone B-cell lymphoma.* Am J Surg Pathol, 2015. **39**(5): p. 644–51.

118. Wang, W. and P. Lin, *Lymphoplasmacytic lymphoma and Waldenstrom macroglobulinaemia: clinicopathological features and differential diagnosis.* Pathology, 2020. **52**(1): p. 6–14.

119. Gertz, M., *Waldenstrom macroglobulinemia: my way.* Leuk Lymphoma, 2013. **54**(3): p. 464–71.

120. Gertz, M.A., *Waldenstrom macroglobulinemia: 2012 update on diagnosis, risk stratification, and management.* Am J Hematol, 2012. **87**(5): p. 503–10.

121. Treon, S.P., *How I treat Waldenstrom macroglobulinemia.* Blood, 2009. **114**(12): p. 2375–85.

122. Girard, L.P., et al., *Immunoglobulin M Paraproteinaemias.* Cancers (Basel), 2020. **12**(6): p. 1688.

12

PHENOTYPIC CLASSIFICATION OF MATURE B-CELL NEOPLASMS

Introduction

The major roles of flow cytometry (FC) in management of patients suspected to have lymphoma are assignment of lineage, determination of the stage of maturation, differentiation between reactive and clonal B-cells, and subclassification of B-cell neoplasm based on aberrant phenotype of B-cells and their forward scatter (FSC) [1–37]. This is especially important in samples from blood, in which there is no tissue available for immunohistochemistry (molecular abnormalities are often not specific for a definite subclassification of neoplastic process, e.g., in chronic lymphocytic leukemia, CLL). The most commonly used markers in evaluation of B-cell neoplasms include CD5, CD10, CD11c, CD19, CD20, CD22, CD23, CD25, CD34, CD38, CD43, CD45, CD79, CD81, CD103, CD200, surface kappa, and surface lambda. The most commonly used markers in evaluation of plasma cell neoplasms include CD19, CD20, CD38, CD45, CD56, CD81, CD117, CD138, CD200, cytoplasmic kappa, and cytoplasmic lambda. In some B-cell neoplasms, especially in those with bright CD10 and CD38 expression, dim or negative CD20 and lack of surface light chain immunoglobulins, the distinction between mature and immature process (B-cell acute lymphoblastic leukemia, B-ALL) requires correlation with CD34 and cytoplasmic staining for TdT, CD22, and CD79a.

Figure 12.1 presents algorithmic approach to the diagnosis of B-cell lymphoproliferations. Based on the immunophenotype, mature B-cell lymphoproliferations can be broadly subdivided into those with specific phenotype (CD5+, CD10+, or CD103+) and those without. The former group includes chronic lymphocytic leukemia/small lymphocytic lymphoma (CLL/SLL, CD5+/CD23+), mantle cell lymphoma (MCL, CD5+), follicular lymphoma (FL, CD10+), Burkitt lymphoma (BL, CD10+), and hairy cell leukemia (HCL, CD25+/CD103+). The group of B-cell lymphoproliferations with non-descript phenotype (CD5−, CD10−, CD103−) includes marginal zone lymphoma (MZL), subset of diffuse large B-cell lymphoma (DLBCL), subset of B-cell prolymphocytic leukemias (B-PLLs), and lymphoplasmacytic lymphoma/Waldenström macroglobulinemia (LPL/WM). Table 12.1 presents the immunophenotypic profile of major types of B-cell lymphoproliferations. Apart from CD5, CD10, and CD103, additional markers which are useful in classification of mature B-cell lymphoproliferations include CD11c, CD23, CD25, CD38, CD71, BCL2, and FMC-7, as well as FSC. Tables 12.1 and 12.2 summarize the major phenotypic characteristics of mature B-cell lymphoproliferations.

Classification of B-cell neoplasms based on CD5 and CD10 expression

CD5+ mature B-cell neoplasms

- CLL/SLL
- Monoclonal B-cell lymphocytosis (MBL) with CLL-like phenotype
- MCL
- Large B-cell lymphoma representing Richter's transformation
- De novo CD5+ DLBCL

- Intravascular large B-cell lymphomas (IVLBLs), subset
- MZL, subset
- Rare cases of lymphoplasmacytic lymphoma (LPL/WM)
- Very rare cases of FL

CD5 expression is most typical for CLL/SLL and MCL. Additionally, large B-cell lymphomas developing in the background of CLL/SLL (Richter's transformation), occasional cases of de novo DLBCL, subset of IVLBLs, and rare cases of MZL and LPL and very few cases of FL may be CD5+ [38–45]. CLL/SLL is characterized by co-expression of CD5 and CD23, negative to dim CD81, positive CD43 and CD200, dim expression of CD20, dim or negative expression of CD22, CD79b and surface light chain immunoglobulins. CD81 is negative or dimly positive (at the same level as normal T-cells). CD11c may be negative, dim or partially positive in CLL/SLL. Atypical CLL/SLL shows either lack of CD23 expression or presence of moderate expression of CD20 and surface light chain immunoglobulins. Among MZLs, CD5 is most often expressed by nodal marginal zone lymphoma (NMZL, 5%–10%) and splenic marginal zone lymphoma (SMZL, 20%) and rarely by mucosa-associated lymphoid tissue lymphoma (MALT type, 1%).

In contrast to CLL/SLL, typical MCL is negative for CD23 and displays moderate to bright expression of both CD20, CD22 and surface light chain immunoglobulins, as well as positive CD81, often positive CD38 and CD43, and negative CD200. CD200 and CD23 expression helps to differentiate between CLL/CLL (both markers positive) and MCL (both markers negative). However, in subset of MCL the phenotype may be abnormal (including positive CD23 and CD200, lack of CD5 or aberrant expression of CD10 expression) and overlap with either CLL or other B-cell lymphoproliferations. CLL cases may also show aberrant phenotype (e.g., moderate CD20, negative CD23 expression) resembling MCL, and therefore final diagnosis requires correlation with morphology, immunohistochemistry, and genetic testing. Immunohistochemistry for cyclin D1 (BCL1) and SOX11, conventional cytogenetics for t(11;14), and/or FISH studies for *CCND1* rearrangement help to establish the diagnosis of MCL. Figure 12.2 compares the flow cytometric differences between CLL and MCL. Table 12.3 compares the phenotype of CLL, atypical CLL and MCL. The scoring systems used to separate CLL from other B-cell lymphoproliferative disorders are discussed in Chapter 13 (in the section of differential diagnosis of CLL).

CD5+ DLBCL may represent a progression of CLL/SLL (Richter's transformation) or develop without prior history of CLL/SLL (de novo CD5+ DLBCL). It differs from both CLL/SLL and typical MCL by large size of the neoplastic cells (high FSC) and often increased Ki-67 index or prominent CD71 expression. Blastoid or pleomorphic variants of MCL, however, may be composed of larger cells which resemble morphologically DLBCL. Immunohistochemical analysis for cyclin D1 (BCL1) and/or cytogenetic/FISH studies for t(11;14)/*CCND1* rearrangement are crucial for a definite subclassification. These tests are also indispensable for the diagnosis of CD5− MCL.

DOI: 10.1201/9781003197935-12

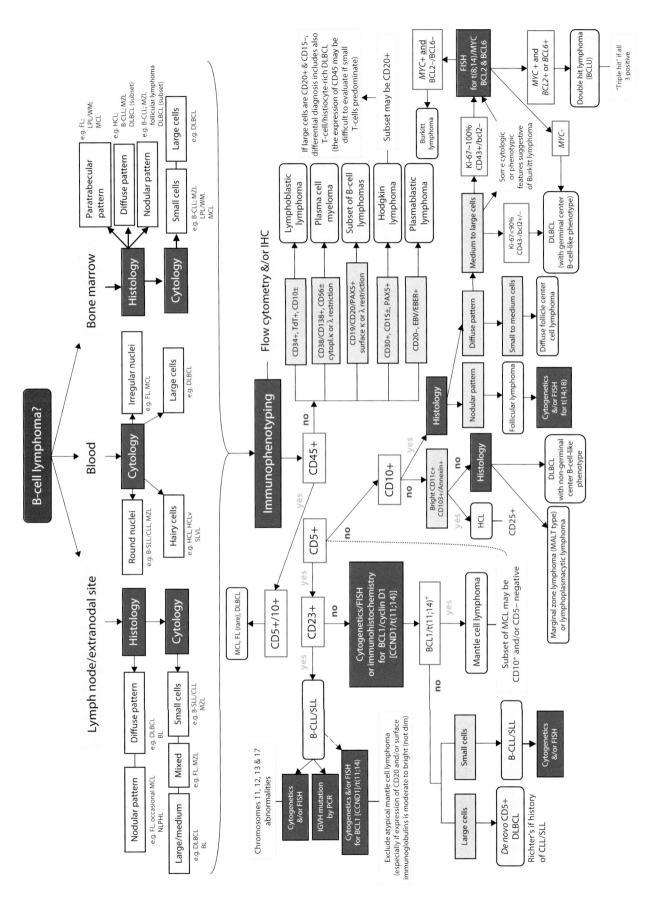

FIGURE 12.1 Algorithm for the diagnosis of B-cell lymphoproliferations.

TABLE 12.1: The Immunophenotypic Profiles of Major Types of Mature B-Cell Neoplasms Composed Mostly of Small to Medium-Sized Cells

	CLL	MCL	MZL^c	HCL	HCL-v	FL	LPL/WM	SDRPL
κ or λ	+^{dim}/(−)	+	+	+	+	+/(−)	+	+
CD5	+	+/(−)	−/(+)	−	−	−	−/(+)	−/(+)
CD10	−	−/(+)	−	−/(+)	−/(+)	+/(−)	−/(+)	−
CD11c	+/−	−	+^{dim}/−	+^{bright}	+^{bright}	−	−	+^{moderate}/(−)
CD19	+	+	+	+	+	+^{dim}	+	+
CD20	+^{dim}/(−)	+	+	+	+	+	+	+
CD23	+/(−)	−/(+)	−/+	−/(+)	−/(+)	−/(+)	−/(+)	−
CD25	−/(+)	−	+/(−)	+	−	−/(+)	+/(−)	−
CD27	+	+	+	−	+	+	+	+
CD38	−/+	+/(−)	+/−	−	−	+/(−)	+/(−)	−
CD43	+	+	+/−	+/(−)	−/(+^{dim})	−/(+)	−	−/(+)
CD45	+	+	+	+	+	+	+	+
CD71	−	−/(+$^{dim/partial}$)	−	−	−	−/+$^{dim/partial}$	−	−
CD79b	−/(+^{dim})^a	+^{moderate}/(−)	+	+^{bright}	+/(−)	+	+	+
CD81	−/+^{dim}	+^{strong}	+/(−)	+^{dim}	+	+^{dim}/−	+/(−)	+/−
CD103	−	−	−	+	+	−	−	−/(+)
CD123	−	−/(+)	+^{dim}/−	+^{bright}	−/(+)	−	−	−/(+)
CD200	+^{bright}	−^{b}	−/(+^{dim})	+^{bright}	−/+^{dim}	−/+^{dim}	+^{dim}/−	+
BCL1	−	+	−	+/−	−/(+)	−	−	−
SOX11	−	+	−	−	−	−	−	−
Genetic changes	*IGVH* mutation, +12, del(13q)	*CCND1* rearrangement, t(11;14)	del(7q) in SMZL *NOTCH* and *KLF2* mutations	*BRAF* mutation	*MAP2K1* mutation	*BCL2* rearrangement, t(14;18)	*MYD88* and *CXCR4* mutations	del(7q), +18

Abbreviations: κ and λ, kappa and lambda surface light chain immunoglobulins; CLL, chronic lymphocytic leukemia; MCL, mantle cell lymphoma; MZL, marginal zone lymphoma; HCL, hairy cell leukemia; HCL-v, hairy cell leukemia variant; FL, follicular lymphoma; LPL/WM, lymphoplasmacytic lymphoma/Waldenström macroglobulinemia; SDRPL, splenic diffuse red pulp B-cell lymphoma; BCL1, B-cell lymphoma 1 (cyclin D1); SMZL, splenic marginal zone lymphoma.

Note: +, positive; (+), rarely positive; − negative; (−), rarely negative.

^{a} Atypical CLL more often positive.

^{b} Rare cases of MCL may be positive for CD200 (4%) and this groups often shows CD23 expression, indolent clinical course, and non-nodal leukemic presentation.

^{c} SMZL is often positive for CD200 and shows bright CD79b (rare cases may be CD103+)

MBL with CLL-like phenotype differs from CLL by the absolute number of clonal B-cells <5 × 10⁹/L. The other less common variants of MBL include MBL with atypical CLL-like phenotype (CD5⁺/CD23⁻CD20⁺⁽ᵈⁱᵐ ᵒʳ ᵐᵒᵈᵉʳᵃᵗᵉ⁾ or CD5⁺/CD23⁺/CD20^bright⁺) and CD5⁻ MBL (non-CLL-type or MZL-like, also termed clonal B-cell lymphocytosis of marginal zone origin, CBL-MZ). CBL-MZ (CD5⁻ MBL) may represent early blood involvement by either SMZL or SDRPl: splenic diffuse red pulp B-cell lymphoma. CBL-MZ are usually negative for *MYD88* mutation, which helps to exclude LPL/WM.

B-PLL entity was deleted from current WHO classification. The introduced splenic B-cell lymphoma/leukemia with prominent nucleoli replaces "hairy cell leukemia variant" and "CD5-negative B-PLL".

A minute subset of benign B-cells in blood, bone marrow (BM), and lymph nodes may express CD5. In adults, majority of circulating B-cells (B-2 cells) are CD5⁻ (they comprise ~10% of lymphocytes), but a minute subset of B-cells expresses CD5. These cells (B-1 cells) can be further subdivided into CD5⁺ transitional B-cells ("bridge" immature B-ells in the BM and mature naïve B-cells in peripheral blood) and CD5⁺ pre-naïve B-cells [46]. The population of benign CD5⁺ B-cells is prominent in fetal and infant circulation, and their number decreases significantly with age. The population of benign circulating CD5⁺ B-cells is more prominent in pediatric population and in patients with regenerating marrow, viral infections, or certain autoimmune disorders.

Phenotypic and molecular characteristics of CD5⁺ B-cell lymphomas:

CLL: CD19⁺, CD20⁺⁽ᵒᶠᵗᵉⁿ ᵈⁱᵐ⁾, CD22⁻ᐟ⁺⁽ᵈⁱᵐ⁾, surface light chain immunoglobulins⁺⁽ᵈⁱᵐ⁾ᐟʳᵃʳᵉˡʸ⁻, CD5⁺, CD23⁺ᐟʳᵃʳᵉˡʸ⁻, CD10⁻, CD38⁺⁽ᵈⁱᵐ ᵒʳ ᵖᵃʳᵗⁱᵃˡ⁾ᐟ⁻, CD43⁺, CD71⁻, CD81⁻ᐟᵈⁱᵐ, CD200⁺ˢᵗʳᵒⁿᵍ, CD11c⁺ᐟ⁻, CD13⁻ᐟʳᵃʳᵉˡʸ⁺, CD2⁻ᐟʳᵃʳᵉˡʸ⁺, cyclin D1 (BCL1)⁻, SOX11⁻

MCL: CD19⁺, CD20⁺, CD22⁺, surface light chain immunoglobulin⁺, CD5⁺ᐟʳᵃʳᵉˡʸ⁻, CD10⁻ᐟʳᵃʳᵉˡʸ⁺, CD11c⁻, CD23⁻, CD38⁺, CD43⁺, CD71⁻ᐟ⁺⁽ᵈⁱᵐ ᵒʳ ᵖᵃʳᵗⁱᵃˡ⁾, CD81⁺, CD200⁻, cyclin D1 (BCL1)⁺, SOX11⁺, t(11;14)/*CCND1*ʳᵉᵃʳʳᵃⁿᵍᵉᵈ

FL: CD19⁺⁽ᵒᶠᵗᵉⁿ ᵈⁱᵐ⁾, CD20⁺, surface light chain immunoglobulin⁺, CD5⁻ᐟʳᵃʳᵉˡʸ⁺, CD10⁺, CD11c⁻, CD23⁻, CD38⁺ᐟʳᵃʳᵉˡʸ⁻, CD43⁻, CD71⁻ᐟ⁺⁽ᵈⁱᵐ ᵒʳ ᵖᵃʳᵗⁱᵃˡ⁾, CD81⁺⁽ᵈⁱᵐ⁾ᐟ⁻, CD200⁻ᐟ⁺⁽ᵈⁱᵐ⁾, t(14;18)/*BCL2*ʳᵉᵃʳʳᵃⁿᵍᵉᵈ

MZL: CD19⁺, CD20⁺, surface light chain immunoglobulin⁺, CD5⁻ᐟʳᵃʳᵉˡʸ⁺, CD10⁻, CD11c⁺ᐟ⁻, CD23⁻ᐟ⁺, CD38⁺ᐟ⁻, CD43⁻ᐟ⁺, CD81⁺ᐟ⁻, CD200⁻ᐟʳᵃʳᵉˡʸ⁺, SMZL may show del(7q)

LPL: CD19⁺, CD20⁺, surface light chain immunoglobulin⁺, CD5⁻ᐟʳᵃʳᵉ ᶜᵃˢᵉˢ⁺, CD10⁻ᐟʳᵃʳᵉˡʸ⁺, CD11c⁻, CD23⁻ᐟʳᵃʳᵉˡʸ⁺, CD38⁺ᐟʳᵃʳᵉˡʸ⁻,

TABLE 12.2: The Immunophenotypic Profiles of Major Types of Mature B-Cell Neoplasms Composed of Medium-Sized to Large Cells

	DLBCL-GCB	DLBCL-ABC	BL	MCL Blastoid	HGBL-R	HGBL NOS	PBL	IVLBL	PEL[a]	PCM	B-ALL
κ and λ	+/(−)	+/(−)	+/(−)	+	+/(−)	+	−/+^{dim}	+	+/(−)	−	−
CD5	−/(+)	−/(+)	−	+/(−)	−	−	−	−	−	−	−
CD10	+	−	+^{bright}	−/(+)	+/(−)	−/+	−/(+)	−	−	−	+^{bright}/(−)
CD11c	−/(+)	−/(+)	−	−	−	−	−	−	−	−	−
CD19	+	+	+	+	+/+^{dim}	+	−	+	−	−	+
CD20	+/+^{dim}	+	+	+	+/+^{dim}	+	−/+^{dim}	+	−	−/(+)	−/(+^{dim})
CD23	−	−	−	−	−	−	−	−	−	− (+)	−
CD25	−/(+)	−/(+)	−	−	−	−	−	−	−	−	−
CD34	−	−	−	−	−	−	−	−	−	−	+/(−)
CD38	+	+^{dim}/(−)	+^{bright}	+	+^{bright}	+	+^{bright}	+/−	+	+^{bright}	+^{bright}
CD43	−/(+^{dim})	+^{dim}/(−)	+^{bright}	+	+/−	+/−	−/(+)	−	−/+	+	+/(−)
CD45	+	+	+	+	+	+	−/(+)	+	+^{dim}/−	−/(+)	−/+^{dim}
CD56	−	−	−	−	−	−	−/+	−	+/−	+/(−)	−/(+)
CD71	+^{dim}/(−)	+/(−)	+^{bright}	+^{dim}/−	+	+	+^{dim}	x	+	+/−	−/+^{dim}
CD79b[b]	+^{moderate}	+	+^{dim}	+/(−)	x	X	−/+^{dim}	x	−	−	x
CD81	+^{dim}/−	+^{dim}/−	+^{bright}	+	+^{bright}	+	x	x	−	−/(+)	+^{dim}
CD103	−^{c}	−^{c}	−	−	−	−	−	−	−	−	−
CD123	−	−	−	−	−	−	−	−	−	−	−
CD200	−/(+^{dim})	−/(+)	−/(+)	−	−/+	−/(+)	x	x	x	+/(−)	+/−
BCL1	−	−	−	+	−	−	−	−	−	−	−
BCL2	+/−	+/−	−	+	+	+/−	−	+	−	+	+
BCL6	+	−/+	+	−	−/+	−/+	−	−	−	−	−
MUM1	−/(+)	+	+	−/+	+	+	+	+/−	+/−	+	−/+
TdT	−	−	−	−	−	−	−	−	−	−	+/(−)
Other features	rarely *MYC*$^{+}$		*MYC*$^{+}$, Ki67~100%	Cyclin D1 (BCL1)$^{+}$, SOX11^{+}, *CCND1*$^{+}$	*MYC*$^{+}$ and *BCL2*$^{+}$ (and/or *BCL6*$^{+}$)		EBER^{+}, high Ki67		HHV8^{+}, EBV^{+}, CD30^{+}		

Abbreviations: κ and λ, kappa and lambda surface light chain immunoglobulins; DLBCL-GCB, diffuse large B-cell lymphoma, germinal center B-cell like; DLBCL-ABC, diffuse large B-cell lymphoma, activated B-cell like; BL, Burkitt lymphoma; HGBL-R, high grade B-cell lymphoma with rearrangement of MYC and BCL2 (and/or BCL6); HGBL-NOS, high grade B-cell lymphoma, not otherwise specified; IVLBL, intravascular large B-cell lymphoma; PBL, plasmablastic lymphoma; PCM, plasma cell myeloma; PEL, primary effusion lymphoma; B-ALL, B-cell acute lymphoblastic leukemia/lymphoma.

Note: +, positive; (+), rarely positive; − negative; (−), rarely negative; x, not available.

a   Solid variant may be positive for B-cell markers.

b   Surface.

c   Rare case of DLBCL may be CD103^{+}.

CD43$^{−}$, CD71$^{−}$, CD81$^{+/−}$, CD200$^{+(dim)/−}$, prominent M protein in serum, *MYD88*^{mutated}, *CXCR4*$^{mutated (subset)}$

DLBCL: FSC^{high}, CD19^{+}, CD20^{+}, surface light chain immunoglobulin^{+}, CD5$^{−/rarely+}$, CD10$^{+/−}$, CD11c$^{−/rarely+}$, CD23$^{−}$, CD25$^{−/rarely+}$, CD38^{+}, CD43$^{−/+}$, CD71$^{+(dim\ or\ rarely\ strong)}$, CD81$^{+(dim)}$, CD200$^{−/rarely\ +(dim)}$, BCL6$^{+/−}$, MUM1$^{+/−}$

CD10^{+} mature B-cell neoplasms

- FL
- BL
- DLBCLs (subset)
- High grade B-cell lymphoma with *MYC* and *BCL2* (and/or *BCL6*) rearrangements (HGBL-R, double or triple hit lymphoma)
- High grade B-cell lymphoma, not otherwise specified (HGBL, NOS), subset

- MCLs, minor subset
- HCLs, minor subset
- LPL, subset
- IVLBLs, subset

CD10 is positive in FL (Figure 12.3), BL, high grade B-cell lymphomas with *MYC* and *BCL2* (and/or *BCL6*) rearrangements (HGBL-R), and subset of DLBCL. Occasional cases of HCL, IVLBL, and MCL (Figure 12.4) may also be CD10^{+} [47–50]. Among benign B-cells, CD10 is expressed by hematogones and reactive follicle center cells. Positive CD10 (especially if bright) and bright expression of CD38 is seen in both mature and immature B-cell neoplasms (FL, DLBCL, BL, HGBL-R, B-ALL).

When analyzed by FC, FL displays moderate CD10 expression (rare cases may be CD10$^{−}$ or show very dim CD10), dim CD19, moderate CD20 and moderate expression of surface light chain immunoglobulins. Rare cases of FL may be negative for surface light chain immunoglobulins. The majority of cases are CD38^{+}.

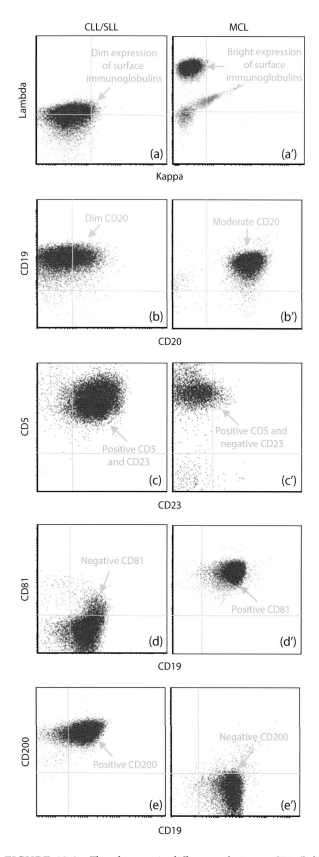

FIGURE 12.2 The phenotypic differences between CLL (left column) and MCL (right column). CLL/SLL differs from MCL by dim expression of surface immunoglobulins (a, a'), dim expression of CD20 (b, b'), positive CD23 (c, c'), negative CD81 (d, d'), and positive CD200 (e, e').

A minor subset of cases is positive for CD23. The expression of CD71 is variable and varies from negative to partial to positive. The expression of CD71 correlates with lymphoma grade [51]. The FSC ranges from low to heterogeneous to high and depends on cellular composition of FL. Primary cutaneous follicle center lymphomas (PCFCCL) with diffuse pattern of infiltrate often lack CD10, whereas those with nodular pattern are usually CD10+.

DLBCL is a heterogeneous group of lymphomas, which can be subdivided into several variants with distinct clinical, morphological, immunophenotypic, or molecular features. DLBCLs without any specific criteria for subdivision are classified as DLBCL, not otherwise specified (NOS). Based on the expression of CD10, BCL6, and MUM1 (IRF4), DLBCL can be divided into germinal center B-cell-like (GCB) and non-germinal center-like ("activated"; ABC) subgroups. DLBCL with GCB-like phenotype is positive for CD10 (>30% of cells) and/or BCL6 (MUM1 is usually not expressed). All other cases are classified as non-germinal center-like type (CD10−/MUM1+). FC analysis of DLBCL may show decreased viability of the sample and/or predominance of reactive elements. The expression of CD19 is usually moderate and CD20 is moderate or bright. FSC is high and CD71 expression is positive.

BL is positive for CD10, CD71, MYC, CD38, CD43, and BCL6, negative for CD5 and BCL2. Bright CD81 is a feature of BL and often distinguishes it from other CD10+ lymphomas. The proliferation fraction determined by Ki-67 approaches 100%. The diagnosis requires confirmation by FISH studies for MYC rearrangements. In addition to BL, also high-grade B-cell lymphomas with MYC and BCL2 (and/or BCL6) rearrangements (HGBL-R) and subset of DLBCL are positive for MYC rearrangement (BL is negative for both BCL2 and BCL6 rearrangements). FCS is increased in BL but lower than in DLBCL. The expression of CD38 is often brighter and expression of CD79a dimmer in BL than in CD10+ DLBCL [11]. In a study by McGowan et al., the percentage of CD71+ cells was higher in BL when compared to DLBCL [11], but based on the earlier study by Wu et al., the CD71 fluorescence intensity did not differ between those two lymphomas [51]. B-cell lymphomas with MYC rearrangement are characterized by bright CD38 expression [52, 53]. HGBL-R differ from CD10+ DLBCL by brighter CD71, CD38, and CD10 and often dimmer CD20. Only minor subset of DLBCL (often with anaplastic or "high-grade" morphology) shows bright expression of both CD38 and CD71. FSC in DLBCL is often homogeneous high while in both BL and HGBL-R is often heterogeneous (variable)

HCL is characterized by bright expression of CD20, CD22 and surface immunoglobulins, negative CD38, positive FMC-7, bright CD11c and co-expression of CD25, CD103, and CD123. Subset of cases may be CD10+. MCLs are usually CD10−, but small subset of cases may co-express CD5 and CD10. Diagnosis is established by identification of t(11;14) [CCND1-IGH rearrangement]. Minor subset of LPL may show aberrant expression of CD10. FC analysis of LPL shows clonal B-cells and clonal plasma cells expressing the same light chain immunoglobulins as clonal B-cells and IgM. Majority of LPLs are positive for MYD88 mutation and are characterized by prominent serum M protein.

Phenotypic and molecular characteristics of CD10+ B-cell lymphomas:

DLBCL: FSC^high, CD19+, CD20+, surface light chain immunoglobulin+, CD5−/rarely+, CD10+/−, CD11c−/rarely+, CD23−, CD25−/rarely+, CD38+, CD43−/+, CD71+(dim or rarely strong), CD81+(dim), CD200−/rarely +(dim), BCL6+/−, MUM1+/−

TABLE 12.3: Differential Diagnosis Between CLL, Atypical CLL (aCLL) and Mantle Cell Lymphoma (MCL)

	κ/λ	CD5	CD10	CD11c	CD20	CD22	CD23	CD38	CD43	CD81	CD200
CLL	+dim/−	+	−	+/−	+dim/−	−/+dim	+	−/+partial	+	−/+dim	+strong
aCLL	+	+	−	+/−	+	+	−/+	−/+partial	+	−/+dim	+strong
MCL	+	+/(−)	−/(+)	−	+	+	−	+/(−)	+	+strong	−a

Notes: +, positive; (+), rarely positive; −, negative; (−), rarely negative.

Dim (or negative) surface light chain immunoglobulins, dim or negative CD20, negative CD22, CD38, CD81, positive (often partial) CD11c and positive CD23 and CD200 are typical for CLL. Atypical cases of CLL may show lack of CD23, moderate surface light chain immunoglobulins, CD20 and CD22, but show negative (or dim) CD81 and strong CD200. MCL differs from both CLL and aCLL by strong expression of CD81, lack of CD200, positive CD38, negative CD11c and moderate expression of surface light chain immunoglobulins, CD20 and CD22.

a   Rare cases of leukemic non-nodal MCL may be positive.

MCL: CD19+, CD20+, surface light chain immunoglobulin+, CD5+, CD10−/rarely+, CD11c−, CD23−, CD38+, CD43+, CD71−/+(dim or partial), CD81+, CD200−, cyclin D1 (BCL1)+, SOX11+, t(11;14)/*CCND1*rearranged

FL: CD19+(often dim), CD20+, surface light chain immunoglobulin+, CD5−, CD10+, CD11c−, CD23−, CD38+/rarely−, CD43−, CD71−/+(dim or partial), CD81+(dim)/−, CD200−/+(dim), t(14;18)/*BCL2*rearranged

LPL: CD19+, CD20+, surface light chain immunoglobulin+, CD5−/rare cases+, CD10−/rarely+, CD11c−, CD13−/rarely+, CD23−/rarely+, CD38+/rarely−, CD43−, CD71−, CD81+/−, CD200+(dim)/−, prominent M protein in serum, *MYD88*mutated, *CXCR4*mutated (subset)

HGBL-R: FSCincreased, CD19+, CD20+ (may be dim), surface light chain immunoglobulin+/rarely−, BCL2+, CD5−, CD10+/rarely−, CD11c−, CD23−, CD25−, CD38+, CD43+/−, CD71+, CD81+,

CD200−, *MYC* and *BCL2* (and/or *BCL6*) rearrangement; Ki-67high

BL: FSCincreased, CD19+, CD20+, surface light chain immunoglobulin+, BCL2−, CD5−, CD10+, CD11c−, CD23−, CD25−, CD38+, CD43+(strong), CD71+(strong), CD81+(strong), CD200−/rarely+(dim), Ki-67~100%, *MYC*rearranged

HCL: CD19+, CD20+, surface light chain immunoglobulin+, CD5−, CD10−/rarely+, CD11c+bright, CD22+bright, CD23−/rarely+, CD25+, CD38−, CD43+(dim)/rarely−, CD71−, CD81+(dim), CD103+, CD123+, CD200+(bright), *BRAF*mutated

CD5+/CD10+ mature B-cell neoplasms

- DLBCL, rare cases
- FL, very rare cases

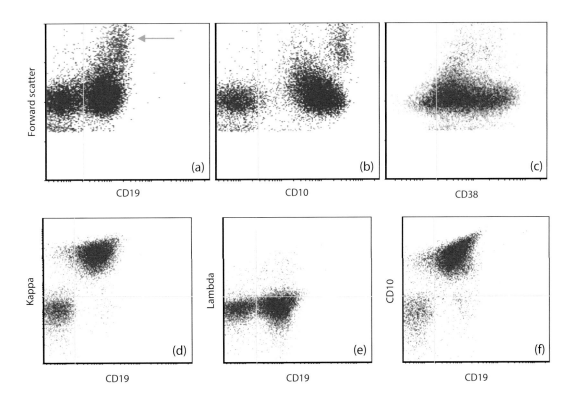

FIGURE 12.3 Follicular lymphoma. Most lymphomatous cells (red dots) have low forward scatter (a) and only minor subset of cells (blue dots, arrow) show increased forward scatter. The expression of CD19 is dim (a), expression of CD10 is strong (b), and the expression of CD38 is variable (c). Majority of FLs show surface light chain immunoglobulin restriction with moderate or bright expression of either kappa or lambda (d–e). Scattergram f shows co-expression of CD19 with CD10.

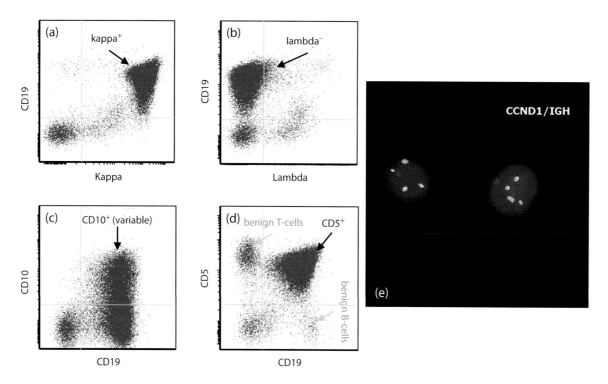

FIGURE 12.4 Mantle cell lymphoma with aberrant expression of CD10. Monoclonal B-cells (a–b) co-express CD10 (c; variable expression) and CD5 (d). FISH studies showed rearrangement of CCND1 and IGH (e; yellow fusion signals).

- MCL, rare cases
- BL, very rare cases

B-cell neoplasms co-expressing both CD5 and CD10 are uncommon and include occasional cases of DLBCL, FL (Figure 12.5), MCL, CLL/SLL, and BL [14, 39, 48]. CD5 and CD10 may be both positive in T-cell lymphoproliferations, e.g., T-lymphoblastic leukemia (T-ALL) and angioimmunoblastic T-cell lymphoma (AITL).

Phenotypic and molecular characteristics of CD5+/CD10+ B-cell lymphomas:

DLBCL: FSC^{high}, CD19$^+$, CD20$^+$, surface light chain immunoglobulin$^+$, CD5$^{-/rarely+}$, CD10$^{+/-}$, CD11c$^{-/rarely+}$, CD23$^-$, CD25$^{-/rarely+}$, CD38$^+$, CD43$^{-/+}$, CD71$^{+(dim\ or\ rarely\ strong)}$, CD81$^{+(dim)}$, CD200$^{-/rarely\ +(dim)}$, BCL6$^{+/-}$, MUM1$^{+/-}$

MCL: CD19$^+$, CD20$^+$, surface light chain immunoglobulin$^+$, CD5$^+$, CD10$^{-/rarely+}$, CD11c$^-$, CD23$^-$, CD38$^+$, CD43$^+$, CD71$^{-/+(dim\ or\ partial)}$, CD81$^+$, CD200$^-$, cyclin D1 (BCL1)$^+$, SOX11$^+$, t(11;14)/*CCND1*^{rearranged}

FL: CD19$^{+(often\ dim)}$, CD20$^+$, surface light chain immunoglobulin$^+$, CD5$^{-/rarely+}$, CD10$^+$, CD11c$^-$, CD23$^-$, CD38$^{+/rarely-}$, CD43$^-$, CD71$^{-/+(dim\ or\ partial)}$, CD81$^{+(dim)/-}$, CD200$^{-/+(dim)}$, t(14; 18)/*BCL2*^{rearranged}

CD5$^-$/CD10$^-$ mature B-cell neoplasms

- MZL
- SMZL
- SDRPL
- CBL-MZ
- LPL/WM
- DLBCL, subset

- HCL
- Hairy cell leukemia variant (splenic B-cell lymphoma/leukemia with prominent nucleoli)
- Plasmablastic lymphoma (PBL)
- IVLBCL
- Rare cases of FL
- Rare cases of MCL

B-cell lymphoproliferations, which are negative for both CD5 and CD10, include MZL (Figure 12.6), LPL/WM, HCL, B-PLL, and DLBCL. Additionally, this group of mature B-cell neoplasms includes rare cases of CD5$^-$ MCL and CD10$^-$ FL. Occasional cases of FL may show discrepant results of CD10 staining by FC and immunohistochemistry (usually CD10$^-$ by FC and CD10$^+$ by immunohistochemistry). Subset of DLBCLs may be CD10$^+$ and/or CD5$^+$.

The diagnosis of HCL is easily confirmed by co-expression of CD25, CD103, and CD123 (all markers are most often strongly positive), but the subclassification of majority of CD5$^-$/CD10$^-$ B-cell lymphoproliferations with leukemic presentation into specific category may be difficult, partially due to absence of accessible tissue for pathological evaluation. In the series of 156 patients with CD5$^-$/CD10$^-$ chronic B-cell lymphoproliferative disorder reported by Goldaniga et al., 30 patients (19.2%) were classified as SMZL (based on splenomegaly, compatible cytomorphology, karyotype, or intrasinusoidal BM pattern), 19 patients (12.2%) were classified as LPL/WM (serum monoclonal component), and the majority of patients remained unclassifiable (median follow-up 51 months; range 6–216 months) [22]. LPL/WM, in contrast to MZL, is often characterized by paratrabecular pattern of the BM involvement, and SMZL shows characteristic intrasinusoidal pattern of BM involvement. High FSC helps to distinguish DLBCL from low grade lymphomas. Among CD5$^-$/CD10$^-$ B-cell lymphoproliferative disorders in blood, bright CD11c expression

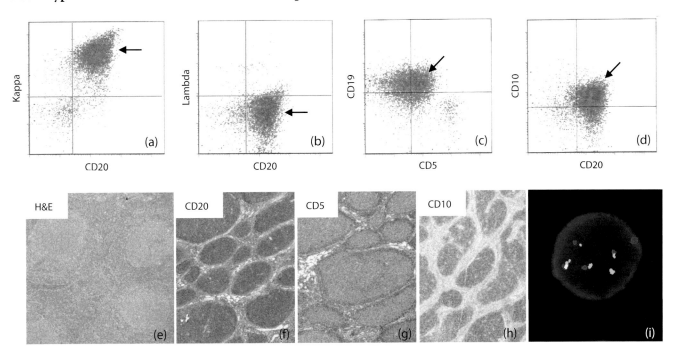

FIGURE 12.5 Follicular lymphoma, unusual case with aberrant CD5 expression. Flow cytometry revealed monoclonal (kappa⁺) B-cells (a–b; arrows) with co-expression of CD5 (c) and CD10 (d). Histology showed nodular infiltrate (e), which by immunohisto-chemistry was positive for CD20 (f), CD5 (g), and CD10 (h). FISH studies confirmed BCL2-IGH rearrangement (i).

is typical for HCL. The variant of HCL (HCL-v), which is CD103⁺ and CD25⁻ shows often bright CD11c, but occasional cases may display moderate expression. Splenic diffuse red pulp small B-cell lymphoma (SDRPL) shows moderate CD11c and MZL, including SMZL is either negative for CD11c or show and partial expression. The expression of CD81 and CD200 is variable in both HCL-v and MZL, but HCL-v often shows stronger expression of CD81 than in MZL of HCL. In HCL and HCL-v, Salem et al. reported an inverse pattern of expression of CD43 and CD81: CD43⁺/CD81ᵈⁱᵐ⁺ in HCL and CD43ᵈⁱᵐ⁺/CD81ᵇʳⁱᵍʰᵗ⁺ in HCL-v [54]. Figure 12.7 compares FC patterns of SMZL and HCL-v. On genetic level, HCL-v often shows mutations of MAP2K1 while

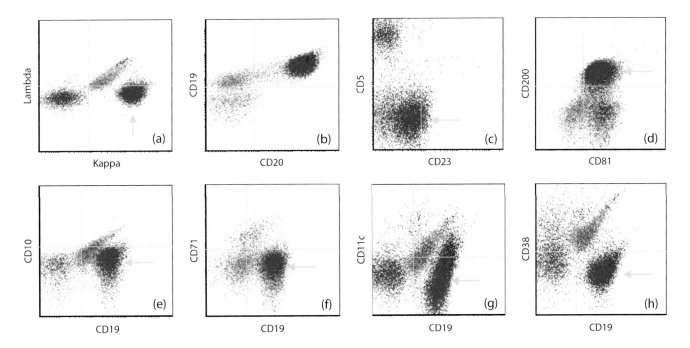

FIGURE 12.6 Marginal zone lymphoma (blood). Clonal B-cells show moderate expression of kappa (a, arrow), moderate to bright expression of both CD19 and CD20 (b), negative CD5 (c, arrow), positive CD81 (d), dim expression of CD200 (d, arrow), negative CD10 (e), negative CD71 (f, arrow), negative CD11c (g, arrow), and negative CD38 (h, arrow).

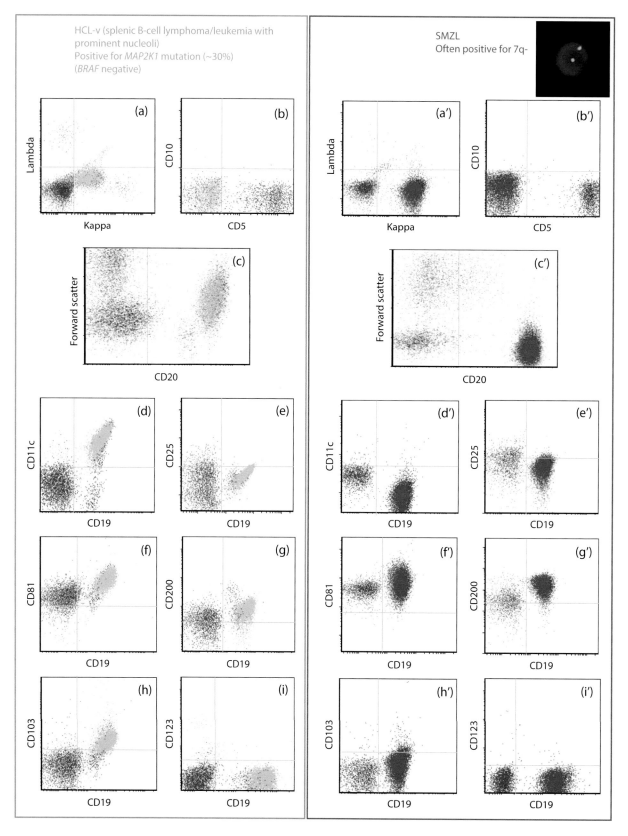

FIGURE 12.7   FC patterns of HCL-v (left; blue dots) and SMZL (right; magenta dots; inset shows FISH analysis with deletion of 7q: red dot represent 7q arm of chromosome 7 and green dots centromere of chromosome 7). Both HCL-v and SMZL show monotypic expression of surface light chain immunoglobulins (a–a′) and non-specific phenotype (CD5⁻, CD10⁻; b–b′). The expression of CD20 is bright in both neoplasms (c–c′), but FSC is higher in HCL-v (c–c′). CD11c is strongly positive in HCL-v (d) and negative in SMZL (d′). The expression of CD25 (e–e′), CD81 (f–f′), and CD200 (g–g′) is similar in both neoplasms. HCL-v differs from SMZL by positive CD103 (h–h′). CD123 is negative in HCL-v and SMZL (i–i′).

SMZL shows deletion7/7q. Phenotypically both neoplasms are often CD5⁻/CD10⁻ with HCL-v being positive for CD103 with higher FSC and stronger expression of both CD11c and CD81, while SMZL show low FSC and is either CD11c⁻ or CD11c^{dim+/partial+} (only minor subset of SMZL may be CD103⁺).

Phenotypic and molecular characteristics of CD5⁻/CD10⁻ B-cell lymphomas:

- **MZL**: CD19⁺, CD20⁺, surface light chain immunoglobulin⁺, CD5^{-/rarely+}, CD10⁻, CD11c^{+/-}, CD23^{-/+}, CD38^{+/-}, CD43^{-/+}, CD81^{+/-}, CD200^{-/rarely+}, SMZL may show del(7q)
- **LPL**: CD19⁺, CD20⁺, surface light chain immunoglobulin⁺, CD5^{-/rare cases+}, CD10^{-/rarely+}, CD11c⁻, CD13^{-/rarely+}, CD23^{-/rarely+}, CD38^{+/rarely-}, CD43⁻, CD71⁻, CD81^{+/-}, CD200^{+(dim)/-}, prominent M protein in serum, *MYD88*^{mutated}, *CXCR4*^{mutated (subset)}
- **B-PLL**: CD19⁺, CD20⁺, surface light chain immunoglobulin⁺, CD5^{-/rarely+}, CD10⁻, CD11c⁻, CD23^{-/rarely+}, CD38⁺, CD43^{-/+}, CD71⁻, CD81⁻, CD200^{+/rarely-}
- **DLBCL**: FSC^{high}, CD19⁺, CD20⁺, surface light chain immunoglobulin⁺, CD5^{-/rarely+}, CD10^{+/-}, CD11c^{-/rarely+}, CD23⁻, CD25^{-/rarely+}, CD38⁺, CD43^{-/+}, CD71^{+(dim or rarely strong)}, CD81^{+(dim)}, CD200^{-/rarely +(dim)}, BCL6^{+/-}, MUM1^{+/-}
- **MCL**: CD19⁺, CD20⁺, surface light chain immunoglobulin⁺, CD5^{+/rarely-}, CD10^{-/rarely+}, CD11c⁻, CD23⁻, CD38⁺, CD43⁺, CD71^{-/+(dim or partial)}, CD81⁺, CD200⁻, cyclin D1 (BCL1)⁺, SOX11⁺, t(11;14)/*CCND1*^{rearranged}
- **HCL**: CD19⁺, CD20⁺, surface light chain immunoglobulin⁺, CD5⁻, CD10^{-/rarely+}, CD11c^{+bright}, CD22^{+bright}, CD23^{-/rarely+}, CD25⁺, CD38⁻, CD43^{+/rarely-}, CD71⁻, CD81^{+(dim)}, CD103⁺, CD123⁺, CD200^{+(bright)}, *BRAF*^{mutated}
- **HCL-v**: CD19⁺, CD20⁺, surface light chain immunoglobulin⁺, CD5⁻, CD10^{-/rarely+}, CD11c^{+bright/rarely-}, CD23^{-/rarely+}, CD25⁻, CD38⁻, CD43^{-/+dim}, CD71⁻, CD81^{+(often strong)}, CD103⁺, CD123^{+/-}, CD200^{-/+(dim)}
- **SDRPL**: surface light chain immunoglobulin⁺, CD5^{-/rarely+}, CD10⁻, CD11c^{-/+}, CD19⁺, CD20⁺, CD22⁺, CD23^{-/rarely+}, CD25⁻, CD38⁻, CD43^{+(dim)/-}, CD45⁺, CD79b^{+(moderate)}, CD81^{+/-}, CD103^{-/rarely+}, CD123^{-/rarely+}, CD200⁺

Additional phenotypic markers in B-cell neoplasms

Surface light chain immunoglobulins (kappa and lambda)

FC analysis of kappa and lambda expression, apart from evaluation of clonality, may also help in further classification of B-cell neoplasm. Dim or negative kappa and lambda expression is typical for CLL/SLL. Subset of DLBCL, FL, BL may also be surface light chain negative. Lack of light chain expression is typical for hematogones and B-ALL. Germinal center cells from follicular hyperplasia may also show diminished expression of light chain with variable kappa and negative to dim lambda, which in rare cases may be confused with clonal CD10⁺ B-cell process (see Chapter 3). B-cells from pleural effusions are often completely surface light chain negative. Mature B lymphocytes exhibit allelic exclusion in which only a single class of light chain, either kappa or lambda, are expressed. However, very rare B-cell neoplasms, especially CLL, may show dual expression of both light chains. Poor separation between kappa⁺/kappa⁻ and lambda⁺/lambda⁻ B-cells, mimicking dual light chain expression is often seen in lymph node samples from patients with human immunodeficiency virus (HIV).

CD11c

CD11c is positive in many B-cell lymphoproliferations. Bright CD11c expression is typical for HCL and HCL variant. Dim to moderate or partial CD11c expression can be seen in CLL/SLL, MZL, and minor subset of DLBCL. SDRPL often shows moderate CD11c (stronger than in MZL) or SMZL. BL, FL, MCL, B-PLL, high grade B-cell lymphoma with MYC and BCL2 (and/or BCL6) rearrangement (HGBL-R) and LPL are most often negative for CD11c.

CD23

CD23 expression is often present on benign B-cells from reactive conditions. Among B-cell lymphoproliferations, CD23 positivity is most typical for B-CLL/SLL. Rare cases of FL, HCL, B-PLL, and MZL may be CD23⁺. MCLs are most often CD23⁻, but rare cases of MCL, especially so-called leukemic non-nodal mantle cell lymphoma (L-NN-MCL) may show phenotype similar to CLL with positive CD23 and CD200, and negative CD81 expression. Positive CD23 in conjunction with weak (or partial) CD5, lack of CD200 and moderate expression of surface light chain immunoglobulins, CD20 and CD22 does not favor the diagnosis of CLL (differential diagnosis should include MZL and other low-grade B-cell lymphoproliferative disorders). Strong expression of CD5, CD23, and CD81 and lack of CD200 should raise the possibility of MCL (especially if CD38 is positive and there is no CD11c expression).

CD25

CD25 expression is not specific for any B-cell lymphoproliferations but helps to differentiate HCL (CD25⁺/CD103⁺/CD123⁺) from HCL-v (CD25⁻/CD103⁺/CD123^{-/+}).

CD30

CD30 is a typical marker for classic Hodgkin lymphoma (cHL) and anaplastic large cell lymphoma (ALCL). In B-cell lymphomas, CD30 is positive in majority of primary mediastinal large B-cell lymphoma (PMBL; up to 80%) and subset of DLBCL (~10%) and PBL (~30%), and occasional cases of IVLBL. Occasional cases of FL may be CD30⁺. Some cases of low-grade B-cell lymphomas (e.g., MZL) may contain scattered large B-cells expressing CD30. Reporting the expression of CD30 is important clinically due to availability of anti-CD30 therapy with immunoconjugate Brentuximab vedotin consisting of a CD30-directed antibody linked to the anti-microtubule agent auristatin.

CD38

CD38 is a transmembrane glycoprotein with a widespread cellular expression and functional activity. The CD38 expression is high in B-cell precursors and in terminally differentiated plasma cells, but low to absent in mature B-cells, where it can be induced by activatory signals. CD38 is often positive (dim to moderate) in AML. Among mature neoplasms, CD38 is often positive in MCL and may be positive in subset of CLL. CD38 is often positive in FL and may be positive in other B- and T-cell lymphoproliferations. T-cell neoplasms, especially anaplastic large cell lymphoma or peripheral T-cell lymphoma and high-grade B-cell lymphomas, such as HGBL NOS, HGBL with rearrangement of *MYC* and *BCL2* also called double hit (DH) or triple hit (TH) lymphoma, and BL often show bright expression of CD38. Generally, bright expression of CD38 is typical for B-cell lymphomas with *MYC* rearrangement, being seen in 70% of B-cell lymphomas with *MYC* rearrangement (both DLBCL with *MYC* rearrangement and HGBL-R), and only in 17% of DLBCL without *MYC* rearrangement [52, 53]. CD38 is positive in subset of HCLs. HCL-v are CD38⁻.

CD39

CD39 expression is weak in BL and FL and strong in DLBCL (much stronger in non-germinal center type when compared to germinal center type) [19].

CD43

Among B-cell lymphoproliferations, CD43 is expressed by CLL/SLL, MCL, BL, subset of MZL, and subset of HCL and HCL-v. Co-expression of CD43 and CD200 is typical for CLL/SLL and co-expression of CD43 with CD81 is typical for MCL. Among DLBCLs, CD43 is often positive in non-germinal center type DLBCL and usually negative (or rarely weak) in germinal center type DLBCL. FL are most often CD43⁻ and BL are usually strongly CD43⁺ (expression of CD43 in BL is stronger than in DLBCL of non-germinal center type) [19].

CD45

The majority of mature B-cell neoplasms are characterized by bright expression of CD45 (in contrast to B-ALL which often shows either negative or dim CD45). Lower level of CD45 expression may be seen in some mature B-cell lymphomas, most often seen in DLBCL and HGBLs, such as BL or HGBL with rearrangement of MYC and BCL2 and/or BCL6 (HGBL-R), also termed DH or TH lymphomas. Apart from dimmer CD45, HGBL-R may show other FC features often associated with "immaturity", such as negative or dim CD20 and/or lack of surface light chain immunoglobulin expression.

CD71

CD71 is an activation marker, which can be considered FC equivalent of tissue staining for Ki-67. It is positive or partially positive in high grade lymphomas (such as BL, DLBCL, PBL, and HGBL-R).

CD81

CD81 is strongly positive in MCL, subset of MZL, HCL-v, and BL, and may be positive in MZL, HCL, DLBCL, FL, and LPL. In HCL, FL, and DLBCL, the expression of CD81 is often dim (comparable to the level of expression in benign T-cells) or variable (from negative to dim). Negative to partially dim CD81 expression may be noted in CLL. Comparison of CD81 and CD200 expression helps in differential diagnosis between CLL, atypical CLL (CD23⁻ and/or CD20strong⁺) and MCL: CLL and atypical CLL show strong CD200 expression and negative or weak CD81 expression, while MCL shows strong CD81 expression and negative CD200.

CD103

CD103 is typically positive in HCL and HCL-v. CD103 may be rarely expressed also in SMZL, SDRPL, and rare cases of DLBCL.

CD200

CD200 is strongly expressed by CLL/SLL but is also positive in SDRPL, HCL, and rare cases of FL, DLBCL, LPL, and MZL. SMZL is more often positive for CD200 when compared to other types of MZLs. Expression of CD200 helps to differentiate CLL (CD200bright⁺) from MCL (CD200⁻) and HCL (CD200bright⁺) from HCL-v (CD200⁻ or dim⁺).

Classification of B-cell neoplasms based on forward scatter (grading)

FSC corresponds to size of lymphocytes and therefore low-grade lymphomas are characterized by low FSC, and large cell lymphomas by high FSC (Figure 12.8).

Mature B-cell neoplasms composed of mostly small to medium-sized cells (Table 12.1):

- CLL/SLL
- MCL, major subset
- B-PLL
- MZL
- LPL/WM
- FL, subset
- HCL
- SBLPN (splenic B-cell lymphoma/leukemia with prominent nucleoli which includes cases previously classified as B-PLL and HCL-v)

Among B-cell lymphoproliferative disorders composed of predominantly small cells, majority are classified as low grade. MCL, however, is considered an aggressive disease, except for its indolent variants (in situ mantle cell neoplasm and L-NN-MCL). FLs are divided into (1) classic FL (cFL), corresponding to prior grade

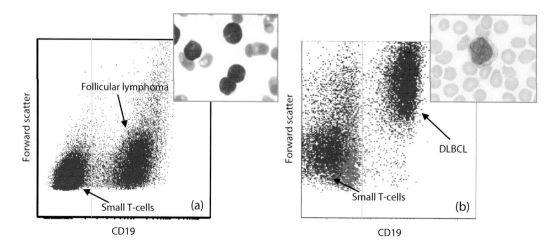

FIGURE 12.8 Comparison of FSC in low grade follicular lymphoma (FL; a) and large B-cell lymphoma (DLBCL; b). Low grade FL show low FSC, which is similar to minimally increased when compared to reactive T-cells (CD19⁻ cells; a). DLBCL is characterized by high FSC (compare to benign CD19⁻ T-cells with low FSC; b). Insets show corresponding smears (Wright-Giemsa, objective ×1000).

1, 2 and 3a FL; follicular large B-cell lymphoma (FLBL) previously termed FL grade 3b and (3) FL with uncommon features (uFL). HCL-v and B-PLL are grouped into splenic B-cell lymphoma/leukemia with prominent nucleoli category in new WHO classification.

Mature B-cell neoplasms composed of mostly medium-sized to large cells (Table 12.2):

- MCL, blastoid and pleomorphic variants
- DLBCL
- FL, subset (high grade variant)
- BL
- HGBL-R
- HGBL, NOS
- PBL
- PEL
- IVLBL
- PMBL
- SBLPN

B-cell lymphoproliferative neoplasms composed of mostly medium-sized or large cells are clinically very heterogeneous with most often characterized by aggressive clinical behavior. The main groups of these neoplasms include DLBCL (and its variants), follicular large B-cell lymphoma (FLBL) PBL, histologic transformation of low grade B-cell lymphomas (including Richter's syndrome), and HGBLs (BL, HGBL-R, HGBL, NOS). Correlation of FSC with expression of CD5 and CD10 helps in differential diagnosis but in most cases, final subclassification is possible based on histomorphology, immunohistochemistry (e.g., MYC, BCL1, MUM1, EBER), and FISH studies (*MYC, BCL2, BCL6,* and *CCND1* rearrangement). Major differential diagnosis of B-cell lymphomas with high FSC and expression of CD5 includes de novo CD5⁺ DLBCL, Richter's syndrome and blastoid or pleomorphic variant of MCL (Figure 12.9). Major differential diagnosis of B-cell lymphomas with high FSC and CD10 expression includes follicular large B-cell lymphoma (FLBL), DLBCL, BL, and HGBL-R. An algorithmic approach to differential diagnosis of HGBLs is presented in Figure 12.10.

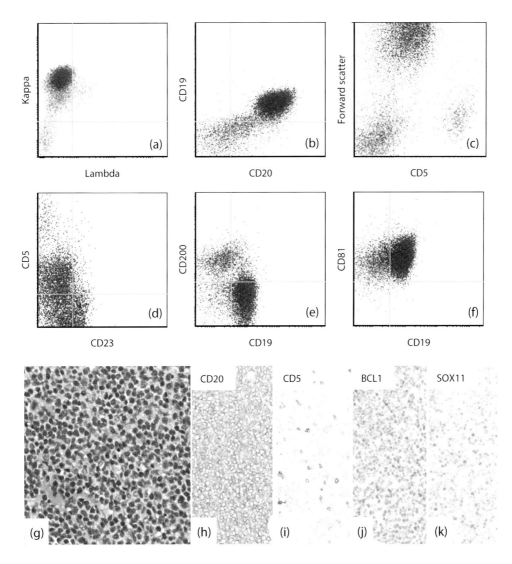

FIGURE 12.9 Pleomorphic variant of MCL. (a–f) Flow cytometry shows clonal B-cells (blue dots) with kappa restriction (a), positive CD19 and CD20 (b), high forward scatter (c), dim CD5 expression (c–d), negative CD23 (d), negative CD200 (e), and dim CD81 (f). (g) Histologic analysis shows diffuse infiltrate of medium to large cells with irregular nuclei. (h–k) Immunohistochemistry shows strong CD20 expression (h), weak CD5 expression (i), positive BCL1 (j), and positive SOX11 (k).

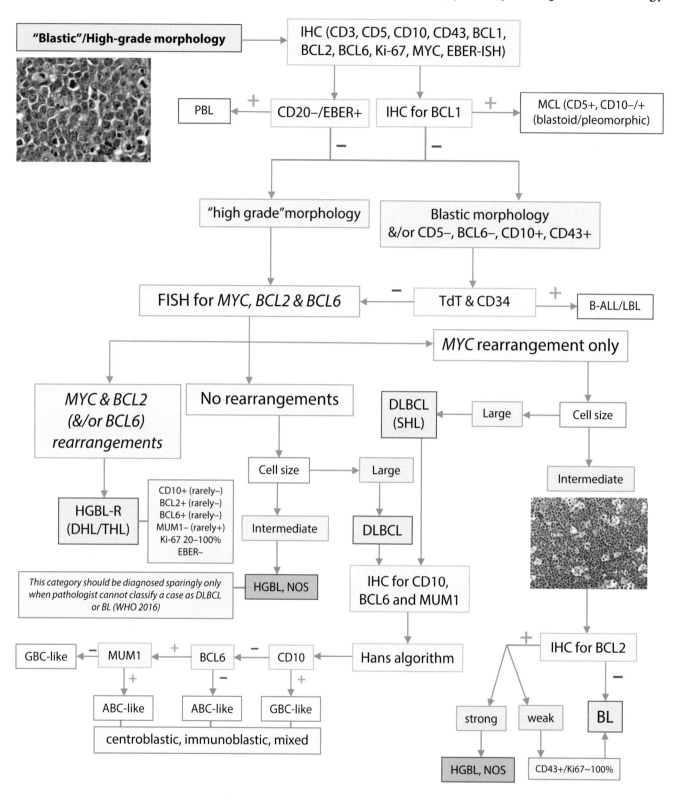

FIGURE 12.10 Algorithmic approach to high grade B-cell lymphomas. *Abbreviations*: ABC, activated B-cell; GCB, germinal center B-cell; HGBL, high grade B-cell lymphoma; HGBL-R, HGBL with rearrangement of MYC and BCL2; BL, Burkitt lymphoma; B-ALL/LBL, acute B-cell lymphoblastic leukemia/lymphoma; DLBCL, diffuse large B-cell lymphoma; IHC, immunohistochemistry; FISH, fluorescence in situ hybridization; SHL, single hit lymphoma; DHT, double hit lymphoma, THL, triple hit lymphoma; PBL, plasmablastic lymphoma.

B-cell neoplasms with plasmacytic differentiation

Most B-cell lymphoproliferations may display plasmacytic differentiation. It is always present in LPL/WM, but majority of other low-grade lymphomas, including MZL, B-CLL/SLL, FL, and DLBCL may also have plasmacytic differentiation. MCL, on the other hand, rarely show plasmacytic differentiation.

B-CLL/SLL is characterized by CD5 and CD23 expression, dim expression of both CD20 and surface light chain immunoglobulins (Figure 12.11). FL is typically CD10+ and therefore can be easily differentiated from both LPL/WM (rarely CD10+) and MZL

(CD10−). The major differential diagnosis among low grade B-cell lymphomas with plasmacytic differentiation is between LPL/WM and MZL, since both display non-specific phenotype without expression of CD5 or CD10 (although occasional cases may be CD5+). It is also worth mentioning that rare cases of FL may be CD10−. Prominent IgM+ plasma cell component, lymphoid cells with plasmacytoid appearance, presence of paratrabecular BM infiltrate, increased mast cells in the BM, high serum M protein and presence of *MYD88* L26P mutation are diagnostic for LPL/WM [55–57]. SMZLs often show intrasinusoidal pattern of BM involvement. Subset of SMZL may show deletion of 7q by cytogenetic and/or FISH analysis.

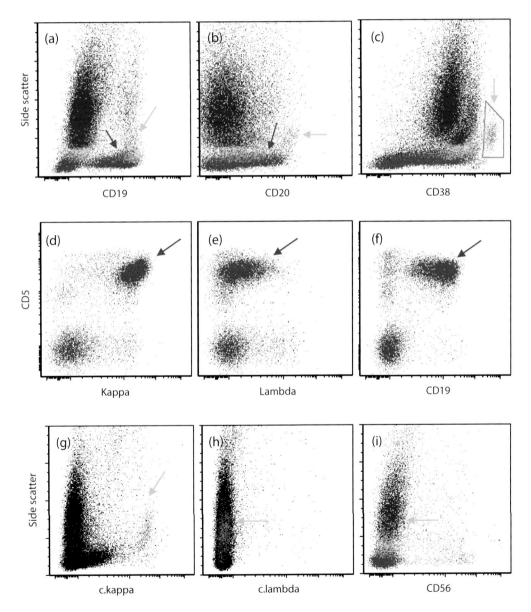

FIGURE 12.11 CLL with plasmacytic differentiation (component) – flow cytometry analysis of the bone marrow aspirate. CLL cells (red dots; red arrows) are positive for CD19 (a, f), CD20 (b; dim expression), CD5 (d–f) and kappa (d). Plasma cells (yellow dots; yellow arrows) show positive CD19 (a), CD20 (b), CD38 (c; bright expression), and cytoplasmic kappa (g). They are negative for CD56 (i).

References

1. Wood, B., *9-color and 10-color flow cytometry in the clinical laboratory*. Arch Pathol Lab Med, 2006. **130**(5): p. 680–90.
2. Wood, B.L., et al., *2006 Bethesda International Consensus recommendations on the immunophenotypic analysis of hematolymphoid neoplasia by flow cytometry: optimal reagents and reporting for the flow cytometric diagnosis of hematopoietic neoplasia*. Cytometry B Clin Cytom, 2007. **72 Suppl 1**: p. S14–S22.
3. Jevremovic, D., et al., *CD5+ B-cell lymphoproliferative disorders: beyond chronic lymphocytic leukemia and mantle cell lymphoma*. Leuk Res, 2010. **34**(9): p. 1235–8.
4. Sandes, A.F., et al., *CD200 has an important role in the differential diagnosis of mature B-cell neoplasms by multiparameter flow cytometry*. Cytometry B Clin Cytom, 2014. **86**(2): p. 98–105.
5. Venkataraman, G., et al., *Characteristic CD103 and CD123 expression pattern defines hairy cell leukemia: usefulness of CD123 and CD103 in the diagnosis of mature B-cell lymphoproliferative disorders*. Am J Clin Pathol, 2011. **136**(4): p. 625–30.
6. DiGiuseppe, J.A. and M.J. Borowitz, *Clinical utility of flow cytometry in the chronic lymphoid leukemias*. Semin Oncol, 1998. **25**(1): p. 6–10.
7. Dunphy, C.H., *Contribution of flow cytometric immunophenotyping to the evaluation of tissues with suspected lymphoma?* Cytometry, 2000. **42**(5): p. 296–306.
8. Tsagarakis, N.J., et al., *Contribution of immunophenotype to the investigation and differential diagnosis of Burkitt lymphoma, double-hit high-grade B-cell lymphoma, and single-hit MYC-rearranged diffuse large B-cell lymphoma*. Cytometry B Clin Cytom, 2020. **98**(5): p. 412–20.
9. Kohnke, T., et al., *Diagnosis of CLL revisited: increased specificity by a modified five-marker scoring system including CD200*. Br J Haematol, 2017. **179**(3): p. 480–87.
10. Stetler-Stevenson, M. and P.R. Tembhare, *Diagnosis of hairy cell leukemia by flow cytometry*. Leuk Lymphoma, 2011. **52 Suppl 2**: p. 11–3.
11. McGowan, P., et al., *Differentiating between Burkitt lymphoma and CD10+ diffuse large B-cell lymphoma: the role of commonly used flow cytometry cell markers and the application of a multiparameter scoring system*. Am J Clin Pathol, 2012. **137**(4): p. 665–70.
12. Tomita, N., et al., *Diffuse large B cell lymphoma without immunoglobulin light chain restriction by flow cytometry*. Acta Haematol, 2009. **121**(4): p. 196–201.
13. Moench, L., et al., *Double- and triple-hit lymphomas can present with features suggestive of immaturity, including TdT expression, and create diagnostic challenges*. Leuk Lymphoma, 2016. **57**(11): p. 2626–35.
14. Craig, F.E. and K.A. Foon, *Flow cytometric immunophenotyping for hematologic neoplasms*. Blood, 2008. **111**(8): p. 3941–67.
15. Tbakhi, A., et al., *Flow cytometric immunophenotyping of non-Hodgkin's lymphomas and related disorders*. Cytometry, 1996. **25**(2): p. 113–24.
16. Borowitz, M.J., *Flow cytometry defended*. Am J Clin Pathol, 2000. **113**(4): p. 596–8.
17. McKinnon, K.M., *Flow cytometry: an overview*. Curr Protoc Immunol, 2018. **120**: p. 5.1.1–5.1.11.
18. D'Archangelo, M., *Flow cytometry: new guidelines to support its clinical application*. Cytometry B Clin Cytom, 2007. **72**(3): p. 209–10.
19. Cardoso, C.C., et al., *The importance of CD39, CD43, CD81, and CD95 expression for differentiating B cell lymphoma by flow cytometry*. Cytometry B Clin Cytom, 2018. **94**(3): p. 451–8.
20. Rawstron, A.C., et al., *Improving efficiency and sensitivity: European Research Initiative in CLL (ERIC) update on the international harmonised approach for flow cytometric residual disease monitoring in CLL*. Leukemia, 2013. **27**(1): p. 142–9.
21. Rawstron, A.C., et al., *Monoclonal B-cell lymphocytosis and chronic lymphocytic leukemia*. N Engl J Med, 2008. **359**(6): p. 575–83.
22. Goldaniga, M., et al., *A multicenter retrospective clinical study of CD5/CD10-negative chronic B cell leukemias*. Am J Hematol, 2008. **83**(5): p. 349–54.
23. Zalcberg, I., et al., *Multidisciplinary diagnostics of chronic lymphocytic leukemia: European Research Initiative on CLL – ERIC recommendations*. Hematol Transfus Cell Ther, 2019. **42**(3): p. 269–74.
24. Baumgarth, N. and M. Roederer, *A practical approach to multicolor flow cytometry for immunophenotyping*. J Immunol Methods, 2000. **243**(1–2): p. 77–97.
25. Kussick, S.J., et al., *Prominent clonal B-cell populations identified by flow cytometry in histologically reactive lymphoid proliferations*. Am J Clin Pathol, 2004. **121**(4): p. 464–72.
26. Borowitz, M.J., et al., *U.S.-Canadian Consensus recommendations on the immunophenotypic analysis of hematologic neoplasia by flow cytometry: data analysis and interpretation*. Cytometry, 1997. **30**(5): p. 236–44.
27. Davis, B.H., et al., *U.S.-Canadian Consensus recommendations on the immunophenotypic analysis of hematologic neoplasia by flow cytometry: medical indications*. Cytometry, 1997. **30**(5): p. 249–63.
28. Seegmiller, A.C., E.D. Hsi, and F.E. Craig, *The current role of clinical flow cytometry in the evaluation of mature B-cell neoplasms*. Cytometry B Clin Cytom, 2019. **96**(1): p. 20–29.
29. Swerdlow, S.H., et al., *The 2016 revision of the World Health Organization classification of lymphoid neoplasms*. Blood, 2016. **127**(20): p. 2375–90.
30. Swerdlow, S.H., Campo, E., Harris, N. L., Jaffe, E. S., Pileri, S. A., Stein, H., et al., ed. WHO classification of tumors of haematopoietic and lymphoid tissues. 2016, IARC: Lyon.
31. Demina, I., et al., *Additional flow cytometric studies for differential diagnosis between Burkitt lymphoma/leukemia and B-cell precursor acute lymphoblastic leukemia*. Leuk Res, 2021. **100**: p. 106491.
32. Shao, H., et al., *Distinguishing hairy cell leukemia variant from hairy cell leukemia: development and validation of diagnostic criteria*. Leuk Res, 2013. **37**(4): p. 401–9.
33. Horna, P., et al., *Flow cytometric analysis of surface light chain expression patterns in B-cell lymphomas using monoclonal and polyclonal antibodies*. Am J Clin Pathol, 2011. **136**(6): p. 954–9.
34. Iancu, D., et al., *Follicular lymphoma in staging bone marrow specimens: correlation of histologic findings with the results of flow cytometry immunophenotypic analysis*. Arch Pathol Lab Med, 2007. **131**(2): p. 282–7.
35. Rosado, F.G., et al., *Immunophenotypic features by multiparameter flow cytometry can help distinguish low grade B-cell lymphomas with plasmacytic differentiation from plasma cell proliferative disorders with an unrelated clonal B-cell process*. Br J Haematol, 2015. **169**(3): p. 368–76.
36. Falay, M., et al., *The role of CD200 and CD43 expression in differential diagnosis between chronic lymphocytic leukemia and mantle cell lymphoma*. Turk J Haematol, 2018. **35**(2): p. 94–98.
37. Wu, D., et al., *Utility of flow cytometry for immunophenotyping double-hit lymphomas*. Cytometry B Clin Cytom, 2013. **84**(6): p. 398.
38. Osuji, N., et al., *T-cell large granular lymphocyte leukemia: a report on the treatment of 29 patients and a review of the literature*. Cancer, 2006. **107**(3): p. 570–8.
39. Barry, T.S., et al., *CD5+ follicular lymphoma: a clinicopathologic study of three cases*. Am J Clin Pathol, 2002. **118**(4): p. 589–98.
40. Kroft, S.H., et al., *De novo CD5+ diffuse large B-cell lymphomas. A heterogeneous group containing an unusual form of splenic lymphoma*. Am J Clin Pathol, 2000. **114**(4): p. 523–33.
41. Matolcsy, A., A. Chadburn, and D.M. Knowles, *De novo CD5-positive and Richter's syndrome-associated diffuse large B cell lymphomas are genotypically distinct*. Am J Pathol, 1995. **147**(1): p. 207–16.
42. Yamaguchi, M., et al., *De novo CD5-positive diffuse large B-cell lymphoma: clinical characteristics and therapeutic outcome*. Br J Haematol, 1999. **105**(4): p. 1133–9.

43. Yamaguchi, M., et al., *De novo CD5⁺ diffuse large B-cell lymphoma: a clinicopathologic study of 109 patients.* Blood, 2002. **99**(3): p. 815–21.

44. Ferry, J.A., et al., *CD5⁺ extranodal marginal zone B-cell (MALT) lymphoma. A low grade neoplasm with a propensity for bone marrow involvement and relapse.* Am J Clin Pathol, 1996. **105**(1): p. 31–7.

45. Ruiz, A., et al., *Extranodal marginal zone B-cell lymphomas of the ocular adnexa: multiparameter analysis of 34 cases including interphase molecular cytogenetics and PCR for Chlamydia psittaci.* Am J Surg Pathol, 2007. **31**(5): p. 792–802.

46. Lee, J., et al., *Identification and characterization of a human CD5⁺ pre-naive B cell population.* J Immunol, 2009. **182**(7): p. 4116–26.

47. Frassoldati, A., et al., *Hairy cell leukemia: a clinical review based on 725 cases of the Italian Cooperative Group (ICGHCL). Italian Cooperative Group for Hairy Cell Leukemia.* Leuk Lymphoma, 1994. **13**(3–4): p. 307–16.

48. Dong, H.Y., et al., *B-cell lymphomas with coexpression of CD5 and CD10.* Am J Clin Pathol, 2003. **119**(2): p. 218–30.

49. Jasionowski, T.M., et al., *Analysis of CD10⁺ hairy cell leukemia.* Am J Clin Pathol, 2003. **120**(2): p. 228–35.

50. Zhang, X., et al., *Comparison of genetic aberrations in CD10⁺ diffused large B-cell lymphoma and follicular lymphoma by comparative genomic hybridization and tissue-fluorescence in situ hybridization.* Cancer Sci, 2004. **95**(10): p. 809–14.

51. Wu, J.M., M.J. Borowitz, and E.G. Weir, *The usefulness of CD71 expression by flow cytometry for differentiating indolent from aggressive CD10⁺ B-cell lymphomas.* Am J Clin Pathol, 2006. **126**(1): p. 39–46.

52. Maleki, A., et al., *Bright CD38 expression is an indicator of MYC rearrangement.* Leuk Lymphoma, 2009. **50**(6): p. 1054–7.

53. Alsuwaidan, A., et al., *Bright CD38 expression by flow cytometric analysis is a biomarker for double/triple hit lymphomas with a moderate sensitivity and high specificity.* Cytometry B Clin Cytom, 2019. **96**(5): p. 368–74.

54. Salem, D.A., et al., *Differential expression of CD43, CD81, and CD200 in classic versus variant hairy cell leukemia.* Cytometry B Clin Cytom, 2019. **96**(4): p. 275–82.

55. Swerdlow, S.H., et al., *The many faces of small B cell lymphomas with plasmacytic differentiation and the contribution of MYD88 testing.* Virchows Arch, 2015. **468**(3): p. 259–75.

56. Gertz, M.A., *Waldenstrom macroglobulinemia: 2012 update on diagnosis, risk stratification, and management.* Am J Hematol, 2012. **87**(5): p. 503–10.

57. Lin, P., et al., *Lymphoplasmacytic lymphoma and other non-marginal zone lymphomas with plasmacytic differentiation.* Am J Clin Pathol, 2011. **136**(2): p. 195–210.

13

MATURE B-CELL LYMPHOPROLIFERATIONS

Chronic lymphocytic leukemia/small lymphocytic lymphoma (CLL/SLL)

SLL/CLL phenotype by flow cytometry: low forward scatter, sIg$^{+(dim)/rarely-}$, CD2$^{-/rarely+}$, CD5$^+$, CD10$^-$, CD11c$^{+(dim/partial)/-}$, CD13$^{-/rarely+}$, CD19$^+$, CD20$^{+(dim)/rarely-}$, CD22$^{-/+(dim)}$, CD23$^{+(rare cases -)}$, CD25$^{-/rarely+}$, CD38$^{-/+(dim/partial)}$, CD43$^{+/rarely-}$, CD45$^{+(moderate\ or\ bright)}$, CD49d$^{-/+}$, CD79a$^+$, CD79b$^{-/+(dim)}$, CD81$^{-/+(dim)}$, CD103$^-$, CD123$^{-/rarely+}$, and CD200$^{+(moderate)}$.

Introduction

Definition of CLL. CLL is a low-grade lymphoproliferative disorder of mature B cells characterized by lymphocytosis ($\geq 5 \times 10^9$/L; >3 months), expression of CD5, CD23, and CD200, and involvement of blood, bone marrow (BM), spleen, and lymph nodes [1]. Patients with clonal CLL-like cells count <5 × 10^9/L and without adenopathy, organomegaly, or other extramedullary disease are classified as monoclonal B-cell lymphocytosis (MBL).

Definition of SLL. SLL is considered a lymphomatous counterpart of CLL involving lymph nodes and extranodal sites with circulating CLL cells count <5 × 10^9/L.

Clinical course and prognostic factors. Clinical course ranges from a very indolent disorder with a normal lifespan to a progressive disease with poor prognosis. Prognostic factors include age, gender, Binet/Rai stage, performance status, β_2-microglobulin, and LDH levels, *ATM*, *IGHV*, *TP53*, *NOTCH1*, *SF3B1* mutational status, chromosomal changes, expression of CD38, CD49d, ZAP70, and response to treatment. The median survival times for patients with 17p deletion, 11q deletion, 12q trisomy, normal karyotype, and 13q deletion as the sole abnormality are 32, 79, 114, 111, and 133 months, respectively [2].

Risk categories [3].

- **High risk:** Patients with *TP53* and/or *BIRC3* abnormalities. Lack of response to purine analogs or short response (<24 months) to prior treatment with fludarabine, cyclophosphamide, and rituximab.
- **Intermediate risk:** Patients with unmutated *IGHV*, 11q deletion, *NOTCH1* and/or *SFB1* mutations, and high β_2-microglobulin.
- **Low risk:** Patients with no prior therapy, +12 and lack of high-risk factors.
- **Very low risk:** Patients with del13q14 only.

Monoclonal B-cell lymphocytosis (MBL)

Definition. MBL is defined by presence of low numbers (<5 × 10^9/L) of circulating monoclonal B-cells in otherwise healthy (asymptomatic) subjects (with no evidence of CLL/other lymphoproliferative disorders, adenopathy, or organomegaly). Clonality is defined by either kappa restriction (κ:λ >3:1), lambda restriction (κ:λ <0.3:1), or >25% surface κ and λ negative B-cells. Some cases may be bi-clonal or tri-clonal.

MBL subtypes:

- CLL-like phenotype (CD5$^+$/CD23$^+$)
- Atypical CLL-like phenotype (CD5$^+$/CD23$^-$)
- Marginal zone lymphoma-like phenotype (MZL-like) or non-CLL-like MBL (CD5$^-$, CD10$^-$), which more recently is designated as clonal B-cell lymphocytosis of marginal zone origin (CBL-MZ)

CLL-like MBL. CLL-like MBL is divided into two categories: high-count MBL and low-count MBL based on a cutoff value of 0.5 × 10^9/L clonal B cells. Low count MBL is defined by blood CLL count <0.5 × 10^9/L and high-count MBL by CLL count ≥0.5 × 10^9/L. The clonal B-cell count is associated with the risk of progression to CLL. Low count MBL (<0.5 × 10^9/L) is very stable over time and is not associated with progression to CLL, while high count MBL could be a premalignant state before the occurrence of CLL. It is postulated that all CLL cases develop from pre-existing MBL. High count MBL with CLL-like phenotype is most often *IGHV* mutated and is characterized by the same genetic changes which occur in CLL (e.g., *NOTCH1*, *SF3B1*, *ATM*, or *TP53* mutations). In MBL, BM shows three infiltration patterns: focal interstitial, nodular (non-paratrabecular), and discrete diffuse lymphocytosis [4]. Figure 13.1 shows an unusual MBL composed of three clones expressing CD5 and partially CD23.

CBL-MZ. CBL-MZ is a recently described entity characterized by the presence of clonal B cells in the blood and/or BM with morphologic and immunophenotypic features consistent with marginal zone derivation in otherwise healthy individuals. CBL-MZ may be associated with IgM paraproteinemia raising the differential diagnosis with Waldenström macroglobulinemia (WM). CBL-MZ is very heterogeneous with mutations not associated with specific lymphoma subtype, including *MYD88* (14%–19%), *BIRC3* (11%), *CCND3* (11%), *NOTCH1* (11%), and *TNFAIP3* (11%), but often show some genetic changes overlapping with splenic marginal zone lymphoma (SMZL) and splenic diffuse red pulp B-cell lymphoma (SDRPL) [5, 6].

Immunophenotype of CLL/SLL

Flow cytometry. Immunophenotypic by flow cytometry (FC) plays crucial role in CLL diagnosis. Phenotypically, CLL is characterized by co-expression of B-cell markers (CD19, CD20, CD79a) with strong expression of CD5, CD23, and often CD43 (Figures 13.2 and 13.3). Other positive markers include CD200, CD11c (often dim or partial), and IgM/IgD (dim). CD10 is not expressed and FMC7, CD22, CD81, and CD79b are usually negative but expression of CD22 may be dimly positive or partial. CD81 is either negative or dim positive (the expression does not exceed the level displayed by benign T-cells). The expression of CD20 and surface immunoglobulins (sIg) by FC analysis is typically dim but may be partial or negative. Rare cases may display aberrant phenotype, e.g., lack of CD23, positive expression of CD2 (~15%), CD4, CD7, CD8, or CD13, and moderate expression of sIg and/or CD20. The expression of CD38 (>30% of clonal cells) or ZAP70 (>20% of clonal cells) is associated with less favorable

DOI: 10.1201/9781003197935-13

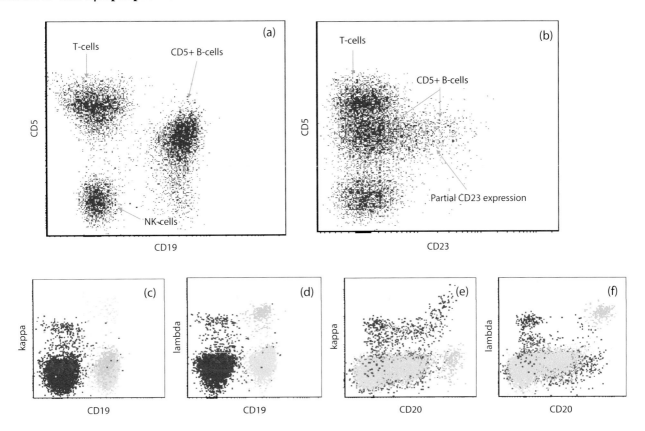

FIGURE 13.1 Monoclonal B-cell lymphocytosis (tri-clonal) with dim CD5 expression and partial CD23 expression (a–b); clone #1 (yellow dots): kappa+, CD19+, CD20+; clone #2 (green dots): lambda+, CD19+, bright CD20+; clone #3 (blue dots): kappa−, lambda−, CD19+, CD20+/− (c–f).

prognosis and often correlates with unmutated *IGHV* status. CD49d expression strongly correlates with a more aggressive disease. Using a ≥30% threshold, CD49d is positive in ~35% of cases [7]. It is not uncommon for CLL to display two or three B-cell clones (kappa+, lambda+, and/or kappa/lambda−) or switch clones during disease progression.

Immunohistochemistry. Prolymphocytes and paraimmunoblasts are positive for Ki-67 and often p53. Large confluent proliferation centers or proliferation centers with high proliferation fraction by Ki-67 are associated with adverse prognosis [8–10]. In minor subset of small lymphocytic lymphoma/chronic lymphocytic leukemia (SLL/CLL) cases, proliferation centers may be BCL1 (cyclin D1) positive without harboring translocation t(11;14) [11].

Morphology

Blood and BM aspirate. CLL cells are small (but minimally larger than benign lymphocytes) with scanty pale cytoplasm, round nuclei, and clumped (coarse) chromatin (Figure 13.4). Occasional smudge cells and larger lymphocytes including prolymphocytes and "paraimmunoblasts" are usually also present. Prolymphocytes are distinguished from small lymphocytes by their relatively larger size, more abundant pale cytoplasm, and prominent central nucleolus (Figure 13.5). Paraimmunoblasts have oval nuclei with large central nucleolus and grayish-blue cytoplasm. CLL with >15% and <55% prolymphocytes defines chronic lymphocytic leukemia/B-cell prolymphocytic leukemia (CLL/B-PLL). B-prolymphocytic leukemia has more than 55% of prolymphocytes. Presence of more than 10% prolymphocytes in

CLL patients and an absolute prolymphocyte count ≥15 × 10⁹/L are associated with less favorable prognosis. T-cell prolymphocytes differ slightly from B-cell prolymphocytes by having often more irregular nuclear contours.

BM biopsy. Patterns of BM involvement by CLL include nodular, interstitial, diffuse, and rarely paratrabecular, but is often mixed. The infiltrate is composed of mostly small lymphocytes with scattered prolymphocytes and paraimmunoblasts. In cases with prominent BM involvement, proliferation centers are often present. Patients with >70% marrow involvement before therapy have a significantly shorter time to progression [12].

Lymph nodes and extranodal sites. SLL in the lymph node shows effacement of the architecture with a characteristic pseudofollicular pattern caused by clusters of prolymphocytes and paraimmunoblasts (proliferation centers) in the background of diffuse small lymphocytic infiltrate. Minority of cases show only minimal number of larger cells creating diffuse pattern without proliferation centers. Occasional cases of SLL show an interfollicular pattern or only partial involvement of the lymph node (Figure 13.6). SLL/CLL frequently involves extranodal sites, including tonsil, liver, spleen, skin, among others. The histomorphologic and immunophenotypic features are like those seen in the lymph nodes (Figure 13.7).

Histologic transformation (HT)

HT of SLL/CLL into a more aggressive neoplasm is referred to as Richter's transformation (or syndrome). Richter's transformation occurs in 2%–12% of patients. The WHO classification recognizes two distinct pathological variants of Richter's transformation,

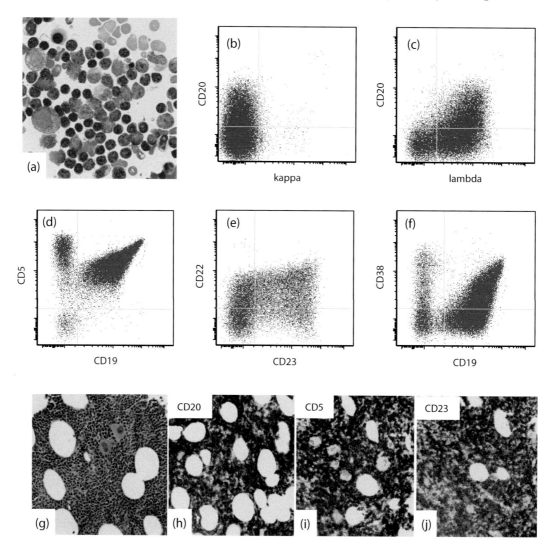

FIGURE 13.2 Chronic lymphocytic leukemia – typical immunophenotypic profile (bone marrow). Bone marrow shows prominent lymphocytosis (a; aspirate smear). Flow cytometry shows dim expression of CD20 (b–c), moderate CD19 and CD5 (d), dim CD22 (e), positive CD23 (e), and dim expression of CD38 (f). Bone marrow biopsy from the same patient shows diffuse BM involvement (g) and positive expression of CD20 (h), CD5 (i), and CD23 (j) by immunohistochemistry.

namely the diffuse large B-cell lymphoma (DLBCL) variant and the classic Hodgkin lymphoma (cHL) variant [1]. Overall, HT of CLL/SLL may be represented by (1) prolymphocytic transformation with predominance of prolymphocytes [13, 14], paraimmunoblastic [15], or CLL with expanded proliferation centers, (2) Hodgkin lymphoma-like transformation [16–20], (3) DLBCL-like transformation [21–27], (4) plasmablastic lymphoma-like transformation, and rarely (5) progression to B-cell acute lymphoblastic leukemia (B-ALL) [28]. HT in the form of DLBCL is commonly clonally related to the founder CLL clone (in >85% of patients with Richter's transformation) but has a poorer outcome than de novo DLBCL and is characterized by chemoresistance and poor survival. The median survival for patients with DLBCL-like Richter's transformation is reported to be around ~6 months and for Hodgkin-like transformation ~30 months. Richter's represented by de novo DLBCL (clonally unrelated to original CLL) is usually managed as regular DLBCL.

Hodgkin variant. Hodgkin variant of Richter syndrome morphologically and immunophenotypically resembles cHL [21, 29–31]. Large neoplastic cells express PAX5, CD15, and CD30, similarly to de novo HL. They may be Epstein-Barr virus (EBV)+ (especially with EBER-ISH staining).

DLBCL variant. Progression of CLL/SLL to DLBCL can present as a localized enlargement of a single lymph node histologically showing DLBCL or increasing generalized adenopathy with rapid deterioration of patient's performance. Morphologic and immunophenotypic features of DLBCL developing after CLL (Richter's syndrome-DLBCL) are similar to de novo DLBCL, but Richter's syndrome-DLBCL differs from de novo DLBCL at molecular levels. Majority of cases show centroblastic morphology with numerous mitoses and apoptotic bodies and focal areas of necrosis. Richter's syndrome associated DLBCL are positive for B-cell markers (CD20, PAX5, CD19, CD22) and are often positive for ZAP70, CD38, and CD49d. They may be positive for CD5 or CD23 and most often

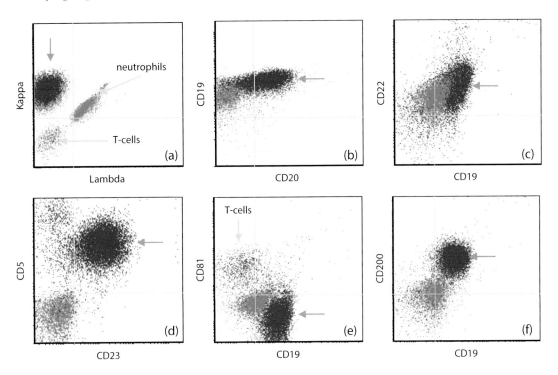

FIGURE 13.3 Typical immunophenotypic profile of CLL. Leukemic B-cells (red dots, arrow) show the following phenotype: clonal expression of surface immunoglobulins (kappa in this case, a), positive CD19 and dimly positive CD20 (b), dimly positive CD22 (c), co-expression of CD5 and CD23 (d), negative CD81 (e), and moderate expression of CD200 (f).

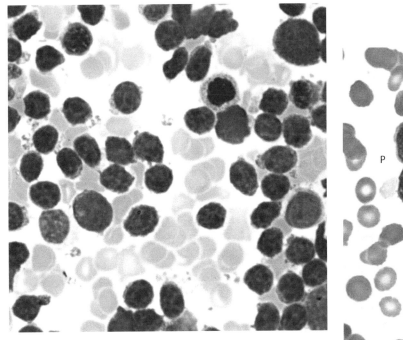

FIGURE 13.4 Chronic lymphocytic leukemia – cytology. Bone marrow aspirate with marked lymphocytosis of small lymphocytes with scanty cytoplasm and small nuclei with dense, clumped nuclear chromatin.

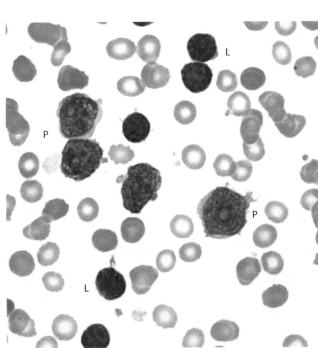

FIGURE 13.5 CLL: small lymphocytes (L) and prolymphocytes (P).

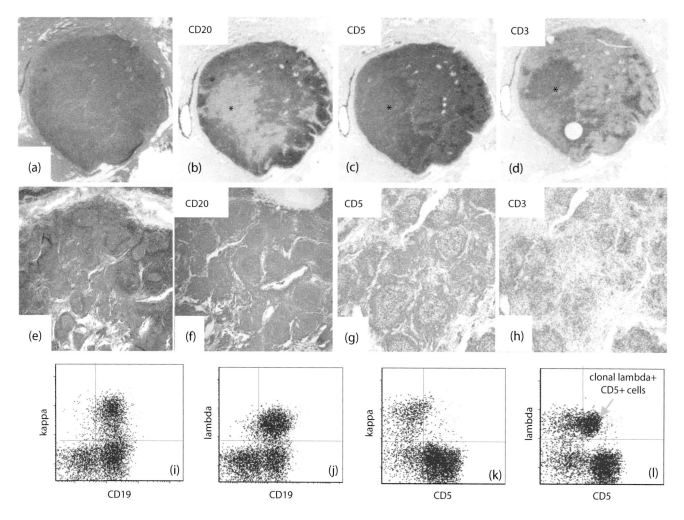

FIGURE 13.6 Small lymphocytic lymphoma – partial involvement of the lymph node (two cases). Case #1 (a–d); (a) Histology (H&E staining). (b–d) Immunohistochemistry. The central, not involved part of the lymph node (*) shows lack of CD20 staining (b), positive CD5 (c, reactive T-cells are slightly darker than neoplastic B-cells), and positive CD3 (d). Neoplastic B-cells at the periphery shows CD20 (b) and CD5 (c) expression and lack of CD3 (d). Case #2; (e) Histology (H&E staining) with follicular hyperplasia. (f–h) Immunohistochemistry. CD20 (f) shows stronger expression by reactive germinal centers. Staining with CD5 (g) and (h) shows interfollicular involvement by SLL. (i–l) Flow cytometry analysis shows lambda⁺ clone expressing CD5 hidden in the mostly polytypic B-cells.

(approximately 80%) show non-germinal center B-cell like phenotype (non-GCB) with negative CD10 and positive MUM1. Figure 13.8 shows FC and morphology of HT of CLL to large B-cell lymphoma, and Figure 13.9 shows FC features of Richter's syndrome in blood.

B-ALL clone and histologic transformation. Rare cases of CLL are complicated by development of B-ALL, with or without concurrent typical large cell transformation to DLBCL. Figure 13.10 presents BM from patient with history of CLL who developed B-ALL and DLBCL in the BM. Such composite B-cell neoplasm may represent either "bi-clonal" Richter's syndrome (B-ALL and DLBCL), or two separate, clonally unrelated processes, B-ALL and typical Richter's (DLBCL). Figure 13.11 shows another example of unusual Richter's transformation in the form of B-ALL. The possibility that some of B-ALL cases following CLL represents de novo acute leukemia rather than Richter's cannot be excluded.

Genetic features

Chromosomal aberrations are identified in >80% of CLL patients. The most frequent chromosomal abnormalities in CLL include trisomy 12, del13q, del(11q)/*ATM*, del(14q), del(6q), and del(17p)/*TP53* [24, 32–34]. Complex karyotype is more often seen as disease progresses. Two major subtypes of CLL can be identified based on the status of immunoglobulin heavy-chain variable region (*IGHV*) (1) CLL with mutated *IGHV*, and (2) CLL with unmutated *IGHV*. Mutational profile in CLL is very heterogeneous, with most mutations clustering around NOTCH1 signaling (*NOTCH1, FBXW7*), BCR and TLR signaling (*EGR2, BCOR, MYD88, TLR2, IKZ3*), MAPK-ERK pathway (*KRAS, NRAS*), NF-κB signaling (*BIRC3, NFKB2, NFKBIE, TRAF2, TRAF3*), chromatin modifiers (*CHD2, SETD2, KMT2D, ASXL1*), cell cycle (*ATM, TP53, CCND2, CDKN1B, CDKN2A*), DNA damage response (*ATM, TP53, POT1*), and RNA splicing and metabolism (*SF3B1, U1, XPO1, DDX3X, RPS15*) [35]. The most common mutations in CLL include *NOTCH1* (17.0%), followed by *SF3B1* (14.1%), *ATM* (11.7%), *TP53* (10.2%), *POT1* (7.0%), *RPS15* (4.4%), *FBXW7* (3.4%), *MYD88* (2.6%), and *BIRC3* (2.3%) [36]. While most mutations lack prognostic significance, *TP53, SF3B1*, and *NOTCH1* mutations are associated with inferior prognosis.

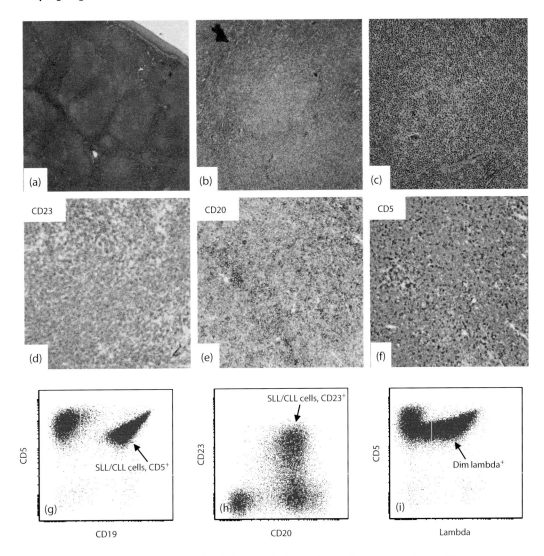

FIGURE 13.7 SLL involving tonsil. H&E sections (a–c) show typical pseudonodular pattern with proliferation centers. SLL cells are positive for CD23 (d), CD20 (e), and CD5 (f) by immunohistochemistry. Flow cytometry analysis (g–i) shows typical immunophenotypic profile with positive CD5 (g–i), CD19 (g), CD20 (h), CD23 (h), and dim lambda expression (i).

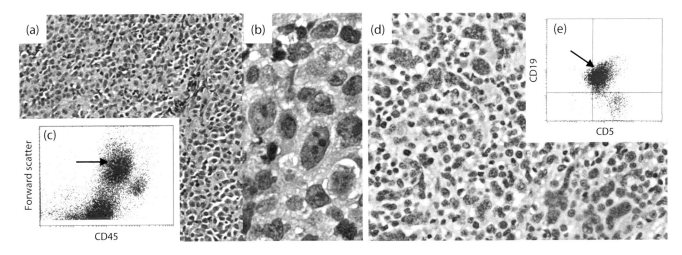

FIGURE 13.8 Richter syndrome. Two cases of large cell transformation (Richter's syndrome) of SLL/CLL (a–c and d–e). (a) Histologic section shows diffuse large cell infiltrate. (b) High magnification shows large lymphocytes with several nucleoli. (c) Flow cytometry reveals predominance of lymphoid cells with increased forward scatter (arrow). Normal (small) lymphocytes with bright CD45 have low forward scatter. (d) Lymph node with highly pleomorphic lymphoid infiltrate which still displays co-expression of CD19 and CD5 by flow cytometric analysis (e).

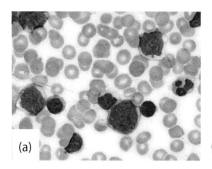 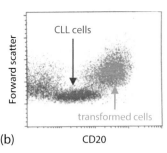 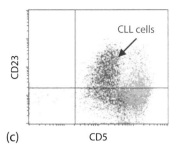

FIGURE 13.9 CLL with large cell transformation – flow cytometry. Atypical large cells (a) show higher forward scatter and brighter expression of CD20, when analyzed by flow cytometry (b, blue dots). Residual CLL cells are CD5 and CD23 positive (c), whereas transformed cells show negative CD23 (c, blue dots).

Disease monitoring

CLL in complete remission (CR) as defined by NCI criteria [37] (<30% lymphocytes in the BM with a morphologically normal trephine biopsy) may show up to 5% of leukemic cells persisting in the BM [38]. In CLL, measurable (minima) residual disease (MRD) has been estimated mainly by FC [38–41] or polymerase chain reaction (PCR)-based techniques, using either consensus PCR or allele-specific PCR [42–45].

Differential diagnosis of CLL/SLL

Flow cytometric differential diagnosis:

- MBL with CLL-like or atypical CLL-like phenotype
- Circulating benign CD5⁺ B-cells
- Mantle cell lymphoma (MCL) including leukemic nonnodal MCL (L-NN-MCL)
- CD5⁺ marginal zone lymphoma (MZL)
- CD5⁺ SMZL
- CD5⁺ DLBCL
- CD5⁺ follicular lymphoma (FL), very rare cases
- Peripheral T-cell lymphoproliferative neoplasms

Differential diagnosis of CLL with Richter's transformation:

- SLL/CLL with prominent proliferation centers
- DLBCL, especially de novo CD5⁺ DLBCL
- cHL
- SBLPN
- T-PLL
- Acute myeloid leukemia (AML) and extramedullary myeloid tumor (EMT)
- Acute lymphoblastic leukemia (ALL)
- Non-hematopoietic tumors (metastatic carcinoma)

Separating CLL from other B-cell lymphoproliferative disorders by FC

The Matutes score (MS) is used to separate CLL from other B-cell lymphoproliferative disorders [46]. Strong expression of CD23, CD5, and weak or absent expression of CD79b (or CD22), FMC7, and surface immunoglobulins translate into 0–5 point score (positivity is defined as ≥20% of the clonal B-cells).

Matutes score (MS):

- Positive CD23: 1 point
- Positive CD5: 1 point
- Weak or absent CD79a (or CD22): 1 point

- Negative FMC7: 1 point
- Weak surface immunoglobulin: 1 point

The MS is effective in separating CLL from non-CLL lymphomas, if the point score is high (4–5 points) or low (0–1 points). However, patient samples with the diagnosis of B-cell lymphoma and an intermediate MS (2–3 points) are often difficult to subclassify [1, 46]. Several authors tried to enhance the diagnostic accuracy of MS by replacing and/or adding additional markers [47–55]. Based on many reports, incorporating CD200 antigen improves the diagnosis of CLL by FC. The European Research Initiative on CLL (ERIC) and European Society for Clinical Cell Analysis (ESCCA) defined "required" and "recommended" antigens for the flow cytometric diagnosis of the B-CLL [53]. The consensus for "required" diagnostic markers include CD19, CD5, CD20, CD23, kappa, and lambda, and for "recommended" markers potentially useful for differential diagnosis include CD43, CD79b, CD81, CD200, CD10, and ROR1. Hoffman et al. proposed adding one point to original MS if mean fluorescence intensity (MFI) values for CD200 and CD43 are above the cutoff [55]. This enhanced MS (MS-e) and the "classical" MS were categorized as high (MS-e 6–7; MS 4–5), intermediate (MS-e 4–5; MS 2–3), and low (MS-e 0–3; MS 0–1). Sensitivity and specificity of the "classical" MS were 82.7% and 98.3% and for the MS-e sensitivity and specificity were 98.8% and 94.7% [55]. These authors showed that integration of CD200 and CD43 into the MS improves the separation of "atypical" CLL cases (MS 2–3) from other B-cell lymphoma types. Sensitivity for CLL diagnosis was significantly better with MS-e compared to "classical" MS without significantly compromising specificity. Strong expression of CD43 and CD200 defined by high MFI is characteristic for CLL with sensitivity of 100% and specificity of 94.7% (only rare cases of large B-cell lymphoma and MZL showed similar pattern).

Enhanced Matutes score (MS-e):

- Positive CD23: 1 point
- Positive CD5: 1 point
- Weak or absent CD79a (or CD22): 1 point
- Negative FMC7: 1 point
- Weak surface immunoglobulin: 1 point
- High MFI of CD200: 1 point

Zhu et al. showed the value of using CD20 expression instead of FMC7 in the MS [56]. D'Arena et al. investigated the value of CD200, CD5, CD22, CD23, CD79b, FMC7, and surface immunoglobulins for the diagnosis of CLL (versus non-CLL) and showed that addition of CD200 improved sensitivity and specificity

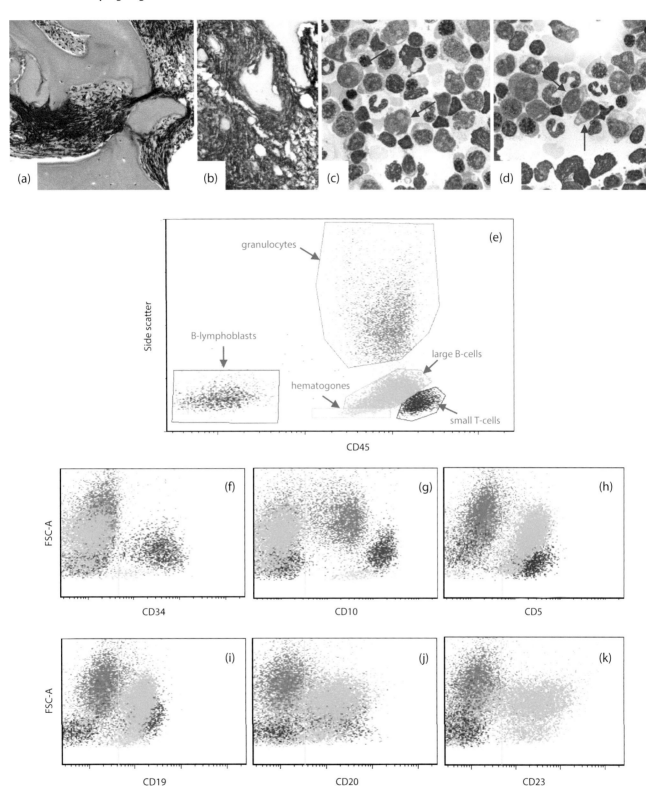

FIGURE 13.10 BM with two B-cell neoplasms (B-ALL and DLBCL) in patient with history of CLL. BM biopsy (a) shows prominent lymphoid infiltrate with crush artifacts, composed of mostly CD20+ B-cells (b). Aspirate smear (c–d) shows maturing marrow elements with highly atypical large lymphoid cells (c, arrows) and blasts (d, arrows), some of which show "hand-mirror" appearance. (e–k) FC analysis shows blasts (maroon dots) with lack of CD45 (e), positive CD34 (f), and CD10 (g; bright expression); hematogones (light blue dots) with partial CD34 expression (f) and positive CD10 (g); large B-cells with bright CD45 (e), negative CD10 (g), positive CD5 (h), CD19 (i), CD20 (j), and CD23 (k). This may represent either unusual bi-clonal Richter's in the form of B-ALL and large B-cell lymphoma or two separate B-cell neoplasms, Richter's (large B-cell lymphoma) and emerging B-ALL (e.g., therapy-related).

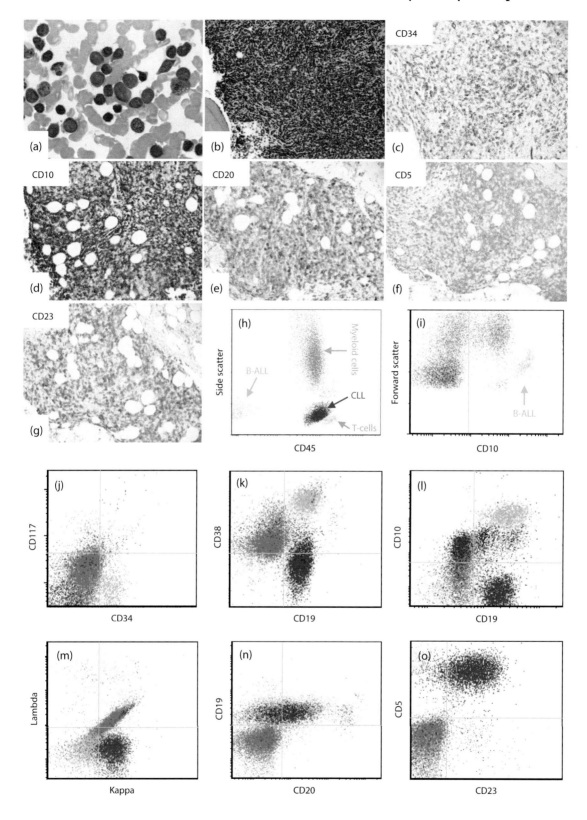

FIGURE 13.11 CLL with unusual Richter's transformation in the form of B-ALL. BM aspirate smear (a) shows CLL cells, lympho-blasts and rare normal marrow elements. Histology (b) shows subtotal BM replacement by lymphoid infiltrate composed of small to medium sized blasts and small lymphocytes. Immunohistochemistry analysis (c–g) shows blasts positive for CD34 (c) and CLL cells partially positive for CD20 (e), positive for CD5 (f) and CD23 (g). Flow cytometry analysis (h–o) shows mixed population of maturing myeloid cells (h, gray dots), CLL cells; h, red dots), normal T-cells (h, blue dots) and CD45⁻ B-ALL blasts (h, green dots). Blasts have slightly increased forward scatter and show bright CD10 expression (i), positive CD34 (j), positive CD19 (k), CD38 (k), and CD10 (l). CLL cells have clonal kappa expression (m) positive CD19 (n), partial CD200 (n), positive CD5 (o), and positive CD23 (o).

TABLE 13.1: Differential Diagnosis between CLL, Atypical CLL, and MCL.

	κ/λ	CD5	CD10	CD11c	CD20	CD22	CD23	CD38	CD43	CD81	CD200
CLL	+^{dim}/−	+	−	+/−	+^{dim}/−	−/+^{dim}	+	−/+^{partial}	+	−/+^{dim}	+^{strong}
aCLL	+	+	−	+/−	+	+	−	−/+^{partial}	+	−/+^{dim}	+^{strong}
MCL	+	+/(−)	−/(+)	−	+	+	−	+/(−)	+	+^{strong}	−^{a}

Notes: +, positive; (+), rarely positive; − negative; (−), rarely negative. Dim (or negative) surface light chain immunoglobulins, dim or negative CD20, negative CD22, CD38, CD81, positive (often partial) CD11c and positive CD23 and CD200 are typical for CLL. Atypical cases of CLL may show lack of CD23, moderate surface light chain immunoglobulins, CD20 and CD22, but show negative (or dim) CD81 and strong CD200. MCL differs from both CLL and call by strong expression of CD81, lack of CD200, positive CD38, negative CD11c and moderate expression of surface light chain immunoglobulins, CD20 and CD22.

^{a}Rare cases of indolent, non-nodal, leukemic MCL may be positive.

compared with the original MS [57]. The substitution of CD79b (modified score #2), surface membrane immunoglobulins (modified score #3), and CD79b and FMC7 (modified score #4) with CD200 showed that only the modified score #4 had both higher sensitivity and higher specificity compared with standard MS [57]. Also study by Mora et al. confirmed improved diagnosis of CLL by adding CD200 into the scoring system (CD200 improved the diagnostic accuracy of MS from 86.7% to 92.5%) [51].

In author's experience, evaluation of expression of CD5, CD10, CD11c, CD20, CD23, CD38, CD81, CD200, and surface immunoglobulins is most helpful in differential diagnosis of CLL versus MCL versus other less common CD5$^+$ B-cell lymphoproliferative. Dim or negative expression of CD20, strong expression of CD23, positive CD11c (even when partial), negative or dim surface immunoglobulins, negative (or partially dim) expression of CD38, strong expression of CD200, lack of CD81 (or expression similar or dimmer than in normal T-cells), and lack of CD10 are most typical for CLL, whereas strong CD20, strong expression of surface light chain immunoglobulins, lack of CD23, positive CD38, negative CD200 (below or at the same level as in T-cells), positive CD81, and positive CD10 (minor subset of cases) are typical for MCL. Regardless of the phenotypic differences, there is a significant overlap between CLL and MCL in occasional cases, especially between CLL and L-NN-MCL and therefore it is highly recommended to follow the FC analysis (at initial work-up) with testing for *CCND1* rearrangement by fluorescence in situ hybridization (FISH) in addition to typical prognostic probes (to definitively exclude or confirm MCL).

MBL with CLL-like or atypical CLL-like phenotype
MBL differs from CLL by <5 × 10^9/L clonal cells in blood (see above). Minor subset of patients with MBL and atypical CLL-like phenotype (CD23$^-$, CD200$^-$, CD81$^+$) may represent an unusual variant of indolent (smoldering) MCL [monoclonal B-cell lymphocytosis with t(11;14)] or L-NN-MCL.

Circulating benign CD5$^+$ B-cells
Circulating B-cells can be subdivided into (1) B-1 B-cells, originating from fetal liver and comprising the majority of B-cells during fetal live and infancy, which include regulatory B-cells (called "Bregs", from B-regulatory) and further subdivided into B-1a (CD5$^+$) and B-1b (CD5$^-$) and (2) conventional B-cells (B-2; ~10% of all circulating lymphocytes) derived from BM, and further subdivided into follicular B-cells and marginal zone B-cells. In healthy adults, CD5$^+$ comprise ~10%–20% of all circulating B-cells. Number of circulating CD5$^+$ B-cells changes in certain disease states or after toxic treatment, but generally decreases with age.

Mantle cell lymphoma (MCL)
The most informative markers for the distinction of CLL, MCL, CD5$^+$ MZL, including atypical cases are MFI values of CD79b,

CD20, CD23, CD43, CD38, CD11c, FMC7, CD200, kappa, and lambda light chain, and their combination [58]. CD23 and CD200 are the most discriminant between CLL and MCL and CD23 plus CD79b between CLL and CD5$^+$ MZL. There is higher intensity of expression of CD23, CD200, CD43, CD11c, and CD5 and lower intensity of expression of CD20, CD79b, FMC7, CD38, CD22, and kappa/lambda light chains in CLL when compared to MCL. CD200 expression in MCL is uncommon (4%); it identifies a subgroup of MCL patients with frequent leukemic non-nodal variant, and an indolent clinical course (L-NN-MCL). Of 43 publications screened, 27 were included in the systematic review (5,764 patients) by Sorigue et al., the median CD200 positivity rate and the percentage of CD200$^+$ patients was 100% and 95% (3,061/3,208) in CLL, 4 and 8% (86/1112) in MCL and 56 and 62% (425/689) in other lymphoproliferative disorders [50]. CD200 was therefore found suboptimal for the differential diagnosis of CLL and disorders other than nodal MCL [50]. ERIC proposed scoring system to differentiate between CD5$^+$ B-cell lymphoproliferative disorders, based on expression of the following markers: CD5, CD23, CD79b, CD20, CD43, CD81, CD10, CD200, and ROR1 [59]. Figure 12.2 (Chapter 12) and Table 13.1 summarize the major phenotypic differences between CLL and MCL.

Prolymphocytic transformation of CLL and T-cell prolymphocytic leukemia (T-PLL)
Typical CLL is composed predominantly of small mature-appearing lymphoid cells with scant cytoplasm, round nuclei, and clumped, condensed chromatin. Some cases may show, however, increased number of prolymphocytes and paraimmunoblasts, requiring differential diagnosis from prolymphocytic transformation, SBLPN or T-PLL. Prolymphocytic transformation of CLL/SLL is defined by CD5-positive non-mantle B-cell neoplasm with >15% prolymphocytes in blood and/or BM. T-PLL is characterized by marked lymphocytosis, generalized adenopathy, hepatosplenomegaly and BM involvement. B-cell prolymphocytes show strong expression of CD20 and surface light chain immunoglobulins and are most often CD5$^-$. T-cell prolymphocytes express pan-T-cell antigens (CD2, CD3, CD5, and CD7), are either CD4 or CD8 positive (minor subset may be dual CD4/CD8 positive or dual CD4/CD8 negative) and lack expression of B-cell markers.

Follicular lymphoma (FL)
FL shows variable proportion of centrocytes and centroblasts. Centrocytes are generally small lymphocytes with cleaved nuclei. Centroblasts are larger non-cleaved lymphocytes with several nucleoli. FL show usually dim CD19, positive CD10 and moderate expression of CD20, and surface light chain immunoglobulins. In contrast to strong expression of CD200 in CLL, the expression of CD200 in FL is either dimly positive or negative. Rare cases of FLs may be surface light chain immunoglobulin negative or

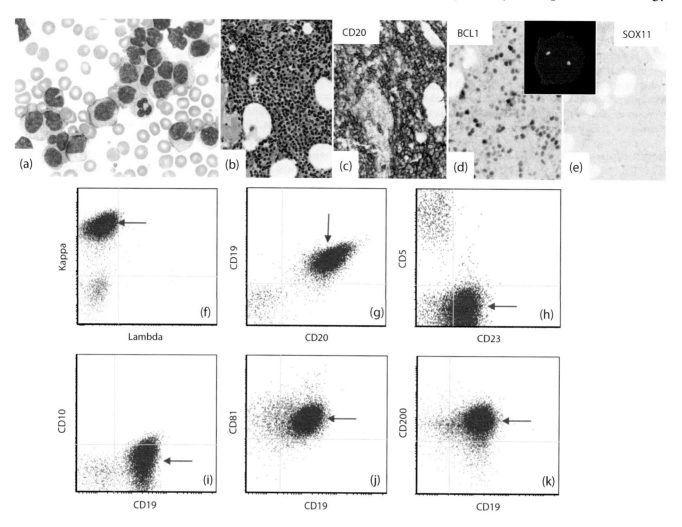

FIGURE 13.13   SBLPN/B-PLL (BM analysis from 76-year-old patient with marked leukocytosis (WBC = 180 k/µL) and mild splenomegaly (no adenopathy and no prior history of lymphoma). (a) Blood smear shows lymphocytosis with cytologic atypia including large nucleoli. (b) BM core biopsy shows diffuse lymphoid infiltrate. (c–d) Immunostaining analysis shows rare cells with expression of BCL1 and negative SOX11 (d–e; inset: FISH is negative for *CCND1* rearrangement, orange = *CCND1*; green = IGH). (f–k) Flow cytometry analysis (BM sample) shows kappa restriction (f), positive CD19 and CD20 (g), negative CD5 and dim CD23 (h), negative CD10 (i), dim CD81 (j), and dim CD200 (k).

T-PLL. Based on morphologic analysis of blood smear, SBLPN/ B-PLL may be confused with acute leukemias. The main differential diagnosis includes MCL, which is diagnosed by presence of t(11;14) translocation [*CCND1* rearrangement] and/or SOX11 expression. Splenic lymphomas of various types, including SMZL and SDRPL as well as FL can undergo prolymphocytoid transformation with more than 55% prolymphocytes in blood mimicking SBLPN/B-PLL [70]. Lymphoblastic leukemias can be easily differentiated form SBLPN/B-PLL by FC showing co-expression of CD19, CD22, CD10, TdT, and CD34 (B-ALL), or CD2, cytoplasmic CD3, CD7, CD34, TdT, and occasionally also CD1a (T-ALL). AMLs are also easily diagnosed by FC with co-expression of blastic markers (CD34, CD117, CD133) with myeloid antigens (CD13, CD33, MPO).

Differential diagnosis of SBLPN/ B-PLL based on immunophenotype

Leukemic cells with CD5 expression (with or without CD23) needs to be differentiated from CLL, CLL/B-PLL (Figure 13.16), MCL, and rarely other B-cell lymphoproliferations with CD5 expression (MZL, DLBCL). SBLPN/B-PLL without CD5 or CD23 expression needs to be differentiated from other B-cell lymphoproliferations

with non-specific phenotype (CD5⁻/CD10⁻), such as CD5⁻ MCL, CD10⁻ FL, DLBCL, MZL, SMZL, LPL/WM, and high-grade B-cell lymphoma (HGBL) with *MYC* and *BCL2* (and/or *BCL6*) rearrangement (HGBL-R, double or triple hit lymphoma). CLL differs from SBLPN/B-PLL but dim, negative, or partial expression of CD20 and dim expression of surface light chain immunoglobulins. FL is most often CD10⁺, MCL shows strong expression of CD5 and CD81, lack of CD23 and CD200, and presence of *CCND1* rearrangement [t(11;14)] and/or SOX11 expression, and BL is CD10⁺ with positive CD43, CD81, CD38 (strong), CD71 and can be confirmed by FISH showing rearranged *MYC*. The differential diagnosis of majority of B-cell lymphoproliferations with non-specific phenotype relies mostly on clinical, laboratory and genetic data. SBLPN/B-PLL is characterized by marked lymphocytosis (often >150 × 10³/µL), a feature rarely seen in MZL, FL, DLBCL, or LPL/WM. Splenomegaly and chromosome 7 abnormalities raise the possibility of SMZL (less often SDRPL). Presence of irregular cytoplasmic borders ("hairy cells"), bright expression of CD11c, and co-expression of CD25 and CD103, is typical for HCL, which on genetic level is associated with *BRAF* mutation. HCL-v is positive for CD103 (without co-expression

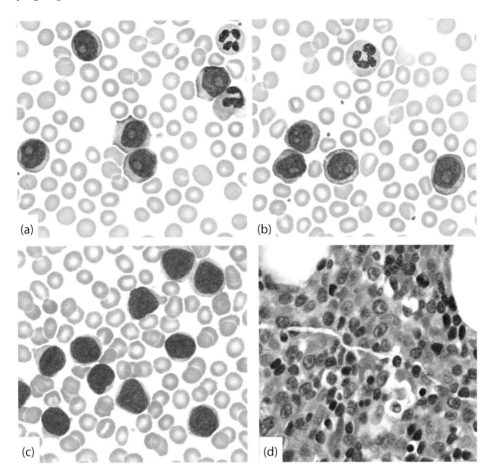

FIGURE 13.14 SBLPN/B-PLL. (a–c) Blood smear shows medium-sized cells with prominent central nucleoli. (d) BM involvement: lymphoid cells with prominent nucleoli.

of CD25) and shows bright CD11c expression. Presence of high serum M protein and *MYD88* mutation with typical cytomorphology showing mixed small lymphocytes, plasmacytoid lymphocytes and rare plasma cells indicates LPL/WM. All cases with prior history of CLL and prominent prolymphocytes are diagnostic as transformed CLL. Figure 13.17 presents an unusual case of prolymphocytoid transformation of FL transforming to HGBL-R with marked lymphocytosis.

Nodal marginal zone lymphoma (MZL)

MZL phenotype by FC: low forward scatter, sIg+, CD5−/rarely+, CD10−, CD11c+/rarely−, CD13−/rarely+, CD19+, CD20+moderate, CD22+, CD23−/rarely+, CD25−, CD38−/rarely+, CD43+/−, CD45+, CD81+/rarely−, CD103−(rarely+), CD123−/rarely+, and CD200+/−

Introduction
MZL is a low grade (indolent) B-cell lymphoma that arises from memory B-cells present normally in the marginal zone of secondary lymphoid tissues, usually in the context of chronic antigenic stimulation due either to infections or autoimmune disorders. MZLs represent approximately 5%–15% of all non-Hodgkin lymphomas in the Western world. This group of lymphomas include nodal marginal zone lymphoma (NMZL), extranodal MZL (or mucosa-associated lymphatic tissue lymphoma; MALT

lymphoma), SMZL, and rare cases of MZL with leukemic presentation. The stomach is the most common site of MALT lymphoma, followed by ocular adnexa, lung, and salivary glands. SMZL accounts for ~20% and NMZL for <10% of cases. The presence of circulating clonal B cells with phenotypic features consistent with a marginal zone origin in the absence of splenomegaly, hepatomegaly, lymphadenopathy, or other symptoms and signs suggestive of an established lymphoma is called CBL-MZ.

NMZL is a low-grade lymphoma with the morphologic and immunophenotypic features similar to extranodal MZL (MALT type) but without splenic or extranodal disease [71–78]. It occurs in peripheral lymph nodes (most commonly in head and neck area) and abdomen, often presents in advanced clinical stage and has more aggressive clinical course than extranodal MZL (MALT type) [1, 72, 75, 77–81]. BM involvement occurs in 30%–40% of patients. Patients with NMZL have lower 5-year overall survival and failure-free survival than patients with MALT lymphoma [78]. Traverse-Glehen et al. found peripheral blood involvement in 23%, anemia in 24%, thrombocytopenia in 10% and presence of serum M component in 33% [80]. In a series of 47 patients with primary NMZL reported by Arcaini et al., 45% had stage IV disease, and 24% had positive Hepatitis C virus serology [72].

Morphology
Lymph nodes. NMZL was earlier divided into two morphologic variants, one resembling nodal involvement by extranodal MZL (MALT type) and the other resembling SMZL [82]. The NMZL is

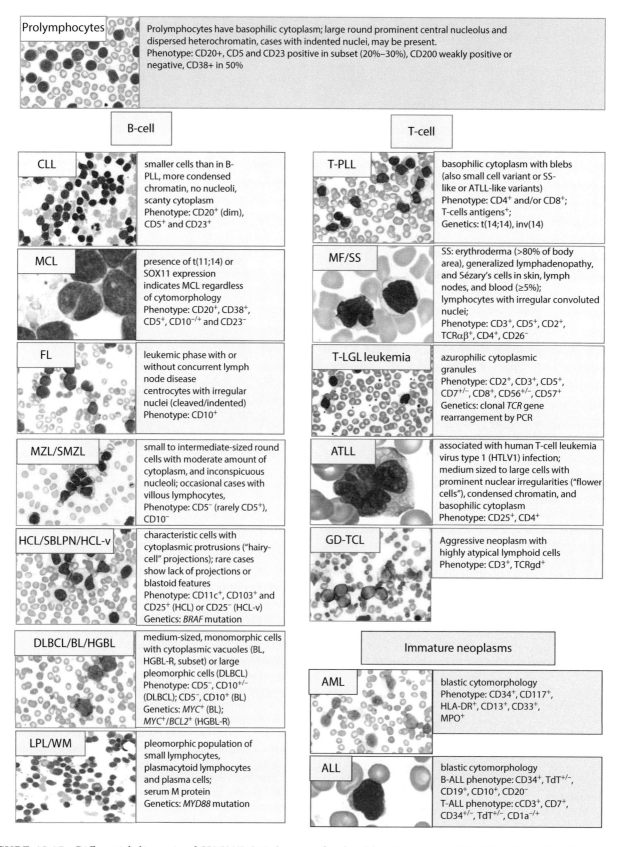

FIGURE 13.15 Differential diagnosis of SBLPN/B-PLL (see text for details). *Abbreviations*: SBLPN, splenic B-cell lymphoma/ leukemia with prominent nucleoli; PLL, prolymphocytic leukemia, CLL, chronic lymphocytic leukemia; FL, follicular lymphoma; MCL, mantle cell lymphoma; MZL, marginal zone lymphoma; SMZL, splenic MZL; HCL, hairy cell leukemia; SBLPN/HCL-v, splenic B-cell lymphoma/hairy cell leukemia variant; DLBCL, diffuse large B-cell lymphoma; BL, Burkitt lymphoma, HGBL-R, high grade B-cell lymphoma with rearranged MYC and BCL2 genes; LPL, lymphoplasmacytic lymphoma; WM, Waldenström macroglobulin-emia; MF, mycosis fungoides; SS, Sézary's syndrome; T-LGL, T large granular lymphocyte; ATLL, adult T-cell lymphoma/leukemia; GD-TCL, gamma/delta T-cell lymphoma/leukemia; AML, acute myeloid leukemia; ALL, acute lymphoblastic leukemia.

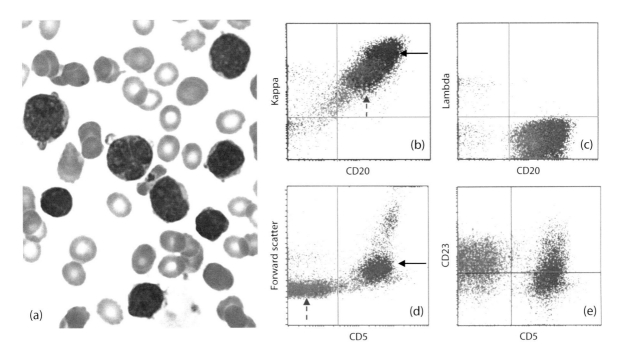

FIGURE 13.16 B-chronic lymphocytic leukemia/prolymphocytic leukemia (B-CLL/PLL). Blood smear (a) shows mixed population of small lymphocytes with dense chromatin and larger cells with prominent nucleoli (prolymphocytes). Flow cytometry analysis (b–e) shows two clonal kappa⁺ (b–c) B-cell populations: small cells with low forward scatter (d; red dots marked with red dotted arrow) and larger cells with higher forward scatter (d; blue dots marked with solid arrow). Larger cells have brighter expression of surface immunoglobulin (b), brighter CD20 (b–c) and positive CD5 (d–e) and CD23 (e). Smaller cells show slightly dimmer kappa (b) and CD20 (b–c), negative CD5 (d), and positive CD23 (e).

currently subdivided according to morphology and immunophenotype into several variants: MALT type (mNMZL), splenic type (sNMZL), floral MZL (fNMZL), and DLBCL with the presence of accompanying MZL lymphoma (DLBCL + MZL) [1, 83–85]. In mNMZL, the lymph node architecture is effaced by a proliferation of lymphoma cells with predominant perisinusoidal, perivascular, and parafollicular distribution. Reactive follicles are seen in most cases and are distinguished from neoplastic cells by intact mantle cuff. The tumor cells have monocytoid appearance with abundant pale cytoplasm and round to irregular nuclei. In sNMZL, tumor cells selectively involve germinal centers or grow near a germinal center without effacing lymph node architecture, mimicking FL. In fNMZL, the expanded and fragmented reactive germinal centers mimic progressive transformation of germinal centers (PTGC). Tumor cells are present in the interfollicular area and may disrupt the follicles. Pediatric NMZL is now considered a provisional clinicopathological entity, with striking predilection for young males and features of fNMZL.

In addition, four architectural patterns can be identified in NMZL (Figure 13.18): diffuse, nodular, interfollicular, and marginal zone (perifollicular) [86]. The diffuse pattern is characterized by sheets of neoplastic cells with effacement of nodal architecture (Figure 13.18). The nodular pattern is characterized by well-formed nodules surrounding and colonizing reactive germinal centers. The nodules are rather sharply demarcated from the uninvolved interfollicular areas. The interfollicular pattern shows the neoplastic B-cells limited to the interfollicular areas with sparing normal secondary follicles and often prominent perivascular/perisinusoidal involvement. The least common, perifollicular pattern is characterized by annular distribution of

the neoplastic cells around uninvolved normal secondary follicles (colonization of germinal centers is minimal or absent), somewhat reminiscent of biphasic pattern in SMZL. Interfollicular and perifollicular patterns show increased number of large cells, when compared to other types. Residual germinal centers are usually preserved but are disrupted. Some cases show prominent colonization of reactive follicles (either complete or partial) with characteristic expansion and disruption of follicular dendritic cell (FDC) meshwork [75]. Residual follicle center cells express CD20, CD10, and BCL6 and are negative for BCL2, whereas neoplastic B-cells infiltrating follicles express CD20, BCL2, and often MUM1.

The lymphoid cells are mostly small to occasionally medium in size with variable admixture of large B-cells with prominent nucleoli (immunoblast-like). In many cases B-cells have a monocytoid appearance with abundant pale or light eosinophilic cytoplasm. Cellular pleomorphism (variable shape and size of neoplastic cells) is seen in majority of cases, and only subset of lymphomas is composed of predominantly small cells with occasional, scattered intermediate-sized cells. Large cell component, usually less than 20% of the infiltrate, can be identified in many cases [86]. Rare cases may show up to 50% large cells, but none of the NMZLs have more than 50% large cell or sheets of large cells [86]. MZL with increased number of large cells (20%–50%) does not behave more aggressively [80]. In contrast to FL, there are no defined criteria for grading of MZL. Transformation to DLBCL is currently diagnosed only if there are sheets of large cells.

Occasional cases of MZL show an plasmacytoid or plasmacytic differentiation and increased number of large cells with high mitotic rate [80]. Presence of extensive plasmacytic differentiation

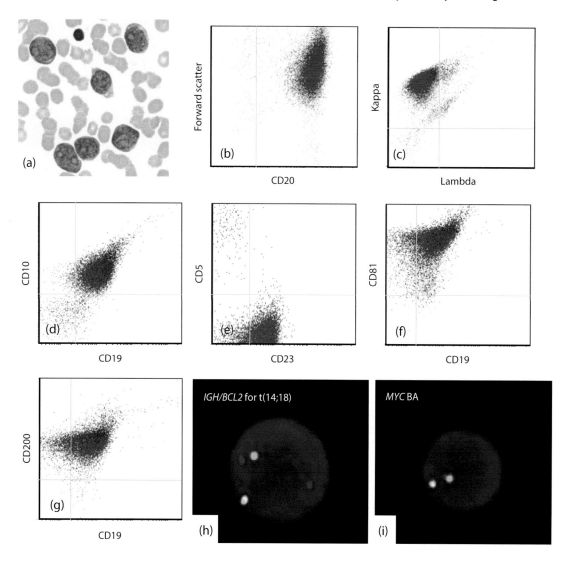

FIGURE 13.17   Prolymphocytoid transformation of FL to HGBL-R. (a) Blood shows marked lymphocytosis (WBC = 140 k/μL) with large lymphoid cells with prominent nucleoli. (b–g) Flow cytometry analysis shows CD20⁺ B-cells with high forward scatter (b), clonal kappa restriction (c), positive CD10 (d), negative CD5 (e), positive CD23 (e) bright CD81 (f), and moderate CD200 (g). (h–i) FISH analysis shows *IGH-BCL2* rearrangement (h, yellow fusion signal indicating *BCL2* rearrangement) and MYC rearrangement (i, break apart probe with normal yellow fusion signal and abnormal orange and green signals indicating *MYC* rearrangement).

pose a problem for differential diagnosis from LPL/WM, nodal plasmacytoma, and IgG4-related lymphadenopathy [87, 88].

Extranodal sites. There is no evidence of involvement of the spleen or other extranodal sites, such as gastrointestinal tract, skin, lung, salivary gland, or ocular adnexa in NMZL.

BM and blood. Blood and BM may be involved by NMZL more frequently than in extranodal MALT lymphomas. The circulating cells are small to intermediate in size and may display monocytoid appearance in blood smear. BM shows usually nodular pattern of involvement. Lymphomatous cells often display monocytoid appearance with admixture of small lymphocytes, plasma cells and occasional lymphocytes with irregular nuclei (centrocyte-like). B-cells predominate but T-cells are also present.

Immunophenotype
The expression of CD20 and surface immunoglobulins is moderate when analyzed by FC (Figures 13.18–13.20). Often, there is dim to moderate expression of CD11c and/or CD43 (21%–50%) [73, 77,

78, 80, 89]. Occasional cases may show bright expression of CD11c (Figure 13.20), prompting the differential diagnosis with HCL or hairy-cell leukemia variant (HCL-v). NMZL is negative for CD103, although CD25 may be occasionally positive. Subset of NMZL cases shows aberrant expression of CD5 or rarely CD13 (Figure 13.21). Minor subset of MZL may show lack of surface immunoglobulin expression (Figure 13.22). CD81 and CD200 are variably expressed in NZML (majority of cases are dimly positive for CD81 and either negative or dimly positive for CD200; Figure 13.22). SMZLs, on the other hand, often show moderate CD200 expression. In the context of CD23, CD81, and CD200 expression, MZLs often resemble benign B-cells. Plasma cells are often monotypic (~30%), a useful parameter in confirming NMZL. Some cases, however, may show increased number of polytypic plasma cells.

Genetic features
Abnormalities identified in more than 15% of patients with non-MALT MZLs included +3/+3q (37%), 7q deletions (31%),

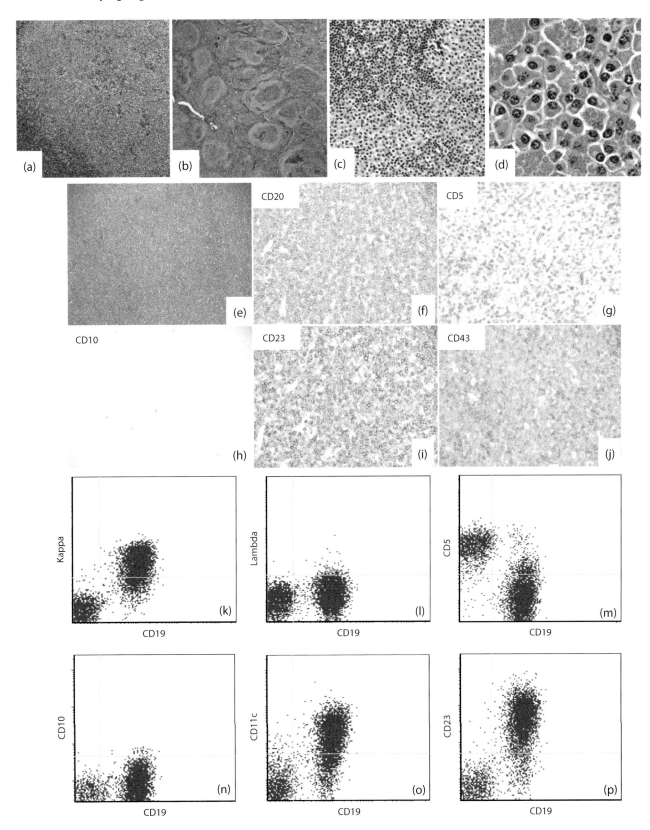

FIGURE 13.18 Histologic features of nodal MZL: (a) diffuse pattern without any residual follicles with reactive germinal centers; (b) perifollicular (marginal) zone pattern; (c) prominent monocytoid appearance of lymphomatous cells; (d) NMZL with extensive plasmacytic differentiation. NMZL with diffuse involvement of the lymph node by small, rather monomorphic lymphoid cells (e). (f–j) Immunohistochemistry staining shows positive CD20 (f), negative CD5 (g), negative CD10 (h), positive CD23 (i), and positive for CD43 (j). Flow cytometric analysis shows clonal B-cells (kappa⁺, k–l) without expression of CD5 (m) or CD10 (n), positive CD11c (o), and positive CD23 (p).

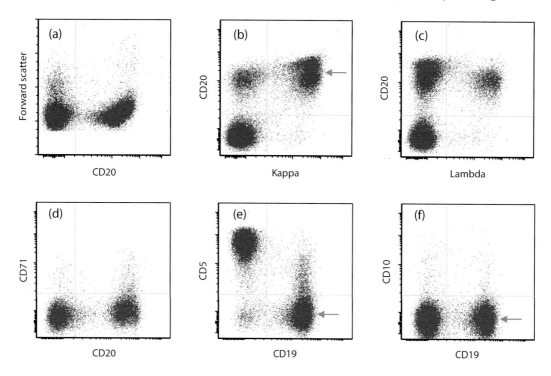

FIGURE 13.19 NMZL – flow cytometry analysis. Flow cytometry analysis shows partial lymph node involvement with CD20⁺ (a–c) monoclonal B-cells (kappa⁺; b, arrow) in the background of polytypic B-cells (kappa⁺ and lambda⁺; b–c). MZL cells are negative for CD71 (d), CD5 (e, arrow), and CD10 (f, arrow).

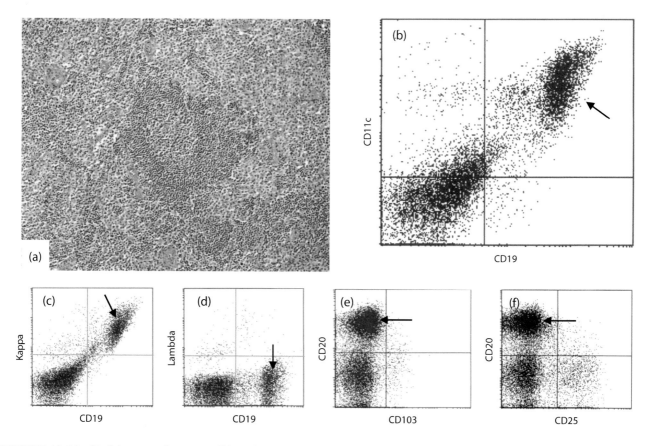

FIGURE 13.20 Nodal marginal zone B-cell lymphoma – flow cytometry. (a) Histology of the lymph node shows residual germinal center surrounded by small lymphocytic infiltrate with plasma cells. Neoplastic B-cells are positive for CD11c (b), kappa immuno-globulins (c–d), and are negative for CD103 (e) and CD25 (f).

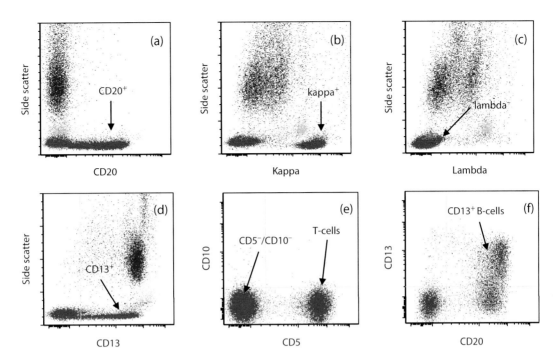

FIGURE 13.21 Marginal zone lymphoma (blood) with aberrant expression of CD13 – flow cytometry (a–d, all events; e–f, lymphocytes only). Monoclonal B-cells express CD20 (a) and kappa (b) and display aberrant expression of CD13 (on subset of monoclonal B-cells with brighter CD20; d, f). CD5 and CD10 are not expressed (e).

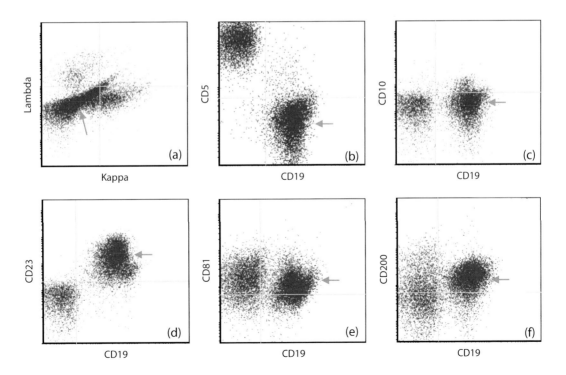

FIGURE 13.22 NMZL with lack of surface immunoglobulin expression – flow cytometry. Lymphomatous cells (arrow) are kappa and lambda negative (a–b; residual benign B-cells are either kappa⁺ or lambda⁺), do not express CD5 (c) or CD10 (d), show dim expression of CD81 and dim expression of CD200.

+18/+18q (28%), 6q deletions (19%), +12/+12q (15%), and 8p deletions (15%) [90]. Trisomy 3/3q, 7q deletions, +18 and +12 were seen in different combinations in more than 30% of patients in comparison to 2% in B-SLL/CLL, 1% in MCL and 7% in FL [90]. Next gene sequencing (NGS) found mutations of *NFKBIE* and *ITPR2* genes in ~8% and ~14% of NMZL [91].

Histologic transformation (HT)

HT is defined by presence of solid or sheet-like proliferation of monotonous, transformed (large) cells. HT of MZL has been reported in 3.2%–14% of patients with a median time to transformation of 13–22 months [27, 92–94]. By PCR-based clonality analysis, HT occurred within 2.5 years after the diagnosis of MZL in patients with clonal relationship, whereas time to aggressive lymphoma was longer in patients identified as clonally-unrelated (most likely secondary) lymphoma (82–202 months), suggesting that HT is an early event in this disease [94]. Histologically, the progression is in the form of DLBCL and only sporadically HL or BL. MZL often shows increased large cells (blasts) [95, 96] and therefore the diagnosis of disease progression (transformation) into DLBCL may be difficult. Usually, the progression of MZL to DLBCL is characterized by clearly identifiable diffuse sheets of large cells that represent at least 50% of the infiltrate. Transformed cells show the phenotype similar to low grade MZL, but some lymphomas are positive for CD10, BCL6, and even p53 or EBV (by EBER-ISH). Ki67 index is most often high (~40%–80%) [97]. The revised WHO classification recommends that ambiguous cases should be diagnoses as DLBCL with a MALT component, rather than using the term "high grade MALT lymphoma" [96].

Differential diagnosis of NMZL lymphoma

- CBL-MZ
- FL
- MCL
- DLBCL
- Lymphoplasmacytic lymphoma (LPL)
- Small lymphocytic lymphoma (SLL)
- Plasma cell neoplasm
- Gamma heavy chain disease (GHCD)
- Hodgkin lymphoma with clusters of monocytoid B-cells
- Peripheral T-cell lymphoma, not otherwise specified (PTCL)
- Secondary lymph node involvement by extranodal MZL (MALT lymphoma)

Clonal B-cell lymphocytosis of marginal zone origin (CBL-MZ)

MBL can be subclassified into three major categories, MBL with CLL-like phenotype, MBL with atypical CLL-like phenotype, and MBL with non-CLL phenotype, also called CBL-MZ or MBL with MZL-like phenotype. CBL-MZ is a recently described entity characterized by the presence of clonal B cells in the blood and/or BM with morphologic and immunophenotypic features consistent with marginal zone derivation in otherwise healthy individuals. CBL-MZ may be associated with IgM paraproteinemia raising the differential diagnosis with WM. CBL-MZ is very heterogeneous with mutations not associated with specific lymphoma subtype, including *MYD88* (14%–19%), *BIRC3* (11%), *CCND3* (11%), *NOTCH1* (11%), and *TNFAIP3* (11%), but often show some genetic changes overlapping with SMZL and SDRPL [5, 6].

SLL/CLL

Small lymphocytic lymphoma (SLL) can be differentiated by presence of proliferation centers (on low power examination of H&E sections) and co-expression of CD5 and CD23. The expression of surface light chain immunoglobulins and CD20 is moderate to bright in NZML and dim (or negative) in SLL/CLL. SLL/CLL differs from NMZL by negative (or very dim) CD81 and positive (often strong) CD200. Plasmacytic differentiation is less common in SLL/CLL than in NMZL. The flow cytometric scoring systems helpful in differentiating CLL/SLL from MZL and other B-cell lymphoproliferations is presented earlier in this chapter (CLL; differential diagnosis).

DLBCL

Important morphologic consideration in the diagnosis of NMZL is its relationship with DLBCL, which is particularly problematic in cases with increased transformed large B cells typical for MZL. Nathwani et al. described progression to DLBCL with more than 20% large cells [76, 77]. Recent data suggest that the presence of increased number of large cells is very common and may approach up to 50% (without sheet formation) [80, 86]. Increased number of scattered large cells should not be confused with sheets of large cells, particularly if the latter is associated with an increase in proliferation (Ki-67 index). Presence of sheets of large cells and/or more than 50% large cells should raise the possibility of progression into DLBCL (DLBCL and NMZL). Kojima et al. recently reported a series of 65 cases of NMZL, of which 20 cases had more than 50% large cells or sheets of large cells and were classified as NMZL and DLBCL [83]. Those cases had significantly worse outcome. The overall criteria for progression of NMZL into DLBCL are not well established, and there is no cutoff for proliferation (Ki-67) to aid in this distinction. By FC analysis, DLBCL differs from NMZL by high forward scatter (FSC) of clonal B-cells. Subset of DLBCL may be CD10+ and majority of DLBCLs are negative for CD11c, CD5, CD23, and CD200.

Follicular lymphoma (FL)

In tissue sections, FL may be difficult to differentiate from MZL, especially in cases of MZL with prominent follicle colonization, or FL with marginal zone differentiation or reversed pattern. The co-expression of CD10, BCL2, and BCL6 by neoplastic cells favors FL, but subset of FL cases may be CD10− or BCL2−. In difficult cases, correlation with FISH and/or PCR testing for *BCL2* rearrangement [t(14;18)] may be needed for final subclassification. Morphologic analysis of the BM core biopsy may also be helpful, as FL often shows prominent paratrabecular lymphoid infiltrate (paratrabecular pattern is not typically seen in MZL). By FC analysis, FLs are characterized by moderate expression of surface immunoglobulins and CD20, dim expression of CD19, positive CD10, negative CD5 and CD11c, and most often negative CD43. FLs often show admixture of residual benign (polytypic) B-cells and many reactive T-cells.

Mantle cell lymphoma (MCL)

MCL differs from MZL by positive CD5, SOX11, and BCL1 (cyclin D1) expression. It most often shows more monomorphic lymphoid infiltrate with scattered histiocytes and without large cell component typical for NMZL. FC analysis in MCL shows moderate expression of CD19, CD20 and surface light chain immunoglobulins. Majority of cases are CD5+, CD23−, CD11c−, CD38+, CD81+ (strong expression), and CD200−. Correlation with genetic studies for *CCND1* rearrangement [t(11;14)] or immunohistochemical analysis for cyclin D1 (BCL1) and SOX11 help to establish the diagnosis of MCL and exclude CD5+ NMZL.

Lymphoplasmacytic lymphoma (LPL)

LPL may be difficult to separate from MZL, especially in blood sample. Both lymphomas display non-specific phenotype (CD5−, CD10−), although minor subset of MZL may be CD5+ and minor subset of LPL may be CD5+ or CD10+. High level of serum IgM protein favors the diagnosis of LPL. Adenopathy is reported in ~15% of LPL and histologic examination shows mixed population of small lymphocytes, plasmacytoid B-cells and plasma cells. In contrast, MZL often shows monocytoid ("clear" cell) appearance of neoplastic B-cells. Analysis of the BM may also be helpful in differential diagnosis of LPL. LPL/WM usually shows interstitial and/or paratrabecular pattern of BM involvement, whereas MZL often displays nodular pattern (paratrabecular pattern is rarely seen in MZL, most often in SMZL). In sample from BM, LPL often show two clonal populations, major B-cell clone, and minor plasma cell clone (plasma cells display the same light chain immunoglobulin restriction as B-cells and are most often IgM+).

Plasma cell neoplasms

Extensive plasmacytic differentiation is often seen in MZL. Lack or very minimal number of B-cells and/or aberrant phenotype of plasma cells (such as expression of BCL1, CD200, CD56, and/or CD117) would favor plasma cell neoplasm. FC analysis may be also helpful. Identification of monoclonal B-cell population and monoclonal plasma cell population (with the same light chain restriction) would favor MZL. Correlation with BM morphology, radiologic imaging data and serum electrophoresis and/or immunofixation may also be helpful.

Gamma heavy chain disease (GHCD)

Lymph node shows polymorphic infiltrate resembling of either MZL or LPL with lymphocytes, plasmacytoid lymphocytes, plasma cells and admixture of large lymphocytes (immunoblasts), histiocytes and eosinophils. Blood may show lymphocytosis of small mature lymphocytes mimicking CLL, or mixture of small lymphocytes and plasmacytoid lymphocytes resembling LPL. Presence of IgG without light chain by immunofixation confirms the diagnosis of GHCD.

Classic Hodgkin lymphoma (cHL)

The presence of reactive monocytoid B-cells can rarely be present in cHL. Neoplastic cells (Reed-Sternberg cells and Hodgkin cells) usually occur outside of the foci of monocytoid B-cells but may be present at the border or even within the monocytoid aggregates.

Peripheral T-cell lymphoma, not otherwise specified (PTCL)

PTCL may show prominent interfollicular (T-zone) pattern of involvement, mimicking MZL. Pleomorphic infiltrate with histiocytes and eosinophils and expression of pan- T-cell antigens (CD2, CD3, CD5, and/or CD7) with CD4 or CD8 restriction establishes the diagnosis of PTCL.

Gastric MZL (MALT lymphoma)

Introduction

MALT lymphoma is the most common type of lymphoma involving the gastrointestinal tract (location in the stomach being the most frequent) [1, 98–101]. Other common sites of involvement include salivary gland, skin, lung, thyroid gland, and orbital area. Gastric MZL (or MALT lymphoma) usually remains localized for long periods within tissue of origin. BM involvement at presentation is uncommon [101, 102]. Disseminated disease including BM involvement appears to be more common in non-gastrointestinal MALT lymphomas [103, 104]. MALT lymphomas harboring t(11;18) are unlikely to transform to a higher-grade lymphoma [105–107], but exceptions may occur. The t(11;18) positive lymphomas usually lack other chromosomal aberrations and microsatellite alterations frequently seen in the translocation-negative MALT lymphomas. Although stomach is the most common site of MALT lymphoma (followed by lung, skin, salivary gland, and ocular adnexa), both small and large intestines (including appendix) may be involved. Intestinal MALT lymphomas are often located in the ileocecal area and the rectum [108–111]. The small intestine is typically involved in patients with immunoproliferative small intestinal disease (IPSID), previously called alpha heavy chain disease [7, 112]. The histologic and immunophenotypic features are similar to MZL at other locations including stomach. Since the reactive lymphoid infiltrate in terminal ileum often shows CD43 expression by benign B-cells, the expression of CD43 cannot be used as a discriminating factor in differential diagnosis between MALT lymphoma and benign lymphoid infiltrate at that location.

Morphology

Gastric MALT (Figures 13.23) shows an expansion of the mucosa and submucosa by atypical B-cell infiltrate which starts around secondary lymphoid follicles (marginal zone pattern) and often spread within mucosa into diffuse pattern [95, 113–116]. Small to medium-sized marginal zone B cells have round to slightly irregular nuclei with inconspicuous nucleoli, moderately dispersed chromatin, and pale cytoplasm, which may display monocytoid features. Monocytoid cells have abundant clear cytoplasm with distinct cell borders. There is often a variable proportion of larger lymphocytes. Some tumors are composed of mostly small lymphocytes with scanty cytoplasm. The neoplastic infiltrate is often accompanied by reactive germinal centers, which are colonized by neoplastic B-cells. In some cases, the follicles are completely replaced by neoplastic marginal zone B-cells, and only focal and disrupted residual FDC meshwork visualized by CD21 and/or CD23 immunostaining shows the areas previously occupied by benign follicles. There is often plasmacytic differentiation subjacent to the surface epithelium, which may or may not be monotypic. Rare cases show predominance of plasma cells resembling extramedullary plasmacytoma rather than B-cell process. Plasma cells may contain Dutcher bodies. *Helicobacter pylori* organisms are frequently found to accompany gastric MALT lymphomas.

Infiltration and destruction of the glandular structures by clusters of neoplastic lymphocytes with formation of lymphoepithelial lesions, although not specific, is an important diagnostic feature of MALT lymphoma (Figure 13.23). Lymphoepithelial lesions are usually defined by ≥3 lymphomatous B-cells within gastric epithelium. The lymphoepithelial lesions can be better visualized with an anti-cytokeratin immunohistochemical stain. Involved epithelium often shows degenerative changes. Presence of scattered individually small lymphocytes within epithelium does not qualify as a lymphoepithelial lesion. Lymphoepithelial lesions along with cytologic atypia, monocytoid features, aberrant CD43 expression and monoclonal plasma cell infiltrate represents major criteria in the diagnosis of MZL. Some of these features are site-dependent [117]. After *H. pylori*-eradication therapy, presence of scattered lymphoid or plasmacytic cells within *lamina propria* or complete lack of lymphoid cells indicate complete histologic remission, whereas presence of lymphoid aggregates or lymphoid nodules in the *lamina propria, muscularis mucosae*, or submucosa indicates probable minimal residual disease [118].

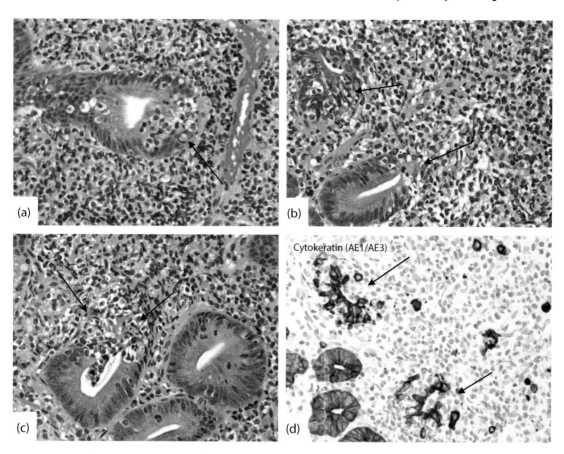

FIGURE 13.23 Gastric marginal zone B-cell lymphoma (MALT-lymphoma) with prominent lymphoepithelial lesions (a–c). The lymphoepithelial lesions can be easily identified by immunohistochemical staining with cytokeratin (d).

Immunophenotype

MZL has a non-specific phenotype (CD5⁻/CD10⁻) with positive expression of B-cell markers (CD19, CD20, CD22, CD79a, and PAX5), BCL2, and IgM (less often IgA or IgG). CD10, CD23, CD103, BCL6, MUM1, and IgD are not expressed. The expression of CD43 is variable. FC shows often dim to moderate expression of CD11c, moderate expression of surface light chain immunoglobulins, and positive (moderate) CD19 and CD20 expression. About 35%–50% of cases display aberrant co-expression of CD43 by neoplastic B-cell, a useful criterion in identifying neoplastic processes. Aberrant CD43 expression is seen most often in MZL of salivary gland, stomach and upper aerodigestive tract [117]. Subset of cases (more often non-gastric, especially in orbital MZL and head and neck area) may be CD5⁺ [119–122]. MALT lymphomas with CD5 expression may have more aggressive clinical behavior and earlier dissemination when compared to CD5⁻ cases [121, 123]. Figure 13.24 presents three examples of MALT lymphomas.

Histological transformation (HT)

There are no definitive criteria for HT in MZL, but HT is usually defined by presence of clearly separated solid or sheet-like proliferation of large cells comprising >20% of the neoplastic population or in mixed (pleomorphic) lymphoid infiltrate, presence of ≥30% large cells (reactive germinal centers must be excluded) [1, 124]. Majority of transformed DLBCLs have centroblastic morphology with the following phenotype: CD10⁺ (9%), BCL6⁺ (59%), MUM1⁺ (38%), MYC⁺ (42%), BCL2⁺ (32%), double BCL2/MYC⁺ (10%), and CD5⁺ (3%) [124]. HT may occur at primary site (54%), lymph node (30%), primary site and lymph node (5%), stomach

(5%), BM (3%), and nasal cavity (1%). Rare cases of concurrent MALT lymphoma and DLBCL have been reported. HT is frequently discovered simultaneously with (70%) and at the primary site of (59%) MALT lymphoma [124]. Patients with MALT lymphoma generally have an indolent clinical course, but HT has been reported to be a risk factor for unfavorable outcome [92]. HT to DLBCL at 10-years occurs in 3%–12% of MALT lymphomas [124, 125]. In the series by Maeshima et al., the risk of HT by 5, 10, and 15 years in 441 patients with MALT lymphoma without DLBCL at initial presentation were 3%, 3%, and 5%, respectively [124]. Ferreri et al. reported that presence of scattered large cells (≤10% of MALT lymphoma) is prognostically irrelevant, whereas compact clusters of large cells (>10% of MALT lymphoma) is associated with worse prognosis [126].

Very rare cases of otherwise typical MALT lymphomas may show scattered Reed-Sternberg and Hodgkin-like cells with the phenotype typical for cHL. It is difficult to determine based on the biopsy of MALT lymphoma site whether this represents HT (similar to Hodgkin-like Richters' transformation in CLL) or separate de novo cHL. Correlation with lymph node status (and biopsy if there is adenopathy) may help in final subclassification.

Genetic features

The t(11;18)(21;q21), which juxtaposes *API2* and *MALT1* genes is the most common translocation detected in the stomach, intestine and lung [98, 127–130]. Other translocations seen in MZL, including t(14;18)(q32;q21), t(3;14)(p14.1;q32), and t(1;14)(p22;q32) are encountered more often at other sites [98, 105, 131–133].

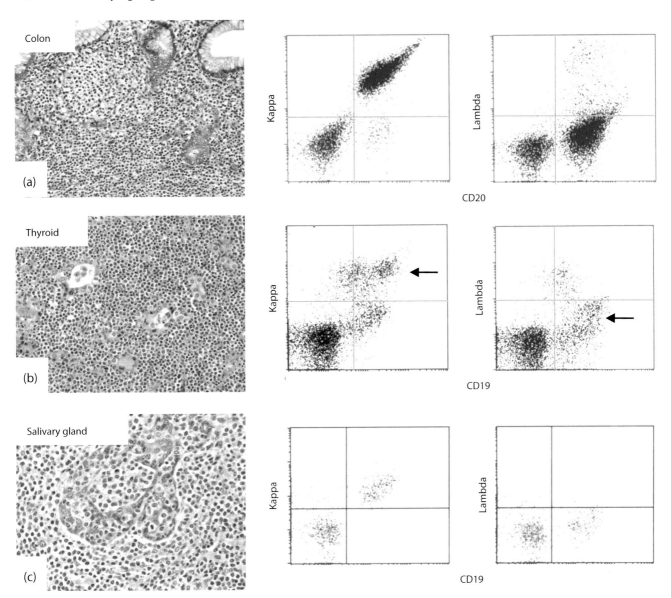

FIGURE 13.24 Extranodal MZL (a, colon; b, thyroid, and c, salivary gland). Flow cytometry (right panels) analysis show kappa⁺ clonal B-cell population with moderate CD19 and CD20 expression.

Splenic marginal zone lymphoma (SMZL)

MZL phenotype by FC: low forward scatter, sIg⁺, CD5$^{-/rarely+}$, CD10⁻, CD11c$^{+(dim)/rarely-}$, CD13$^{-/rarely+}$, CD19⁺, CD20$^{+moderate}$, CD22⁺, CD23$^{-/rarely+}$, CD25⁻, CD38$^{-/rarely+}$, CD43$^{+/-}$, CD45⁺, CD81⁺, CD103$^{-/rarely+}$, CD123$^{-/rarely+}$, and CD200$^{+/rarely-}$

Introduction
There are three different types of MZLs: extranodal MZL of mucosa-associated lymphoid tissue (MALT lymphoma), SMZL, and NMZL [1]. In spleen, according to WHO classification, the main types of primary splenic B-cell lymphomas include SMZL, HCL, splenic diffuse red pulp small B-cell lymphoma (SDRPL), and splenic B-cell lymphoma/leukemia with prominent nucleoli (SBLPN). [1, 134]. SMZL is an indolent B-cell lymphoma involving splenic white pulp with focal infiltration of the red pulp,

usually involving also splenic hilar lymph nodes, BM, and blood [1, 135–138]. SMZL is a disease of elderly with median age at presentation of 65 years (range 30–90). The disease presents as an incidental finding (most patients are asymptomatic) or with symptoms of splenic enlargement, cytopenia (most often anemia or thrombocytopenia), or lymphocytosis. Circulating lymphoma cells in blood are detected in 57%–68% of cases [139, 140]. Majority of cases have BM involvement and roughly a third have liver involvement. Serum paraproteinemia is observed in 10%–28% of cases but is usually minimal. Approximately 70% of SMZLs exhibit heterozygous deletion in 7q22-36. Some patient experience autoimmune manifestations including autoimmune hemolytic anemia or immune thrombocytopenia.

SMZL is an indolent extranodal B-cell lymphoma with the reported median survival of 78%–84% at 5 years and median overall survival time exceeding 10 years [141–144]. In a subset of patients (approximately third of cases), however, the disease follows an aggressive course [139]. Those patients are more likely to have the 7q31 deletion,

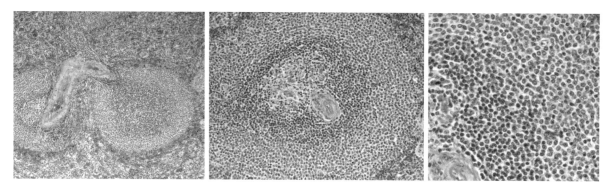

FIGURE 13.25   SMZL with characteristic biphasic pattern (histology at low intermediate and high magnification).

lack of *IGHV* somatic mutation, or both [145]. The parameters predictive of shorter cause-specific survival (univariate analysis) included hemoglobin levels <12 g/dL, albumin levels <3.5 g/dL, International Prognostic Index (IPI) scores of 2–3, LDH levels above normal, age >60 years, unmutated *IGVH* genes, platelet counts <100×10^9/L, and no splenectomy at diagnosis [79, 144]. In the same study, values that maintained a negative influence on cause-specific survival in multivariate analysis were hemoglobin level less <12 g/dL, LDH level greater than normal, and albumin level <3.5 g/dL [79]. Splenectomy remains one of the first line options in patients fit for surgery, and amongst chemotherapy, purine analogues, in particular fludarabine in combination or not with Rituximab and Rituximab alone have a greater efficacy than alkylating agents in terms of achieving better quality of response and longer progression free survival; therefore these agents are recommended particularly in patients who are not candidates for surgery or relapse after splenectomy [146].

Morphology

Spleen. SMZL involves the white pulp of the spleen and usually has spillover into the red pulp (Figure 13.25). Spleen is enlarged (usually >300–400 g). Low power magnification shows either nodular pattern or diffuse involvement. In the nodular pattern, prominent nodules of white pulp are composed of residual germinal centers surrounded by expanded marginal zone with either small lymphocytes or cells with abundant pale ("clear") cytoplasm (monocytoid features). The follicles are often colonized by neoplastic B-cells, which eventually lead to follicle regression. The involvement of white pulp may create either biphasic or monophasic patterns. In the biphasic pattern, the central (dark) portion of the nodule is composed of small round

lymphocytes that infiltrate and often replace the residual germinal centers with complete obliteration of mantle zone and the outer (paler) portion is composed of slightly larger cells with moderate amount of pale (clear) cytoplasm. The biphasic pattern is also seen with presence of residual follicles which are surrounded by expanded marginal zone with monocytoid (clear) B-cells. This classical biphasic pattern is most common, but some of cases are composed of either predominantly small lymphocytes with round nuclei (inner zone type) or marginal (outer) zone type with monocytoid features [98, 147]. Besides small lymphocytes and monocytoid B-cells, few scattered medium-sized and large cells may be noted. Plasma cell differentiation may be present. The red pulp infiltration which is usually limited is composed of either small lymphocytes or marginal zone type cells, which occasionally form small nodules and, when more prominent, may involve the sinuses. Presence of clusters or sheets of large lymphoid cells should raise the possibility of large cell transformation into DLBCL (histological transformation; HT).

Blood. Circulating lymphocytes in patients with SMZL consist of small- to medium-sized lymphocytes with a round nuclei, condensed chromatin, and basophilic cytoplasm with polar short villi ("villous" lymphocytes). Prominent villous projections lead to designation of some SMZLs as splenic lymphoma with villous lymphocytes. Some lymphocytes may be irregular with nuclear clefts or abundant pale cytoplasm that resembles monocytes. Cells with plasmacytoid features may be also seen.

Bone marrow (BM). BM is very often involved in SMZL showing usually prominent intrasinusoidal pattern of involvement (Figure 13.26), although interstitial and nodular patterns may also occur (with many cases showing mixture of several

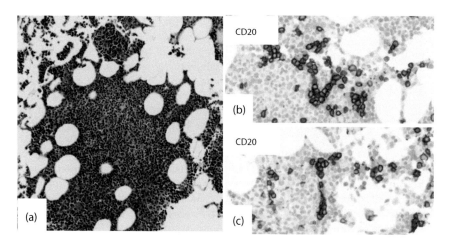

FIGURE 13.26   Bone marrow involvement by SMZL– nodular and intrasinusoidal pattern (a, H&E staining; b–c, CD20 staining).

patterns). Mixed intrasinusoidal/interstitial pattern is observed in 37%, predominantly nodular pattern combined with other types is observed in 28%, interstitial in 9%, diffuse in 6%, and pure intrasinusoidal pattern in 9% [148]. In contrast to FL or LPL, paratrabecular pattern is not typical for MZL involving BM but may be occasionally seen in SMZL. Lymphoid cells are small to medium-sized often with pale cytoplasm.

Immunophenotype

SMZL is positive for B-cell markers (CD19, CD20, CD22, CD79a), FMC7, CD24, BCL2, surface IgM (or less often IgD), and light chain immunoglobulins, and in most cases is negative for CD5, CD23, CD43, CD103 and CD123. DBA44 (CD76) may be expressed (60%) [148]. The expression of both surface light chain immunoglobulins, CD79b and CD20 is moderate when analyzed by FC. Majority of cases show non-specific phenotype without expression of CD5 or CD10, but minor subset of cases may be CD5+. Co-expression of CD5 and CD23 is rare in SMZL. CD10 is negative and most cases are negative for CD103. The expression of CD81 is usually positive and CD200 is also often positive (in contrast to MZL in other locations). Subset of cases may be positive for CD27, CD35, CD43, and surface IgD. SMZL show CD11c expression more often than non-splenic MZLs [149]. The expression of CD11c is positive in most cases and is either dim, dim to moderate or partial, and only rarely as bright as seen in HCL or HCL-v. CD5+ SMZLs show higher lymphocytosis, diffuse BM involvement, more frequently trisomy 3/3q, deletion 6q, and trisomy 18 without influence on prognosis [150–153]. They may be CD23+ (33%) and dimly CD38+ and are usually CD11c- and CD25- [152]. CD5+ SMZL may show discordant phenotypic profile between blood (FC) and spleen (immunohistochemistry). This may be due to variable sensitivity of the two methodologies and/or different epitopes of CD5 detected by FC and immunohistochemistry [98, 153]. Rare cases of SMZL may show aberrant expression of CD13, similarly to other low grade B-cell lymphoproliferations [150, 154, 155]. Ki-67 index is low (<10%). Rare cases of SMZL express CD103 [136, 156] or CD123. Some of the published data reported co-expression of CD103 and CD123 being 100% specific for HCL [157]. Figure 11.7 (Chapter 11) shows flow cytometric, cytogenetic, and morphologic features of SMZL involving the BM.

Genetic features

Trisomies of chromosomes 3 and 18, deletions at 6q23, deregulation of nuclear factor kappa B, and chromatin remodeling genes are frequent events in all 3 types of MZL (SMZL, MALT lymphoma, and NMZL), they differ in the presence of recurrent translocations, mutations affecting the NOTCH pathway, and the transcription factor Kruppel-like factor 2 (KLF2) or the receptor-type protein tyrosine phosphatase delta (PTPRD). There is no genetic abnormality specific for SMZL, but majority of cases show abnormal karyotype (~70%) [151]. The chromosomal abnormalities identified in SMZL include del (6q), del(7q32), del(10) (q22q24), del(17p), add(8)(q24), add(3q), add(5q), add(12p), add (9q), t(2;22), t(8;22), or trisomy 3 [145, 151, 158–161]. In the series reported by Hernandez et al. the most frequent gains involved 3q (31%), 5q (28%), 12q and 20q (24% each), 9q (21%), and 4q (17%), while losses were observed in 7q (14%) and 17p (10%) [162]. In the series reported by Vega et al., common chromosomal abnormalities included deletions involving 7q and 14q, and gains of 9p [161]. In series reported by Watkins et al., comparative genomic hybridization identified 7q32 deletion as the most frequent copy number change (44%), followed by gains of 3q (32%), 8q (12%), 9q34 (20%), 1p23-24 (8%), and chromosome 8 (12%), and losses of 6q (16%), 8p (12%), and 17p (8%) [163]. Complex chromosomal abnormalities have been reported in more than 50% of cases. They include gains of 3/3q (15%–32%), trisomy 18 (8%–12%), trisomy 12 (5%–20%), and deletion of 7q32 (21%–44%) [146, 164, 165]. Immunoglobulin gene translocations have been reported in 7%–21% of SMZL and include t((9;14)(p13;q32), t(3;14)(q27;q32), t(14;19)(q32;p13), t(14;19)(q32;q13), t(6;14)(p21;q32), and t(2;7) (p11;q21-22). Genotypic profile of SMZL is similar to NMZL. Mutations reported in SMZL include NOTCH1, NOTCH2, BIRC3, TNFAIP3, TRAF3, IKBKB, MYD88, CD79B, and CARD11. MYD88 mutations, characteristic of LPL occur in ~5% of SMZL.

Differential diagnosis of SMZL

Immunophenotypic (flow cytometric) differential diagnosis of splenic B-cell lymphomas is presented in Table 13.2.

Differential diagnosis of SMZL includes:

- MCL
- LPL
- SDRPL, SBLPN (HCL-v)
- HCL
- DLBCL
- Gamma heavy-chain disease (GHCD)
- CBL-MZ

HCL and SBLPN/HCL-v

HCL and SBLPN/HCL-v can be differentiated from SMZL by their diffuse pattern of infiltration, and more monomorphic appearance of lymphoid cells (SMZL often shows nodular pattern of splenic involvement with biphasic cytology). In contrast to SMZL, HCL and SBLPN/HCL-v are positive for CD103 and show bright expression of CD11c (most cases of SMZL are CD103 negative, but rare cases may be positive). In FC analysis, HCL is characterized by the strong expression of three markers: CD11c, CD25, and CD103. On genetic level, HCL is positive for BRAF mutation, which is not identified in SDRPL and SMZL. SBLPN/HCL-v shows bright CD11c and positive CD103, but in contrast to HCL is negative for CD25. The expression of CD11c is negative or dim (partial) in SMZL and the expression of CD81 is often brighter in SBLPN/HCL-v than in SMZL. There may be significant overlap in clinical and phenotypic features of SBLPN/HCL-v, SDRPL, and SMZL and differential diagnosis based on FC alone may be difficult. Peripheral blood smear in SBLPN/HCL-v show lymphocytosis of small to medium-sized cells with clumped chromatin, basophilic cytoplasm and characteristic broad-based villous projections and prominent nucleoli. The cytologic features of SMZL are heterogeneous with mixture of small to medium-sized lymphocytes with round nuclei and condensed chromatin and occasional cytoplasmic villi. The villi in SMZL are usually short and thin. Some of the cells may display plasmacytoid appearance. Mutational prolife of SMZL and HCL-v is different. SBLPN/HCL-v shows frequently mutation of MAP2K1 (50%) and none of the mutations found in SMZL. Figure 12.7 in Chapter 12 compares FC findings in SMZL and SBLPN/HCL-v.

Mantle cell lymphoma

The biphasic pattern of infiltration, typical for SMZL is not unique, as it can be sometimes seen in other low-grade lymphomas [166, 167]. The infiltrate of MCL is usually more monotonous than in SMZL and it stains for BCL1 (cyclin D1) and SOX11. By

TABLE 13.2: Differential Diagnosis of Splenic B-Cell Lymphomas

	SMZL	CLL	MCL	HCL	SBLPN/HCL-v	FL	LPL/WM	SDRPL
K and λ	+	+^{dim}/(−)	+	+	+	+/(−)	+	+
CD5	−/(+)	+	+/(−)	−	−	−	−/(+)	−/(+)
CD10	−	−	−/(+)	−/(+)	−/(+)	+	−/(+)	−
CD11c	+$^{dim/partial}$/−	+/−	−	+^{bright}	+^{bright}	−/(+)	−	+^{moderate}/(−)
CD20	+	+^{dim}/(−)	+	+	+	+	+	+
CD23	−/+	+/(−)	−/(+)	−/(+)	−/(+)	−/(+)	−/(+)	−
CD25	−/+	−/(+)	−	+^{moderate}	−	−/(+)	−/+	−
CD43	+/−	+	+	+/−	−/+^{dim}	−/(+)	−	−/(+)
CD81	+/(−)	−/+^{dim}	+^{moderate}	+^{dim}	+	+^{dim}/−	+/(−)	+/−
CD103	−/(+)	−	−	+	+/−	−	−	−/(+)
CD123	−/(+^{dim})	−	−/(+)	+^{bright}	−/(+)	−	−	−/(+)
CD200	+/(−)	+^{bright}	−	+^{bright}	+^{dim}	+^{dim}/−	+^{dim}/−	+
BCL1	−	−	+	+/−	−/(+)	−	−	−
SOX11	−	−	+	−	−	−	−	−
IgD	+/(−)	+	+	+	+	+/−	−	+/−
Monocytopenia	−	−	−	+	−	−	−	−
Spleen histology	White pulp expansion, biphasic pattern	White pulp involvement with spill to red pulp, diffuse small lymphocytic infiltrate with proliferation centers	White pulp involvement	Diffuse red pulp with atrophic white pulp, red blood cell lakes	Diffuse red pulp involvement, no white pulp follicles	Nodular pattern with white pulp involvement	White and red pulp involvement by small lymphocytes, plasmacytoid lymphocytes, and plasma cells	Diffuse red pulp involvement
Genetic changes	del(7q) *NOTCH2* and *KLF2* mutations	*IGHV* mutation +12, del(13q)	t(11;14) *CCND1* rearrangement	*BRAF* mutation	*MAP2K1* mutation	t(14;18) *BCL2* rearrangement	*MYD88* and *CXCR4* mutations	del(7q), +18

Abbreviations: κ/λ, surface light chain immunoglobulins; SMZL, splenic marginal zone lymphoma; CLL, chronic lymphocytic leukemia; MCL, mantle cell lymphoma; HCL, hairy cell leukemia; SBLPN/HCL-v (splenic B-cell lymphoma/leukemia with prominent nucleoli/hairy cell leukemia variant); FL, follicular lymphoma; DLBCL, diffuse large B-cell lymphoma; SDRPL, splenic diffuse red pulp B-cell lymphoma.

Notes: + positive; (+), rarely positive; −, negative; (−), rarely negative.

FC, MCL is characterized by expression of CD5 (most cases), lack of CD11c, positive CD38, negative CD23 and CD200, and strong expression of CD81. Rare cases of MCL may be CD5− or show co-expression of CD5 with CD10. MCL shows rearrangement of *CCND1* reflecting t(11;14).

Lymphoplasmacytic lymphoma

Cases of SMZL with prominent plasmacytic differentiation need to be differentiated from LPL/WM. LPL is morphologically heterogeneous and can be difficult to differentiate from MZL with plasmacytic differentiation. LPL shows white and red pulp involvement by small lymphocytes, lymphoplasmacytic cells and mature plasma cells. Follicles may be present and are often regressed. Typical for SMZL biphasic pattern or monocytoid features are not seen in LPL. The serum monoclonal protein is higher in LPL/WM than in SMZL (2.0 g/dL and 0.95 g/dL, respectively) [168]. In the BM, SMZL shows either nodular or more often intrasinusoidal pattern of involvement, whereas LPL/WM usually shows interstitial and/or paratrabecular pattern. Distinction between SMZL and LPL/WM in the BM may be difficult, because SMZL may also show plasmacytic differentiation, paratrabecular component and both entities show non-specific phenotype (CD5−/CD10−). Minor subset of LPL may be CD5+ or CD10+ (SMZL are rarely CD5 but do not show CD10 expression).

Presence of prominent paratrabecular pattern of infiltrate, high serum M protein levels, lymphoplasmacytoid cells with Dutcher bodies and *MYD88* and/or *CXCR4* mutation would indicate LPL/WM, while mostly intrasinusoidal pattern of BM involvement, deletion 7q, lack of *MYD88* or *CXCR4* mutations and low level of serum M protein would indicate SMZL.

Splenic diffuse red pulp small B-cell lymphoma (SDRPL)

SDRPL is characterized by predominantly red pulp involvement by a monomorphic population of small lymphocytes. The phenotype and cytology of SDRPL are similar to SMZL (CD5−, CD10−, BCL2+, CD23−, DBA44+/−, CD11c+/−, Annexin-A1−, and CD43−), although SMZL may be CD23+. Most cases of SDRPL are CD103−, but CD103 is more often positive in SDRPL than in SMZL. Some cases have reactive hyperplastic follicles in the white pulp isolated in the middle of a diffuse monomorphic infiltrate [166]. HCL-v, SDRPL, and SMZL are disorders with overlapping features; however, the prognosis is better in SMZL. Survival at 5-year is significantly worse in HCL-v (57%) compared with 84% in SMZL [144]. Differential diagnosis between SDRPL and SMZL may be difficult if based only on FC features. Morphologic examination of spleen in often essential in confirming the diagnosis of SDRPL with characteristic diffuse infiltration of the splenic red pulp, which contrast to the usual white pulp involvement and biphasic pattern by SMZL. In a series published by Traverse-Glehen, phenotypic feature favoring SMZL over SDRPL include aberrant expression of CD5 and/or CD23, positive CD38 and lack of CD103 and CD123 expression [169]. Baseggio et al. proposed to use scoring system based on the expression of CD11c, CD22, CD76, CD38, and CD27 to improve the differential diagnosis between SDRPL and SMZL [170]. In their series, SDRPL showed strong CD22 and strong CD11c expression, positive CD103 in 33%, positive CD25 in 3% and dimly positive CD123 in in 15% (no cases co-expressed CD123 and CD103) [170]. The expression of three markers (CD25, CD103, and CD123) was discriminatory between SDRPL and HCL, but not between SDRPL and SMZL. In the same series, the expression of CD11c was observed in 49%, 100%, and 100% of SMZL, SDRPL, and HCL, respectively [170]. In addition, the MFI of CD11c and CD22 helped in differential diagnosis between HCL, SDRPL, and SMZL: HCL showed the highest MFI of CD11c and CD22, and SMZL showed the lowest fluorescence intensity (SDRPL had intermediate values between those two diseases). Thus dim expression of CD11c is typical for SMZL, moderate expression for SDRPL and very bright expression for HCL [170].

Diffuse large B-cell lymphoma (DLBCL)
Since most of the disease-related deaths in SMZL are associated with HT to DLBCL, sample be carefully analyzed for the number of large lymphoid cells and patients have to be followed to exclude large cell transformation. HT into DLBCL occurs between 12 and 85 months after diagnosis of SMZL and most frequently involves peripheral lymph nodes [97].

Gamma heavy-chain disease (GHCD)
There is no specific histological pattern. Most frequently the infiltrate is pleomorphic lymphoplasmacytic proliferation mainly seen in BM and lymph nodes. Some cases present with a predominantly plasmacytic proliferation mimicking plasmacytoma or lymphocytosis of small mature lymphocytes mimicking CLL. GHCD may also involve blood showing mixture of small lymphocytes, plasmacytoid lymphocytes and plasma cells at various proportions. Occasional cases show presence of large cells (immunoblasts), histiocytes, and eosinophils. The most common site of extranodal involvement is the skin, although involvement of thyroid and parotid, oropharynx, and gastrointestinal tract has been reported. Immunofixation electrophoresis (IFE) helps to establish the diagnosis by revealing IgG without light chain.

Marginal zone lymphoma with blood and/or BM involvement

The recent World Health Organization (WHO) classification recognizes three subtypes of MZL: extranodal MZL of MALT, primary cutaneous MZL, pediatric MZL, SMZL, and NMZL. Those categories of MZLs may progress to blood and/or BM involvement. A minor subset of SMZL with leukemic blood involvement and "prolymphocytic" cytology is now classified as splenic B-cell lymphoma/leukemia with prominent nucleoli (SBLPN).

Morphology
Blood involvement is noted in up to 40% of MZL cases, most often in leukemic subtype (~100%), followed by SMZL (~50%), and less often in nodal variant of MZL (~10%) [140].

BM involvement is present in ~70% of the cases, less frequently in the nodal subtype (43% compared with 80%–100% in other subtypes) [140].

Flow cytometry
The phenotypic features are similar to NMZL or SMZL (see preceding texts).

Clonal B-cell lymphocytosis of marginal zone origin (CBL-MZ, monoclonal B-cell lymphocytosis with marginal zone-like phenotype, MBL-MZL-like)
MBL is defined by presence of low numbers (<5×10^9/L) of circulating monoclonal B-cells in otherwise healthy (asymptomatic) subjects (with no evidence of CLL/other lymphoproliferative disorders, adenopathy or organomegaly). Clonality is defined by either kappa restriction (κ:λ >3:1); lambda restriction (κ:λ <0.3:1) or >25% surface κ and λ negative B-cells. Some cases may be bi-clonal or tri-clonal. MBL may show (1) CLL-like phenotype (CD5+/CD23+), (2) atypical CLL-like phenotype (CD5+/CD23−), and (3) MZL-like phenotype (MZL-like) or non-CLL-like MBL (CD5−, CD10−), which is more recently designated as CBL-MZ. Clonal B-cell lymphocytosis of marginal zone type (CBL-MZ) is a recently described entity characterized by the presence of clonal B cells in the blood and/or BM with morphologic and immunophenotypic features consistent with marginal zone derivation in otherwise healthy individuals. CBL-MZ may be associated with IgM paraproteinemia raising the differential diagnosis with WM. CBL-MZ is very heterogeneous with mutations not associated with specific lymphoma subtype, including *MYD88* (14%–19%), *BIRC3* (11%), *CCND3* (11%), *NOTCH1* (11%), and *TNFAIP3* (11%), but often show some genetic changes overlapping with SMZL and SDRPL [5, 6]. Unlike CLL-like MBL which may precede the development of CLL, there is no defined cut-off in the clonal B-cell lymphocyte count for discriminating CBL-MZ from MZL. Only a minority (15%–20%) of patients will eventually progress to an overt lymphoma, most often MZL [171].

Splenic B-cell lymphoma/leukemia with prominent nucleoli/hairy cell leukemia variant (SBLPN/HCL-v)

SBLPN/HCL-v phenotype by FC: sIg+, CD5−/rarely+, CD10−/rarely+, CD11c+(moderate/bright), CD19+, CD20+, CD22+, CD23−, CD25−, CD38−, CD43−, CD45+, CD79b+(dim), CD81+(often strong), CD103+, CD123−/rarely+(dim), and CD200−/rarely+.

Introduction
SBLPN/HCL-v is a rare B-cell disorder which accounts for ~10% of HCL cases and presents with splenomegaly, leukocytosis (lymphocytosis) and cytopenias without monocytopenia (monocytopenia is typical for HCL) [1, 172–178]. Subset of patients has abdominal or retroperitoneal lymphadenopathy and 28% of patients have hepatomegaly [178]. SBLPN/HCL-v includes cases of B-cell chronic lymphoproliferative disorders that resemble classic HCL but exhibit variant clinical features (such as leukocytosis, presence of monocytes, cells with prominent nucleoli, cells with blastic or convoluted nuclei and/or absence of irregular cytoplasmic borders), variant immunophenotype (i.e., absence of CD25 expression, annexin A1, or TRAP), and resistance to conventional HCL therapy (i.e., lack of response to cladribine). SBLPN/HCL-v is not biologically related to HCL. SBLPN/HCL-v frequently involves spleen, BM, and blood. Middle-aged to elderly patients are affected with slight male predominance (median age

is 79 years; range, 50–89). Patients have indolent course with a long survival time. Treatment with Rituxan and anti-CD22 immunotoxin is highly effective. It shares some clinical and phenotypic features with SMZL (splenic lymphoma with villous lymphocytes) and SDRPL but not with classic HCL [179].

Morphology

Blood and bone marrow aspirate. Cytologically, the leukemic cells are predominantly medium- to large with abundant basophilic cytoplasm with villous projections, regular nuclear borders, and distinct nucleolus (minor subset of cases has inconspicuous nucleoli and rare case shows no nucleoli). The cytologic features are intermediate between HCL or SDRPL cells. Highly atypical nuclear features (e.g., blastoid appearance, clefted nuclei, and prominent nucleoli are seen in rare cases, mostly at the time of relapse [178]).

Bone marrow core biopsy. The pattern of BM involvement is more reminiscent of SMZL with mild infiltrate (predominantly intrasinusoidal or interstitial) and a good hematopoietic reserve [136]. Some cases show a mixture of intrasinusoidal and interstitial pattern and rarely nodular pattern or prominent diffuse infiltrate. Paratrabecular marrow involvement is not reported in SBLPN/HCL-v. In majority of cases there is no significant reticulin fibrosis, but many cases show focal reticulin fibrosis (diffuse reticulin fibrosis seen in HCL is rarely seen in SBLPN/HCL-v).

Spleen. In the spleen the infiltrate involves the red pulp with morphologic features overlapping with SDRPL and HCL. Similar to HCL, SBLPN/HCL-v involves red pulp and can form blood lakes.

Immunophenotype

The immunophenotype (Figure 13.27) shows a mature B-cell phenotype with expression of B-cell antigens (CD19, CD20, CD22, and CD79b), CD11c (100%), and CD103, but in contrast to classical HCL, the SBLPN/HCL-v cells are negative for CD25 and annexin-1 (some case may show faint partial CD25 expression, but never as strong as seen in HCL). The CD123 may be positive in SBLPN/HCL-v (usually dim), but majority of cases are negative. The expression of CD20, CD22, and surface light chain immunoglobulins (by FC) is bright. CD11c is usually moderate to bright. Majority of SBLPN/HCL-v cases are negative for CD43 and positive for CD79b. The expression of CD81 is positive (often strong but may be dim) and CD200 is variable, and may be negative.

Genetic features

MAP2K1 gene mutations are observed in one-third of cases.

Differential diagnosis of SBLPN/HCL-v

Differential diagnosis includes:

- SMZL
- SDRPL
- HCL
- Other low-grade B-cell lymphomas.

HCL and SBLPN/HCL-v rarely show abnormal karyotype (e.g., del17p, +12), whereas SMZL has abnormal karyotype in 80% (+3, +18, del7q) and SDRPL in ~30% (+3, del7q). It is suggested that SMZL, SBLPN/HCL-v, and SDRPL may represent overlapping entities. In contrast to HCL, SBLPN/HCL-v is negative for V600E *BRAF* mutations [180–183]. When analyzed by FC, HCL shows bright expression of CD20, CD22, CD11c, and CD123, often positive CD43 and CD79b, dim expression of CD81 and is always strongly positive for CD25. In series reported by Salem et al., the

expression of both CD43 and CD81 tended to show an inverse pattern when comparing HCL (CD43+, CD81dim+) with SBLPN/ HCL-v (CD43dim+, CD81bright+) [175]. When compared to HCL, SBLPN/HCL-v is negative for CD25, usually negative or dim for CD43, negative or dimly positive for CD123, and shows brighter expression of CD81. CD200 is dimmer in SBLPN/HCL-v than in HCL. Also, aberrant expression of CD10 is seen more often in HCL than in SBLPN/HCL-v. CD11c in SMZL is either negative or dim to partially positive and in SDRPL is most often moderate. SMZL are most often negative for CD103 and CD123 by FC, although dim or partial CD103 or CD123 may be occasionally seen. Differential diagnosis between SBLPN/HCL-v, SMZL, and SDRPL may be difficult because of the overlapping morphologic, genetic, and immunophenotypic features. In contrast to SMZL and SDRPL, SBLPN/HCL-v are strongly positive for CD103 by FC and often show bright (or moderate to bright) CD11c expression (Figure 12.7 in Chapter 7). The expression of CD200 is usually dim or negative in HCL-v and moderate in SMZL (other MZLs usually show negative or dim CD200). The definite diagnosis between SBLPN/HCL-v, SDRPL and SMZL may require a comprehensive immunophenotyping and spleen histology for final diagnosis. Presence of MAP2K1 mutation would support the diagnosis of SBLPN/HCL-v. The chromosomal abnormalities described in SDRPL are similar to those described in SMZL (7q deletion, partial trisomy 3q, and complete trisomy 18) [136].

Hairy cell leukemia (HCL)

HCL phenotype by FC: sIg+, CD5−, CD10−/rarely+, CD11c+(bright), CD19+, CD20+, CD22+bright, CD23−/rarely+, CD25+, CD38−, CD43+/−, CD45+, CD79b+(moderate), CD81+(dim), CD123+(bright), and CD200+bright.

Introduction

HCL is an indolent chronic B-cell lymphoproliferative disorder of mature lymphocytes with abundant cytoplasm with "hairy" projections, characterized by diffuse BM involvement, splenic red pulp involvement, monocytopenia, and pancytopenia (or less often anemia and neutropenia) [1, 177, 180, 181, 183–195]. *BRAF* V600E mutation, detected in ~90% of the cases, is described as a driver mutation [177, 180, 181, 183, 196–198]. A variant lacking CD25, annexin A1, TRAP, and the *BRAF* V600E mutation, called SBLPN/HCL-v, is more aggressive and is classified as a separate disease [1]. HCL affects predominantly middle-aged and elderly men (males to females ratio is between 4:1 and 5:1; median age at diagnosis is 55–60 years) and comprises ~2%–3% of all adult leukemias in the United States [189, 199]. Patients present with symptoms of anemia, infections and/or abdominal discomfort related to splenomegaly. Splenomegaly, hepatomegaly and intra-abdominal adenopathy are present in 60%–70%, 40%–50%, and 15%–20% of patients, respectively [172]. Leukemic cells have characteristic cytomorphology (hairy-like cytoplasmic protrusions) and immunophenotype (CD11c+bright/CD25+/CD103+). Factors associated with worse prognosis include high WBC count, low hemoglobin levels, and prominent splenomegaly.

Morphology

HCL involves predominantly the BM and spleen and presents with leukopenia and monocytopenia. HCL may infiltrate skin, liver, and less often lymph nodes.

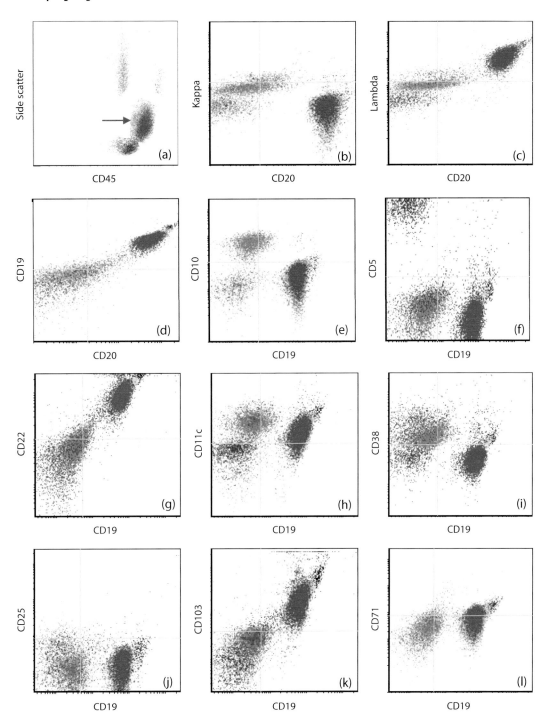

FIGURE 13.27 SBLPN/HCL-v. Leukemic cells (magenta dots, arrow) are characterized by bright CD45 and increased side scatter (a), bright CD20 (b–d), bright surface light chain immunoglobulin expression (b–c), moderate CD19 (d), negative CD10 (e), negative CD5 (f), moderate CD22 (g), moderate CD11c (h), negative CD38 (i), negative CD25 (j), positive CD103 (k), and negative to partially dim CD71 (l).

Blood and bone marrow aspirate. Neoplastic cells are medium-sized (slightly larger than small lymphocytes) with pale cytoplasm with characteristic villous cytoplasmic projections (Figure 13.28). The nuclei are oval and often reniform or bean-shaped central nuclei and clumped (granular) or evenly dispersed chromatin, inconspicuous nucleoli, and smooth nuclear membrane. Occasional cases of HCL may display unusual cytology, including blastoid features or highly irregular nuclei.

Bone marrow core biopsy. In the BM, the leukemic infiltrate is always interstitial or diffuse, rather monotonous without formation of well-defined aggregates and is accompanied by reticulin fibrosis (Figure 13.29). In some cases, BM is hypocellular with subtle infiltrate which can be best visualized with CD20 immunostaining. The most common pattern is an interstitial infiltrate, which tends to preserve the marrow adipose tissue. HCL infiltrate may induce an extravasation of red blood cells (similar to

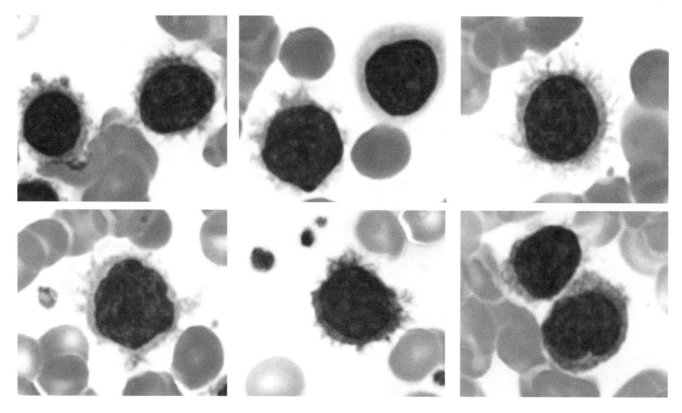

FIGURE 13.28   Hairy cell leukemia – cytology (blood smear of several cases of HCL).

pattern observed in spleen), with creation of blood lakes. The neo-plastic cells have abundant pale cytoplasm with distinct borders and central nucleus, giving rise to so-called fried-egg or honey-comb appearance. The HCL infiltrate is often, especially in early phase of the disease, due to widely spaced small lymphoid cells with pale cytoplasm which blend into residual normal marrow element making their identification difficult on H&E sections. Immunohistochemical staining with CD20 helps to identify leu-kemic cells and establish the degree of BM involvement, which often is underestimated on H&E examination alone.

Lymph node. Involvement of the lymph nodes by HCL is uncom-mon and is most often observed in abdominal and retroperitoneal areas, and only sporadically in peripheral lymph node. Lymph node infiltration is predominantly paracortical with sparing of

follicles (Figure 13.30). Sinuses are typically intact. The infiltrate may extend into surrounding adipose tissue. The leukemic cells are medium sized with pale cytoplasm and irregular nuclei.

Spleen. The splenic histology of HCL is very distinctive. Spleen shows atrophic white pulp and prominent red pulp infiltration by a uniform population of cytologically monotonous mononuclear cells that expanded the red pulp cords, with formation of typical blood lakes consisting of hemorrhage surrounded by hairy cells with clear cytoplasm [98].

Immunophenotype

HCL has characteristic immunophenotype. FC analysis of blood or BM shows lymphoid cells with increased side scatter (SSC) and bright CD45 expression, placing leukemic cells in the "monocytic"

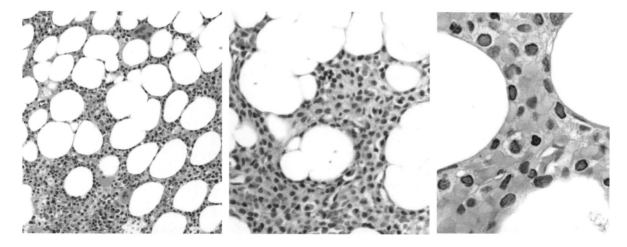

FIGURE 13.29   HCL – histology (BM): interstitial infiltrate (low, intermediate and high magnification).

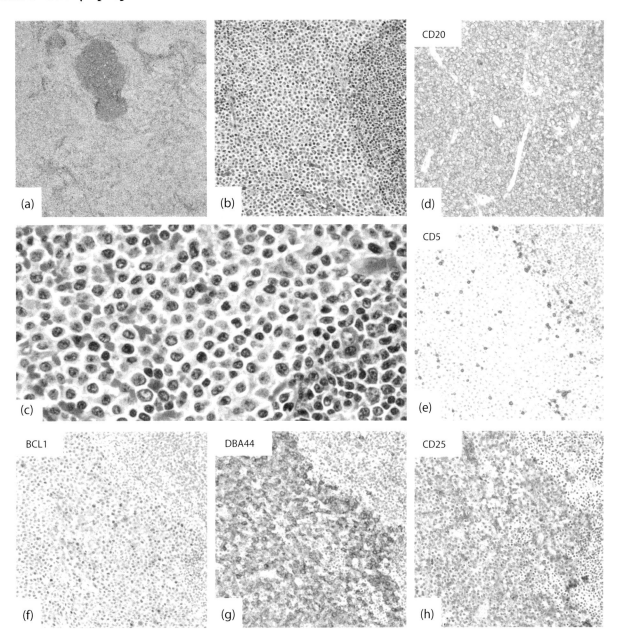

FIGURE 13.30 Hairy cell leukemia – lymph node. (a) Low magnification shows prominent perifollicular/paracortical infiltrate. (b–c) Higher magnification shows atypical lymphoid cells with moderate amount of pale cytoplasm and irregular nuclei. Hairy cell leukemia cells are positive for CD20 (d), negative for CD5 (e) and positive for bcl-1 (f), DBA44 (g), and CD25 (h).

region on CD45 versus SSC, bright expression of CD11c, CD19, CD20, CD22, CD43, CD76, CD200, and surface immunoglobulins (kappa or lambda), positive CD25, CD81 (dim), CD103, and CD123 (Figures 13.31 and 13.32). Hairy cells are usually negative for CD5, CD10, CD23, CD27, and CD38. The expression of both CD11c and CD22 is much brighter in HCL than in SBLPN/HCL-v, SMZL, or SDRPL. Occasional cases of HCL may be CD5+ (Figure 13.33), CD10+ (Figure 13.34), surface light chain immunoglobulin negative (Figure 13.35) or show aberrant expression of CD2 (Figure 13.35). Majority of HCL cases are positive for CD43 (dim), CD79b, CD81 (dim expression), and CD200 (bright expression). By immunohistochemistry analysis HCL often show positive expression of Annexin A1 (staining may be suboptimal in decalcified core biopsy) and BCL1 (without *CCND1* rearrangement). The expression of CD200

is often brighter in HCL than in SBLPN/HCL-v, and the expression of CD81 is dimmer in HCL than in HCL-v [175].

Measurable (minimal) residual disease (MRD)

MRD is defined as identification of persistent HCL after treatment using immunophenotypic analysis, immunohistochemistry staining, or DNA PCR in the absence of disease detectable by morphologic criteria. Multicolor FC (e.g., CD11c, CD25, CD103, CD123, and CD20) is highly sensitive and specific for detecting low levels of hairy cell in either blood or BM (detection limit estimated at 0.003%–0.05%) [200]. Down regulation of cyclin D1 and CD25 has been reported in patients following *BRAF* inhibitor therapy and assessment of these antigens should not be used in this context when evaluating for MRD.

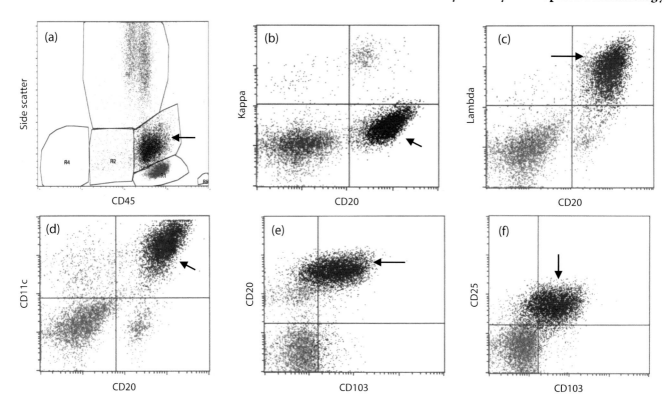

FIGURE 13.31 Hairy cell leukemia – flow cytometry (FC). delete this part FC analysis shows increased orthogonal side scatter (a; SSC, arrow), which places the cells in the "monocytic region", above normal lymphocytes (red dots). HCL cells show moderate to bright expression of CD20 (b–e), surface immunoglobulin (lambda, c), bright expression of CD11c (d), and co-expression of CD25 and CD103 (e–f).

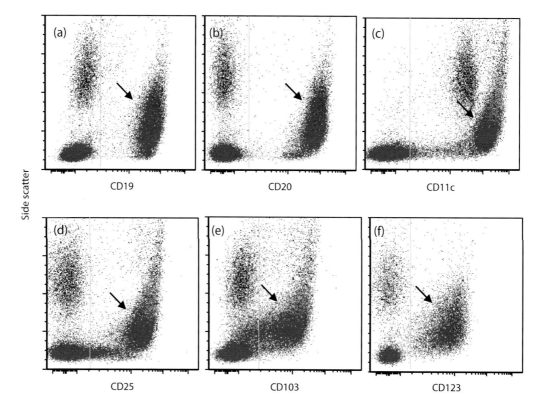

FIGURE 13.32 HCL – flow cytometry analysis (blood). HCL cells (arrow) are strongly positive for CD19 (a), CD20 (b), CD11c (c), CD25 (d), CD103 (e), and CD123 (f).

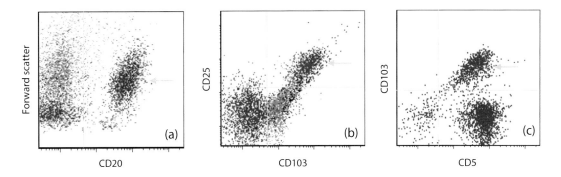

FIGURE 13.33 HCL with aberrant expression of CD5. FC analysis shows show bright CD20⁺ HCL cells (a, arrow) with co-expression of CD25 and CD103 (b) and aberrant expression of CD5 (c; gated on lymphocytes only).

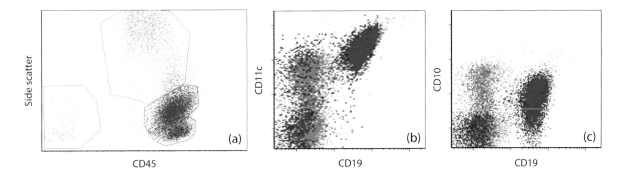

FIGURE 13.34 HCL with aberrant expression of CD10. FC analysis of BM shows leukemic cells with bright CD45 and increased side scatter (a, blue dots), kappa restriction (b–c), bright CD10 expression (d).

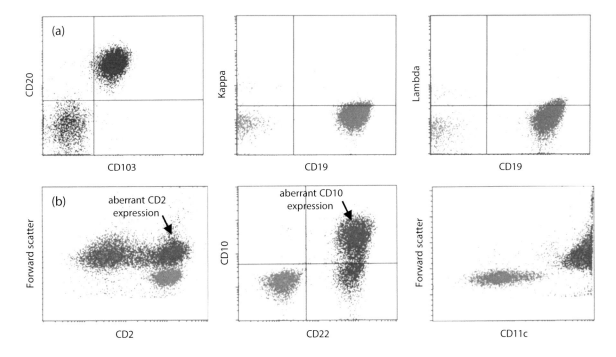

FIGURE 13.35 Hairy cell leukemia (HCL) with no detectable surface immunoglobulins (a) and HCL with aberrant (partial) CD2 expression and aberrant CD10 expression (b).

Genetic features

Cytogenetics studies in HCL are rare. HCL usually have mutated *IGVH* genes and have no consistent or specific chromosome abnormalities. Clonal chromosomal aberrations are reported in 25%–44% of patients and include +1p, +5q13-q31 (~20%), del(7q22-q35) (~6%), +12, chromosome 14 abnormalities, complex abnormalities (including chromosomes 1, 6, 7, 8, and 17), del(17)(q25), and t(11;20)(q13;q11) [201–208]. Deletion of *p53/TP53* has also been reported [202]. *BRAF* V600E mutations are a genetic hallmark of HCL. It can be detected in 80%–90% of cases. This specific point mutation is exceedingly rare in other peripheral B-cell neoplasms [180–182, 209]. In *BRAF*+ HCL cases, other mutations can be found in 33% (*KLF2, CDKN1B, NOTCH1, ARID1B,* and *CREBBP*) [174]. Absence of the BRAF gene mutation is reported in up to 10%–20% of patients with HCL and could constitute a subgroup of HCL patients with a poor prognosis. In those patients, the possibility of a mutation in exon 11 (F468C, D449E) should be excluded [198].

Differential diagnosis of HCL

Based on FC, differential diagnosis of HCL includes:

- SBLPN/HCL-v
- MZL
- SMZL
- Chronic lymphocytic leukemia/small lymphocytic lymphoma (CLL/SLL)
- B-PLL
- T-cell prolymphocytic leukemia (T-PLL)
- SDRPL
- FL in leukemic phase
- MCL

Based on CD103 expression, differential diagnosis of HCL includes:

- Enteropathy-associated T-cell lymphoma (EATL)
- Monomorphic epitheliotropic intestinal T-cell lymphoma (MEITL)
- SMZL
- SBLPN/HCL-v
- SDRPL

Based on cytology (blood smear), differential diagnosis of HCL includes:

- SBLPN/HCL-v
- SDRPL
- SMZL
- B-PLL
- T-PLL
- FL
- MCL
- CLL

SBLPN/HCL-v

Lymphocytes of SBLPN/HCL-v have centrally located nucleus with usually prominent nucleolus, abundant cytoplasm with homogeneously distributed hairy projections. In contrast to HCL, cells from SBLPN/HCL-v tend to be more irregular and may have more prominent nucleoli. Unlike HCL, there is no monocytopenia in SBLPN/HCL-v. By FC analysis, SBLPN/HCL-v differs from HCL by lack of CD25 expression and on molecular level by lack of *BRAF*

mutation. Phenotypically, SBLPN/HCL-v similarly to HCL shows bright expression of CD20 and CD22, positive (often bright) CD11c, and positive CD103, but in contrast to HCL lacks CD25 expression. The expression of CD123 in SBLPN/HCL-v is dim (40%) or negative (60%), whereas in HCL is brightly positive and homogenous [176]. Both HCL and SBLPN/HCL-v may show aberrant expression of CD5 (2% and 3%), CD2 (2% and 9%), CD13 (0.5% and 3%), and CD10 (12%–14% and 3%). The analysis of the expression of CD43, CD79b, and CD81 also helps in differential diagnosis between HCL and SBLPN/HCL-v. HCL is characterized by variable CD43, dimmer CD81, and positive CD79b, whereas SBLPN/HCL-v lacks CD43 expression (or is dimly positive), has brighter CD81, and dim CD79b [175]. The expression of CD200 is brighter in HCL and variable (often dim) in SBLPN/HCL-v. Non HCL B-cell lymphoproliferations, including HCL-v are invariably negative for *BRAF*-V600E. The intensity of expression of CD43 and CD200 is higher in HCL when compared to SBLPN/HCL-v, while intensity of CD81 is lower in HCL than in SBLPN/HCL-v [175]. Figure 13.36 compares flow cytometric features between HCL, SMZL, and SBLPN/HCL-v.

SMZL

The cytologic appearance of SMZL (or splenic lymphoma with villous lymphocytes) in blood varies from small mantle-zone-like lymphocytes, marginal-zone cells, villous lymphocytes, or more pleomorphic pattern with scattered larger (blastoid) forms. The hallmark of SMZL is the presence of medium sized cells with irregularly distributed short membrane villi. Villi distribution, as well as the nuclear characteristics of chromatin and nucleolus are distinct from those of HCL cells. The SMZL cells are usually larger than the lymphocytes found in CLL, with diameters comparable with those of prolymphocytes. A minor subset of SMZL with leukemic blood involvement and "prolymphocytic" cytology is classified as SBLPN. The nuclei are round or ovoid, sometimes eccentric, with a clumped chromatin pattern, and in half the cases 40%–90% of these lymphocytes showed a single prominent nucleolus, sometimes surrounded by heterochromatin, or associated with the nuclear membrane, or both, as is usually seen in prolymphocytes [210]. In most SMZL cases there is 3% and 12% of plasmacytoid cells, which are characterized by a more pronounced cytoplasmic basophilia, and a clear perinuclear zone corresponding to the Golgi apparatus [210]. In HCL and SBLPN/HCL-v hairy projections are homogeneously distributed which contrasts with the preferential polar localization of short and thin villi, or of the few, long, broad based projections characteristic of SMZL lymphocytes [211].

Rare cases of SMZL may be CD103+. Both HCL and SMZL are strongly positive for B-cell markers and usually do not express CD5 or CD10 (rare cases of HCL may be CD10+ or CD5+ and minor subset of SMZL may show aberrant expression of CD5). Majority of SMZLs are CD25−. The expression of CD11c and CD22 is very bright in HCL and the expression of CD22 in SMZL is moderate and expression of CD11c is negative or dim. Positive CD25, bright CD11c, positive CD103, bright CD22, positive CD123 and lack of CD38 are typical for HCL, while negative or dim CD11c, moderate CD22, positive CD38 and lack of CD103 and CD123 are typical for SMZL [170]. Minor subset of SMZL cases may be CD103+ and subset of cases may be CD38−. Figure 13.36 compares flow cytometric features between HCL, SMZL, and SBLPN/HCL-v.

SDRPL

The phenotype and cytology of SDRPL are similar to SMZL (CD5−, CD10−, BCL2+, CD23−, DBA44+/−, CD11c+/−, Annexin-A1−, and CD43−), although SMZL may be CD23+. Subset of SDRPL is

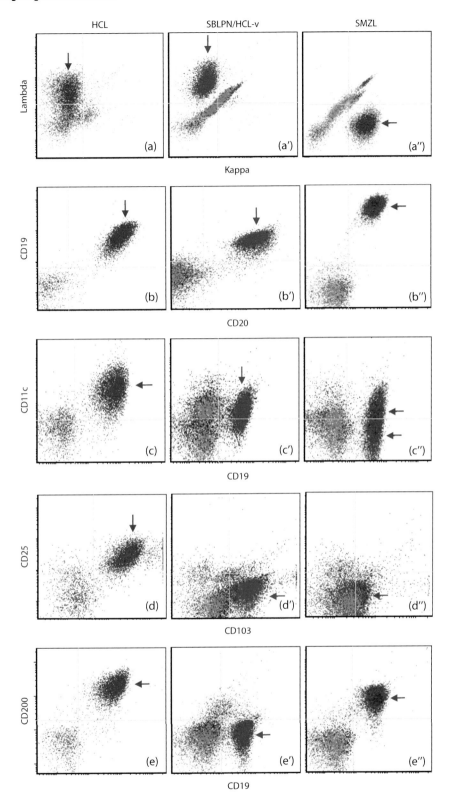

FIGURE 13.36 Comparison of flow cytometry characteristics of HCL (left column, red dots), HCL-v (middle column, blue dots), and SMZL (right column, red dots). All three disorders show moderate expression of surface light chain immunoglobulins (a–a″) and moderate to bright expression of CD19 and CD20 (b–b″). HCL is characterized by bright expression of CD11c (c), while the expression of CD11c in SBLPN/HCL-v is moderate (c′) and negative to partially dim in SMZL (c″). HCL and SBLPN/HCL-v are positive for CD103 (d–d′) and SMZL shows negative to minimally dimly positive CD103 (d″). CD25 expression is positive only in HCL (d). SBLPN/HCL-v are always CD25⁻ (d′), while SMZL are either negative (d″) or positive (not shown). CD200 is strongly expressed in HCL (e) and is negative in SBLPN/HCL-v (e′). The expression of CD200 in MZLs are usually negative or dimly positive, but SMZL often shows moderate CD200 (e″).

CD103+, but expression of CD25 and CD123 is only rarely present. The expression of CD11c and CD22 are dimmer in SDRPL than in HCL [170]. Rare cases of SDRPL may be CD38+, while HCL is CD38-.

EATL and MEITL

EATL and MEITL display aberrant expression of CD103+. Analysis of B- and T-cell markers helps to differentiate T-cell lymphoproliferations from HCL.

B-cell prolymphocytic leukemia (B-PLL). B-PLL is a rare malignancy usually involving blood, BM, and spleen, characterized by marked lymphocytosis with lymphoid cells characterized by prominent nucleoli. B-PLL shows strong expression of B-cells markers by FC, usually negative CD5 and CD23, and differs from HCL by lack of CD103 expression. *BRAF* mutations, typical for HCL, have been reported in sporadic cases of CLL, but not in B-PLL.

Leukemic mantle cell lymphoma (MCL). Occasional cases of MCL may present with lymphocytosis in blood, mimicking either CLL or B-PLL. L-NN-MCL characteristically involves BM, peripheral blood, and spleen, and is composed often of small round lymphocytes (similar to CLL) [1, 212–215]. It follows a rather indolent course with a wait and watch approach [1]. Phenotypically, L-NN-MCL variant is more often CD5-, SOX11-, and/or CD200+, when compared to classic MCL [212–215]. MCL is characterized by irregular (indented) nuclei, co-expression of CD5 (without CD23) and presence of *CCND1* rearrangement by FISH [corresponding to t(11;14) by metaphase cytogenetics].

T-cell prolymphocytic leukemia (T-PLL). The leukemic cells from T-PLL are medium sized with either round (oval), or very irregular nuclei (somewhat reminiscent of Sézary's cells). They have single prominent nucleolus and basophilic cytoplasm. Immunophenotyping by FC shows expression of pan-T cell markers (CD2, CD4, CD5, and CD7). Majority of cases are CD4+ (most often) but CD8+ and dual CD4+/CD8+ or dual CD4-/CD8- expression may occur. CD25 is variably expressed, but there is no expression of B-cell markers.

CLL. CLL is characterized by rather monotonous small mature lymphoid cells with round nuclei with condensed chromatin, scant cytoplasm, and variable proportion of prolymphocytes. By FC immunophenotyping they show co-expression of CD5 and CD23 and are negative for CD103. The expression of CD11c is either dim, negative, or partial and never as bright as seen in HCL.

Splenic diffuse red pulp small B-cell lymphoma (SDRPL)

> SDRPL phenotype by FC: sIg+, CD5-/rarely+, CD10-, CD11c-/+, CD19+, CD20+, CD22+, CD23-/rarely+, CD25-, CD38-, CD43+(dim)/-, CD45+, CD79b+(moderate), CD81+/-, CD103-/rarely+, CD123-/rarely+, and CD200+.

Introduction

SDRPL is an uncommon lymphoma with diffuse pattern of involvement of the splenic red pulp, BM sinusoids and peripheral blood by small monomorphous basophilic B lymphocytes often with villous cytoplasm [1, 134, 148, 216–219]. It is currently a provisional WHO entity included within the group of splenic B-cell lymphoma/leukemia, unclassifiable (together with HCL-v) [1]. All cases are diagnosed at advanced stage with spleen, BM, and blood involvement [218]. Rare cases with skin involvement have

been reported. Clinical findings (splenomegaly, lymphocytosis without pancytopenia) are reminiscent of SMZL and HCL-v [148, 169, 220]. Men are affected more often than women. The most frequent chromosomal changes include chromosome 7q deletion, complete trisomy 18, and partial trisomy 3q [169]. This is indolent but incurable disease with good response after splenectomy. Complication in the form of transformation to B-PLL in patients with SDRPL has been reported [70, 221]. Diagnosis of SDRPL relies mostly on immunophenotyping, morphologic analysis of spleen and BM, and exclusion of other lymphoma types.

Morphology

Blood. Blood smear shows a homogeneous infiltrate of small to medium sized cells with round or oval nuclei, sometimes eccentrically placed, and dense and clumped chromatin, basophilic with characteristic broad based, unevenly distributed cytoplasmic expansions (villous projections) [218]. Only rare cases may display prominent nucleoli. Many cases may show pale or eosinophilic cytoplasm with plasmacytoid features.

Spleen. Spleen shows diffuse involvement of the red pulp, with both cord and sinusoid infiltration and characteristic intrasinusoidal aggregates (pattern similar to HCL and SBLPN/HCL-v). White pulp is most often also replaced or atrophic and shows only occasional residual follicles. Some lymphoplasmacytoid cells can be observed on blood smear or in the spleen.

Bone marrow. BM aspirate shows small lymphocytes with villous processes (similar to those seen in blood smear). BM core biopsy infiltrate is often subtle on H&E sections. It shows characteristic intrasinusoidal involvement, which occasionally can be accompanied by interstitial or nodular infiltration. No paratrabecular pattern has been reported. Reticulin fibrosis is minimal. Presence of a significant percentage of medium to large cells with a prominent nucleolus suggests progression (transformation).

Immunophenotype

Flow cytometry. Neoplastic B-cells are positive for CD19, CD20 (strong expression), CD22 (strong expression) and are negative for CD5, CD10, and CD25. Occasional cases may show partial and dim expression of CD43 or CD103 [170]. CD103 and CD123 are positive in subset of cases (~40% and ~15%, respectively). Only sporadic cases have been reported to be CD25+. FC analysis shows occasional expression of CD5 or CD23 (without co-expression) [218]. CD200 is positive. There is no consensus about CD11c expression in SDRPL. Some series reported moderate CD11c expression, whereas other noted lack of CD11c [1, 169, 217]. Baseggio et al. proposed a scoring system using the intensity of expression of CD11c, CD22, CD38, and CD27 to better differentiate between SDRPL and SMZL [170]. In that series, SDRPL cases showed strong expression of CD22 (100%), strong expression of CD11c (97%), and occasional expression of CD103 (33%) or CD123 (15%). No cases co-expressed CD103 with CD123, and only rare cases were positive for CD38 (3%), while CD27 was positive in 20%.

Immunohistochemistry. Lymphoma cells in SDRPL express B-cell markers (CD19, CD20, CD22, CD79a, PAX5), BCL2, and DBA44, and are negative for CD5, CD10, CD23, CD43, BCL1 (cyclin D1), BCL6, MUM1, and annexin-A1 [148, 217, 218].

Genetic features

SDRPL shows del 7(q), partial trisomy 3q, trisomy 18, and del17p [169]. It does not have *BRAF V600E* mutation, but may show *NOTCH1, NOTCH2, TP53, MAPK1, CCND3,* or rarely *MYD88* mutations.

Differential diagnosis of SDRPL

- CLL
- SMZL
- HCL
- LPL/WM
- SBLPN/HCL-v
- B-PLL

CLL

CLL has characteristic FC pattern with dim expression of surface light immunoglobulins, dim CD20 (maybe negative or partial), co-expression of CD5 and CD23, positive CD200, and negative CD81. The infiltrate is composed of small mature round lymphocytes with scanty cytoplasm with typical proliferation centers containing increased number of prolymphocytes or paraimmunoblasts. In contrast to red pulp involvement by SDRPL, CLL is mainly limited to white pulp involvement.

SMZL

The circulating cell morphology and the pattern of spleen involvement are clearly distinct. The villous expansions of SDRPL are distinct from the short and thin cytoplasmic expansions of the villous cells usually observed in SMZL. The spleen histology is also distinct: SMZL involves mostly white pulp and shows follicular replacement, biphasic cytology, and marginal zone infiltration, whereas SDRPL involves red pulp without marginal zone expansion or biphasic features. The immunophenotype by FC shows occasional expression of CD103 and absence of expression of CD24, CD38, and CD27 in SDRPL [170]. Majority of SMZL cases are CD103−, whereas SDRPL may be positive in up to 33%. The expression of CD11c is not always helpful in differential diagnosis between those two entities, but often shows moderate expression of CD11c while SMZL is either negative or dimly positive for CD11c. In case when the distinction between SMZL and SDRPL is difficult, WHO classification recommended to diagnose splenic B-cell lymphoma/leukemia, unclassifiable.

HCL

SDRPL shares with HCL some common features, such as the male predominance, the massive congested red pulp pattern with sometimes blood lakes, the rarity of clonal chromosomal abnormalities, the expression of classical HCL markers (i.e., CD11c, CD103, and CD123). However, unlike SDRPL, HCL affects younger patients and can be distinguished by presence of severe pancytopenia, including monocytopenia, BM fibrosis, cytomorphology, and immunophenotypic profile. The cytoplasmic expansions in SDRPL are shorter and larger with a less abundant and more basophilic cytoplasm and a polar distribution around the cell contrasting with the circumferential distribution observed in hairy cells [218]. The chromatin pattern, in peripheral blood and spleen, is quite distinct in most cases, and the cytoplasm presents straight boundaries. The large blood lakes are inconstant and less extensive. The intensity of expression of CD11c, CD103, and CD123 are much lower in SDRPL than in HCL. Annexin-A1, CD25, and BCL1 typically detected by immunohistochemistry in HCL are absent in SDRPL. BM infiltration in SDRPL displays neither massive fibrosis, nor diffuse interstitial infiltration and granulocytic hypoplasia, characteristic of HCL. Analysis for *BRAF* mutation could help in the differential diagnosis and needs to be analyzed in borderline cases, as its presence would indicate HCL [180, 222].

SBLPN/HCL-v

SDRPL and SBLPN/HCL-v have a very similar clinicopathological presentation and the differential diagnosis is not easy [169, 173]. Peripheral blood smears are distinct from SMZL and HCL, but close to SDRPL, showing a homogeneous infiltrate of small to medium sized cells with clumped chromatin, basophilic cytoplasm, and characteristic broad-based villous projections, with an uneven distribution in a high proportion of cells. However, the nucleolus described as small or not visible in SDRPL is prominent in SBLPN/HCL-v. The spleen section shows a monomorphic diffuse infiltrate, predominant in the congestive red pulp with atrophic white pulp [218]. Small blood lakes can be observed. The BM infiltrate shows a variable cellularity and mild fibrosis with predominantly intrasinusoidal lymphoid infiltrate, which can be accompanied by interstitial or nodular infiltration. The immunophenotype is distinct from SMZL and HCL with moderate to bright expression of CD11c and CD22, low expression of CD103, but absence of CD25 and Annexin-1 expression in SBLPN/HCL-v [218].

LPL/WM

Due to frequent "plasmacytoid" appearance of lymphomatous cells, SDRPL may be confused with LPL/WM. SDRPL is not associated with presence of serum paraprotein or polymorphous composition of cells ranging from small lymphocytes, plasmacytoid cells with basophilic cytoplasm to mature plasma cells typical for LPL/WM. In contrast to LPL/WM, CD38 is only rarely seen in SDRPL. Presence of significant serum monoclonal protein (M protein), monotypic plasma cells by immunohistochemistry or FC analysis, paratrabecular pattern of BM involvement, and *MYD88* mutation help to confirm the diagnosis of LPL/WM.

SBLPN

Presence of prominent nucleoli or development of prolymphocytic transformation reported in rare cases of SDRPL prompt differential diagnosis with SBLPN. In contrast to SBLPN, most cases of SDRPL present without blood lymphocytosis, and show characteristic villous projections.

Lymphoplasmacytic lymphoma (LPL)

LPL phenotype by FC: sIg+, CD5−/rarely+, CD10−/rarely+, CD11c−, CD19+, CD20+, CD22+, CD23−/rarely+, CD25+/(−), CD38+/rarely−, CD43−, CD45+, CD79b−, CD81+(dim)/rarely−, CD103−, CD123−, and CD200+dim/−. Clonal B-cells are often accompanied by clonal CD19+/CD45+/CD56−/IgM+ plasma cells.

Introduction

Definition. LPL is defined as a low grade B-cell neoplasm composed of a mixture of small lymphocytes, lymphocytes with plasmacytoid features and plasma cells, which does not fulfill the criteria for any of the other small B-cell lymphoid neoplasm [1, 223–229]. The proportion of these three elements is variable and one cell type can be predominant. In over 95% of LPL cases, the malignant clone produces an IgM paraprotein consistent with WM. However, in the remaining LPL cases, the malignant clone can produce IgG or IgA, light chains alone, or be nonsecretory. WM represents most LPL cases, whereas LPL of non-WM type is rare and mainly composed of cases without BM involvement and/or absence of IgM protein.

Clinical features. LPL/WM occurs most frequently in adult Caucasian patients with a median age in the seventh decade and is less common in Asian and African American populations. LPL most commonly involves BM and blood whereas lymph node and spleen are only involved in subset of patients. Monoclonal paraprotein (usually IgM) is often present but is not required for the diagnosis of LPL. In most patients, adenopathy develops slowly over many years. Extramedullary sites may be involved as well, although most of these cases represent MZL with plasmacytic differentiation. The most common extramedullary sites include lymph nodes, soft tissue, spleen, skin, lung, tonsil, gastrointestinal (GI) tract, and liver [230]. IgM gammopathies may lead to hyperviscosity, BM replacement by LPL infiltrate, cold agglutinin disease, amyloid deposition, cryoglobulinemia or coagulopathy, neuropathy, renal damage, cutaneous infiltrates/Schnitzler's syndrome, leukemic blood involvement, or organomegaly. Some patients have more lymphomatous manifestation with adenopathy or extranodal infiltrates.

Pathogenesis The identification of *MYD88* L265P gene mutation has been a major advance in the diagnosis of patients with LPL/WM [228, 231, 232]. *MYD88* can be mutated also in subset of cases of non-IgM LPL. Patients with IgM monoclonal gammopathy of uncertain significance (MGUS) have a greater than 200-fold increased risk of developing WM. Therefore, IgM MGUS is considered a precursor of WM. Progression from IgM MGUS to smoldering WM followed by overt WM has been reported.

Waldenström macroglobulinemia. WM is currently defined as LPL with BM involvement and an IgM monoclonal paraprotein of any concentration [1, 225, 226, 233, 234]. Less than 5% of cases is associated with IgA or IgG gammopathy (rare nonsecretory LPL have also been reported). To establish the diagnosis of WM it is necessary to demonstrate an IgM monoclonal protein, along with histologic evidence of infiltration of the BM by lymphoplasmacytic cells (there is no minimal percentage of BM infiltration or a minimal serum IgM level). Clinical manifestations of the disease include fatigue due to anemia, hepatomegaly (20%), splenomegaly (15%), and adenopathy (15%) [235]. In advanced disease patients may acquire anemia and hyperviscosity syndrome. WM has a chronic, indolent course with a highly variable prognosis. The median survival ranges from 5 to 6 years. The second malignancy

in patients with WM is observed in 10%, histological transformation (HT) in 3% and rapid rise of M-component in 6% of patients.

IgM monoclonal gammopathy of uncertain significance (IgM MGUS). IgM MGUS is defined as a serum IgM monoclonal protein (M protein) <3 g/dL, with a lymphoplasmacytic lymphoid infiltrate in BM <10% but without anemia, hyperviscosity, lymphadenopathy, hepatosplenomegaly, or any end-organ damage [229, 231, 236–238]. IgM MGUS may progress to LPL, amyloidosis, other B-cell lymphoproliferations or rarely IgM PCM.

Smoldering WM. Smoldering WM is defined clinically as having a serum monoclonal IgM protein of ≥3 g/dL and/or ≥10% BM lymphoplasmacytic infiltrate but no evidence of end-organ damage (anemia, constitutional symptoms, hyperviscosity, lymphadenopathy, or hepatosplenomegaly). In a series reported by Kyle et al., 71% progressed to symptomatic WM requiring treatment, one to primary amyloidosis, and one to lymphoma (total, 75%) [236, 239]. The cumulative probability of progression to symptomatic WM, amyloidosis, or lymphoma was 6% at 1 year, 39% at 3 years, 59% at 5 years, and 68% at 10 years. The major risk factors for progression were percentage of lymphoplasmacytic cells in the BM, size of the serum M-spike, and the hemoglobin value.

Morphology

Bone marrow (BM). LPL/WM is characterized by mixture of small lymphocytes, lymphocytes with plasmacytoid features (lymphoplasmacytoid variant) and plasma cells (Figure 13.37). Rare cases show more pleomorphic cellular composition with increased number of large cells (polymorphous variant; see also histologic transformation below). Plasma cells may contain Dutcher bodies (intranuclear inclusions) or Russell bodies (intracytoplasmic inclusions). Dutcher bodies are conspicuous in majority of cases. BM involvement by LPL may be interstitial (intertrabecular), nodular, paratrabecular (Figure 13.38), diffuse or mixed. Majority of cases show prominent paratrabecular component. There is often increased number of mast cells, especially at the periphery of lymphoid infiltrates. Presence of follicles with preserved FDCs and lymphoid cells with abundant pale cytoplasm is not typical for LPL/WM and would favor the diagnosis of MZL. Occasional cases of LPL may be associated with systemic or localized amyloidosis.

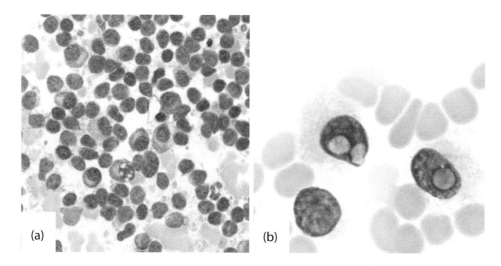

(a)   (b)

FIGURE 13.37   Lymphoplasmacytic lymphoma (bone marrow aspirate). typical mixture of small lymphocytes, plasmacytoid lymphocytes and plasma cells (a). Many plasma cells show Dutcher bodies (intranuclear inclusions; b).

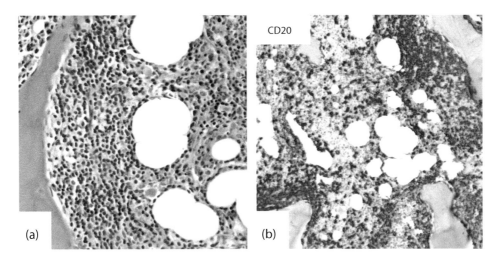

FIGURE 13.38   LPL – paratrabecular BM involvement (a, histology; b, immunohistochemistry). CD20 immunostaining shows prominent paratrabecular accumulation of lymphoid cells (b).

Blood. A leukemic blood involvement by LPL can occur de novo or during progression of the disease. Blood film shows lymphocytosis of small lymphocytes with occasional plasmacytoid cells and/or plasma cells (Figure 13.39). Rare cases may be characterized by increased number of prolymphocytes (usually reflecting prolymphocytic transformation). Testing for *MYD88* mutation is helpful to confirm the diagnosis of LPL.

Crystal storing histiocytosis. Rare cases of LPL/WM (and multiple myeloma) may be associated with crystal-storing histiocytosis, a rare disorder characterized by accumulation of histiocytes that have phagocytized an abnormal crystalline immunoglobulin. The intracellular crystal formation is almost always accompanied by the expression of kappa light chains [240–245]. Patients usually present with marked paraproteinemia and symptoms of hyperviscosity, as well as symptoms related to involvement of specific organs. Multi-organ involvement with symptoms similar to other storage diseases has been reported.

Lymph nodes. Histological findings of LPL in lymph nodes are variable, ranging from cases with preserved architecture to cases with complete distortion of architecture. In most typical cases, the architecture is rather preserved with patent sinuses, small or hyperplasic residual germinal centers and proliferation of lymphomatous cells in medullary, interfollicular, or paracortical areas. In other cases, LPL shows a diffuse growth pattern with extension to perinodal adipose tissue. Cytologically, there is a proliferation of three types of cells, small lymphocytes, plasmacytoid lymphocytes and plasma cells. The latter often contain prominent intranuclear inclusions (Dutcher bodies), which are PAS+. Apart from Dutcher bodies, increased mast cells and hemosiderin deposition may also be seen. WM in lymph nodes typically does not show a marginal zone growth pattern. Monocytoid cells can be seen in rare cases but are less prominent than in MZL. Based on the cellular composition, three histological variants have been described: lymphoplasmacytoid type (composed of mostly small lymphocytes), lymphoplasmacytic (composed of a mixture of lymphocytes and plasma cells), and polymorphous type, characterized by an increased number of large cells (at least 5%) [230]. The polymorphous variant is associated with increased chromosomal abnormalities and an aggressive clinical behavior and may represent an early phase of progression into DLBCL. Some cases of LPL show increased number of epithelioid histiocytes.

Other sites. In other organs, there is often a diffuse proliferation of a mixture of lymphocytes and plasma cells. In spleen, the lymphoplasmacytic infiltrate may be diffuse and/or nodular with involvement of red pulp, white pulp, or the junction of the red and white pulp [230].

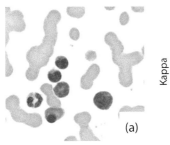 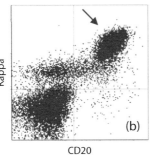 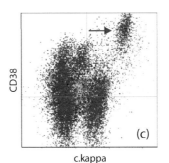 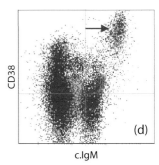

FIGURE 13.39   LPL (*MYD88*+) with blood involvement. (a) Blood smear with small lymphocytes and occasional plasma cells. (b–d) Flow cytometry analysis shows clonal B-cells with CD20 and kappa expression (b, arrow) and smaller population of clonal plasma cells with bright CD38 (c–d), cytoplasmic kappa expression (c, arrow) and c.IgM expression (d, arrow).

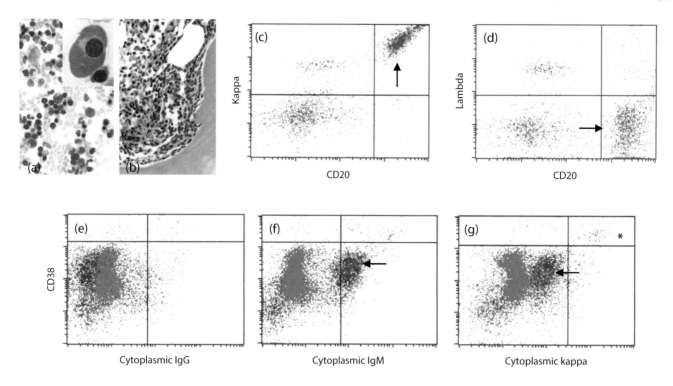

FIGURE 13.40 Lymphoplasmacytic lymphoma. (a) Aspirate smear with lymphocytes, plasmacytoid lymphocytes and plasma cells (*inset*: flame cell). (b) Core biopsy with atypical paratrabecular lymphoid aggregate. (c–g) FC analysis shows clonal B-cells and clonal plasma cells. B-cells (arrow) display strong expression of surface immunoglobulins (kappa, c–d) and dim to moderate expression of cytoplasmic IgM (f). Plasma cells (*) are relatively rare. They have bright expression of cytoplasmic IgM (f, compare with cytoplasmic IgG on display e) and bright cytoplasmic kappa (g).

Immunophenotype

Due to frequent paratrabecular involvement of the BM by LPL, number of clonal B-cells and plasma cells may be low when analyzed by FC. FC shows two distinct clonal populations, predominant population of clonal B-cells and usually much smaller population of clonal plasma cells. B-cells in LPL show moderate and clonal expression surface immunoglobulin light chains, moderate to bright expression of CD19 and CD20, dim expression of CD22, dim to moderate expression of cytoplasmic IgM, and bright CD45, and are usually negative for CD5, CD10, and CD103 (Figures 13.39 and 13.40). CD38 is variably expressed on B-cells, and when positive, is dimmer than in plasma cells. Some LPLs may be positive for CD5 (Figure 13.41), CD10 (Figure 13.42), CD11c, CD23, CD25, and CD43. The expression of CD5 is seen in ~6% and CD10 in ~2% of LPL/WM. Morice et al. reported CD5 expression in 43% of cases and CD23 expression in 52% of cases, both usually with only partial expression [246], but other reports show only very rare CD5+ or CD10+ cases [247]. EBV staining is negative. BCL1 (cyclin D1) is negative. TCL1 is positive in 75% of cases and is associated with a poorer prognosis [248]. LPL of non-WM type shows a similar immunophenotype except for expression of IgG or IgA instead of IgM. The accompanying plasma cell population is usually smaller and is negative for surface immunoglobulins, brightly positive for cytoplasmic immunoglobulins (of the same isotype as B-cells), brightly positive for CD38 and CD138, most often positive for cytoplasmic IgM, and often positive for CD19, CD27, and CD45 and negative for CD56 and CD117. By immunohistochemistry, plasma cells often express PAX5. Occasional cases may show a minor polytypic plasma cells in

addition to clonal plasma cell population. Non-IgM LPLs are clinically and pathologically heterogeneous and often harbor *MYD88* L265P mutation (43%), albeit at lower rate than classical IgM+ LPL/WM [249]. *MYD88* status does not correlate with any specific pathologic or clinical manifestations in this group. Aberrant expression of CD13 by LPL has been reported [250]. Rare cases are either IgG+ or IgA+ (Figure 13.43). The non-IgM type of LPL may show variable loss or decreased CD19 and CD45 by plasma cells. Blood involvement is characterized by presence of clonal B-cells with non-specific phenotype (CD5−, CD10−). Circulating clonal plasma cells are rarely identified but may be present.

Histologic transformation (HT)

HT occurs in 1%–19% of patients with LPL/WM, usually as DLBCL and only sporadically as BL or cHL [251, 252]. It is more common in women with the median age of 56 years (range 42–80 years) [230]. In LPL cases involving lymph nodes large cells are relatively few (more often seen in polymorphous type) and predominance of large cells either in BM or extramedullary sites (including lymph nodes), especially when occurring in sheets indicate either HT to large cell lymphoma or a diagnosis other than LPL. Occasional cases of LPL are followed by cHL or display prolymphocytic transformation.

Genetic features

There are no specific chromosomal changes in LPL. The 6q deletions are most common chromosomal abnormalities and are present in 30%–60% of patients [253, 254]. The 6q deletion is associated with adverse prognosis [254]. Subset of cases shows

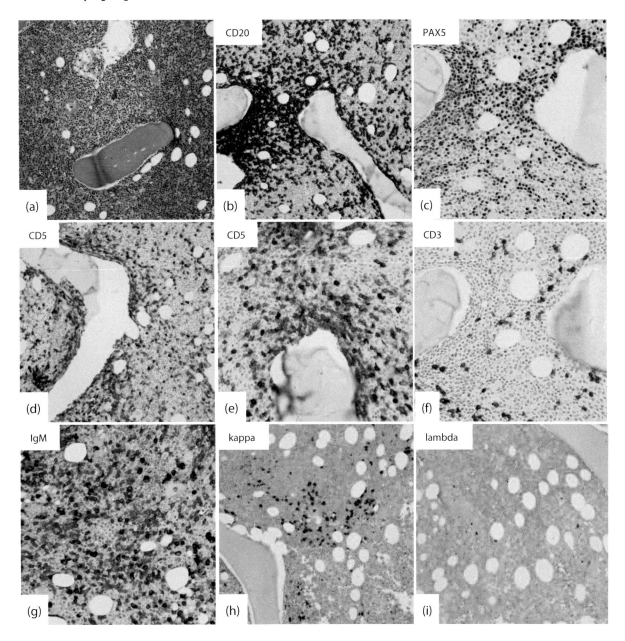

FIGURE 13.41 LPL with partial CD5 expression – immunohistochemistry. The BM core biopsy shows atypical interstitial and paratrabecular lymphoid infiltrate (a). Lymphoid cells are positive for CD20 (b) and PAX5 (c) and display aberrant expression of CD5 (d–e; two different areas, compare with CD3 staining on f). Plasma cells are positive for IgM (g) and kappa (h–i).

complex karyotypic abnormalities. The t(9;14)(p13;q32) occurs in subset of patients. This translocation involves the *PAX5* gene on chromosome 9, which encodes a B-cell specific transcription factor involved in the control of B-cell proliferation and differentiation. Presence of abnormal cytogenetic findings, e.g., −8 or del(6q) correlates with poor prognosis [255]. *MYC*, *CCND1*, and BCL2 rearrangements are characteristically absent in WM. Lack of *IGH* translocations differentiates WM from multiple myeloma and many lymphomas including FL, MCL, and DLBCL. WM does not have the t(9;14)(p13;q32) translocation, but often have deletions of 6q21 (21%–55%) [253, 256]. On the other hand, no 6q deletions can be found in IgM+ MGUS samples and therefore presence of 6q- helps to distinguish WM from IgM+ MGUS [257].

NGS has revealed recurring somatic mutations in LPL/WM, including *MYD88* (95%–97%), *CXCR4* (30%–40%), *ARID1A* (17%), and *CD79B* (8%–15%). Majority of LPL/WM are characterized by presence of *MYD88* L265P mutations [228, 231, 232, 258, 259]. *MYD88* is detected less frequently in non-IgM LPL type (40%) [249]. The *MYD88* gene is located at chromosome 3q22.2 and encodes an adaptor protein in the interleukin-1 (IL-1) and toll-like receptor pathways. The primary consequence of *MYD88* mutation is NF-κB activation via Bruton tyrosine kinase and other molecules. Although highly prevalent in LPL/WM, *MYD88* has been described in other lymphomas, including 70% of primary DLBCL of central nervous system (CNS) and testicular DLBCL, 50% of cutaneous DLBCL, leg type and 24% of ABC type of DLBCL, NOS [260]. Occasional CLL/SLL and SMZL cases also carry *MYD88* mutations [261–265].

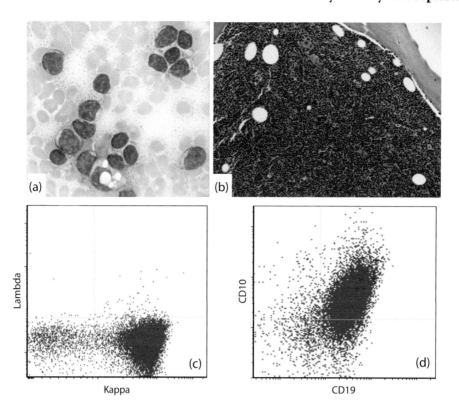

FIGURE 13.42 LPL (IgG⁺) with aberrant expression of CD10 (FISH analysis was negative for BCL2, BCL6, and MYC rearrangements; molecular studies showed *MYD88* mutation). (a) Aspirate smear with prominent lymphocytosis. (b) BM core biopsy with diffuse lymphoid infiltrate of mostly small lymphocytes (immunostaining with CD138 showed only rare monotypic plasma cells). (c–d) FC analysis shows clonal (kappa⁺) B-cells (c) with CD10 expression (d).

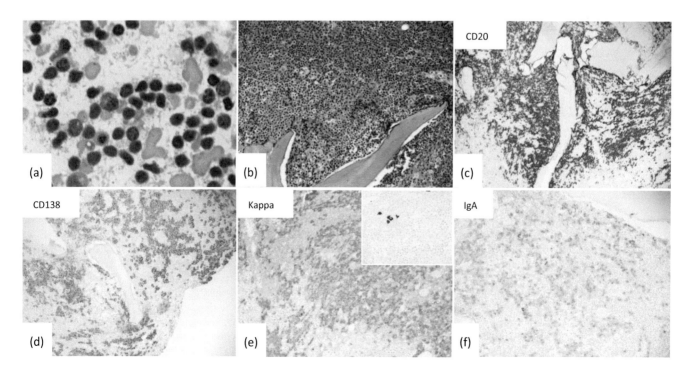

FIGURE13.43 IgA⁺ LPL. (a) Aspirate smear with lymphocytosis with occasional plasma cells. (b). Core biopsy shows atypical paratrabecular lymphoid infiltrate. (c–f) Immunohistochemistry. B-cells are CD20⁺ (c) and plasma cells are CD138 (d), kappa⁺ (e, inset lambda staining), and IgA⁺ (f).

Differential diagnosis of LPL

The differential diagnosis of B-cell and plasma cell neoplasms associated with IgM gammopathies can be challenging and require multimethodology approach using serum protein electrophoresis (SPEP), IFE, serum free light chain (SFLC) assays, molecular testing (*MYD88* and *CXCR4* mutations), FC of analysis of blood and/or BM, FISH studies, radiologic imaging, and morphologic correlation. The most common cause of IgM paraproteinemia is LPL/WM, but considerations include also other B-cell lymphomas and plasma cell neoplasms.

Differential diagnosis of LPL includes:

- CBL-MZ
- IgM$^+$ monoclonal gammopathy of undetermined potential (MGUS)
- MZL with plasmacytic differentiation
- SMZL
- SDRPL
- MCL with plasmacytic differentiation
- PCM
- CLL/SLL with plasmacytic differentiation
- Other B-cell lymphomas with plasmacytic differentiation
- Gamma$^+$ heavy-chain disease
- Reactive lymphoplasmacytic infiltrates including IgG4 related disease

CBL-MZ. MBL is defined by presence of low numbers (<5×10^9/L) of circulating monoclonal B-cells in otherwise healthy (asymptomatic) subjects (with no evidence of CLL/other lymphoproliferative disorders, adenopathy or organomegaly). Clonality is defined by either kappa restriction (κ:λ >3:1), lambda restriction (κ:λ <0.3:1), or >25% surface κ and λ negative B-cells. Some cases may be bi-clonal or tri-clonal. MBL may show (1) CLL-like phenotype (CD5$^+$/CD23$^+$), (2) atypical CLL-like phenotype (CD5$^+$/CD23$^-$ or cases with bright expression of CD20 and surface light chain immunoglobulins), and (3) MZL-like phenotype (MZL-like) or non-CLL-like MBL (CD5$^-$, CD10$^-$), which is more recently designated as CBL-MZ. CBL-MZ is characterized by the presence of clonal B cells in the blood and/or BM with morphologic and immunophenotypic features consistent with marginal zone derivation in otherwise healthy individuals. CBL-MZ may be associated with IgM paraproteinemia raising the differential diagnosis with WM. CBL-MZ is very heterogeneous with mutations not associated with specific lymphoma subtype, including *MYD88* (14%–19%), *BIRC3* (11%), *CCND3* (11%), *NOTCH1* (11%), and *TNFAIP3* (11%), but often show some genetic changes overlapping with SMZL and SDRPL [5, 6].

IgM$^+$ MGUS

IgM$^+$ MGUS is defined by a serum paraprotein concentration <3g/dL, BM lymphoplasmacytic infiltration <10% and lack of anemia, constitutional symptoms, hyperviscosity, lymphadenopathy, or hepatosplenomegaly [229, 231, 236–238]. IgM$^+$ MGUS is regarded as precursor lesion that carries a risk of progression at 1% per year to either WM, AL amyloidosis or rarely IgM PCM. More than 50% of IgM$^+$ MGUS cases have *MYD88* mutation, Distinguishing IgM$^+$ MGUS from WM is mainly based on the degree of BM involvement and the clinical presentation.

Mantle cell lymphoma (MCL) with plasmacytic differentiation

MCL show specific phenotype (in most cases) with co-expression of B-cell markers with CD5 and CD43. They are positive for BCL1

(cyclin D1) and SOX11. Only minor subset of LPL shows aberrant CD5 expression, but in contrast to MCL, LPL is negative for BCL1 (cyclin D1) and SOX11 and does not carry t(11;14)/*CCND1*.

Follicular lymphoma (FL) with plasmacytic differentiation

Occasional cases of FL show monocytoid or plasmacytic differentiation. Nodular pattern, co-expression of CD10, BCL2 and BCL6 by lymphomatous cells, lack of *MYD88* mutation, and presence of t(14;18) [*BCL2* rearrangement] indicate the diagnosis of FL.

Marginal zone lymphoma

Morphology. MZLs, both nodal and extranodal, may show prominent plasmacytic differentiation. MZL involving the BM often are accompanied by follicles with dendritic cells, feature not typical for LPL/WM. Lymphomatous cells in MZL often display monocytoid appearance with abundant pale (clear) cytoplasm. The distinction between LPL/WM and MZL is not always possible, and some cases may need to be classified as a small B-cell lymphoma with plasmacytic differentiation. Lymphomatous cells in LPL are more monotonous mostly small with some cells showing plasmacytic differentiation (lymphoplasmacytoid cells), and plasma cells showing Dutcher bodies, whereas MZL shows heterogeneous population of lymphoid cell, including some transformed large cells or prominent monocytoid features. In lymph node, preferential paracortical, medullar or interfollicular involvement with obvious plasmacytic differentiation, patent sinuses, presence of Dutcher bodies, increased number of mast cells and hemosiderin deposit would favor LPL, whereas prominent monocytoid differentiation, marked reactive follicular hyperplasia, a marginal zone growth patterns as well as disrupted FDC meshwork would favor the diagnosis of NMZL. In the BM, MZL shows nodular or interstitial infiltrate while LPL often has interstitial, paratrabecular or diffuse infiltrate. Presence of the *MYD88* gene mutation is now considered an essential biomarker for distinguishing LPL/WM from MZL, as it is observed only rarely in patients with the latter disease.

Immunophenotype. B-cells in both LPL/WM and MZL are typically negative for CD5, CD10, and CD23, but subset of both lymphomas may show aberrant CD5 expression and rare cases of LPL/WM are CD10$^+$. CD138 expression may be useful in establishing the diagnosis, since the differences between MZL and LPL regarding the intensity and the percentage of CD138$^+$ cells are significant and correlate with serum IgM level [266]. FDC meshwork highlighted by CD21 and/or CD23 immunostains is seen more often in MZL, although it can be present in LPL. Subset of LPL/WM cases may be positive for CD13, while other B-cell lymphomas are most often CD13$^-$. Expression of PAX5 by plasma cells is seen more often in LPL/WM than in MZL. CD25 is positive in most cases of LPL/WM but only in 50% of MZL. In a series reported by Kyrtsonis et al., 60% of LPL/WM cases expressed CD138 in contrast to 18% of SMZL patients [266]. Patients with extranodal MZL (MALT lymphoma) can have a serum IgM paraprotein, but the differential diagnosis between MALT lymphoma and LPL/WM involving extranodal sites is seldom a problem, as LPL/WM rarely has extranodal involvement at the time of initial presentation.

Genetic features. LPL has not been shown to harbor the t(11;18), t(1;14), or t(14;18) translocations that are frequently observed in MALT lymphomas. MYD88 is mutated in most LPL/WM cases.

Splenic marginal zone lymphoma (SMZL)

The differential diagnosis between WM and SMZL can be challenging [17]. Splenomegaly, serum paraproteinemia and *MYD88* mutation may be present in both disorders. Patients with SMZL may have a serum monoclonal protein, but in much smaller titers than in LPL and marked hyperviscosity and hypergammaglobulinemia are uncommon. Presence of prominent isolated splenomegaly without concurrent lymphadenopathy or extensive BM involvement, lack of *MYD88*, and lack of high levels of serum M protein would favor the diagnosis of SMZL, as splenomegaly is usually a late stage finding in LPLWM, *MYD88* is only rarely positive (<10%) in SMZL and serum monoclonal protein in SMZL most often show low titers. In a series reported by Arcaini et al., the median serum level of monoclonal protein was 2.0 g/dL in LPL/WM and 0.95 g/dL in SMZL [168]. Splenomegaly, typical feature of SMZL is seen in 10%–15% of patients with LPL/WM.

BM morphology. SMZL shows either characteristic intrasinusoidal (most often) or less often nodular pattern of BM involvement, whereas LPL/WM displays interstitial, nodular, and paratrabecular pattern. The BM analysis from patients with LPL/WM and patients with SMZL showed that patients with SMZL had a higher percentage of intrasinusoidal infiltration (70%) and a more frequent nodular pattern, whereas patients with LPL/WM tended to have interstitial distribution and paratrabecular component. Follicular dendritic meshwork highlighted by CD21 or CD23 immunostaining is more often present in MZL, although these can be rarely seen in LPL. Intermediate/high intensity of CD138 expression was observed in 47% of WM while it is low in all SMZL patients.

Blood smears. In contrast to increased white cell count and lymphocytosis commonly seen in SMZL, patients with LPL/WM less commonly present with lymphocytosis. Morphologically, lymphocytes in LPL/WM are monotonous, small and have little cytoplasm (except for lymphoplasmacytic cells). In contrast, lymphocytes in SMZL often have relatively more cytoplasm with polar villi or are more variable in size. The hallmark of SMZL is the presence of medium sized cells with irregularly distributed short membrane villi. Villi distribution, as well as the nuclear characteristics of chromatin and nucleolus are distinct from those of HCL cells. The SMZL cells are usually larger than the lymphocytes found in CLL, with diameters comparable with those of prolymphocytes. The nuclei are round or ovoid, sometimes eccentric, with a clumped chromatin pattern, and in half the cases 40%–90% of these lymphocytes showed a single prominent nucleolus, sometimes surrounded by heterochromatin, or associated with the nuclear membrane, or both, as is usually seen in prolymphocytes [210]. In most SMZL cases there is 3% and 12% of plasmacytoid cells, which are characterized by a more pronounced cytoplasmic basophilia, and a clear perinuclear zone corresponding to the Golgi apparatus [210].

Splenic diffuse red pulp B-cell lymphoma (SDRPL)

SDRPL is rare disorder presenting with leukemic blood involvement, splenomegaly and BM involvement. The lymphomatous cells display morphology similar to MZL, with clear (pale) cytoplasm and often plasmacytoid features, or rarely plasmacytic differentiation. Phenotype of clonal B-cells is non-specific, without CD5 or CD10 expression. Genetic changes may include mutations of *CCND3*, *NOTCH1*, *TP53*, *BRAF*, and *SF3B1*. In contrast to LPL, *MYD88* is not mutated in SDRPL.

SLL/CLL

SLL/CLL may present with paraprotein in the serum, and therefore may mimic WM. Rare CLL cases have *MYD88* mutation. Cytomorphologic features (predominance of small lymphocytes with scanty cytoplasm and nuclei with mature compact chromatin

without nucleoli), clinical presentation (lymphadenopathy and/or lymphocytosis), and immunophenotype (CD5+/CD23+, dim CD20, dim expression of surface immunoglobulins, strongly positive CD200 and negative CD81) help to diagnose B-CLL/SLL rather than LPL/WM (B-cells in LPL/WM show moderate CD20 and surface immunoglobulins, and most often lack both CD5 and CD23). Some atypical CLL cases may have dim/partial to negative CD5 with brighter expression of B-cell markers and surface light chain immunoglobulins, resembling LPL/WM. Presence of proliferation centers by morphology is diagnostic for CLL.

Plasma cell myeloma (PCM)

IgM PCM is a rare entity representing approximately 0.5% of all PCM. It needs to be distinguished from malignant neoplasms of B cells with plasmacytic differentiation such as WM and MZL with plasmacytic differentiation. The distinction between IgM+ PCM, IgM+ MGUS, smoldering (indolent) WM, and LPL/WM is based on cytologic features, immunophenotype, cytogenetics/FISH, clinical features, and radiologic imaging findings. Diagnostic criteria for IgM PCM are similar to typical (non-IgM) PCM (see Chapter 17 for details). PCM is characterized by pure plasma cell infiltrate (without admixture of small lymphocytes or plasmacytoid lymphocytes) and typical radiologic findings (e.g., lytic bone lesions). In some cases of LPL/WM, especially after treatment, plasma cells can predominate, thus raising the differential diagnosis with PCM. Morphologically, plasma cells in WM show a low histological grade, are small and mature. In PCMs, plasma cells show a spectrum of histologic grades, from small mature to large and pleomorphic with distinct nucleoli (plasmablastic features). Plasma cells in LPL/WM and PCM differ immunophenotypically. Plasma cells in LPL/WM have some immunophenotypic overlap with B-cells, often being positive for CD19 and CD45, as well as CD27 (50%) and CD81, but negative for CD56 and CD117. In contrast, PCMs are most often negative for CD19, CD45, CD27, and CD81, and show aberrant expression of CD56, CD117, and/or CD200. *MYD88* mutation is positive in LPL/WM but negative in PCM. Rare cases of concurrent PCM and LPL/WM have been reported. In contrast to PCMs, plasma cell component of LPL is negative for CD56 and CD117.

Gamma heavy-chain disease (GHCD)

There is no specific histological pattern in GHCD. Most frequently the infiltrate is pleomorphic lymphoplasmacytic proliferation mainly seen in BM and lymph nodes [1]. Some cases present with a predominantly plasmacytic proliferation mimicking plasmacytoma or lymphocytosis of small mature lymphocytes mimicking CLL. GHCD may also involve blood showing mixture of small lymphocytes, plasmacytoid lymphocytes and plasma cells at various proportions. Occasional cases show presence of large cells (immunoblasts), histiocytes and eosinophils [1]. The most common site of extranodal involvement is the skin, although involvement of thyroid and parotid, oropharynx, and gastrointestinal tract has been reported. IFE helps to establish the diagnosis by revealing IgG without light chain.

Reactive lymphoplasmacytic infiltrates

Significant plasma cells or plasmacytoid infiltrate can accompany many reactive processes in lymph node. Reactive lymphoid and/or lymphoplasmacytic infiltrates show mixture of B- and T-cells, plasma cells, and other inflammatory cells. The nodal architecture is mostly preserved, and both B-cells and plasma cells do not display significant cytologic atypia or aberrant phenotype. Plasma cells and B-cells are polytypic by either immunohistochemistry or

FC. Infectious etiology may be associated with hepatitis C, cytomegalovirus, human immunodeficiency virus, infectious mononucleosis, toxoplasmosis, or syphilis, sometimes leading to clonal or oligoclonal lymphoplasmacytic proliferations. Other causes of prominent lymphoplasmacytic infiltrate are Castleman's disease, Rosai-Dorfman disease, and IgG4 related disease (IgG4-RD). IgG4-RD is characterized by dense lymphoplasmacytic inflammatory infiltrate with increased numbers of IgG4$^+$ plasma cells, increased eosinophils; storiform pattern of fibrosis; and obliterative vasculitis but various other morphologic changes may be present including PTGC, follicular hyperplasia or inflammatory pseudotumor pattern. IgG4$^+$ plasma cells comprise >100/high power field (HPF) and the IgG4/IgG ratio is >40% [87, 88].

Follicular lymphoma

FL phenotype by FC: sIg$^{+/rarely-}$, CD5$^{-/rarely+}$, CD10$^{+/rarely-}$, BCL2$^{+/rarely-}$, CD11c$^-$, CD19$^{+(often\ dim)}$, CD20$^+$, CD22$^+$, CD23$^{-/rarely+}$, CD25$^-$, CD38$^{+/rarely-}$, CD43$^{-/rarely+}$, CD45$^+$, CD81^{+dim}, CD103$^-$, CD123$^{-/rarely+}$, and CD200$^{variable\ (+/-)}$.

Introduction
FL is one of the most common type of malignant lymphoma in adults and is defined as a B-cell neoplasm of follicle center cell origin which usually displays a nodular pattern of growth, t(14;18)(q32;q21) by cytogenetic (or FISH) and co-expression of CD10, BCL2, and BCL6 by FC and/or immunohistochemistry [1, 267–272]. Current WHO classification distinguishes 3 major subtypes of FL: classic FL (cFL; known previously as FL grade1,2 or 3a), follicular large B-cell lymphoma (FLBL; classified previously s FL, grade 3b), and FL with uncommon features (uFL). FL is composed of a variable proportion of small and large centrocytes (cleaved cells) and centroblasts (large non-cleaved cells). The t(14;18) alone is not sufficient to cause lymphoma, as 50%–70% of healthy individual have detectable levels of this translocation in blood [273–275].

Prognosis of FL
FL is a heterogeneous group of tumors with variable course, but the majority of cases have an indolent and slowly progressive clinical course with relatively long median survival, good response to initial treatment and a continuous pattern of relapses, sometimes followed by HT into DLBCL or HGBL [276–282].

Stage. Prognosis is closely related to the extent of the disease at the time of diagnosis. The International Prognostic Index for FL (FLIPI) is a strong predictor of outcome [282]. Approximately 65% of patients are in stage III or IV at the time of diagnosis [283]. Long-term survival is relatively high when the disease is diagnosed in stages I or II [284]. With current therapy the expected median survival is approximately 8–10 years [276].

Grade. Grading of FL (pertinent only to cFL) is no longer mandatory (updated WHO classification). Grade 3 FL with diffuse areas >25% (now recognized as areas of DLBCL) have a worse prognosis than purely follicular cases [285, 286].

Genetics. The presence of more than six chromosomal breaks and a complex karyotype has been shown to associated with a poor outcome; in addition, del 6q23-26, del17p, and mutations in *TP53* as well as −1p, −12, +18p, +Xp confer a worse prognosis and a shorter time to transformation [287, 288]. Genetic changes associated with worse prognosis include *BCL6* rearrangements, *MYC* abnormalities, 1p36 deletions, *TP53* mutations, *MLL2* and *EZH2* mutations, and *CDKN2A* deletions.

Location. The survival rate is higher in extranodal FL than in nodal FL. Patients with primary cutaneous FL have a more favorable long-term prognosis than those with equivalent nodal disease [289]. FLs in non-cutaneous extranodal sites have similarly favorable outcome [290]. Majority of extranodal FLs do not harbor t(14;18) [289, 290]. In FL of the gastrointestinal tract, the estimated 5-year disease-free survival was 62%, and the median disease-free survival is 69 months [291].

Morphology: Lymph nodes
In the lymph node (Figure 13.44), there is effacement of the architecture by a nodular or nodular and diffuse proliferation of small-cleaved cells (small centrocytes) admixed with variable number of large cells (centroblasts) [272, 292, 293]. The number of centroblasts defines the grade of FL. Centrocytes are small- to medium-sized lymphocytes with irregular nuclear contours (cleaved cells), condensed chromatin and scant cytoplasm. Centroblasts are large cells (usually ≥3 times that of a resting lymphocyte) with round to oval nuclei, multiple peripherally located nucleoli and variable amount of distinct cytoplasm. FDCs may resemble centroblasts, but in contrast to centroblasts have dispersed, nearly clear chromatin with a single eosinophilic nucleolus, more prominent nuclear membrane, and indistinct cytoplasm. The non polarized follicular nodules are usually tightly packed with a back-to-back arrangement and have comparable size and shape, which differ from florid follicular hyperplasia. The neoplastic follicles most often lack a well-defined mantle zone, polarization, or tingible-body macrophages. Occasional cases show a vague nodularity, nodules of variable size or shape. High grade FL may have a starry sky pattern, which together with lack of BCL2 expression imitates a reactive process.

Morphologic variants of FL (Figure 13.45) include:

- Floral variant (follicles with irregular borders reminiscent of a floral design; two patterns: macrogerminal and microgerminal)
- Diffuse variant (diffuse infiltrate of mostly small cells with CD10 expression)
- Monocytoid variant (FL with marginal zone differentiation; FL with reversed pattern)
- FL with prominent sclerosis
- Signet-ring cell variant
- FL with Reed-Sternberg like cells
- Epithelioid variant (FL with numerous granulomas)
- FL with extensive plasmacytic differentiation
- FL with Castleman-like changes (hyaline vascular variant with increased vascularity)
- FL with blastoid features (many cells resemble blasts)
- In situ follicular neoplasia (ISFN, discussed in separate section)
- ISFN-like variant (numerous follicles with very bright expression of both CD10 and BCL2)
- FL with partial lymph node involvement

Morphology: Bone marrow and blood
Many patients with FL have stage IV disease with BM and often blood involvement ("leukemic" phase). BM is involved by systemic FL in 30%–80% of cases. Peripheral blood smear shows atypical lymphocytes (centrocytes) with irregular nuclei or prominent nuclear cleavage and scanty cytoplasm (Figure 13.46). Larger lymphocytes (centroblasts) may be seen in various proportions, depending on stage and grade of the disease. In BM, FL lymphoma typically shows prominent paratrabecular pattern of involvement,

prominent nodular pattern

vague nodular pattern

nodules of different sizes

irregular nodules

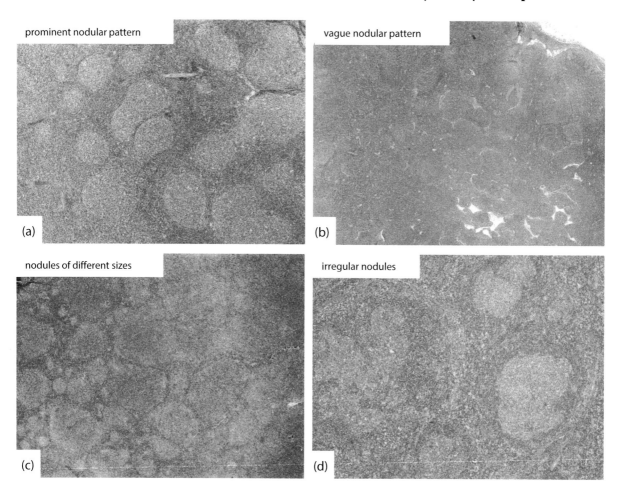

(a)   (b)

(c)   (d)

FIGURE 13.44   Follicular lymphoma (FL) – lymph node. (a) FL with prominent nodular pattern. (b) FL with vague nodularity. (c) FL with nodules of different sizes. (d) FL with irregular nodules.

but nodular or interstitial infiltrates may be also seen (Figure 13.47). Due to predominantly paratrabecular location of involvement and their association with FDC meshwork, the neoplastic cells often do not aspirate well which leads to false negative FC analysis. The immunostaining of the BM, apart from B-cells (CD19+/CD20+) shows also very often increased number of small, reactive T-cells (CD3+/CD5+), obscuring the neoplastic B-cells. The immunostaining with CD10 and BCL6 is often suboptimal in the decalcified sections and those markers often appear either downregulated or negative in the BM core biopsy samples. BM biopsy performed after treatment (R-CHOP) may show atypical paratrabecular infiltrate composed exclusively of reactive T-cells. Discrepancy between the grade of nodal and BM compartments is not uncommon. Approximately 10%–25% of patients with low grade FL in BM have grade 3 FL or DLBCL in other tissues [294]. Discordance between the BM morphology and other tissue sites is observed in 24.9% of B-cell lymphomas and is most often seen with FL or DLBCL [294]. In a British series of 345 patients with NHL for whom both LN and BM biopsy were available, only 8 patients with FL were found to have discordant marrow disease by histology, all of which were classified as DLBCL [295].

Immunophenotype of FL

Immunophenotypically, FLs are most often positive for CD45, B-cell markers (CD19, CD20, CD22, CD79a, OCT2, BOB1, and PAX5), CD10, BCL2, and BCL6 (Figure 13.48). Most cases are

negative for CD43. The expression of BCL2 is usually dimmer than in residual benign small T-cells. Some cases, however, show strong BCL2 positivity. This is especially common in cases with partial involvement by FL or ISFN. FLs, even those with distinct nodular architecture, may show a significant proportion of CD10+ B-cells (with or without BCL6 expression) in the interfollicular areas. Presence of interfollicular spread of neoplastic cells does not constitute a diffuse pattern of FL [1]. Subset of FL may be negative for CD10 and/or BCL2 (Figure 13.49). Very few cases of FL may show aberrant expression of CD5. The expression of CD5 has been associated with a higher rate of transformation to DLBCL and shorter progression-free survival [296–300]. BCL2 negative tumors are usually of higher grade. Lack of both BCL2 and CD10 expression is often observed in FL without t(14;18) and with *BCL6* rearrangement [301, 302]. Additional markers indicating germinal center phenotype include LMO2, HGAL, and GCET1 [303–305]. CD21 and CD23 are helpful in identifying the FDC meshwork which are often more irregular than those seen in benign follicles. Subset of FLs, especially diffuse variant is CD23+.

Ki-67. Mirroring the centroblast count, Ki-67 increases with grade. Classic FLs have a Ki-67 rate <20%, while FLBLs have >70% positivity. Minor subset of tumors shows discrepant grade and Ki-67 rate, when cFLs show high Ki-67 index [1, 272].

Flow cytometry (FC). FC analysis (Figures 13.50 and 13.51) shows monotypic expression of surface light chain immunoglobulins

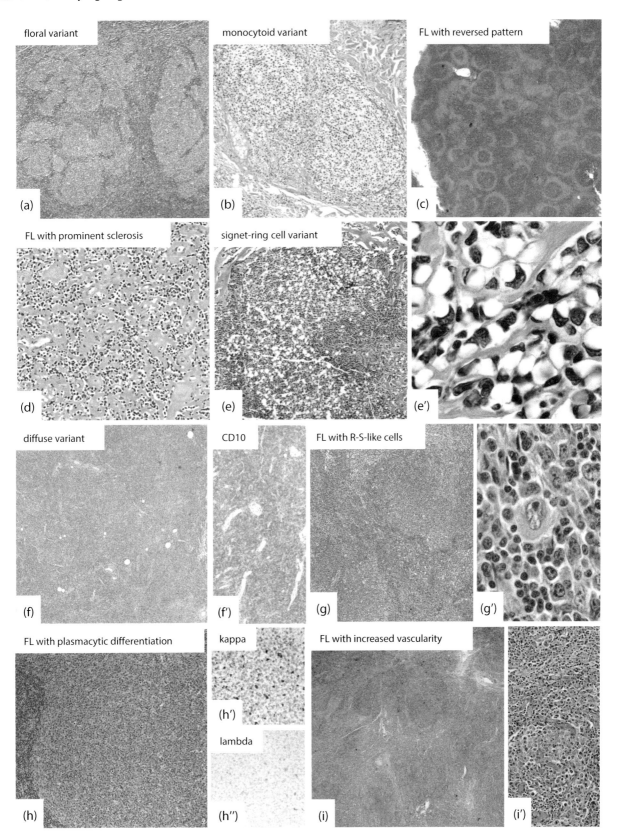

FIGURE 13.45 Morphologic variants of FL. (a) Floral variant. (b) FL with pale (clear) cytoplasm (monocytoid B-cell appearance). (c) Reversed pattern. (d) FL with prominent sclerosis, obliterating nodular architecture. (e–e') Signet ring cell variant (low and high magnification). (f–f') Diffuse variant of FL. (g–g') FL with Reed-Sternberg-like cells. (h–h'') FL with prominent plasmacytic differentiation. (i–i') FL with increased vascularity.

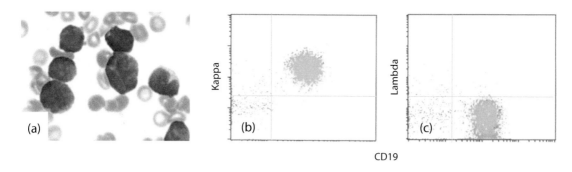

FIGURE 13.46 Leukemic peripheral blood involvement by follicular lymphoma (a, blood smear). Flow cytometry (b–c) shows clonal expression of kappa light chain immunoglobulin.

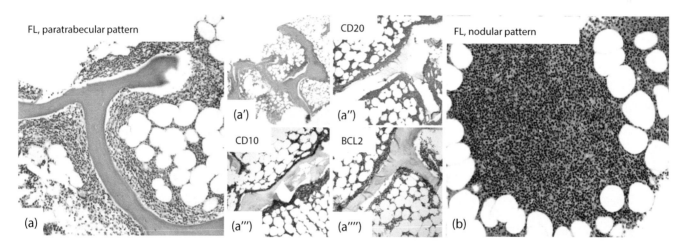

FIGURE 13.47 Follicular lymphoma – patterns of bone marrow involvement. (a) Characteristic paratrabecular pattern of involvement with lymphomatous cells expressing CD20, CD10, and BCL2 (a′, low magnification; a″ CD20 immunostaining; a‴ CD10 immunostaining; a⁗ BCL2 immunostaining). (b) Nodular bone marrow involvement.

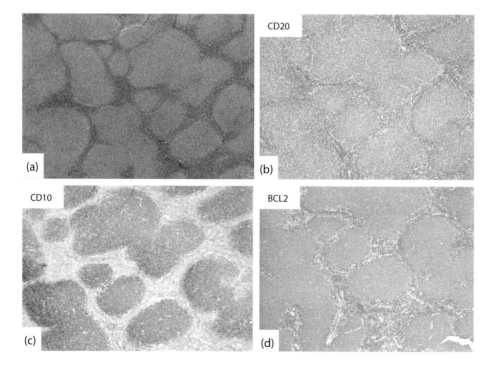

FIGURE 13.48 Follicular lymphoma (FL) – immunohistochemistry. Typical FL (a) is positive for CD20 (b), CD10 (c), and BCL2 (d).

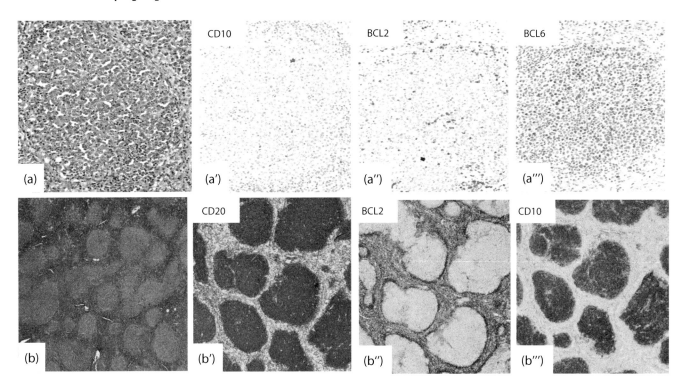

FIGURE 13.49 (a) FLBL with unusual lack of CD10 (a′) and BCL2 (a″). BCL6 is positive (a‴). (b) Classic FL with positive CD20 (b′), lack of BCL2 (b″) and strong CD10 (b‴).

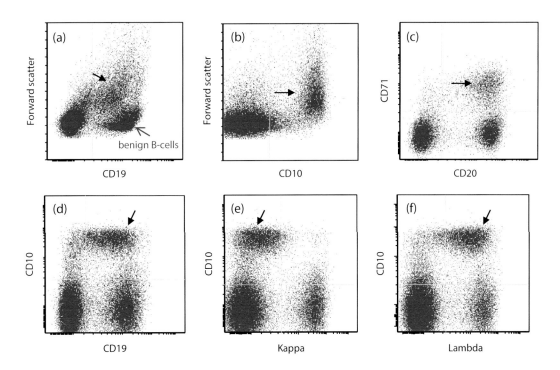

FIGURE 13.50 Follicular lymphoma – flow cytometry analysis. Neoplastic B-cells (black arrow) show increased forward scatter (a–b), dim expression of CD19 (a; compare with benign B-cells), positive CD10 (b; d–f) and positive CD71 (c). CD10+ population is lambda positive (compare e–f). Increased forward scatter and positive CD71 is usually associated with FLBL (cFLs show low forward scatter and negative CD71).

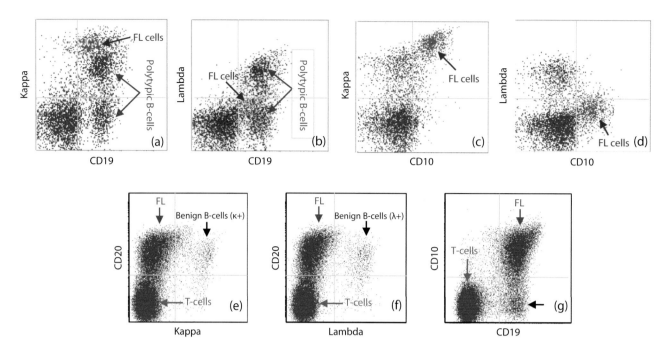

FIGURE 13.51   Follicular lymphoma – flow cytometry. (a–d) Analysis of lymph node with FL shows polytypic B-cells (red dots; red arrows), clonal B-cells (blue dots; blue arrow) and reactive T-cells (CD19⁻). The lymphomatous cells show dim CD19 (a–b) and bright kappa (a). Clonal B-cells show expression of CD10 (c–d). In another example (e–g) follicular lymphoma cells (red arrow) are surface light chain immunoglobulin negative (e–f) and show positive CD10 expression (g). Rare polytypic B-cells show kappa and lambda expression (e–f, black arrow). Numerous T-cells (blue arrow) are also noted (kappa, lambda and CD19 negative; e–g).

(κ or λ), moderate to bright expression of CD20, dim expression of CD19 and positive expression of CD10 and BCL2. In many cases FC reveals two B-cell populations: a neoplastic population with monotypic expression of surface immunoglobulins and a subpopulation of residual benign (polytypic) B-cells, as well as increased number of reactive T-cells. Dim expression of CD19 and co-expression of CD10 and BCL2 usually confirm malignant process in these cases. Rare cases of FL show aberrant expression of CD5 (Figure 13.52), CD30, or CD43. A subset of FL may be negative for surface light chain immunoglobulins (Figure 13.53). Similar to discrepancy in morphologic features (grade) between primary nodal site and BM, also the phenotype may differ between primary and secondary sites, i.e., different CD10 expression (positive versus negative) or

different expression of light chain immunoglobulins (Figure 13.54). The phenotypic difference may be observed at the time of diagnosis or at the time of relapse.

Immunophenotypic variants of FL:

- BCL2⁻ FL
- CD10⁻/MUM1⁺ FL
- EBV⁺ FL

BCL2⁻ FL. Co-expression of BCL2 with CD10 and BCL6 is abnormal and indicates lymphoma. The frequency of BCL2 expression varies depending on the grade of FL. Although low grade FLs stain positively for BCL2 in 85%–90% of cases, grade 3 FLs stain

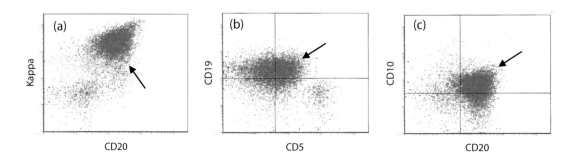

FIGURE 13.52   FL with aberrant expression of CD5. Flow cytometry (a–c) shows monoclonal (kappa⁺) B-cell population co-expressing CD5 (b) and CD10 (c).

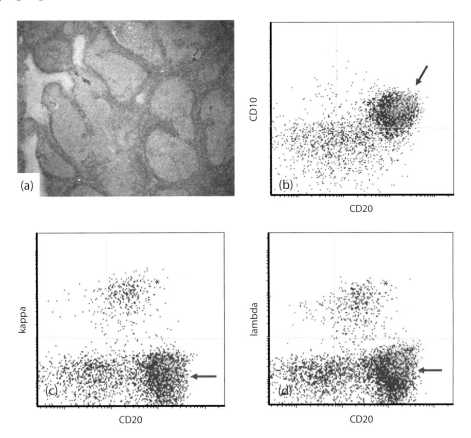

FIGURE 13.53 FL with lack of surface light chain immunoglobulin expression. (a) Histology with atypical nodular proliferation. (b–d) Flow cytometry shows co-expression of CD20 with CD10 (b, arrow), and lack of both kappa (c) and lambda (d) expression. Rare polytypic B-cells are noted (*).

positively in only 50%–70% of cases [306–308]. BCL2 negativity should not be used to exclude a diagnosis of FL if the other features are present [270].

CD10⁻/MUM1⁺ FL. Similar to BCL2, CD10 expression by immunohistochemistry can also be scant or absent, which is more frequently observed in the setting of grade 3 FL [306, 308–311]. Rare FLs show unusual phenotype with lack of CD10 and strong MUM1 expression. CD10⁻/MUM1⁺ FLs (when compared to typical CD10⁺/MUM1⁻ FLs) occur more often in the elderly (67.0 versus 58.7 years), have more often higher grade (3a or 3b) morphology (91% versus 17%), diffuse proliferation (59% versus 19%), lack *BCL2/IGH* translocation (5% versus 92.5%), and show often *BCL6* gene abnormalities (translocation or amplification) [312]. Strong MUM1 expression is also seen in large B-cell lymphoma with *IRF4* rearrangement. Those lymphomas occur more often in younger patient and have predilection to Waldeyer's ring or cervical lymph nodes. They are CD10⁺.

EBV⁺ FL. EBV⁺ FL is rare (~2.5% of FLs) [313, 314]. Majority of patients with EBV⁺ FL progress to a higher-grade FL or to DLBCL [313, 315].

Grading of FL

FL was graded based on the proportion of centroblasts (small and large) in ten neoplastic follicles per 40× high-power microscopic field (HPF; Figure 13.55). Current WHO classification eliminated the need for FL grading: all cases previously categorized as grade, 1, 2 and 3a are now called classic FL while cases

previously graded as 3b are now termed follicular large B-cell lymphoma (FLBL). Cases of cFL (grade 3a) with focal diffuse growth pattern may be termed "DLBCL with follicular lymphoma". [1].

Flow cytometry and FL grade

Analysis of FSC and CD71 can help to differentiate between low grade FLs with majority of cells displaying low FSC (Figure 13.56) and lack of CD71 expression, from high grade FLs showing increased FSC (Figure 13.57) and positive CD71 (the expression of CD71 may be partial). The expression of CD200 is often negative in high grade FL (similar to DLBCLs).

DLBCL component. Any area of DLBCL in an FL should be reported as the primary diagnosis, with the estimate of the proportion of DLBCL and FL component. Since the cytomorphologic features often vary among follicles, the whole lymph node must be sampled and carefully evaluated. Centroblasts need to be differentiated from other large cells such as histiocytes, endothelial cells, FDCs and large centrocytes. It is also necessary to exclude any areas with diffuse large cell infiltrate.

Genetic features of FL

The t(14;18)(q32;q21) is the cytogenetic hallmark of FL. It occurs in 90% of cases [288, 316, 317]. The translocation results in the juxtaposition of the *BCL2* oncogene into the *IGH* heavy chain locus on chromosome 14, leading to its overexpression. Chromosomal breakpoints mainly occur at two different sites on chromosome 18:

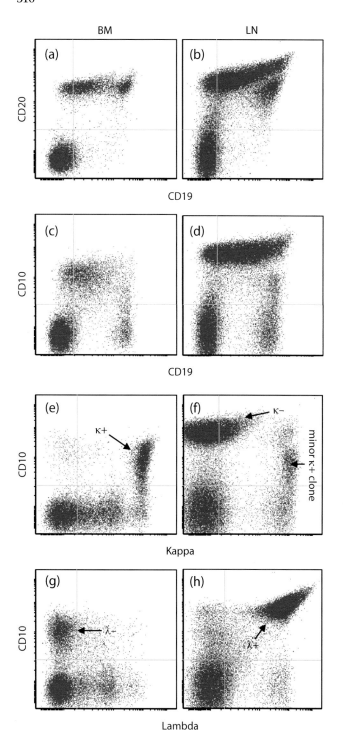

FIGURE 13.54 Follicular lymphoma – concurrent flow cytometry analysis of the bone marrow (BM; left column) and lymph node (LN; right column) showing discrepant phenotype of clonal cells between those two sites. Both populations are CD19+ (a–b), CD20+ (a–b), and CD10+ (c–h), but clonal B-cells is the BM are kappa+ (e) and show moderate intensity of CD10 expression (c), whereas clonal B-cells in the lymph node are mostly lambda+ (h) with only minor population being kappa+ (f), and show bright CD10 expression (d).

Major Breakpoint Region (MBR) and minor cluster region (mcr), which account for 80% and 10% of translocations, respectively [318]. Approximately 10% of FL cases lack t(14;18), but show other chromosomal abnormalities [319]. Subset of FL shows translocations involving *BCL6* gene, often without concurrent *BCL2* rearrangement. FLs without t(14;18)(q32;q21) and with *BCL6* rearrangement are usually characterized by prominent nodular architecture, higher frequency of grade 3 morphology, monocytoid component, weak or absent CD10 and BCL2 expression and increased Ki-67 proliferation index, but there are no significant differences regarding age, performance status, BM involvement or overall survival when compared to FL with t(14;18) [271, 311, 320–322]. Other genetic events include loss of 1p, 6q, 10q, and 17p and gains of 1q, 6p, 7, 12, 18, and X.

FL with MYC and BCL2 (and/or BCL6) rearrangement (double-hit or triple-hit FL). Rare cases of otherwise typical FL with classic morphologic and immunophenotypic features may show rearrangements of *MYC* with *BCL2* (and/or *BCL6*), as seen in double-hit lymphomas [HGBL with *MYC* and *BCL2* (and/or *BCL6*) rearrangements; HGBL-R]. Those unusual cases of FL are not classified as HGBL-R, when both morphology and phenotype at typical for FL. Regardless of histological grade, FL with *MYC* and *BCL2* (and/or *BCL6*) rearrangements have more aggressive clinical course than typical FL without *MYC* and *BCL2* (and/or *BCL6*) rearrangements [323].

Histologic transformation (HT)

Progression refers to recurrence of FL after therapy, without evolution to a more aggressive lymphoma. HT is a histological shift, most often to DLBCL with few cases transforming to HGBL or B-cell acute lymphoblastic leukemia/lymphoma (B-ALL/LBL). Approximately 30% of FLs undergo transformation, but the frequency of transformation varies (depending on detection methods and definitions) between 10% and 60% and is associated with a poor prognosis [27, 324]. Morphologically, progression of FL is characterized by loss of nodular growth pattern, increased number of centroblasts (HT from cFL to FLBL), and presence of sheets of large cells, either centroblasts or immunoblasts (HT to DLBCL) [283, 325–327]. HT to BL, HGBL, HGBL-R (Figure 13.58), plasmablastic lymphoma (PBL), and B-ALL/LBL (Figure 13.59) are much less common [269, 328–331]. HT is also accompanied by decreased number of T-cells and lack of FDCs. Transformed lymphomatous cells are positive for B-cell markers, CD10, BCL6, LMO2, and BCL2. Ki-67 index is high. Occasional cases may be CD30+ and/or p53+. The progression into HGBL is rare and has been reported more often in women in the 5th to 7th decade of life [27, 332]. The transformed component often involves extranodal sited and may be present synchronously or metachronously with FL [332, 333]. Morphologically, these tumors resemble BL with starry-sky pattern, frequent mitoses, and apoptotic cells. Lymphomatous cells are positive for B-cell markers and may be positive for CD10, BCL6, BCL2, and MUM1. Ki-67 index varies from 50% to 100%. Occasion cases may lack surface immunoglobulin expression when analyzed by FC. Progression into high grade lymphoma with blastoid morphology (B-ALL/LBL, blastoid FL, or blastoid unclassified B-cell lymphoma) occurs more often in men in their 4th to 7th decade of life. Lymphomatous cells appear immature with fine chromatin, nucleoli, and many mitotic figures. They are positive for CD19, PAX5, CD22, CD79a, and occasionally CD20 and in most cases also for CD10, BCL2, and TdT

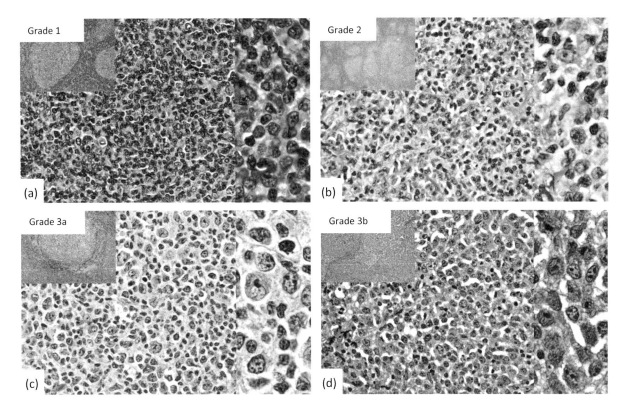

FIGURE 13.55 Follicular lymphoma (FL) – grading. (a) Low grade FL (grade 1) is composed predominantly of small cells with irregular nuclei. (b) Intermediate grade FL (grade 2) has mixture of small (centrocytes) and larger (centroblasts) lymphocytes. (c–d) High grade FL (grade 3) has predominantly large lymphocytes. Depending on the presence of few scattered small lymphocytes grade 3 FL can be subdivided into 3a (small cells present) and 3b (small cells absent). Grade 1, 2 and 3a are now classified as cFL and grade 3b FL is now classified as FLBL.

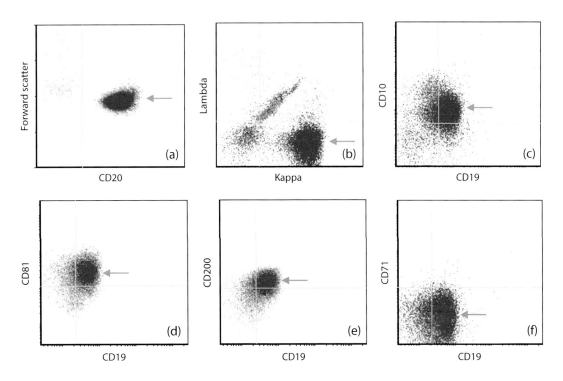

FIGURE 13.56 Flow cytometry of low-grade follicular lymphoma (histologically grade 1–2 of 3). Lymphomatous cells display low forward scatter (a, arrow), positive CD20 (a), kappa restriction (b), positive CD10 (c), dim CD81 (d) and CD200 (e), and negative CD71 (f).

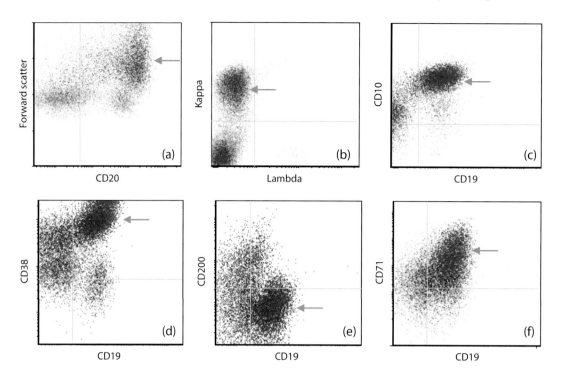

FIGURE 13.57 Flow cytometry of FLBL. Lymphomatous cells display high forward scatter (a, blue dots, arrow), positive CD20 (a), kappa restriction (b), positive CD10 (c), bright CD81 (d), negative CD200 (e), and positive CD71 (f).

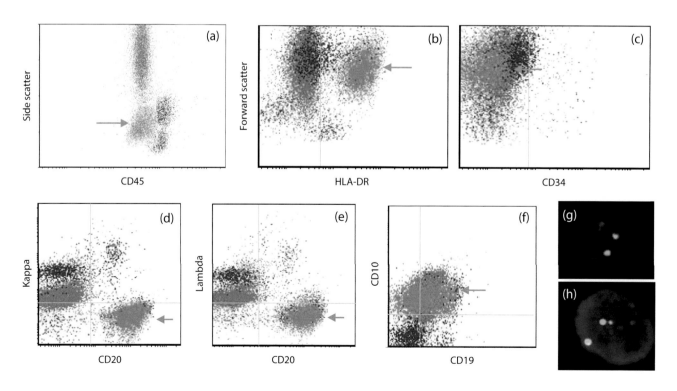

FIGURE 13.58 FL with transformation to HGBL-R (double-hit lymphoma). Patient with history of FL. Flow cytometry of blood (a–f) shows neoplastic cells (orange dots, arrow) with moderate CD45 expression (a), high forward scatter (b), positive HLA-DR (b), negative CD34 (c), bright CD20 (d–e), lack of surface light chain immunoglobulins expression (d–e), dimly positive CD19 (f), and positive CD10 (f). FISH studies show *MYC* rearrangement (g; break-apart probe showing one orange, one green and one fusion) and *BCL2-IGH* rearrangement (h; one green, one orange and two yellow fusion signals).

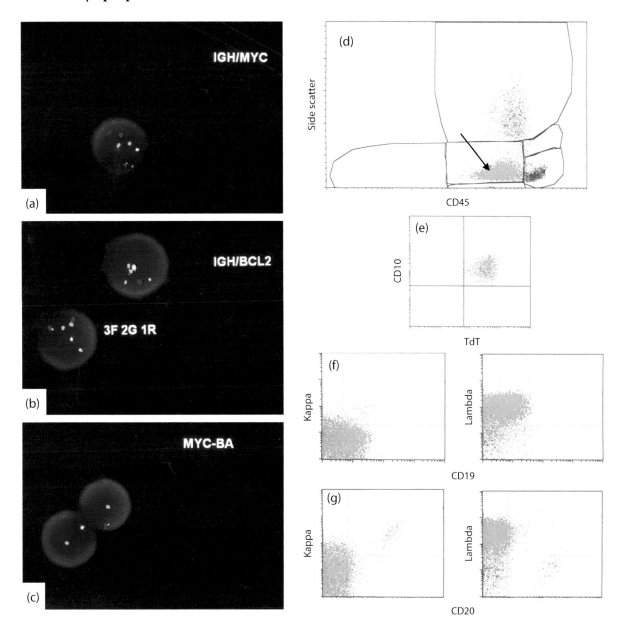

FIGURE 13.59 Blastic transformation of FL. (a–c) FISH analysis showing *MYC* rearrangement (a), *BCL2* rearrangement (b) and break-apart dual color with split signals (c; red and green split signals; yellow, normal signal). (d–g) Flow cytometry analysis shows leukemic cells in blastic region (d; arrow, green dots) co-expressing CD10 and TdT (e) with clonal lambda expression (f–g), dim CD19 (f), and negative CD20 (g).

[334]. Transformed cells lose the expression of BCL6 and may be surface immunoglobulin negative. Similarly to de novo B-ALL, some case may be negative for CD45 and positive for pan-myeloid markers (CD13, CD33). Ki67 index is generally high (~90%).

Differential diagnosis of FL
Flow cytometric differential diagnosis of FL include:

- Reactive follicular hyperplasia
- DLBCL (germinal center B-cell like type)
- BL
- HGBL with *MYC* and *BCL2* (and/or *BCL6*) rearrangement (HGBL-R)
- AITL

- Peripheral T-cell lymphoma with T-follicular helper phenotype (PTCL-TFH)
- MCL
- LPL
- HCL

Reactive follicular hyperplasia
The flow cytometric distinction between FL and follicular hyperplasia may be occasionally difficult, especially when the latter shows significant number of CD10⁺ B-cells. Benign lymph node (Figure 13.60) shows polytypic B-cells with dim expression of CD23, CD81, and CD200 and occasional CD10⁺ cells. Reactive lymph node with follicular hyperplasia shows typically two B-cell

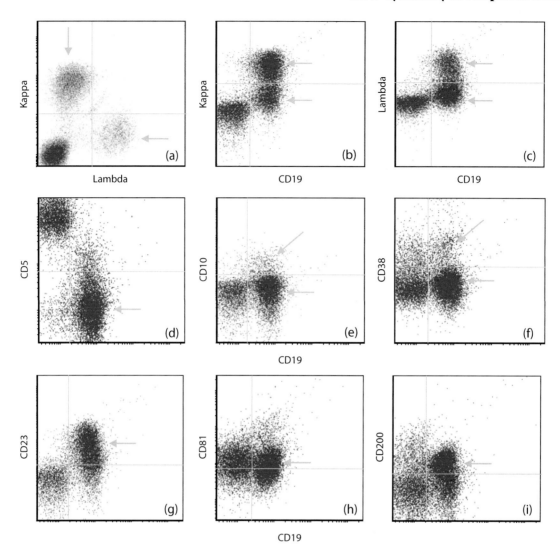

FIGURE 13.60 Benign lymph node. Flow cytometry analysis shows polytypic B-cells (a–c, arrows) which are mostly CD5⁻ (d). Rare B-cells express CD10 (e) and CD38 (f). Majority of show dim expression of CD23 (g), CD81 (h), and CD200 (i).

populations (Figures 13.61 and 13.62): CD10⁺ germinal center cells and CD10⁻ B-cells. The latter are characterized by distinct kappa⁺ and lambda⁺ populations, moderate CD19 and CD20 expression, positive CD23 and negative CD71 expression. Germinal center cells show variable (heterogeneous) expression of both kappa and lambda (often with kappa slightly brighter than lambda), brighter CD20, slightly brighter CD19, negative CD23, and positive (dim or partial) CD71. Some cases show distinct kappa⁺ (or less often lambda⁺, especially in children and young patients) B-cells with bright CD20 and CD10 expression mimicking a clonal population (Figure 13.62). The brighter expression of kappa by CD10⁺ B-cell population in follicular hyperplasia may be misinterpreted as clonal cells representing FL, especially in cases with predominance of CD10⁺ B-cells such as in florid follicular hyperplasia or when FC sample such as fine needle aspirate represents predominantly reactive germinal center. Additionally, since the expression of both kappa and lambda by CD10⁺ reactive germinal center cells is dimmer than in CD10⁻ B-cells, the FC findings may be misinterpreted as surface negative cells, a feature often seen in FLs. Admixture of benign B-cells (sometimes predominant) in many cases of FL is yet another factor contributing to difficulties

in differential diagnosis between FL and follicular hyperplasia by FC. Several FC features helps to distinguish reactive follicular hyperplasia from FLs. In contrast to clonal B-cells, benign germinal center cells have heterogeneous ("smeary" or variable) expression of surface immunoglobulins (Figures 13.61 and 13.62). Lymphomatous cells from FL show distinct (cohesive) cluster of clonal B-cells without variable or "smeary" pattern or are surface immunoglobulin-negative. Occasional cases of FL may show dim expression of surface immunoglobulins, in which identification of clonal cells may be difficult. The expression of CD19 is often dim in FL. In benign B-cells, the expression of CD19 is usually moderate to bright. The expression of CD10 is often brighter in FL than in reactive germinal center cells and the expression of CD38 is often dimmer in FL when compared to reactive germinal center cells. Typical FL shows co-expression of CD10 and BCL2 in contrast to reactive CD10⁺ germinal center cells which are BCL2⁻. However, subset of FL, may be BCL2⁻ (more often in high grade FL). The morphologic and immunohistochemical evaluation of original sample should follow FC for final diagnosis. FISH studies for t(14;18)/*IGH-BCL2* and/or molecular test (PCR) for B-cell clonality may be needed in difficult cases.

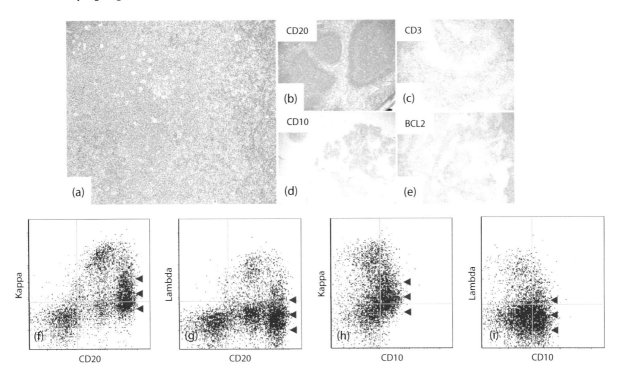

FIGURE 13.61 Flow cytometry (FC) of florid follicular hyperplasia (a, H&E; b–e, immunohistochemistry; f–i, flow cytometry). Reactive lymph node with florid follicular hyperplasia (a; H&E section) shows numerous large CD20+ follicles (b) with scattered CD3+ T-cells (c) and irregular CD10+ germinal centers (d) which are BCL2– (e). FC shows two distinct B-cell populations, one with moderate CD20 and second (predominant) population with bright CD20 expression (f–g; red arrowheads). Those bright CD20+ B-cells represent CD10+ germinal centers cells. They show dim CD10 expression (h–i) and typically a "smeary" expression of surface light chain immunoglobulins with kappa usually brighter than lambda (f–i). This pattern should not be confused with a clonal (kappa+) B-cell population in the background of polytypic B-cells.

DLBCL, BL, and HGBL-R

Increased FSC of lymphomatous cells suggests FLBL, which needs to be differentiated from DLBCL, BL, and HGBL-R. The final subclassification requires correlation with histomorphology and molecular testing for *MYC*, *BCL2*, and *BCL6* rearrangement. Typical BLs are positive for B-cell markers, CD10, CD38 (bright), CD43, CD71, CD81, and negative for BCL2, CD11c, CD23, CD25, and CD200. DLBCLs (germinal center B-cell like), except for CD10 expression are positive for B-cell markers, CD38 (dim to moderate), BCL2 (majority), and usually positive for CD81 (dim), while CD43 and CD200 are often negative.

Other CD10+ B-cell lymphoproliferations

MCL often has a nodular pattern and is positive for B-cell makers, CD5, CD43, and BCL1 (cyclin D1). Positive CD5, CD43, SOX11, and BCL1 (cyclin D1) expression distinguishes MCL from FL. Subset of MCL may be CD5– and even CD10+ and therefore immunohistochemical staining for BCL1 (cyclin D1) and SOX11, and cytogenetic/FISH studies for t(11;14)/*CCND1* rearrangement are often necessary to establish the correct diagnosis. Rare cases of LPL may be CD10+. Lack of t(14;18) [*BCL2/IGH*] and presence of *MYD88* mutations helps to diagnose LPL. Rare cases of HCL may be CD10+. By FC analysis HCL is characterized by bright expression of CD11c and co-expression of CD25 and CD103. On molecular level, HCL is usually positive for *BRAF* mutation.

CD10+ T-cell lymphomas

The revised WHO classification of hematolymphoid tumors introduced a category of nodal lymphoma with T follicular helper cell (TFH) phenotype, which includes AITL, follicular T-cell lymphoma (FTCL), and nodal peripheral T-cell lymphoma with T follicular helper phenotype (PTCL-TFH) [1, 96]. FTCL involves lymph node follicles resembling morphologically follicular B-cell lymphoma (FL). Both FTCL and PTCL-TFH were previously classified under the umbrella of PTCL. The WHO criteria specifically state that the expression of at least two TFH markers is required for the diagnosis of PTCL-TFH. TFH markers include CD10, BCL6, CXCL13, PD1 (CD279), ICOS, SAP (SLAM-associated protein), CXCR5, MAF (c-MAF), and CD200. AITL is the classic form of T-cell lymphoma of TFH origin, with diagnostic criteria that remain essentially unchanged from prior 2008 WHO classification. Both AITL and PTCL-TFH have similar phenotype, gene expression profile and common mutation in *TET2*, *DNMT3A*, and *RHOA* genes [335–342]. Cutaneous T-cell lymphomas expressing TFH markers are excluded from this category (WHO).

Differential diagnosis of FL in the BM biopsy (based on paratrabecular pattern):

- MCL
- LPL/WM
- CLL (rare cases)
- DLBCL
- Peripheral T-cell lymphomas (PTCL), especially AITL

Apart from FL, differential diagnosis of paratrabecular lymphoid infiltrates includes DLBCL, LPL/WM, MCL (Figure 13.63), PTCL, occasional cases of AITL or ALCL, and rare cases of CLL.

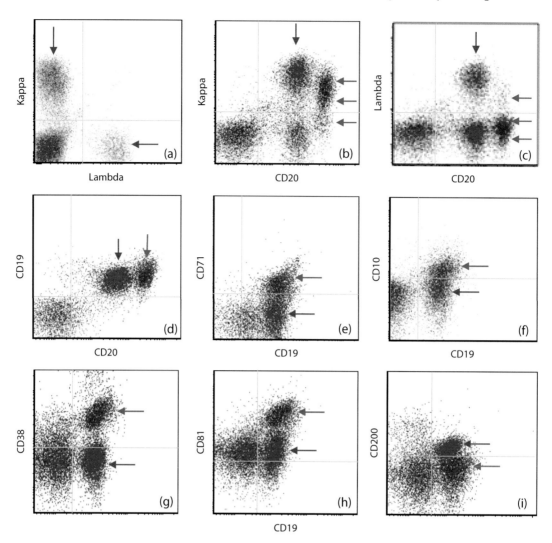

FIGURE 13.62   Reactive lymph node with florid follicular hyperplasia showing distinct kappa⁺ B-cells mimicking clonal population. Flow cytometry shows polytypic, kappa⁺ and lambda⁺ B-cells (a–c) with distinct two populations, one with moderate CD20 expression of polytypic kappa and lambda expression (b–c, red dots/red arrows) and another with brighter CD20 and predominantly kappa expression (blue dots/blue arrows). The bright CD20⁺ germinal center cells (blue dots/blue arrows) show moderate expression of CD19 (d), dim CD71 (e), dim CD10 (f), bright CD38 (g), bright CD81 (h), and negative CD200 (i).

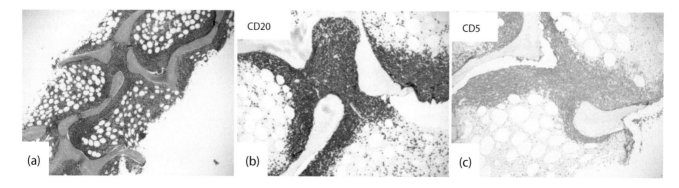

FIGURE 13.63   MCL with prominent paratrabecular BM involvement (a, histology; b, CD20 immunostaining; c, CD5 immunostaining).

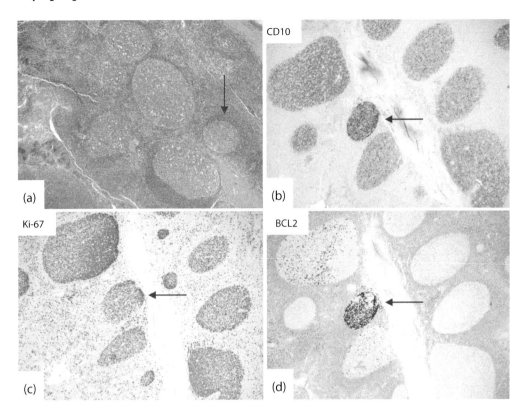

FIGURE 13.64 Tonsil with ISFN. (a) Histology shows mostly reactive germinal centers. One neoplastic follicle (arrow) shows bright expression of CD10 (b), positive Ki-67 without overt polarization (c), and bright expression of BCL2 (d).

In situ follicular B-cell neoplasm (ISFN)

ISFN (WHO classification; Figures 13.64 and 13.65) is often discovered incidentally and comprise isolated scattered follicles colonized by monoclonal t(14;18)+ B-cells over-expressing BCL2 and CD10 within an otherwise uninvolved lymph node [1, 274, 343–346]. ISFNs are often associated with prior or synchronous FL. Further evaluation reveals evidence of FL at another site in about half of the patients, but the risk of progression to clinically significant lymphoma is not yet fully known for these focal lesions. The challenge is to distinguish true ISFN from lymph nodes with partial involvement by FL, which more often progress to overt lymphoma. Jegalian et al. compared FL in situ with partial involvement by FL [343]. In ISFN the lymphoid architecture was intact, with patent sinuses, preserved paracortex/interfollicular regions, and scattered follicles with well-defined mantle zones. Both BCL2 and CD10 were strongly expressed, Ki-67 fraction was low, and CD10+/BCL2+ cells were confined to the germinal centers (often without replacing the entire follicle) [343]. In partial involvement of the lymph node by FL (<25%), the involved follicles were typically larger than uninvolved follicles within the same lymph node. The mantle zones were sometimes attenuated or disrupted, and the margin between the follicle center and the cuff was often blurred. Staining with BCL2 and CD10 was variable and generally less intense than in FL in situ [343]. In addition, single cells positive for CD10 and BCL2 were sometimes observed in the interfollicular area. In ISFN higher levels of circulating t(14;18)+ lymphocytes (>10⁻⁴ of total cells) indicate a higher risk for FL [347].

ISFN without overt lymphoma has indolent clinical course and requires follow-up without treatment. ISFN with synchronous FL is treated as typical (overt) FL. ISFN may precede FL or other lymphomas (e.g., DLBCL, MCL, SMZL, and classical HL) by years. In a series

reported by Jegalian et al., of 24 cases in which ISFN was the only lesion identified, 3 patients (12%) were identified on further clinical evaluation to have FL at another site, either before or at the of biopsy. One patient develop FL at 29 months, and 20 of 24 (83%) of patients did not develop evidence of FL during follow-up (median 41 months) [343]. In five patients ISFN was diagnosed in a lymph node containing a histologically unrelated type of lymphoma (composite). In patients with partial involvement by FL, the risk for subsequent FL is greater. At clinical staging or within 6 months of diagnosis, 6 of 17 (35%) patients with partial involvement by FL develop FL, most often in the same LN region [343]. Three additional patients were diagnosed with FL between 13 and 72 months after original diagnosis of partial involvement by FL. Six patients with partial involvement by FL treated by local radiation therapy or rituximab remained free of clinically evident disease (median follow-up 51.5 months) [343].

Pediatric-type follicular lymphoma (PTFL)

The pediatric variant of FL (pediatric-type follicular lymphoma, PTFL) is a newly recognized variant of FL (WHO classification) occurring in lymph nodes of children and young adults (18–30 years old) [1, 96, 348–352]. It affects males more commonly than females. PTFL usually presents with localized disease (usually in the head and neck area), high histological grade, and the lack of BCL2 protein expression and t(14;18) [1]. Majority of cases are localized and may not require treatment other than excision. PTFL has an excellent prognosis with sustained CR achieved in most cases after systemic therapy [350]. PFL do not relapse or progress even when treated by excision alone [350]. Although PTFL was initially identified in pediatric patients, it was subsequently found to occur also in young adults and more rarely in older patients.

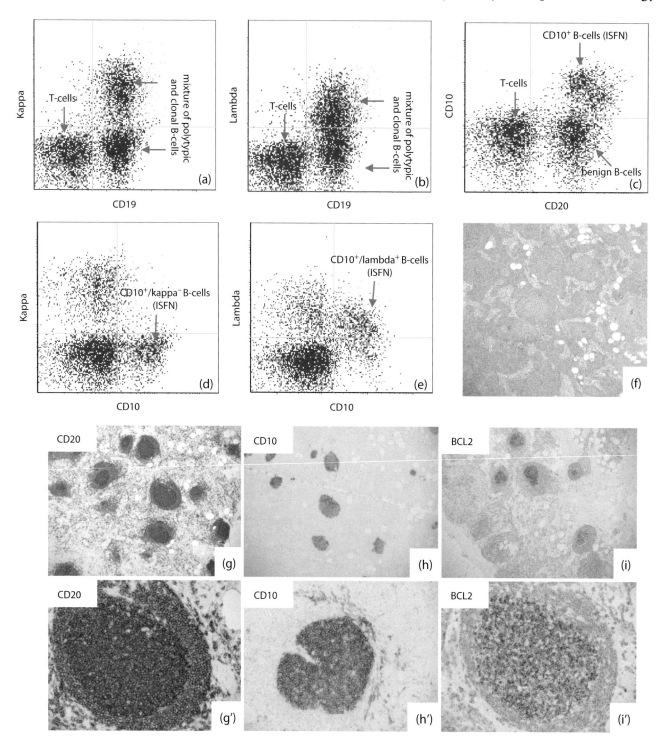

FIGURE 13.65 ISFN. (a–e) Flow cytometry shows predominant population of benign (polytypic) B-cells (a–b), T-cells (a) and minor population of CD10⁺ B-cells (c). Analysis of CD10 versus kappa and lambda (d–e) shows clonal CD10⁺ B-cells with dim lambda expression. (f) Histology of the lymph node shows scattered lymphoid aggregates. (g–i) Immunohistochemistry (low and high magnification) shows strong expression of CD20 (g–g′), CD10 (h–h′), and BCL2 (i–i′) by neoplastic B-cells.

Morphology of PTFL

Morphologically (Figure 13.66), PTFL is characterized by high grade, high proliferation fraction (Ki-67) and large irregular follicles with increased number of cells with blastoid follicular center cells [267, 348, 350, 351, 353]. Many nodal cases show a distinctive serpiginous pattern. In lymph node, blastoid cell predominate with fine chromatin and regular oval to round nuclei, and typical centroblasts with peripheral membrane-bound nucleoli or centrocytes are seen sporadically [353]. Due to lack of typical centroblasts and centrocytes, PTFLs are not graded. The blastoid cells have round to oval nuclei, finely clumped chromatin, small nucleoli, and scant cytoplasm [353]. There is often abundant

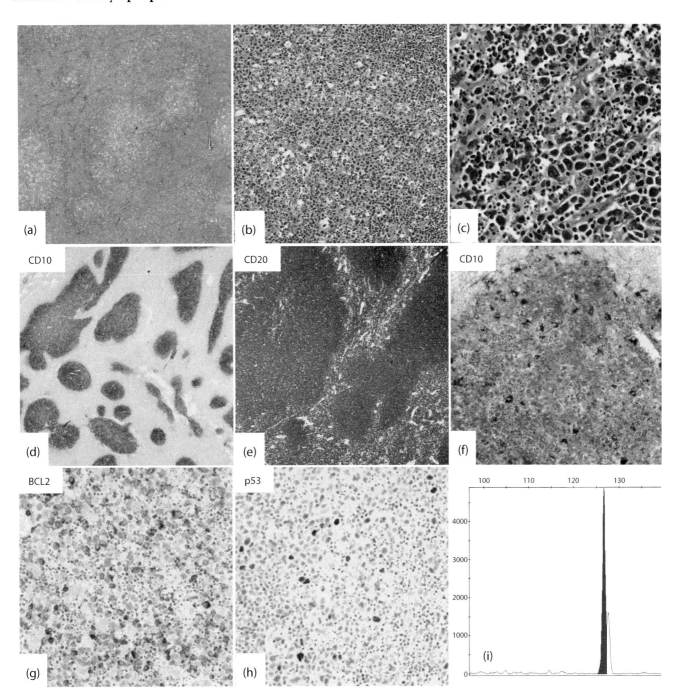

FIGURE 13.66 Pediatric-type follicular lymphoma (PTFL). Inguinal lymph node from 7-year-old patient shows atypical nodular infiltrate (a–b) composed highly atypical large cells (c). Nodular pattern is visualized by CD10 staining (d; low magnification) and CD20 (e; intermediate magnification). Lymphomatous cells are positive for CD10 (f), negative for BCL2 (g) and positive for p53 (h). Molecular studies (PCR) confirmed clonal rearrangement of *IGH* gene (i).

apoptosis with associated tingible-body macrophages leading to starry-sky pattern. Only rare cases of PTFL show grade 1–2 of 3 histomorphology. The category of PTFL excludes cases with diffuse areas (foci of DLBCL). The lymph nodes may be only partially involved, which in conjunction with presence of starry-sky appearance cause difficulties in differential diagnosis from reactive process. Marginal zone differentiation has been described in PTFL, though the monocytoid cells are often restricted to a thin rim around the neoplastic follicles and lack significant interfollicular spread [353]. Plasma cells are infrequent. Presence of any

diffuse pattern with high grade cytology exclude the diagnosis of PTFL and constitutes a diagnosis of DLBCL [272].

Immunophenotype of PTFL

PTFL are strongly positive for B-cell markers, CD10, FOXP-1, and BCL6. Majority of cases are negative for BCL2. BCL2 expression, when present is dim [353]. Rare cases may be positive for MUM1, especially in lymphomas located in the Waldeyer's ring [353]. CD5 is rarely expressed. Ki-67 expression is often high and lacks polarization in the neoplastic follicles. The IgD stain shows thin and attenuated mantle zone in PTFL. The staining with T$_{FH}$ marker, PD1 (CD279) shows more abundant PD1$^+$ T-cells in reactive follicles with higher number of cells in the light zone (polarization) and lack of polarization in the distribution of PD1$^+$ T-cells and their tendency to accumulate at the periphery of the nodules [353]. FLs in young adults most often display morphologic, immunophenotypic, and genetic features typical for usual FL.

Genetic features
PTFL is negative for *BCL2*, *BCL6*, *IRF4*, and *MYC* rearrangements.

Differential diagnosis of PTFL

- Florid follicular hyperplasia
- Pediatric MZL
- FL
- Large B-cell lymphoma with *IRF4* rearrangement
- Duodenal type FL

Pediatric MZLs are very infrequent but should also be included in diagnostic considerations. Differential diagnosis may be difficult event with application of additional testing such as FC and PCR. The clonal B-cell populations may be identified by FC or PCR in histologically reactive lymphoid proliferations [354]. Presence of 'starry-sky" pattern is not specific for reactive hyperplasia, as it is often seen in high grade FL, including majority of PTFL. Presence of monotonous population of blastoid cells without polarization (on H&E section or with Ki-67, BCL6, or PD-1 staining) and lack of typical centrocytes and centroblasts help to identify PTFL [353]. PCR for detection of a clonal B-cell population, although not 100% specific, appears to be sensitive test in PTFL, especially with multiple primer sets [355].

The distinction between PTFL and typical FL is important in order to avoid unnecessary treatment in the former. Majority of typical FL are BCL2$^+$, whereas PTFL are CD10$^+$, BCL6$^+$, and BCL2$^-$. On genetic levels, PTFL is characterized by lack of *BCL2* and *BCL6* rearrangement and frequent mutations of *MAP2K1* and *TNFSF14* [349].

Large B-cell lymphoma with *IRF4* rearrangement, which also occur most commonly in children and young adults is considered a distinct WHO entity (large B-cell lymphoma with *IRF4* rearrangement) [96]. Those lymphomas occur usually in Waldeyer's ring and/or cervical lymph nodes. They affect patients of a wide age range (4–79 years), with a median age of 12 years. They may have follicular, follicular, and diffuse or diffuse growth pattern and are often diagnosed as DLBCL with or without FL component. Immunophenotypically, they are positive for MUM1 and BCL6 and more than half of the cases express BCL2 and CD10. Rare cases may be CD5$^+$. FISH studies show *IRF4* rearrangement

(majority of cases) with or without *BCL6* rearrangement. There is no *BCL2* rearrangement. Despite the aggressive histologic appearance and complex genetic landscape, patients with large B-cell lymphoma with *IRF4* rearrangement usually have favorable outcome and therefore it is important in cases of large B-cell lymphomas with strong expression of MUM1 and expression of germinal center markers (CD10 and/or BCL6) involving head and neck or Waldeyer's ring to assess for the presence of *IRF4* by FISH.

Primary cutaneous follicle center lymphoma (PCFCL)
PCFCL is composed of follicle center B-cells including centrocytes and variable numbers of centroblasts with follicular, follicular, and diffuse, or diffuse growth patterns [1, 356–360]. By definition, there is no systemic or nodal involvement at the time of diagnosis. It has a characteristic clinical presentation with solitary or grouped plaques and tumors, preferentially located on the scalp or forehead, less often on the trunk, and only rarely on the leg. Approximately 15% of PCFCLs have multifocal skin involvement. Histologically PCFCL shows perivascular or periadnexal to diffuse infiltrates in the dermis which are separated do not involve the epidermis and are separated from it by a grenz zone. The tumors have follicular, follicular and diffuse or diffuse architecture, with the diffuse pattern being the most common [357, 361, 362]. The neoplastic cells express CD20 and other B-cell markers (CD19, CD22, CD79a, PAX5). Absence of detectable surface immunoglobulins is common, especially in tumors with diffuse population of large follicle center cells. Of follicle center markers, PCFCL is BCL6$^+$, but CD10 expression is often negative (CD10 expression is observed in cases with a nodular growth pattern but is negative in lymphomas with diffuse pattern). MUM1/IRF4, FOX-P1, CD5, and CD43 are negative in majority of cases. PCFCL are mostly BCL2$^-$ but some cases may show faint BCL2 staining (usually in a minority of neoplastic B-cells). Strong BCL2/CD10 co-expression is suggestive of cutaneous involvement by systemic FL. Figure 13.67 shows PCFCL with CD10 expression involving scalp from 38-year-old patient and Figure 13.68 shows composite lymphoma (PCFCL and SLL) involving scalp from 71-year-old patient.

Mantle cell lymphoma (MCL)

MCL phenotype by FC: sIg$^{+(moderate)}$, CD2$^-$, CD5$^{+/rarely-}$, CD10$^{-/rarely+}$, CD11c$^-$, CD19$^+$, CD20$^{+(moderate/bright)}$, CD22$^+$, CD23$^{-/(rare\ cases\ +)}$, CD25$^-$, CD38$^{+/rarely-}$, CD43$^{+/rarely-}$, CD45$^{+(bright)}$, CD49d$^{-/+}$, CD79a$^+$, CD79b$^{+(bright)}$, CD81$^{+strong}$, CD103$^-$, CD123$^{-/rarely+}$, and CD200$^-$.

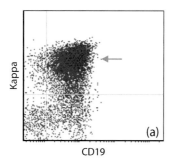 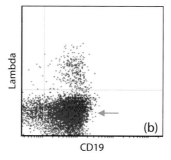 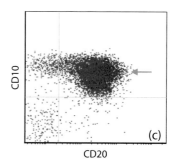

FIGURE 13.67 PCFCL. Flow cytometry of scalp lesion from 38-year-old patient showing clonal kappa$^+$ B-cell population (a–b, arrow) with CD10 expression (c).

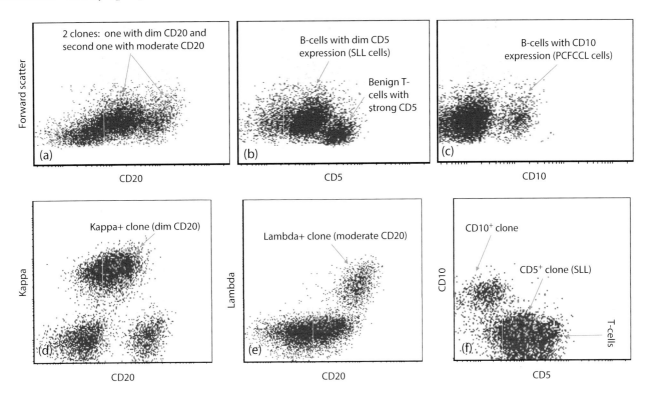

FIGURE 13.68 Composite lymphoma (PCFCL and small lymphocytic lymphoma) involving scalp from 71-year-old patient. Larger SLL clone shows dim expression of CD20 (a), dim CD5 (b), negative CD10 (c), and moderate kappa expression (d). Minor PCFCCL clone shows moderate CD20 (a), negative CD5 (b), positive CD10 (c), and moderate expression of lambda (e). Benign (reactive) T-cells show brighter expression of CD5 when compared to SLL cells (b and f).

Introduction

MCL is a CD5+ mature B-cell lymphoma of small to medium-sized lymphocytes with irregular (indented) nuclei characterized by BCL1 (cyclin D1) expression and translocation t(11;14)(q13;q32), leading to rearrangement between *CCND1* gene coding for the cyclin D1 and *IGH* gene [1, 213, 363–366]. MCL has distinct immunophenotypic profile: CD5+/CD20+/CD23−/BCL1+/SOX11+. MCL is characterized by disseminated disease, with most patients presenting with stage III or IV disease, lymphadenopathy, hepatosplenomegaly, and BM and blood involvement. The gastrointestinal tract is frequently involved (most often in the form of microscopic infiltrate, but occasionally also in the form of lymphomatous polyposis). BM involvement is observed in 50%–80%, hepatosplenomegaly in 30%–60%, B-symptoms in 50% and extranodal involvement in 20% of patients [283, 367–369]. Very rare cases of MCL have been reported to lack BCL1 (cyclin D1) expression and *CCND1* rearrangement; those cases have the molecular prolife typical for MCL, are positive for SOX11 and CD5 and in 55% carry *CCND2* translocations [370, 371]. According to the 2016 WHO classification, there are two major variants of MCL: classic MCL which affects the lymph nodes and extra nodal sites, and L-NN-MCL, which involves the BM, blood, and spleen [1, 213, 372].

Prognosis

MCL is typically an aggressive disease with poor outcomes. Non-nodal presentation, predominantly hypermutated *IGHV*, lack of genomic complexity, and absence of SOX11 expression identify specific subtype of indolent MCL with excellent outcomes

that might be managed more conservatively than typical (classic) MCL [373]. Parameters associated with poor prognosis or shorter survival include poor performance status, splenomegaly, B-symptoms, leukocyte count >10 × 10⁹/L, high LDH level, blastoid/pleomorphic histology, and high/intermediate or high risk IPI, complex karyotype, *MYC* translocation, unmutated *IGHV* status and CNS involvement [366, 369]. The most consistently reported adverse histopathological prognostic parameter is a high mitotic rate (>20/10hpf, >50/mm²) [374, 375]. A high proportion of Ki-67 positive cells (>40%–60%) in non-BM tissue is also an adverse prognostic indicator [374, 376]. The three groups with different Ki-67 index of <10%, 10%–29%, and ≥30% show significantly different overall survival in patients treated with CHOP as well as in patients treated with CHOP in combination with anti-CD20 therapy (R-CHOP) [377, 378].

Smoldering MCL. Cases with lack of B-symptoms, white blood cell count <30 × 10⁹/L, Ki-67 in non BM tissue <30%, non-blastoid/pleomorphic histomorphology, spleen <20cm, lymph node diameter <3cm, low MCL-IPI score, non-nodal leukemic presentation, absence of *TP53* or *NOTCH1/2* mutations and absence of 17p deletion or *MYC* translocation have been termed smoldering MCL [215, 366, 372, 379]. Other clinicopathological variants with indolent presentation include MBL with t(11;14), L-NN-MCL (with positive expression of CD200 and CD23 and negative expression of CD5 and CD38) and in-situ MCL [379].

Morphology

Lymph nodes. Histology reveals a monomorphic lymphoid infiltrate with scattered histiocytes (Figure 13.69). The lymphomatous

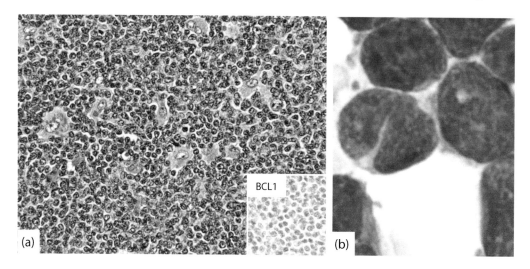

FIGURE 13.69   Mantle cell lymphoma (MCL) – histology and cytology. Histologic examination (a) shows diffuse lymphoid infiltrate composed of lymphocytes with irregular nuclear contours. Note the presence of histiocytes, often present in MCL [*inset*: BC1 immunostaining with positive nuclei]. Cytologic analysis (b) shows irregular nuclear outlines (cleaved nuclei).

infiltrate may be diffuse, with a mantle zone distribution or nodular. The nuclei are characteristically irregular or cleaved, best visualized in cytologic smears. MCL with mantle zone growth pattern may be difficult to diagnose without immunohistochemical staining for BCL1. This pattern is usually seen in areas of partially involved lymph nodes that otherwise show the most common nodular or diffuse involvement by the tumor [365]. The observation of this pattern in isolated lymph nodes in occasional patients with an indolent clinical course suggest that is represent the initial infiltration of the lymph node by the tumor [365, 380, 381].

Extranodal involvement. MCL usually present with advanced disease, including generalized lymphadenopathy and BM involvement, and a with a tendency for extranodal involvement, most often in the gastrointestinal tract, followed by spleen, Waldeyer's ring and less often other locations (e.g., nasopharynx, salivary gland, skin, ocular adnexa, CNS; Figure 13.70). An extranodal involvement is seen in majority of patients, and in 30%–50% of the patients is seen in more than two extranodal sites [365]. An extranodal presentation without apparent nodal involvement is observed in only 4%–15% of cases [365]. MCL in the gastrointestinal tract is the second most common type of lymphoma composed of small cells behind MALT lymphoma. It may present as (1) subtle infiltrate detected on histologic examination or (2) less often, but more typical (although not specific) in the form of a polypoid nodular growth (lymphomatous polyposis). The involvement of the gastrointestinal tract may represent either primary or secondary lymphoma. MCL in gastrointestinal tract usually involves the ileocecal region and large intestine, but often disseminates to the other parts and mesenteric lymph nodes. In spleen MCL usually involves white pulp with variable expansion into red pulp, similar to SMZL with biphasic pattern (small cells in the center and larger cells with more abundant cytoplasm at the periphery).

BM involvement. The BM involvement (Figure 13.71) may be diffuse, nodular, and/or paratrabecular. Occasional cases display intrasinusoidal involvement). BCL1 (cyclin D1) immunohistochemistry helps to confirm BM involvement, but the immunostaining in the decalcified trephine core biopsy material may be sometimes suboptimal or even falsely negative.

Special MCL variants

Apart from classic MCL, several morphologic and clinical variants are recognized by WHO classification [1].

Leukemic non-nodal MCL (L-NN-MCL). L-NN-MCL characteristically involves the BM, peripheral blood, and the spleen, and is composed often of small round lymphocytes (similar to CLL) [1, 212–215]. It follows a rather indolent course with a wait and watch approach [1]. Despite indolent clinical behavior, L-NN-MCL might transform to a more aggressive disease. Phenotypically, L-NN-MCL variant is more often CD5⁻, SOX11⁻, and/or CD200⁺, when compared to classic MCL [212–215].

In situ mantle cell neoplasm (IS-MCN). Recently, BCL1⁺ (cyclin D1⁺) B cell infiltrate with MCL phenotype (Figures 13.72 and 13.73) in the mantle zones of reactive-appearing lymphoid follicles or in colonic mucosa has been described and was termed in situ mantle cell neoplasm (formerly: MCL in situ). IS-MCN is an extremely rare phenomenon and represents either an early MCL (no overt lymphoma identified elsewhere) or an overt lymphoma (confirmed by morphologic and immunophenotypic analysis of concurrent tissues at different location) [268, 382–386]. The t(11;14) translocation is the primary event facilitating the transformation of a B lymphocyte that would initially colonize and expand the mantle cell area of the lymphoid follicles as seen in IS-MCN [365]. Patients with IS-MCL and no overt lymphoma, should be followed up very closely [268].

Small cell variant. This variant is composed of small round lymphocytes reminiscent of CLL.

Marginal zone-like variant. This variant shows presence of monocytoid-like cells with abundant pale cytoplasm.

Blastoid and pleomorphic variants. The pleomorphic variant (Figure 13.74a) shows a heterogeneous population of larger cells with irregular nuclei, and blastoid variant (Figure 13.74b) is characterized by lymphoblast-like cells, high mitotic rate (at least 20–30/10hpf), high Ki-67 index (>40%), occasional starry-sky pattern and prominent nucleoli. The growth pattern of blastoid variants is usually diffuse, less frequently nodular, and rarely exhibits mantle zone pattern [387]. An "in-situ" pattern of blastoid MCL has not been observed. Blastoid variant of MCL show more often lack of CD5 expression when compared to classical type. Blastoid morphology is associated with a high proliferation,

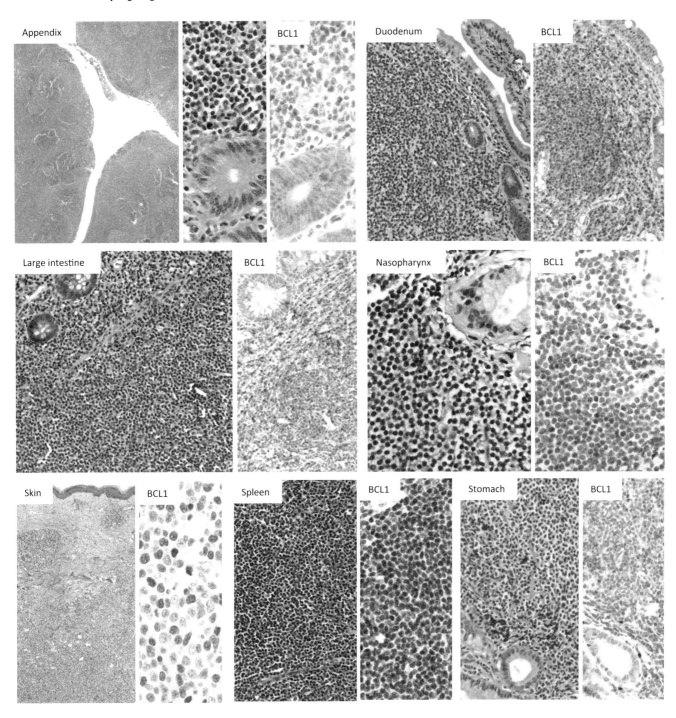

FIGURE 13.70 Extranodal MCL.

as measured by the Ki-67 index. Blastoid MCLs are characterized by a high level of c-MYC expression despite the fact that *MYC* translocations are rare [387, 388]. Blastoid and pleomorphic variants occur usually de novo and less frequently in patients with previous diagnosis of "classic" MCL [389]. The switch from classical to blastoid morphology may occur in subset of patients during the course of the disease, whereas an inverse pattern of evolution is observed in rare cases [390, 391].

Prolymphocytoid-like variant. An unusual variant of MCL with "prolymphocytoid-like" transformation may be rarely seen, showing two cell types: small lymphocytes with irregular nuclei

and inconspicuous nucleoli surrounded by larger cells with nucleoli and a geographic-like distribution [392]. Both populations are positive for CD20, CD5, and BCL1 (cyclin D1), but larger cells display dimmer CD20 staining, brighter CD5 staining and are positive for Ki-67 and p53.

Immunophenotype
Immunohistochemistry
Phenotypically, typical MCL is CD5+ and CD23−, shows nuclear expression of cyclin D1 (BCL1, ~100%), nuclear expression of SOX11 (100%), and is positive for CD20 and other B-cell markers

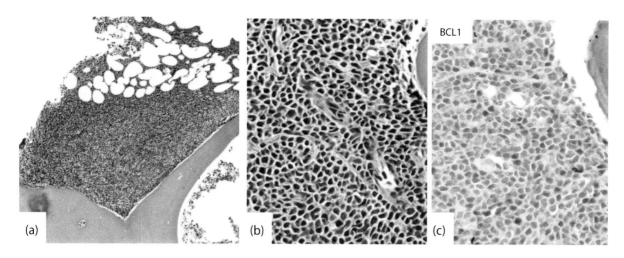

FIGURE 13.71 Mantle cell lymphoma – BM (paratrabecular pattern). (a) Histology of BM core biopsy shows a dense paratrabecular lymphoid infiltrate. (b) Higher magnification displays nuclear contour irregularities. (c) Neoplastic lymphocytes are positive for BCL1.

(BOB1, CD22, CD79, PAX5, OCT2), CD43, and BCL2 without expression of germinal center cell markers (Figure 13.75).

Flow cytometry

FC shows small to intermediate cells based on FSC with moderate expression of CD20 and surface immunoglobulins, positive CD5, negative CD23 and CD200, positive CD81, negative to dim (partial) CD71, and often positive CD38 (Figures 13.76 and 13.77). The expression of CD11c is usually negative. The cells express relatively intense surface IgM/IgD. Occasional cases may display an unusual phenotype such as lack of CD5 (Figure 13.78), aberrant expression of CD10 (Figure 13.79) or aberrant expression of CD23

(Figure 13.80). CD23⁺ MCL is associated with better outcome when compared to typical CD23⁻ MCL. With 57-month median follow-up, the 4-year event-free and overall survival rates for CD23⁺ MCLs were 45% and 75%, respectively, compared to 19% and 51% for CD23⁻ MCL [393]. Blastoid and pleomorphic variants of MCL show increased FSC and are often CD71⁺ (Figures 13.81 and 13.82).

SOX11⁻ MCL. Compared with patients with SOX11⁺ MCL, SOX11⁻ MCL is characterized by more frequent leukemic non-nodal disease, classic morphology, more frequent expression of CD23 and CD200, and a lower Ki67 index [394]. CD10 and/or BCL6 expression has been reported in subset of MCL (10%–12%) [395, 396]. 35% of MCL cases express MUM1, more often in cases

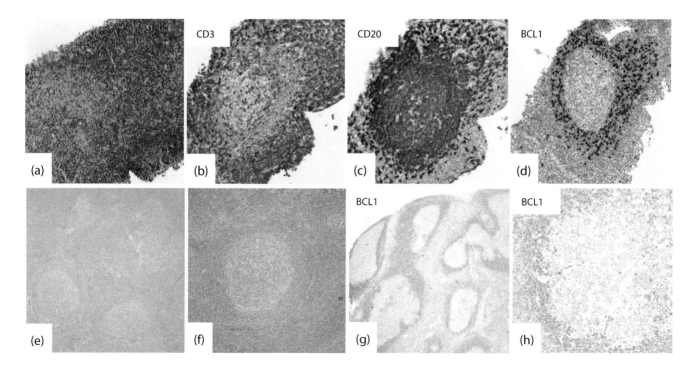

FIGURE 13.72 In situ mantle cell neoplasm (two cases). (a–d) Case #1. (a) Histologic section shows "reactive" looking lymphoid infiltrate composed of mostly small cells. (b–d) Immunohistochemistry shows CD3⁺ (b), CD20⁺ (c), and BCL1⁺ (d) subtle infiltrate around reactive germinal center. (e–h) Case #2. (e–f) Histologic section (low and higher magnification) shows lymph node with reactive follicles. Staining with BCL1 (cyclin D1; g–h) helps to differentiate between reactive follicular hyperplasia and early MCL.

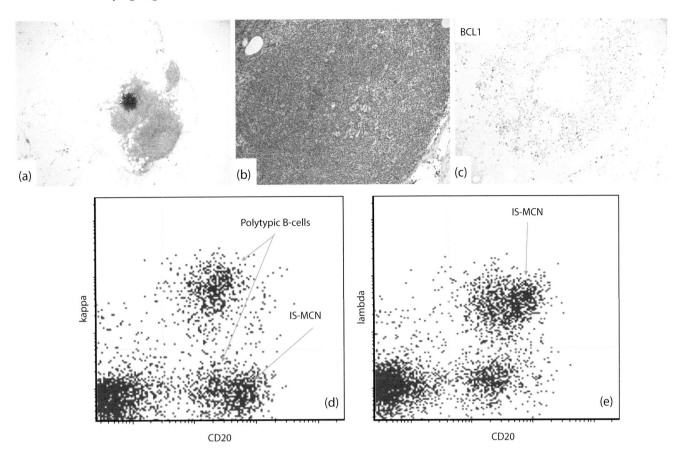

FIGURE 13.73 In situ mantle cell neoplasm (lymph node). (a) Minute fragment of lymph node (H&E section, ×20; with reactive germinal centers (b, H&E section ×100) and focal infiltrate by BCL1⁺ mantle cells (c); FC analysis (d–e) shows a minute lambda⁺ clonal population with bright CD20 expression in the background of mostly polytypic B-cells.

expressing also BCL6 (67%) [396]. At least one-third of the reported cases of CD10⁺ MCL have been blastoid or pleomorphic variants.

BCL1⁻ MCL. Minor subset of MCL without BCL1 (cyclin D1) expression and *CCND1* rearrangement has been identified, more often in blastoid variant. Genomic profile identical to BCL1⁺ MCL and positive SOX11 staining confirms the diagnosis of MCL.

Genetic features

Cytogenetics and FISH. MCL is characterized by t(11;14) leading to the fusion between *CCND1* on 11q13 and *IGH* on 14q32 [397]. Virtually all cases demonstrate the t(11;14) translocation by using FISH. Many cases of MCL have additional cytogenetic abnormalities and often complex karyotype [398–402]. The most common

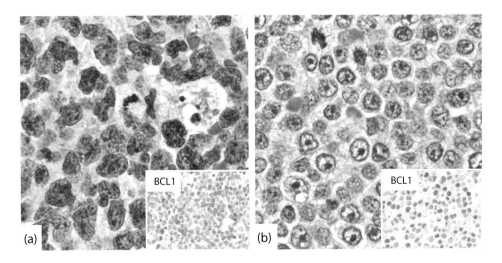

FIGURE 13.74 Aggressive variants of mantle cell lymphoma. (a) Pleomorphic variant of mantle cell lymphoma with irregular nuclei and few inconspicuous nucleoli. (b) Blastoid variant with monomorphic features and prominent nucleoli.

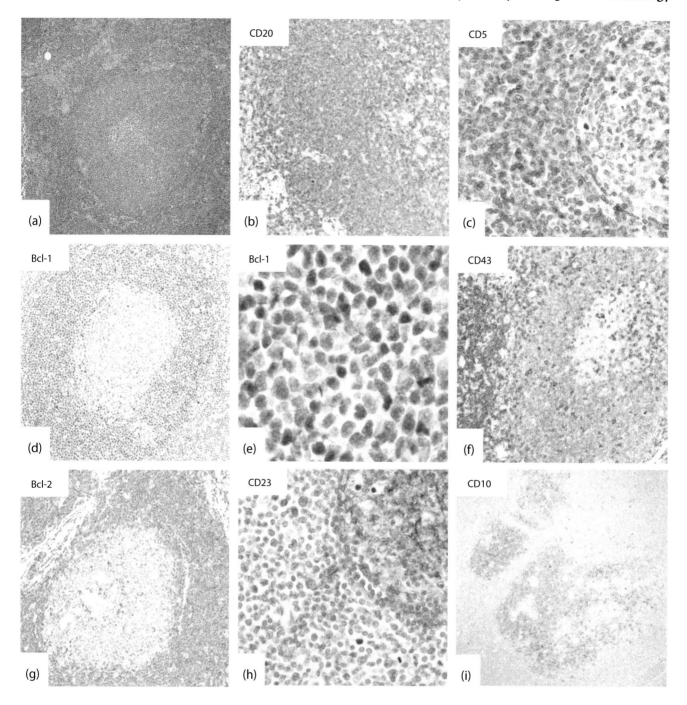

FIGURE 13.75 Mantle cell lymphoma (MCL) with classic mantle zone pattern. Neoplastic B-cells surround benign (residual) germinal center (a; H&E section). Lymphomatous cells express CD20 (b), CD5 (c), BCL1 (d–e, low and high magnification), CD43 (f), and BCL2 (g), and are negative for CD23 (h) and CD10 (i).

cytogenetic aberrations in MCL include 13q14 deletion, followed by 17p deletion and +12. In a series reported by Perry-Jones et al., 81% cases had at least one abnormality in addition to t(11;14) [402]. Trisomy 12 and deletions at 6q21 and 13q14 are associated with poorer prognosis [402, 403]. Cases with *TP53* deletion are more likely to have splenomegaly and marked leukocytosis (>30 × 10⁹/L) and less likely adenopathy than those without deletion and cases with deletions at 11q23 and 6q21 are associated with extranodal disease [402]. Complex karyotype is associated with

poor prognosis [404]. Although both leukemic and nodal MCL show similar genomic patterns of losses (involving 6q, 11q22-q23, 13q14, and 17p13) and gains (affecting 3q and 8q), genomic loss of chromosome 8p occurs more frequently in patients with leukemic disease (79% versus 11%) [405].

Next gene sequencing (NGS). The most frequently mutated genes in MCL at the time of diagnosis include *ATM* (~43%), *TP53* (~27%), *CDKN2A* (~24%), *CCND1* (~20%), *NSD2* (~15%), *KMT2A* (~9%), *S1PR1* (~8%), and *CARD11* (~8%) [406]. When comparing the

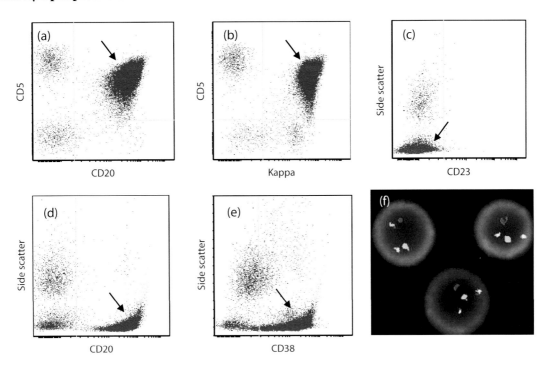

FIGURE 13.76 Mantle cell lymphoma – flow cytometry (blood). Lymphomatous cells display moderate expression of CD20 (a, d) and kappa (b), positive CD5 (a–b), negative CD23 (c), and positive CD38 (e). FISH studies performed on blood sample confirms the diagnosis of MCL by positive rearrangement of *CCND1* (f; yellow fusion signal).

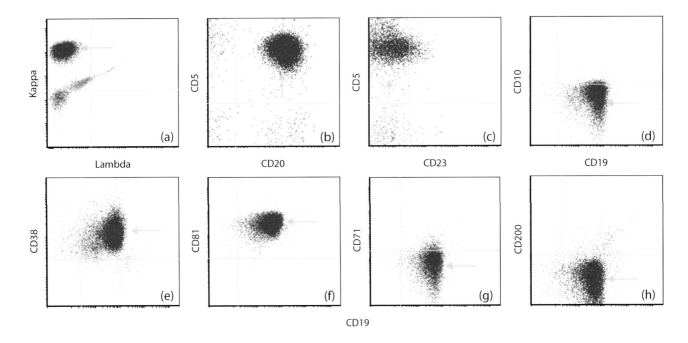

FIGURE 13.77 MCL – typical flow cytometry pattern. MCL is characterized by moderate expression of surface immunoglobulins (a) and CD20 (b), positive CD5 (b–c), negative CD23 (c), negative CD10 (d), positive CD38 (e), positive CD81 (f), negative CD71 (g), and negative CD200 (h).

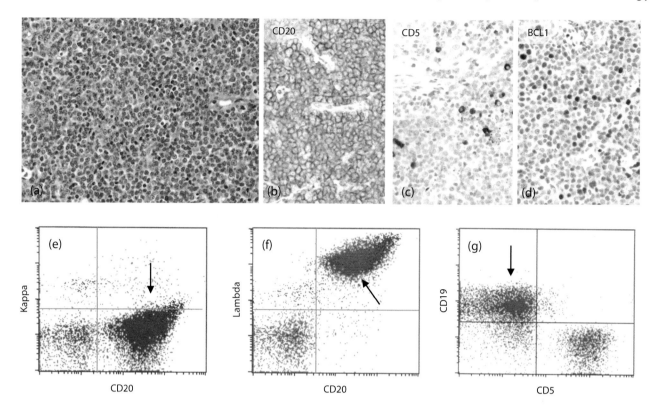

FIGURE 13.78 CD5-negative mantle cell lymphoma (a, histology). Neoplastic cells are positive for CD20 (b) and BCL1 (d); they lack CD5 (c). (e–g) Flow cytometry analysis (e–g) shows positive CD19, CD20 and lambda, and negative CD5. CD5-negative MCL comprise approximately 11% of all MCL cases.

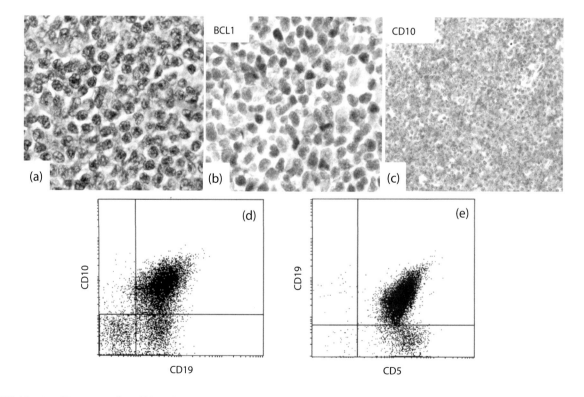

FIGURE 13.79 CD10+ mantle cell lymphoma (MCL). (a) histology; (b–c) immunohistochemistry; (d–e) flow cytometry. MCL cells express BCL1 (b) and co-express CD5 and CD10 (c–e).

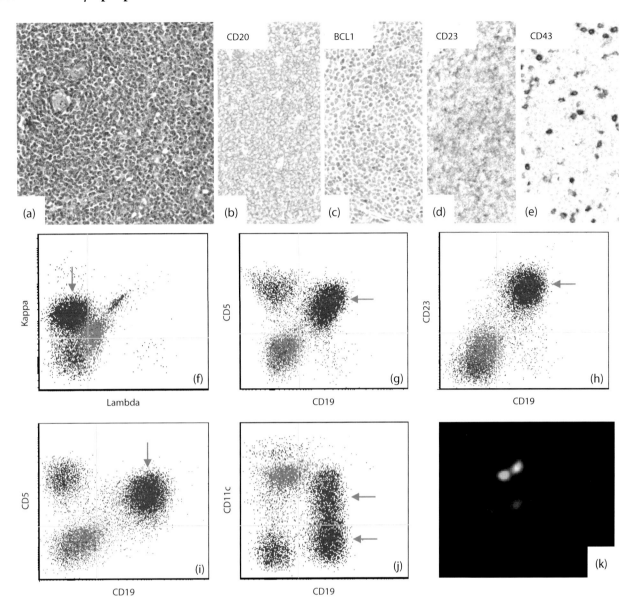

FIGURE 13.80 Mantle cell lymphoma with aberrant CD23 expression (two cases). (a–e) Spleen. Histology shows atypical lymphoid infiltrate (a). (b–e) Immunohistochemistry. Lymphomatous cells express CD20 (b), BCL1 (c), and CD23 (d) and are negative for CD43 (e). (f–k) Blood. Flow cytometry analysis shows kappa restriction (f), co-expression of CD19 with CD5 and CD23 (g–i), and partial expression of CD11c (j). (k) FISH analysis shows *IGH/CCND1* rearrangement: one green (*IGH*), one orange (*CCND1*) and one yellow fusion signal.

mutational status at diagnosis (baseline) and at disease progression, Hill et al. noted the highest mutational frequency difference (>5%) in the following genes: *TP53, ATM, KMT2A, MAP3K14, BTK, TRAF2, CHD2, TLR2, ARID2, RIMS2, NOTCH2, TET2, SPEN, NSD2, CARD11, CCND1, SP14, CDKN2A,* and *S1PR1* [406].

Differential diagnosis of MCL

Differential diagnosis of MCL based on CD5 expression:

- SLL/CLL
- MBL with CLL-like phenotype
- MBL with atypical CLL-like phenotype
- De novo CD5⁺ DLBCL
- SBLPN

- MZL with aberrant CD5 expression
- SMZL with aberrant CD5 expression
- LPL/WM with aberrant CD5 expression
- FL with aberrant CD5 expression (very rare cases)
- HCL with aberrant CD5 expression (very rare cases)

Differential diagnosis of MCL based on CD5 and CD10 co-expression:

- AITL
- Peripheral T-cell lymphoma with follicular T-helper phenotype (PTCL-TFH)
- FTCL
- FL, rare cases
- DLBCL, rare cases

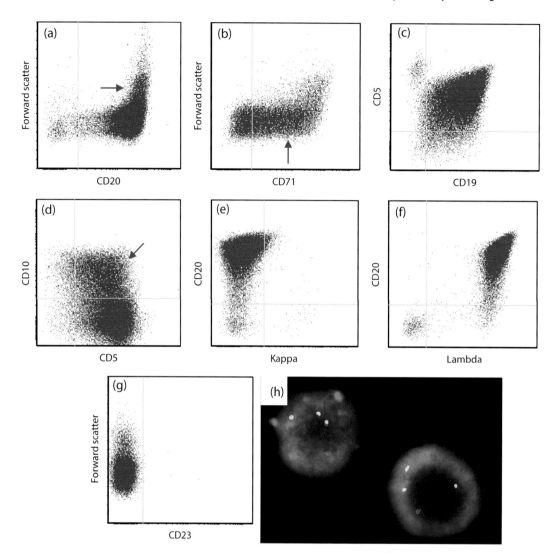

FIGURE 13.81 Blastoid variant of MCL – flow cytometry and FISH studies. Lymphomatous cells have increased forward scatter (a, arrow). They are positive for CD20 (a), partially CD71 (b, arrow), CD5 (c–d), partially CD10 (d; arrow), lambda (e–f) and are negative for CD23 (g). FISH studies (h) showed rearrangement of *CCND1* (red) and *IGH* (green) giving yellow fusion signals.

Differential diagnosis of leukemic non-nodal MCL (L-NN-MCL):

- MBL with CLL-like phenotype
- MBL with atypical CLL-like phenotype
- MCL (classic type in leukemic phase)
- SBLPN
- MZL with aberrant CD5 expression
- SMZL with aberrant CD5 expression

Occasional cases of MCL (both classic type and L-NN-MCL) present with marked lymphocytosis imitating prolymphocytes or acute leukemias. Majority of cases with numerous prolymphocytes in blood represent MCL with leukemic blood involvement. CLL and MBL with CLL-like phenotype most often show dim expression of CD20 and surface light chain immunoglobulins, as well as co-expression of CD5 with CD23. Other B-cell lymphoprolifera-tions usually lack CD5 expression, but occasional cases of MZL, SMZL or even LPL/WM may be CD5+. FISH studies for *CCND1*

rearrangement are usually necessary to differentiate MCL from other B-cell lymphoproliferations, as both MCL and other B-cell process may show phenotypic overlap (e.g., lack of CD5 in MCL, positive CD23 in MCL, presence of CD5 in MZL, SMZL, and LPL/ WM). Acute leukemias can be easily differentiated from MCL by FC analysis showing expression of CD19, CD22, CD10, TdT and CD34 (B-ALL), CD2, cytoplasmic CD3, CD7, CD34, TdT and occa-sionally also CD1a (T-ALL), CD34, CD117, CD133. CD13, CD33, and MPO (AML) or CD4, CD56, and CD123 (blastic plasmacytoid dendritic cell neoplasm, BPDCN). Tables 12.1 and 12.2 in Chapter 12 summarize flow cytometric features of major types of B-cell lymphoproliferative disorders.

Small lymphocytic lymphoma/chronic lymphocytic leukemia (SLL/CLL)

SLL is characterized by proliferation centers and predominance of small round lymphoid cells mixed with occasional prolymphocytes and paraimmunoblasts. In contrast to MCL, majority of SLL show dim expression of surface light chain immunoglobulin and CD20

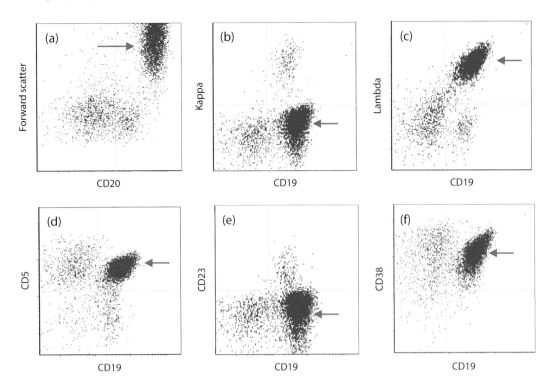

FIGURE 13.82 Large cell (pleomorphic) variant of mantle cell lymphoma involving lung. The lymphomatous cells (blue dots; blue arrow) show high forward scatter (a), bright CD20 expression (a), moderate CD19 (b–f), moderate lambda (c), positive CD5 (d), negative CD23 (e), and positive CD38 (f).

and positive CD23. They lack BCL1 expression, although positive expression BCL1 without t(11;14)/CCND1 rearrangement has been reported in expanded proliferation centers in some SLL cases [11]. Subset of MCL may display aberrant phenotype, including lack of CD5, positive CD10 and/or positive CD23 expression. In all cases of CD23+ MCL, CD23 expression is dim or partial, unlike moderate to bright CD23 expression observed in SLL/CLL. Patients with CD23+ MCL often have an elevated leukocyte count, BM involvement, stage 4 disease, and a leukemic presentation [215]. CD23+ MCL is also more often positive for CD200 (17% versus 4.6%) and less commonly positive for SOX11 when compared to CD23− MCL [215].

Figure 12.2 (Chapter 12) and Table 13.1 summarize the major phenotypic differences between CLL and MCL. CLL is characterized by dim expression of CD20, dim expression of surface light chain immunoglobulins (occasional cases may be kappa and lambda negative), co-expression of CD5 with CD23, often positive CD11c, negative or dimly positive CD81 and positive CD200, while MCL shows moderate expression of CD20 and surface light chain immunoglobulins, lack of CD23 and CD11c, positive CD38, negative CD200, and bright expression of CD81. Figure 13.83 compares the phenotype of CD23+ MCL with CLL. Presence of BCL1 and/or SOX11 expression by immunohistochemistry or CCND1 rearrangement by FISH studies helps to establish the diagnosis of MCL with an unusual phenotype. FC scoring systems used to differentiate CLL, atypical CLL, MCL, and other low-grade B-cell lymphoproliferations are discussed at the beginning of this chapter (CLL, differential diagnosis).

Monoclonal B-cell lymphocytosis (MBL) with CLL-like or atypical CLL-like phenotype

MBL is defined by presence of low numbers (<5 × 10⁹/L) of circulating monoclonal B-cells in otherwise healthy (asymptomatic) subjects (with no evidence of CLL/other lymphoproliferative disorders, adenopathy or organomegaly). MBL with CLL-like phenotype shows phenotypic characteristics of CLL with dim expression of CD20 and surface light chain immunoglobulins, co-expression of CD5, CD23, CD200, and often CD11c. MBL with atypical CLL-like phenotype may resemble phenotypically either MCL or other B-cell lymphoproliferations with aberrant CD5 expression. Identification of CCND1 rearrangement by FISH studies helps to confirm the diagnosis of MCL or L-NN-MCL.

Marginal zone lymphoma (MZL)

Rare cases of MCL from lymph nodes and extranodal sites (gastrointestinal tract, salivary gland, spleen, other) may show unusual monocytoid appearance mimicking MZL (MALT lymphoma). In spleen, MCL may even show typical for SMZL biphasic pattern with smaller lymphocytes in the white pulp and larger lymphocytes with more abundant cytoplasm ("monocytoid" cells) at the periphery. In contrast to MZL, MCL is most often CD5 positive and shows BCL1 and/or SOX11 expression. The phenotype of MZL and SMZL with aberrant CD5 expression may overlap with MCL when analyzed by FC. Positive CD11c, dim CD81, positive CD200 and lack of CD38 and CD43 would favor MZL or SMZL, but often FISH studies for CCND1 are needed for final subclassification, especially if morphologic tissue is not available for histologic and immunohistochemical analysis.

Follicular lymphoma (FL)

FL are CD5−, CD10+, BCL6+ and do not express BCL1. Both FL and MCL may present with leukemic blood involvement with overlapping cytologic features (Figure 13.84). Approximately 10% of MCL is CD10+ and very rare cases of FL may be CD5+. FC (CD5

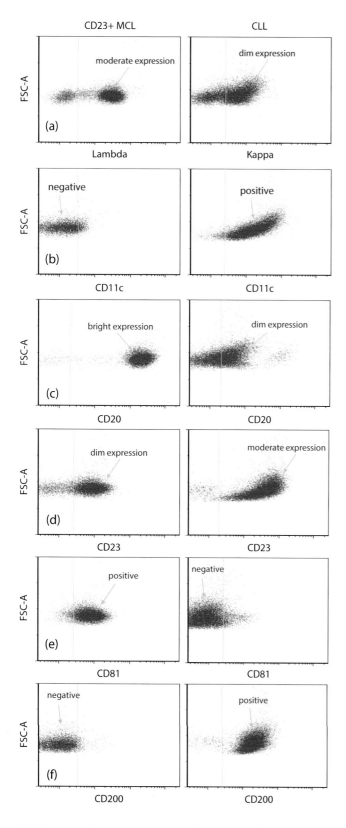

FIGURE 13.83 Flow cytometry features of CD23⁺ MCL and CLL. MCL differs from CLL by stronger expression of surface immunoglobulins (a), lack of CD11c (b), bright expression of CD20 (c), positive CD81 (e), and lack of CD200 (f). Only minor subset of MCL shows CD23 expression imitating CLL (d).

versus CD10 expression), immunohistochemical staining for BCL1 (cyclin D1) and SOX11, and genetic studies (*CCND1* versus *BCL2* rearrangement) help to reach correct diagnosis.

Hairy cell leukemia (HCL)

MCL composed of medium sized cells with abundant pale cytoplasm with irregular cytoplasmic borders may resemble cytologically MZL or HCL. Rare cases of HCL may display aberrant expression of CD5. HCL can be diagnosed by FC by characteristic bright CD11c and co-expression of CD25, CD103, CD123, and CD200 (MCL is most often negative for CD11c and does not express CD103, CD123, and CD200).

Splenic B-cell lymphoma/leukemia with prominent nucleoli (SBLPN)

SBLPN is associated with lymphocytosis and characteristic cytologic features of leukemic cells showing prominent central nucleolus. Phenotypically they are often CD5⁻, but subset of cases may be CD5⁺ with or without CD23 expression. In contrast to MCL, SBLPN show negative or dim CD81, positive CD200 (most cases) brighter expression of CD79b, and infrequent CD43 expression. There is no BCL1 or SOX11 expression by immunohistochemistry or t(11;14) [cases with t(11;14)/*IGH-CCND1* rearrangements are classified as leukemic variant of MCL].

T-cell prolymphocytic leukemia (T-PLL) and other mature T-cell lymphomas

Mature T-cell lymphoproliferations including T-PLL apart from CD5 expression are positive for other pan T-cell antigens (CD2, CD3, and/or CD7) and are either CD4⁺ or CD8⁺ (some tumors may be dual CD4/CD8⁻).

T-cell lymphomas with CD10 expression

Subset of MCL shows co-expression of CD5 and CD10, which is also seen in T-cell lymphomas with follicular T-helper phenotype (TFH), including AITL, FTCL, and PTCL-TFH. Lack of B-cell markers and positive expression of surface or cytoplasmic CD3 indicate T-cell process.

Diffuse large B-cell lymphoma (DLBCL)

DLBCL are most often CD5⁻, and may be positive for CD10, BCL6, and/or MUM1. DLBCL with CD5 expression represents either de novo CD5⁺ DLBCL or Richter's syndrome. Lack of BCL1 (cyclin D) or SOX11 allows to exclude CD5⁻ and CD5⁺ DLBCL from blastoid or pleomorphic variant of MCL.

Burkitt lymphoma (BL) and high-grade B-cell lymphomas (HGBLs)

BL shows co-expression of CD10, BCL6, and MYC, high Ki-67 index (close to 100%) and lacks CD5 and BCL1 expression. HGBLs are subdivided into HGBL with *MYC* and *BCL2* (and/or *BCL6*) rearrangement (HGBL-R) and HGBL, not otherwise specified. (HGBL, NOS). Their differential diagnosis is presented in Chapter 12 (Figure 12.8) and further in this chapter in sections "Burkitt lymphoma" and "High grade B-cell lymphomas".

Extramedullary myeloid tumor (EMT)

Acute leukemic infiltrate outside BM (EMT) shows blastic cytomorphology with expression of blastic markers (CD34/CD117/CD133) and myeloid markers (CD13, CD33, MPO) or monocytic markers (CD14, CD64, CD68, and/or muramidase). Monoblastic leukemias are often CD56⁺.

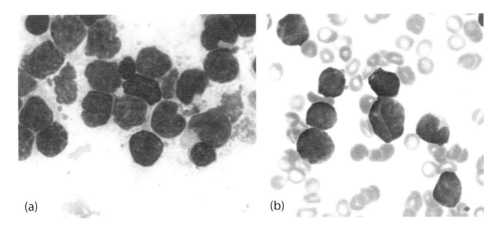

FIGURE 13.84 Cytologic features of mantle cell lymphoma (a) and follicular lymphoma (b) in blood smear.

Blastic plasmacytoid dendritic cell neoplasm (BPDCN)

BPDCN has characteristic phenotype: CD4[+], CD56[+], and CD123[+]. It usually presents with skin lesion with progression to leukemic blood and BM involvement. B-cell markers are negative.

Precursor B- and T-cell acute lymphoblastic leukemia/lymphoma (B-ALL/LBL, T-ALL/LBL)

Some cases of MCL with leukemic blood involvement show blastic feature mimicking cytologically ALL. Precursor neoplasms are positive for blastic markers (CD34 and/or TdT). B-ALL/LBLs are positive for CD19 and often shows bright expression of CD10. T-ALL/LBLs are positive for pan T-cell markers (especially CD7), often lack surface CD3 (when analyzed by FC) and show either dual CD4/CD8 positive or dual CD4/CD8 negative expression.

Plasma cell myeloma (PCM)

PCM or plasmacytomas are positive for CD138 and MUM1, negative for CD5, and in most cases also negative for CD19, CD20, PAX5, CD81, and CD45. Subset of PCMs may express CD56 (70%–80%), CD200 (60%–70%), and/or CD117 (30%). MCLs are positive for CD19, CD20, CD5, CD81, and CD45 and negative for CD200, CD56, and CD117. FC analysis shows presence of clonal B-cell population expressing surface kappa or lambda immunoglobulins in MCL (plasma cells are positive for cytoplasmic light chain immunoglobulins). In BM sample, evaluation of aspirate smears often helps to differentiate between PCM and MCL, but subset of cases may show overlapping cytologic features between those two entities (e.g., lymphoid appearance of plasma cells or plasmacytoid appearance of MCL).

Diffuse large B-cell lymphoma (DLBCL)

DLBCL phenotype by FC: FSC[high], sIg[+/rarely−], CD5[−/rarely+], CD10[+/−], BCL2[+/rarely−], CD11c[−/rarely+], CD19[+], CD20[+], CD22[+], CD23[−], CD25[−], CD34[−], CD38[+], CD43[−/rarely+], CD45[+], CD71[+], CD79b[+], CD81[−/dim+], CD103[−], CD200[−/rarely+]

Introduction

DLBCL is the most common type of lymphoma, with an annual US incidence of >25,000 cases (it accounts for approximately one third of the total number of adult non-Hodgkin lymphoma

patients). DLBCL may occur in nodal and extranodal sites and is characterized by a marked degree of morphologic, genetic, and clinical heterogeneity [1, 407–413]. WHO classification divides DLBCL into several morphologic and clinical variants (Figure 13.85): DLBCL, not otherwise specified (centroblastic, immunoblastic, and anaplastic variants), T-cell/histiocyte-rich large B-cell lymphoma (THRLBL), primary large B-cell lymphoma of CNS, EBV[+] DLBCL, and primary cutaneous large B-cell lymphoma, leg type (C-DLBCL-LT), with the centroblastic variant being the most frequent type (>80%). Other lymphomas of large B-cells include primary mediastinal large B-cell lymphoma (PMBL), intravascular large B-cell lymphoma (IVLBCL), lymphomatoid granulomatosis (LyG), ALK[+] large B-cell lymphoma, PBL, large B-cell lymphoma arising in HHV8-associated multicentric Castleman's disease and primary effusion lymphoma (PEL). Majority of DLBCL are positive for CD45 and B-cell markers (CD19, CD20, CD22, CD79a, and PAX5). Subset of DLBCL expresses CD5 (de novo CD5[+] DLBCL).

Based on the gene expression profiling, DLBCL is be subdivided into germinal center B-cell-like (GCB), activated B-cell-like (ABC), and PMBL [414–416]. The prognosis is worse for patients with ABC-like DLBCL than for those with GCB-like subtype when treated with conventional chemotherapy. Surrogates of the molecular markers have been developed using immunohistochemistry (Figure 13.86), including algorithms proposed by Hans et al. (CD10, BCL6, and MUM1/IRF4), Muris et al. (CD10, MUM1/IRF4, and BCL2), Colomo et al. (MUM1/IRF4, CD10, and BCL6), Tally (CD10, GCET1, MUM1, and FOXP1), Visco-Young (CD10, FOXP1, BCL6), and Choi et al. (GCET1, MUM1/IRF4, CD10, FOXP1, and BCL6) [417–421]. Review of several immunohistochemical algorithms by Hwang et al., showed excellent concordance of Hans, Choi, and Visco-Young algorithms which could reliably separate GCB-like from non-GCB-like DLBCL [422]. An algorithm proposed by Choi correlated with the genetic expression profiling classification with 93% concordance and showed its prognostic relevance (3-year survival of 87% for GCB-like DLBCL and 44% for ABC-like DLBCL) [417]. Based on the algorithm proposed by Hans, the 5-year overall survival for GCB-like group was 75% compared with only 34% for ABC-like group [418].

Morphology
Lymph nodes

DLBCL is composed of sheets of medium-sized to large cells displaying centroblastic, immunoblastic and less often "anaplastic"

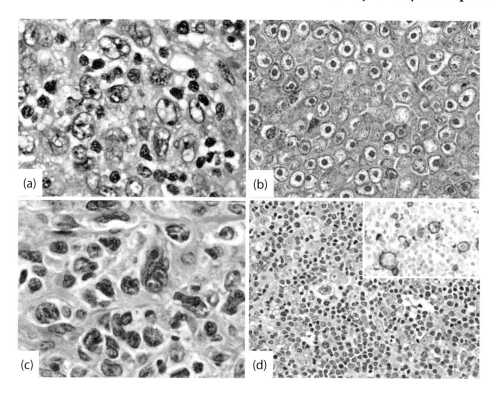

FIGURE 13.85 DLBCL: centroblastic (a), immunoblastic (b), anaplastic (c), and T-cell-rich (d; *inset*: CD20 immunostaining showing scattered large B-cells).

cytomorphology. Many cases show mixture of centroblasts and immunoblasts.

DLBCL, centroblastic. DLBCL with centroblastic morphology (centroblastic variant; Figure 13.87) is a most common variant. It is composed of medium-sized to large cells with vesicular nuclei, irregular (clumped) chromatin, and several nucleoli located at the periphery close to the nuclear membrane, often antiparallel to the long axis of the cell. The nuclei may be irregular. Centroblasts (and large cell variants of centrocytes) comprise the majority of the total cell population. The cytoplasm is either amphophilic or basophilic. Centroblastic variant of DLBCL is usually of germinal center-B-cell-like subtype with neoplastic cells being positive for CD45, B-cell markers and often BCL6 and CD10.

DLBCL, immunoblastic. The immunoblasts, based on classical definition given by Lennert and Feller, are large blastic cells with small to medium-sized rim of basophilic/amphophilic cytoplasm, large nuclei with fine chromatin and a prominent singular central nucleolus [423]. DLBCL with immunoblastic morphology (immunoblastic variant; Figure 13.88) is comprised of predominantly of immunoblasts (>90%), but many cases show also variable (occasionally significant) population of cells with plasmacytoid or plasmablastic features. Those cells are smaller than immunoblasts, have more abundant and deeper basophilic cytoplasm and an eccentric nucleus. In contrast to centroblastic lymphoma, typical centroblasts and large cell variants of centrocytes (large cells with irregular nuclei) comprise <10% of the entire infiltrate. Neoplastic cells (both immunoblasts and plasmablastic/plasmacytoid cells) are strongly positive for CD45 and B-cell markers (including CD20), and are negative for TdT, CD34, CD138, CD56, EMA, and BCL1 (cyclin D1). Typical PBLs are CD20⁻.

DLBCL, anaplastic. Anaplastic variant of DLBCL shows marked pleomorphism of tumor cells which may resemble Hodgkin cells, Reed-Sternberg cells, carcinoma cells, or hallmark cells of anaplastic

large T-cell lymphoma (ALCL). Large B-cells tend to form cohesive clusters with characteristic intrasinusoidal distribution. Neoplastic cells are positive for at least some B-cell markers and are negative for cytokeratin, EMA, ALK, S100, pan-T antigens, and CD15. CD45 may be negative, and many cases are CD30⁺. The term ALCL is restricted to large T-cell lymphoma, which is unrelated to the anaplastic variant of DLBCL (*see* Chapter 24). Anaplastic features may be also present in CD30⁺ DLBCL with THRLBL features and gray zone lymphoma (GZL) with features intermediate between cHL and DLBCL.

T-cell/histiocyte-rich large B-cell lymphoma

THRLBL is a rare variant of DLBCL composed of scattered large B-cells and a predominance of reactive elements, such as small T-cells and histiocytes [1]. Neoplastic large B-cells represent a minority of the neoplasm (up to 10%), usually as single cells that do not form aggregates or sheets. The background is composed of reactive T lymphocytes and histiocytes with very few small reactive B lymphocytes. THRLBL affects lymph nodes with frequent involvement of BM, spleen, and liver. THRLBL is uncommon and represents <5% of DLBCLs. Liver, BM, and spleen are more often involved than in typical DLBCL. More than half of the patients present with an advanced stage disease. Patients respond poorly to therapy and overall survival at 3 years ranges from 46% to 72%.

The lymph node architecture is completely disrupted, although some cases may show vague nodularity (Figure 13.89). Scattered large neoplastic cells are surrounded by a prominent pleomorphic inflammatory background. The neoplastic B-cells do not form aggregates or solid sheets and are rather haphazardly distributed. According to WHO classification, this lymphoma is morphologically characterized by <10% of large neoplastic B-cells in a background of abundant host T-cells and frequently (non-epithelioid) histiocytes. Lymphoma cells may resemble centroblasts, immunoblasts, LP cells (lymphocyte predominant cells), or Hodgkin

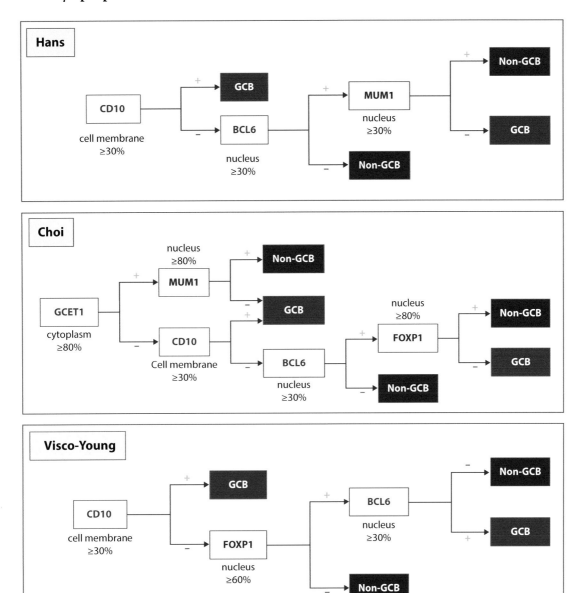

FIGURE 13.86 Immunophenotypic algorithms for subclassification of DLBCL.

cell (Reed-Sternberg cells). T lymphocyte rosettes around tumor cells, typical for NLPHL, are absent.

Bone marrow

Approximately 10%–25% of patients with DLBCL present with BM involvement at the time of initial diagnosis. BM involvement may be concordant (both primary site and BM shows DLBCL) or discordant in which BM shows involvement by a low-grade lymphoma. The patterns of involvement differ, ranging from interstitial, nodular, paratrabecular, or diffuse. Some studies have shown that patients with DLBCL and concordant BM involvement have an inferior overall survival compared with those with discordant BM involvement.

Immunophenotype

DLBCLs usually express CD45 and pan-B-cell antigens, such as CD19, CD20, CD22, CD79a, BOB1, OCT2, and PAX5. Terminally differentiated DLBCL such as immunoblastic or PBLs and DLBCL treated with anti-CD20 antibodies (Rituximab) may lack the expression of CD20. Expression of BCL2, a protein involved in control of apoptosis, is observed in 40%–50% of DLBCL. DLBCL with negative BCL2 and positive CD10, BCL6, and CD43 need to be differentiated form BL, and DLBCL with strong expression of both BCL2 and CD10 needs to be differentiated from HGBL with rearrangement of *MYC* and *BCL2* (HGBL-R, double hit lymphoma). BCL6 and CD10, stage specific markers of germinal center cell differentiation, are expressed by subset of DLBCL (BCL6

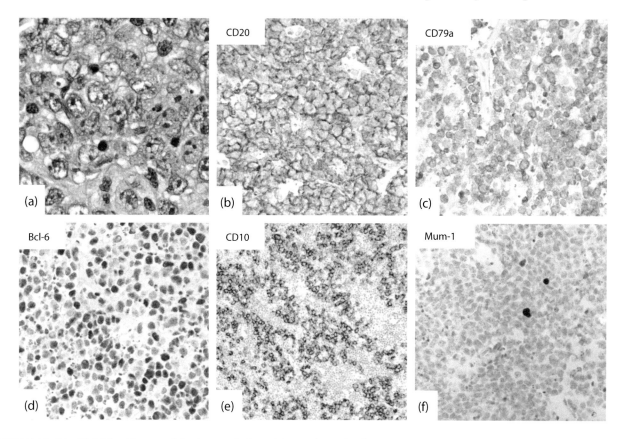

FIGURE 13.87   DLBCL with centroblastic morphology. (a) Histology; (b–f) Immunohistochemistry. Lymphomatous cells express CD20 (b), CD79a (b), BCL6 (d), CD10 (e), and are negative for MUM1 (f).

in ~60% and CD10 in ~40%). CD30 is expressed in 14%–21% of DLBCL and is associated with unique gene expression profiling, non-germinal-center origin and favorable prognosis [424, 425]. Both PMBL and anaplastic variant of DLBCL are often CD30$^+$. MUM1 is expressed by ~40% of cases. A small subset of DLBCL (<10%) expresses CD5 (de novo CD5$^+$ DLBCL) or CD43 (20%). De novo CD5$^+$ DLBCL is diagnosed when there is no history of B-CLL/SLL and no evidence of BCL1/t(11;14) (either by immunohistochemistry or cytogenetic/FISH) [426–429]. Rare cases of

DLBCL may show aberrant expression of CD56. They often co-express CD10 [430].

Phenotypic sub-categories. Based on the expression of CD10, BCL6 and MUM1/IRF4, DLBCL can be subdivided by Hans algorithm into germinal center-like (GCB) and non-germinal center-like (non-GCB) subgroups (Figure 13.86) [418]. Cases with CD10 expression by >30% of cells and BCL6$^+$/MUM1$^-$ cases (regardless of CD10 status) are regarded as GCB-like, and all other cases are regarded as non-GCB type [418].

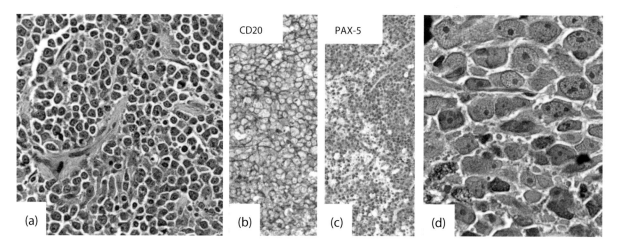

FIGURE 13.88   Diffuse large B-cell lymphoma (DLBCL) – immunoblastic variant. (a) Lymph node with diffuse large cell lymphoid infiltrate. Neoplastic cells are positive for CD20 (b) and PAX5 (c). High magnification shows large monomorphic cells with prominent central nuclcoli (d).

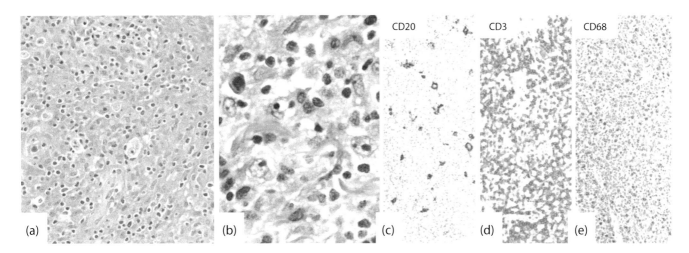

FIGURE 13.89 THRLBL. (a–b) Low and high magnifications show scattered large cells in the background of small lymphocytes and histiocytes. Lymphomatous cells are positive for CD20 (c). T-cells express CD3 (d) and histiocytes express CD68 (e).

Flow cytometry. Due to selective drop-out of neoplastic cells, FC analysis in DLBCL may not detect clonal B-cell population or show predominance of reactive elements and only minor clonal population (Figure 13.90). This false negative FC results are more common in HGBLs and in cases with prominent necrosis. In cases with low number of neoplastic cells (e.g., THRLBL) or DLBCL with prominent fibrosis (e.g., PMBL), FC results are often falsely negative. In successful analysis, FC reveals clonal B-cell population with high FSC and often positive CD38 and CD71 expression (Figure 13.91). Figure 13.92 shows example of DLBCL with GBC-like phenotype and Figure 13.93 shows CD10⁻ DLBCL. High FSC displayed by clonal B-cells helps to differentiate it from low grade FL. Differential diagnosis includes high grade FL, BL, and HGBL-R. The expression of CD19 and CD20 is heterogeneous on FC analysis, but often DLBCL shows strong expression of all B-cell markers and co-expression of CD38 (Figure 13.94). In a series reported by Johnson et al., a total of 43 of 272 (16%) samples had reduced CD20 expression by FC; of these, 35 (13%) had bright CD19 expression. The latter had a markedly inferior survival when treated with cyclophosphamide, doxorubicin, vincristine, and prednisone (CHOP) or rituximab-CHOP (R-CHOP) [431]. Rare cases of DLBCL show aberrant expression of CD7 (Figure 13.95) or very rarely CD3.

Genetic features

Chromosomal aberrations in DLBCL are common (~50%) and often complex. The most frequent chromosomal change involves the *BCL6* gene at 3q27; other translocations involve *MYC* and *BCL2* genes. The chromosomal translocations of 3q27 involving the locus of the *BCL6* gene, are the most characteristic and common genetic abnormalities occurring in 30% to 40%. Approximately 5%–17% of DLBCLs harbor an *MYC* rearrangement [432–434]. Those lymphomas are usually diagnosed in older patients and are often characterized by high proliferation rate (high Ki-67 index) and starry-sky pattern, which may resemble BL. Mutations in the *TP53* gene leading to a functionally defective protein have been detected in about 20% of DLBCL and are associated with drug resistance, shorter disease-free survival, shorter survival and generally a more aggressive clinical course and poor outcome [435]. The p53 is detected in DLBCL in 30%–40% of cases by immunohistochemistry [435]. Patients with extra copies of *MYC*, *BCL2*, and/or *BCL6* (but no rearrangement) have worse prognosis than DLBCL without genetic changes involving *MYC*, *BCL2*, or *BCL6* [436].

Based on molecular studies, DLBCL is divided into GCB, ABC, and molecular high grade (MHG) [411, 414, 437, 438]. DLBCL with GCB signature have higher overall survival compared to

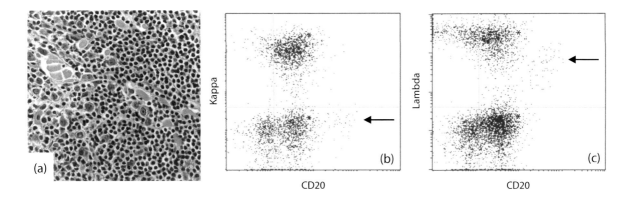

FIGURE 13.90 Large B-cell lymphoma. Tissue section (a) shows atypical large lymphoid cells in the background of small lymphocytes. Flow cytometry (b–c) reveals only rare neoplastic cells (arrow); benign (polytypic) B-cells predominate (*).

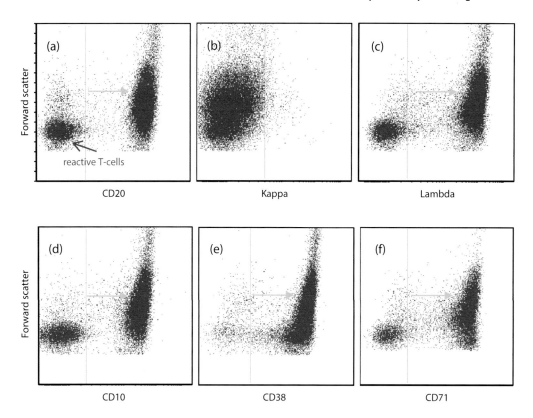

FIGURE 13.91 DLBCL – flow cytometry (lymph node). Neoplastic B-cells show increased forward scatter (a–f, black arrow; compare with residual reactive T-cells, red arrow). Lymphomatous cells express CD20 (a; bright expression), lambda (c), CD10 (d), CD38 (e), and CD71 (f).

patients with DLBCL with ABC or primary mediastinal B-cell lymphoma signature on treatment with CHOP or R-CHOP regimens [414, 415, 439–441]. GCB-DLBCL is characterized by mutations in the apoptosis pathway including BCL2. The GCB group shows t(14;18) translocation, CD10 expression, c-REL amplification and evidence of ongoing somatic hypermutation in the immunoglobulin variable heavy genes (IGVH). The t(14;18) (q32;q21) translocation involving the BCL2 gene and the amplification of the c-REL locus on chromosome 2p have been detected almost exclusively in GCB-like DLBCL. The t(14;18) is present in 45% of GCB-DLBCL and only in 8% of ABC-DLBCL [442]. The ABC subtype of DLBCL remains the least curable form of this malignancy despite recent advances in therapy. Constitutive nuclear factor (NF)-kappa B and JAK kinase signaling promotes malignant cell survival in these lymphomas. Similar function is attributed to L265P mutation in the MYD88 gene, which has been identified recently in 29% of ABC type of DLBCL [443].

In addition to the subtypes of DLBCL based on molecular features, other genes have been implicated in prognosis of DLBCL including c-MYC (proto-oncogene in chromosome 8q24), BCL2 oncogene on chromosome 18q21), BCL6 (transcriptional repressor on chromosome 3q27), MYD88, NOTCH2, and NOTCH1. DLBCLs which show overexpression of MYC and BCL2 (≥40% and >50%, respectively by IHC) are called double expressor lymphomas (DELs) and are associated with an intermediate prognosis to up-front R-CHOP. DEL lymphomas occur primarily in the ABC subtype, whereas double-hit lymphomas with concurrent translocation of MYC and BCL2 are found primarily in GCB subtype.

In addition to the subtypes of DLBCL based on molecular features, other genes have been implicated in prognosis of DLBCL including c-MYC (proto-oncogene in chromosome 8q24), BCL2 oncogene on chromosome 18q21), BCL6 (transcriptional repressor on chromosome 3q27), MYD88, NOTCH2, and NOTCH1. DLBCLs which show overexpression of MYC and BCL2 (≥40% and >50%, respectively by IHC) are called DEL and are associated with an intermediate prognosis to up-front R-CHOP. DEL lymphomas occur primarily in the ABC subtype, whereas double-hit lymphomas with concurrent translocation of MYC and BCL2 are found primarily in GCB subtype.

Genetic subtypes by Schmitz et al. [410]:

- MCD subtype (MYD88 and CD79B mutations)
- BN2 subtype (BCL6 fusions and NOTCH2 mutations)
- N1 subtype (NOTCH1 mutations)
- EZB subtype (EZH2 mutations and BCL2 translocations)

Genetic subtypes by Chapuy et al. [408]:

- C1 subtype (BCL6 translocations with NOTCH 2 or SPEN mutations) [similar to BN2]
- C2 subtype (biallelic inactivation of TP53, 9p21.3/CDKN2A and associated genomic instability)
- C3 subtype (BCL2 translocations and genetic alterations disrupting the epigenetic regulators EZH2, CREBBP, or KMT2D) [similar to EZB]

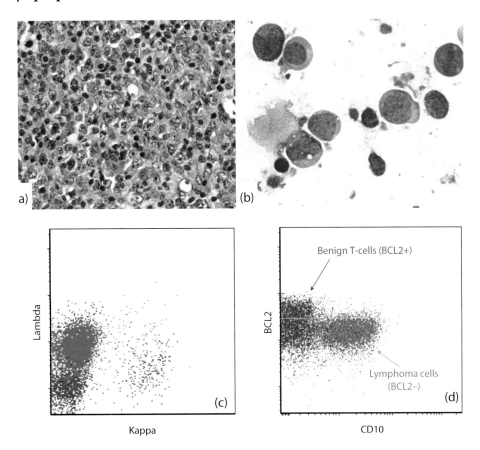

FIGURE 13.92 DLBCL with GCB-like phenotype and negative BCL2. (a) Histomorphology. (b) Touch smear cytology showing large atypical lymphoid cells. (c–d) FC analysis showing clonal lambda⁺ B-cells (c; blue dots) expressing CD10 (d). BCL2 is negative (d). FISH studies in this cases showed only *BCL6* rearrangement (both *MYC* and *BCL2* were negative).

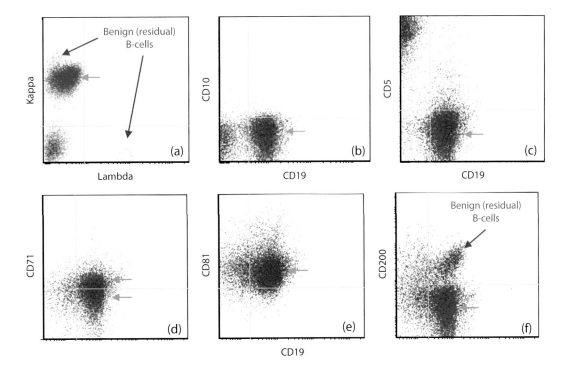

FIGURE 13.93 DLBCL (ABC-like). Clonal B-cells (kappa⁺, a, blue arrow) are negative for CD10 (b) and CD5 (c), show negative to partially dim CD71 (d), dim CD81 (e) and negative CD200 (f). Rare benign (polytypic) B-cells are also noted (red dots, red arrows).

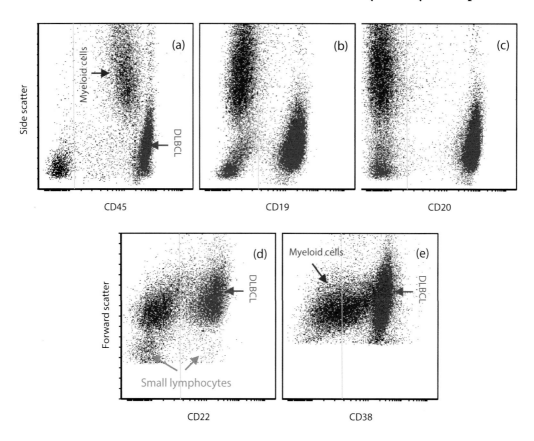

FIGURE 13.94 DLBCL – bone marrow. Lymphomatous cells display bright CD45 (a), moderate CD19 (b), bright CD20 (c), moderate CD22 (d), and moderate CD38 (e). The forward scatter is increased (d–e), being higher than in granulocytes/maturing myeloid precursors (purple dots).

- C4 subtype (alterations in *BCR/PI3K*, *JAK/STAT*, and *BRAF* pathway components and multiple histones)
- C5 subtype (*MYD88* and *CD79B* mutations) [similar to MCD]

Genetic subtypes by Lacy et al. [444]:

- MYD88 subtype (MYD88, PIM1, CD79B, ETV6, CDKN2A mutations)
- BCL2 subtype (BCL2 translocation and EZH2, CREBBP, TNFRSF14, KMT2D mutations)
- SOCS1/SGK1 subtype (SOCS1, CD83, NFKBIA, HIST1H1E mutations)
- TET2/SGK1 subtype (TET2, BRAF, SGK1, ID3 mutations)
- NOTCH2 subtype (NOTCH2, BCL10, TNFAIP3, CCND3, SPEN mutations)
- unclassified subtype/NEC (a default category, containing cases that could not be classified elsewhere and cases with no mutations)

Genetic subtypes by Zhang et al. [445]:

- MYC-trans signature with *MYC* translocation
- BCL2-trans signature with *BCL2* translocation
- BCL6-trans signature with *BCL6* translocation
- MC signature with *MYD88* and/or *CD79B* mutations

Molecular-pathological correlation. The subtypes characterized by genetic alterations of *BCL2*, *NOTCH2*, and *MYD88* showed good, intermediate, and poor prognosis, respectively.

The *SOCS1/SGK1* subtype showed biological overlap with primary mediastinal B-cell lymphoma with excellent prognosis. The impact of *TP53* mutation varied with genomic subtype, conferring no effect in the NOTCH2 subtype and poor prognosis in MYD88 subtype [444]. MYD88 (C5 or MCD) subtype is associated with poor prognosis, ABC-like DLBCL and contains the majority of primary CNS and primary testicular DLBCLs. BCL2 (C3 or EZB) subtype is associated with good prognosis and GCB-type DLBCL. Mutational profile is shared with FL. SOCS1/SGK1 (or C4) subtype is associated with most favorable prognosis, represented predominantly by GCB-like type and shares genetic features with PMBL. TET2/SGK1 is similar to SOCS1/SGK1 but differs by addition of *TET2* and *BRAF* mutations and lack of *SOCS1* and *CD83*. It is associated with favorable prognosis. NOTCH2 (or C1, BN2) subtype is not associated with any cell of origin and shares mutational similarity with MZL.

Differential diagnosis of DLBCL
Marginal zone lymphoma (MZL)
The presence of increased number of large cells is very common in NMZL and may approach up to 50% (without sheet formation) [80, 86]. In contrast to DLBCL, MZL with increased large cells shows majority of B-cells with low FSC, negative CD38 and lack of CD71.

Mantle cell lymphoma (MCL)
Blastoid and pleomorphic variants of MCL mimic DLBCL. Diagnostic difficulties may also arise because subset of MCL may be CD5⁻ or CD10⁺, and subset of DLBCL may be CD5⁺, thus displaying overlapping immunophenotypic profile between

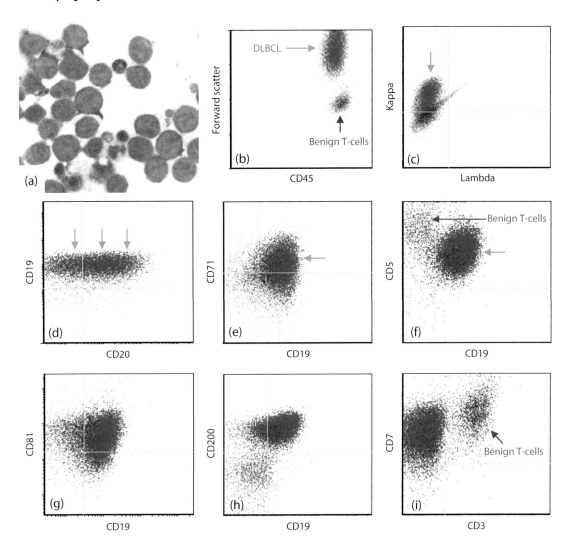

FIGURE 13.95 DLBCL of the testis with aberrant expression of CD5 and CD7. Tumor cells show centroblastic cytomorphology (a, touch imprint). By flow cytometry analysis, they are characterized by high forward scatter (b, blue arrow), bright CD45 expression (b), kappa restriction (c), positive CD19 (d), variable expression of CD20 (d), positive CD71 (e), positive CD5 (f; residual benign T-cells show brighter CD5 expression), positive CD81 (g), and positive CD200 (h). Comparison of CD3 versus CD7 expression shows that clonal B-cells have slightly dimmer expression of CD7 when compared to benign T-cells (i).

those two entities. Correlation with histomorphology, immuno-histochemistry (BCL1, SOX11), and FISH studies (*CCND1* rearrangement) is required to differentiate DLBCL from MCL with overlapping immunophenotypic features (e.g., increased FSC and CD5 expression).

Follicular lymphoma (FL)
Low grade FL shows low FSC and can be easily differentiated from DLBCL. However, high grade FL shows overlapping FC features with DLBCL (CD10 expression, high FSC, CD38 expression, positivity for CD71) and therefore definite subclassification should be established based on histomorphology, immunohistochemistry, and FISH studies.

Burkitt lymphoma (BL)
Subset of DLBCL may share phenotypic features with BL (co-expression of CD10, CD43, and CD71, and lack of BCL2 expression). Bright expression of CD10, CD38, and CD81, dim CD79b, lack of BCL2 and positive CD43 favor BL over DLBCL. When compared to BL, DLBCL usually displays dimmer CD10 and CD38, dim or negative CD81, negative CD43 and is often BCL2+. The expression of CD71 is positive in both BL and DLBCL and may be very high in some cases of DLBCL (Figure 13.96, see also Figure 10.8 in Chapter 10), while is usually dim or variable in BL. The majority of BL shows bright expression of CD38 (82%), whereas only 17% of *MYC*- DLBCL show bright CD38 [446]. FSC is higher in DLBCL than in BL. The final subclassification requires correlation with histomorphology and FISH analysis (including *BCL2*, *BCL6*, and *MYC* probes).

High grade B-cell lymphoma with MYC and BCL2 rearrangement (HGBL-R)
HGBL-R shows strong expression of B-cell markers and surface light chain immunoglobulins and often bright CD10 and BCL2 expression. Minor subset of HGBL-R may be CD10-. The expression of CD38 and CD81 is often brighter in HGBL-R than in DLBCL. Analysis of CD43, CD71, and CD200 is often not helpful in differential diagnosis between those two lymphomas as the

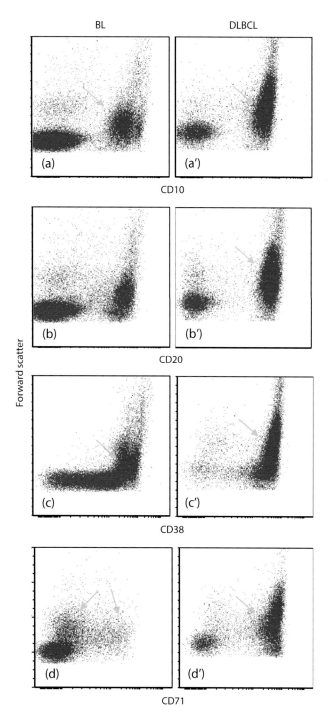

FIGURE 13.96 Comparison of FC analysis of BL (left column) and DLBCL (GCB-like; right column). When compared to BL, DLBCL differs by higher forward scatter (a–d; a'–d'). Both BL and DLBCL with germinal center B-cell phenotype express CD10 (a, a'), CD20 (b–b') and CD38 (c–c'). The expression of CD71 is brighter in DLBCL than in BL (d–d').

frequency of expression and its intensity is variable. Because of the overlapping immunophenotypic features between DLBCL, MCL (blastoid and pleomorphic variants), BL, and HGBL-R it is necessary to correlate with histomorphology and FISH studies (*MYC, BCL2, CCND1,* and *BCL6* rearrangements) for final sub-classification in all large B-cell lymphomas identified by FC.

Plasmablastic lymphoma (PBL)

PBL is characterized by diffuse proliferation of large cells with plasmablastic, immunoblastic and/or plasmacytic features. PBLs are most often CD20⁻ and usually positive for plasma cell markers (CD38, CD138), often with aberrant CD56 expression.

Specific variants of DLBCL

Variants of DLBCL include CD5⁺ DLBCL, T-cell/histiocyte rich large B-cell lymphoma (THRLBL); ALK⁺ large B-cell lymphoma; PBL; IVLBCL; large B-cell lymphoma with IRF4 rearrangement; PMBL; primary cutaneous DLBCL, leg type; primary DLBCL of the CNS; DLBCL associated with chronic inflammation; LyG; PEL; HHV8⁺ DLBCL, EBV⁺ DLBCL, and EBV⁺ mucocutaneous ulcer [1, 407].

De novo CD5⁺ diffuse large B-cell lymphoma

CD5 is a pan-T-cell marker (a cell surface glycoprotein) expressed by T-cells, naïve B-cells, and certain B-cell lymphomas, mainly SLL/CL and MCL. It is also present in de novo CD5⁺ DLBCL. Other T-cell markers are rarely expressed by B-cell lymphomas. Among 501 B-cell lymphoma cases analyzed by Tsuyama et al., 92 cases were positive for T-cell marker(s), including DLBCL (23%), MCL (100%), CLL (100%), MZL (5%), IVLBCL (100%), FL (0.7%), and low grade lymphoma unclassifiable (21%) [447]. Apart from CD5, other T-cell markers (CD2, CD4, CD7, and CD8) are only rarely expressed by DLBCL (5%) [447]. De novo CD5⁺ DLBCL is known to have phenotypically and genotypically different characteristics than CD5⁻ DLBCL. Its reported frequency is from 5% to 22% [426–429, 448, 449]. It differs from MCL by negative nuclear expression of cyclin D1 and SOX11 and lack of t(11;14)/*CCND1* rearrangement. Histomorphology of de novo CD5⁺ DLBCL is similar to DLBCL. Majority of cases (~70%) belong to ABC category. Subset of tumors co-expresses CD10, BCL6, and MUM1. Figure 13.97 presents de novo CD5⁺ DLBCL.

Intravascular large B-cell lymphoma (IVLBCL)

IVLBCL (angiotropic lymphoma; Figure 13.98) is a distinct subtype of extranodal DLBCL characterized by proliferation of large lymphomatous cells within the lumina of small to medium-sized vessels [1, 407, 450–453]. The IVLBCL is an aggressive and usually disseminated disease (Ann Arbor stage IV in 68% of cases) that predominantly affects elderly patients (median age 67–70 years, range: 34–90) with B symptoms (55%–76%), anemia and/or thrombocytopenia (63%–84%), hepatosplenomegaly (77%), BM involvement (75%), high serum LDH level (86%), and hemophagocytosis (61%) [454, 455]. Emergence of IVLBCL following small B-cell lymphoma or DLBCL has been reported. Based on clinical presentation, major variants of IVLBCL include classic, cutaneous, and hemophagocytic syndrome-associated variants [1, 407, 453]. The hemophagocytic syndrome-associated form has been reported mostly in Asian countries and the median patient age is 66 years [453]. This patient group has the shortest OS [453]. The cutaneous variant has disease confined to skin; patients tend to be younger and are more often female [453]. The involved sites include: BM (32%–66%), brain (40%), skin (40%), liver (17%–26%), spleen (16%–26%), kidney (21%), endocrine glands (16%), lung (16%), prostate (16%), heart (11%), lymph nodes (11%), gastrointestinal tract (8%), uterus (8%), gallbladder (3%), and sporadically other organs [451, 454–456]. Leukemic blood involvement is infrequent (5%–11%) [450, 451, 456]. Patients with disease limited to the skin ("cutaneous variant"; 26% of cases) are invariably

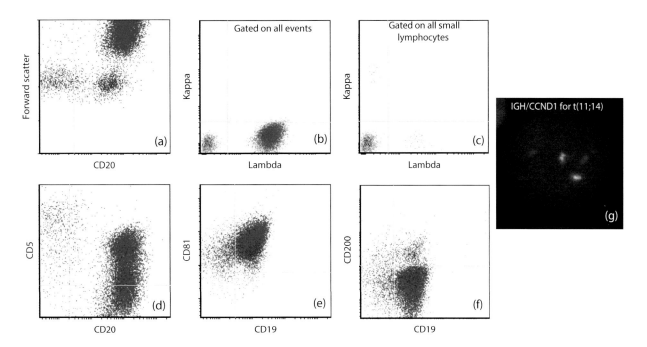

FIGURE 13.97 Lymph node with de novo CD5⁺ DLBCL. (a–f) Flow cytometry shows major population of large B-cells (blue dots) with high forward scatter and positive CD20 (a) and residual small lymphocytes with low forward scatter (red dots). Large B-cells show lambda restriction (b), while small B-cells are polytypic (c). Lymphomatous cells are positive for CD5 (d; partial expression) and CD81 (e), and negative for CD200 (f). FISH for *CCND1/IGH* shows two green signals (*IGH*) and two red signals (*CCND1*) indicating lack of *CCND1* rearrangement (g). Lack of history of CLL or small clonal CD5⁺ B-cells excludes Richter's transformation.

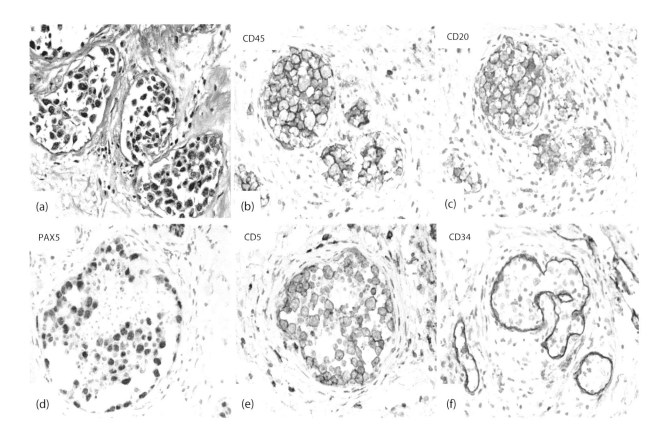

FIGURE 13.98 Intravascular large B-cell lymphoma (IVLBCL; bladder). (a) Histology shows large atypical lymphoid cells within large vascular space. (b–f) Immunohistochemistry. Tumor cells are positive for CD45 (b), CD20 (c), PAX5 (d), and CD5 (e). CD34 staining shows vessel wall (f).

females with a normal platelet count, and exhibit a significantly better outcome than the remaining patients [455]. The tumor cells display mature B-cell phenotype expressing CD45, CD20, and other B-cell markers. The expression of CD20 is strong but rare CD20⁻ cases have been reported. Majority of cases show a non-germinal center phenotype with MUM1 expression (75%–80%) [454]. Rare cases may be positive for CD30, display GCB phenotype with CD10/BCL6 immunoreactivity (CD10 and BCL6 expression was noted in 13%–22% and 22%–26%, respectively) [454, 457]. Recent series by Matsue et al. did not report CD10 expression in IVLBCL [451]. There is aberrant CD5 expression in significant proportion of cases (38%–47%) [451, 452, 454], more often than in DLBCL.

Primary diffuse large B-cell lymphoma of the central nervous system (CNS)

Primary CNS lymphomas comprise 5%–7% of primary brain tumors. They occur in immunosuppressed patients, especially those with AIDS or those who have received solid organ transplants and are uncommon in immunocompetent patients. Most primary CNS lymphomas in immunocompetent patients are categorized as DLBCL. Unlike HIV-associated primary CNS lymphomas, DLBCL developing in immunocompetent patients are not associated with EBV and occur usually over the age of 50 years. Differential diagnosis includes systemic lymphomas involving brain or transformation of low-grade lymphomas (e.g., MZL involving brain, spinal cord, or orbital area). The tumor cells are positive for B-cell markers, CD45, MUM1 and usually BCL6. DLBCL with GCB-like phenotype (CD10⁺ or CD10⁻/MUM1⁻/BCL6⁺) are less common. Subset of tumors may co-express CD56 (Figure 13.99).

Primary mediastinal large B-cell lymphoma (PMBL)

Primary mediastinal (thymic) large B-cell lymphoma (PMBL) is subtype of DLBCL. PMBL accounts for approximately 5% of aggressive lymphomas and has a predilection for young women,

bulky disease in the anterior-superior mediastinum, high LDH levels and frequent intrathoracic extension to adjacent organs such as pleura, pericardium, and lung [416, 458–475]. Extrathoracic dissemination or BM involvement are uncommon. Clinically, PMBL resembles cHL. It is of thymic origin [476, 477]. PMBCL has a relatively favorable clinical outcome, with a 5-year survival rate of 64% compared with 46% for other DLBCL patients [416].

On histologic examination there is a diffuse infiltrate, which in many cases shows characteristic fibrosis separating individual tumor cells. The lymphomatous cells may vary in size and shape, but medium-sized to large cells with round or oval nuclei predominate. They often have abundant pale to clear cytoplasm. Although the tumor grows diffusely, collagenous fibrosis compartmentalizing the tumor cells is frequently observed, mimicking nodules. Residual thymic tissue may be seen, usually in larger biopsy specimens.

Phenotypically, tumor cells are positive for CD45, B-cell markers (PAX5, CD19, CD20, CD22, CD79a, OCT2, and BOB1), and usually BCL6 (95%), CD23, p63, CD30, MYC (65%), and MUM1 (95%). There is variable expression of BCL2 (65%) and CD83 (40%), but CD10 is only expressed in 25%. The expression of CD30 is usually heterogeneous. There is no immunoreactivity with CD21. CD5 and CD138 are negative. PAX5 and CD20 are strongly positive. A characteristic finding in PMBL, unlike other DLBCL, is the expression of CD23, myelin and lymphocyte protein (MAL) and programmed cell death ligand PD-L1 and PD-L2 [464, 478–481]. MAL and CD200 are positive in 72% and 81%, respectively. Expression of BCL6 was reported more frequently in PD-L1⁺ than in PD-L1⁻ PMBL [475]. Rare cases of PMBCL may show non-specific BCL1 expression with copy number gains of *CCND1* but without rearrangement [482].

In an FC series reported by Cherian et al., neoplastic cells of PMLBCL displayed a B cell immunophenotype (CD19⁺/CD20⁺), bright CD40, lack immunoglobulin light chains, CD10, and CD15; frequent positivity for CD30 and positive CD71 and CD95 in all cases [483].

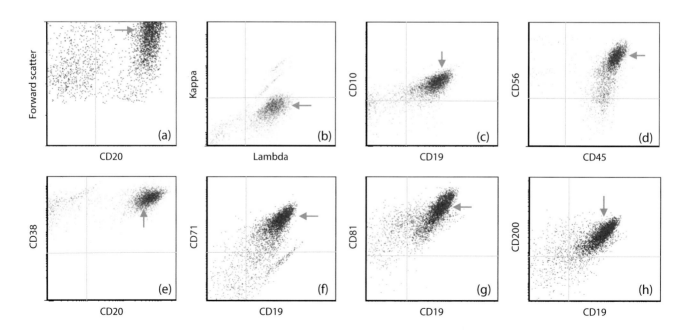

FIGURE 13.99 Primary DLBCL of CNS. Lymphomatous cells (blue dots, arrow) show high forward scatter and bright CD20 expression (a), lambda restriction (b), and are positive for CD10 (c), CD56 (d), CD38 (e), CD71(f), CD81 (g), and CD200 (h).

Burkitt lymphoma (BL)

BL phenotype by FC: $FSC^{increased}$, $sIg^{+/rarely-}$, $CD5^{-/rarely+}$, $CD10^{+bright}$, $BCL2^-$, $CD11c^-$, $CD19^+$, $CD20^+$, $CD22^+$, $CD23^-$, $CD25^-$, $CD34^-$, $CD38^{+bright}$, $CD43^{+strong}$, $CD45^+$, $CD71^+$, $CD79b^{+dim}$, $CD81^{+moderate\ to\ bright}$, $CD103^-$, $CD200^{-/(may\ be\ dimly+)}$, and TdT^-

Introduction

BL is an aggressive B-cell lymphoma with mature germinal center B-cell phenotype characterized by a bulky disease, common extranodal location, high degree of proliferation (Ki-67 index approaching 100%), frequent leukemic presentation, and the deregulation of the *MYC* gene most often due to t(8;14)(q24.1;q32) [1, 484–488]. It can present as lymphoma or leukemia. Three epidemiological variants of BL are recognized: (1) endemic, (2) sporadic (spontaneous), and (3) associated with immunodeficiency (HIV). Adult patients with sporadic or immunodeficiency-associated BL typically present with extranodal disease. The endemic variant is most often observed in children aged 4–7 with frequent involvement of the mandible and maxilla and abdominal organs, especially kidneys. BM involvement is rare. BL is associated with malaria endemicity and EBV is found in almost all cases. The sporadic BL occurs mainly in older children and young adults and presents as abdominal disease (60%–80%), followed by head and neck, including lymph nodes, oropharynx, tonsils, and sinuses. Involvement of the jaw is rare. Significant subset of BL is associated with EBV infection (endemic and HIV-associated forms). A leukemic phase can be observed in patients with bulky disease, but only rare cases present purely as leukemia with blood and BM involvement. With the current chemotherapy regimens, the overall survival rate is approximately 90% in children and 50%–70% in adults [489–492]. Algorithmic approach to the diagnosis of BL and HGBLs is presented in Figure 13.100 and Figure 12.8 in Chapter 12.

Morphology

Cytomorphology. Cytologically (Figure 13.101), BL is characterized by atypical lymphoid cells with increased nuclear/cytoplasmic ratio, vacuolated and basophilic cytoplasm, medium-sized round monomorphic nuclei (comparable to nuclei of histiocytes) with granular or stippled chromatin and several paracentrally located basophilic nucleoli. In cases with "atypical" morphology, nucleoli may be more prominent and nuclei more pleomorphic or exhibit plasmacytoid features.

Lymph nodes. BL is characterized by relatively monotonous, cohesive, diffuse infiltrate of medium-sized cells with numerous mitoses (>10/HPF), apoptotic cells, and scattered macrophages with engulfed apoptotic bodies, creating a "starry-sky" appearance (Figure 13.102). Rare cases may show slightly more pleomorphic infiltrate with larger cells.

BM. BM maybe involved with or without leukemic presentation. The predominant pattern of involvement is diffuse infiltrate by "blastoid" cells with vacuolated cytoplasm and round or oval nuclei (Figure 13.103). Figure 13.104 shows Burkitt leukemia with prominent involvement of BM.

Extranodal location. Extranodal sites are involved more often than lymph nodes and include jaws or orbit bones (endemic BL), abdominal organs (especially ileocecal region and kidneys), breast, and retroperitoneal area. The histomorphologic features are similar regardless of location (Figure 13.105) and include starry-sky pattern and monomorphic infiltrate of medium-sized cells. Areas of necrosis are often present.

Immunophenotype

Immunohistochemistry. Tumor cells in BL are positive for CD45, B-cell markers (PAX5, BOB1, OCT2, CD19, CD20, CD22, and CD79a), CD10, CD43, CD71, MYC, and BCL6. They lack BCL2 expression. CD21 expression is variable and is more often associated with the endemic form. Blastic markers (TdT and CD34) are negative. Majority of BLs are CD5$^-$. The proliferation index determined by Ki-67 staining approaches 100%. BL in immunocompromised patient is often EBV/EBER positive.

Flow cytometry. FC analysis shows clonal B-cell population with moderate to bright expression of CD20 and surface immunoglobulins, positive CD10, CD38 (strong), CD43 (strong), CD71, CD79b (dim), and CD81 (strong), increased FSC and negative BCL2 (Figures 13.106 and 13.107). Rare cases of BL may be surface light chain immunoglobulins negative or show aberrant expression of CD5 (Figure 13.108). The expression of CD71 is often strong but may be dim or partial in some cases. The majority of BL shows bright expression of CD38 (82%), whereas only 17% of *MYC*$^-$ DLBCL show bright CD38 [446]. Bright expression of CD38 is also typical for HGBLs with *MYC* and *BCL2* (and/or *BCL6*) rearrangements (HGBL-R), but bright CD38 expression in conjunction with bright CD10 (>80%), negative (low) BCL2 and high Ki-67 by FC is characteristic of BL and helps to differentiate it from single hit DLBCL (*MYC*$^+$ DLBCL) and HGBL-R [446, 493].

Genetic features

Majority of BL cases have t(8;14)(q24;q32) (Figure 13.109), resulting in the juxtaposition of the *MYC* oncogene (on chromosome 8q24) with *IGH* heavy chain locus (on chromosome 14). This is seen in 70%–80% of cases. Remaining cases have either t(2;8)(p11;q24) or t(8;22)(q24;q11.2), that juxtapose *MYC* to the immunoglobulin light chain genes, kappa (*IGK*) on 2p11 and lambda (*IGL*) on 22q11, respectively [494]. The *MYC* deregulation [t(8;14)] is not specific for BL, and can also be detected in approximately 15% of DLBCL as well as in secondary precursor B-lymphoblastic leukemia/lymphoma, aggressive lymphoma transforming from FL, and in some cases of HGBLs and PCM [330, 495–502]. The differential diagnosis between BL and DLBCL is very important from clinical point of view since the treatment and prognosis of two diseases differs.

Differential diagnosis of BL

Differential diagnosis of BL includes:

- FL
- DLBCL
- HGBL with *MYC* and *BCL2* rearrangement (HGBL-R, double-hit lymphoma)
- HGBL, NOS
- PBL
- Florid follicular hyperplasia
- MCL, blastoid variant
- B-ALL/LBL
- T-cell acute lymphoblastic leukemia/lymphoma (T-ALL/LBL)

Follicular lymphoma (FL)

The FSC in FL depends on the subtype but is usually lower than in BL. FLBL may have increased FSC comparable to DLBCL. Typical FL shows dim CD19 expression, dim to moderate CD38, lack of

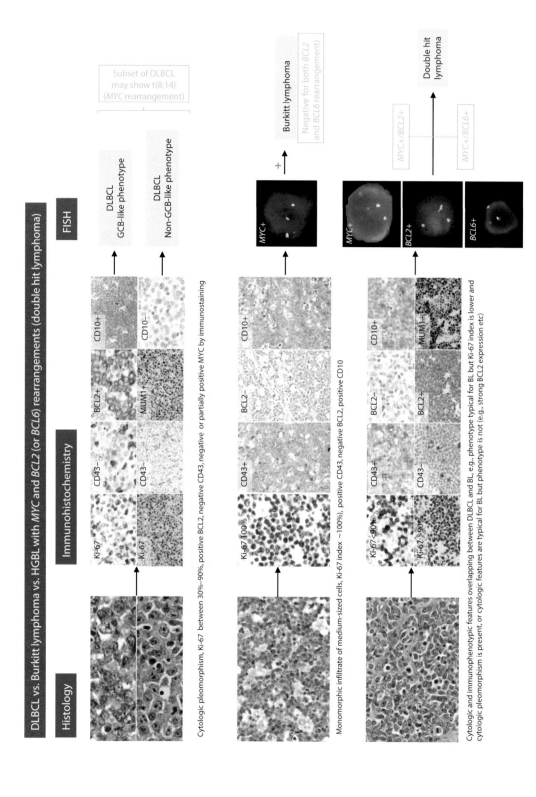

FIGURE 13.100 Algorithm for differential diagnosis of Burkitt lymphoma versus DLBCL versus HGBL with MYC and BCL2 (ad/or BCL6) rearrangements. HGBL with MYC and BCL2 (double hit lymphoma) is diagnosed with rearrangement of *MYC* and *BCL2* or *MYC* and *BCL6*, and triple hit lymphoma is diagnosed with rearrangement of all three genes (*MYC, BCL2, and BCL6*). Presence of *BCL2* and *BCL6* rearrangement without *MYC* does not qualify as double hit lymphoma.

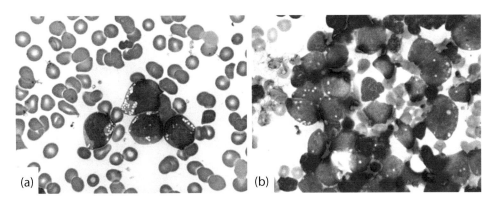

FIGURE 13.101 Burkitt lymphoma: Blood smear (a) and touch smear from the lymph node (b) shows highly atypical lymphoid cells with increased nuclear/cytoplasmic ratio, vacuolated, basophilic cytoplasm, slightly granular chromatin and several small nucleoli.

CD43 expression and positive BCL2. In rare cases of CD43+ FL, the expression of this marker is dimmer when compared to BL. Strong expression of CD81 is typical for BL (in FL the expression of CD81 is either dim or negative). Positive expression of CD95 favors the diagnosis of FL, as CD95 is usually negative in BL [503]. Subset of FLs, especially FLBL may be BCL2 negative, shows stronger CD38 expression and increased FSC making it difficult to differentiate from BL (and DLBCL) based on FC analysis alone.

Correlation with histomorphology and FISH studies (*MYC* and *BCL2* probes) is necessary for definite subclassification. Cardoso et al. compared the expression of CD39, CD43, CD81, and CD95 in BL and FL, and showed similar intensity of expression of CD39, brighter expression of CD43 and CD81 in BL, and lower expression of CD95 in BL [503]. McGowan et al. reported much stronger expression of CD38, CD43, and CD71 in BL when compared to FL [504].

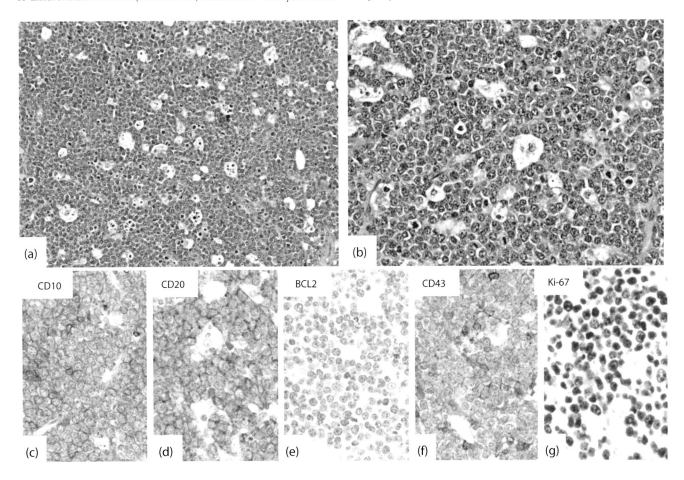

FIGURE 13.102 Burkitt lymphoma. (a–c) Lymph node: low magnification shows diffuse lymphoid infiltrate with scattered histiocytes creating "starry-sky" pattern (a); high magnification shows medium sized monomorphic lymphomatous cells with increased nuclear-cytoplasmic ratio (b). Tingible body macrophages are present. (c–g) Immunohistochemistry reveals the typical phenotype: positive expression of CD10 (c), CD20 (d), and CD43 (f) and negative staining with BCL2 (h). Proliferation index as determined by staining with Ki-67 (MIB-1) approaches 100% (i).

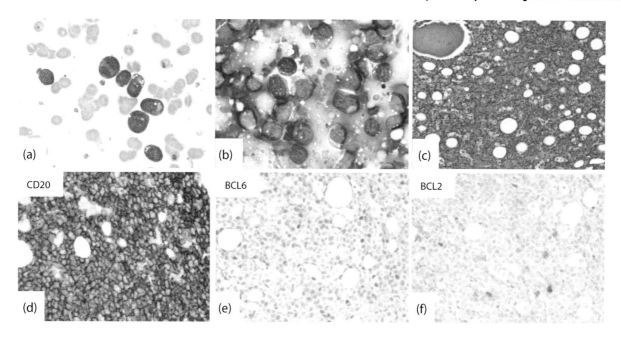

FIGURE 13.103 BL: diffuse BM involvement. Aspirate smear (a) and touch smear (b) shows typical cytomorphologic features of BL. Histologic section (c) shows diffuse replacement of BM by atypical lymphoid infiltrate. Tumor cells are positive for CD20 (d) and BCL6 (e), and do not express BCL2 (f).

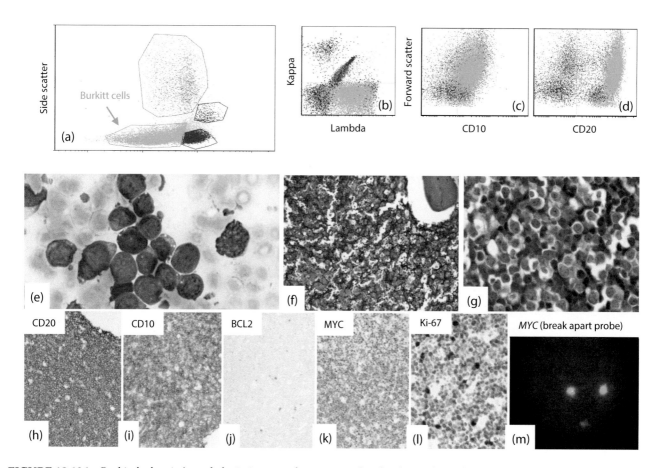

FIGURE 13.104 Burkitt leukemia (morphologic, immunophenotypic and molecular analysis of blood and BM from 45-year-old patient). FC analysis showed 25% clonal B-cells in blood with low side scatter, dim to moderate expression of CD45 (a, green dots), monotypic lambda expression (b), positive CD10 (c), and bright CD20 (d). Aspirate smear (e) shows atypical cells with blastoid appearance. Histologic section from core biopsy (f–g, low and high power) shows diffuse infiltrate by monotonous medium-sized lymphoid cells. Immunohistochemistry analysis (h–l) shows positive CD20 (h) and CD10 (i), negative BCL2 (j), strong expression of MYC (>90%, k), and high Ki-67 index (l). FISH analysis (m) shows one green, one orange, and one yellow/green/orange fusion signal indicative of a chromosomal break in the *MYC* locus.

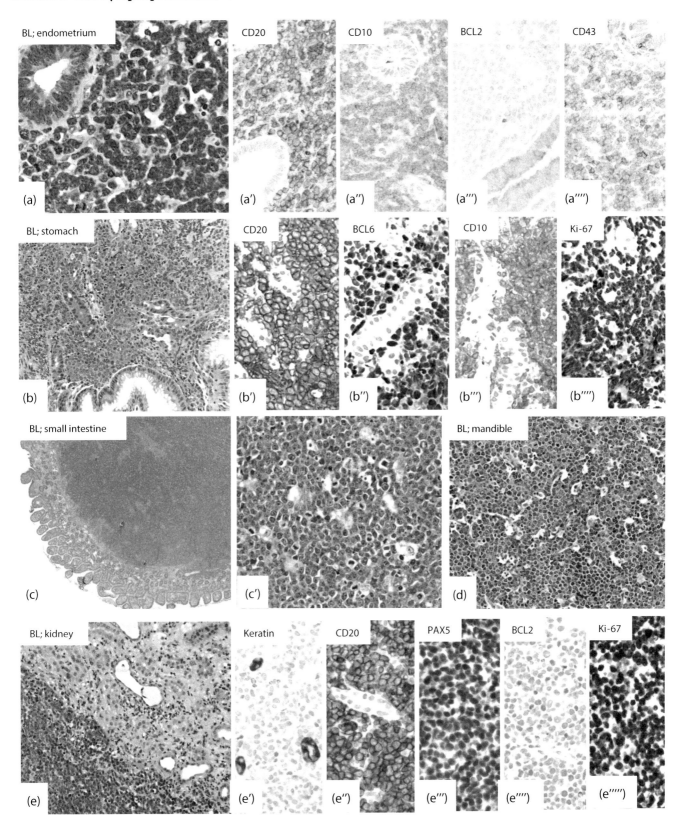

FIGURE 13.105 Extranodal BL. (a) BL – endometrium. (a) Dense monomorphic lymphoid infiltrate with somewhat "blastoid" appearance composed of medium-sized cells with high nuclear-cytoplasmic ratio. Tumor cells are positive for CD20 (a′), CD10 (a″), negative for BCL2 (a‴), and positive for CD43 (a⁗). (b) BL – stomach, expressing CD20 (b′), BCL6 (b″), CD10 (b‴), and Ki-67 (b⁗). (c) BL – small intestine (low and high magnification). (d) BL – mandible. (e) BL – kidney. Tumor cells are negative for keratin (e′), express CD20 (e″), and PAX5 (e‴), are negative for BCL2 (e⁗) and show strong Ki-67 staining (e⁗′).

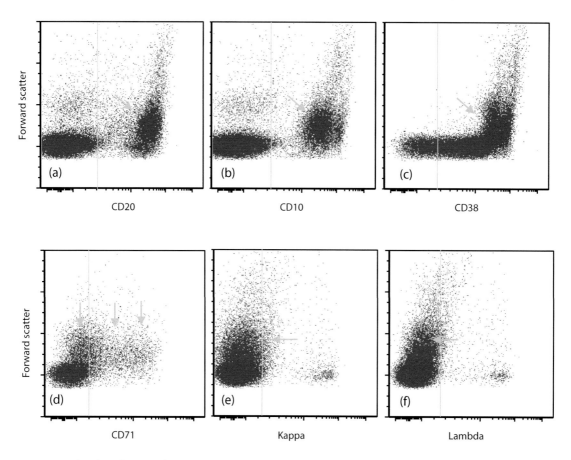

FIGURE 13.106   Burkitt lymphoma – flow cytometry (lymph node). Neoplastic B-cells show increased forward scatter (a–f, arrow), positive CD20 (a), CD10 (b), CD38 (c), CD71 (d; partial), and do not express surface light chain immunoglobulins (e–f).

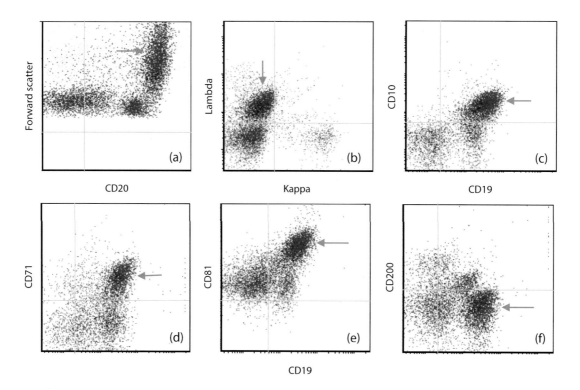

FIGURE 13.107   BL. Lymphomatous cells (blue dots, arrow) show increased forward scatter (a), bright CD20 expression (a), lambda restriction (b), and positive expression of CD10 (c), CD71 (d), and CD81 (c). CD200 is negative (f).

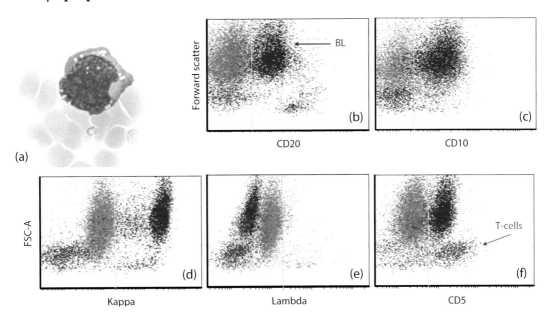

FIGURE 13.108 BL with unusual CD5 expression (43-year-old man with mediastinal mass and circulating "blasts"). Blood smear shows highly atypical lymphoid cells (a). FC analysis shows B-cells with high forward scatter and positive expression of CD20 (b), CD10 (c), kappa (d; compare with lambda, e), and CD5 (f).

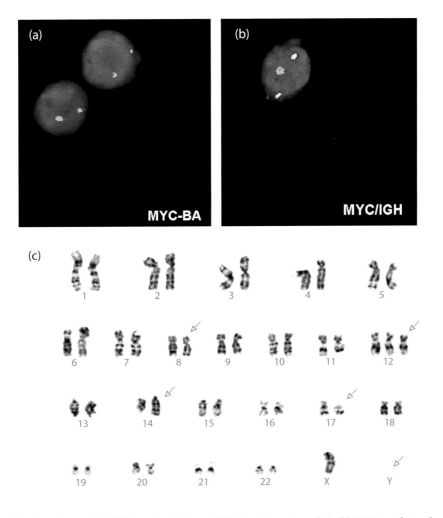

FIGURE 13.109 Burkitt lymphoma. (a) FISH analysis for c-*MYC* (break-apart probe); (b) FISH analysis shows *MYC-IGH* fusion. (c) Conventional cytogenetics shows complex changes including t(8;14).

DLBCL

Differential diagnosis of BL includes DLBCLs which may resemble BL morphologically or phenotypically. DLBCL usually shows more pleomorphic infiltrate without starry-sky appearance, composed of centroblasts, immunoblasts or cells with cytologic features overlapping between centroblasts or immunoblasts. In addition, the majority of DLBCL do not show co-expression of CD10 and CD43 without BCL2 expression. However, subset of DLBCL may display the phenotype similar to BL (CD10+, CD43+, BCL2−, and BCL6+). On FC analysis, BL differs from CD10+ DLBCL by lower FSC, dimmer CD79b expression, brighter CD43 expression, lack of BCL2 and strong CD81 expression. Higher expression of CD71 in BL than in DLBCL mirrors Ki-67 index on tissue sections (it approaches 100% in BL, whereas in DLBCL is most often <90%), but subset of BL shows partial or dim CD71 and subset of DLBCL show very bright CD71 expression. CD200 is usually negative or less often dimly positive in BL and variably expressed in DLBCL. McGowan et al. evaluated 9 FC parameters including forward and SSC, mean fluorescent intensity (MFI) for CD20, CD10, CD38, CD79b, CD43, and CD71; and the percentage of neoplastic cells positive for CD71 and reported that the FSC, MFIs of CD10, CD43, CD79b, and CD71, and percent of CD71 cells were significantly different between BL and CD10+ DLBCL [504]. Their 5-point scoring system (FSC, %CD71, and MFIs of CD43, CD79b, and CD71) were helpful in the differential diagnosis between BL and DLBCL [504]. Schniederjan et al. reported significantly lower expression of CD44 and CD54 in BL compared with CD10+ DLBCL [505]. Cardoso et al. showed stronger expression of CD39 and dimmer expression of CD43 and CD81 by DLBCL cells when compared to BL [503].

Florid follicular hyperplasia

In needle core biopsy specimens, differential diagnosis includes reactive processes with follicular hyperplasia. In a minute biopsy, large hyperplastic follicle may resemble BL cytologically and immunophenotypically (CD10+ and BCL2−). Reactive germinal centers differ from BL by showing polarization with dark and light zones. The former is composed of centroblasts and the latter shows predominance of centrocytes and FDCs. The polarization is best visualized by staining with Ki-67 or PD1. In difficult cases, larger (excisional) biopsy should be recommended. FC analysis in lymph node with florid follicular hyperplasia may show CD10+ B-cell population with kappa excess (or less often lambda excess) mimicking clonal process. Low FSC, lack or partially dim CD71 expression, negative CD43 and the presence of a major polytypic B-cell population point toward the diagnosis of reactive process.

HGBL, NOS (high grade B-cell lymphoma, not otherwise specified)

HGBL, NOS is a rare variant of B-cell lymphoma, which does not fulfill the criteria for neither BL, HGBL-R nor DLBCL. It may resemble morphologically DLBCL, BL or B-ALL. In BL-like cases, there is no *MYC* rearrangement, allowing to exclude the diagnosis of BL. Figure 13.110 shows very unusual case of composite HGBL with BL and HGBL, NOS components (37-year-old male patient with adrenal mass).

HGBL-R [high grade B-cell lymphoma with MYC and BCL2 rearrangement; double hit lymphoma]

HGBL-R may morphologically and immunophenotypically resemble BL but differs from it by rearrangement of *BCL2* or

BCL6 (double-hit lymphoma) or both *BCL2* and *BCL6* (triple hit lymphoma) in addition to *MYC* rearrangement. BL shows only *MYC* rearrangement. Subset of HGBL-R may resemble morphologically DLBCL, but often show strong expression of both BCL2 and CD10 (the expression of MYC by immunohistochemistry does not always correlate with genetic *MYC* rearrangement status), and therefore it is recommended to perform FISH analysis for *MYC*, *BCL2*, and *BCL6* in all DLBCL cases.

Burkitt-like lymphoma with 11q aberration

Burkitt-like lymphoma with 11q aberration is a provisional WHO entity [1]. In contrast to BL, it is negative for *MYC* rearrangement. Phenotypically, Burkitt-like lymphomas with 11q aberration are positive for CD20, CD10, and CD38 (dim), negative for BCL2 and CD43 and occasional positive for CD56 [506]. On FC analysis, Burkitt-like lymphoma with 11q aberration differs from BL by dimmer expression of CD38, stronger expression of CD45 and presence of CD16, CD56, and CD8 [506].

PBL

Overlapping features between BL and PBL include frequent extranodal location, history of HIV infection, starry-sky pattern on histologic examination, and MYC and EBV co-expression by immunophenotyping. BL is composed of smaller lymphoid when compared to immunoblastic or plasmablastic variant of PBL. PBL are most often CD45− (minor subset of cases may be dimly CD45+), do not express B-cell markers (CD19, CD20, PAX5) and are positive for plasma cell markers (MUM1, CD38, CD138) and often CD56, whereas BLs are positive for CD45, CD19, CD20, CD79a, PAX5, CD10, and BCL6. Ki-67 index is high in both entities (100% in BL and often >90% in PBL).

MCL

Subset of MCL may be CD10+ and/or display cytomorphologic features similar to BL (blastoid MCL. MCL differs from BL by positive CD5 expression (in majority of cases), lower Ki-67 index, positive BCL1 (cyclin D1), positive SOX11, presence of t(11;14)/*CCND1* rearrangement, and negative *MYC* rearrangement.

B-ALL

B-ALL may be distinguished from BL by positive expression of blastic markers (e.g., CD34 or TdT) and lack of the expression of CD20 and surface immunoglobulins. Both BL and B-ALL show strong expression of CD10, CD38, CD44, and CD43. The expression of CD58 is higher in BL than in B-ALL [507]. The expression of CD81 is brighter in BL than in B-ALL, and the expression of CD200 is more often positive in B-ALL than in BL.

T-ALL

T-ALL/LBL is distinguished by lack of B-cell markers and presence of one or more pan-T antigens (especially CD7 and cytoplasmic CD3) and expression of TdT, CD1a, and/or CD34.

High-grade B-cell lymphomas

HGBL includes two types of aggressive mature B-cell lymphomas, HGBL with *MYC* and *BCL2* (with/without *BCL6*) rearrangements (HGBL-R, "double hit" or "triple hit" lymphoma, DHL/THL), and HGBL, not otherwise specified (HGBL, NOS) [1, 96, 508].

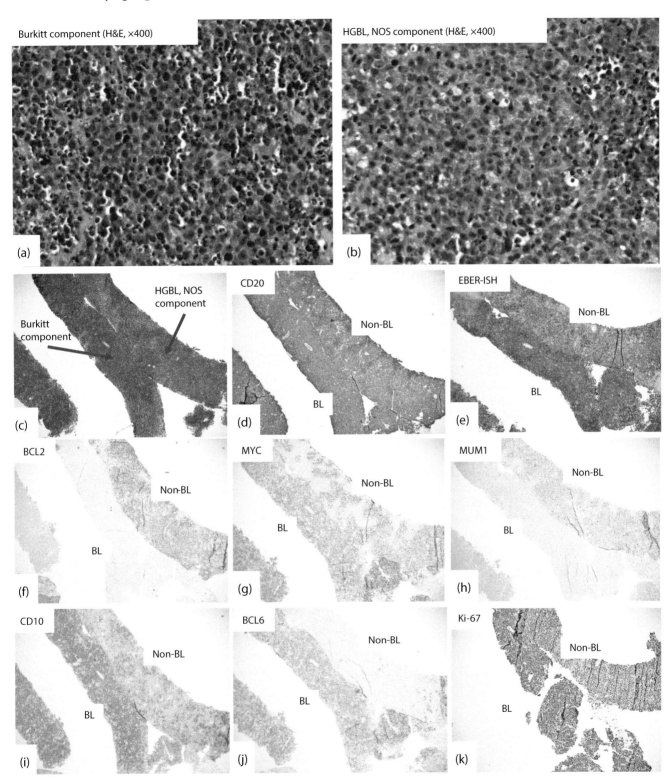

FIGURE 13.110 Composite high-grade B-cell lymphoma: Burkitt lymphoma (BL) and high-grade B-cell lymphoma, NOS. (a–c) Histology with monomorphic infiltrate with starry sky appearance. The BL cells are slightly smaller than non-BL (compare a and b). (c) Low poser shows several core biopsy, some of which show Burkitt lymphoma component (BL) and some non-Burkitt lymphoma component (non-BL). (d–k) Immunohistochemistry shows different phenotype of two components of this composite lymphoma, BL is positive for CD20 (d), EBC (e), MYC (g), CD10 (I, strong expression), BCL6 (j) and Ki-67 (k), while BCL2 (f) and MUM1 (h) are negative. Non-BL component is positive for CD20 (d), EBV (e), BCL2 (f), MYC (g, partial expression), MUM1 (h), CD10 (I, dim expression), and Ki-67 (k). The expression of BCL6 is negative (g).

High-grade B-cell lymphoma with *MYC* and *BCL2* with/without *BCL6* rearrangements (HGBL-R, double/triple hit lymphoma)

HGBL-R phenotype by FC: FSC^increased, sIg^+ (often dim)/rarely−, CD5−, CD10^+bright/rarely−, BCL2^+, CD11c−, CD19^+, CD20^+(may be dim), CD22^+, CD23−, CD25−, CD34−, CD38^+bright, CD43^+/−, CD45^+, CD71^+, CD81^+, CD103−, CD123−, CD200^−/+, and TdT−

Prior (2016) WHO guidelines for tumors of hematopoietic and lymphoid tissues classified this type of tumor in a new category named HGBL with rearrangements of *MYC* and *BCL2* and/or *BCL6*, also called "double-hit" (DHL) or "triple-hit" lymphoma (THL) [1, 508]. Among them, approximately 65% of patients are classified as *MYC/BCL2* type DHL; 14% as *MYC/BCL6* type DHL; and the remaining 21% of patients as THL [509]. Updated (2022) WHO classifies tumors with MYC and BCL2 rearrangements as DLBCL/high-grade B-cell lymphoma with MYC and BCL2 rearrangements. Cases with dual MYC and BCL6 rearrangements are now classified as DLBCL, NOS or HGBL, NOS.

Cases with MYC and BCL2 protein co-expression but without genetic rearrangement of *BCL2* and *MYC* are called "double-expressor" lymphoma (DEL). DELs account for 19%–34% of DLBCL cases [510]. Similarly, current Previous studies showed that DEL is associated with a poor outcome intermediate between those of DHL and DLBCL after treatment with R-CHOP [511]. The cases with concurrent *MYC* and *CCND1* rearrangement are classified as aggressive variants of MCL based on the premise that t(11;14) (q13;q32)/*CCND1-IGH* is a founder abnormality [1, 508].

HGBL with *MYC* and *BCL2* rearrangements (HGBL-R, double-hit lymphoma) represents a very aggressive lymphoma with morphologic and immunophenotypic features overlapping between BL and DLBCL [96, 432, 484, 512–515]. Cases with similar morphologic and phenotypic features, but without *MYC* rearrangement are classified as HGBL, not otherwise specified (HGBL, NOS) [96]. Cases of DLBCLs with concurrent *MYC* and *BCL2* and/or *BCL6* gene abnormalities other than typical DHL/THL [e.g., DLBCL with *MYC* rearrangement and *BCL2* and/or *BCL6* extra copies or DLBCL with *MYC* extra copies and *BCL2* and/or *BCL6* rearrangement/extra copies] do not belong to DHL or THL category and are sometimes termed atypical DHL/THL [436].

Morphology

HGBL-R are morphologically and phenotypically heterogeneous with overlapping features between DLBCL or BL. Blastoid morphology is seen more often in HGBL, NOS, rather than HGBL-R. HGBL-Rs show diffuse lymphoid infiltrate with starry sky pattern, mitotic figures, and prominent apoptosis (Figures 13.111 and 13.112). Necrotic areas are usually present and may be prominent. The cells are medium sized to large. Approximately half of cases show diffuse large cell infiltrate with some pleomorphism, resembling DLBCL, and the rest show more monotonous infiltrate of medium-sized cells with starry-sky pattern with numerous mitoses resembling BL.

Four morphological variants of HGBL-R are recognized [508]:

- DLBCL-like variant (centroblastic features with intermediate to large cells with vesicular chromatin, two to four membrane-bound nucleoli and moderate amount of cytoplasm)
- DLBCL versus BL like variant (previously designated as B-cell lymphoma, unclassifiable with features intermediate between DLBCL and BL)

- BL-like variant (monotonous infiltrate of intermediate-sized cells, scanty cytoplasm, finely clumped chromatin and two to three nucleoli)
- Lymphoblast-like variant (rarest variant with intermediate-sized cells, fine chromatin and indistinct nucleoli)

Immunophenotype

Phenotypically, HGBLs usually have a germinal center phenotype, almost always express BCL2 and have high Ki-67 index (approx. 90%) [432, 515]. B-cell markers (CD19, CD20, CD22, CD79a, and PAX5) are positive. Majority of cases show monoclonal expression of surface immunoglobulins, but some cases (double-hit lymphomas) may be surface immunoglobulin negative. Most HGBL-R have germinal center phenotype with expression of CD10 (90%–100%) and BCL6 (75%–100%). MUM1 is detected in subset of cases. BCL2 protein is detected in up to 95% [432]. MYC expression is noted in 67%–100% of cases [508]. The proliferation (Ki-67) index is generally high (~90%), but reported cases have the index between 20% and 100%. Majority of cases have strong expression of CD71 and co-expression of CD10 and BCL2 by FC (Figures 13.111 and 13.112). Surface light chain immunoglobulin expression by FC is often decreased and can be absent in 20% of cases [446]. Bright CD38 expression (CD38^bright) analyzed either qualitatively or semi-quantitatively is more common in DH/THL (56%) than in *MYC*− DLBCL (17%) but less common compared to *MYC*+ lymphomas (82%), indicating that CD38^bright can serve as a biomarker for DH/THL [446]. The BCL2 positivity in cases that otherwise might be classified as BL should raise the possibility of a double-hit lymphoma with both *MYC* and *BCL2* translocations. DLBCL with *MYC* and *BCL6* rearrangement are often CD10^+ and BCL2− and may express MUM1/IRF4 [513]. Rare cases are positive for *BCL2*, *MYC*, and *BCL6* rearrangement (triple-hit lymphomas; Figure 13.113). The T-cell markers (CD2, CD3, and CD7) are negative, but rare cases can be CD5^+.

Differential diagnosis of HGBL-R

DLBCL. DLBCL with MYC and BCL2 overexpression by immunohistochemistry (so-called double expressor DLBCL) but without *MYC* and *BCL2* rearrangement are not classified as double hit lymphomas (immunohistochemistry analysis should not be used as a surrogate for genetic results).

Burkitt lymphoma. Distinguishing features of HGBL-R from BL includes expression of BCL2, MUM1/IRF4, Ki-67 <95%, and absence of EBV-EBER. BL differs from HGBL-R by lack both *BCL2* and *BCL6* rearrangements. Monotonous infiltrate of medium sized cells with "starry-sky" pattern, negative BCL2 immunostaining, Ki-67~100% and *IGH-MYC* rearrangement (simple karyotype) favor BL. Presence of more pleomorphic infiltrate, positive BCL2 immunostaining, *IGH-MYC* rearrangement with concurrent *BCL2* (and/or *BCL6*) rearrangement and Ki-67<95% favor BCLU, whereas positive BCL2 immunostaining, Ki-67 <90%, negative *MYC* rearrangement and positive *BCL2* or *BCL6* rearrangement favor DLBCL.

Double hit follicular lymphoma. FL with typical histomorphology and double hit (rearrangement) are classified as FL and not HGBL-R (double hit lymphoma). FL having both *MYC* and *BCL2* translocations without high-grade transformation (double-hit FL) is extremely rare. Double-hit FLs tend to be high-grade (grade 3) with high *MYC* positivity, and the frequency of *MYC/IGH* fusion higher than that of HGBLs with *MYC* and *BCL2* and/or *BCL6* rearrangements [516].

Follicular lymphoma (FL) transforming to high grade lymphoma. Most commonly, HT from FL manifests as a DLBCL, not

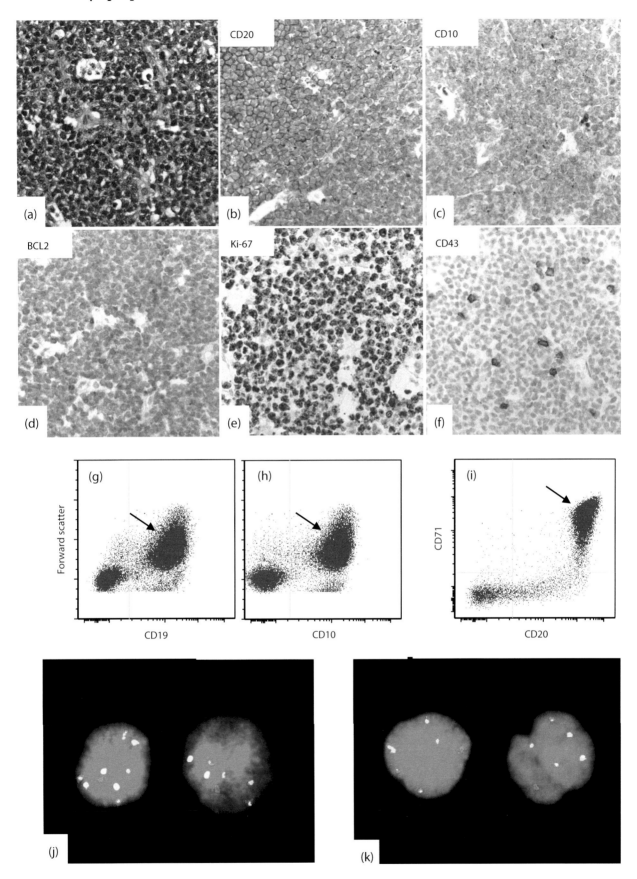

FIGURE 13.111 HGBL-R (double hit lymphoma): lymphoid cells are positive for CD20 (b), CD10 (c), and BCL2 (d; dim expression). The proliferation fraction is high (<90%; e). CD43 is not expressed (f). Flow cytometry shows B-cells with increased forward scatter (g–h), positive CD19 (g), CD10 and CD71 (i). FISH studies revealed rearrangement *MYC-IGH* (j) and *IGH-BCL2* (k).

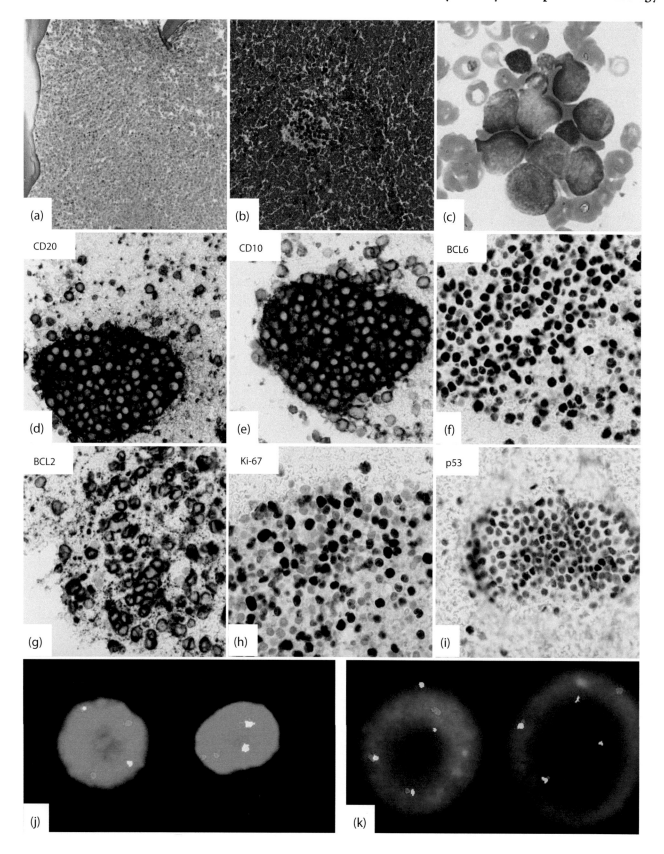

FIGURE 13.112   HGBL-R (double hit) with extensive BM involvement. Core biopsy (a) shows complete BM replacement by necrotic lymphoma. Clot section (b) shows aggregates of highly atypical, viable lymphoid cells. Aspirate smear (c; oil magnification) shows group of neoplastic cells with "blastoid" appearance. Immunohistochemistry stainings (clot) show positive CD20 (d), CD10 (e), BCL6 (f), BCL2 (g), and p53 (i). Majority of cells express Ki-67 (h). FISH analysis showed rearrangement of *MYC* (j; break-apart probe) and *BCL2* (*IGH-BCL2* probe).

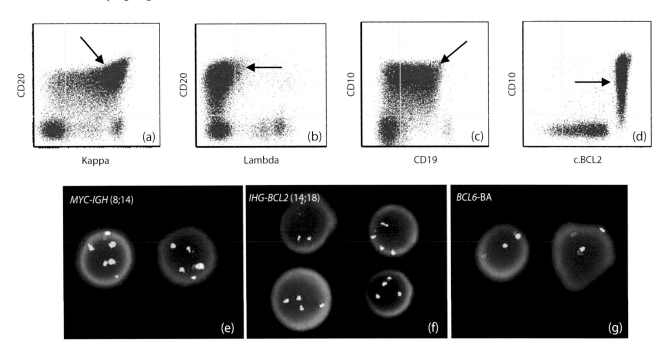

FIGURE 13.113 Triple hit lymphoma (71-year-old patient with adenopathy and lymphocytosis). Flow cytometry analysis (a–c) shows monoclonal B-cell population (arrows) with expression of CD20 (a–b), kappa (a), CD10 (c), and BCL2 (d). FISH studies showed rearrangement of *MYC* (e; *MYC*, red; *IGH*, green; centromere 8, blue), *BCL2* (f; *IGH*, green; *BCL2*, red), and *BCL6* (g; break-apart probe).

otherwise specified (DLBCL, NOS). Less frequently, HT may result in an HGBL with *MYC* and *BCL2* and/or *BCL6* gene rearrangements. In extremely rare cases, HT results in both the intermediate DLBCL and BL phenotypes and exhibits lymphoblastic features, in which case the WHO recommends that this morphological appearance should be noted [1]. Most reported cases of lymphoblastic transformation of FL are double hit (i.e., carry both *MYC* and *BCL2* gene rearrangement). While the prognosis of lymphoblastic transformation with double-hit is slightly worse than that of de novo double-hit lymphoma, it is unclear whether the lymphoblastoid morphology or the double-hit nature of this transformation confers a worse prognosis than what would be expected from a typical transformation of FL to DLBCL. Lymphoblastic transformation is characterized by expression of TdT, loss of BCL6, variable loss of immunoglobulin light chain, and persistence of PAX-5, BCL2, and CD10 [334]. Double-hit lymphoma derived from FL is classified as germinal center B-cell (GCB) lymphoma.

Double/triple hit B-cell lymphomas with TdT expression (B-ALL with MYC and BCL2 rearrangement; high-grade TdT+ blastic B-cell lymphoma/leukemia). Rare HGBLs with double or triple hit express TdT, and based on current WHO recommendation those cases are classified as B-cell acute lymphoblastic lymphoma/leukemia, although some authors suggest to use term high-grade TdT+ blastic B-cell lymphoma/leukemia, as lack of other features of immaturity, presence of monotypic surface immunoglobulin by FC, partial BCL6 expression and double/triple-hit genetics indicate a mature B-cell lymphoma [1, 508, 517]. Patients with double hit B-ALL most often present with large abdominal and/or retroperitoneal masses and diffuse BM replacement by sheets of blasts [27, 518]. Blasts are medium to large and may show prominent cytoplasmic vacuoles especially in double hit cases. Tumor cells are positive for TdT, CD10, CD19, negative or partially positive for CD34, negative or partially dimly positive for CD20 and negative for surface immunoglobulins [518]. Some of

these neoplasms may represent transformation of prior low-grade lymphoma (e.g., FL). In some of these neoplasms FC may show a mature B-cell lymphoma component and BM core biopsy may show peri- to paratrabecular infiltrate of small cells in addition to "blasts" [518]. De novo B-ALL with *BCL2* rearrangement [t(14;18) (q32;q21)] has also been reported [334, 518–523]. These tumors may be indistinguishable morphologically and immunophenotypically from FL with lymphoblastic transformation.

Double-hit events are extremely rare in B-ALL, especially in pediatric patients or young adults. In adult population they often represent progression from FL [330, 334, 518, 524]. *MYC* rearrangement is rarely observed in B-ALL/LBL in the absence of the t(14;18) *IGH/BCL2* rearrangement. Since 1980, only 13 cases of B-ALL/LBL with isolated *MYC* rearrangement were reported [525–531]. Like other B-ALL/LBLs, most of the cases occur in pediatric patients and only three cases were reported in adults. In a study of 5280 cases of pediatric ALL, only five (<0.1%) with isolated *MYC* rearrangement were identified [525]. Geyer et al. published a series of 7 patients with TdT+ B-lymphoblastic transformation of FL [334]. In that series, the authors raise the possibility that patients presenting with de novo double-hit B-LBL may have a pre-existing low-grade FL masked by the higher-grade process. TdT positivity was reported in subset of patients with DHL or THL by Moench et al. [532]. One of the cases was positive for TdT but expressed monotypic surface light chain, bright CD45 and CD20, and had a centroblastic morphology, favoring a mature neoplasm, one case showed blastic morphology but mature FC immunophenotype and two cases represented transformation of FL.

In a serious reported by Ok et al., the groups of TdT+ lymphomas included [508, 517]:

- de novo HGBL with *MYC*, *BCL2*, and/or *BCL6* rearrangements (double-hit or triple-hit lymphoma) with TdT expression (including cases of de novo composite lymphomas in which there were components of DLBCL and TdT+ blastic B-cell lymphoma)

- FL transformed to DHL with TdT expression (TdT-positive aggressive B-cell lymphoma arising in patients who previously had FL)
- initial relapse of FL to TdT− aggressive B-cell lymphoma, followed by relapses in which the neoplasm acquired TdT expression; and
- mature B-cell lymphomas that acquired TdT expression at relapse (this group included one case of EBV+ DLBCL and one case of pleomorphic variant MCL).

FC immunophenotypic analysis shows an immature B-cell immunophenotype (CD10+, CD19+, TdT+, surface Ig−) and immunohistochemistry shows high expression of MYC and BCL2. In three B-ALL cases described by Li et al., flow cytometric analysis showed dim CD45, positive CD10, CD19, TdT, and dim to absent CD20 (one of the cases showed lambda chain restriction) [533]. In a series by Moench et al., FC dim CD45, absence of CD20 or surface light chain, or expression of TdT suggesting of immature phenotype.

All patients show complex karyotypes associated with 8q24 abnormalities in the form of t(8;9)(q24;p13) or t(8;14)(q24;q32) and t(14;18)(q32;q21) [517, 534]. B-ALL cases with MYC rearrangement appear to represent a distinct biological phenomenon, in which a *MYC* translocation may be acquired at an immature stage of differentiation, in which the tumor cells still express TDT and lack a mature B-cell phenotype.

Atypical double (or triple) hit lymphoma (atypical DHL/THL) and double/triple extra copies lymphoma (DECL/TECL)

Cases of DLBCLs with concurrent *MYC* and *BCL2* and/or BCL6 gene abnormalities other than typical DHL/THL [e.g., DLBCL with *MYC* rearrangement and *BCL2* and/or *BCL6* extra copies or *DLBCL* with *MYC* extra copies and BCL2 and/or BCL6 rearrangement/extra copies] do not belong to DHL or THL and are sometimes termed atypical DHL/THL [436]. Quesada et al. defined double/triple extra copies lymphoma (DECL/TECL) as tumors with extra copies of *MYC* and *BCL2* and/or *BCL6* and tumors with extra *MYC* copies and concomitant rearrangements of *BCL2* and/or *BCL6*. They found that patients with DECL/TECL showed a similar poor clinical outcome as that of patients with DHL/THL [535]. Li et al. defined atypical DHL as all tumors with concurrent *MYC* and *BCL2* abnormalities other than coexisting translocations, and patients with atypical DHL had similar clinical outcomes to patients with DHL [536]. Huang et al. expanded the definition of atypical DHL/THL to include all patients with concurrent *MYC* and *BCL2* and/or *BCL6* abnormalities except DHL/THL [436]. Patients with atypical DHL/THL predicted poor outcome.

High-grade B-cell lymphoma, not otherwise specified (HGBL, NOS)

HGBL, NOS is an aggressive B-cell lymphoma that lack morphologic, immunophenotypic and genetic features typical for DLBCL, HGBL-R or BL [1]. HGBL, NOS, share some morphological or immunophenotypical features with both DLBCL and BL, hence the other designation of "gray zone" lymphoma [1, 96, 512, 537]. WHO classification states that this category should be used sparingly only when pathologist cannot classify a case as DLBCL or BL [1]. Cases of otherwise typical DLBCL, NOS harboring *MYC* translocation should be classified as DLBCL, NOS.

Morphology

HGBL, NOS is exceedingly rare and diagnosed only after exclusion of DLBCL, BL, and HGBL-R (DHL/THL). HGBL, NOS may morphologically resemble BL (monomorphic BL-like HGBL, NOS), DLBCL (pleomorphic DLBCL-like HGBL, NOS) or lymphoblastic lymphoma (blastoid HGBL, NOS Figure 13.114). BL-like variant displays diffuse infiltrate of medium-sized cells with starry-sky pattern, many mitoses, and many apoptotic cells. Rare mature B-cell lymphomas with blastoid appearance are negative for TdT, *CCND1* rearrangement [t(11;140] and negative for double *MYC* and *BCL2* rearrangement [96].

Immunophenotype

HGBL, NOS are positive for CD20 and BCL6, negative for MUM1/IRF, while the expression of CD10 and MYC varies (cases with *MYC* rearrangement are positive for MYC immunostaining). Proliferation fraction (Ki-67 index) is variable, but usually high. TdT and CD34 are negative in all cases of HGBL, NOS.

Genetic features

MYC rearrangement is present in 20%–35% of cases. Cases with a *BCL2* rearrangement and increase copy number or high-level amplification of *MYC* have been reported [536, 538, 539].

Differential diagnosis of HGBL, NOS

HGBL is rare and diagnosed only cases do not fulfill criteria for the diagnosis of BL, DLBCL, or HGBL-R (DHL/THL). HGBL, NOS with BL-like morphology may resemble BL morphologically, but atypical immunophenotype including strong BCL2 expression and/or lack of CD10 expression, and complex karyotype or lack of *MYC* rearrangement support HGBL, NOS [508, 517]. Majority of HGBLs are either DHL or THL. See differential diagnosis of BL and HGBL-R, above.

Plasmablastic lymphoma (PBL)

PBL phenotype by FC: FSC^high, sIg+/rarely+, CD5−/rarely+, CD10−/rarely+, CD11c−, CD19−, CD20−/+(dim), CD23−, CD25−, CD30−/+, CD34−, CD38+bright, CD43−/rarely+, CD45−/rarely+, CD56+/−, CD71+dim, CD79b−/+dim, CD103−, CD117−/rarely+, CD200+/−

Introduction

PBL is rare, aggressive, post-germinal center B-cell neoplasm that usually occurs in the setting of immunosuppression due to human immunodeficiency virus (HIV) infection [1]. PBL is composed of diffuse infiltrate of CD20− immunoblastic or plasmablastic cells which display plasma cell-like phenotype (CD38+, CD138+, MUM1+). PBL represents approximately 3% of HIV related lymphomas [407, 540–543]. The male:female ratio varies with clinical context; there is a male predominance, up to 7:1 in HIV-positive patients. These neoplasms can occur also in patients following allogeneic transplant and in patients with other forms of immunodeficiency. In addition, a subset of elderly patients may develop PBL, presumably attributable to physiological immunosenescence. PBLs are predominantly seen in extranodal sites especially oral cavity, but are also reported in various mucosal sites, skin, soft tissue, bone, and rarely in lymph nodes. At presentation, 90% of patients have extranodal involvement, 69% present with advanced stage disease and 27% had oral involvement [544]. Disseminated

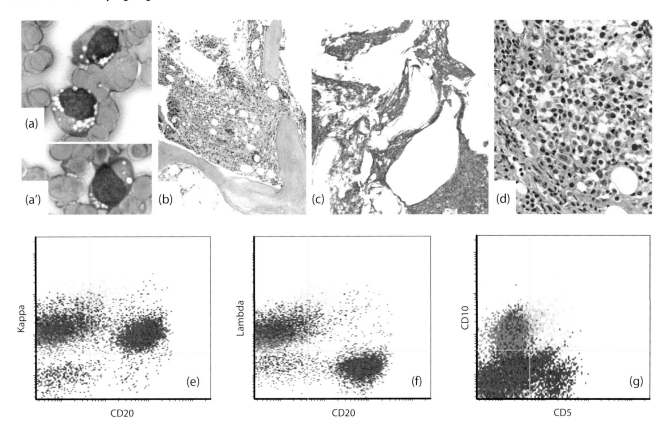

FIGURE 13.114 HGBL, NOS (BM involvement). Aspirate smear (a) show highly atypical lymphoid cells with blastoid appearance. Core biopsy of the BM (b–d) shows prominent involvement by atypical CD20+ (c) B-cell infiltrate with paratrabecular pattern progressing to diffuse pattern. FC analysis (e–g) shows clonal kappa+ (e–f) B-cells without CD5 or CD10 expression (g).

presentation is not uncommon. The cytomorphologic features resemble immunoblastic variant of DLBCL, PCM with plasmablastic features, precursor B- and T-cell lymphoblastic lymphomas, and immature myeloid neoplasms. Apart from HIV+ patients, PBL may occur in transplant recipients (post-transplant lymphoproliferative disorder) and in HIV− patients as HT of low-grade lymphoma (e.g., CLL or FL). [545, 546]. PBL is often associated with *MYC-IGH* rearrangement [544, 547]. The median overall survival is 11 months, regardless of the intensity of chemotherapy [544, 548].

Morphology

Typical PBL (oral mucosa type) shows diffuse and monotonous infiltrate composed of immunoblast-like or plasmablast-like cells with variable degrees of plasmacytic differentiation (Figures 13.115 and 13.116). Infiltrates are diffuse with effacement of the architecture of nodal or extranodal site with confluent areas of necrosis. Plasmablast-like cells are large with abundant pale-basophilic cytoplasm, slightly eccentric nucleus, and immunoblastic-like cells are have large oval to round vesicular nuclei with open chromatin and prominent central nucleoli. Similarly to other high-grade tumors, mitoses, tingible body macrophages, and apoptotic cells are easily identified, and many cases show a "starry-sky" pattern. Cases of PBL with plasmacytic differentiation show variable numbers of cells with plasmacytic differentiation and monoclonal light chain expression (Figure 13.117). PBLs located in sites other than oral mucosa tend to show more plasmacytic differentiation with basophilic cytoplasm, paranuclear hof and eccentric large nuclei. In contrast to plasma cell neoplasms, there are no Dutcher or Russell bodies.

Bone marrow. In rare cases of BM involvement (Figure 13.118), there are sheets of atypical large cells with plasmablastic or immunoblastic morphology, many mitoses, and apoptotic cells with or without plasmacytic differentiation. Areas of necrosis are often present. Cases with plasmacytic differentiation show more mature plasma cells with eccentric nuclei, inconspicuous nucleoli, and paranuclear hofs.

Immunophenotype

The phenotype is similar to plasma cell tumors. Most B-cell markers are negative, but CD79a may be positive in 40% of cases. Plasma cell-associated markers, including MUM1/IRF-4, VS38, CD38, CD138, BLIMP-1, and XBP-1 are usually positive. BOB1 or OCT2 are positive in most cases, MYC is positive in up to 100%, EMA in ~60%, p53 in ~50%, BCL2 in ~33%, CD30 in ~33%, CD56 in ~25%, CD10 in 20%–40%, and BCL6 in ~20% [407, 549, 550]. CD45 is most often negative, but minor subset of cases may be dim CD45+. ALK, BCL1 (cyclin D1), and HHV8 are negative. Subset of cases may show aberrant expression of T-cell markers (CD3, CD4, or CD7). In situ hybridization for EBV encoded RNA (EBER-ISH) is positive in about 70% of cases (HIV-associated cases are more often EBV positive than non-HIV cases). Figures 13.114–13.117 illustrate the major phenotypic characteristics of PBL. Cytoplasmic light and heavy chain immunoglobulins are most often negative, but may be positive, especially in cases with plasmacytic differentiation. Ki67 index is high (usually >90%). In contrast to PCM, PBL is most often CD117−. Figure 13.119 shows PBL with unusual CD45 expression and aberrant CD117 expression.

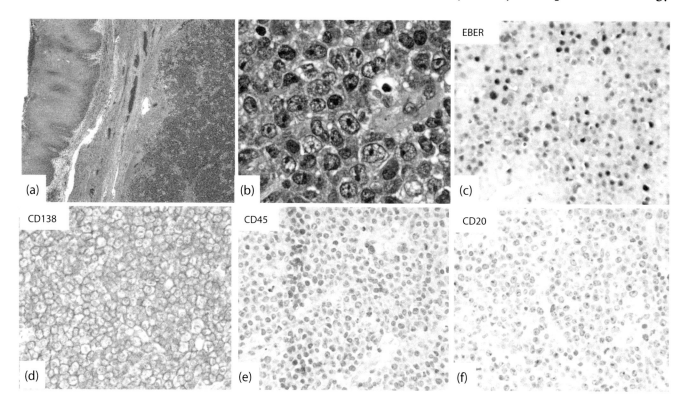

FIGURE 13.115 Plasmablastic lymphoma, oral mucosa. (a–b) histology (a, low power; b, high power); (c–f) immunohistochemistry: lymphomatous cells are positive for EBER (c) and CD138 (d), and negative for CD45 (e) and CD20 (f).

Differential diagnosis of PBL

The morphology can be quite variable with features of plasma cell differentiation (eccentrically placed nucleus, abundant cytoplasm, and prominent nucleolus) present in only some cases. In most other cases, PBL is indistinguishable from several other large cell lymphomas in the absence of an extensive immunophenotype analysis.

Main differential diagnosis of PBL includes:

- PCM
- ALK⁺ large B cell lymphoma
- DLBCL
- BL
- PEL
- Large cell lymphoma arising in HHV-8 associated multicentric Castleman's disease
- Immunodeficiency-associated lymphoproliferative disorders
- Extranodal NK/T-cell lymphoma, nasal type (ENKTL)
- EMT
- Acute leukemias (in cases with BM involvement)

DLBCL

Positive expression of EBER, frequent expression of CD56, EMA and lack of CD20, PAX5, CD45, and BCL6 helps to distinguish PBL from DLBCL. Subset of PBLs may be BCL6⁺ or dimly CD45⁺, and rare cases of DLBCL may be CD20⁻.

PCM

PBL and PCM have similar phenotype: both tumors are usually negative for CD45 and B-cell markers (CD19, CD20, PAX5), positive for plasma cell markers (CD38, CD138, and MUM1), and often express CD56. Rare cases of both PBL and PCM may be CD45⁺. PBL are often positive for MYC and negative for CD117, whereas

PCM are often positive for CD117 and negative for MYC. EBER expression is the major factor in differential diagnosis; it is positive in PBL and negative in PCM. PBL usually involves extranodal sites and rarely spreads to BM. Presence of serum monoclonal protein (M protein), BM involvement and radiologic imaging showing lytic bone lesions would indicate the diagnosis of PCM rather than PBL.

BL

Despite starry-sky pattern, high Ki67 index, EBV and MYC expression shared by both BL and PBL, BL differs from PBL by positive expression of CD45 and B-cell makers (CD19, CD20, PAX5) and lack of CD56 and EMA expression. Presence of CD10 and BCL6 would favor the diagnosis of BL (BCL6 is only rarely positive in PBL and CD10 is positive in PBL in approximately 50% of cases), whereas presence of plasma cell markers (MUM1, CD38, CD138) and CD56 would favor the diagnosis of PBL.

ALK⁺ large B-cell lymphoma

This rare lymphoma is more common in younger patients and children and differs from PBL by frequent involvement of lymph nodes, intrasinusoidal growth pattern and positive expression of ALK and CD45. Similar to PBL, ALK⁺ large B-cell lymphomas are usually CD20⁻.

B-ALL/LBL

Precursor B-cell acute lymphoblastic lymphoma/leukemia differs by expression of CD19, CD22, CD34, CD45, CD79a, TdT, and often bright CD10, as well as negative EBER.

T-ALL/LBL

Precursor T-lymphoblastic lymphoma/leukemia differs by positive cytoplasmic CD3, CD7, CD34, TdT, and negative EBER.

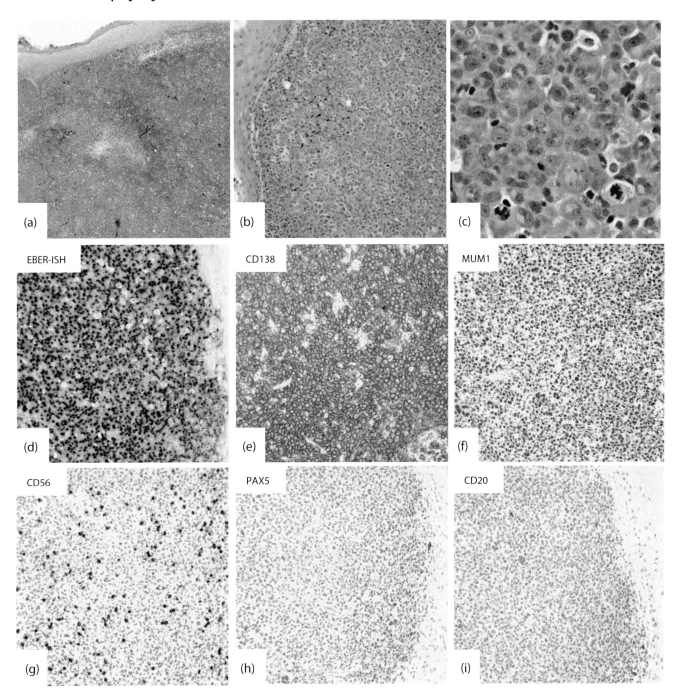

FIGURE 13.116   PBL of the buccal mucosa. Histologic section (a–c; different magnifications) shows diffuse highly atypical infiltrate composed of large cells with irregular nuclei, scanty cytoplasm and several prominent nucleoli. Tumor cells express EBV/EBER (by ISH; d), CD138 (e), MUM1 (f), and are negative for CD56 (g), PAX5 (h), and CD20 (i).

PEL

Kaposi's sarcoma-associated herpesvirus, the viral agent of Kaposi's sarcoma, is associated with two lymphoproliferative disorders: PEL and multicentric Castleman's disease. PEL is characterized by large "anaplastic" and/or "immunoblastic" cells with abundant basophilic cytoplasm with occasional vacuoles, pleomorphic nuclei, and nucleoli. PEL is characterized by peculiar phenotype, somewhat similar to PBL and plasma cell tumors. The lymphoma cells are positive for HHV8, CD45 (>80%) usually dim, CD38 (up to 100%), CD138 (35%–75%), MUM1 (up to 100%), CD43, EMA, HLA-DR, and CD30 (>50%). They are usually

negative for CD19, CD20, CD22, cytoplasmic CD79a, surface and cytoplasmic light chain kappa and lambda immunoglobulins, CD56, CD81, and CD117.

Large B-cell lymphoma arising in Kaposi sarcoma-associated virus positive multicentric Castleman's disease

A variant of PBL may occur in the setting of multicentric Castleman's disease. They occur in lymph nodes and spleen and frequently involve blood. The neoplastic cells form vague nodules which are surrounded by polytypic plasma cells. Lymphomatous

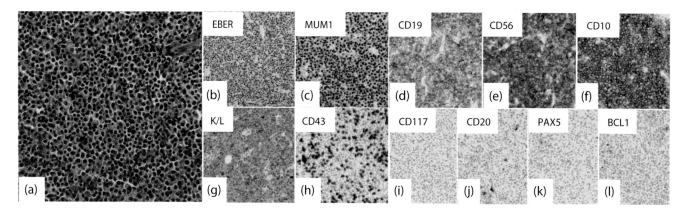

FIGURE 13.117   PBL with plasmacytic differentiation (a, histologic section). Tumor cells express EBV/EBER (by ISH; b), MUM1 (c), CD19 (d), CD56 (e), CD10 (f), and lambda (g; dual kappa and lambda staining with kappa brown and lambda red); they are negative for CD43 (h), CD117 (i), CD20 (j), PAX5 (k), and BCL1 (cyclin D1; l).

cells have immunoblastic morphology are positive for CD20 (dim), CD45, HHV-8, and lambda immunoglobulins and negative for CD30 and EBV.

ENKTL
ENKTL, which is EBV/EBER⁺, is composed of either small, intermediate, or large cells (often shows mixture of small and large cells) differs from PBL by expression of CD2, cytoplasmic CD3, and cytotoxic markers.

HHV8⁺ multicentric Castleman disease
This disorder frequently involves lymph node and/or spleen, is HHV8⁺, EBER/EBV⁻, CD20⁺, and often lambda⁺.

EMT
Positive expression of blastic markers (CD34, CD117), myeloid antigens (MPO, CD13, CD33) or monocytic markers (CD14, CD64, muramidase) in conjunction with lack of plasma cell markers and EBV help to differentiate between EMT and PBL.

EBV⁺ tumors
Apart from PBL, EBV is positive in EBV-associated reactive changes, posttrasplant lymphoproliferations, EBV⁺ DLBCL, LyG, cHL, BL, B-immunoblasts in AITL, ENKTL, methotrexate-induces EBV-associated B-cell lymphoproliferative disorder and nasopharyngeal carcinoma.

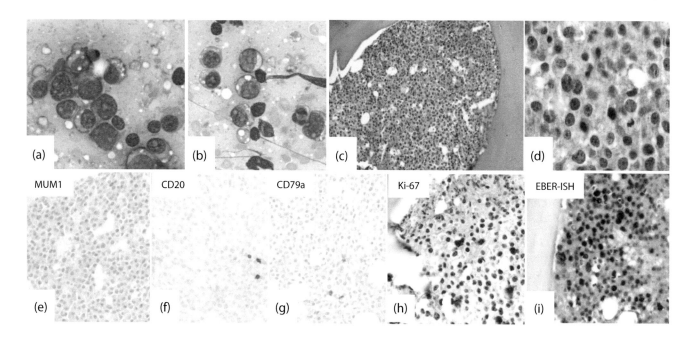

FIGURE 13.118   PBL involving BM. (a–b) Aspirate smear shows highly atypical mononuclear cells with blastoid features (plasmablasts) with macronucleoli, fine chromatin and abundant basophilic cytoplasm with occasional vacuoles. Some cells resemble more mature plasma cells. (c–d) Histology shows diffuse BM involvement (low and high power). (e–i) Immunohistochemistry. PBL cells show the following phenotype: MUM1⁺ (e), CD20⁻ (f), CD79a⁻ (g), Ki-67⁺ (h), and EBV⁺ (i).

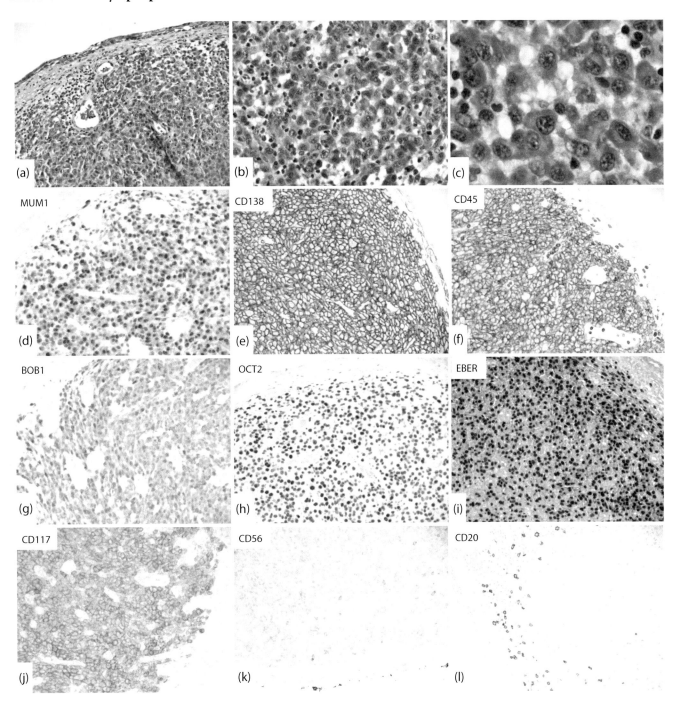

FIGURE 13.119 PBL (presenting as nasal polyp). (a–c) Histology (low, intermediate and high power). (d–l) Immunohistochemistry. Tumor cells are positive for MUM1 (d), CD138 (e), CD45 (f), BOB1 (g), OCT2 (h), EBV (i), CD117 (j), and weakly positive for CD56 (k). CD20 is negative (l).

Primary effusion lymphoma (PEL)

PEL phenotype by FC: FSC^{high}, sIg$^{+/rarely-}$, CD5$^-$, CD10$^-$, CD11c$^-$, CD19$^-$, CD20$^-$, CD22$^-$, CD23$^-$, CD25$^-$, CD34$^-$, CD38$^+$, CD43$^{-/+}$, CD45$^{+dim/-}$, CD79b$^-$, CD81$^-$, CD103$^-$

PEL is an aggressive lymphoma associated with Kaposi sarcoma-associated herpesvirus (KSHV; human herpesvirus 8; HHV8),

which occurs most commonly in younger HIV-infected patients or older patients [1, 407, 548, 551–555]. Immunosuppression related to age and comorbidities (especially organ transplantation) may also predispose to PEL. Morphologically, PEL is characterized by large "anaplastic", "plasmablastic", and/or "immunoblastic" cells with abundant basophilic cytoplasm with occasional vacuoles, pleomorphic nuclei, and nucleoli. Kaposi sarcoma herpesvirus (KSHV) is the etiologic agent, and ~80% of tumors are coinfected with EBV. Given this common viral etiology, patients with PEL may have concurrent Kaposi sarcoma and/or multicentric Castleman disease (KSHV-MCD). More recently, solid lymphomas not associated with lymphomatous effusion have been found in HIV-seropositive and HIV-seronegative patients. Tumors with cytomorphologic and immunophenotypic features of PEL may occur in locations other than body cavities (extracavitary PEL): gastrointestinal tract, skin, lung, scrotum, and CNS [542, 556–558]. These tumors have similar morphology to PEL or PBL, express KSHV (HHV8), are often positive for CD30 and frequently lack lineage specific markers (null cell phenotype). PEL usually remains localized.

Morphology

Tumor cells are large with either immunoblastic (round nuclei with central prominent nucleoli), anaplastic (highly pleomorphic and hyperchromatic cells) or plasmablastic features (eccentric nuclei with abundant cytoplasm and perinuclear hof) (Figures 13.120–13.122). Cytoplasm is densely basophilic and moderate to abundant and may contain vacuoles. Nuclei are large and often irregular with prominent nucleoli. Histology (either cell block preparations or pleural biopsy) reveals large closely packed neoplastic cells with abundant

cytoplasm, large nuclei with coarse unevenly distributed chromatin and prominent nucleoli.

Immunophenotype

PEL is characterized by peculiar phenotype, somewhat similar to PBL and plasma cell tumors. The lymphoma cells are positive for HHV8, CD45 (>80%) usually dim, CD38 (up to 100%), CD138 (35%–75%), MUM1 (up to 100%), CD43, EMA, HLA-DR, and CD30 (>50%). They are usually negative for CD19, CD20, CD22, cytoplasmic CD79a, surface and cytoplasmic light chain kappa and lambda immunoglobulins, CD56, CD81, and CD117. Aberrant expression of pan-T-cell markers (CD3, CD5, or CD7) is often seen in PEL [552, 559, 560]. Other B-cell markers, such as BOB1 and OCT2 are often positive and occasional tumors express CD20 and CD79a. Strong nuclear staining for HHV8 is helpful in establishing the diagnosis (Figures 13.120–13.122). These neoplasms have ABC/non-GCB immunophenotype. PD-1 expression have been reported in up to 50% of cases. Aberrant T-cell antigen expression can be observed, including CD45RO, CD7 and CD4. CD10, CD15, and BCL6 are negative. EBER by ISH is usually positive, especially in HIV setting.

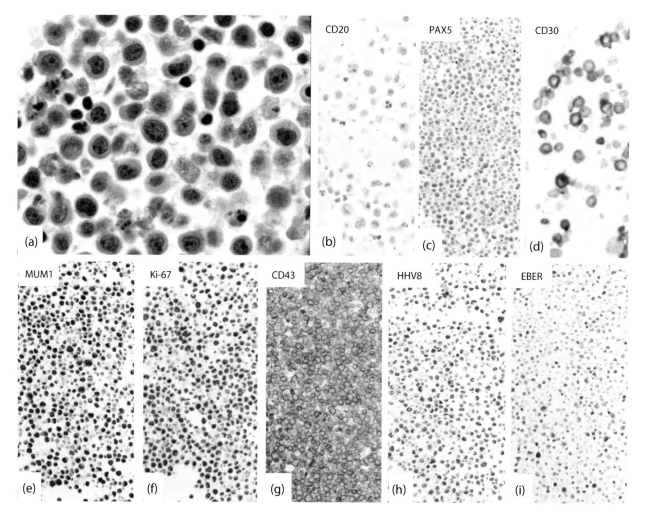

FIGURE 13.120 PEL – immunohistochemistry. (a) Cell block preparation shows large atypical lymphoid cells. (b–d) Immunohistochemistry. Tumor cells are negative for CD20 (b) and PAX5 (c), and are positive for CD30 (d), MUM1 (e), Ki-67 (f), CD43 (g), HHV-8 (h), and EBER (i).

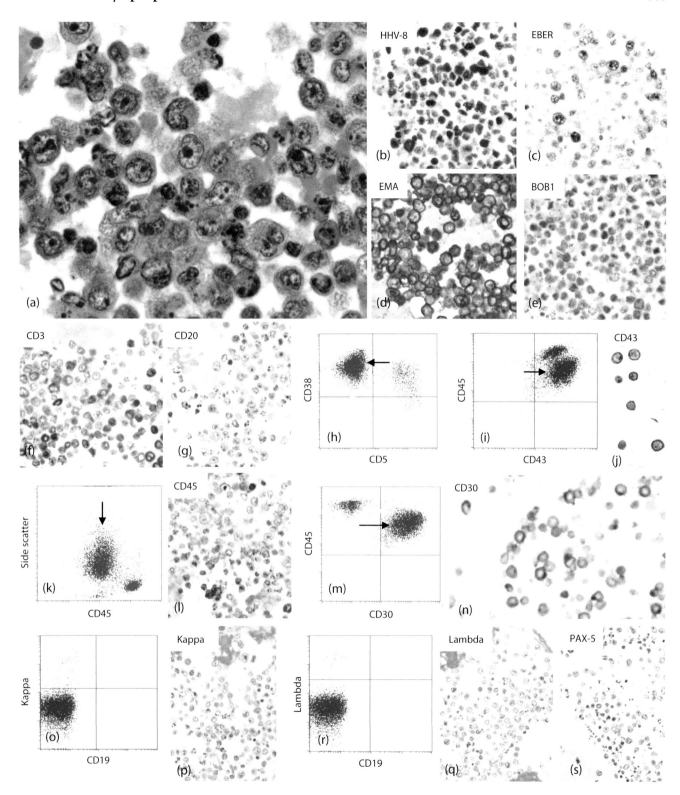

FIGURE 13.121 Primary effusion lymphoma (PEL). Lymphomatous cells are large with irregular nuclei and prominent nucleoli (a). Flow cytometry and immunohistochemical staining (cell block) showed tumor cells positive for HHV-8 (b), EBER (c), EMA (d), BOB1 (e), and CD3 (f), negative for CD20 (g), positive for CD38 (h), CD45 (i–k), CD43 (i–j), CD30 (m–n) and negative for kappa (o–p), lambda (r–q) and PAX5 (s).

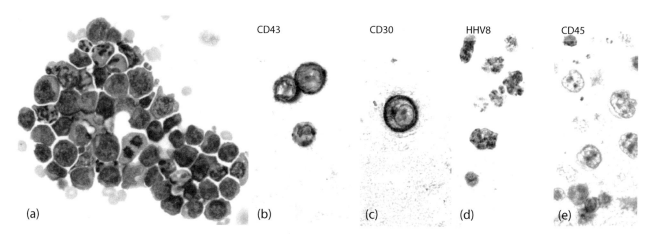

CD43   CD30   HHV8   CD45

(a)   (b)   (c)   (d)   (e)

FIGURE 13.122 Primary effusion lymphoma – cytology (cytospin preparation) and immunohistochemistry. The tumor cells are large and pleomorphic with increased nuclear-cytoplasmic ratio, basophilic cytoplasm and irregular nuclei (a) and express CD43 (b), CD30 (c), HHV8 (d) and lack CD45 (e). Immunocytochemical staining was performed on smears.

Extracavitary PEL more often express CD20 an CD79a and is less likely positive for CD45 and CD138.

Extracavitary PEL
Extracavitary PELs have been reported in lymph nodes, retroperitoneum, skin, spleen, and heart [552]. In lymph node intrasinusoidal involvement is common.

Differential diagnosis of PEL
Differential diagnosis of PEL includes DLBCLs, especially with predominantly immunoblastic cytomorphology, HGBLs, PBL, plasma cell neoplasms, ALCL and other large T-cell lymphomas, mesothelioma, and poorly differentiated carcinoma. Table 12.2 (Chapter 12) shows major phenotypic differences between PEL and other large cell lymphomas. Plasma cell tumors differ by positive staining with cytoplasmic immunoglobulins and lack of HHV8 and EBER. ALCL can be excluded by lack of ALK, pan-T antigens (except CD3) and positive HHV8 and EBER. Metastatic carcinoma and mesothelioma are distinguished by the expression of epithelial markers. Lack of keratin expression helps to exclude carcinomatous involvement of the serous cavities. Majority of cases are also positive for EBV (detected by EBER).

HHV8 is associated with several other distinct lymphoproliferative disorders, apart from PEL: multicentric Castleman's disease, multicentric Castleman's disease-associated PBL, and HHV8+/EBV+ germinotropic lymphoproliferative disorder. Differential diagnosis of PEL includes metastatic carcinoma, pyothorax-associated primary lymphoma, systemic large B-cell lymphoma, and ALCL.

HHV8-negative effusion-based lymphomas resembling PEL have been reported in the literature [553]. Patients are older, generally HIV-negative and not immunosuppressed, frequently hepatitis C positive and often have an underlying medical condition leading to fluid overload [553]. Lymphomatous cells are positive for B-cell markers and often display germinal center phenotype (with CD10 and BCL6 expression), have high proliferation index and may be positive for EBV. EBV is positive in nearly 30% of cases [553].

References

1. Swerdlow, S.H., Campo, E., Harris, N. L., Jaffe, E. S., Pileri, S. A., Stein, H., et al., ed. *WHO classification of tumors of haematopoietic and lymphoid tissues*. 2016, IARC: Lyon.
2. Dohner, H., et al., *Genomic aberrations and survival in chronic lymphocytic leukemia*. N Engl J Med, 2000. **343**(26): p. 1910–6.
3. Rossi, D., et al., *Integrated mutational and cytogenetic analysis identifies new prognostic subgroups in chronic lymphocytic leukemia*. Blood, 2013. **121**(8): p. 1403–12.
4. Randen, U., et al., *Bone marrow histology in monoclonal B-cell lymphocytosis shows various B-cell infiltration patterns*. Am J Clin Pathol, 2013. **139**(3): p. 390–5.
5. Defrancesco, I., et al., *Targeted next-generation sequencing reveals molecular heterogeneity in non-chronic lymphocytic leukemia clonal B-cell lymphocytosis*. Hematol Oncol, 2020. **38**(5): p. 689–97.
6. Kalpadakis, C., et al., *Detection of L265P MYD-88 mutation in a series of clonal B-cell lymphocytosis of marginal zone origin (CBL-MZ)*. Hematol Oncol, 2017. **35**(4): p. 542–7.
7. Strati, P., et al., *CD49d associates with nodal presentation and subsequent development of lymphadenopathy in patients with chronic lymphocytic leukaemia*. Br J Haematol, 2017. **178**(1): p. 99–105.
8. Gradowski, J.F., et al., *Chronic lymphocytic leukemia/small lymphocytic lymphoma with cyclin D1 positive proliferation centers do not have CCND1 translocations or gains and lack SOX11 expression*. Am J Clin Pathol, 2012. **138**(1): p. 132–9.
9. Gibson, S.E., et al., *Proliferation centres of chronic lymphocytic leukaemia/small lymphocytic lymphoma have enhanced expression of MYC protein, which does not result from rearrangement or gain of the MYC gene*. Br J Haematol, 2015. **175**(1): p. 173–5.
10. Gine, E., et al., *Expanded and highly active proliferation centers identify a histological subtype of chronic lymphocytic leukemia ("accelerated" chronic lymphocytic leukemia) with aggressive clinical behavior*. Haematologica, 2010. **95**(9): p. 1526–33.
11. Teixeira Mendes, L.S., et al., *Cyclin D1 overexpression in proliferation centres of small lymphocytic lymphoma/chronic lymphocytic leukaemia*. J Clin Pathol, 2017. **70**(10): p. 899–902.
12. Oudat, R., et al., *Significance of the levels of bone marrow lymphoid infiltrate in chronic lymphocytic leukemia patients with nodular partial remission*. Leukemia, 2002. **16**(4): p. 632–5.
13. Kjeldsberg, C.R. and J. Marty, *Prolymphocytic transformation of chronic lymphocytic leukemia*. Cancer, 1981. **48**(11): p. 2447–57.
14. Enno, A., et al., *'Prolymphocytoid' transformation of chronic lymphocytic leukaemia*. Br J Haematol, 1979. **41**(1): p. 9–18.
15. Pugh, W.C., J.T. Manning, and J.J. Butler, *Paraimmunoblastic variant of small lymphocytic lymphoma/leukaemia*. Am J Surg Pathol, 1988. **12**(12): p. 907–17.
16. Ohno, T., et al., *Origin of the Hodgkin/Reed-Sternberg cells in chronic lymphocytic leukemia with "Hodgkin's transformation"*. Blood, 1998. **91**(5): p. 1757–61.

17. Williams, J., et al., *Chronic lymphocytic leukemia with coexistent Hodgkin's disease. Implications for the origin of the Reed-Sternberg cell.* Am J Surg Pathol, 1991. **15**(1): p. 33–42.

18. Brecher, M. and P.M. Banks, *Hodgkin's disease variant of Richter's syndrome. Report of eight cases.* Am J Clin Pathol, 1990. **93**(3): p. 333–9.

19. Momose, H., et al., *Chronic lymphocytic leukemia/small lymphocytic lymphoma with Reed-Sternberg-like cells and possible transformation to Hodgkin's disease. Mediation by Epstein-Barr virus.* Am J Surg Pathol, 1992. **16**(9): p. 859–67.

20. Kanzler, H., et al., *Hodgkin and Reed-Sternberg-like cells in B-cell chronic lymphocytic leukemia represent the outgrowth of single germinal-center B-cell-derived clones: potential precursors of Hodgkin and Reed-Sternberg cells in Hodgkin's disease.* Blood, 2000. **95**(3): p. 1023–31.

21. Tsimberidou, A.M. and M.J. Keating, *Richter syndrome: biology, incidence, and therapeutic strategies.* Cancer, 2005. **103**(2): p. 216–28.

22. Wiernik, P.H., *Second neoplasms in patients with chronic lymphocytic leukemia.* Curr Treat Options Oncol, 2004. **5**(3): p. 215–23.

23. Ansell, S.M., et al., *Epstein-Barr virus infection in Richter's transformation.* Am J Hematol, 1999. **60**(2): p. 99–104.

24. Bea, S., et al., *Genetic imbalances in progressed B-cell chronic lymphocytic leukemia and transformed large-cell lymphoma (Richter's syndrome).* Am J Pathol, 2002. **161**(3): p. 957–68.

25. Harousseau, J.L., et al., *Malignant lymphoma supervening in chronic lymphocytic leukemia and related disorders. Richter's syndrome: a study of 25 cases.* Cancer, 1981. **48**(6): p. 1302–8.

26. Travis, L.B., et al., *Second cancers following non-Hodgkin's lymphoma.* Cancer, 1991. **67**(7): p. 2002–9.

27. Agbay, R.L., et al., *High-grade transformation of low-grade B-cell lymphoma: pathology and molecular pathogenesis.* Am J Surg Pathol, 2016. **40**(1): p. e1–e16.

28. Torelli, U.L., et al., *Simultaneously increased expression of the c-myc and mu chain genes in the acute blastic transformation of a chronic lymphocytic leukaemia.* Br J Haematol, 1987. **65**(2): p. 165–70.

29. Tsimberidou, A.M., et al., *Hodgkin transformation of chronic lymphocytic leukemia: the M. D. Anderson Cancer Center experience.* Cancer, 2006. **107**(6): p. 1294–302.

30. Tsimberidou, A.M. and M.J. Keating, *Richter's transformation in chronic lymphocytic leukemia.* Semin Oncol, 2006. **33**(2): p. 250–6.

31. Tsimberidou, A.M., et al., *Clinical outcomes and prognostic factors in patients with Richter's syndrome treated with chemotherapy or chemoimmunotherapy with or without stem-cell transplantation.* J Clin Oncol, 2006. **24**(15): p. 2343–51.

32. Dierlamm, J., et al., *Genetic abnormalities in chronic lymphocytic leukemia and their clinical and prognostic implications.* Cancer Genet Cytogenet, 1997. **94**(1): p. 27–35.

33. Foon, K.A., K.R. Rai, and R.P. Gale, *Chronic lymphocytic leukemia: new insights into biology and therapy.* Ann Intern Med, 1990. **113**(7): p. 525–39.

34. Oscier, D.G., et al., *Multivariate analysis of prognostic factors in CLL: clinical stage, IGVH gene mutational status, and loss or mutation of the p53 gene are independent prognostic factors.* Blood, 2002. **100**(4): p. 1177–84.

35. Delgado, J., et al., *Chronic lymphocytic leukemia: from molecular pathogenesis to novel therapeutic strategies.* Haematologica, 2020. **105**(9): p. 2205–17.

36. Tausch, E., et al., *Prognostic and predictive impact of genetic markers in patients with CLL treated with obinutuzumab and venetoclax.* Blood, 2020. **135**(26): p. 2402–12.

37. Cheson, B.D., et al., *National Cancer Institute-sponsored Working Group guidelines for chronic lymphocytic leukemia: revised guidelines for diagnosis and treatment.* Blood, 1996. **87**(12): p. 4990–7.

38. Rawstron, A.C., et al., *Quantitation of minimal disease levels in chronic lymphocytic leukemia using a sensitive flow cytometric assay improves the prediction of outcome and can be used to optimize therapy.* Blood, 2001. **98**(1): p. 29–35.

39. Moreton, P., et al., *Eradication of minimal residual disease in B-cell chronic lymphocytic leukemia after alemtuzumab therapy is associated with prolonged survival.* J Clin Oncol, 2005. **23**(13): p. 2971–9.

40. Robertson, L.E., et al., *Response assessment in chronic lymphocytic leukemia after fludarabine plus prednisone: clinical, pathologic, immunophenotypic, and molecular analysis.* Blood, 1992. **80**(1): p. 29–36.

41. Esteve, J., et al., *Stem cell transplantation for chronic lymphocytic leukemia: different outcome after autologous and allogeneic transplantation and correlation with minimal residual disease status.* Leukemia, 2001. **15**(3): p. 445–51.

42. Provan, D., et al., *Eradication of polymerase chain reaction-detectable chronic lymphocytic leukemia cells is associated with improved outcome after bone marrow transplantation.* Blood, 1996. **88**(6): p. 2228–35.

43. Milligan, D.W., et al., *Results of the MRC pilot study show autografting for younger patients with chronic lymphocytic leukemia is safe and achieves a high percentage of molecular responses.* Blood, 2005. **105**(1): p. 397–404.

44. Pfitzner, T., et al., *A real-time PCR assay for the quantification of residual malignant cells in B cell chronic lymphatic leukemia.* Leukemia, 2000. **14**(4): p. 754–66.

45. Bottcher, S., et al., *Comparative analysis of minimal residual disease detection using four-color flow cytometry, consensus IgH-PCR, and quantitative IgH PCR in CLL after allogeneic and autologous stem cell transplantation.* Leukemia, 2004. **18**(10): p. 1637–45.

46. Matutes, E., et al., *The immunological profile of B-cell disorders and proposal of a scoring system for the diagnosis of CLL.* Leukemia, 1994. **8**(10): p. 1640–5.

47. Falay, M., et al., *The role of CD200 and CD43 expression in differential diagnosis between chronic lymphocytic leukemia and mantle cell lymphoma.* Turk J Haematol, 2018. **35**(2): p. 94–8.

48. Kohnke, T., et al., *Diagnosis of CLL revisited: increased specificity by a modified five-marker scoring system including CD200.* Br J Haematol, 2017. **179**(3): p. 480–7.

49. Lesesve, J.F., et al., *Combination of CD160 and CD200 as a useful tool for differential diagnosis between chronic lymphocytic leukemia and other mature B-cell neoplasms.* Int J Lab Hematol, 2015. **37**(4): p. 486–94.

50. Sorigue, M., et al., *Positive predictive value of CD200 positivity in the differential diagnosis of chronic lymphocytic leukemia.* Cytometry B Clin Cytom, 2019. **98**(5): p. 441–8.

51. Mora, A., et al., *CD200 is a useful marker in the diagnosis of chronic lymphocytic leukemia.* Cytometry B Clin Cytom, 2019. **96**(2): p. 143–8.

52. Palumbo, G.A., et al., *CD200 expression may help in differential diagnosis between mantle cell lymphoma and B-cell chronic lymphocytic leukemia.* Leuk Res, 2009. **33**(9): p. 1212–6.

53. Rawstron, A.C., et al., *Reproducible diagnosis of chronic lymphocytic leukemia by flow cytometry: an European Research Initiative on CLL (ERIC) & European Society for Clinical Cell Analysis (ESCCA) Harmonisation project.* Cytometry B Clin Cytom, 2018. **94**(1): p. 121–8.

54. Sandes, A.F., et al., *CD200 has an important role in the differential diagnosis of mature B-cell neoplasms by multiparameter flow cytometry.* Cytometry B Clin Cytom, 2014. **86**(2): p. 98–105.

55. Hoffmann, J., et al., *Determination of CD43 and CD200 surface expression improves accuracy of B-cell lymphoma immunophenotyping.* Cytometry B Clin Cytom, 2020. **98**(6): p. 476–82.

56. Zhu, J., et al., *Holding on to the Matutes score while dropping FMC7: new opportunity from standardised approaches in multiparameter flow cytometry.* Br J Haematol, 2020. **190**(4): p. e255–8.

57. D'Arena, G., et al., *CD200 included in a 4-marker modified Matutes score provides optimal sensitivity and specificity for the diagnosis of chronic lymphocytic leukaemia.* Hematol Oncol, 2018. **36**: p. 543–6.

58. Starostka, D., et al., *Quantitative assessment of informative immunophenotypic markers increases the diagnostic value of immunophenotyping in mature CD5-positive B-cell neoplasms.* Cytometry B Clin Cytom, 2018. **94**(4): p. 576–87.

59. Zalcberg, I., et al., *Multidisciplinary diagnostics of chronic lymphocytic leukemia: European Research Initiative on CLL - ERIC recommendations.* Hematol Transfus Cell Ther, 2019. **42**(3): p. 269–74.

60. Del Giudice, I., et al., *B-cell prolymphocytic leukemia and chronic lymphocytic leukemia have distinctive gene expression signatures.* Leukemia, 2009. **23**(11): p. 2160–7.

61. Dearden, C., *How I treat prolymphocytic leukemia*. Blood, 2012. **120**(3): p. 538–51.

62. Shvidel, L., et al., *B-cell prolymphocytic leukemia: a survey of 35 patients emphasizing heterogeneity, prognostic factors and evidence for a group with an indolent course*. Leuk Lymphoma, 1999. **33**(1–2): p. 169–79.

63. Del Giudice, I., et al., *IgVH genes mutation and usage, ZAP-70 and CD38 expression provide new insights on B-cell prolymphocytic leukemia (B-PLL)*. Leukemia, 2006. **20**(7): p. 1231–7.

64. Krishnan, B., E. Matutes, and C. Dearden, *Prolymphocytic leukemias*. Semin Oncol, 2006. **33**(2): p. 257–63.

65. Lens, D., et al., *p53 abnormalities in B-cell prolymphocytic leukemia*. Blood, 1997. **89**(6): p. 2015–23.

66. Lens, D., et al., *Frequent deletions at 11q23 and 13q14 in B cell prolymphocytic leukemia (B-PLL)*. Leukemia, 2000. **14**(3): p. 427–30.

67. Crisostomo, R.H., J.A. Fernandez, and W. Caceres, *Complex karyotype including chromosomal translocation (8;14) (q24;q32) in one case with B-cell prolymphocytic leukemia*. Leuk Res, 2007. **31**(5): p. 699–701.

68. Ruchlemer, R., et al., *B-prolymphocytic leukaemia with t(11;14) revisited: a splenomegalic form of mantle cell lymphoma evolving with leukaemia*. Br J Haematol, 2004. **125**(3): p. 330–6.

69. Kuriakose, P., et al., *Translocation (8;14)(q24;q32) as the sole cytogenetic abnormality in B-cell prolymphocytic leukemia*. Cancer Genet Cytogenet, 2004. **150**(2): p. 156–8.

70. Hoehn, D., et al., *Splenic B-cell lymphomas with more than 55% prolymphocytes in blood: evidence for prolymphocytoid transformation*. Hum Pathol, 2012. **43**(11): p. 1828–38.

71. Adrada, B.E., et al., *Breast implant-associated anaplastic large cell lymphoma: sensitivity, specificity, and findings of imaging studies in 44 patients*. Breast Cancer Res Treat, 2014. **147**(1): p. 1–14.

72. Arcaini, L., et al., *Primary nodal marginal zone B-cell lymphoma: clinical features and prognostic assessment of a rare disease*. Br J Haematol, 2007. **136**(2): p. 301–4.

73. Camacho, F.I., et al., *Nodal marginal zone lymphoma: a heterogeneous tumor: a comprehensive analysis of a series of 27 cases*. Am J Surg Pathol, 2003. **27**(6): p. 762–71.

74. Nakamura, S. and M. Ponzoni, *Marginal zone B-cell lymphoma: lessons from Western and Eastern diagnostic approaches*. Pathology, 2020. **52**(1): p. 15–29.

75. Naresh, K.N., *Nodal marginal zone B-cell lymphoma with prominent follicular colonization - difficulties in diagnosis: a study of 15 cases*. Histopathology, 2008. **52**(3): p. 331–9.

76. Nathwani, B.N., et al., *Marginal zone B-cell lymphoma: a clinical comparison of nodal and mucosa-associated lymphoid tissue types. Non-Hodgkin's Lymphoma Classification Project*. J Clin Oncol, 1999. **17**(8): p. 2486–92.

77. Nathwani, B.N., et al., *Nodal monocytoid B-cell lymphoma (nodal marginal-zone B-cell lymphoma)*. Semin Hematol, 1999. **36**(2): p. 128–38.

78. Traverse-Glehen, A., et al., *Nodal marginal zone B-cell lymphoma: a diagnostic and therapeutic dilemma*. Oncology (Williston Park), 2012. **26**(1): p. 92–9, 103–4.

79. Arcaini, L., et al., *Nongastric marginal-zone B-cell MALT lymphoma: prognostic value of disease dissemination*. Oncologist, 2006. **11**(3): p. 285–91.

80. Traverse-Glehen, A., et al., *A clinicopathological study of nodal marginal zone B-cell lymphoma. A report on 21 cases*. Histopathology, 2006. **48**(2): p. 162–73.

81. Mollejo, M., et al., *Monocytoid B cells. A comparative clinical pathological study of their distribution in different types of low-grade lymphomas*. Am J Surg Pathol, 1994. **18**(11): p. 1131–9.

82. Campo, E., et al., *Primary nodal marginal zone lymphomas of splenic and MALT type*. Am J Surg Pathol, 1999. **23**(1): p. 59–68.

83. Kojima, M., et al., *Clinical implications of nodal marginal zone B-cell lymphoma among Japanese: study of 65 cases*. Cancer Sci, 2007. **98**(1): p. 44–9.

84. Karube, K., et al., *A "floral" variant of nodal marginal zone lymphoma*. Hum Pathol, 2005. **36**(2): p. 202–6.

85. Pileri, S. and M. Ponzoni, *Pathology of nodal marginal zone lymphomas*. Best Pract Res Clin Haematol, 2017. **30**(1–2): p. 50–55.

86. Salama, M.E., et al., *Immunoarchitectural patterns in nodal marginal zone B-cell lymphoma: a study of 51 cases*. Am J Clin Pathol, 2009. **132**(1): p. 39–49.

87. Cheuk, W., et al., *Lymphadenopathy of IgG4-related sclerosing disease*. Am J Surg Pathol, 2008. **32**(5): p. 671–81.

88. Sato, Y., et al., *Systemic IgG4-related lymphadenopathy: a clinical and pathologic comparison to multicentric Castleman's disease*. Mod Pathol, 2009. **22**(4): p. 589–99.

89. Kojima, M., et al., *Nodal marginal zone B-cell lymphoma associated with Sjogren's syndrome: a report of three cases*. Leuk Lymphoma, 2007. **48**(6): p. 1222–4.

90. Callet-Bauchu, E., et al., *Cytogenetic analysis delineates a spectrum of chromosomal changes that can distinguish non-MALT marginal zone B-cell lymphomas among mature B-cell entities: a description of 103 cases*. Leukemia, 2005. **19**(10): p. 1818–23.

91. Koh, J., et al., *Discovery of novel recurrent mutations and clinically meaningful subgroups in nodal marginal zone lymphoma*. Cancers (Basel), 2020. **12**(6): p. 1669.

92. Meyer, A.H., et al., *Transformation and additional malignancies are leading risk factors for an adverse course of disease in marginal zone lymphoma*. Ann Oncol, 2014. **25**(1): p. 210–5.

93. Xing, K.H., et al., *Outcomes in splenic marginal zone lymphoma: analysis of 107 patients treated in British Columbia*. Br J Haematol, 2015. **169**(4): p. 520–7.

94. Kiesewetter, B., et al., *Transformed mucosa-associated lymphoid tissue lymphomas: a single institution retrospective study including polymerase chain reaction-based clonality analysis*. Br J Haematol, 2019. **186**(3): p. 448–59.

95. Bacon, C.M., M.Q. Du, and A. Dogan, *Mucosa-associated lymphoid tissue (MALT) lymphoma: a practical guide for pathologists*. J Clin Pathol, 2007. **60**(4): p. 361–72.

96. Swerdlow, S.H., et al., *The 2016 revision of the World Health Organization classification of lymphoid neoplasms*. Blood, 2016. **127**(20): p. 2375–90.

97. Camacho, F.I., et al., *Progression to large B-cell lymphoma in splenic marginal zone lymphoma: a description of a series of 12 cases*. Am J Surg Pathol, 2001. **25**(10): p. 1268–76.

98. Wotherspoon, A.C., *Extranodal and splenic small B-cell lymphoma*. Mod Pathol, 2013. **26 Suppl 1**: p. S29–41.

99. Isaacson, P.G., *Gastric MALT lymphoma: from concept to cure*. Ann Oncol, 1999. **10**(6): p. 637–45.

100. Starostik, P., et al., *Gastric marginal zone B-cell lymphomas of MALT type develop along 2 distinct pathogenetic pathways*. Blood, 2002. **99**(1): p. 3–9.

101. Zucca, E., et al., *The gastric marginal zone B-cell lymphoma of MALT type*. Blood, 2000. **96**(2): p. 410–9.

102. Isaacson, P.G., et al., *Long-term follow-up of gastric MALT lymphoma treated by eradication of H. pylori with antibodies*. Gastroenterology, 1999. **117**(3): p. 750–1.

103. Thieblemont, C., et al., *Mucosa-associated lymphoid tissue lymphoma is a disseminated disease in one third of 158 patients analyzed*. Blood, 2000. **95**(3): p. 802–6.

104. Zinzani, P.L., et al., *Nongastrointestinal low-grade mucosa-associated lymphoid tissue lymphoma: analysis of 75 patients*. J Clin Oncol, 1999. **17**(4): p. 1254.

105. Ott, G., et al., *The t(11;18)(q21;q21) chromosome translocation is a frequent and specific aberration in low-grade but not high-grade malignant non-Hodgkin's lymphomas of the mucosa-associated lymphoid tissue (MALT-) type*. Cancer Res, 1997. **57**(18): p. 3944–8.

106. Rosenwald, A., et al., *Exclusive detection of the t(11;18)(q21;q21) in extranodal marginal zone B cell lymphomas (MZBL) of MALT type in contrast to other MZBL and extranodal large B cell lymphomas*. Am J Pathol, 1999. **155**(6): p. 1817–21.

107. Dierlamm, J., et al., *Detection of t(11;18)(q21;q21) by interphase fluorescence in situ hybridization using API2 and MLT specific probes*. Blood, 2000. **96**(6): p. 2215–8.

108. Barth, T.F., et al., *Molecular-cytogenetic comparison of mucosa-associated marginal zone B-cell lymphoma and large*

B-cell lymphoma arising in the gastro-intestinal tract. Genes Chromosomes Cancer, 2001. **31**(4): p. 316–25.

109. Hawkes, E.A., A. Wotherspoon, and D. Cunningham, *Diagnosis and management of rare gastrointestinal lymphomas.* Leuk Lymphoma, 2012. **53**(12): p. 2341–50.

110. Oh, S.Y., et al., *Intestinal marginal zone B-cell lymphoma of MALT type: clinical manifestation and outcome of a rare disease.* Eur J Haematol, 2007. **79**(4): p. 287–91.

111. Kohno, S., et al., *Clinicopathological analysis of 143 primary malignant lymphomas in the small and large intestines based on the new WHO classification.* Histopathology, 2003. **43**(2): p. 135–43.

112. Grogg, K.L., et al., *Nodular pulmonary amyloidosis is characterized by localized immunoglobulin deposition and is frequently associated with an indolent B-cell lymphoproliferative disorder.* Am J Surg Pathol, 2013. **37**(3): p. 406–12.

113. Zukerberg, L.R., et al., *Lymphoid infiltrates of the stomach. Evaluation of histologic criteria for the diagnosis of low-grade gastric lymphoma on endoscopic biopsy specimens.* Am J Surg Pathol, 1990. **14**(12): p. 1087–99.

114. Isaacson, P.G., *Gastrointestinal lymphomas of T- and B-cell types.* Mod Pathol, 1999. **12**(2): p. 151–8.

115. Isaacson, P.G. and J. Spencer, *The biology of low grade MALT lymphoma.* J Clin Pathol, 1995. **48**(5): p. 395–7.

116. Isaacson, P.G. and M.Q. Du, *MALT lymphoma: from morphology to molecules.* Nat Rev Cancer, 2004. **4**(8): p. 644–53.

117. Rawal, A., et al., *Site-specific morphologic differences in extranodal marginal zone B-cell lymphomas.* Arch Pathol Lab Med, 2007. **131**(11): p. 1673–8.

118. Copie-Bergman, C., et al., *Proposal for a new histological grading system for post-treatment evaluation of gastric MALT lymphoma.* Gut, 2003. **52**(11): p. 1656.

119. Dronca, R.S., et al., *CD5-positive chronic B-cell lymphoproliferative disorders: diagnosis and prognosis of a heterogeneous disease entity.* Cytometry B Clin Cytom, 2010. **78 Suppl 1**: p. S35–41.

120. Jevremovic, D., et al., *CD5⁺ B-cell lymphoproliferative disorders: beyond chronic lymphocytic leukemia and mantle cell lymphoma.* Leuk Res, 2010. **34**(9): p. 1235–8.

121. Wenzel, C., et al., *CD5 expression in a lymphoma of the mucosa-associated lymphoid tissue (MALT)-type as a marker for early dissemination and aggressive clinical behaviour.* Leuk Lymphoma, 2001. **42**(4): p. 823–9.

122. Jaso, J., et al., *CD5-positive mucosa-associated lymphoid tissue (MALT) lymphoma: a clinicopathologic study of 14 cases.* Hum Pathol, 2012. **43**(9): p. 1436–43.

123. Ferry, J.A., et al., *CD5⁺ extranodal marginal zone B-cell (MALT) lymphoma. A low grade neoplasm with a propensity for bone marrow involvement and relapse.* Am J Clin Pathol, 1996. **105**(1): p. 31–7.

124. Maeshima, A.M., et al., *Clinicopathological features of histological transformation from extranodal marginal zone B-cell lymphoma of mucosa-associated lymphoid tissue to diffuse large B-cell lymphoma: an analysis of 467 patients.* Br J Haematol, 2016. **174**(6): p. 923–31.

125. Zucca, E., et al., *Gastric marginal zone lymphoma of MALT type: ESMO Clinical Practice Guidelines for diagnosis, treatment and follow-up.* Ann Oncol, 2013. **24 Suppl 6**: p. vi144–8.

126. Ferreri, A.J., et al., *Prognostic significance of the histopathologic recognition of low- and high-grade components in stage I-II B-cell gastric lymphomas.* Am J Surg Pathol, 2001. **25**(1): p. 95–102.

127. Inagaki, H., et al., *Gastric MALT lymphomas are divided into three groups based on responsiveness to Helicobacter Pylori eradication and detection of API2-MALT1 fusion.* Am J Surg Pathol, 2004. **28**(12): p. 1560–7.

128. Liu, H., et al., *T(11;18) is a marker for all stage gastric MALT lymphomas that will not respond to H. pylori eradication.* Gastroenterology, 2002. **122**(5): p. 1286–94.

129. Ye, H., et al., *Variable frequencies of t(11;18)(q21;q21) in MALT lymphomas of different sites: significant association with CagA strains of H pylori in gastric MALT lymphoma.* Blood, 2003. **102**(3): p. 1012–8.

130. Ye, H., et al., *High incidence of t(11;18)(q21;q21) in Helicobacter pylori-negative gastric MALT lymphoma.* Blood, 2003. **101**(7): p. 2547–50.

131. Dierlamm, J., et al., *The apoptosis inhibitor gene API2 and a novel 18q gene, MLT, are recurrently rearranged in the t(11;18)(q21;q21) associated with mucosa-associated lymphoid tissue lymphomas.* Blood, 1999. **93**(11): p. 3601–9.

132. Murga Penas, E.M., et al., *Translocations t(11;18)(q21;q21) and t(14;18)(q32;q21) are the main chromosomal abnormalities involving MLT/MALT1 in MALT lymphomas.* Leukemia, 2003. **17**(11): p. 2225–9.

133. Streubel, B., et al., *Variable frequencies of MALT lymphoma-associated genetic aberrations in MALT lymphomas of different sites.* Leukemia, 2004. **18**(10): p. 1722–6.

134. Suzuki, T., et al., *Clinicopathological analysis of splenic red pulp low-grade B-cell lymphoma.* Pathol Int, 2020. **70**(5): p. 280–6.

135. Franco, V., A.M. Florena, and E. Iannitto, *Splenic marginal zone lymphoma.* Blood, 2003. **101**(7): p. 2464–72.

136. Matutes, E., et al., *Splenic marginal zone lymphoma proposals for a revision of diagnostic, staging and therapeutic criteria.* Leukemia, 2008. **22**(3): p. 487–95.

137. Arcaini, L., D. Rossi, and M. Paulli, *Splenic marginal zone lymphoma: from genetics to management.* Blood, 2016. **127**(17): p. 2072–81.

138. Geyer, J.T., S. Prakash, and A. Orazi, *B-cell neoplasms and Hodgkin lymphoma in the spleen.* Semin Diagn Pathol, 2021. 38(2): p. 125–34.

139. Chacon, J.I., et al., *Splenic marginal zone lymphoma: clinical characteristics and prognostic factors in a series of 60 patients.* Blood, 2002. **100**(5): p. 1648–54.

140. Berger, F., et al., *Non-MALT marginal zone B-cell lymphomas: a description of clinical presentation and outcome in 124 patients.* Blood, 2000. **95**(6): p. 1950–6.

141. Parry-Jones, N., et al., *Prognostic features of splenic lymphoma with villous lymphocytes: a report on 129 patients.* Br J Haematol, 2003. **120**(5): p. 759–64.

142. Mulligan, S.P., et al., *Splenic lymphoma with villous lymphocytes: natural history and response to therapy in 50 cases.* Br J Haematol, 1991. **78**(2): p. 206–9.

143. Troussard, X., et al., *Splenic lymphoma with villous lymphocytes: clinical presentation, biology and prognostic factors in a series of 100 patients. Groupe Francais d'Hematologie Cellulaire (GFHC).* Br J Haematol, 1996. **93**(3): p. 731–6.

144. Hockley, S.L., et al., *The prognostic impact of clinical and molecular features in hairy cell leukaemia variant and splenic marginal zone lymphoma.* Br J Haematol, 2012. **158**(3): p. 347–54.

145. Algara, P., et al., *Analysis of the IgV(H) somatic mutations in splenic marginal zone lymphoma defines a group of unmutated cases with frequent 7q deletion and adverse clinical course.* Blood, 2002. **99**(4): p. 1299–304.

146. Matutes, E., *Splenic marginal zone lymphoma with and without villous lymphocytes.* Curr Treat Options Oncol, 2007. **8**(2): p. 109–16.

147. Papadaki, T., et al., *Splenic marginal-zone lymphoma: one or more entities? A histologic, immunohistochemical, and molecular study of 42 cases.* Am J Surg Pathol, 2007. **31**(3): p. 438–46.

148. Ponzoni, M., et al., *Bone marrow histopathology in the diagnostic evaluation of splenic marginal-zone and splenic diffuse red pulp small B-cell lymphoma: a reliable substitute for spleen histopathology?* Am J Surg Pathol, 2012. **36**(11): p. 1609–18.

149. Kost, C.B., J.T. Holden, and K.P. Mann, *Marginal zone B-cell lymphoma: a retrospective immunophenotypic analysis.* Cytometry B Clin Cytom, 2008. **74**(5): p. 282–6.

150. Kojima, M., et al., *Characteristics of CD5-positive splenic marginal zone lymphoma with leukemic manifestation; clinical, flow cytometry, and histopathological findings of 11 cases.* J Clin Exp Hematop, 2010. **50**(2): p. 107–12.

151. Salido, M., et al., *Cytogenetic aberrations and their prognostic value in a series of 330 splenic marginal zone B-cell lymphomas: a multicenter study of the Splenic B-Cell Lymphoma Group.* Blood, 2010. **116**(9): p. 1479–88.

152. Baseggio, L., et al., *CD5 expression identifies a subset of splenic marginal zone lymphomas with higher lymphocytosis: a clinicopathological, cytogenetic and molecular study of 24 cases.* Haematologica, 2010. **95**(4): p. 604–12.

153. Giannouli, S., et al., *Splenic marginal zone lymphomas with peripheral CD5 expression.* Haematologica, 2004. **89**(1): p. 113–4.

154. Kampalath, B., M.P. Barcos, and C. Stewart, *Phenotypic heterogeneity of B cells in patients with chronic lymphocytic leukemia/small lymphocytic lymphoma.* Am J Clin Pathol, 2003. **119**(6): p. 824–32.

155. Morabito, F., et al., *Expression of myelomonocytic antigens on chronic lymphocytic leukemia B cells correlates with their ability to produce interleukin 1.* Blood, 1987. **70**(6): p. 1750–7.

156. Ocio, E.M., et al., *Immunophenotypic and cytogenetic comparison of Waldenstrom's macroglobulinemia with splenic marginal zone lymphoma.* Clin Lymphoma, 2005. **5**(4): p. 241–5.

157. Venkataraman, G., et al., *Characteristic CD103 and CD123 expression pattern defines hairy cell leukemia: usefulness of CD123 and CD103 in the diagnosis of mature B-cell lymphoproliferative disorders.* Am J Clin Pathol, 2011. **136**(4): p. 625–30.

158. Sole, F., et al., *Splenic marginal zone B-cell lymphomas: two cytogenetic subtypes, one with gain of 3q and the other with loss of 7q.* Haematologica, 2001. **86**(1): p. 71–7.

159. Viaggi, S., et al., *Uncommon cytogenetic findings in a case of splenic marginal zone lymphoma with aggressive clinical course.* Cancer Genet Cytogenet, 2004. **148**(2): p. 133–6.

160. Ott, M.M., et al., *Marginal zone B-cell lymphomas (MZBL) arising at different sites represent different biological entities.* Genes Chromosomes Cancer, 2000. **28**(4): p. 380–6.

161. Vega, F., et al., *Splenic marginal zone lymphomas are characterized by loss of interstitial regions of chromosome 7q, 7q31.32 and 7q36.2 that include the protection of telomere 1 (POT1) and sonic hedgehog (SHH) genes.* Br J Haematol, 2008. **142**(2): p. 216–26.

162. Hernandez, J.M., et al., *Novel genomic imbalances in B-cell splenic marginal zone lymphomas revealed by comparative genomic hybridization and cytogenetics.* Am J Pathol, 2001. **158**(5): p. 1843–50.

163. Watkins, A.J., et al., *Splenic marginal zone lymphoma: characterization of 7q deletion and its value in diagnosis.* J Pathol, 2010. **220**(4): p. 461–74.

164. Novara, F., et al., *High-resolution genome-wide array comparative genomic hybridization in splenic marginal zone B-cell lymphoma.* Hum Pathol, 2009. **40**(11): p. 1628–37.

165. Baro, C., et al., *New chromosomal alterations in a series of 23 splenic marginal zone lymphoma patients revealed by Spectral Karyotyping (SKY).* Leuk Res, 2008. **32**(5): p. 727–36.

166. Piris, M.A., A. Arribas, and M. Mollejo, *Marginal zone lymphoma.* Semin Diagn Pathol, 2011. **28**(2): p. 135–45.

167. Piris, M.A., et al., *A marginal zone pattern may be found in different varieties of non-Hodgkin's lymphoma: the morphology and immunohistology of splenic involvement by B-cell lymphomas simulating splenic marginal zone lymphoma.* Histopathology, 1998. **33**(3): p. 230–9.

168. Arcaini, L., et al., *Distinctive clinical and histological features of Waldenstrom's macroglobulinemia and splenic marginal zone lymphoma.* Clin Lymphoma Myeloma Leuk, 2011. **11**(1): p. 103–5.

169. Traverse-Glehen, A., et al., *Splenic red pulp lymphoma with numerous basophilic villous lymphocytes: a distinct clinicopathologic and molecular entity?* Blood, 2008. **111**(4): p. 2253–60.

170. Baseggio, L., et al., *Relevance of a scoring system including CD11c expression in the identification of splenic diffuse red pulp small B-cell lymphoma (SRPL).* Hematol Oncol, 2011. **29**(1): p. 47–51.

171. Xochelli, A., et al., *Clonal B-cell lymphocytosis exhibiting immunophenotypic features consistent with a marginal-zone origin: is this a distinct entity?* Blood, 2014. **123**(8): p. 1199–206.

172. Catovsky, D., et al., *Hairy cell leukemia (HCL) variant: an intermediate disease between HCL and B prolymphocytic leukemia.* Semin Oncol, 1984. **11**(4): p. 362–9.

173. Cessna, M.H., et al., *Hairy cell leukemia variant: fact or fiction.* Am J Clin Pathol, 2005. **123**(1): p. 132–8.

174. Maitre, E., et al., *New generation sequencing of targeted genes in the classical and the variant form of hairy cell leukemia highlights mutations in epigenetic regulation genes.* Oncotarget, 2018. **9**(48): p. 28866–76.

175. Salem, D.A., et al., *Differential expression of CD43, CD81, and CD200 in classic versus variant hairy cell leukemia.* Cytometry B Clin Cytom, 2019. **96**(4): p. 275–82.

176. Shao, H., et al., *Distinguishing hairy cell leukemia variant from hairy cell leukemia: development and validation of diagnostic criteria.* Leuk Res, 2013. **37**(4): p. 401–9.

177. Troussard, X. and E. Cornet, *Hairy cell leukemia 2018: update on diagnosis, risk-stratification, and treatment.* Am J Hematol, 2017. **92**(12): p. 1382–90.

178. Angelova, E.A., et al., *Clinicopathologic and molecular features in hairy cell leukemia-variant: single institutional experience.* Mod Pathol, 2018. **31**(11): p. 1717–32.

179. Hockley, S.L., et al., *Higher expression levels of activation-induced cytidine deaminase distinguish hairy cell leukemia from hairy cell leukemia-variant and splenic marginal zone lymphoma.* Leukemia, 2010. **24**(5): p. 1084–6.

180. Arcaini, L., et al., *The BRAF V600E mutation in hairy cell leukemia and other mature B-cell neoplasms.* Blood, 2012. **119**(1): p. 188–91.

181. Tiacci, E., et al., *BRAF mutations in hairy-cell leukemia.* N Engl J Med, 2011. **364**(24): p. 2305–15.

182. Xi, L., et al., *Both variant and IGHV4-34-expressing hairy cell leukemia lack the BRAF V600E mutation.* Blood, 2012. **119**(14): p. 3330–2.

183. Andrulis, M., et al., *Application of a BRAF V600E mutation-specific antibody for the diagnosis of hairy cell leukemia.* Am J Surg Pathol, 2012. **36**(12): p. 1796–800.

184. Hoffman, M.A., *Clinical presentations and complications of hairy cell leukemia.* Hematol Oncol Clin North Am, 2006. **20**(5): p. 1065–73.

185. Bouroncle, B.A., *Thirty-five years in the progress of hairy cell leukemia.* Leuk Lymphoma, 1994. **14 Suppl 1**: p. 1–12.

186. Federico, M., et al., *Hairy cell leukemia: the Italian Cooperative Group experience.* Leukemia, 1992. **6 Suppl 4**: p. 147–8.

187. Frassoldati, A., et al., *Hairy cell leukemia: a clinical review based on 725 cases of the Italian Cooperative Group (ICGHCL). Italian Cooperative Group for Hairy Cell Leukemia.* Leuk Lymphoma, 1994. **13**(3–4): p. 307–16.

188. Goodman, G.R., K.J. Bethel, and A. Saven, *Hairy cell leukemia: an update.* Curr Opin Hematol, 2003. **10**(4): p. 258–66.

189. Swords, R. and F. Giles, *Hairy cell leukemia.* Med Oncol, 2007. **24**(1): p. 7–15.

190. Else, M., et al., *Long-term follow-up of 233 patients with hairy cell leukaemia, treated initially with pentostatin or cladribine, at a median of 16 years from diagnosis.* Br J Haematol, 2009. **145**(6): p. 733–40.

191. Grever, M.R., *How I treat hairy cell leukemia.* Blood, 2010. **115**(1): p. 21–8.

192. Sherman, M.J., C.A. Hanson, and J.D. Hoyer, *An assessment of the usefulness of immunohistochemical stains in the diagnosis of hairy cell leukemia.* Am J Clin Pathol, 2011. **136**(3): p. 390–9.

193. Tadmor, T., et al., *The BRAF-V600E mutation in hematological malignancies: a new player in hairy cell leukemia and Langerhans cell histiocytosis.* Leuk Lymphoma, 2012. **53**(12): p. 2339–40.

194. Grever, M.R., et al., *Consensus guidelines for the diagnosis and management of patients with classic hairy cell leukemia.* Blood, 2017. **129**(5): p. 553–60.

195. Kreitman, R.J. and E. Arons, *Update on hairy cell leukemia.* Clin Adv Hematol Oncol, 2018. **16**(3): p. 205–15.

196. Badalian-Very, G., et al., *Recurrent BRAF mutations in Langerhans cell histiocytosis.* Blood, 2010. **116**(11): p. 1919–23.

197. Langabeer, S.E., et al., *Correlation of the BRAF V600E mutation in hairy cell leukaemia with morphology, cytochemistry and immunophenotype.* Int J Lab Hematol, 2012. **34**(4): p. 417–21.

198. Tschernitz, S., et al., *Alternative BRAF mutations in BRAF V600E-negative hairy cell leukaemias.* Br J Haematol, 2014. **165**(4): p. 529–33.

199. Goodman, G.R., et al., *Extended follow-up of patients with hairy cell leukemia after treatment with cladribine.* J Clin Oncol, 2003. **21**(5): p. 891–6.

200. Ravandi, F., et al., *Eradication of minimal residual disease in hairy cell leukemia.* Blood, 2006. **107**(12): p. 4658–62.

201. Sambani, C., et al., *Clonal chromosome rearrangements in hairy cell leukemia: personal experience and review of literature*. Cancer Genet Cytogenet, 2001. **129**(2): p. 138–44.

202. Vallianatou, K., et al., *p53 gene deletion and trisomy 12 in hairy cell leukemia and its variant*. Leuk Res, 1999. **23**(11): p. 1041–5.

203. Sole, F., et al., *Cytogenetic findings in five patients with hairy cell leukemia*. Cancer Genet Cytogenet, 1999. **110**(1): p. 41–3.

204. Ishida, F., et al., *Hairy cell leukemia with translocation (11;20) (q13;q11) and overexpression of cyclin D1*. Leuk Res, 1999. **23**(8): p. 763–5.

205. Sucak, G.T., et al., *del(17)(q25) in a patient with hairy cell leukemia: a new clonal chromosome abnormality*. Cancer Genet Cytogenet, 1998. **100**(2): p. 152–4.

206. Cawley, J.C., *The pathophysiology of the hairy cell*. Hematol Oncol Clin North Am, 2006. **20**(5): p. 1011–21.

207. Dierlamm, J., et al., *Chromosomal gains and losses are uncommon in hairy cell leukemia: a study based on comparative genomic hybridization and interphase fluorescence in situ hybridization*. Cancer Genet Cytogenet, 2001. **128**(2): p. 164–7.

208. Andersen, C.L., et al., *A narrow deletion of 7q is common to HCL, and SMZL, but not CLL*. Eur J Haematol, 2004. **72**(6): p. 390–402.

209. Verma, S., et al., *Rapid detection and quantitation of BRAF mutations in hairy cell leukemia using a sensitive pyrosequencing assay*. Am J Clin Pathol, 2012. **138**(1): p. 153–6.

210. Melo, J.V., et al., *Splenic B cell lymphoma with circulating villous lymphocytes: differential diagnosis of B cell leukaemias with large spleens*. J Clin Pathol, 1987. **40**(6): p. 642–51.

211. Melo, J.V., et al., *Splenic B cell lymphoma with "villous" lymphocytes in the peripheral blood: a disorder distinct from hairy cell leukemia*. Leukemia, 1987. **1**(4): p. 294–8.

212. Chapman-Fredricks, J., et al., *Progressive leukemic non-nodal mantle cell lymphoma associated with deletions of TP53, ATM, and/or 13q14*. Ann Diagn Pathol, 2014. **18**(4): p. 214–9.

213. Jain, A.G., et al., *Leukemic non-nodal mantle cell lymphoma: diagnosis and treatment*. Curr Treat Options Oncol, 2019. **20**(12): p. 85.

214. Sakhdari, A., et al., *TP53 mutations are common in mantle cell lymphoma, including the indolent leukemic non-nodal variant*. Ann Diagn Pathol, 2019. **41**: p. 38–42.

215. Saksena, A., et al., *CD23 expression in mantle cell lymphoma is associated with CD200 expression, leukemic non-nodal form, and a better prognosis*. Hum Pathol, 2019. **89**: p. 71–80.

216. Martinez, D., et al., *NOTCH1, TP53, and MAP2K1 mutations in splenic diffuse red pulp small B-cell lymphoma are associated with progressive disease*. Am J Surg Pathol, 2016. **40**(2): p. 192–201.

217. Kanellis, G., et al., *Splenic diffuse red pulp small B-cell lymphoma: revision of a series of cases reveals characteristic clinico-pathological features*. Haematologica, 2010. **95**(7): p. 1122–9.

218. Traverse-Glehen, A., et al., *Splenic diffuse red pulp small-B cell lymphoma: toward the emergence of a new lymphoma entity*. Discov Med, 2012. **13**(71): p. 253–65.

219. Mollejo, M., et al., *Splenic small B-cell lymphoma with predominant red pulp involvement: a diffuse variant of splenic marginal zone lymphoma?* Histopathology, 2002. **40**(1): p. 22–30.

220. Behdad, A. and N.G. Bailey, *Diagnosis of splenic B-cell lymphomas in the bone marrow: a review of histopathologic, immunophenotypic, and genetic findings*. Arch Pathol Lab Med, 2014. **138**(10): p. 1295–301.

221. Cheng, W.Y., et al., *Development of B-cell prolymphocytic leukemia in a patient with splenic diffuse red pulp small B-cell lymphoma*. Leuk Lymphoma, 2018. **59**(8): p. 1990–3.

222. Tiacci, E., et al., *Simple genetic diagnosis of hairy cell leukemia by sensitive detection of the BRAF-V600E mutation*. Blood, 2012. **119**(1): p. 192–5.

223. Wang, W. and P. Lin, *Lymphoplasmacytic lymphoma and Waldenstrom macroglobulinaemia: clinicopathological features and differential diagnosis*. Pathology, 2020. **52**(1): p. 6–14.

224. Gertz, M., *Waldenstrom macroglobulinemia: my way*. Leuk Lymphoma, 2013. **54**(3): p. 464–71.

225. Gertz, M.A., *Waldenstrom macroglobulinemia: 2012 update on diagnosis, risk stratification, and management*. Am J Hematol, 2012. **87**(5): p. 503–10.

226. Treon, S.P., *How I treat Waldenstrom macroglobulinemia*. Blood, 2009. **114**(12): p. 2375–85.

227. Treon, S.P. and Z.R. Hunter, *A new era for Waldenstrom macroglobulinemia: MYD88 L265P*. Blood, 2013. **121**(22): p. 4434–6.

228. Treon, S.P., et al., *Genomic landscape of Waldenstrom macroglobulinemia*. Hematol Oncol Clin North Am, 2018. **32**(5): p. 745–52.

229. Girard, L.P., et al., *Immunoglobulin M paraproteinaemias*. Cancers (Basel), 2020. **12**(6): p. 1688.

230. Lin, P., et al., *Waldenstrom macroglobulinemia involving extramedullary sites: morphologic and immunophenotypic findings in 44 patients*. Am J Surg Pathol, 2003. **27**(8): p. 1104–13.

231. Xu, L., et al., *MYD88 L265P in Waldenstrom macroglobulinemia, immunoglobulin M monoclonal gammopathy, and other B-cell lymphoproliferative disorders using conventional and quantitative allele-specific polymerase chain reaction*. Blood, 2013. **121**(11): p. 2051–8.

232. Poulain, S., et al., *MYD88 L265P mutation in Waldenstrom macroglobulinemia*. Blood, 2013. **121**(22): p. 4504–11.

233. Dimopoulos, M.A., et al., *Update on treatment recommendations from the Fourth International Workshop on Waldenstrom's Macroglobulinemia*. J Clin Oncol, 2009. **27**(1): p. 120–6.

234. Vijay, A. and M.A. Gertz, *Waldenstrom macroglobulinemia*. Blood, 2007. **109**(12): p. 5096–103.

235. Dimopoulos, M.A. and A. Anagnostopoulos, *Waldenstrom's macroglobulinemia*. Best Pract Res Clin Haematol, 2005. **18**(4): p. 747–65.

236. Kyle, R.A., et al., *IgM monoclonal gammopathy of undetermined significance (MGUS) and smoldering Waldenstrom's macroglobulinemia (SWM)*. Clin Lymphoma Myeloma Leuk, 2011. **11**(1): p. 74–6.

237. Kyle, R.A. and S.V. Rajkumar, *Monoclonal gammopathy of undetermined significance*. Clin Lymphoma Myeloma, 2005. **6**(2): p. 102–14.

238. Rajkumar, S.V., et al., *International Myeloma Working Group updated criteria for the diagnosis of multiple myeloma*. Lancet Oncol, 2014. **15**(12): p. e538–48.

239. Kyle, R.A., et al., *IgM monoclonal gammopathy of undetermined significance and smoldering Waldenstrom's macroglobulinemia*. Clin Lymphoma Myeloma, 2009. **9**(1): p. 17–8.

240. de Lastours, V., et al., *Bone involvement in generalized crystal-storing histiocytosis*. J Rheumatol, 2006. **33**(11): p. 2354–8.

241. Jones, D., et al., *Crystal-storing histiocytosis: a disorder occurring in plasmacytic tumors expressing immunoglobulin kappa light chain*. Hum Pathol, 1999. **30**(12): p. 1441–8.

242. Llobet, M., et al., *Massive crystal-storing histiocytosis associated with low-grade malignant B-cell lymphoma of MALT-type of the parotid gland*. Diagn Cytopathol, 1997. **17**(2): p. 148–52.

243. Papla, B., et al., *Generalized crystal-storing histiocytosis as a presentation of multiple myeloma: a case with a possible pro-aggregation defect in the immunoglobulin heavy chain*. Virchows Arch, 2004. **445**(1): p. 83–9.

244. Pock, L., D. Stuchlik, and J. Hercogova, *Crystal storing histiocytosis of the skin associated with multiple myeloma*. Int J Dermatol, 2006. **45**(12): p. 1408–11.

245. Swerdlow, S.H., et al., *The many faces of small B cell lymphomas with plasmacytic differentiation and the contribution of MYD88 testing*. Virchows Arch, 2015. **468**(3): p. 259–75.

246. Morice, W.G., et al., *Novel immunophenotypic features of marrow lymphoplasmacytic lymphoma and correlation with Waldenstrom's macroglobulinemia*. Mod Pathol, 2009. **22**(6): p. 807–16.

247. Lin, P. and L.J. Medeiros, *Lymphoplasmacytic lymphoma/Waldenstrom macroglobulinemia: an evolving concept*. Adv Anat Pathol, 2005. **12**(5): p. 246–55.

248. Lemal, R., et al., *TCL1 expression patterns in Waldenstrom macroglobulinemia*. Mod Pathol, 2016. **29**(1): p. 83–8.

249. King, R.L., et al., *Lymphoplasmacytic lymphoma with a non-IgM paraprotein shows clinical and pathologic heterogeneity and may harbor MYD88 L265P mutations.* Am J Clin Pathol, 2016. **145**(6): p. 843–51.

250. Raimbault, A., et al., *CD13 expression in B cell malignancies is a hallmark of plasmacytic differentiation.* Br J Haematol, 2019. **184**(4): p. 625–33.

251. Lin, P., et al., *Diffuse large B-cell lymphoma occurring in patients with lymphoplasmacytic lymphoma/Waldenstrom macroglobulinemia. Clinicopathologic features of 12 cases.* Am J Clin Pathol, 2003. **120**(2): p. 246–53.

252. Ling, S., et al., *Transformation and progression of Waldenstrom's macroglobulinemia following cladribine therapy in two cases: natural evolution or iatrogenic causation?* Am J Hematol, 2006. **81**(2): p. 110–4.

253. Schop, R.F., et al., *Waldenstrom macroglobulinemia neoplastic cells lack immunoglobulin heavy chain locus translocations but have frequent 6q deletions.* Blood, 2002. **100**(8): p. 2996–3001.

254. Chang, H., et al., *Prognostic relevance of 6q deletion in Waldenstrom's macroglobulinemia: a multicenter study.* Clin Lymphoma Myeloma, 2009. **9**(1): p. 36–8.

255. Mansoor, A., et al., *Cytogenetic findings in lymphoplasmacytic lymphoma/Waldenstrom macroglobulinemia. Chromosomal abnormalities are associated with the polymorphous subtype and an aggressive clinical course.* Am J Clin Pathol, 2001. **116**(4): p. 543–9.

256. Terre, C., et al., *Trisomy 4, a new chromosomal abnormality in Waldenstrom's macroglobulinemia: a study of 39 cases.* Leukemia, 2006. **20**(9): p. 1634–6.

257. Schop, R.F., et al., *6q deletion discriminates Waldenstrom macroglobulinemia from IgM monoclonal gammopathy of undetermined significance.* Cancer Genet Cytogenet, 2006. **169**(2): p. 150–3.

258. Hunter, Z.R., et al., *The genomic landscape of Waldenstrom macroglobulinemia is characterized by highly recurring MYD88 and WHIM-like CXCR4 mutations, and small somatic deletions associated with B-cell lymphomagenesis.* Blood, 2014. **123**(11): p. 1637–46.

259. Hunter, Z.R., et al., *Insights into the genomic landscape of MYD88 wild-type Waldenstrom macroglobulinemia.* Blood Adv, 2018. **2**(21): p. 2937–46.

260. Yu, X., et al., *MYD88 L265P Mutation in Lymphoid Malignancies.* Cancer Res, 2018. **78**(10): p. 2457–62.

261. Martinez-Trillos, A., et al., *Mutations in TLR/MYD88 pathway identify a subset of young chronic lymphocytic leukemia patients with favorable outcome.* Blood, 2014. **123**(24): p. 3790–6.

262. Baliakas, P., et al., *Recurrent mutations refine prognosis in chronic lymphocytic leukemia.* Leukemia, 2015. **29**(2): p. 329–36.

263. Baliakas, P., et al., *Prognostic relevance of MYD88 mutations in CLL: the jury is still out.* Blood, 2015. **126**(8): p. 1043–4.

264. Martinez-Trillos, A., et al., *Clinical impact of MYD88 mutations in chronic lymphocytic leukemia.* Blood, 2016. **127**(12): p. 1611–3.

265. Martinez-Lopez, A., et al., *MYD88 (L265P) somatic mutation in marginal zone B-cell lymphoma.* Am J Surg Pathol, 2015. **39**(5): p. 644–51.

266. Kyrtsonis, M.C., et al., *CD138 expression helps distinguishing Waldenstrom's macroglobulinemia (WM) from splenic marginal zone lymphoma (SMZL).* Clin Lymphoma Myeloma Leuk, 2011. **11**(1): p. 99–102.

267. Agrawal, R. and J. Wang, *Pediatric follicular lymphoma: a rare clinicopathologic entity.* Arch Pathol Lab Med, 2009. **133**(1): p. 142–6.

268. Carbone, A. and A. Santoro, *How I treat: diagnosing and managing "in situ" lymphoma.* Blood, 2011. **117**(15): p. 3954–60.

269. Casulo, C., W.R. Burack, and J.W. Friedberg, *Transformed follicular non-Hodgkin lymphoma.* Blood, 2015. **125**(1): p. 40–7.

270. Choi, S.M., B.L. Betz, and A.M. Perry, *Follicular lymphoma diagnostic caveats and updates.* Arch Pathol Lab Med, 2018. **142**(11): p. 1330–40.

271. Leich, E., et al., *Follicular lymphomas with and without translocation t(14;18) differ in gene expression profiles and genetic alterations.* Blood, 2009. **114**(4): p. 826–34.

272. Randall, C. and Y. Fedoriw, *Pathology and diagnosis of follicular lymphoma and related entities.* Pathology, 2020. **52**(1): p. 30–9.

273. Mamessier, E., et al., *Nature and importance of follicular lymphoma precursors.* Haematologica, 2014. **99**(5): p. 802–10.

274. Mamessier, E., et al., *Early lesions of follicular lymphoma: a genetic perspective.* Haematologica, 2014. **99**(3): p. 481–8.

275. Schuler, F., et al., *Prevalence and frequency of circulating t(14;18)-MBR translocation carrying cells in healthy individuals.* Int J Cancer, 2009. **124**(4): p. 958–63.

276. Horning, S.J., *Natural history of and therapy for the indolent non-Hodgkin's lymphomas.* Semin Oncol, 1993. **20**(5 Suppl 5): p. 75–88.

277. Advani, R., S.A. Rosenberg, and S.J. Horning, *Stage I and II follicular non-Hodgkin's lymphoma: long-term follow-up of no initial therapy.* J Clin Oncol, 2004. **22**(8): p. 1454–9.

278. Bastion, Y., et al., *Follicular lymphomas: assessment of prognostic factors in 127 patients followed for 10 years.* Ann Oncol, 1991. **2 Suppl 2**: p. 123–9.

279. Bastion, Y. and B. Coiffier, *Is the International Prognostic Index for Aggressive Lymphoma patients useful for follicular lymphoma patients?* J Clin Oncol, 1994. **12**(7): p. 1340–2.

280. Coiffier, B., et al., *Prognostic factors in follicular lymphomas.* Semin Oncol, 1993. **20**(5 Suppl 5): p. 89–95.

281. Davies, A.J., et al., *Transformation of follicular lymphoma to diffuse large B-cell lymphoma proceeds by distinct oncogenic mechanisms.* Br J Haematol, 2007. **136**(2): p. 286–93.

282. Solal-Celigny, P., et al., *Follicular lymphoma international prognostic index.* Blood, 2004. **104**(5): p. 1258–65.

283. Feller, A.C., Diebold, J., Histopathology of nodal and extranodal non-Hodgkin's lymphomas. 3rd ed. 2004, Springer-Verlag: Berlin, Heidelberg.

284. Brittinger, G., et al., *Clinical and prognostic relevance of the Kiel classification of non-Hodgkin lymphomas results of a prospective multicenter study by the Kiel Lymphoma Study Group.* Hematol Oncol, 1984. **2**(3): p. 269–306.

285. Rodriguez, J., et al., *Follicular large cell lymphoma: an aggressive lymphoma that often presents with favorable prognostic features.* Blood, 1999. **93**(7): p. 2202–7.

286. Hans, C.P., et al., *A significant diffuse component predicts for inferior survival in grade 3 follicular lymphoma, but cytologic subtypes do not predict survival.* Blood, 2003. **101**(6): p. 2363–7.

287. Levine, E.G. and C.D. Bloomfield, *Cytogenetics of non-Hodgkin's lymphoma.* J Natl Cancer Inst Monogr, 1990(10): p. 7–12.

288. Tilly, H., et al., *Prognostic value of chromosomal abnormalities in follicular lymphoma.* Blood, 1994. **84**(4): p. 1043–9.

289. Goodlad, J.R., et al., *Primary cutaneous follicular lymphoma: a clinicopathologic and molecular study of 16 cases in support of a distinct entity.* Am J Surg Pathol, 2002. **26**(6): p. 733–41.

290. Goodlad, J.R., et al., *Extranodal follicular lymphoma: a clinicopathological and genetic analysis of 15 cases arising at non-cutaneous extranodal sites.* Histopathology, 2004. **44**(3): p. 268–76.

291. Shia, J., et al., *Primary follicular lymphoma of the gastrointestinal tract: a clinical and pathologic study of 26 cases.* Am J Surg Pathol, 2002. **26**(2): p. 216–24.

292. Hollowood, K. and J.R. Goodlad, *Follicular lymphomas.* Histopathology, 1996. **29**(2): p. 195.

293. Miller, T.P., et al., *Follicular lymphomas: do histologic subtypes predict outcome?* Hematol Oncol Clin North Am, 1997. **11**(5): p. 893–900.

294. Arber, D.A. and T.I. George, *Bone marrow biopsy involvement by non-Hodgkin's lymphoma: frequency of lymphoma types, patterns, blood involvement, and discordance with other sites in 450 specimens.* Am J Surg Pathol, 2005. **29**(12): p. 1549–57.

295. Sovani, V., et al., *Bone marrow trephine biopsy involvement by lymphoma: review of histopathological features in 511 specimens and correlation with diagnostic biopsy, aspirate and peripheral blood findings.* J Clin Pathol, 2014. **67**(5): p. 389–95.

296. Li, Y., et al., *CD5-positive follicular lymphoma: clinicopathologic correlations and outcome in 88 cases.* Mod Pathol, 2015. **28**(6): p. 787–98.

297. Mayson, E., J. Saverimuttu, and K. Cartwright, *CD5-positive follicular lymphoma: prognostic significance of this aberrant marker?* Intern Med J, 2014. **44**(4): p. 417–22.

298. Miyaoka, M., et al., *Composite Follicular Lymphoma and CD5-Positive Nodal Marginal Zone Lymphoma.* J Clin Exp Hematop, 2016. **56**(1): p. 55–8.

299. Miyoshi, H., et al., *CD5-positive follicular lymphoma characterized by CD25, MUM1, low frequency of t(14;18) and poor prognosis.* Pathol Int, 2014. **64**(3): p. 95–103.

300. Sekiguchi, Y., et al., *CD5-positive follicular lymphoma: a case report and literature review.* Intern Med, 2011. **50**(8): p. 899–904.

301. Jardin, F., et al., *Follicle center lymphoma is associated with significantly elevated levels of BCL-6 expression among lymphoma subtypes, independent of chromosome 3q27 rearrangements.* Leukemia, 2002. **16**(11): p. 2318–25.

302. Skinnider, B.F., et al., *Bcl-6 and Bcl-2 protein expression in diffuse large B-cell lymphoma and follicular lymphoma: correlation with 3q27 and 18q21 chromosomal abnormalities.* Hum Pathol, 1999. **30**(7): p. 803–8.

303. Goteri, G., et al., *Comparison of germinal center markers CD10, BCL6 and human germinal center-associated lymphoma (HGAL) in follicular lymphomas.* Diagn Pathol, 2011. **6**: p. 97.

304. Montes-Moreno, S., et al., *Gcet1 (centerin), a highly restricted marker for a subset of germinal center-derived lymphomas.* Blood, 2008. **111**(1): p. 351–8.

305. Natkunam, Y., et al., *Expression of the human germinal center-associated lymphoma (HGAL) protein, a new marker of germinal center B-cell derivation.* Blood, 2005. **105**(10): p. 3979–86.

306. Horn, H., et al., *Follicular lymphoma grade 3B is a distinct neoplasm according to cytogenetic and immunohistochemical profiles.* Haematologica, 2011. **96**(9): p. 1327–34.

307. Maeshima, A.M., et al., *Prognostic implications of histologic grade and intensity of Bcl-2 expression in follicular lymphomas undergoing rituximab-containing therapy.* Hum Pathol, 2013. **44**(11): p. 2529–35.

308. Wahlin, B.E., et al., *Clinical significance of the WHO grades of follicular lymphoma in a population-based cohort of 505 patients with long follow-up times.* Br J Haematol, 2012. **156**(2): p. 225–33.

309. Eshoa, C., et al., *Decreased CD10 expression in grade III and in interfollicular infiltrates of follicular lymphomas.* Am J Clin Pathol, 2001. **115**(6): p. 862–7.

310. Bosga-Bouwer, A.G., et al., *Follicular lymphoma grade 3B includes 3 cytogenetically defined subgroups with primary t(14;18), 3q27, or other translocations: t(14;18) and 3q27 are mutually exclusive.* Blood, 2003. **101**(3): p. 1149–54.

311. Guo, Y., et al., *Low-grade follicular lymphoma with t(14;18) presents a homogeneous disease entity otherwise the rest comprises minor groups of heterogeneous disease entities with Bcl2 amplification, Bcl6 translocation or other gene aberrances.* Leukemia, 2005. **19**(6): p. 1058–63.

312. Karube, K., et al., *CD10-MUM1⁺ follicular lymphoma lacks BCL2 gene translocation and shows characteristic biologic and clinical features.* Blood, 2007. **109**(7): p. 3076–9.

313. Mackrides, N., et al., *Epstein-Barr virus-positive follicular lymphoma.* Mod Pathol, 2017. **30**(4): p. 519–29.

314. Mackrides, N., et al., *Prevalence, clinical characteristics and prognosis of EBV-positive follicular lymphoma.* Am J Hematol, 2019. **94**(2): p. E62–4.

315. Chapman, J.R., et al., *Unusual variants of follicular lymphoma: case-based review.* Am J Surg Pathol, 2020. **44**(3): p. 329–39.

316. Yunis, J.J., et al., *Distinctive chromosomal abnormalities in histologic subtypes of non-Hodgkin's lymphoma.* N Engl J Med, 1982. **307**(20): p. 1231–6.

317. Cheung, K.J., et al., *High resolution analysis of follicular lymphoma genomes reveals somatic recurrent sites of copy-neutral loss of heterozygosity and copy number alterations that target single genes.* Genes Chromosomes Cancer, 2010. **49**(8): p. 669–81.

318. Lee, M.S., *Molecular aspects of chromosomal translocation t(14;18).* Semin Hematol, 1993. **30**(4): p. 297–305.

319. Horsman, D.E., et al., *Follicular lymphoma lacking the t(14;18)(q32;q21): identification of two disease subtypes.* Br J Haematol, 2003. **120**(3): p. 424–33.

320. Jardin, F., et al., *Follicular lymphoma without t(14;18) and with BCL-6 rearrangement: a lymphoma subtype with distinct pathological, molecular and clinical characteristics.* Leukemia, 2002. **16**(11): p. 2309–17.

321. Cook, J.R., *Paraffin section interphase fluorescence in situ hybridization in the diagnosis and classification of non-Hodgkin lymphomas.* Diagn Mol Pathol, 2004. **13**(4): p. 197–206.

322. Guo, Y., et al., *Bcl2-negative follicular lymphomas frequently have Bcl6 translocation and/or Bcl6 or p53 expression.* Pathol Int, 2007. **57**(3): p. 148–52.

323. Ziemba, J.B., et al., *Double-Hit and Triple-Hit Follicular Lymphoma.* Am J Clin Pathol, 2020. **153**(5): p. 672–85.

324. Lossos, I.S. and R.D. Gascoyne, *Transformation of follicular lymphoma.* Best Pract Res Clin Haematol, 2011. **24**(2): p. 147–63.

325. Bastion, Y., et al., *Incidence, predictive factors, and outcome of lymphoma transformation in follicular lymphoma patients.* J Clin Oncol, 1997. **15**(4): p. 1587–94.

326. Ersboll, J., et al., *Follicular low-grade non-Hodgkin's lymphoma: long-term outcome with or without tumor progression.* Eur J Haematol, 1989. **42**(2): p. 155–63.

327. Horning, S.J. and S.A. Rosenberg, *The natural history of initially untreated low-grade non-Hodgkin's lymphomas.* N Engl J Med, 1984. **311**(23): p. 1471–5.

328. Lee, J.T., D.J. Innes, Jr., and M.E. Williams, *Sequential bcl-2 and c-myc oncogene rearrangements associated with the clinical transformation of non-Hodgkin's lymphoma.* J Clin Invest, 1989. **84**(5): p. 1454–9.

329. Natkunam, Y., et al., *Blastic/blastoid transformation of follicular lymphoma: immunohistologic and molecular analyses of five cases.* Am J Surg Pathol, 2000. **24**(4): p. 525–34.

330. de Jong, D., et al., *Activation of the c-myc oncogene in a precursor-B-cell blast crisis of follicular lymphoma, presenting as composite lymphoma.* N Engl J Med, 1988. **318**(21): p. 1373–8.

331. Kroft, S.H., et al., *Precursor B-lymphoblastic transformation of grade I follicle center lymphoma.* Am J Clin Pathol, 2000. **113**(3): p. 411–8.

332. Hwang, Y.Y., et al., *Atypical Burkitt's lymphoma transforming from follicular lymphoma.* Diagn Pathol, 2011. **6**: p. 63.

333. Xu, X., et al., *Double-hit and triple-hit lymphomas arising from follicular lymphoma following acquisition of MYC: report of two cases and literature review.* Int J Clin Exp Pathol, 2013. **6**(4): p. 788–94.

334. Geyer, J.T., et al., *Lymphoblastic transformation of follicular lymphoma: a clinicopathologic and molecular analysis of 7 patients.* Hum Pathol, 2015. **46**(2): p. 260–71.

335. Prieto-Torres, L., et al., *Large cells with CD30 expression and Hodgkin-like features in primary cutaneous marginal zone B-cell lymphoma: a study of 13 cases.* Am J Surg Pathol, 2019. **43**(9): p. 1191–202.

336. Huang, Y., et al., *Peripheral T-cell lymphomas with a follicular growth pattern are derived from follicular helper T cells (TFH) and may show overlapping features with angioimmunoblastic T-cell lymphomas.* Am J Surg Pathol, 2009. **33**(5): p. 682–90.

337. Pileri, S.A., *Follicular helper T-cell-related lymphomas.* Blood, 2015. **126**(15): p. 1733–4.

338. Agostinelli, C., et al., *Peripheral T cell lymphomas with follicular T helper phenotype: a new basket or a distinct entity? Revising Karl Lennert's personal archive.* Histopathology, 2011. **59**(4): p. 679–91.

339. Dobay, M.P., et al., *Integrative clinicopathological and molecular analyses of angioimmunoblastic T-cell lymphoma and other nodal lymphomas of follicular helper T-cell origin.* Haematologica, 2017. **102**(4): p. e148–51.

340. Rodriguez-Pinilla, S.M., et al., *Peripheral T-cell lymphoma with follicular T-cell markers.* Am J Surg Pathol, 2008. **32**(12): p. 1787–99.

341. Lemonnier, F., et al., *Recurrent TET2 mutations in peripheral T-cell lymphomas correlate with TFH-like features and adverse clinical parameters.* Blood, 2012. **120**(7): p. 1466–9.

342. Palomero, T., et al., *Recurrent mutations in epigenetic regulators, RHOA and FYN kinase in peripheral T cell lymphomas.* Nat Genet, 2014. **46**(2): p. 166–70.

343. Jegalian, A.G., et al., *Follicular lymphoma in situ: clinical implications and comparisons with partial involvement by follicular lymphoma.* Blood, 2011. **118**(11): p. 2976–84.

344. Pillai, R.K., U. Surti, and S.H. Swerdlow, *Follicular lymphoma-like B cells of uncertain significance (in situ follicular lymphoma) may infrequently progress, but precedes follicular lymphoma, is associated with other overt lymphomas and mimics follicular lymphoma in flow cytometric studies.* Haematologica, 2013. **98**(10): p. 1571–80.

345. Oishi, N., S. Montes-Moreno, and A.L. Feldman, *In situ neoplasia in lymph node pathology.* Semin Diagn Pathol, 2018. **35**(1): p. 76–83.

346. Ogata, S., et al., *Clinicopathological features of in situ follicular neoplasm and relations with follicular lymphoma in Japan.* Ann Hematol, 2020. **99**(2): p. 241–53.

347. Roulland, S., et al., *t(14;18) Translocation: a predictive blood biomarker for follicular lymphoma.* J Clin Oncol, 2014. **32**(13): p. 1347–55.

348. Lorsbach, R.B., et al., *Clinicopathologic analysis of follicular lymphoma occurring in children.* Blood, 2002. **99**(6): p. 1959–64.

349. Louissaint, A., Jr., et al., *Pediatric-type nodal follicular lymphoma: a biologically distinct lymphoma with frequent MAPK pathway mutations.* Blood, 2016. **128**(8): p. 1093–100.

350. Louissaint, A., Jr., et al., *Pediatric-type nodal follicular lymphoma: an indolent clonal proliferation in children and adults with high proliferation index and no BCL2 rearrangement.* Blood, 2012. **120**(12): p. 2395–404.

351. Agostinelli, C., et al., *Novel markers in pediatric-type follicular lymphoma.* Virchows Arch, 2019. **475**(6): p. 771–9.

352. Attarbaschi, A., et al., *Rare non-Hodgkin lymphoma of childhood and adolescence: a consensus diagnostic and therapeutic approach to pediatric-type follicular lymphoma, marginal zone lymphoma, and nonanaplastic peripheral T-cell lymphoma.* Pediatr Blood Cancer, 2020. **67**(8): p. e28416.

353. Liu, Q., et al., *Follicular lymphomas in children and young adults: a comparison of the pediatric variant with usual follicular lymphoma.* Am J Surg Pathol, 2013. **37**(3): p. 333–43.

354. Kussick, S.J., et al., *Prominent clonal B-cell populations identified by flow cytometry in histologically reactive lymphoid proliferations.* Am J Clin Pathol, 2004. **121**(4): p. 464–72.

355. Berget, E., et al., *Detection of clonality in follicular lymphoma using formalin-fixed, paraffin-embedded tissue samples and BIOMED-2 immunoglobulin primers.* J Clin Pathol, 2011. **64**(1): p. 37–41.

356. Skala, S.L., B. Hristov, and A.C. Hristov, *Primary cutaneous follicle center lymphoma.* Arch Pathol Lab Med, 2018. **142**(11): p. 1313–21.

357. Cerroni, L., et al., *Primary cutaneous follicle center cell lymphoma with follicular growth pattern.* Blood, 2000. **95**(12): p. 3922–8.

358. Golling, P., et al., *Primary cutaneous B-cell lymphomas – clinicopathological, prognostic and therapeutic characterisation of 54 cases according to the WHO-EORTC classification and the ISCL/EORTC TNM classification system for primary cutaneous lymphomas other than mycosis fungoides and Sézary syndrome.* Leuk Lymphoma, 2008. **49**(6): p. 1094–103.

359. Swerdlow, S.H., et al., *Cutaneous B-cell lymphoproliferative disorders: report of the 2011 society for hematopathology/European association for haematopathology workshop.* Am J Clin Pathol, 2013. **139**(4): p. 515–35.

360. Wilcox, R.A., *Cutaneous B-cell lymphomas: 2013 update on diagnosis, risk-stratification, and management.* Am J Hematol, 2013. **88**(1): p. 73–6.

361. Kempf, W., et al., *Primary cutaneous B-cell lymphomas.* J Dtsch Dermatol Ges, 2012. **10**(1): p. 12–22; quiz 23.

362. Willemze, R., et al., *WHO-EORTC classification for cutaneous lymphomas.* Blood, 2005. **105**(10): p. 3768–85.

363. Banks, P.M., et al., *Mantle cell lymphoma. A proposal for unification of morphologic, immunologic, and molecular data.* Am J Surg Pathol, 1992. **16**(7): p. 637–40.

364. Campo, E., M. Raffeld, and E.S. Jaffe, *Mantle-cell lymphoma.* Semin Hematol, 1999. **36**(2): p. 115–27.

365. Jares, P. and E. Campo, *Advances in the understanding of mantle cell lymphoma.* Br J Haematol, 2008. **142**(2): p. 149–65.

366. Jain, P. and M. Wang, *Mantle cell lymphoma: 2019 update on the diagnosis, pathogenesis, prognostication, and management.* Am J Hematol, 2019. **94**(6): p. 710–25.

367. Pittaluga, S., et al., *Mantle cell lymphoma: a clinicopathological study of 55 cases.* Histopathology, 1995. **26**(1): p. 17–24.

368. Meusers, P., et al., *Multicentre randomized therapeutic trial for advanced centrocytic lymphoma: anthracycline does not improve the prognosis.* Hematol Oncol, 1989. **7**(5): p. 365–80.

369. Bosch, F., et al., *Mantle cell lymphoma: presenting features, response to therapy, and prognostic factors.* Cancer, 1998. **82**(3): p. 567–75.

370. Fu, K., et al., *Cyclin D1-negative mantle cell lymphoma: a clinico-pathologic study based on gene expression profiling.* Blood, 2005. **106**(13): p. 4315–21.

371. Salaverria, I., et al., *CCND2 rearrangements are the most frequent genetic events in cyclin D1(–) mantle cell lymphoma.* Blood, 2013. **121**(8): p. 1394–402.

372. Hu, Z., et al., *CD200 expression in mantle cell lymphoma identifies a unique subgroup of patients with frequent IGHV mutations, absence of SOX11 expression, and an indolent clinical course.* Mod Pathol, 2018. **31**(2): p. 327–36.

373. Fernandez, V., et al., *Genomic and gene expression profiling defines indolent forms of mantle cell lymphoma.* Cancer Res, 2010. **70**(4): p. 1408–18.

374. Tiemann, M., et al., *Histopathology, cell proliferation indices and clinical outcome in 304 patients with mantle cell lymphoma (MCL): a clinicopathological study from the European MCL Network.* Br J Haematol, 2005. **131**(1): p. 29–38.

375. Argatoff, L.H., et al., *Mantle cell lymphoma: a clinicopathologic study of 80 cases.* Blood, 1997. **89**(6): p. 2067–78.

376. Katzenberger, T., et al., *The Ki67 proliferation index is a quantitative indicator of clinical risk in mantle cell lymphoma.* Blood, 2006. **107**(8): p. 3407.

377. Determann, O., et al., *Ki-67 predicts outcome in advanced-stage mantle cell lymphoma patients treated with anti-CD20 immunochemotherapy: results from randomized trials of the European MCL Network and the German Low Grade Lymphoma Study Group.* Blood, 2008. **111**(4): p. 2385–7.

378. Klapper, W., et al., *Ki-67 as a prognostic marker in mantle cell lymphoma-consensus guidelines of the pathology panel of the European MCL Network.* J Hematop, 2009. **2**(2): p. 103–11.

379. Ye, H., et al., *Smoldering mantle cell lymphoma.* J Exp Clin Cancer Res, 2017. **36**(1): p. 185.

380. Espinet, B., et al., *Clonal proliferation of cyclin D1-positive mantle lymphocytes in an asymptomatic patient: an early-stage event in the development or an indolent form of a mantle cell lymphoma?* Hum Pathol, 2005. **36**(11): p. 1232–7.

381. Nodit, L., et al., *Indolent mantle cell lymphoma with nodal involvement and mutated immunoglobulin heavy chain genes.* Hum Pathol, 2003. **34**(10): p. 1030–4.

382. Adam, P., et al., *Incidence of preclinical manifestations of mantle cell lymphoma and mantle cell lymphoma in situ in reactive lymphoid tissues.* Mod Pathol, 2012. **25**(12): p. 1629–36.

383. Aqel, N., et al., *In-situ mantle cell lymphoma—a report of two cases.* Histopathology, 2008. **52**(2): p. 256–60.

384. Edlefsen, K.L., et al., *Early lymph node involvement by mantle cell lymphoma limited to the germinal center: report of a case with a novel "follicular in situ" growth pattern.* Am J Clin Pathol, 2011. **136**(2): p. 276–81.

385. Neto, A.G., et al., *Colonic in situ mantle cell lymphoma.* Ann Diagn Pathol, 2012. **16**(6): p. 508–14.

386. Wilcox, R.A., *Cutaneous T-cell lymphoma: 2011 update on diagnosis, risk-stratification, and management.* Am J Hematol, 2011. **86**(11): p. 928–48.

387. Dreyling, M., et al., *Update on the molecular pathogenesis and clinical treatment of mantle cell lymphoma: report of the 11th annual conference of the European Mantle Cell Lymphoma Network.* Leuk Lymphoma, 2013. **54**(4): p. 699–707.

388. Dai, B., et al., *B-cell receptor-driven MALT1 activity regulates MYC signaling in mantle cell lymphoma.* Blood, 2017. **129**(3): p. 333–46.

389. Dreyling, M., W. Klapper, and S. Rule, *Blastoid and pleomorphic mantle cell lymphoma: still a diagnostic and therapeutic challenge!* Blood, 2018. **132**(26): p. 2722–9.

390. Pott, C., et al., *Blastoid variant of mantle cell lymphoma: late progression from classical mantle cell lymphoma and quantitation of minimal residual disease*. Eur J Haematol, 2005. **74**(4): p. 353–8.

391. Vogt, N. and W. Klapper, *Variability in morphology and cell proliferation in sequential biopsies of mantle cell lymphoma at diagnosis and relapse: clinical correlation and insights into disease progression*. Histopathology, 2013. **62**(2): p. 334–42.

392. Smith, M.D., et al., *Case report: mantle cell lymphoma, prolymphocytoid variant, with leukostasis syndrome*. Mod Pathol, 2004. **17**(7): p. 879–83.

393. Kelemen, K., et al., *CD23+ mantle cell lymphoma: a clinical pathologic entity associated with superior outcome compared with CD23- disease*. Am J Clin Pathol, 2008. **130**(2): p. 166–77.

394. Xu, J., et al., *SOX11-negative mantle cell lymphoma: clinicopathologic and prognostic features of 75 patients*. Am J Surg Pathol, 2019. **43**(5): p. 710–6.

395. Dong, H.Y., et al., *B-cell lymphomas with coexpression of CD5 and CD10*. Am J Clin Pathol, 2003. **119**(2): p. 218–30.

396. Gualco, G., et al., *BCL6, MUM1, and CD10 expression in mantle cell lymphoma*. Appl Immunohistochem Mol Morphol, 2010. **18**(2): p. 103–8.

397. Williams, M.E., S.H. Swerdlow, and T.C. Meeker, *Chromosome t(11;14)(q13;q32) breakpoints in centrocytic lymphoma are highly localized at the bcl-1 major translocation cluster*. Leukemia, 1993. **7**(9): p. 1437–40.

398. Espinet, B., et al., *Translocation (11;14)(q13;q32) and preferential involvement of chromosomes 1, 2, 9, 13, and 17 in mantle cell lymphoma*. Cancer Genet Cytogenet, 1999. **111**(1): p. 92–8.

399. Wlodarska, I., et al., *Secondary chromosome changes in mantle cell lymphoma*. Haematologica, 1999. **84**(7): p. 594–9.

400. Bentz, M., et al., *t(11;14)-positive mantle cell lymphomas exhibit complex karyotypes and share similarities with B-cell chronic lymphocytic leukemia*. Genes Chromosomes Cancer, 2000. **27**(3): p. 285–94.

401. Allen, J.E., et al., *Identification of novel regions of amplification and deletion within mantle cell lymphoma DNA by comparative genomic hybridization*. Br J Haematol, 2002. **116**(2): p. 291–8.

402. Parry-Jones, N., et al., *Cytogenetic abnormalities additional to t(11;14) correlate with clinical features in leukaemic presentation of mantle cell lymphoma, and may influence prognosis: a study of 60 cases by FISH*. Br J Haematol, 2007. **137**(2): p. 117–24.

403. Cuneo, A., et al., *13q14 deletion in non-Hodgkin's lymphoma: correlation with clinicopathologic features*. Haematologica, 1999. **84**(7): p. 589–93.

404. Cuneo, A., et al., *Cytogenetic profile of lymphoma of follicle mantle lineage: correlation with clinicobiologic features*. Blood, 1999. **93**(4): p. 1372–80.

405. Martinez-Climent, J.A., et al., *Loss of a novel tumor suppressor gene locus at chromosome 8p is associated with leukemic mantle cell lymphoma*. Blood, 2001. **98**(12): p. 3479–82.

406. Hill, H.A., et al., *Genetic mutations and features of mantle cell lymphoma: a systematic review and meta-analysis*. Blood Adv, 2020. **4**(13): p. 2927–38.

407. Sukswai, N., et al., *Diffuse large B-cell lymphoma variants: an update*. Pathology, 2019. **52**(1): p. 53–67.

408. Chapuy, B., et al., *Molecular subtypes of diffuse large B cell lymphoma are associated with distinct pathogenic mechanisms and outcomes*. Nat Med, 2018. **24**(5): p. 679–90.

409. Said, J.W., *Aggressive B-cell lymphomas: how many categories do we need?* Mod Pathol, 2013. **26 Suppl 1**: p. S42–56.

410. Schmitz, R., et al., *Genetics and pathogenesis of diffuse large B-cell lymphoma*. N Engl J Med, 2018. **378**(15): p. 1396–407.

411. Sha, C., et al., *Molecular high-grade B-cell lymphoma: defining a poor-risk group that requires different approaches to therapy*. J Clin Oncol, 2019. **37**(3): p. 202–12.

412. Tang, H., et al., *Clinicopathologic significance and therapeutic implication of de novo CD5+ diffuse large B-cell lymphoma*. Hematology, 2019. **24**(1): p. 446–54.

413. Tousseyn, T. and C. De Wolf-Peeters, *T cell/histiocyte-rich large B-cell lymphoma: an update on its biology and classification*. Virchows Arch, 2011. **459**(6): p. 557–63.

414. Alizadeh, A.A., et al., *Distinct types of diffuse large B-cell lymphoma identified by gene expression profiling*. Nature, 2000. **403**(6769): p. 503–11.

415. Rosenwald, A., et al., *The use of molecular profiling to predict survival after chemotherapy for diffuse large-B-cell lymphoma*. N Engl J Med, 2002. **346**(25): p. 1937–47.

416. Rosenwald, A., et al., *Molecular diagnosis of primary mediastinal B cell lymphoma identifies a clinically favorable subgroup of diffuse large B cell lymphoma related to Hodgkin lymphoma*. J Exp Med, 2003. **198**(6): p. 851–62.

417. Choi, W.W., et al., *A new immunostain algorithm classifies diffuse large B-cell lymphoma into molecular subtypes with high accuracy*. Clin Cancer Res, 2009. **15**(17): p. 5494–502.

418. Hans, C.P., et al., *Confirmation of the molecular classification of diffuse large B-cell lymphoma by immunohistochemistry using a tissue microarray*. Blood, 2004. **103**(1): p. 275–82.

419. Colomo, L., et al., *Clinical impact of the differentiation profile assessed by immunophenotyping in patients with diffuse large B-cell lymphoma*. Blood, 2003. **101**(1): p. 78–84.

420. Muris, J.J., et al., *Immunohistochemical profiling of caspase signaling pathways predicts clinical response to chemotherapy in primary nodal diffuse large B-cell lymphomas*. Blood, 2005. **105**(7): p. 2916–23.

421. Meyer, P.N., et al., *Immunohistochemical methods for predicting cell of origin and survival in patients with diffuse large B-cell lymphoma treated with rituximab*. J Clin Oncol, 2011. **29**(2): p. 200–7.

422. Hwang, H.S., et al., *High concordance of gene expression profiling-correlated immunohistochemistry algorithms in diffuse large B-cell lymphoma, not otherwise specified*. Am J Surg Pathol, 2014. **38**(8): p. 1046–57.

423. Lennert, K. and Mohri, N., *Histopathology of Non-Hodgkin's lymphomas*. 1992, Springer Verlag: New York.

424. Campuzano-Zuluaga, G., et al., *Frequency and extent of CD30 expression in diffuse large B-cell lymphoma and its relation to clinical and biologic factors: a retrospective study of 167 cases*. Leuk Lymphoma, 2013. **54**(11): p. 2405–11.

425. Hu, S., et al., *CD30 expression defines a novel subset of diffuse large B-cell lymphoma with favorable prognosis and distinct gene expression signature: a report from The International DLBCL Rituximab-CHOP Consortium Program Study*. Blood, 2013. **121**(14): p. 2715–24.

426. Kroft, S.H., et al., *De novo CD5+ diffuse large B-cell lymphomas. A heterogeneous group containing an unusual form of splenic lymphoma*. Am J Clin Pathol, 2000. **114**(4): p. 523–33.

427. Matolcsy, A., A. Chadburn, and D.M. Knowles, *De novo CD5-positive and Richter's syndrome-associated diffuse large B cell lymphomas are genotypically distinct*. Am J Pathol, 1995. **147**(1): p. 207–16.

428. Yamaguchi, M., et al., *De novo CD5-positive diffuse large B-cell lymphoma: clinical characteristics and therapeutic outcome*. Br J Haematol, 1999. **105**(4): p. 1133–9.

429. Yamaguchi, M., et al., *De novo CD5+ diffuse large B-cell lymphoma: a clinicopathologic study of 109 patients*. Blood, 2002. **99**(3): p. 815–21.

430. Weisberger, J., W. Gorczyca, and M.C. Kinney, *CD56-positive large B-cell lymphoma*. Appl Immunohistochem Mol Morphol, 2006. **14**(4): p. 369–74.

431. Johnson, N.A., et al., *Diffuse large B-cell lymphoma: reduced CD20 expression is associated with an inferior survival*. Blood, 2009. **113**(16): p. 3773–80.

432. Aukema, S.M., et al., *Double-hit B-cell lymphomas*. Blood, 2011. **117**(8): p. 2319–31.

433. Horn, H., et al., *MYC status in concert with BCL2 and BCL6 expression predicts outcome in diffuse large B-cell lymphoma*. Blood, 2013. **121**(12): p. 2253–63.

434. Horn, H., et al., *Diffuse large B-cell lymphomas of immunoblastic type are a major reservoir for MYC-IGH translocations*. Am J Surg Pathol, 2015. **39**(1): p. 61–6.

435. Gascoyne, R.D., *Pathologic prognostic factors in diffuse aggressive non-Hodgkin's lymphoma*. Hematol Oncol Clin North Am, 1997. **11**(5): p. 847–62.

436. Huang, S., et al., *Prognostic impact of diffuse large B-cell lymphoma with extra copies of MYC, BCL2 and/or BCL6: comparison with double/triple hit lymphoma and double expressor lymphoma.* Diagn Pathol, 2019. **14**(1): p. 81.

437. Wright, G., et al., *A gene expression-based method to diagnose clinically distinct subgroups of diffuse large B cell lymphoma.* Proc Natl Acad Sci U S A, 2003. **100**(17): p. 9991–6.

438. Painter, D., et al., *Cell-of-origin in diffuse large B-cell lymphoma: findings from the UK's population-based Haematological Malignancy Research Network.* Br J Haematol, 2019. **185**(4): p. 781–4.

439. Lossos, I.S., et al., *Ongoing immunoglobulin somatic mutation in germinal center B cell-like but not in activated B cell-like diffuse large cell lymphomas.* Proc Natl Acad Sci U S A, 2000. **97**(18): p. 10209–13.

440. Huang, J.Z., et al., *The t(14;18) defines a unique subset of diffuse large B-cell lymphoma with a germinal center B-cell gene expression profile.* Blood, 2002. **99**(7): p. 2285–90.

441. Alizadeh, A.A., et al., *Towards a novel classification of human malignancies based on gene expression patterns.* J Pathol, 2001. **195**(1): p. 41–52.

442. Poulsen, C.B., et al., *Microarray-based classification of diffuse large B-cell lymphoma.* Eur J Haematol, 2005. **74**(6): p. 453–65.

443. Ngo, V.N., et al., *Oncogenically active MYD88 mutations in human lymphoma.* Nature, 2011. **470**(7332): p. 115–9.

444. Lacy, S.E., et al., *Targeted sequencing in DLBCL, molecular subtypes, and outcomes: a Haematological Malignancy Research Network report.* Blood, 2020. **135**(20): p. 1759–71.

445. Zhang, W., et al., *Novel bioinformatic classification system for genetic signatures identification in diffuse large B-cell lymphoma.* BMC Cancer, 2020. **20**(1): p. 714.

446. Alsuwaidan, A., et al., *Bright CD38 expression by flow cytometric analysis is a biomarker for double/triple hit lymphomas with a moderate sensitivity and high specificity.* Cytometry B Clin Cytom, 2019. **96**(5): p. 368–74.

447. Tsuyama, N., et al., *Clinical and prognostic significance of aberrant T-cell marker expression in 225 cases of de novo diffuse large B-cell lymphoma and 276 cases of other B-cell lymphomas.* Oncotarget, 2017. **8**(20): p. 33487–500.

448. Xu-Monette, Z.Y., et al., *Clinical and biological significance of de novo CD5+ diffuse large B-cell lymphoma in Western countries.* Oncotarget, 2015. **6**(8): p. 5615–33.

449. Yamaguchi, M., et al., *De novo CD5+ diffuse large B-cell lymphoma: results of a detailed clinicopathological review in 120 patients.* Haematologica, 2008. **93**(8): p. 1195–202.

450. Ponzoni, M., et al., *Definition, diagnosis, and management of intravascular large B-cell lymphoma: proposals and perspectives from an international consensus meeting.* J Clin Oncol, 2007. **25**(21): p. 3168–73.

451. Matsue, K., et al., *Diagnosis of intravascular large B cell lymphoma: novel insights into clinicopathological features from 42 patients at a single institution over 20 years.* Br J Haematol, 2019. **187**(3): p. 328–36.

452. Masaki, Y., et al., *Intravascular large B cell lymphoma: proposed of the strategy for early diagnosis and treatment of patients with rapid deteriorating condition.* Int J Hematol, 2009. **89**(5): p. 600–10.

453. Ponzoni, M., E. Campo, and S. Nakamura, *Intravascular large B-cell lymphoma: a chameleon with multiple faces and many masks.* Blood, 2018. **132**(15): p. 1561–7.

454. Murase, T., et al., *Intravascular large B-cell lymphoma (IVLBCL): a clinicopathologic study of 96 cases with special reference to the immunophenotypic heterogeneity of CD5.* Blood, 2007. **109**(2): p. 478–85.

455. Ferreri, A.J., et al., *Intravascular lymphoma: clinical presentation, natural history, management and prognostic factors in a series of 38 cases, with special emphasis on the 'cutaneous variant'.* Br J Haematol, 2004. **127**(2): p. 173–83.

456. Ponzoni, M. and A.J. Ferreri, *Intravascular lymphoma: a neoplasm of 'homeless' lymphocytes?* Hematol Oncol, 2006. **24**(3): p. 105–12.

457. Yegappan, S., et al., *Angiotropic lymphoma: an immunophenotypically and clinically heterogeneous lymphoma.* Mod Pathol, 2001. **14**(11): p. 1147–56.

458. Cazals-Hatem, D., et al., *Primary mediastinal large B-cell lymphoma. A clinicopathologic study of 141 cases compared with 916 nonmediastinal large B-cell lymphomas, a GELA ("Groupe d'Etude des Lymphomes de l'Adulte") study.* Am J Surg Pathol, 1996. **20**(7): p. 877–88.

459. Zinzani, P.L., et al., *Primary mediastinal large B-cell lymphoma with sclerosis: a clinical study of 89 patients treated with MACOP-B chemotherapy and radiation therapy.* Haematologica, 2001. **86**(2): p. 187–91.

460. Tsang, P., et al., *Molecular characterization of primary mediastinal B cell lymphoma.* Am J Pathol, 1996. **148**(6): p. 2017–25.

461. Traverse-Glehen, A., et al., *Mediastinal gray zone lymphoma: the missing link between classic Hodgkin's lymphoma and mediastinal large B-cell lymphoma.* Am J Surg Pathol, 2005. **29**(11): p. 1411–21.

462. Todeschini, G., et al., *Primary mediastinal large B-cell lymphoma (PMLBCL): long-term results from a retrospective multicentre Italian experience in 138 patients treated with CHOP or MACOP-B/VACOP-B.* Br J Cancer, 2004. **90**(2): p. 372–6.

463. Savage, K.J., et al., *The molecular signature of mediastinal large B-cell lymphoma differs from that of other diffuse large B-cell lymphomas and shares features with classical Hodgkin's lymphoma.* Blood, 2003. **102**: p. 3871–9.

464. Pileri, S.A., et al., *Primary mediastinal B-cell lymphoma: high frequency of BCL-6 mutations and consistent expression of the transcription factors OCT-2, BOB.1, and PU.1 in the absence of immunoglobulins.* Am J Pathol, 2003. **162**(1): p. 243–53.

465. Paulli, M., et al., *Mediastinal B-cell lymphoma: a study of its histomorphologic spectrum based on 109 cases.* Hum Pathol, 1999. **30**(2): p. 178–87.

466. Moller, P., et al., *Primary mediastinal clear cell lymphoma of B-cell type.* Virchows Arch A Pathol Anat Histopathol, 1986. **409**(1): p. 79–92.

467. Higgins, J.P. and R.A. Warnke, *CD30 expression is common in mediastinal large B-cell lymphoma.* Am J Clin Pathol, 1999. **112**(2): p. 241–7.

468. Gorczyca, W., et al., *Flow cytometry in the diagnosis of mediastinal tumors with emphasis on differentiating thymocytes from precursor T-lymphoblastic lymphoma/leukemia.* Leuk Lymphoma, 2004. **45**(3): p. 529–38.

469. Davis, R.E., R.F. Dorfman, and R.A. Warnke, *Primary large-cell lymphoma of the thymus: a diffuse B-cell neoplasm presenting as primary mediastinal lymphoma.* Hum Pathol, 1990. **21**(12): p. 1262–8.

470. Chadburn, A. and G. Frizzera, *Mediastinal large B-cell lymphoma vs classic Hodgkin lymphoma.* Am J Clin Pathol, 1999. **112**(2): p. 155–8.

471. Barth, T.F., F. Leithauser, and P. Moller, *Mediastinal B-cell lymphoma, a lymphoma type with several characteristics unique among diffuse large B-cell lymphomas.* Ann Hematol, 2001. **80** Suppl 3: p. B49–53.

472. Barth, T.F., et al., *Mediastinal (thymic) large B-cell lymphoma: where do we stand?* Lancet Oncol, 2002. **3**(4): p. 229–34.

473. Boleti, E. and P.W. Johnson, *Primary mediastinal B-cell lymphoma.* Hematol Oncol, 2007. **25**(4): p. 157–63.

474. Hutchinson, C.B. and E. Wang, *Primary mediastinal (thymic) large B-cell lymphoma: a short review with brief discussion of mediastinal gray zone lymphoma.* Arch Pathol Lab Med, 2011. **135**(3): p. 394–8.

475. Yamamoto, W., et al., *Clinicopathological analysis of mediastinal large B-cell lymphoma and classical Hodgkin lymphoma of the mediastinum.* Leuk Lymphoma, 2012. **54**(5): p. 967–72.

476. Isaacson, P.G., A.J. Norton, and B.J. Addis, *The human thymus contains a novel population of B lymphocytes.* Lancet, 1987. **2**(8574): p. 1488–91.

477. Hofmann, W.J., F. Momburg, and P. Moller, *Thymic medullary cells expressing B lymphocyte antigens.* Hum Pathol, 1988. **19**(11): p. 1280–7.

478. Gentry, M., et al., *Performance of a commercially available MAL antibody in the diagnosis of primary mediastinal large B-cell lymphoma.* Am J Surg Pathol, 2017. **41**(2): p. 189–94.

479. Dorfman, D.M., A. Shahsafaei, and M.A. Alonso, *Utility of CD200 immunostaining in the diagnosis of primary mediastinal large B cell lymphoma: comparison with MAL, CD23, and other markers.* Mod Pathol, 2012. **25**(12): p. 1637–43.

480. Shi, M., et al., *Expression of programmed cell death 1 ligand 2 (PD-L2) is a distinguishing feature of primary mediastinal (thymic) large B-cell lymphoma and associated with PDCD1LG2 copy gain.* Am J Surg Pathol, 2014. **38**(12): p. 1715–23.

481. Chen, B.J., et al., *PD-L1 expression is characteristic of a subset of aggressive B-cell lymphomas and virus-associated malignancies.* Clin Cancer Res, 2013. **19**(13): p. 3462–73.

482. Chen, B.J., et al., *Cyclin D1-positive mediastinal large B-cell lymphoma with copy number gains of CCND1 gene: a study of 3 cases with nonmediastinal disease.* Am J Surg Pathol, 2019. **43**(1): p. 110–20.

483. Cherian, S. and J.R. Fromm, *Evaluation of primary mediastinal large B cell lymphoma by flow cytometry.* Cytometry B Clin Cytom, 2018. **94**(3): p. 459–67.

484. Bellan, C., et al., *Burkitt lymphoma versus diffuse large B-cell lymphoma: a practical approach.* Hematol Oncol, 2010. **28**(2): p. 53–6.

485. Casulo, C. and J.W. Friedberg, *Burkitt lymphoma- a rare but challenging lymphoma.* Best Pract Res Clin Haematol, 2018. **31**(3): p. 279–84.

486. Cogliatti, S.B., et al., *Diagnosis of Burkitt lymphoma in due time: a practical approach.* Br J Haematol, 2006. **134**(3): p. 294–301.

487. Hummel, M., et al., *A biologic definition of Burkitt's lymphoma from transcriptional and genomic profiling.* N Engl J Med, 2006. **354**(23): p. 2419–30.

488. Jaffe, E.S., et al., *Burkitt's lymphoma: a single disease with multiple variants. The World Health Organization classification of neoplastic diseases of the hematopoietic and lymphoid tissues.* Blood, 1999. **93**(3): p. 1124.

489. Murphy, S.B., et al., *Results of treatment of advanced-stage Burkitt's lymphoma and B cell (SIg+) acute lymphoblastic leukemia with high-dose fractionated cyclophosphamide and coordinated high-dose methotrexate and cytarabine.* J Clin Oncol, 1986. **4**(12): p. 1732–9.

490. Patte, C., et al., *Therapy of Burkitt and other B-cell acute lymphoblastic leukaemia and lymphoma: experience with the LMB protocols of the SFOP (French Paediatric Oncology Society) in children and adults.* Baillieres Clin Haematol, 1994. **7**(2): p. 339–48.

491. Patte, C., et al., *The Societe Francaise d'Oncologie Pediatrique LMB89 protocol: highly effective multiagent chemotherapy tailored to the tumor burden and initial response in 561 unselected children with B-cell lymphomas and L3 leukemia.* Blood, 2001. **97**(11): p. 3370–9.

492. Blum, K.A., G. Lozanski, and J.C. Byrd, *Adult Burkitt leukemia and lymphoma.* Blood, 2004. **104**(10): p. 3009–20.

493. Tsagarakis, N.J., et al., *Contribution of immunophenotype to the investigation and differential diagnosis of Burkitt lymphoma, double-hit high-grade B-cell lymphoma, and single-hit MYC-rearranged diffuse large B-cell lymphoma.* Cytometry B Clin Cytom, 2020. **98**(5): p. 412–20.

494. Boxer, L.M. and C.V. Dang, *Translocations involving c-myc and c-myc function.* Oncogene, 2001. **20**(40): p. 5595–610.

495. Sigaux, F., et al., *Malignant lymphomas with band 8q24 chromosome abnormality: a morphologic continuum extending from Burkitt's to immunoblastic lymphoma.* Br J Haematol, 1984. **57**(3): p. 393–405.

496. Ladanyi, M., et al., *MYC rearrangement and translocations involving band 8q24 in diffuse large cell lymphomas.* Blood, 1991. **77**(5): p. 1057–63.

497. Nishida, K., et al., *The Ig heavy chain gene is frequently involved in chromosomal translocations in multiple myeloma and plasma cell leukemia as detected by in situ hybridization.* Blood, 1997. **90**(2): p. 526–34.

498. Kramer, M.H., et al., *Clinical relevance of BCL2, BCL6, and MYC rearrangements in diffuse large B-cell lymphoma.* Blood, 1998. **92**(9): p. 3152–62.

499. Akasaka, T., et al., *Molecular and clinical features of non-Burkitt's, diffuse large-cell lymphoma of B-cell type associated with the c-MYC/immunoglobulin heavy-chain fusion gene.* J Clin Oncol, 2000. **18**(3): p. 510–18.

500. Nakamura, N., et al., *The distinction between Burkitt lymphoma and diffuse large B-Cell lymphoma with c-myc rearrangement.* Mod Pathol, 2002. **15**(7): p. 771–6.

501. Barth, T.F., et al., *Homogeneous immunophenotype and paucity of secondary genomic aberrations are distinctive features of endemic but not of sporadic Burkitt's lymphoma and diffuse large B-cell lymphoma with MYC rearrangement.* J Pathol, 2004. **203**(4): p. 940–5.

502. Haralambieva, E., et al., *Clinical, immunophenotypic, and genetic analysis of adult lymphomas with morphologic features of Burkitt lymphoma.* Am J Surg Pathol, 2005. **29**(8): p. 1086–94.

503. Cardoso, C.C., et al., *The importance of CD39, CD43, CD81, and CD95 expression for differentiating B cell lymphoma by flow cytometry.* Cytometry B Clin Cytom, 2018. **94**(3): p. 451–8.

504. McGowan, P., et al., *Differentiating between Burkitt lymphoma and CD10+ diffuse large B-cell lymphoma: the role of commonly used flow cytometry cell markers and the application of a multiparameter scoring system.* Am J Clin Pathol, 2012. **137**(4): p. 665–70.

505. Schniederjan, S.D., et al., *A novel flow cytometric antibody panel for distinguishing Burkitt lymphoma from CD10+ diffuse large B-cell lymphoma.* Am J Clin Pathol, 2010. **133**(5): p. 718–26.

506. Rymkiewicz, G., et al., *A comprehensive flow-cytometry-based immunophenotypic characterization of Burkitt-like lymphoma with 11q aberration.* Mod Pathol, 2018. **31**(5): p. 732–43.

507. Demina, I., et al., *Additional flow cytometric studies for differential diagnosis between Burkitt lymphoma/leukemia and B-cell precursor acute lymphoblastic leukemia.* Leuk Res, 2021. **100**: p. 106491.

508. Ok, C.Y. and L.J. Medeiros, *High-grade B-cell lymphoma: a term re-purposed in the revised WHO classification.* Pathology, 2020. **52**(1): p. 68–77.

509. Landsburg, D.J., et al., *Impact of oncogene rearrangement patterns on outcomes in patients with double-hit non-Hodgkin lymphoma.* Cancer, 2016. **122**(4): p. 559–64.

510. Rosenthal, A. and A. Younes, *High grade B-cell lymphoma with rearrangements of MYC and BCL2 and/or BCL6: double hit and triple hit lymphomas and double expressing lymphoma.* Blood Rev, 2017. **31**(2): p. 37–42.

511. Green, T.M., et al., *Immunohistochemical double-hit score is a strong predictor of outcome in patients with diffuse large B-cell lymphoma treated with rituximab plus cyclophosphamide, doxorubicin, vincristine, and prednisone.* J Clin Oncol, 2012. **30**(28): p. 3460–7.

512. Hasserjian, R.P., et al., *Commentary on the WHO classification of tumors of lymphoid tissues (2008): "Gray zone" lymphomas overlapping with Burkitt lymphoma or classical Hodgkin lymphoma.* J Hematop, 2009. **2**(2): p. 89–95.

513. Pillai, R.K., et al., *Double-hit B-cell lymphomas with BCL6 and MYC translocations are aggressive, frequently extranodal lymphomas distinct from BCL2 double-hit B-cell lymphomas.* Am J Surg Pathol, 2013. **37**(3): p. 323–32.

514. Snuderl, M., et al., *B-cell lymphomas with concurrent IGH-BCL2 and MYC rearrangements are aggressive neoplasms with clinical and pathologic features distinct from Burkitt lymphoma and diffuse large B-cell lymphoma.* Am J Surg Pathol, 2010. **34**(3): p. 327–40.

515. Wu, D., et al., *"Double-Hit" mature B-cell lymphomas show a common immunophenotype by flow cytometry that includes decreased CD20 expression.* Am J Clin Pathol, 2010. **134**(2): p. 258–65.

516. Miyaoka, M., et al., *Clinicopathological and genomic analysis of double-hit follicular lymphoma: comparison with high-grade B-cell lymphoma with MYC and BCL2 and/or BCL6 rearrangements.* Mod Pathol, 2018. **31**(2): p. 313–26.

517. Ok, C.Y., et al., *High-grade B-cell lymphomas with TdT expression: a diagnostic and classification dilemma.* Mod Pathol, 2019. **32**(1): p. 48–58.

518. Loghavi, S., J.L. Kutok, and J.L. Jorgensen, *B-acute lymphoblastic leukemia/lymphoblastic lymphoma.* Am J Clin Pathol, 2015. **144**(3): p. 393–410.

519. Mufti, G.J., et al., *Common ALL with pre-B-cell features showing (8;14) and (14;18) chromosome translocations.* Blood, 1983. **62**(5): p. 1142–6.

520. Carli, M.G., et al., *Lymphoblastic lymphoma with primary splenic involvement and the classic 14;18 translocation.* Cancer Genet Cytogenet, 1991. **57**(1): p. 47–51.

521. Kramer, M.H., et al., *De novo acute B-cell leukemia with translocation t(14;18): an entity with a poor prognosis.* Leukemia, 1991. **5**(6): p. 473–8.

522. Nacheva, E., et al., *C-MYC translocations in de novo B-cell lineage acute leukemias with t(14;18)(cell lines Karpas 231 and 353).* Blood, 1993. **82**(1): p. 231–40.

523. Subramaniyam, S., et al., *De novo B lymphoblastic leukemia/lymphoma in an adult with t(14;18)(q32;q21) and c-MYC gene rearrangement involving 10p13.* Leuk Lymphoma, 2011. **52**(11): p. 2195–9.

524. Kobrin, C., et al., *Molecular analysis of light-chain switch and acute lymphoblastic leukemia transformation in two follicular lymphomas: implications for lymphomagenesis.* Leuk Lymphoma, 2006. **47**(8): p. 1523–34.

525. Navid, F., et al., *Acute lymphoblastic leukemia with the (8;14) (q24;q32) translocation and FAB L3 morphology associated with a B-precursor immunophenotype: the Pediatric Oncology Group experience.* Leukemia, 1999. **13**(1): p. 135–41.

526. Komrokji, R., et al., *Burkitt's leukemia with precursor B-cell immunophenotype and atypical morphology (atypical Burkitt's leukemia/lymphoma): case report and review of literature.* Leuk Res, 2003. **27**(6): p. 561–6.

527. Meznarich, J., et al., *Pediatric B-cell lymphoma with lymphoblastic morphology, TdT expression, MYC rearrangement, and features overlapping with Burkitt lymphoma.* Pediatr Blood Cancer, 2016. **63**(5): p. 938–40.

528. Hassan, R., et al., *Burkitt lymphoma/leukaemia transformed from a precursor B cell: clinical and molecular aspects.* Eur J Haematol, 2008. **80**(3): p. 265–70.

529. Gupta, A.A., et al., *Occurrence of t(8;22)(q24.1;q11.2) involving the MYC locus in a case of pediatric acute lymphoblastic leukemia with a precursor B cell immunophenotype.* J Pediatr Hematol Oncol, 2004. **26**(8): p. 532–4.

530. Higa, B., et al., *Precursor B-cell acute lymphoblastic leukaemia with FAB L3 (i.e., Burkitt's leukaemia/lymphoma) morphology and co-expression of monoclonal surface light chains and TdT: report of a unique case and review of the literature.* Pathology, 2009. **41**(5): p. 495–8.

531. Slavutsky, I., et al., *Variant (8;22) translocation in lymphoblastic lymphoma.* Leuk Lymphoma, 1996. **21**(1–2): p. 169–72.

532. Moench, L., et al., *Double- and triple-hit lymphomas can present with features suggestive of immaturity, including TdT expression, and create diagnostic challenges.* Leuk Lymphoma, 2016. **57**(11): p. 2626–35.

533. Li, Y., et al., *B lymphoblastic leukemia/lymphoma with Burkitt-like morphology and IGH/MYC rearrangement: report of 3 cases in adult patients.* Am J Surg Pathol, 2018. **42**(2): p. 269–76.

534. Liu, W., et al., *De Novo MYC and BCL2 double-hit B-cell precursor acute lymphoblastic leukemia (BCP-ALL) in pediatric and young adult patients associated with poor prognosis.* Pediatr Hematol Oncol, 2015. **32**(8): p. 535–47.

535. Quesada, A.E., et al., *Increased MYC copy number is an independent prognostic factor in patients with diffuse large B-cell lymphoma.* Mod Pathol, 2017. **30**(12): p. 1688–97.

536. Li, S., et al., *B-cell lymphomas with concurrent MYC and BCL2 abnormalities other than translocations behave similarly to MYC/BCL2 double-hit lymphomas.* Mod Pathol, 2015. **28**(2): p. 208–17.

537. Li, J., et al., *High-grade B-cell lymphomas, not otherwise specified: a study of 41 cases.* Cancer Manag Res, 2020. **12**: p. 1903–12.

538. Lin, P., et al., *Prognostic value of MYC rearrangement in cases of B-cell lymphoma, unclassifiable, with features intermediate between diffuse large B-cell lymphoma and Burkitt lymphoma.* Cancer, 2012. **118**(6): p. 1566–73.

539. Perry, A.M., et al., *B-cell lymphoma, unclassifiable, with features intermediate between diffuse large B-cell lymphoma and Burkitt lymphoma: study of 39 cases.* Br J Haematol, 2013. **162**(1): p. 40–49.

540. Delecluse, H.J., et al., *Plasmablastic lymphomas of the oral cavity: a new entity associated with the human immunodeficiency virus infection.* Blood, 1997. **89**(4): p. 1413–20.

541. Brown, R.S., et al., *Plasmablastic lymphoma: a new subcategory of human immunodeficiency virus-related non-Hodgkin's lymphoma.* Clin Oncol (R Coll Radiol), 1998. **10**(5): p. 327–9.

542. Colomo, L., et al., *Diffuse large B-cell lymphomas with plasmablastic differentiation represent a heterogeneous group of disease entities.* Am J Surg Pathol, 2004. **28**(6): p. 736–47.

543. Gaidano, G., et al., *Molecular histogenesis of plasmablastic lymphoma of the oral cavity.* Br J Haematol, 2002. **119**(3): p. 622–8.

544. Castillo, J.J., et al., *Human immunodeficiency virus-associated plasmablastic lymphoma: poor prognosis in the era of highly active antiretroviral therapy.* Cancer, 2012. **118**(21): p. 5270–7.

545. Borenstein, J., F. Pezzella, and K.C. Gatter, *Plasmablastic lymphomas may occur as post-transplant lymphoproliferative disorders.* Histopathology, 2007. **51**(6): p. 774–7.

546. Castillo, J.J., M. Bibas, and R.N. Miranda, *The biology and treatment of plasmablastic lymphoma.* Blood, 2015. **125**(15): p. 2323–30.

547. Bogusz, A.M., et al., *Plasmablastic lymphomas with MYC/IgH rearrangement: report of three cases and review of the literature.* Am J Clin Pathol, 2009. **132**(4): p. 597–605.

548. Montes-Moreno, S., C. Montalban, and M.A. Piris, *Large B-cell lymphomas with plasmablastic differentiation: a biological and therapeutic challenge.* Leuk Lymphoma, 2012. **53**(2): p. 185–94.

549. Loghavi, S., et al., *Stage, age, and EBV status impact outcomes of plasmablastic lymphoma patients: a clinicopathologic analysis of 61 patients.* J Hematol Oncol, 2015. **8**: p. 65.

550. Laurent, C., et al., *Immune-checkpoint expression in Epstein-Barr virus positive and negative plasmablastic lymphoma: a clinical and pathological study in 82 patients.* Haematologica, 2016. **101**(8): p. 976–84.

551. Ammari, Z.A., et al., *Diagnosis and management of primary effusion lymphoma in the immunocompetent and immunocompromised hosts.* Thorac Cardiovasc Surg, 2013. **61**(4): p. 343–9.

552. Courville, E.L., et al., *Diverse clinicopathologic features in human herpesvirus 8-associated lymphomas lead to diagnostic problems.* Am J Clin Pathol, 2014. **142**(6): p. 816–29.

553. Alexanian, S., et al., *KSHV/HHV8-negative effusion-based lymphoma, a distinct entity associated with fluid overload states.* Am J Surg Pathol, 2013. **37**(2): p. 241–9.

554. Chen, Y.B., A. Rahemtullah, and E. Hochberg, *Primary effusion lymphoma.* Oncologist, 2007. **12**(5): p. 569–76.

555. Tong, L.C., et al., *Subclassification of lymphoproliferative disorders in serous effusions: a 10-year experience.* Cancer Cytopathol, 2012. **121**(5): p. 261–70.

556. Beaty, M.W., et al., *A biphenotypic human herpesvirus 8-associated primary bowel lymphoma.* Am J Surg Pathol, 1999. **23**(8): p. 992–4.

557. Oksenhendler, E., et al., *High incidence of Kaposi sarcoma-associated herpesvirus-related non-Hodgkin lymphoma in patients with HIV infection and multicentric Castleman disease.* Blood, 2002. **99**(7): p. 2331–6.

558. Carbone, A. and A. Gloghini, *KSHV/HHV8-associated lymphomas.* Br J Haematol, 2008. **140**(1): p. 13–24.

559. Pan, Z.G., et al., *Extracavitary KSHV-associated large B-Cell lymphoma: a distinct entity or a subtype of primary effusion lymphoma? Study of 9 cases and review of an additional 43 cases.* Am J Surg Pathol, 2012. **36**(8): p. 1129–40.

560. Li, M.F., et al., *Human herpesvirus 8-associated lymphoma mimicking cutaneous anaplastic large T-cell lymphoma in a patient with human immunodeficiency virus infection.* J Cutan Pathol, 2012. **39**(2): p. 274–8.

14

PLASMA CELL NEOPLASMS

Plasma cell myeloma (PCM)

PCM phenotype by flow cytometry: CD10[−/rarely+], CD19[−/rarely+], CD20[−/rarely dim+], cytoplasmic kappa+ or cytoplasmic lambda+, CD27−, CD33[−/rarely+], CD38[+bright], CD45−, CD56[+/less often−], CD81[−/dim+], CD117[+/less often−], CD138[+bright], CD200[+/less often−], HLA-DR[−/rarely+]

Introduction

Plasma cell myeloma (PCM) is a clonal late B-cell disorder in which malignant plasma cells expand and accumulate in the bone marrow (BM) resulting in cytopenias, bone resorption (lytic bone lesions; Figure 14.1) and production of serum monoclonal protein (M protein) [1–4]. Majority of patients with myeloma evolve from pre-malignant stage (MGUS; monoclonal gammopathy of undetermined significance) [5–7]. MGUS is present in over 3% of the population above the age of 50 years and progresses to myeloma or related neoplasms at a rate of 1% per year.

The diagnosis and subclassification of the various plasma cell neoplasms relies on correlation of radiologic imaging and laboratory data (M-protein type and amount) with morphologic, cytogenetic, phenotypic, and molecular findings. Based on International Myeloma Working Group and WHO guidelines, plasma cell neoplasms have been divided into MGUS, smoldering (asymptomatic) plasma cell myeloma (SPCM), solitary plasmacytoma of bone, and symptomatic PCM [1, 8]. Minor subset of patients with PCM has true nonsecretory disease and has no evidence of M protein in the serum. The subtypes of myeloma are largely defined by the specific genetic and cytogenetic aberrations. POEMS syndrome is a rare paraneoplastic disorder associated with an underlying plasma cell neoplasm and polyneuropathy, organomegaly, endocrinopathy, monoclonal protein, and skin changes [9–13].

Diagnostic criteria for symptomatic PCM [1]:

- BM clonal plasma cells (≥10%) or plasmacytoma and ≥1 of the following myeloma-defining events:
  - End-organ damage attributable to the plasma cell proliferation (hypercalcemia >11 mg/dL, renal insufficiency, anemia; ≥1 osteolytic bone lesions)
  - ≥1 of the following: clonal BM plasma cells ≥60%, an involved to uninvolved serum free light chain ratio ≥100 or >1 focal lesion on MRI imaging [14–16]

Prognosis

Clinical outcomes of myeloma are highly heterogeneous and range from indolent (smoldering) to aggressive disseminated disease with leukemic blood involvement with survival ranging from a few days to more than 10 years [17–23]. Numerous prognostic factors are associated with poor prognosis in PCM, including advanced clinical stage, old age, poor performance status and/or comorbidities, extensive BM involvement, immature

(plasmablastic) morphology, BM failure (anemia, thrombocytopenia), high serum level of β$_2$-microglobulin, deletion of 17p13, hypodiploid karyotype, high number of circulating plasma cells, and increased plasma cell labeling index/high S-phase [24–32].

Based on several prognostic factors, PCM patients can be broadly categorized into standard, intermediate, and high risk for disease relapse, morbidity, and mortality. Patients without adverse genetic changes, low β$_2$-microglobulin (<3.5 mg/L) and serum albumin ≥3.5 g/dL are considered low risk. PCMs with one of adverse genetic changes [del(17p), t(4;14), t(14;16), and t(14;20)], primary plasma cell leukemia (PCL), β$_2$-microglobulin ≥5.5 mg/L, patient specific factors (such as old age, poor performance status, and co-morbidities) are considered high-risk (with survival <3 years). All other patients are considered intermediate risk [4, 33–37].

Smoldering plasma cell myeloma (SPCM)

SPCM is an asymptomatic disease which can be positioned between a mostly premalignant MGUS and active PCM [15, 32, 38]. It accounts for ~8%–20% of newly diagnosed myeloma cases. SPCM, which might have been also described as "indolent" myeloma or asymptomatic myeloma, meets the criteria for PCM (≥10% plasma cells in BM or M protein ≥30 g/L), but patients do not show significant symptoms (end organ damage), including lytic bone lesions (or osteoporosis with compression fracture), symptomatic hyperviscosity, anemia (hemoglobin 2 g/dL below normal or <10 g/dL), hypercalcemia, amyloidosis, >2 bacterial infections/12 months, or renal failure [3, 7, 10, 14, 39].

Diagnostic criteria for SPCM:

- M-protein in serum at myeloma levels (>30 g/L; IgG or IgA) and/or 10%–60% clonal plasma cells in BM
- No related organ or tissue impartment (end organ damage or bone lesions, hypercalcemia, renal insufficiency, anemia, bone lesions, amyloidosis, recurrent infections)

IgM MGUS

Patients with IgM monoclonal protein >30 g/L and/or BM lymphoplasmacytic cells >10% and no evidence of anemia, constitutional symptoms, lymphadenopathy or hepatosplenomegaly are classified as smoldering lymphoplasmacytic lymphoma (LPL) [3, 7, 40]. IgM MGUS is defined by a serum IgM paraprotein <30 g/L, BM lymphoplasmacytic infiltrate <10% and no evidence of anemia, constitutional symptoms, organomegaly or end-organ damage.

Morphology

Cytology. Cytologic features of PCM vary from mature forms resembling benign plasma cells to highly atypical, immature (plasmablastic), and pleomorphic ("anaplastic") cells (Figure 14.2). Mature plasma cells are round or oval with abundant basophilic cytoplasm, perinuclear cytoplasmic clearing (hof) and an eccentric nucleus with clumped chromatin creating "clock-face" ("cartwheel") pattern. Binucleation or multinucleation is

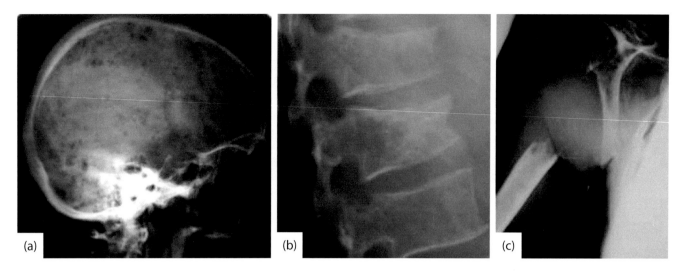

FIGURE 14.1 PCM: radiograph of the skull demonstrating lytic bone lesions (a), radiograph of the vertebrae demonstrating compressive fracture (b), and radiograph of the humerus with pathologic fracture (c).

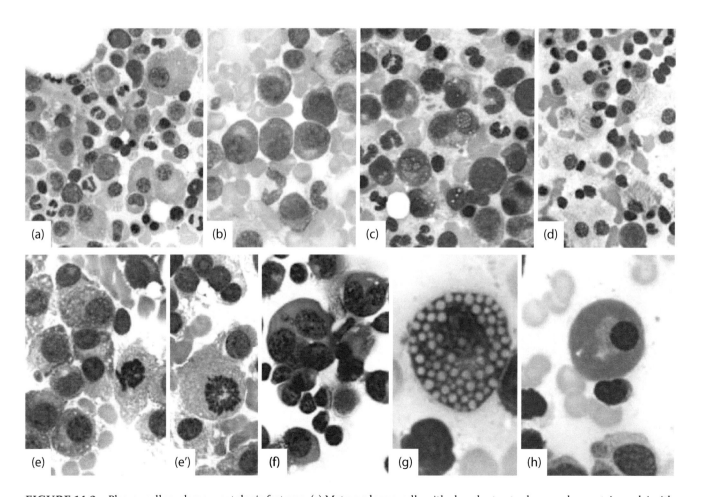

FIGURE 14.2 Plasma cell myeloma – cytologic features. (a) Mature plasma cells with abundant cytoplasm and eccentric nuclei with clumped chromatin; (b) Plasma cells with mild anisocytosis and inconspicuous nucleoli; (c) Plasma cells with intranuclear inclusions; (d) plasma cells with crystalloid cytoplasm mimicking Gaucher cells; (e, e′) Atypical plasma cells with prominent nucleoli and mitotic figures; (f) Multinucleated cells; (g) Mott cell with numerous cytoplasmic vacuoles; (g) "flame" cell.

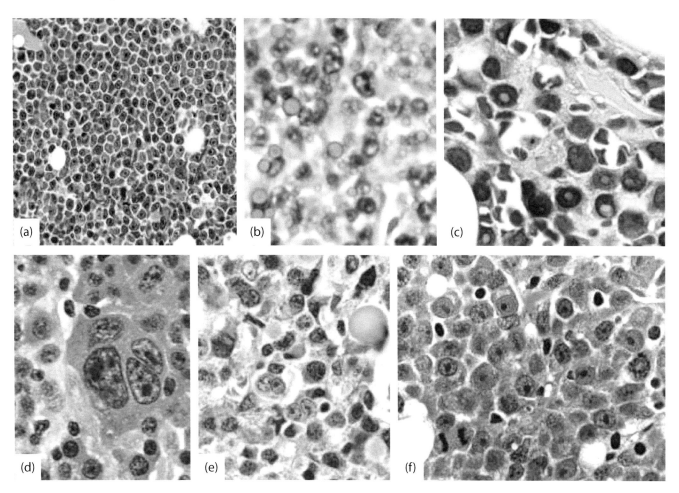

FIGURE 14.3 Plasma cell myeloma – histologic features. (a) Diffuse plasma cell infiltrate completely replacing bone marrow elements. (b) Russell bodies. (c) Dutcher bodies. (d–e) Anaplastic (immature) variants of plasma cell myeloma (two cases). Note prominent nuclear pleomorphism, hyperchromasia, macronucleoli, and multinucleation. (f) Plasma cell myeloma with prominent nucleoli and mitotic figures.

common. Plasmablastic features include fine reticulin chromatin pattern without clumping, large nucleus (>10 μm), prominent nucleolus (>2 μm), and scant cytoplasm (less than one half of the nuclear area) with no or minute hof region. Other cytologic variations of plasma cells include Mott cells ("bunch of grapes" appearance due to multiple blue cytoplasmic vacuoles), Russell bodies (red round cytoplasmic hyaline inclusions), pseudo-Gaucher cells (increased cytoplasmic crystals/fibrils), Dutcher bodies ("intranuclear" inclusions), Touton-like multinucleated giant cells, flame cells (irregular accumulation of red-colored immunoglobulins in cytoplasm), and lymphoplasmacytic-like small plasma cells. Dutcher and Russell bodies are both intra-cytoplasmic inclusions due to accumulation of immunoglobulin (Dutcher bodies invaginate into or overlie the nucleus whereas Russell bodies are seen within the cytoplasm). In blood smear PCMs often is associated with characteristic rouleaux formation of red blood cells.

Histology. Morphologic analysis of the BM core biopsy plays important role in the diagnosis of PCM, allowing for enumeration of plasma cells and analysis of growth pattern and cytologic atypia. On histologic examination (Figure 14.3) plasma cells may occur as subtle interstitial infiltrate, in clusters or as

a diffuse infiltrate replacing normal BM elements. The distribution of plasma cells in BM may vary in the same biopsy, from areas with hardly identifiable plasma cells to areas with sheets of plasma cells approaching 100% of marrow cellularity. This heterogeneous distribution of plasma cells may contribute (in part) to frequent discrepancy between the number of plasma cells seen in BM aspirate smears (or flow cytometry [FC] sample) and an actual number of plasma cells in BM, as represented by core biopsy. Some PCMs show prominent cytoplasmic inclusions (Russell bodies) or "intranuclear" inclusions (Dutcher bodies). Immature PCMs exhibit marked pleomorphism with multinucleation, prominent nucleoli, and mitotic figures (plasmablastic or anaplastic features). Some PCM are composed of small plasma cells mimicking lymphocytes or lymphoplasmacytic cells.

Immunohistochemistry

PCMs are positive for CD38, CD43, CD138, light and heavy chain immunoglobulins, MUM1/IRF4, OCT2, and BOB1 (Figure 14.4). They often show aberrant expression of CD56, CD117, EMA, and/or BCL1 (cyclin D1).

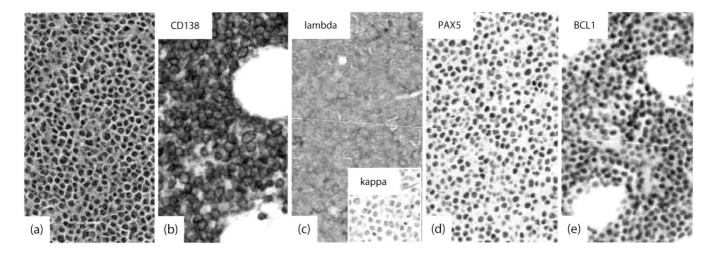

FIGURE 14.4   Plasma cell myeloma – immunohistochemistry. Plasma cells (a) express CD138 (b), lambda (c), PAX-5 (d), and BCL1 (cyclin D1; e).

Flow cytometry

Introduction

FC is an integral part of the evaluation and management of plasma cell neoplasms including diagnosis, prognostic stratification, monitoring of response to therapy (evaluation of minimal residual disease, MRD) and more recently identification of potential therapeutic targets expressed by plasma cells. Similar to the aspirate smears, FC usually underestimates the number of plasma cell when compared to slide-based morphological evaluation (core biopsy). The reason for this is multifactorial, including uneven distribution of plasma cell infiltrate in the BM, hemodilution during aspiration procedure, adherence of plasma cells to bone spicules and/or fat particles, loss of plasma cells during aspiration and sample preparation for FC, loss of surface expression of CD138 and CD38 because of cell processing prior to FC, and/or shedding of CD38/CD138 related to decreased cellular viability. The study by Cogbill et al. showed a mean aspirate plasma cell percent of 32.9 (±23.2%) which decreased in both the cytospin (10.9%) and by FC (8.2%) [41].

Panel selection

The antibody panel selected for analysis of plasma cell neoplasms should include both surface and cytoplasmic markers and markers which can identify clonal B-cell population, clonal plasma cell population and aberrant phenotype of both B-cells and plasma cells: CD5, CD10, CD19, CD20, CD27, CD45, CD56, CD81, CD117, CD138, CD200, surface and cytoplasmic light chain immunoglobulins (kappa and lambda), and cytoplasmic heavy chain immunoglobulins (IgG, IgM, and IgA). The phenotypic markers are described in Chapter 7.

Benign plasma cells

Plasma cells are identified by FC using CD38 and CD138 antibodies. CD38 is a relatively broadly expressed marker, present in immature CD34+ precursors, including myeloblasts, lymphoblasts, B-cell progenitors (hematogones), monocytes, NK-cells, and in subset of activated B-cells and T-cells. During B-cell maturation, CD38 expression is remarkably high in B-lineage committed precursors and gradually decreases on immature B-lymphocytes in BM to become fully negative in naïve B-cells

[42, 43]. Mature activated B-cells start expressing CD38 again, with high levels typically seen on germinal center B-cells and later further maturation to memory cells is associated with down-regulation of CD38 expression, while progression to plasma cells is associated with high level of expression. The intensity of expression of CD38 by plasma cells is much higher than that seen in all other hematopoietic cells and therefore CD38 is considered as one of the most reliable marker for the identification of plasma cells by FC [44]. CD138 is another marker with bright expression on plasma cells. Down-regulation of CD138 expression may be observed on aged sample as well as on samples exposed to heparin [45, 46].

Benign plasma cells have bright expression of CD38 and are most often positive for CD138, CD19, CD27, CD43, and CD81, dimly positive for CD45, and negative for CD20, CD22, surface immunoglobulins, CD56, CD117, CD200, and HLA-DR (Figure 14.5). Occasionally, subset of benign plasma cells may be CD56+ or CD45-. The expression of CD19 is usually heterogeneous with minor subset of plasma cells being negative (up to 30%). Similarly, small subset of benign plasma cells may be negative for CD45 and CD81, and positive for CD56 (6%–9% of plasma cells in normal BM samples are CD56+). The pattern of expression of CD19, CD45, CD56, and CD81 reflects different stages of plasma cell maturation, with major subpopulation being CD19+, CD45+, CD81+, and CD56- gradually progressing to minor CD19-/CD56-, and CD19-/CD56+ subpopulations [45, 47–51]. Schouweiler et al. showed considerable immunophenotypic heterogeneity of benign (polytypic) plasma cells with uniformly positive CD19 and CD27, uniformly negative CD117 expression, and variable expression of CD28 and CD56 (42% cases showed atypical expression of CD28 and/or CD56) [52].

Summary of the immunophenotype of benign plasma cells:

- CD19+(heterogenous expression)
- CD20-
- CD22-
- CD27+
- CD38+(bright)
- CD45+(heterogenous expression)
- CD56-/rare cells+
- CD81+

Plasma Cell Neoplasms

383

- CD117⁻
- CD138^{+(bright)}
- CD200⁻
- cytoplasmic κ and λ: polytypic pattern
- surface κ⁻ and λ⁻

Myeloma associated phenotype (MAP)

Malignant plasma cells retain the expression of CD38 and CD138, but the phenotype of myeloma plasma cells (MAP, myeloma associate phenotype) differs from that of benign plasma cells by restricted expression of either κ or λ light chain immunoglobulins and aberrant expression of CD19, CD20, CD27, CD28, CD33, CD45, CD54, CD56, CD81, CD117, and/or CD200 (Figures 14.6–14.8). Immunophenotyping by FC in most cases of PCM shows monotypic expression of cytoplasmic immunoglobulins, low (or less often variable to high) side scatter (SSC), high or variable forward scatter (FSC), negative CD45, negative CD19, negative CD27, positive CD38, and positive CD138 (see Table 14.1). Some cases may display high SSC (Figure 14.9). In contrast to benign plasma cells, neoplastic plasma cells are most often CD19⁻/CD27⁻/CD45⁻ and often display aberrant

expression of CD56, CD117, and CD200. Rare cases show positive CD19, CD20, and CD45 (Figure 14.10), positive CD10, positive CD27 (Figure 14.11), and positive CD33 (Figure 14.7). PCM with immature (plasmablastic) morphology, positive CD45, CD56, CD4, and/or CD117 may mimic both cytologically or phenotypically acute myeloid leukemia (AML) or blastic plasmacytoid dendritic cell neoplasm (BPDCN; Figure 14.12). Occasional cases may show loss of CD38 or CD138 expression (Figure 14.13). When compared to normal plasma cells, myeloma cells usually show weaker CD38 and stronger CD138 expression. Expression of CD23 (Figure 14.14) seen in 10% of PCM is associated with t(11;14) [approx. 40% of t(11;14)⁺ PCM cases are CD23⁺]. PCM composed of small cells with lymphocytic appearance are often CD20⁺, BCL1⁺, and CD45⁺ (Figure 14.14). In contrast to lymphoid cells (e.g., LPL or chronic lymphocytic leukemia), those PCM cases are CD19⁻ and HLA-DR⁻ and display often aberrant expression of CD56 and/or CD117. The expression of surface immunoglobulins is usually negative in PCM, but occasional cases display dim expression of light chains. IgG is most common heavy chain expressed by PCM, followed by IgA, no heavy chain, IgM, and IgD (Figure 14.15).

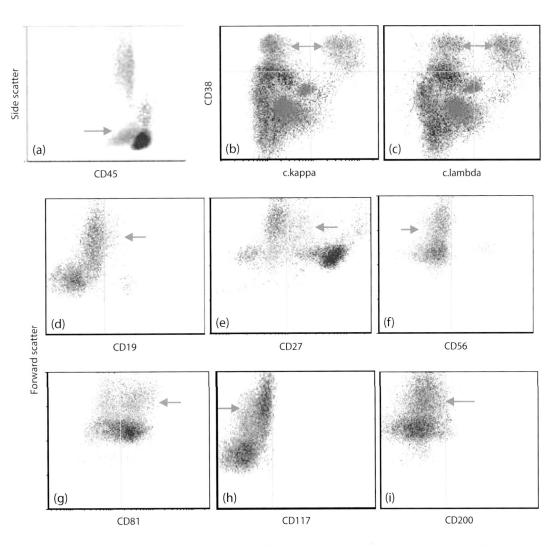

FIGURE 14.5 Benign plasma cells – flow cytometry (blood). Benign plasma cells (orange dots, arrow), are positive for CD45 (a), show polytypic expression of cytoplasmic light chain immunoglobulins (b–c), and are most often dimly CD19⁺ (d), CD27⁺ (e), CD56⁻ (f), CD81⁺ (g), CD17⁻ (h), and CD200⁻ (i).

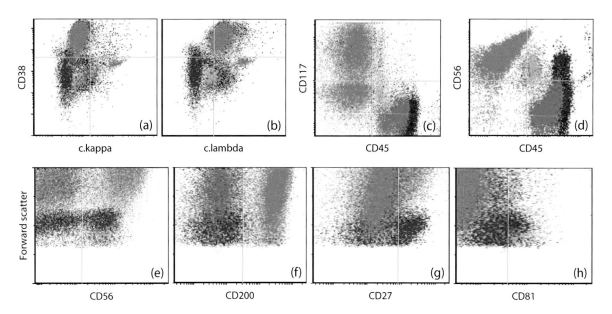

FIGURE 14.6 PCM – flow cytometry. Plasma cells (orange dots) show clonal expression of cytoplasmic lambda (a–b), bright expression of CD38 (a–b) and typical aberrant phenotype associated with plasma cell myeloma with negative CD45 (c–d), positive CD117 (d; partial expression), positive CD56 (e–f), negative CD27 (f), and negative CD81 (i).

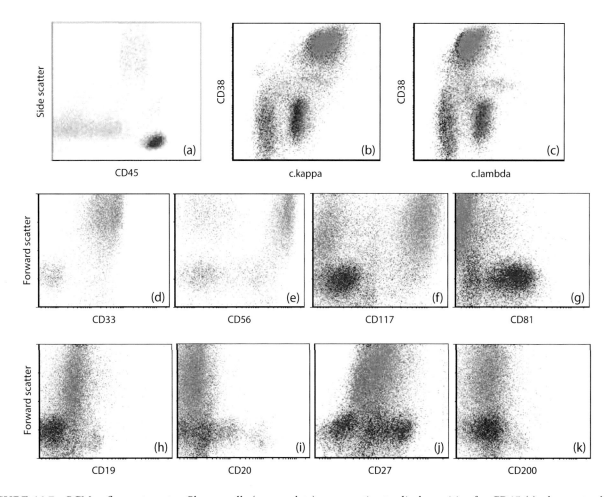

FIGURE 14.7 PCM – flow cytometry. Plasma cells (orange dots) are negative to dimly positive for CD45 (a), show cytoplasmic kappa restriction (b–c) and aberrant expression of CD33 (d), CD56 (e), and CD117 (f). The expression of CD81 (g), CD19 (h), CD20 (i), and CD27 (j) is negative (as seen in most plasma cell neoplasms). Many plasma cell myelomas display aberrant (positive) expression of CD200, but presented case is CD200⁻ (k).

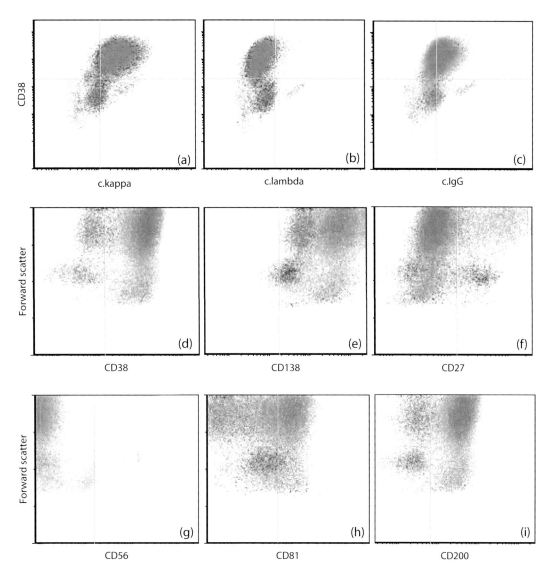

FIGURE 14.8 PCM – flow cytometry. Plasma cells (orange dots) show cytoplasmic kappa restriction (a–b), positive cytoplasmic IgG (c), bright expression of CD38 (d) and CD138 (f), negative to partially positive CD27 (f), negative CD56 (g), positive CD81 (h), and positive CD200 (i).

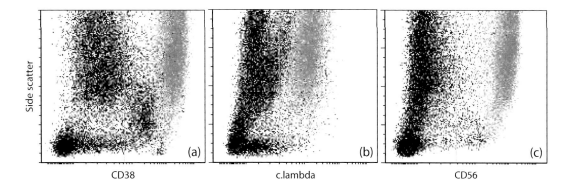

FIGURE 14.9 Plasma cell myeloma with unusual high side scatter (a–c; orange dots), bright CD38 (a), bright cytoplasmic lambda (b), and bright CD56 (c).

TABLE 14.1: Phenotypic Differences between Benign and Malignant Plasma Cells

Marker	Benign Plasma Cells	PCM
c. κ and c. λ	Polytypic Pattern	Monotypic Expression
CD10	−	−/(+)
CD13	−	−/(+)
CD19	+[v]	−/(+)
CD20	−	−/+
CD22	−	−/+
CD23	−	−/+
CD27	+[bright]	−/+[dim]
CD28	+	+/−
CD33	−	−/(+)
CD38	+[bright]	+
CD45	+[v]	−/(+)
CD56	−	+/(−)
CD81	+	+/−
CD117	−	+/−
CD138	+[bright]	+
CD200	−/(+)	+/(−)
BCL1	−	+/−
PAX5	−	−/+

Abbreviations: +, positive; + bright positive; (+), rarely positive; −, negative; (−), rarely negative; v, variable expression.

Summary of myeloma associated phenotype (MAP):

- CD19− [(97%)]
- CD20+dim [(17–30%)]
- CD27− or dim+ [(40%–68%)]
- CD33+ [(18%)]
- CD38+dim [(80%)]
- CD45− [(73–89%)]
- CD56+ [(60–86%)]
- CD81− or dim+ [(55%–86%)]
- CD117+ [(30%–60%)]
- CD200+ [(>70%)]
- CD10+ [(rare cases)]
- HLA-DR+ [(rare cases)]
- CD138− [(rare cases)]

Number of clonal plasma cells reported by FC is usually an underestimate and correlates with sample quality [53]. Cytoplasm of plasma cells is delicate and the destruction of cells during sample preparation may contribute to under-representation of plasma cells by FC. The study by Cogbill et al. showed a mean aspirate plasma cell percent of 32.9 (±23.2%) which decreased in both the cytospin (10.9%) and by FC (8.2%) [41].

Biclonal PCM and PCM with dual expression of light immunoglobulins

Minor subset of PCMs (~2%) produces more than one paraprotein, one population producing kappa and separate subset producing lambda (Figures 14.16 and 14.17). These myeloma cases are classified as biclonal PCM [54–57]. Myelomas producing two separate heavy chain immunoglobulins have also been reported. Very few PCMs may show dual expression of light chain immunoglobulins (κ and λ) in a single clonal plasma cell population positivity (Figure 14.18) [58].

PCM with expression of only light chains

About 15% of patients have light chain myeloma. In this type of myeloma, the myeloma cells secrete only light chain protein and no heavy chains [47, 59, 60].

Phenotype and maturation stage

Based on the expression of CD19 and CD81, Paiva et al. proposed dividing plasma cells into fully differentiated (CD19−/CD81−), intermediately differentiated (CD19−/CD81+), and less differentiated (CD19+/CD81+) [61]. In normal BM samples, CD19+/CD81+ plasma cells predominate over CD19−/CD81+ and CD19−/CD81− subsets. In PCM, the differentiation stage was associated with prognosis with CD19+/CD81+ PCM having poor prognosis and lower overall survival (OS) [61].

Phenotype and prognosis

Based on CD117 and CD28 expression, Mateo et al. identified three risk categories: poor risk (CD28+/CD117−), intermediate risk (CD28−/CD117− or CD117+/CD28+), and good risk (CD28−/CD117+) [62]. CD45 expression correlates with the proliferation rate of myeloma cells [63–65]. Apart from CD45 expression, proliferating myeloma cells are characterized by CD11a+/BCL2dim+ phenotype [65]. CD45+ status was recently reported as an independent predictor of inferior OS among newly diagnosed patients with PCM [66]. Based on study by Arana et al., negative impact of CD19 (when positive in ≥50% clonal plasma cells) and, particularly CD45 (when positive in ≥25% clonal plasma cells) was only significant in elderly patients [67]. In the same study, the favorable effect of CD117 expression (when positive in ≥50% of clonal plasma cells) was only significant in transplant-eligible patients treated without proteasome inhibitors and/or immune modulators [67]. CD56 is the marker expressed by majority of PCMs in the BM, and lack of CD56 expression is associated with fewer osteolytic lesions and a poorer prognosis. The patterns of expression of CD38, CD81, and CD138 were of prognostic value in all therapeutic protocols. Patients with aberrantly low expression of CD38 and/or CD138 had worse prognosis compared to patients with bright expression. Presence of ≥25% CD81+ plasma cells identified a subset of patients with inferior survival [67]. Aberrantly low expression of CD38 together with reactivity for CD81 (≥25% positive plasma cells) in the absence of homogeneous expression of CD117 (<50% positive plasma cells) identified a subset of patients that had significantly inferior progression-free survival (22 versus 35 months) and OS (43 versus 76 months) [67]. The CD38lowCD81+CD117− phenotype was related to significantly higher rates of early relapses and was identified as the most powerful combination to discriminate patients with inferior outcomes. The CD138highCD38highCD19− phenotypic profile emerged as the most powerful combination to define a subset of patients that displayed significantly superior PFS and OS, and this phenotypic profile remained significant even in MRD+ patients [67].

Targeted therapy

Daratumumab and SLAMF7 (elotuzumab) targeting CD38 and signaling lymphocytic activation molecule F7, respectively, are being tried in treatment of relapsed and refractory PCM. However, both antigens are also expressed on other normal tissues including hematopoietic lineages and immune effector cells, which may limit their long-term clinical use. B cell maturation antigen (BCMA), a transmembrane glycoprotein in the tumor necrosis factor receptor superfamily 17 (TNFRSF17), is expressed

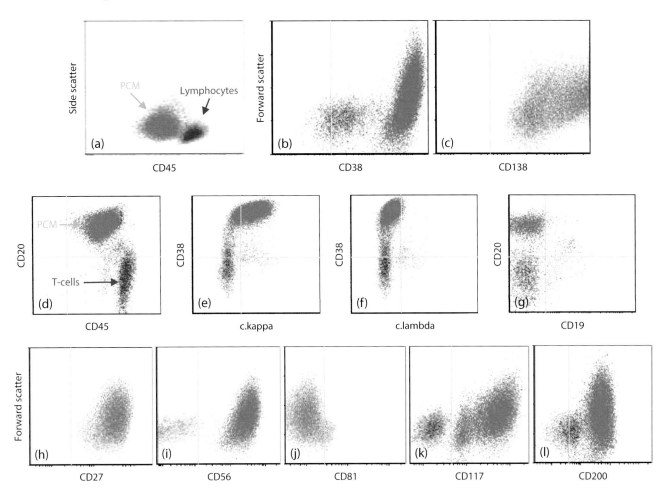

FIGURE 14.10 PCM – flow cytometry. Plasma cells (blue dots) display aberrant (positive) expression of CD45 (a), normal (bright) expression of CD38 (b) and CD138 (c), aberrant expression of CD20 (d), monotypic kappa restriction (e–f), negative CD19 (g), aberrant positivity for CD27 (h) and CD56 (i), lack of CD81 (j), and positive expression of CD117 (k) and CD200 (l).

at significantly higher levels in PCM but not on other normal tissues (except normal plasma cells), and anti-BCMA antibody-drug conjugate showed clinical responses in patients who failed at least three prior lines of therapy, including an anti-CD38 antibody, a proteasome inhibitor, and an immunomodulatory agent. In addition, BCMA is an antigen targeted by chimeric antigen receptor (CAR) T-cells, which have already shown significant clinical activities in patients with refractory PCMs who have undergone at least three prior treatments, including a proteasome inhibitor and an immunomodulatory agent.

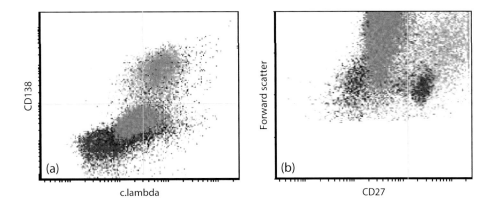

FIGURE 14.11 PCM with unusual CD27 expression. Plasma cells (orange dots) are monotypic (lambda⁺; a) and show positive CD27 expression (b).

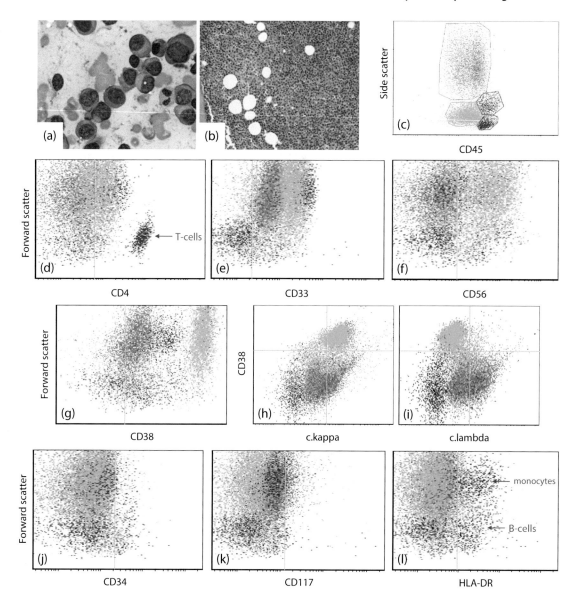

FIGURE 14.12 Plasma cell myeloma with immature (plasmablastic) cytomorphology. Blastic morphology (a, BM aspirate smear; b, BM core biopsy) in conjunction with positive CD45 (c), CD4 (d, dim), CD33 (e), and CD56 (f) mimic acute myeloid leukemia or blastic plasmacytoid dendritic cell neoplasm (BPDCN). Bright expression of CD38 (g), monotypic expression of cytoplasmic light chain immunoglobulins (h–i), and lack of CD34 (j), CD117 (k) and HLA-DR (k) helps to exclude both AML and BPDCN and establish the diagnosis of PCM.

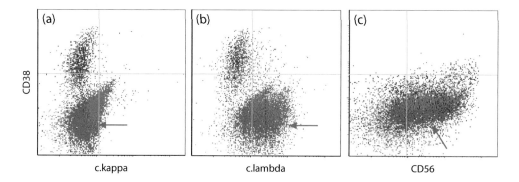

FIGURE 14.13 Plasma cell myeloma with aberrant lack of CD38 expression (a–c; arrow), lambda restriction (b) and positive CD56 (c). Activated T-cells and NK-cells are CD38+ (a–b; red dots).

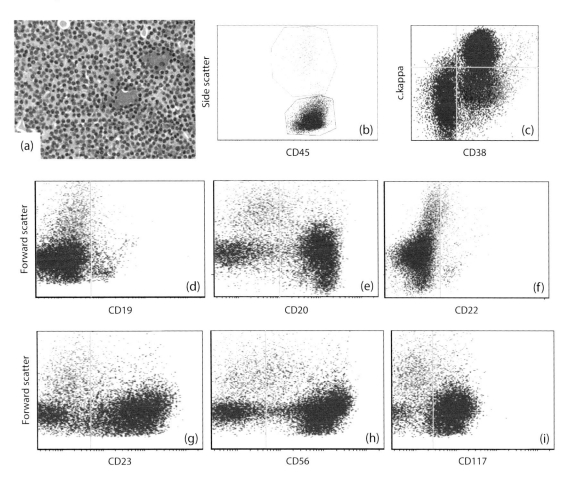

FIGURE 14.14 PCM – FC analysis. This "lymphocytic" variant of PCM (a) shows bright CD45 expression (b), bright CD38 (c) and cytoplasmic kappa expression (c), negative CD19 (d), positive CD20 (e), negative CD22 (f) and positive CD23 (g), CD56 (h), and CD117 (i).

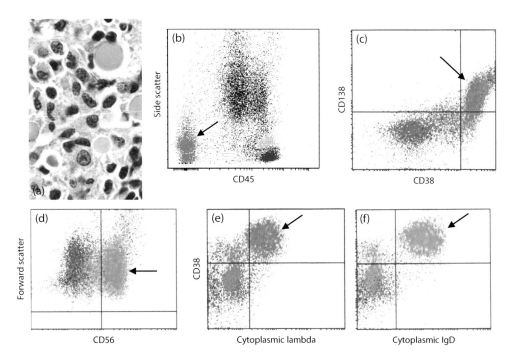

FIGURE 14.15 Plasma cell myeloma – flow cytometry. Plasma cells (histology section of the bone marrow, a) are negative for CD45 (b), positive for CD38/CD138 (c) and CD56 (d) and show clonal expression of lambda and IgD (e–f).

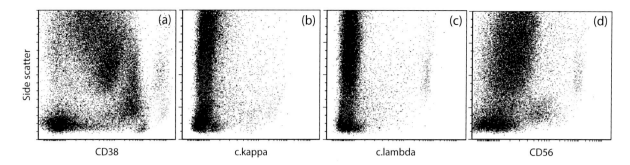

FIGURE 14.16 Biclonal plasma cell myeloma. Both kappa⁺ (orange dots) and lambda⁺ (purple dots) populations are CD38⁺ (a). Monoclonal kappa⁺ plasma (b) have low side scatter and negative to dim CD56 (d), whereas monoclonal lambda⁺ plasma cells (c) have high scatter and bright CD56 expression (d).

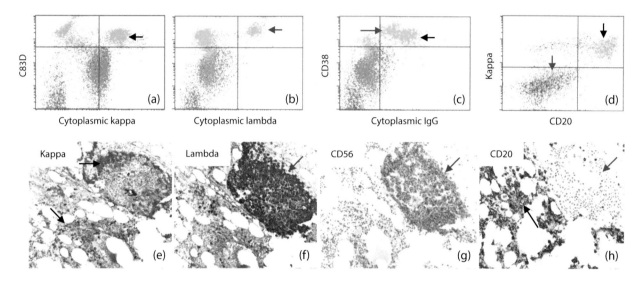

FIGURE 14.17 Biclonal plasma cell myeloma. Flow cytometry shows two population of neoplastic IgG⁺ plasma cells: larger population express cytoplasmic kappa (a; black arrow) and smaller population express cytoplasmic lambda (b; red arrow). Both population show bright expression of CD38, but careful evaluation reveals that kappa⁺ population has slightly dimmer CD38 when compared to lambda⁺ cells (compare a and b). The difference in the intensity of CD38 expression is more evident on panel c showing expression of cytoplasmic IgG versus CD38: kappa⁺ cells (black arrow) and lambda⁺ cells (red arrow) express IgG (there was no expression of other heavy chain immunoglobulins). Kappa⁺ cells are positive for CD20 (d). Bone marrow core biopsy (e–h) confirmed flow cytometry findings: two plasma cell populations are evident. Kappa⁺ cells are occur individually and in small clusters (black arrows), whereas lambda⁺ cells form large aggregate (red arrow). Lambda⁺ population has strong expression of CD56 (g) and is CD20⁻ (h).

IgM⁺ PCM

True IgM myeloma is rare (<0.5% of all myeloma patients). IgM⁺ PCMs express CD38, CD138, MUM1, and IgM without evidence of a definable B-cell component either by morphology or immunophenotyping (rare B-cells may be present by they are polyclonal by FC). IgM PCMs are usually negative for CD20, CD56, and CD117, and may show aberrant expression of CD19, CD45, and PAX5 [68]. The t(11;14) translocations (associated with positive expression of cyclin D1) are identified in majority of cases [68, 69]. IgM⁺ myeloma may be associated with an inferior outcome compared with IgG/IgA cases.

Measurable (minimal) residual disease (MRD)

MRD can be identified by FC analysis, DNA sequencing assay (next generation sequencing, NGS) or allele-specific oligonucleotide quantitative PCR (ASOqPCR) on BM aspirates [70–78].

Despite the use of highly effective drug combinations, next generation MRD techniques have recently demonstrated that great fraction of the patients still remains MRD⁺ after treatment [70, 76, 79]. The detection of MRD by FC is recognized as a sensitive and rapid approach to evaluate treatment efficacy that predicts progression-free (PFS) and OS [45, 53, 70, 80–85]. The achievement of complete response (CR) after high-dose therapy/autologous stem cell transplantation (HDT/ASCT) is a surrogate for prolonged survival in PCM; however, patients who lose their CR status within 1 year of HDT/ASCT (unsustained CR) have poor prognosis. Thus, the identification of these patients is highly relevant [86].

The sensitivity of conventional 4-6-color FC MRD (<10⁻⁴) remains lower than that of ASOqPCR and NGS (<10⁻⁴–10⁻⁶). More recent studies have shown that 8-color or 10-color FC assays have an increased sensitivity (limit of detection; LOD) between <10⁻⁴ and <10⁻⁵, leading to a significantly improved prediction of outcome [78, 87, 88]. The EuroFlow consortium

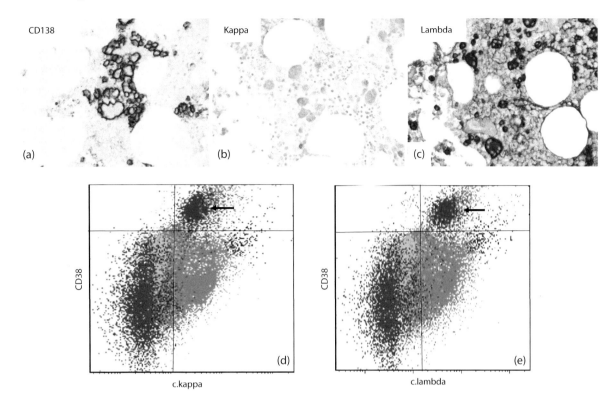

FIGURE 14.18 PCM with unusual co-expression of kappa and lambda. (a–c) Immunohistochemistry. (d–e) FC analysis. Highly atypical plasma cells (including multinucleated giant plasma cells) are strongly positive for CD138 (a) and positive for kappa (b, d) and lambda (c, e). This unusual co-expression of kappa and lambda was confirmed by electrophoresis analysis of serum and urine.

developed next generation flow cytometry (NGFC) assay, which consists of two standardized FC tubes with eight antibodies each including 8-color surface antibody only tube and 8-color mixed surface and cytoplasmic antibody tube [70], while investigators from Memorial Sloan Kettering Cancer Center developed a single tube, 10-color method with results comparable to EuroFlow [89]. It is well known that the immunophenotype of blasts in AML may change between the diagnosis and relapse due to subclonal selection/evolution, which has important consequences for MRD detection [90]. In PCM, the shift in antigen expression during MRD assessment takes place in a small subset of patients (17%) and mostly involves CD81 [67]. Analysis of MRD in PCM by FC relies on the identification of MAP (see above). In FC analysis of MRD in PCM by Flores-Montero et al. (EuroFlow protocol), eight markers which contributed most frequently to discriminate between benign and neoplastic plasma cells included: CD19 (97% of cases), CD45 (89%); CD56 (86%); CD81 (86%), c.λ (73%); CD27 (71%); CD117 (60%); and c.κ (56%) [70].

National Comprehensive Cancer Network (NCCN) and EuroNet guidelines for MRD analysis in PCM (www.nccn.org; [45, 70, 87, 89]):

- No single marker alone can distinguish normal (reactive) plasma cells from neoplastic cells.
- Intracellular (cytoplasmic; c.) light chain evaluation does not provide additional information in >97% of patients and therefore it is not necessary to use c.κ and c.λ in routine MRD panels. However, c.κ and c.λ light chain staining may be helpful to clarify atypical findings in some cases and therefore a separate tube with light chain immunoglobulin

may be appropriate in MRD analysis. The c.κ:c.λ ratio must be interpreted with caution since a skewed c.κ:c.λ ratio does not necessarily indicate residual disease.

- If laboratory chooses to construct their own panel, the panel must contain CD19, CD38, CD138, and CD45 in each tube and CD27, CD56, CD81, and CD117 must be included.
- There is no need for isotype control, because in an adequate BM specimen there are suitable internal positive and negative control for all markers: mature and precursor B-cells can be used as positive control for CD19, CD45, CD38, CD27, and CD81; myeloid precursors and mast cells can be used as control for CD117, and NK-cells can be used as control for CD56. Nucleated red blood cells can be distinguished for plasma cells by being negative for CD19, CD38, CD138, CD81, CD56, and CD81.
- By using a consensus panel at diagnosis and during follow-up, neoplastic plasma cells from virtually every PCM could be identified as being phenotypically aberrant.
- The FC panel should provide information about sample viability and quality (to confirm that events represent BM and sample is not hemodiluted). Nevertheless, in hypocellular and/or hemodiluted samples, analysis of a high number of PC is often difficult; in such cases, following recently consensus recommendations by the European Myeloma Network information about a minimum of 100 neoplastic PC should be acquired. In parallel, the quality of the BM aspirate can be assessed according to the presence of nucleated red blood cells (CD45-), and mast cells (CD117+bright) and the absence of any of this cell populations could indicate a nonrepresentative BM (e.g., highly

contaminated with PB). This procedure (double-step acquisition), together with the usage of additional multiple staining provides the basis for the accurate immunophenotypic characterization of PC and subsequent discrimination between phenotypically aberrant (clonal) and normal/reactive (polyclonal) PC.

- FC panel for myeloma and MRD should be able to identify presence of significant population of mast cells (bright CD117, high SSC), hematogones (bright CD38, positive CD19, dim to moderate CD45, low FSC), myeloblasts (CD117+ and moderate CD45 expression), and/or assessment of neutrophilic maturation (CD45 versus SSC).
- BM sample must be insulated against excessive temperature changes during shipment and storage. Shipment at room temperature (RT) has been validated as acceptable.
- Specimens should be labeled with date and time of collection and processed as soon as possible. 48-hours cut-off for specimen age is acceptable, however samples should not be rejected if they exceeded 48-hours in cases of irreplaceable sample.
- Sample with <85% viability should be reported with a statement indicating that the viability is suboptimal for testing.
- Consensus group support pre-lysis protocol: the entire sample can be gently pre-lysed by incubating with 155 nM ammonium chloride, 10 nM potassium bicarbonate and 0.2 nM EDTA for 10 min at RT at a ratio of 1:9 (volume of sample: volume of lysing solution). Ficoll Hypaque enrichment must never be used.
- Absolute minimum for MRD is 500,000 cells. Higher number of events is mandatory for best practice, and it is therefore recommended to acquire 2 million total cells. If less than 2 million total cells are collected and there is no MRD identified, report should state that number of events collected was less than recommended (<2 million).
- 8- or 10-color FC approach measuring a total of 10 antigens is recommended *The FC by EuroFlow is an eight-color two tube approach, which has been extensively validated. The two-tube approach improves reliability, consistency, and sensitivity because of the acquisition of a greater number of cells. The eight-color technology is widely available globally and NGFC method has already been adopted in many flow laboratories worldwide.*
- Use of lyophilized mixture of antibodies is preferable as it reduces time, errors and costs.
- Sensitivity of detection is 1 plasma cell in 10^5 nucleated cells or higher.
- EDTA tubes are recommended as heparin may interfere with the expression of certain markers (especially CD138).
- Gating should be based on combined CD45, CD38, CD138, FSC, and SSC parameters, and those markers should be present in each tube.
- CD38 is a bright marker and should be combined with less intense fluorochrome (e.g., FITC) to avoid compensation problems with more sensitive fluorochromes such as BV421, PE, PECy7, or APC.
- CD138 is dim markers and should be combined with more sensitive fluorochromes of intermediate or bright intensity (HV450, BV421, APC, or PE).

In recent studies, suboptimal CD138-PacO reagent was replaced by CD138-BV421; suboptimal CD81-APC H7 by CD81-APC C750, suboptimal CD27-PerCP Cy5.5 by CD27-BV510, suboptimal

CD45-PacB by CD45-PerCPCy5.5 and suboptimal c.λ-APC H7 by c. λ-APC C750 [70].

- 3rd tube may be used to assess viability: Fixable Live Dead reagent, CD38, CD138, and CD45.
- If MRD panel is also used for regular analysis for PCMs, 4th tube will be needed to exclude B-cell lymphoma: CD20, surface κ (s. κ), surface λ (s. λ), CD19, CD3, CD45, CD38, and CD138. Alternatively, 8-color two tube panels may be replaced with 10-color two tube panels, which will include CD20, s.κ, and s.λ in addition to plasma cell markers.
- Overall, bulk-lysis procedures are associated with acquisition of a significantly greater number of cells versus the conventional BD FACS Lysing Solution. However, all bulk-lysis conditions but that using low bovine serum albumin (0.5% bovine serum albumin) and FACS-lysing-fixation step showed a significantly higher proportion of debris and dead cells versus FACS-lyse protocols. Therefore, the bulk-lysis procedure including a FACS-lysing-fixation step and 0.5% bovine serum albumin is recommended as the reference SOP [70].
- Abnormal plasma cell population is identified by aberrant phenotype (with/without specific software for automatic abnormal plasma cells identification) [70, 85]. The immunophenotypic markers include: CD38, CD138, CD19, CD45, CD56, CD81, c.κ, c.λ, CD27, and CD117.

Response criteria for PCM by NCCN guidelines:

- Relapse from CR (to be used only if the endpoint is disease-free survival) [any one or more of the following]:
  - reappearance of serum or urine M-protein by immunofixation or electrophoresis
  - development of ≥5% plasma cells in the BM
  - appearance of any other sign of progression (i.e., new plasmacytoma, lytic bone lesion, or hypercalcemia)
- Relapse from MRD negative (to be used only if the endpoint is disease-free survival) [one or more of the following criteria]:
  - loss of MRD negative state (evidence of clonal plasma cells on FC or NGS (next generation sequencing), or positive imaging study for recurrence of myeloma)
  - reappearance of serum or urine M-protein by immunofixation or electrophoresis
  - development of >5% clonal plasma cells in BM
  - appearance of any other sign of progression (i.e., new plasmacytoma, lytic bone lesion or hypercalcemia)
- Flow MRD-negative:
  - Absence of phenotypically aberrant clonal plasma cells by FC on BM aspirates using EuroFlow standard operation procedure for MRD detection in multiple myeloma (or validated equivalent method) with a minimum sensitivity of 1 plasma cell in 10^5 nucleated cells or higher [86, 91]

Differential diagnosis of PCM

Immunophenotypic differential diagnosis of PCM includes:

- Reactive plasmacytosis
- Heavy chain diseases (HCDs)
- Bright CD38+ tumors

- B-cell lymphomas, subset (usually of high grade)
- T-cell lymphomas, subset
- AML, subset
- Acute lymphoblastic leukemia (ALL), subset
- CD45⁻ tumors
  - B-cell acute lymphoblastic leukemia (B-ALL)
  - Metastatic carcinoma, rhabdomyosarcoma or melanoma
  - AML, rare cases
  - ALK⁺ large B-cell lymphoma (ALK⁺ LBCL)
  - Plasmablastic lymphoma (PBL)
  - Acute erythroid leukemia (AEL)
  - T-cell prolymphocytic leukemia (T-PLL), subset
  - Diffuse large B-cell lymphoma (DLBCL), rare cases
  - Anaplastic large cell lymphoma (ALCL) rare cases
- CD56⁺ tumors
  - AML, especially with monocytic differentiation
  - BPDCN
  - Peripheral T-cell lymphomas (PTCLs), subset
  - DLBCL (especially extranodal), rare cases
  - Extranodal T/NK-cell lymphoma, nasal type (ENKTL)
  - Monomorphic epitheliotropic intestinal T-cell lymphoma (MEITL)
  - Enteropathy-associated T-cell lymphoma (EATL), subset
  - Hepatosplenic T-cell lymphoma (HSTL)
  - Primary cutaneous gamma delta T-cell lymphoma (PCGD-TCL)
  - Small cell carcinoma and melanoma
- CD33⁺ tumors
  - AML
  - Myeloid neoplasms
- CD117⁺ tumors
  - AML
  - AEL
  - Systemic mastocytosis (SM)
  - Non-hematopoietic tumors (carcinoma, gastrointestinal stromal tumor [GIST], melanoma)
- BCL1⁺ tumors
  - Mantle cell lymphoma (MCL)
- Castleman's disease
- IgG4 disease
- MGUS
- Lymphoplasmacytic lymphoma/Waldenström macroglobulinemia (LPL/WM)
- Marginal zone lymphoma (MZL) and other B-cell lymphomas with extensive plasmacytic differentiation

Morphologic (cytologic) differential diagnosis of PCM includes (Figure 14.19):

- Metastatic carcinoma
- AML
- AEL
- B-cell lymphomas with plasmablastic morphology (PBL, primary effusion lymphoma, ALK⁺ large B-cell lymphoma)
- BPDCN

Benign plasma cells. The phenotypic differences between neoplastic and benign plasma cells are discussed in the flow cytometry section (above).

Heavy chain diseases. Heavy chain disease (HCD) is a family of rare, systemic syndromes defined as a neoplasm of lymphocytes, plasmacytoid lymphocytes, and plasma cells characterized by the production of an abnormally truncated heavy chain protein that lacks associated light chains [10, 92, 93]. Pathological diagnosis of underlying diseases includes B-cell lymphoma, chronic lymphocytic leukemia, plasmacytoma, and plasma cell proliferative disorder. There are three types of HCD, defined by the class of immunoglobulin heavy chain produced: IgA (α-HCD), IgG (γ-HCD), and IgM (μ-HCD). Alpha-HCD is the most common and usually occurs as intestinal malabsorption in a young adult from a country of the Mediterranean area. Gamma HCD, also called Franklin disease, has a heterogeneous clinical and pathologic presentation with three patterns: (1) generalized lymphoma, (2) lymphoma limited to the BM (referred to in the literature as localized medullary disease), or (3) with localized extranodal disease.

CD45⁻ tumors. Lack of CD45 expression is not specific for PCM. Among hematopoietic tumors, CD45 is negative and subset of acute B-ALL, occasional cases of AML (including acute monoblastic leukemia), ALK⁺ large B-cell lymphoma (ALK⁺ LBCL), PBL, AEL, subset of T-PLL and rare cases of DLBCL and ALCL. Non-hematopoiesis tumors, such as carcinoma, melanoma, or rhabdomyosarcoma are CD45 and may show positive expression of CD56 and/or CD117. Figure 14.20 shows B-ALL with negative CD45, partial (dim) expression of CD56 and positive CD38 mimicking PCM. B-ALL differs from PCM by co-expression of CD19, CD10, CD34, and/or TdT and lack of expression of light and heavy chain immunoglobulins.

CD38⁺ tumors. CD38 is a transmembrane glycoprotein with a widespread cellular expression and functional activity. The CD38 expression is high in B-cell precursors and in terminally differentiated plasma cells, but low to absent in mature B-cells, where it can be induced by activatory signals. CD38 is often positive (dim to moderate) in AML. Among mature neoplasms, CD38 is often positive in MCL and may be positive in subset of chronic lymphocytic leukemia (CLL), follicular lymphoma (FL) and often in other B- and T-cell lymphoproliferations, especially of high grade (Burkitt lymphoma, high grade B-cell lymphoma, ALCL). CD38 is positive in subset of hairy cell leukemia (HCL).

CD56⁺ tumors. CD56 expression is noted in tumors of NK-cell lineage, and in many hematopoietic and non-hematopoietic tumors, including AML, especially with monocytic differentiation, BPDCN, subset of PTCLs, and rare cases of DLBCL (especially extranodal). Among extranodal T-cell lymphomas, CD56 is positive in ENKTL, MEITL, subset of EATL, HSTL, and PCGD-TCL. Small cell carcinoma and melanoma are also often CD56⁺.

CD33⁺ tumors. Rare PCM, usually less differentiated express CD33, which in conjunction with often positive CD117 prompt differential diagnosis of AML and other myeloid neoplasms. Lack of CD45, HLA-DR, and CD34 in conjunction with bright CD38 and presence of cytoplasmic light chain immunoglobulin restriction and cytomorphology helps to diagnose PCM.

BCL1⁺ tumors. BCL1 (cyclin D1) is expressed by MCL, HCL, and subset of PCM. In HCL, there is no *CCND1* rearrangement. Occasional cases of SLL/CLL may show BCL1 expression by prominent proliferation centers (not associated with *CCND1* rearrangement).

CD117⁺ tumors. CD117 (c-kit gene product) is positive in the majority of AMLs, subset of carcinomas and malignant melanomas, mast cell disease, AEL, and GISTs.

Monoclonal gammopathy of undetermined significance (MGUS). MGUS differs from PCM by serum monoclonal protein level <30 g/L, clonal BM plasma cells <10%, and absence of end-organ damage such as hypercalcemia, renal insufficiency, anemia, and bone lesions.

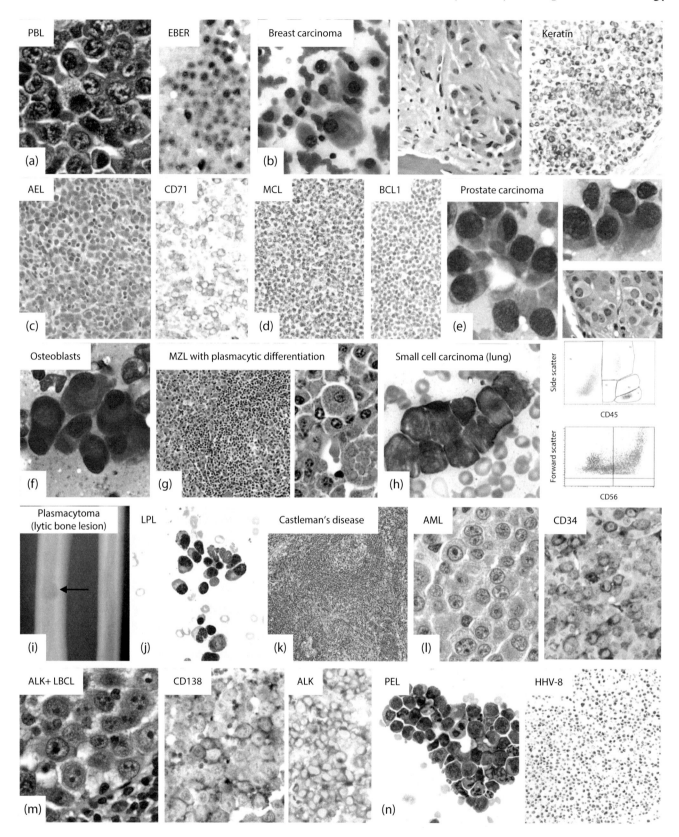

FIGURE 14.19 PCM – differential diagnosis. (a) Plasmablastic lymphoma (PBL). (b) Metastatic breast carcinoma (bone marrow aspirate smear, histology, and immunostaining for cytokeratin). (c) Acute erythroid leukemia (AEL). (d) Mantle cell lymphoma (MCL). (e) Metastatic adenocarcinoma (prostate). (f) Osteoblasts. (g) MZL with extensive plasmacytic differentiation. (h) Metastatic small cell carcinoma. (i) Solitary plasmacytoma. (j) Lymphoplasmacytic lymphoma (LPL). (k) Castleman's disease (plasma cell type). (l) AML. (m) Large B-cell lymphoma with ALK expression. (n) Primary effusion lymphoma (PEL).

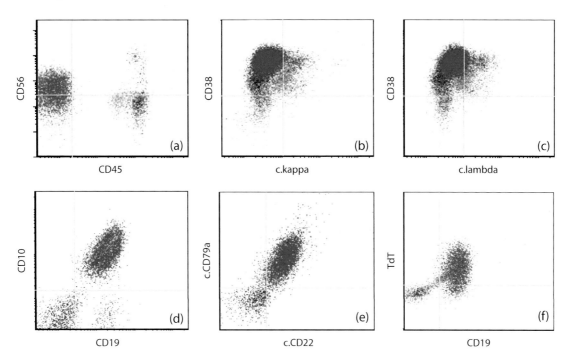

FIGURE 14.20 B-ALL with negative CD45 and partial expression of CD56. B-lymphoblasts (blue dots) show negative CD45 (a) and dim CD56 (a), mimicking PCM. Lack of cytoplasmic light chain immunoglobulin expression (b–c), and co-expression of CD19 (d), CD10 (d), cytoplasmic CD22 and CD79a (e), and TdT (f) confirms the diagnosis of B-ALL.

Lymphoplasmacytic lymphoma/Waldenström macroglobulinemia (LPL/WM). The distinction between IgM⁺ PCM, IgM⁺ MGUS, smoldering (indolent) WM, and LPL/WM is based on cytologic features, immunophenotype, cytogenetics/FISH, clinical features, and radiologic imaging findings. PCM is characterized by pure plasma cell infiltrate (without admixture of small lymphocytes or plasmacytoid lymphocytes) and typical radiologic findings (e.g., lytic bone lesions). In some cases of LPL/WM, especially after treatment, plasma cells can predominate, thus raising the differential diagnosis with PCM. Morphologically, plasma cells in WM show a low histological grade, are small and mature, often with intranuclear inclusions and gradual transition from small lymphocytes into plasma cells. The latter may have a "flame cell" appearance often associated with the IgA isotype. In PCMs, plasma cells show a spectrum of histologic grades, from small mature to large and pleomorphic with distinct nucleoli (plasmablastic features). Plasma cells in LPL/WM and PCM differ immunophenotypically. Plasma cells in LPL/WM have some immunophenotypic overlap with B-cells, often being positive for CD19 and CD45, as well as CD27 (50%) and CD81, but negative for CD56 and CD117. In contrast, PCMs are most often negative for CD19, CD45, CD27, and CD81, show aberrant expression of CD56 and/or CD117 and positive CD200. *MYD88* mutation is positive in LPL/WM but negative in PCM. Rare cases of concurrent PCM and LPL/WM have been reported.

B-cell lymphomas with plasmacytic differentiation. Malignant lymphomas with extensive plasmacytic differentiation may be indistinguishable morphologically from plasma cell neoplasms, especially when plasma cells predominate (e.g., after treatment which eliminated the B-cell component or in limited biopsy specimens which reflects plasma cell-rich areas). LPL and other types of B-cell lymphomas, especially marginal zone B-cell lymphoma can be differentiated from plasma cell neoplasms by

demonstration of a clonal B-cell component with monotypic expression of the same light chain immunoglobulin. Marginal zone B-cell lymphoma differs by clinical presentation and lack of a significant serum M-protein. Occasional cases of MZLs may be difficult to distinguish from extraosseous plasmacytoma.

Differential diagnosis of IgM⁺ PCM:

- LPL/WM
- IgM⁺ MGUS

IgM⁺ PCM. IgM⁺ PCM needs to be differentiated from LPL/WM and IgM MGUS. IgM⁺ MGUS is defined by a serum paraprotein concentration <3 g/dL, BM lymphoplasmacytic infiltration <10% and lack of anemia, constitutional symptoms, hyperviscosity, lymphadenopathy, or hepatosplenomegaly [16, 94–97]. IgM⁺ MGUS is regarded as precursor lesion that carries a risk of progression at 1% per year to either WM, AL amyloidosis, or rarely IgM PCM. More than 50% of IgM⁺ MGUS cases have *MYD88* mutation. Distinguishing IgM⁺ MGUS from WM is mainly based on the degree of BM involvement and the clinical presentation. IgM⁺ PCM is characterized by pure plasma cell infiltrate (without admixture of small lymphocytes or plasmacytoid lymphocytes) and typical radiologic findings (e.g., lytic bone lesions). In some cases of LPL/WM, especially after treatment, plasma cells can predominate, thus raising the differential diagnosis with PCM. Morphologically, plasma cells in WM show a low histological grade, are small and mature. In PCMs, plasma cells show a spectrum of histologic grades, from small mature to large and pleomorphic with distinct nucleoli (plasmablastic features). Plasma cells in LPL/WM and PCM differ immunophenotypically. Plasma cells in LPL/WM have some immunophenotypic overlap with B-cells, often being positive for CD19 and CD45, as well as CD27 (50%) and CD81, but negative for CD56 and CD117. In contrast,

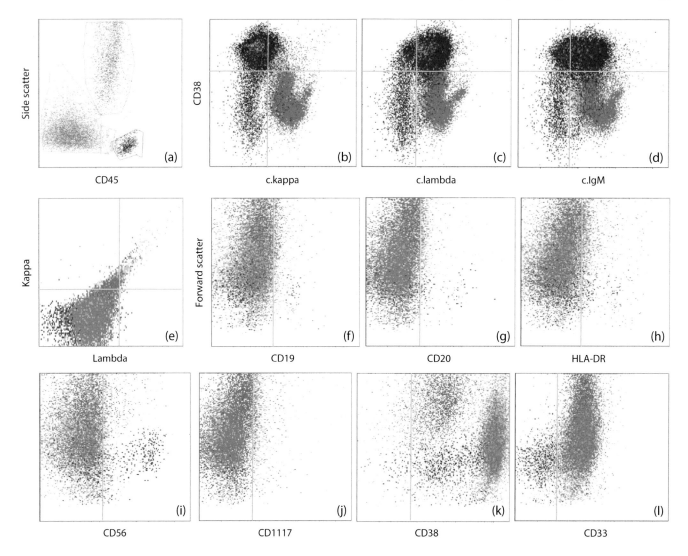

FIGURE 14.21 IgM⁺ PCM. Neoplastic plasma cells (orange dots represent FC analysis with surface antibodies and brown dots represent FC with cytoplasmic antibodies) show lack of CD45 (a), monotypic expression of cytoplasmic lambda (b–c), positive cytoplasmic IgM (d), negative expression of surface light chain immunoglobulins (e), CD19 (f), CD20 (g), HLA-DR (h), CD56 (i), CD117 (j), bright CD38 (k), and aberrant positivity for CD33 (l). Lack of CD45, CD19, CD20, HLA-DR, and surface light chain immunoglobulins excludes B-cell lymphoma.

PCMs are most often negative for CD19, CD45, CD27, and CD81, show aberrant phenotype (e.g., aberrant expression of CD33, CD56, and/or CD117) and positive CD200. *MYD88* mutation is positive in LPL/WM but negative in PCM. Rare cases of concurrent PCM and LPL/WM have been reported. Figure 14.21 presents IgM⁺ PCM with aberrant expression of CD33.

Plasmacytoma

Plasmacytoma is a localized collection of monoclonal plasma cells without the evidence of systemic plasma cell neoplasm. Plasmacytoma may be localized in the bone (solitary bone plasmacytoma) or in soft tissues, such as upper aerodigestive tract, skin, salivary gland, or thyroid (Figure 14.22). In a series of 116 patients with SBP reported by Dingli et al., the median age at diagnosis was 60 years (range, 26–93) with male predominance (70%) and M protein was detected in 64% (median 5 g/L; range, 0–30 g/L) [98]. The common presentation of SBP is in the axial

skeleton, whereas the extramedullary plasmacytoma is usually seen in the head and neck.

Monoclonal gammopathy of undetermined significance

MGUS is defined by the presence of a monoclonal protein in serum (<30 g/L), BM plasma cells <10% without lytic bone lesions and myeloma-related organ (tissue) damage (anemia, hypercalcemia, bone lesions, or renal failure), and absence of B-cell lymphoproliferations (e.g. Waldenström macroglobulinemia, B-CLL, primary amyloidosis, plasmacytoma) [3, 5, 7, 99–103]. Asymptomatic myeloma is defined by M-protein in serum >30 g/L and/or BM clonal plasma cells >10% without myeloma-related organ or tissue impairment (including bone lesions or symptoms).

The IgM MGUS is defined as serum IgM <30 g/L, BM lymphoplasmacytic infiltrate <10% and no evidence of anemia, constitutional symptoms, hyperviscosity, lymphadenopathy, or

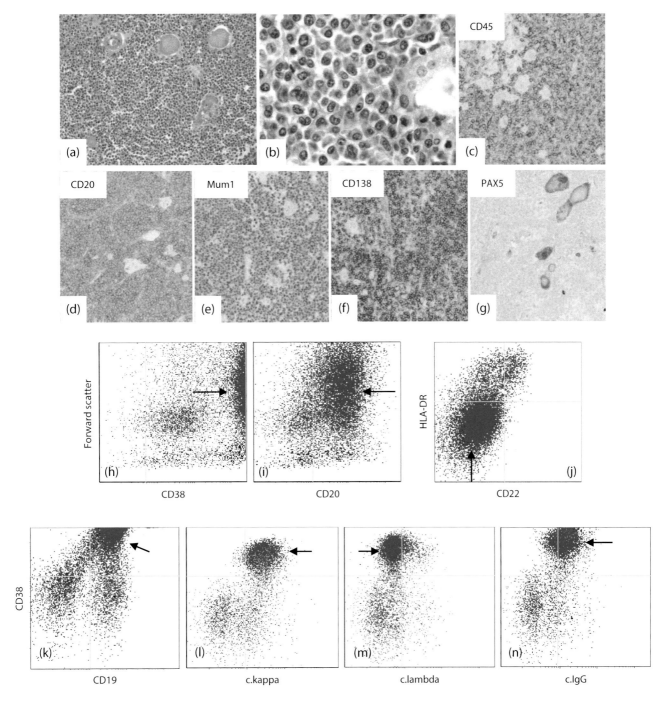

FIGURE 14.22 Plasmacytoma of the thyroid. Histologic section shows prominent atypical plasma cell infiltrate (a–b), which by immunohistochemistry are positive for CD45 (c), CD20 (d), MUM1 (e), and CD138 (f), and do not express PAX5 (g). Flow cytometry analysis (h–n) showed plasma cells (arrow) with bright CD38 expression (h), positive CD20 (i) negative CD22 (j) and HLA-DR (j), positive CD38 (k–n), positive CD19 (k), cytoplasmic kappa restriction (l–m), positive IgG (n), surface markers (h–k), and cytoplasmic markers (l–n).

hepatosplenomegaly [3, 5, 7]. The prevalence of MGUS is ~5% among persons 70 years of age or older and 7.5% among those 85 years of age or older [104]. Based on the international criteria, patients with MGUS have serum monoclonal protein level <30 g/L, <10% plasma cells in BM and no clinical manifestation related to monoclonal gammopathy [8, 105]. Majority of patients (70%) have the level of protein <10 g/L. In the Mayo

clinic series, IgG was the most common immunoglobulin (69%), followed by IgM (17%), and IgA (11%), and the concentration of monoclonal immunoglobulin was less than 10 g/L in 63.5% and at least 20 g/L in only 4.5% [104]. The POEMS syndrome (poly-neuropathy, organomegaly, endocrinopathy, serum monoclonal protein, and skin changes) has median survival of 165 months, independent of the number of syndrome features, bone lesions, or plasma cells at diagnosis [13]. Additional features of the syndrome often develop, but the complications of classic PCM are rare.

Diagnostic criteria for MGUS

- Serum monoclonal protein <30 g/L
- Clonal BM plasma cells <10%
- Absence of end-organ damage such as hypercalcemia, renal insufficiency, anemia, and bone lesions

Diagnostic criteria for IgM MGUS

- Serum IgM monoclonal protein <30 g/L
- Clonal BM lymphoplasmacytic infiltrate <10%
- Absence of end-organ damage such as hypercalcemia, renal insufficiency, anemia, and bone lesions

Prognosis

MGUS is a premalignant plasma-cell proliferative disorder with the median survival rate only slightly shorter than that of a comparable US population associated life-long risk of progression to multiple myeloma, WM, and primary amyloidosis [106]. Risk of progression of MGUS to plasma cell malignancy is indefinite and persists even after more than 30 years of follow-up, with no reliable predictors of malignant evolution [107]. Majority of patients with myeloma evolve from MGUS, but in many patients this premalignant stage is not recognized clinically [3, 5, 7, 40]. In subset of patients, an intermediate stage between MGUS and myeloma is called smoldering PCM.

Progression

Patients with MGUS of IgM class progress to LPL/WM, B-CLL, and other lymphomas, whereas patients with IgG or IgA MGUS progress to PCM, plasmacytoma, or primary amyloidosis. The cumulative risk of progression to myeloma or other lymphoproliferative disorders is 10% at 10 years, 21% at 20 years, and 26% at 25 years. The overall risk of progression is 1% per year and the risk remains even after 25 years. The majority of patients with MGUS die from causes other than transformation [103]. Long term follow-up of (241) patients with MGUS revealed progression to multiple myeloma or related disorders in 27% of patients; 6% patients were alive without evidence of the disease, and the remaining patients died without evidence of multiple myeloma or a related disorder [108]. The average risk of progression of patients with an IgM MGUS is 1.5% per year [109]. The risk of progression at 10 years ranges from 12% to 17% and at 20 years from 25% to 34% [6, 39, 100, 108, 110]. The percentage of neoplastic plasma cells within the all BM plasma cell compartment ≥95% is associated with higher risk of progression from MGUS to PCM [111].

Immunophenotype

FC often shows two populations of plasma cells, one polyclonal with normal immunophenotype (CD38$^{bright+}$, CD19$^+$, CD56$^-$) and second monoclonal population with an aberrant phenotype, most often CD19$^-$/CD56$^+$ or CD19$^-$/CD56$^-$. The monoclonal population may exhibit weaker expression of CD38 and other aberrant antigen expression (negative to weak CD45, CD117 expression, lack of CD138, positive CD20). Jerez et al. showed that an increased ratio of abnormal to normal plasma cells in BM as the main independent prognostic variable in patients with MGUS: values of 4 or higher defined a group at high risk of progression and values of 0.20 or lower were associated with immune disorders or chronic infections [112].

Plasma cell leukemia

Plasma cell leukemia (PCL) is defined by circulating clonal plasma cells (>2 × 10^9/L or ≥20% of leukocyte differential count) [10, 113–122]. Plasma cells are often present in other locations, including spleen, liver, effusions, and cerebrospinal fluid (CSF). PCL may be present at the time of diagnosis (primary PCL) or represent leukemic transformation of end-stage PCM (secondary PCL). The dissemination of tumor cells out of the BM is associated with loosing dependence of BM microenvironment and acquiring the protection against apoptosis and immune surveillance. In primary PCL, neoplastic plasma cells already have the genetic abnormalities, which in more typical myeloma cases accumulate gradually as disease progresses from MGUS to myeloma to finally PCL.

Genetic changes

The t(11;14) is the most prevalent *IGH* translocation in primary PCL [122–126]. The frequencies of t(4;14) and t(14;16) are similar in both primary and secondary PCL and are higher compared with newly diagnosed PCM. In both primary and secondary PCL the frequency of poor-risk chromosomal abnormalities such as del(17p), del(13q), del(1p21), amp(1q21) and *MYC* rearrangements is markedly higher compared with newly diagnosed PCM [123–125, 127].

Morphology and phenotype

Peripheral blood smear shows circulating plasma cells and typically leukoerythroblastosis [124]. Plasma cells display various morphology with either normal-appearing plasma cells, lymphoplasmacytoid features or highly atypical immature forms. In some cases, plasma cells may resemble lymphocytes and require FC analysis for definite diagnosis. Phenotypically PCL is similar to PCM, but tumor cells from primary PCL have reduced expression of CD56, are less often positive for CD71, CD117 and HLA-DR, but more likely express CD19, CD20, CD23, and CD45 [114, 115, 117, 121, 128, 129]. Compared to IgG or IgA myeloma, a higher proportion of light chain only, IgD, or IgE myeloma present as PCL. Figures 14.23 and 14.24 show examples of PCL.

Prognosis

Detection of myeloma cells in blood (circulating myeloma cells) by FC in patients with PCM is a marker of active disease of high-risk. The prognosis of patients with PCL is poor, and is associated with a median survival of 7–12 months, based on retrospective series of conventionally treated patients (without use of novel agents or ASCT) [116, 130]. Presence of hypodiploidy, complex karyotype, del(13q), del(17p), del(1q), or amp(1q) is associated with reduced OS [119]. Of 246 patients undergoing autologous stem-cell transplantation (ASCT) analyzed by Dingli et al., 95 had myeloma cells in blood [98]. CR rates after transplantation were 32% and 36% for patients with and without circulating myeloma cells, respectively and OS were 33.2 and 58.6 months, respectively. On multivariate analysis, circulating myeloma cells remained independent of cytogenetics and disease status at time of transplantation [98]. Taking into account both cytogenetic and presence of myeloma cells in blood, patients with neither, one, or both parameters had a median OS of 55, 48, and 21.5 months and a median time to progression of 22, 15.4, and 6.5 months, respectively [98]. Using a receiver operating characteristics, Gonsalves et al. showed that presence of ≥400 cells (per 150,000 collected events) by FC was associated with high-risk disease with shorter median time-to-next treatment (14 months versus 26 months) and OS (32 months versus not reached) in patients with newly diagnosed PCM [131]. Introduction of novel agents, such as proteasome inhibitors

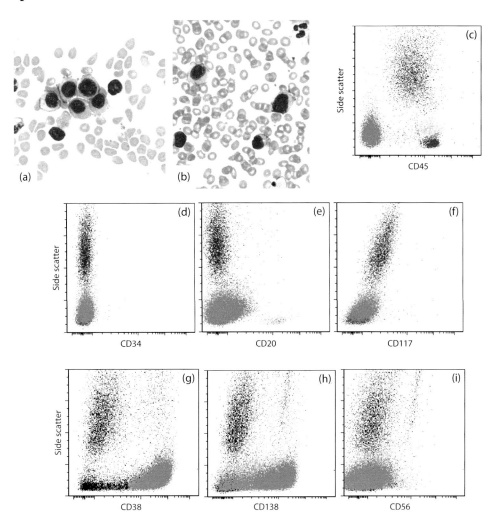

FIGURE 14.23 Plasma cell leukemia. (a–b) Blood smear with circulating plasma cells with prominent atypia (immature features) mimicking acute (monoblastic leukemia). (c–i) Flow cytometry revealed the following phenotype of plasma cells (orange dots): CD45− (c), CD34− (d), CD20− (e), CD117− (f), CD38+ (g), CD138+ (h), and CD56− (i). Plasma cells were monoclonal (lambda+; not shown).

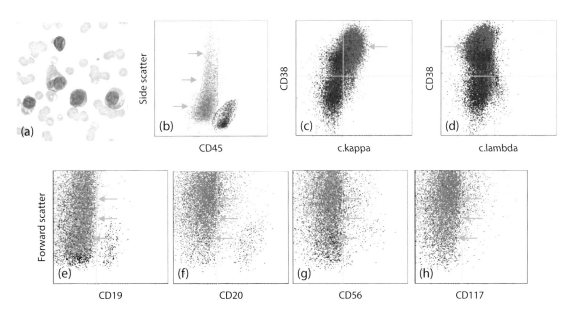

FIGURE 14.24 Plasma cell leukemia. (a) Blood smear with circulating plasma cells. (b–h) Flow cytometry shows plasma cells with positive CD45 (b) and variable although mostly low side scatter (b; arrows), kappa restriction (c–d), and negative expression of CD19 (d), CD20 (e), CD56 (f), and CD117 (h).

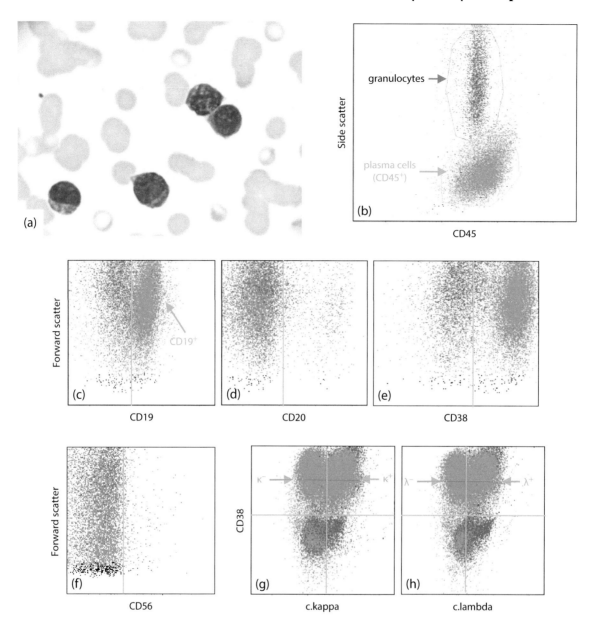

FIGURE 14.25 Prominent (reactive) plasmacytosis in blood from a 25-year-old patient with AITL. Plasma cells comprise >50% cells in peripheral blood and display cytologic atypia (a). They are CD45⁺ (b), CD19⁺ (c), CD20⁻ (d), CD38⁺ (e; bright expression), and CD56⁻ (f). Staining with cytoplasmic kappa and lambda confirmed benign (polytypic) nature of plasma cells (g–h).

and immunomodulatory drugs, as well as stem cell transplantation in the treatment of PCL improve survival to a range of 22–38 months [113, 118–120, 132].

Differential diagnosis of PCL
Reactive plasmacytosis in blood
Very prominent polytypic blood plasmacytosis mimicking PCL can be seen in blood in many conditions, including patients with viral infections (HIV, hepatitis, parvovirus infections), staphylococcal sepsis, tuberculosis, treatment with intravenous immunoglobulins, drug reactions, and autoimmune disorders, mononucleosis-like reaction, sickle cell disease, and in certain malignancies, especially angioimmunoblastic T-cell lymphoma (AITL, Figure 14.25) [133–135]. In most cases of reactive plasmacytosis in blood the plasma cell count does not exceed 10%.

References

1. Swerdlow, S.H., et al., ed. *WHO classification of tumors of haematopoietic and lymphoid tissues.* 2016, IARC: Lyon.
2. Fonseca, R., et al., *International Myeloma Working Group molecular classification of multiple myeloma: spotlight review.* Leukemia, 2009. **23**(12): p. 2210–21.
3. Kyle, R.A. and S.V. Rajkumar, *Monoclonal gammopathy of undetermined significance and smoldering multiple myeloma.* Hematol Oncol Clin North Am, 2007. **21**(6): p. 1093–113, ix.
4. Usmani, S.Z., et al., *Defining and treating high-risk multiple myeloma.* Leukemia, 2015. **29**(11): p. 2119–25.
5. Kyle, R.A., et al., *Prevalence of monoclonal gammopathy of undetermined significance.* N Engl J Med, 2006. **354**(13): p. 1362–9.
6. Kyle, R.A., et al., *A long-term study of prognosis in monoclonal gammopathy of undetermined significance.* N Engl J Med, 2002. **346**(8): p. 564–9.

7. Rajkumar, S.V., M.Q. Lacy, and R.A. Kyle, *Monoclonal gammopathy of undetermined significance and smoldering multiple myeloma.* Blood Rev, 2007. **21**(5): p. 255–65.

8. International, M.W.G., *Criteria for the classification of monoclonal gammopathies, multiple myeloma and related disorders: a report of the International Myeloma Working Group.* Br J Haematol, 2003. **121**(5): p. 749–57.

9. Li, J. and D.B. Zhou, *New advances in the diagnosis and treatment of POEMS syndrome.* Br J Haematol, 2013. **161**(3): p. 161.

10. Swerdlow, S.H., Campo, E., Harris, N. L., Jaffe, E. S., Pileri, S. A., Stein, H., et al., ed. WHO classification of tumors of haematopoietic and lymphoid tissues. 2008, IARC: Lyon.

11. Decaux, O., et al., *Systemic manifestations of monoclonal gammopathy.* Eur J Intern Med, 2009. **20**(5): p. 457–61.

12. Dispenzieri, A., *POEMS syndrome: update on diagnosis, risk-stratification, and management.* Am J Hematol, 2012. **87**(8): p. 804–14.

13. Dispenzieri, A., et al., *POEMS syndrome: definitions and long-term outcome.* Blood, 2003. **101**(7): p. 2496–506.

14. Dispenzieri, A., et al., *Smoldering multiple myeloma requiring treatment: time for a new definition?* Blood, 2013. **122**(26): p. 4172–81.

15. Rajkumar, S.V., O. Landgren, and M.V. Mateos, *Smoldering multiple myeloma.* Blood, 2015. **125**(20): p. 3069–75.

16. Rajkumar, S.V., et al., *International Myeloma Working Group updated criteria for the diagnosis of multiple myeloma.* Lancet Oncol, 2014. **15**(12): p. e538–48.

17. Barlogie, B., et al., *Plasma cell myeloma—new biological insights and advances in therapy.* Blood, 1989. **73**(4): p. 865–79.

18. Kyle, R.A., *Why better prognostic factors for multiple myeloma are needed.* Blood, 1994. **83**(7): p. 1713–6.

19. Drach, J., et al., *Interphase fluorescence in situ hybridization identifies chromosomal abnormalities in plasma cells from patients with monoclonal gammopathy of undetermined significance.* Blood, 1995. **86**(10): p. 3915–21.

20. Avet-Loiseau, H., et al., *Oncogenesis of multiple myeloma: 14q32 and 13q chromosomal abnormalities are not randomly distributed, but correlate with natural history, immunological features, and clinical presentation.* Blood, 2002. **99**(6): p. 2185–91.

21. Fonseca, R., et al., *Myeloma and the t(11;14)(q13;q32); evidence for a biologically defined unique subset of patients.* Blood, 2002. **99**(10): p. 3735–41.

22. Shaughnessy, J., Jr., et al., *Cyclin D3 at 6p21 is dysregulated by recurrent chromosomal translocations to immunoglobulin loci in multiple myeloma.* Blood, 2001. **98**(1): p. 217–23.

23. Boersma-Vreugdenhil, G.R., et al., *The recurrent translocation t(14;20)(q32;q12) in multiple myeloma results in aberrant expression of MAFB: a molecular and genetic analysis of the chromosomal breakpoint.* Br J Haematol, 2004. **126**(3): p. 355–63.

24. Rajkumar, S.V. and P.R. Greipp, *Prognostic factors in multiple myeloma.* Hematol Oncol Clin North Am, 1999. **13**(6): p. 1295–314, xi.

25. Rajkumar, S.V., et al., *Cytogenetic abnormalities correlate with the plasma cell labeling index and extent of bone marrow involvement in myeloma.* Cancer Genet Cytogenet, 1999. **113**(1): p. 73–7.

26. Rajkumar, S.V., et al., *Beta2-microglobulin and bone marrow plasma cell involvement predict complete responders among patients undergoing blood cell transplantation for myeloma.* Bone Marrow Transplant, 1999. **23**(12): p. 1261–6.

27. Fonseca, R., et al., *Clinical and biologic implications of recurrent genomic aberrations in myeloma.* Blood, 2003. **101**(11): p. 4569–75.

28. Smadja, N.V., et al., *Hypodiploidy is a major prognostic factor in multiple myeloma.* Blood, 2001. **98**(7): p. 2229–38.

29. Shaughnessy, J., et al., *Continuous absence of metaphase-defined cytogenetic abnormalities, especially of chromosome 13 and hypodiploidy, ensures long-term survival in multiple myeloma treated with Total Therapy I: interpretation in the context of global gene expression.* Blood, 2003. **101**(10): p. 3849–56.

30. Soverini, S., et al., *Cyclin D1 overexpression is a favorable prognostic variable for newly diagnosed multiple myeloma patients treated with high-dose chemotherapy and single or double autologous transplantation.* Blood, 2003. **102**(5): p. 1588–94.

31. Gonsalves, W.I., et al., *Trends in survival of patients with primary plasma cell leukemia: a population-based analysis.* Blood, 2014. **124**(6): p. 907–12.

32. Waxman, A.J., et al., *Classifying ultra-high risk smoldering myeloma.* Leukemia, 2015. **29**(3): p. 751–3.

33. Avet-Loiseau, H., *Ultra high-risk myeloma.* Hematology Am Soc Hematol Educ Program, 2010. **2010**: p. 489–93.

34. Palumbo, A., et al., *Revised international staging system for multiple myeloma: a report from International Myeloma Working Group.* J Clin Oncol, 2015. **33**(26): p. 2863–9.

35. Jekarl, D.W., et al., *Impact of genetic abnormalities on the prognoses and clinical parameters of patients with multiple myeloma.* Ann Lab Med, 2013. **33**(4): p. 248–54.

36. Hebraud, B., et al., *Role of additional chromosomal changes in the prognostic value of t(4;14) and del(17p) in multiple myeloma: the IFM experience.* Blood, 2015. **125**(13): p. 2095–100.

37. Pawlyn, C., et al., *Coexistent hyperdiploidy does not abrogate poor prognosis in myeloma with adverse cytogenetics and may precede IGH translocations.* Blood, 2015. **125**(5): p. 831–40.

38. Neben, K., et al., *Progression in smoldering myeloma is independently determined by the chromosomal abnormalities del(17p), t(4;14), gain 1q, hyperdiploidy, and tumor load.* J Clin Oncol, 2013. **31**(34): p. 4325–32.

39. Cesana, C., et al., *Prognostic factors for malignant transformation in monoclonal gammopathy of undetermined significance and smoldering multiple myeloma.* J Clin Oncol, 2002. **20**(6): p. 1625–34.

40. Kyle, R.A., et al., *Review of 1027 patients with newly diagnosed multiple myeloma.* Mayo Clin Proc, 2003. **78**(1): p. 21–33.

41. Cogbill, C.H., et al., *Morphologic and cytogenetic variables affect the flow cytometric recovery of plasma cell myeloma cells in bone marrow aspirates.* Int J Lab Hematol, 2015. **37**(6): p. 797–808.

42. Quijano, S., et al., *Association between the proliferative rate of neoplastic B cells, their maturation stage, and underlying cytogenetic abnormalities in B-cell chronic lymphoproliferative disorders: analysis of a series of 432 patients.* Blood, 2008. **111**(10): p. 5130–41.

43. Perez-Andres, M., et al., *Human peripheral blood B-cell compartments: a crossroad in B-cell traffic.* Cytometry B Clin Cytom, 2010. **78 Suppl 1**: p. S47–S60.

44. Orfao, A., et al., *A new method for the analysis of plasma cell DNA content in multiple myeloma samples using a CD38/propidium iodide double staining technique.* Cytometry, 1994. **17**(4): p. 332–9.

45. Flores-Montero, J., et al., *Immunophenotype of normal vs. myeloma plasma cells: toward antibody panel specifications for MRD detection in multiple myeloma.* Cytometry B Clin Cytom, 2016. **90**(1): p. 61–72.

46. Jourdan, M., et al., *The myeloma cell antigen syndecan-1 is lost by apoptotic myeloma cells.* Br J Haematol, 1998. **100**(4): p. 637–46.

47. Robillard, N., et al., *Immunophenotype of normal and myelomatous plasma-cell subsets.* Front Immunol, 2014. **5**: p. 137.

48. Cannizzo, E., et al., *Multiparameter immunophenotyping by flow cytometry in multiple myeloma: the diagnostic utility of defining ranges of normal antigenic expression in comparison to histology.* Cytometry B Clin Cytom, 2010. **78**(4): p. 231–8.

49. Paiva, B., et al., *Clinical significance of CD81 expression by clonal plasma cells in high-risk smoldering and symptomatic multiple myeloma patients.* Leukemia, 2012. **26**(8): p. 1862–9.

50. Pojero, F., et al., *Old and new immunophenotypic markers in multiple myeloma for discrimination of responding and relapsing patients: The importance of "normal" residual plasma cell analysis.* Cytometry B Clin Cytom, 2015. **88**(3): p. 165–82.

51. Peceliunas, V., et al., *Six color flow cytometry detects plasma cells expressing aberrant immunophenotype in bone marrow of healthy donors.* Cytometry B Clin Cytom, 2011. **80**(5): p. 318–23.

52. Schouweiler, K.E., N.J. Karandikar, and C.J. Holman, *Immuno-phenotypic heterogeneity of polytypic plasma cells and the impact on myeloma minimal residual disease detection by multiparameter flow cytometry.* Cytometry B Clin Cytom, 2019. **96**(4): p. 310–8.

53. Rawstron, A.C., et al., *Report of the European Myeloma Network on multiparametric flow cytometry in multiple myeloma and related disorders.* Haematologica, 2008. **93**(3): p. 431–8.

54. Garcia-Garcia, P., et al., *Biclonal gammopathies: retrospective study of 47 patients.* Rev Clin Esp (Barc), 2015. **215**(1): p. 18–24.

55. Chen, Z.W., et al., *Biclonal IgD and IgM plasma cell myeloma: a report of two cases and a literature review.* Case Rep Hematol, 2013. **2013**: p. 293150.

56. Gu, H.J., et al., *Biclonal plasma cell myeloma with the simultaneous appearance of both secretory lambda and nonsecretory kappa monoclonal light chains.* Clin Chem Lab Med, 2017. **55**(1): p. e21–e24.

57. Mullikin, T.C., et al., *Clinical characteristics and outcomes in biclonal gammopathies.* Am J Hematol, 2016. **91**(5): p. 473–5.

58. Jiang, A.S., et al., *Plasma cell myeloma with dual expression of kappa and lambda light chains.* Int J Clin Exp Pathol, 2018. **11**(9): p. 4718–23.

59. Heaney, J.L.J., et al., *Diagnosis and monitoring for light chain only and oligosecretory myeloma using serum free light chain tests.* Br J Haematol, 2017. **178**(2): p. 220–30.

60. Nishio, Y., et al., *Light-chain plasma cell myeloma caused by 14q32/IGH translocation and loss of the other allele.* Int J Hematol, 2019. **109**(5): p. 572–7.

61. Paiva, B., et al., *Differentiation stage of myeloma plasma cells: biological and clinical significance.* Leukemia, 2017. **31**(2): p. 382–92.

62. Mateo, G., et al., *Prognostic value of immunophenotyping in multiple myeloma: a study by the PETHEMA/GEM cooperative study groups on patients uniformly treated with high-dose therapy.* J Clin Oncol, 2008. **26**(16): p. 2737–44.

63. Pope, B., et al., *The bone marrow plasma cell labeling index by flow cytometry.* Cytometry, 1999. **38**(6): p. 286–92.

64. Fujii, R., et al., *MPC-1-CD49e- immature myeloma cells include CD45+ subpopulations that can proliferate in response to IL-6 in human myelomas.* Br J Haematol, 1999. **105**(1): p. 131–40.

65. Robillard, N., C. Pellat-Deceunynck, and R. Bataille, *Phenotypic characterization of the human myeloma cell growth fraction.* Blood, 2005. **105**(12): p. 4845–8.

66. Gonsalves, W.I., et al., *The prognostic significance of CD45 expression by clonal bone marrow plasma cells in patients with newly diagnosed multiple myeloma.* Leuk Res, 2016. **44**: p. 32–39.

67. Arana, P., et al., *Prognostic value of antigen expression in multiple myeloma: a PETHEMA/GEM study on 1265 patients enrolled in four consecutive clinical trials.* Leukemia, 2018. **32**(4): p. 971–8.

68. Feyler, S., et al., *IgM myeloma: a rare entity characterized by a CD20-CD56-CD117- immunophenotype and the t(11;14).* Br J Haematol, 2008. **140**(5): p. 547–51.

69. Avet-Loiseau, H., et al., *14q32 Translocations discriminate IgM multiple myeloma from Waldenstrom's macroglobulinemia.* Semin Oncol, 2003. **30**(2): p. 153–5.

70. Flores-Montero, J., et al., *Next Generation Flow for highly sensitive and standardized detection of minimal residual disease in multiple myeloma.* Leukemia, 2017. **31**(10): p. 2094–103.

71. Puig, N., et al., *Critical evaluation of ASO RQ-PCR for minimal residual disease evaluation in multiple myeloma. A comparative analysis with flow cytometry.* Leukemia, 2014. **28**(2): p. 391–7.

72. Sarasquete, M.E., et al., *Minimal residual disease monitoring in multiple myeloma: a comparison between allelic-specific oligonucleotide real-time quantitative polymerase chain reaction and flow cytometry.* Haematologica, 2005. **90**(10): p. 1365–72.

73. Ladetto, M., et al., *Real-Time polymerase chain reaction of immunoglobulin rearrangements for quantitative evaluation of minimal residual disease in multiple myeloma.* Biol Blood Marrow Transplant, 2000. **6**(3): p. 241–53.

74. Puig, N., et al., *Kappa deleting element as an alternative molecular target for minimal residual disease assessment by real-time quantitative PCR in patients with multiple myeloma.* Eur J Haematol, 2012. **89**(4): p. 328–35.

75. Puig, N., et al., *The use of CD138 positively selected marrow samples increases the applicability of minimal residual disease assessment by PCR in patients with multiple myeloma.* Ann Hematol, 2013. **92**(1): p. 97–100.

76. Martinez-Lopez, J., et al., *Prognostic value of deep sequencing method for minimal residual disease detection in multiple myeloma.* Blood, 2014. **123**(20): p. 3073–9.

77. Bal, S., et al., *Challenges and opportunities in the assessment of measurable residual disease in multiple myeloma.* Br J Haematol, 2019. **186**(6): p. 807–19.

78. Royston, D.J., et al., *Single-tube 10-fluorochrome analysis for efficient flow cytometric evaluation of minimal residual disease in plasma cell myeloma.* Am J Clin Pathol, 2016. **146**(1): p. 41–9.

79. de Tute, R.M., et al., *Minimal residual disease following autologous stem cell transplant in myeloma: impact on outcome is independent of induction regimen.* Haematologica, 2016. **101**(2): p. e69–e71.

80. Fukumoto, K., et al., *Prognostic impact of immunophenotypic complete response in patients with multiple myeloma achieving better than complete response.* Leuk Lymphoma, 2016: p. 1–7.

81. Arroz, M., et al., *Consensus guidelines on plasma cell myeloma minimal residual disease analysis and reporting.* Cytometry B Clin Cytom, 2015. **90**(1): p. 31–9.

82. Rawstron, A.C., et al., *Minimal residual disease assessed by multi-parameter flow cytometry in multiple myeloma: impact on outcome in the Medical Research Council Myeloma IX Study.* J Clin Oncol, 2013. **31**(20): p. 2540–7.

83. Rawstron, A.C., et al., *Minimal residual disease in myeloma by flow cytometry: independent prediction of survival benefit per log reduction.* Blood, 2015. **125**(12): p. 1932–5.

84. Rawstron, A.C., B. Paiva, and M. Stetler-Stevenson, *Assessment of minimal residual disease in myeloma and the need for a consensus approach.* Cytometry B Clin Cytom, 2016. **90**(1): p. 21–5.

85. Stetler-Stevenson, M., et al., *Consensus guidelines for myeloma minimal residual disease sample staining and data acquisition.* Cytometry B Clin Cytom, 2016. **90**(1): p. 26–30.

86. Paiva, B., et al., *High-risk cytogenetics and persistent minimal residual disease by multiparameter flow cytometry predict unsustained complete response after autologous stem cell transplantation in multiple myeloma.* Blood, 2012. **119**(3): p. 687–91.

87. Paiva, B., et al., *Minimal residual disease monitoring and immune profiling in multiple myeloma in elderly patients.* Blood, 2016. **127**(25): p. 3165–74.

88. Rawstron, A.C., et al., *Measuring disease levels in myeloma using flow cytometry in combination with other laboratory techniques: Lessons from the past 20 years at the Leeds Haematological Malignancy Diagnostic Service.* Cytometry B Clin Cytom, 2016. **90**(1): p. 54–60.

89. Roshal, M., et al., *MRD detection in multiple myeloma: comparison between MSKCC 10-color single-tube and EuroFlow 8-color 2-tube methods.* Blood Adv, 2017. **1**(12): p. 728–32.

90. Zeijlemaker, W., J.W. Gratama, and G.J. Schuurhuis, *Tumor heterogeneity makes AML a "moving target" for detection of residual disease.* Cytometry B Clin Cytom, 2014. **86**(1): p. 3–14.

91. Kumar, S., et al., *International Myeloma Working Group consensus criteria for response and minimal residual disease assessment in multiple myeloma.* Lancet Oncol, 2016. **17**(8): p. e328–e346.

92. Fermand, J.P., et al., *Gamma heavy chain "disease": heterogeneity of the clinicopathologic features. Report of 16 cases and review of the literature.* Medicine (Baltimore), 1989. **68**(6): p. 321–35.

93. Ria, R., F. Dammacco, and A. Vacca, *Heavy-chain diseases and myeloma-associated Fanconi syndrome: an update.* Mediterr J Hematol Infect Dis, 2018. **10**(1): p. e2018011.

94. Kyle, R.A., et al., *IgM monoclonal gammopathy of undetermined significance (MGUS) and smoldering Waldenstrom's macroglobulinemia (SWM).* Clin Lymphoma Myeloma Leuk, 2011. **11**(1): p. 74–76.

95. Kyle, R.A. and S.V. Rajkumar, *Monoclonal gammopathy of undetermined significance.* Clin Lymphoma Myeloma, 2005. **6**(2): p. 102–14.

96. Xu, L., et al., *MYD88 L265P in Waldenstrom macroglobulinemia, immunoglobulin M monoclonal gammopathy, and other B-cell lymphoproliferative disorders using conventional and quantitative allele-specific polymerase chain reaction.* Blood, 2013. **121**(11): p. 2051–8.

97. Girard, L.P., et al., *Immunoglobulin M paraproteinaemias.* Cancers (Basel), 2020. **12**(6): 1688.

98. Dingli, D., et al., *Immunoglobulin free light chains and solitary plasmacytoma of bone.* Blood, 2006. **108**(6): p. 1979–83.

99. Hanamura, I., et al., *Frequent gain of chromosome band 1q21 in plasma-cell dyscrasias detected by fluorescence in situ hybridization: incidence increases from MGUS to relapsed myeloma and is related to prognosis and disease progression following tandem stem-cell transplantation.* Blood, 2006. **108**(5): p. 1724–32.

100. Montoto, S., J. Blade, and E. Montserrat, *Monoclonal gammopathy of undetermined significance.* N Engl J Med, 2002. **346**(26): p. 2087–8; author reply 2087–8.

101. Perez-Andres, M., et al., *Clonal plasma cells from monoclonal gammopathy of undetermined significance, multiple myeloma and plasma cell leukemia show different expression profiles of molecules involved in the interaction with the immunological bone marrow microenvironment.* Leukemia, 2005. **19**(3): p. 449–55.

102. Schop, R.F., et al., *6q deletion discriminates Waldenstrom macroglobulinemia from IgM monoclonal gammopathy of undetermined significance.* Cancer Genet Cytogenet, 2006. **169**(2): p. 150–3.

103. Bird, J., et al., *UK Myeloma Forum (UKMF) and Nordic Myeloma Study Group (NMSG): guidelines for the investigation of newly detected M-proteins and the management of monoclonal gammopathy of undetermined significance (MGUS).* Br J Haematol, 2009. **147**(1): p. 22–42.

104. Kyle, R.A. and S.V. Rajkumar, *Monoclonal gammopathy of undetermined significance.* Br J Haematol, 2006. **134**(6): p. 573–89.

105. Kyle, R.A., *Monoclonal gammopathy of undetermined significance. Natural history in 241 cases.* Am J Med, 1978. **64**(5): p. 814–26.

106. Landgren, O., et al., *Monoclonal gammopathy of undetermined significance (MGUS) consistently precedes multiple myeloma: a prospective study.* Blood, 2009. **113**(22): p. 5412–7.

107. Kyle, R.A. and S.V. Rajkumar, *Multiple myeloma.* N Engl J Med, 2004. 351(18): p. 1860–73.

108. Kyle, R.A., et al., *Long-term follow-up of 241 patients with monoclonal gammopathy of undetermined significance: the original Mayo Clinic series 25 years later.* Mayo Clin Proc, 2004. **79**(7): p. 859–66.

109. Kyle, R.A., et al., *Long-term follow-up of IgM monoclonal gammopathy of undetermined significance.* Blood, 2003. **102**(10): p. 3759–64.

110. Pasqualetti, P., et al., *The natural history of monoclonal gammopathy of undetermined significance. A 5- to 20-year follow-up of 263 cases.* Acta Haematol, 1997. **97**(3): p. 174–9.

111. Perez-Persona, E., et al., *New criteria to identify risk of progression in monoclonal gammopathy of uncertain significance and smoldering multiple myeloma based on multiparameter flow cytometry analysis of bone marrow plasma cells.* Blood, 2007. **110**(7): p. 2586–92.

112. Jerez, A., et al., *Bone-marrow immunophenotypic analysis allows the identification of high risk of progression and immune condition-related monoclonal gammopathy of undetermined significance.* Ann Med, 2009. **47**(7): p. 547–58.

113. van de Donk, N.W., et al., *How I treat plasma cell leukemia.* Blood, 2012. **120**(12): p. 2376–89.

114. Pellat-Deceunynck, C., et al., *The absence of CD56 (NCAM) on malignant plasma cells is a hallmark of plasma cell leukemia and of a special subset of multiple myeloma.* Leukemia, 1998. **12**(12): p. 1977–82.

115. Kraj, M., et al., *Flow cytometric immunophenotypic characteristics of 36 cases of plasma cell leukemia.* Leuk Res, 2011. **35**(2): p. 169–76.

116. Dimopoulos, M.A., et al., *Primary plasma cell leukaemia.* Br J Haematol, 1994. **88**(4): p. 754–9.

117. Costello, R., et al., *Primary plasma cell leukaemia: a report of 18 cases.* Leuk Res, 2001. **25**(2): p. 103–7.

118. Drake, M.B., et al., *Primary plasma cell leukemia and autologous stem cell transplantation.* Haematologica, 2010. **95**(5): p. 804–9.

119. Pagano, L., et al., *Primary plasma cell leukemia: a retrospective multicenter study of 73 patients.* Ann Oncol, 2011. **22**(7): p. 1628–35.

120. Usmani, S.Z., et al., *Primary plasma cell leukemia: clinical and laboratory presentation, gene-expression profiling and clinical outcome with Total Therapy protocols.* Leukemia, 2012. **26**(11): p. 2398–405.

121. Garcia-Sanz, R., et al., *Primary plasma cell leukemia: clinical, immunophenotypic, DNA ploidy, and cytogenetic characteristics.* Blood, 1999. **93**(3): p. 1032–7.

122. Johnson, M.R., et al., *Primary plasma cell leukemia: morphologic, immunophenotypic, and cytogenetic features of 4 cases treated with chemotherapy and stem cell transplantation.* Ann Diagn Pathol, 2006. **10**(5): p. 263–8.

123. Avet-Loiseau, H., et al., *Cytogenetic and therapeutic characterization of primary plasma cell leukemia: the IFM experience.* Leukemia, 2012. **26**(1): p. 158–9.

124. Tiedemann, R.E., et al., *Genetic aberrations and survival in plasma cell leukemia.* Leukemia, 2008. **22**(5): p. 1044–52.

125. Avet-Loiseau, H., et al., *Prognostic significance of copy-number alterations in multiple myeloma.* J Clin Oncol, 2009. **27**(27): p. 4585–90.

126. Gutierrez, N.C., et al., *Differences in genetic changes between multiple myeloma and plasma cell leukemia demonstrated by comparative genomic hybridization.* Leukemia, 2001. **15**(5): p. 840–5.

127. Chang, H., et al., *Genetic aberrations including chromosome 1 abnormalities and clinical features of plasma cell leukemia.* Leuk Res, 2009. **33**(2): p. 259–62.

128. Pellat-Deceunynck, C., et al., *Adhesion molecules on human myeloma cells: significant changes in expression related to malignancy, tumor spreading, and immortalization.* Cancer Res, 1995. **55**(16): p. 3647–53.

129. Buda, G., et al., *CD23 expression in plasma cell leukaemia.* Br J Haematol, 2010. **150**(6): p. 724–5.

130. Noel, P. and R.A. Kyle, *Plasma cell leukemia: an evaluation of response to therapy.* Am J Med, 1987. **83**(6): p. 1062–8.

131. Gonsalves, W.I., et al., *Quantification of clonal circulating plasma cells in relapsed multiple myeloma.* Br J Haematol, 2014. **167**(4): p. 500–5.

132. D'Arena, G., et al., *Frontline chemotherapy with bortezomib-containing combinations improves response rate and survival in primary plasma cell leukemia: a retrospective study from GIMEMA Multiple Myeloma Working Party.* Ann Oncol, 2012. **23**(6): p. 1499–502.

133. Nagoshi, H., et al., *Clinical manifestation of angioimmunoblastic T-cell lymphoma with exuberant plasmacytosis.* Int J Hematol, 2013. **98**(3): p. 366–74.

134. Ahsanuddin, A.N., R.K. Brynes, and S. Li, *Peripheral blood polyclonal plasmacytosis mimicking plasma cell leukemia in patients with angioimmunoblastic T-cell lymphoma: report of 3 cases and review of the literature.* Int J Clin Exp Pathol, 2011. **4**(4): p. 416–20.

135. Gawoski, J.M. and W.W. Ooi, *Dengue fever mimicking plasma cell leukemia.* Arch Pathol Lab Med, 2003. **127**(8): p. 1026–7.

15

PHENOTYPIC CLASSIFICATION OF MATURE T/NK-CELL LYMPHOPROLIFERATIONS

Introduction

T-cell lymphomas are diverse group of lymphoid neoplasms manifesting heterogeneous clinical, histologic, immunophenotypic, and cytogenetic features [1–29]. T-cell lymphomas represent approximately 10% of all non-Hodgkin lymphomas in Western countries. The classification of T-cell lymphoma is based largely on the histomorphologic features and clinical parameters.

Diagnostic process

The diagnosis of T-cell proliferations by flow cytometry (FC) may be difficult, especially at the early stages of the disease and in certain types of lymphomas with prominent admixture of reactive elements (e.g., nodal TFH cell lymphoma, angioimmunoblastic-type, AITL). Detection of clonal rearrangements of T-cell receptor loci γ, δ, and β (*TCRG, TCRD, TCRB*) by polymerase chain reaction (PCR) may be very helpful in the diagnostic process. Presence of human T-cell lymphoma virus type 1 (HTLV-1) is associated with risk for adult T-cell leukemia/lymphoma (ATLL). Detection of anaplastic lymphoma kinase (ALK) by immunohistochemistry or t(2;5)$^{ALK/NPM}$ by fluorescence in situ hybridization (FISH) helps to diagnose anaplastic large cell lymphoma (ALCL) (ALK$^+$). Other chromosomal abnormalities present in specific T-cell lymphoproliferations include isochromosome 7q typical for hepatosplenic T-cell lymphoma (HSTL), often showing also trisomy 8, and inversion of chromosome 14/t(14;14) seen in T-cell prolymphocytic leukemia (T-PLL). Identification of atypical T-cells by FC is presented in Chapter 5. Figure 15.1 presents the algorithmic approach to the diagnosis of mature T- and NK-cell neoplasms, and Table 15.1 presents the FC phenotype of major types of mature T-cell lymphoproliferations based on the series of the author's >400 cases.

T-cell neoplasms with predominantly nodal distribution

Predominantly nodal distribution is characteristic for AITL, peripheral T-cell lymphoma, not otherwise specified (PTCL, NOS), and ALCL. Figure 15.2 shows the algorithmic approach to the diagnosis of nodal T/NK-cell lymphomas.

T-cell neoplasms with predominantly extranodal distribution

Extranodal location is seen in mycosis fungoides (MF), cutaneous ALCL, extranodal NK/T-cell lymphoma, nasal type (ENKTL), enteropathy-associated T-cell lymphoma (EATL), HSTL, and subcutaneous panniculitis-like T-cell lymphoma (SPTL). Figure 15.3 shows preferential involvement by cutaneous lymphomas based on body area.

T-cell neoplasms with leukemic blood involvement

Leukemic blood involvement is typical for T-PLL, T-cell large granular lymphocyte (T-LGL) leukemia (T-LGLL), and leukemic variant of ATLL. Subset of other mature T-cell neoplasms may present with leukemic blood involvement, including PTCL and ALCL.

Prognosis

Majority of T-cell lymphoproliferative disorders are aggressive with only MF and cutaneous ALCL frequently following indolent course. Response to conventional therapy generally is poor. New treatment modalities, including purine analogs, monoclonal antibodies (Campath), and stem cell transplantation, offer improved response rates and better remissions [25]. Based on survival analysis, three distinct prognostic subgroups of T-cell neoplasms can be distinguished: favorable (cutaneous ALCL; T-LGLL, 5-year overall survival 78%); intermediate (PTCL, ALCL, and AITL), 5-year overall survival 35%–43%; unfavorable (extranodal NK/T-cell lymphoma, nasal type, and EATL), 5-year overall survival 22%–24%.

Classification of major categories of mature peripheral T-cell lymphoproliferations

- T-PLL
- T-large granular lymphocytes leukemia (T-LGLL)
- Chronic NK-cell lymphoproliferative disorder of NK-cells (CLPD-NK)
- Aggressive NK-cell leukemia (ANKL)
- Adult T-cell lymphoma/leukemia (ATLL)
- PTCL, NOS
- ALCL
- Nodal T-follicular helper (TFH) cell lymphoma: (1) angioimmunoblastic-type, AITL; (2) follicular-type, FTCL; and (3) nodal TFH cell lymphoma, NOS (PTCL-TFH)
- ENKTL
- MF and Sézary's syndrome (SS)
- Lymphomatoid papulosis (LyP)
- Primary cutaneous anaplastic large cell lymphoma (C-ALCL)
- Primary cutaneous gamma/delta T-cell lymphoma (PCGD-TCL)
- HSTL
- Monomorphic epitheliotropic intestinal T-cell lymphoma (MEITL)
- EATL
- SPTL

Nodal T-cell lymphomas with CD10 expression (T-cell lymphomas with T follicular helper phenotype)

The revised WHO classification of hematolymphoid tumors introduced a category of nodal lymphoma with T follicular helper (TFH) cell phenotype, which includes AITL, FTCL, and nodal PTCL with T follicular helper phenotype (PTCL-TFH) [1, 30]. CD10 expression is seen in 70%–90% of AITL (with samples from blood or BM showing less frequent CD10 expression when compared to lymph nodes). FTCL involves lymph node follicles resembling morphologically follicular B-cell lymphoma (FL). The WHO criteria specifically state that the expression of at least two TFH markers is required for the diagnosis of PTCL-TFH. TFH

DOI: 10.1201/9781003197935-15

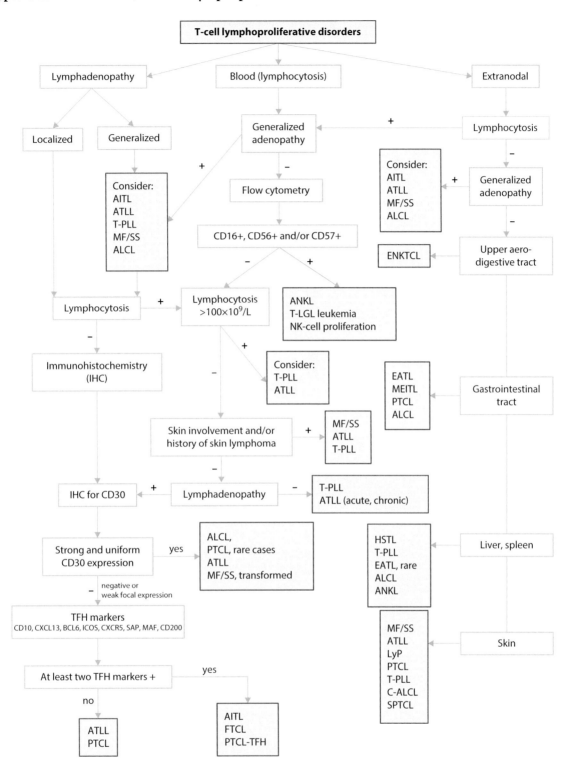

FIGURE 15.1 Algorithmic approach to the diagnosis of T-cell lymphomas. *Abbreviations*: ATLL, adult T-cell lymphoma/leukemia; AITL, angioimmunoblastic T-cell lymphoma; ALCL, anaplastic large cell lymphoma; ANKL, aggressive NK-cell leukemia; EATL, enteropathy-associated T-cell lymphoma; HSTL, hepatosplenic T-cell lymphoma; LGL, large granular lymphocyte; LyP, lymphomatoid papulosis; MEITL, monomorphic epitheliotropic intestinal T-cell lymphoma; MF, mycosis fungoides; PTCL, peripheral T-cell lymphoma; SS, Sézary's syndrome; TFH, SPTCL, subcutaneous panniculitis-like T-cell lymphoma; T follicular helper; T-PLL, T-cell prolymphocytic leukemia.

TABLE 15.1: Phenotype of Major Types of Mature T and NK-Cell Neoplasms

	CD2	s.CD3	CD5	CD7	CD4/CD8	Other Markers
T-PLL	+	+/(−)	+/(−)	+/(−)	CD4+ (61%) CD8+ (23%) CD4+/CD8+ (14%) CD4−/CD8− (5%)	c.TCL+, CD117+ in rare cases (most often CD8+)
T-LGLL	+	+	+/(−)	+/−	CD4+ (10%) CD8+ (74%) CD4+/CD8+ (8%) CD4−/CD8− (8%)	CD16+/−, CD56+/−, CD57+/(−)
NK-LGLL	+	−	−	+/−	Often dual CD4/CD8−	CD16+/−, CD56+/(−), CD57+/−
MF/SS	+/(−)	+/(−)	+/−	−/(+)	CD4+/(−) CD8−/(+)	CD25+/−, CD26−
ATLL	+/(−)	+/−	+/(−)	−	CD4+	CD25+strong, CD26−
ALCL	+/−	−/+	−/+	−/(+)	CD4+/− CD8−/+ Rarely dual CD4/CD8+ or CD4/CD8−	CD30+strong, ALK1+/−, EMA+/−, CD43+, TIA1+, granzyme B+
PTCL	+/(−)	+/−	+/−	−/+	CD4+/−, CD8−/+ Rarely dual CD4/CD8+ or CD4/CD8−	CD30−/+, CD56−/(+)
SPTCL	+	+	−	−	CD8+	TIA1+, granzyme B+, CD56−
AITL	+/(−)	−/+	+	−/+	CD4+	At least two TFH markers+ (CD10, BCL6, CXCL13, PD1, ICOS, SAP, CCR5, c-MAF and CD200), CD10+ in 70%–90% of cases
FTCL	+	+/−	+	−/+	CD4+	At least two TFH markers+ (CD10, BCL6, CXCL13, PD1, ICOS, SAP, CCR5, c-MAF and CD200)
PTCL-TFH	+	+/−	+	+/−	CD4+	At least two TFH markers+ (CD10, BCL6, CXCL13, PD1, ICOS, SAP, CCR5, c-MAF and CD200)
HSTL	+/(−)	+	−/(+)	+/(−)	CD4−/CD8− Rarely CD8+	TCRγδ+ (rare cases are TCRαβ+), TIA1+, granzyme B−, perforin−, CD16−/+, CD56+/−, CD57−
EATL	+/−	+	−/(+)	+	CD4−/CD8− Rarely CD4+ or CD8+	CD103+, CD30+/−, CD56−/+, TIA1+ (80%)
MEITL	+/−	+	−/(+)	+	CD8+/(−) CD4−/CD8−	CD103+/−, CD30−/(+), CD56+, EBER−, TIA1+, granzyme B−/+, perforin−/+, CD20−/(+)
ENKTL	+	−	−	−/+	CD4−/CD8−	TIA1+, CD56+, granzyme B+, CD25+/−, EBV/EBER+

Abbreviations: TFH, T-follicular helper; T-PLL, T-cell prolymphocytic leukemia; T-LGLL, T-cell large granular lymphocyte leukemia; NK-LGLL, NK-cell large granular lymphocyte leukemia (chronic lymphoproliferative disorder of NK-cells); MF, mycosis fungoides; SS, Sézary's syndrome; ATLL, adult T-cell lymphoma/leukemia; ALCL, anaplastic large cell lymphoma; PTCL, peripheral T-cell lymphoma; SPTCL, subcutaneous panniculitis-like T-cell lymphoma; AITL, angioimmunoblastic T-cell lymphoma; PTCL-TFH, nodal peripheral T-cell lymphoma with T follicular helper phenotype; FTCL, follicular T-cell lymphoma; HSTL, Hepatosplenic T-cell lymphoma; EATL, enteropathy-associated T-cell lymphoma; MEITL, monomorphic epitheliotropic intestinal T-cell lymphoma; ENKTL, extranodal NK/T-cell lymphoma, nasal type.
Note: +, positive; (+), rarely positive; −, negative; (−), rarely negative.

markers include CD10, BCL6, CXCL13, PD1 (CD279), ICOS, SAP (SLAM-associated protein), CXCR5, MAF (c-MAF), and CD200. AITL is the classic form of T-cell lymphoma of TFH origin, with diagnostic criteria that remain essentially unchanged from prior 2008 WHO classification. Both AITL and PTCL-TFH have similar phenotype, gene expression profile, and common mutation in *TET2*, *DNMT3A*, and *RHOA* genes [11, 31–37]. Cutaneous T-cell lymphomas expressing TFH markers are excluded from this category (WHO).

T-cell lymphoproliferations with CD30 expression

CD30 is expressed in ALK+ ALCL (100%), ALK− ALCL (100%), C-ALCL (100%), large cells in EATL (>50%), LyP (60%–100%), pagetoid reticulosis (a variant of MF, 100%), MF with large cell transformation, SS, PTCL, and ATLL. Minor population of CD30+ large T-cells is frequently present in other T-cell lymphomas, especially AITL. T-cell lymphomas with strong and uniform expression of CD30 include ALCL (both ALK+ and ALK−), ATLL, primary C-ALCL, breast-implant-associated ALCL, MF with large cell transformation and rare cases of PTCL, NOS, and ENKTL. T-cell lymphomas with focal, variable, or weak expression of CD30 include AITL and subset of PTCL, EATL, ENKTL, and MEITL. Both ALK+ ALCL and PTCL may undergo rapid progression to leukemic blood involvement with prominent leukocytosis. Those cases need to be differentiated from ATLL, T-PLL, and MF/SS. Strong expression of CD30 and high forward scatter would favor the diagnosis of ALCL. PTCL usually displays more heterogeneous or partial CD30 expression. MF/SS and ATLL show CD4 expression with lack of CD26 (ATLL is also strongly positive for CD25). T-PLL, in contrast to other T-cell neoplasms,

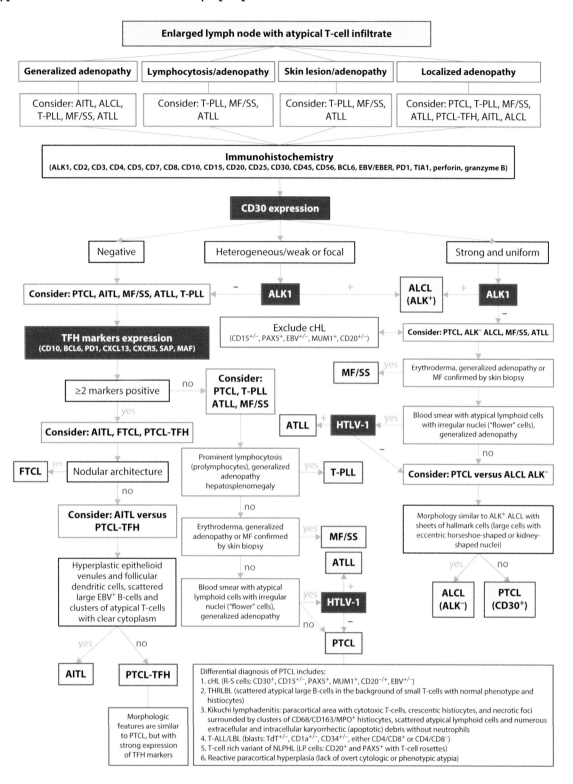

FIGURE 15.2 Algorithmic approach to lymph node with atypical T-cell infiltrate. *Abbreviations*: AITL, angioimmunoblastic T-cell lymphoma; ALCL, anaplastic large cell lymphoma; ATLL, adult T-cell lymphoma/leukemia; cHL, classic Hodgkin lymphoma; FTCL, follicular T-cell lymphoma; LP cells, large cells from NLPHL; MF, mycosis fungoides; NLPHL, nodular lymphocyte predominant Hodgkin lymphoma; PLL, prolymphocytic leukemia; PTCL, peripheral T-cell lymphoma; SS, Sézary's syndrome; T-ALL, T-cell acute lymphoblastic leukemia; T-LBL, T-cell acute lymphoblastic lymphoma, TFH, T-follicular helper.

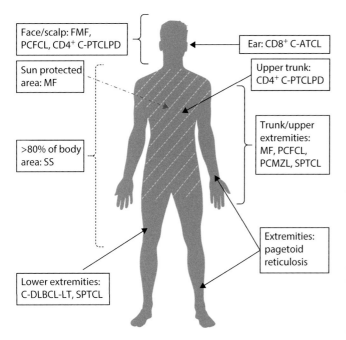

FIGURE 15.3 Preferential involvement by cutaneous lymphomas based on body area. *Abbreviations*: MF, mycosis fungoides; FMF, folliculotropic MF; CD8+ C-ATLC, primary cutaneous acral CD8+ T-cell lymphoma; CD4+ C-PTCLPD, primary cutaneous CD4+ small/medium pleomorphic T-cell lymphoproliferative disorder; PCFCL, primary cutaneous follicle center lymphoma; PCMZL, primary cutaneous marginal zone lymphoma; SPTCL, subcutaneous panniculitis-like T-cell lymphoma; SS, Sézary's syndrome; C-DLBCL-LT, cutaneous diffuse large B-cell lymphoma, leg type.

often displays normal expression of all T-cell antigens. Figure 15.4 shows leukemic blood involvement by acute form of ATLL with partial CD30 expression.

T-cell lymphoproliferations with CD25 expression

Strong expression of CD25 is most characteristic for ATLL, but dimmer, heterogeneous, or partial expression of CD25 may be seen in other T-cell lymphoproliferations. CD25 is often expressed by ALCL. Subset of PTCLs may be CD25+, whereas AITL and HSTL are usually CD25-.

T-cell lymphoproliferations with CD56 expression

CD56 is expressed by natural killer (NK) cells and a subset of T-cells and monocytes. Its expression is well recognized not only in hematolymphoid malignancies of NK-cell lineage but also in subset of T-cell neoplasms, including LyP, ENKTL, MEITL, EATL (subset), HSTL, and PCGD-TCL.

Additional phenotypic markers in T-cell lymphoproliferations

CD4 and CD8
AITL, ATLL, and SS/MF are mostly CD4+. Majority of T-PLL (~61%), PTCL (~62%), and ALCL (~69%) express CD4, but they may be also CD8+, dual CD4/CD8+, or dual CD4/CD8-. CD8+ T-cell neoplasms include the majority of T-LGL leukemias, panniculitis-like T-cell

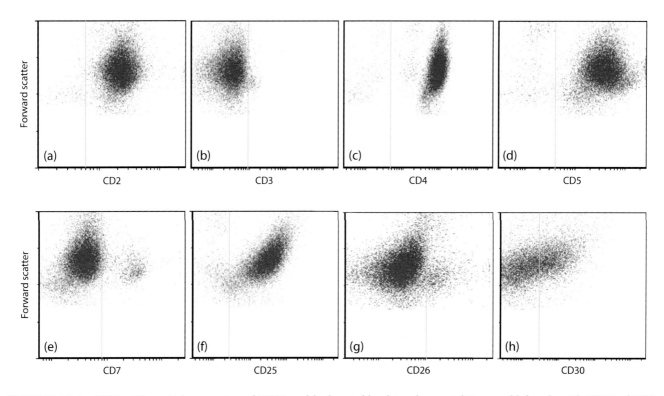

FIGURE 15.4 ATLL with partial expression of CD30 and leukemic blood involvement (63-year-old female with WBC of 34k). Neoplastic T-cells show the following phenotype: CD2+ (a), surface CD3- (b), CD4+ (c), CD5+ (d), CD7- (e), CD25+ (f), CD26+ (g), and CD30+ (partial; g).

lymphomas, and EATLs. Occasional cases of PTCL (~8%), T-PLL (~23%), and ALCL (~19%), as well as rare cases of HSTL (20%) are CD8+. Co-expression of CD4 and CD8 may be seen in very minute subset of benign T-cell in blood (average: 0.2%; range: 0%–2.3%; SD: 0.32) and/or bone marrow (average: 0.13%; range: 0%–2.7%; SD: 0.56). It is unusual in peripheral T-cell disorders, and most often indicates T-ALL/LBL. In the sample from mediastinum, dual CD4/CD8 expression is seen in thymocytes (either from thymic hyperplasia or thymoma). Among mature (peripheral) T-cell neoplasms, dual CD4/CD8 expression is observed in ~11% of T-PLL, ~4% of PTCL, ~3% of ALCL, and ~8% of T-LGL leukemia. CD4−/CD8− phenotype is uncommon in mature T-cell lymphoproliferations: EATL (~7%), NK-cell LGL leukemia (~68%), extranodal T/NK-cell lymphoma (nasal type), HSTL (~80%), non-hepatosplenic γδ T-cell lymphoma, followed by PTCL (~26%), T-PLL (~5%), ALCL (~9%), and T-LGL leukemia (~7%).

CD5-negative T-cell lymphoproliferations
Lack of CD5 expression is most typical for HSTL, EATL, MEITL, and ALCL. See Table 15.2.

Positive expression of all pan-T-cell antigens (CD2, CD3, CD5, and CD7)
Positive expression of all pan-T-cell antigens is most often seen in T-PLL (~73%), T-LGLL (~53%), followed by AITL (~28%) and PTCL (~23%). See Table 4.3 in Chapter 4 and Table 15.2.

Negative expression of all pan-T-cell antigens (CD2, CD3, CD5, and CD7)
Complete lack of T-cell antigen expression is seen in subset of ALCL (~18%) and EATL/MEITL (14%).

CD45-negative T-cell lymphoproliferations
Loss of CD45 expression is seen in subset of T-PLL, PTCL, and ALCL. See Table 4.5 in Chapter 4.

NK-cell markers (CD16, CD56, and CD57)
CD16 is often expressed by T-LGL leukemia, NK-cell proliferations, and HSTL. CD57 is expressed by NK cells and subset of T-cells. It is positive on T-LGL leukemia, subset of NK-cell neoplasms, and rare precursor T-cell lymphoblastic leukemias.

CD26
The analysis of CD26 is useful in evaluation patients with MF, which show loss of CD26 expression in 92% of cases of transformed MF [38]. Circulating neoplastic T-cells from patients with MF (Sézary's syndrome) can be identified by FC by their loss of CD26 expression. Similar to cutaneous T-cell lymphomas involving blood, also ATLL cells are CD26− [39, 40].

CD103
EATL is often CD103+ MEITL may be also CD103+.

CD15
Only very rare cases PTCLs (including ALCL and PTCL) display aberrant CD15 expression [41].

Epstein-Barr virus (EBV)
EBV, also called human herpes virus 4 (HHV-4), is a member of herpes family and is one of the most common viruses in human beings. EBV is a latent γ-herpesvirus that infects more than 90% of population. Primary lytic infection occurs in the oropharynx and may be asymptomatic or present as infectious mononucleosis. EBV is highly immunogenic and during primary infection causes a vigorous humoral and cellular immune response. The EBV life cycle is biphasic, with phases of lytic replication and latency.

EBV-associated T-cell disorders include:

- Systemic EBV+ T-cell lymphoma of childhood (STCLC)
- ANKL
- ENKTL
- Primary EBV+ nodal T/NK-cell lymphoma (nodal TNKL)
- FTCL, rare cases
- PTCL, NOS, rare cases
- Posttransplant T-cell lymphoproliferations
- Chronic active EBV infection of T- and NK-cell type, systemic and cutaneous forms

TABLE 15.2: Frequency (%) of Antigen Expression in Peripheral (Mature/Post-Thymic) T-Cell Neoplasms

	AITL (n=40)	ALCL (n=33)	ATLL (n=22)	EATL/ MEITL (n=7)	HSTL (n=18)	MF/SS (n=29)	NK-LGLL (n=35)	PTCL (n=111)	T-LGLL (n=106)	T-PLL (n=66)
CD2+	90%	67%	92%	86%	83%	93%	100%	90%	98%	95%
CD3+	68%	30%	75%	86%	100	96%	3%	65%	100%	91%
CD5+	100%	42%	96%	14%	17%	86%	0	84%	75%	97%
CD7+	48%	27%	0	0	89%	38%	89%	48%	66%	86%
All 4 T-cell antigens+	28%	9%	0	14%	17%	31%	0	23%	53%	73%
CD4+	100%	70%	100	0	0	94%	0	61%	10%	61%
CD8+	0	18%	0	86%	17%	6%	31%	9%	74%	23%
CD4/CD8+	0	3%	0	0	0	0	0	4%	8%	14%
CD4/CD8−	0	9%	0	14%	83%	3.7	69%	26%	8%	5%
CD56+	5%	12%	0	71%	94%	0	63%	10%	33%	7%
CD57+	0	0	0	0	7%	0	63%	6%	96%	5%
CD10+	80%	0	0	0	0	0	0	0	0	0
CD117+	0	0	0	0	0	0	0	0	0	15%
CD45+	100%	97%	100%	100%	100%	100%	100%	96%	100%	91%

Abbreviations: n, number of cases; PTCL, peripheral T-cell lymphoma; AITL, angioimmunoblastic T-cell lymphoma; ALCL, anaplastic large cell lymphoma; ATLL, adult T-cell lymphoma/leukemia; T-PLL, T-cell prolymphocytic leukemia; T-LGL, T-cell large granular lymphocyte leukemia; NK-LGL, NK-cell large granular lymphocyte leukemia; MF/SS, mycosis fungoides/Sézary's syndrome; HSTL, hepatosplenic T-cell lymphoma.

All these conditions can present with EBV-associated hemophagocytic lymphohistiocytosis (EBV-HLH).

References

1. Swerdlow, S.H., Campo, E., Harris, N.L., Jaffe, E.S., Piler, i S.A., Stein, H. and Thiele, J., ed. *WHO classification of tumors of haematopoietic and lymphoid tissues*. 2016, IARC: Lyon.

2. Takatsuki, K., et al., *Clinical diversity in adult T-cell leukemia-lymphoma*. Cancer Res, 1985. **45**(9 Suppl): p. 4644s–45s.

3. Miyashiro, D. and J.A. Sanches, *Cutaneous manifestations of adult T-cell leukemia/lymphoma*. Semin Diagn Pathol, 2020. **37**(2): p. 81–91.

4. Wilcox, R.A., *Cutaneous T-cell lymphoma: 2011 update on diagnosis, risk-stratification, and management*. Am J Hematol, 2011. **86**(11): p. 928–48.

5. Zettl, A., et al., *Enteropathy-type T-cell lymphoma*. Am J Clin Pathol, 2007. **127**(5): p. 701–6.

6. Tsang, W.Y. and J.K. Chan, *Epstein-Barr virus and T-cell lymphoma*. Histopathology, 1994. **25**(5): p. 501–2.

7. Hue, S.S., et al., *Epstein-Barr virus-associated T- and NK-cell lymphoproliferative diseases: an update and diagnostic approach*. Pathology, 2020. **52**(1): p. 111–27.

8. Dupuis, J., et al., *Expression of CXCL13 by neoplastic cells in angioimmunoblastic T-cell lymphoma (AITL): a new diagnostic marker providing evidence that AITL derives from follicular helper T cells*. Am J Surg Pathol, 2006. **30**(4): p. 490–4.

9. Jhuang, J.Y., et al., *Extranodal natural killer/T-cell lymphoma, nasal type in Taiwan: a relatively higher frequency of T-cell lineage and poor survival for extranasal tumors*. Hum Pathol, 2015. **46**(2): p. 313–21.

10. Li, S., et al., *Extranodal NK/T-cell lymphoma, nasal type: a report of 73 cases at MD Anderson Cancer Center*. Am J Surg Pathol, 2013. **37**(1): p. 14–23.

11. Pileri, S.A., *Follicular helper T-cell-related lymphomas*. Blood, 2015. **126**(15): p. 1733–4.

12. Soderquist, C.R. and G. Bhagat, *Gastrointestinal T- and NK-cell lymphomas and indolent lymphoproliferative disorders*. Semin Diagn Pathol, 2020. **37**(1): p. 11–23.

13. Vega, F., L.J. Medeiros, and P. Gaulard, *Hepatosplenic and other gammadelta T-cell lymphomas*. Am J Clin Pathol, 2007. **127**(6): p. 869–80.

14. Ferreri, A.J., S. Govi, and S.A. Pileri, *Hepatosplenic gamma-delta T-cell lymphoma*. Crit Rev Oncol Hematol, 2012. **83**(2): p. 283–92.

15. Yamaguchi, M., *Hepatosplenic gamma delta T-cell lymphoma: difficulty in diagnosis*. Intern Med, 2004. **43**(2): p. 83–4.

16. Bossard, C., et al., *Immunohistochemistry as a valuable tool to assess CD30 expression in peripheral T-cell lymphomas: high correlation with mRNA levels*. Blood, 2014. **124**(19): p. 2983–6.

17. Loghavi, S., et al., *Immunophenotypic and diagnostic characterization of angioimmunoblastic T-cell lymphoma by advanced flow cytometric technology*. Leuk Lymphoma, 2016: p. 1–9.

18. Tian, S., et al., *Monomorphic epitheliotropic intestinal T-cell lymphoma may mimic intestinal inflammatory disorders*. Int J Immunopathol Pharmacol, 2019. **33**: p. 2058738419829387.

19. Hwang, S.T., et al., *Mycosis fungoides and Sezary syndrome*. Lancet, 2008. **371**(9616): p. 945–57.

20. Song, S.X., et al., *Mycosis fungoides: report of the 2011 society for hematopathology/European association for haematopathology workshop*. Am J Clin Pathol, 2013. **139**(4): p. 466–90.

21. Kwong, Y.L., *Natural killer-cell malignancies: diagnosis and treatment*. Leukemia, 2005. **19**(12): p. 2186–94.

22. Jaffe, E.S., *Pathobiology of peripheral T-cell lymphomas*. Hematology Am Soc Hematol Educ Program, 2006: p. 317–22.

23. Jaffe, E.S., et al., *The pathologic spectrum of adult T-cell leukemia/lymphoma in the United States. Human T-cell leukemia/lymphoma virus-associated lymphoid malignancies*. Am J Surg Pathol, 1984. **8**(4): p. 263–75.

24. Weisenburger, D.D., et al., *Peripheral T-cell lymphoma, not otherwise specified: a report of 340 cases from the International Peripheral T-cell Lymphoma Project*. Blood, 2011. **117**(12): p. 3402–8.

25. Dearden, C.E. and F.M. Foss, *Peripheral T-cell lymphomas: diagnosis and management*. Hematol Oncol Clin North Am, 2003. **17**(6): p. 1351–66.

26. Cook, L.B., et al., *Revised adult T-cell leukemia-lymphoma international consensus meeting report*. J Clin Oncol, 2019. **37**(8): p. 677–87.

27. Willemze, R., et al., *Subcutaneous panniculitis-like T-cell lymphoma: definition, classification, and prognostic factors: an EORTC Cutaneous Lymphoma Group Study of 83 cases*. Blood, 2008. **111**(2): p. 838–45.

28. Mioduszewska, O., *T-cell lymphomas*. Arch Geschwulstforsch, 1979. **49**(8): p. 685–93.

29. Dearden, C.E., *T-cell prolymphocytic leukemia*. Clin Lymphoma Myeloma, 2009. **9 Suppl 3**: p. S239–S243.

30. Swerdlow, S.H., et al., *The 2016 revision of the World Health Organization classification of lymphoid neoplasms*. Blood, 2016. **127**(20): p. 2375–90.

31. Prieto-Torres, L., et al., *Large cells with CD30 expression and Hodgkin-like features in primary cutaneous marginal zone B-cell lymphoma: a study of 13 cases*. Am J Surg Pathol, 2019. **43**(9): p. 1191–202.

32. Huang, Y., et al., *Peripheral T-cell lymphomas with a follicular growth pattern are derived from follicular helper T cells (TFH) and may show overlapping features with angioimmunoblastic T-cell lymphomas*. Am J Surg Pathol, 2009. **33**(5): p. 682–90.

33. Agostinelli, C., et al., *Peripheral T cell lymphomas with follicular T helper phenotype: a new basket or a distinct entity? Revising Karl Lennert's personal archive*. Histopathology, 2011. **59**(4): p. 679–91.

34. Dobay, M.P., et al., *Integrative clinicopathological and molecular analyses of angioimmunoblastic T-cell lymphoma and other nodal lymphomas of follicular helper T-cell origin*. Haematologica, 2017. **102**(4): p. e148–51.

35. Rodriguez-Pinilla, S.M., et al., *Peripheral T-cell lymphoma with follicular T-cell markers*. Am J Surg Pathol, 2008. **32**(12): p. 1787–99.

36. Lemonnier, F., et al., *Recurrent TET2 mutations in peripheral T-cell lymphomas correlate with TFH-like features and adverse clinical parameters*. Blood, 2012. **120**(7): p. 1466–9.

37. Palomero, T., et al., *Recurrent mutations in epigenetic regulators, RHOA and FYN kinase in peripheral T cell lymphomas*. Nat Genet, 2014. **46**(2): p. 166–70.

38. Maitre, E., et al., *Usefulness of flow cytometry for the detection of cutaneous localization in malignant hematologic disorders*. Cytometry B Clin Cytom, 2019. **96**(4): p. 283–93.

39. Jones, D., et al., *Absence of CD26 expression is a useful marker for diagnosis of T-cell lymphoma in peripheral blood*. Am J Clin Pathol, 2001. **115**(6): p. 885–92.

40. Kelemen, K., et al., *The usefulness of CD26 in flow cytometric analysis of peripheral blood in Sezary syndrome*. Am J Clin Pathol, 2008. **129**(1): p. 146–56.

41. Gorczyca, W., et al., *CD30-positive T-cell lymphomas co-expressing CD15: an immunohistochemical analysis*. Int J Oncol, 2003. **22**(2): p. 319–24.

16

MATURE T/NK-CELL LYMPHOPROLIFERATIVE DISORDERS

T-cell prolymphocytic leukemia (T-PLL)

T-PLL phenotype by flow cytometry: CD2$^{+/-}$, CD3$^{+/-}$, CD4$^+$ (less often CD8$^+$, CD4/CD8$^+$ or CD4/CD8$^-$), CD5$^{+/-}$, CD7$^{+/-}$, CD25$^-$, CD26$^+$, CD45$^{+/rarely-}$, CD56$^-$, CD57$^-$, CD81$^+$, CD117$^{-/rarely+}$, CD200$^-$

Introduction

T-cell prolymphocytic leukemia (T-PLL) is a rare mature (post-thymic) T-cell lymphoproliferative disorder (T-LPD) which affects adults with median age of 64 years, occurs more frequently in men, and is characterized by aggressive clinical course and poor outcome [1–4]. The World Health Organization (WHO) classification defines T-PLL as aggressive T-cell leukemia of proliferating small to medium sized T-lymphocytic cells with prominent nucleoli, that despite their post-thymic origin and mature phenotype are called T-prolymphocytes [1, 2, 4–7]. The principal disease characteristics are B-symptoms, organomegaly (especially splenomegaly and lymphadenopathy), anemia, thrombocytopenia, and prominent (often rapidly increasing) lymphocytosis in blood ($>100 \times 10^9$/L) with involvement of bone marrow (BM). Nodal and extranodal presentation is also frequent, including involvement of the skin, liver, pleural or peritoneal cavities, and central nervous system (CNS) [1, 8]. Skin manifestations include nodules, maculopapular rash, or, rarely, erythroderma. Peripheral edema, particularly periorbital and/or conjunctival occurs relatively frequently in T-PLL [9, 10]. There is no association with human T-cell lymphotropic viruses (HTLV-I/II) [11]. Prior to the use of pentostatin and alemtuzumab in clinical protocols, outcome for T-PLL patients was exceedingly poor (median survival <1 year).

Morphology

Blood. In the blood film, leukemic cells have scanty basophilic cytoplasm without cytoplasmic granules and prominent nucleolus (Figure 16.1). In a subset of cases the nucleolus may be inconspicuous, resembling B-CLL cells or irregular resembling "flower" or Sézary's cells.

The main cytomorphologic variants of T-PLL [1, 2, 5, 8, 12]:

- Medium-sized cell variant (75% of cases) with a high nuclear/cytoplasmic ratio, moderately condensed chromatin, a single visible nucleolus, and a slightly basophilic cytoplasm without granules but typically demonstrating cytoplasmic protrusions (blebs)
- Small cell variant (20% of cases) with condensed chromatin and a nucleolus that is invisible by light microscopy
- Cerebriform variant (5% of cases) with irregular nuclei similar to the cerebriform nuclei found in Sézary's cells of mycosis fungoides (MF)

Bone marrow. BM involvement (Figure 16.2) is usually characterized by prominent interstitial or diffuse lymphoid infiltrate but may be subtle or nodular. Reticulin fibrosis is increased.

Lymph nodes. T-PLL involvement of the lymph node is usually paracortical with preserved follicles and patent sinusoids but may be diffuse with total effacement of lymph node architecture (Figure 16.3). Leukemic cells are medium sized with nucleoli and frequent mitotic figures. Small cell infiltrate without prominent nucleoli (reminiscent of CLL) may be also present in subset of T-PLL cases.

Spleen. The spleen shows dense white and red pulp infiltration by small to medium-sized cells with nucleoli. Prominent white pulp infiltrate of follicles and marginal zone, with atrophic residual germinal centers creates vague nodular pattern. The lymphoid infiltrate in both portal areas and within sinusoids and cords may extend to capsule and perisplenic adipose tissue.

Effusions. Effusions may develop during the course of the disease but may be also seen at diagnosis. Cytologic features are similar to those observed in blood.

Skin. T-PLL often involves the skin (with a predilection to face and ears). The skin biopsies demonstrate a largely superficial but non-epidermotropic, angiocentric, and periadnexal lymphocytic infiltrate with accompanying hemorrhage. In some cases, T-PLL shows diffuse replacement of the dermis or prominent subcutaneous nodules.

Immunophenotype

Immunophenotypic analysis by immunohistochemistry or flow cytometry (FC) shows expression of CD45, pan-T antigens (CD2, CD3, CD5, CD7) and lack of expression of B-cell markers, HLA-DR, CD1a, TdT, and CD34 (Figures 16.4–16.6). Positive expression of all pan-T-cell makers is seen in 73% with normal expression (either moderate or bright) in 52% of cases (Figures 16.6 and 16.7); feature rarely seen in other T-cell lymphoproliferations. CD3 and CD7 are most often missing. In 61% of cases the T-PLL are CD4$^+$, in 23% they are CD8$^+$, in 14% they co-express CD4/CD8 (Figure 16.6) and in the remaining 5% they are CD4/CD8$^-$. Majority of cases shows moderate/bright expression of CD45. Rare cases of T-PLL may be CD45 negative (Figure 16.8) or show negative CD45 only on subset of cells (Figure 16.9). Subset of cases with CD8 expression often shows aberrant expression of CD117 (Figure 16.9). Overall, CD117 expression is seen in 15% of T-PLL. The CD52 antigen is expressed at high density on the malignant T-cells, CD25 is most often negative, CD26 and CD81 are positive, and CD200 is usually negative (Figure 16.10). Rare cases may be HLA-DR$^+$ (Figure 16.11). Many cases show overexpression of TCL1. Table 16.1 summarizes the phenotype of T-PLL.

Genetic features

T-PLL is genetically characterized by the presence of complex karyotypes in majority of cases (70%–80%) with recurrent alterations involving chromosomes 8, 11, and 14 including inv(14)(q11;q32), t(14;14)(q11;q32), and i(8)(q10) [13]. Consistent chromosomal translocations involving the T-cell receptor (TCR) gene and one of two protooncogenes (*TCL1* and *MTCP-1*) are seen in most cases and are likely to be involved in the pathogenesis of the disorder. Rearrangements involving *TCL1* (T-cell leukemia/lymphoma1) family genes *TCL1A*, *MTCP1* (mature

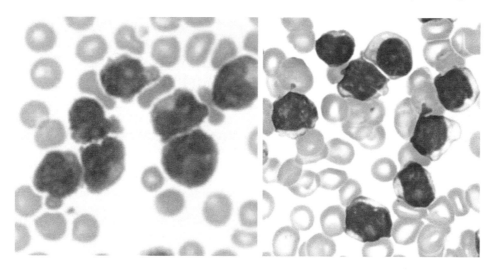

FIGURE 16.1   T-prolymphocytic leukemia (T-PLL) – peripheral blood films. Small to medium-sized lymphocytes with scanty basophilic cytoplasm and irregular nuclei with nucleoli predominate.

T-cell proliferation), or *TCL1B* (alias *TCL1/MTCP1*-like 1 [*TML1*]), are relatively specific for T-PLL and are present in more than 90% of cases, either as inv(14)(q11q32) or t(14;14)(q11;q32) (involving *TCL1A* or *TCL1B*), or t(X;14)(q28;q11) (involving *MTCP1*; mature T-cell proliferation). Detection of aberrant TCL1 protein expression via FC or immunohistochemistry is more sensitive than cytogenetics and represents a diagnostic hallmark. The translocations involving chromosome 14 juxtapose the locus of the *TCRAB* gene with the *TCL1* and *TCL1b* genes at 14q32 (Figure 16.12). Chromosome 14 abnormalities are often accompanied by complex karyotype (Figure 16.13). Comparative genomic hybridization (CGH) of T-PLL showed that chromosomal regions most often over-represented were 8q (75%), 5p (62%), and 14q (37%), as well as 6p and 21 (both 25%), while the chromosomal regions most often underrepresented were 8p and 11q (75%), 13q (37%), and 6q, 7q, 16q, 17p, and 17q (25%) [14].

Differential diagnosis of T-PLL
Blood and BM
Algorithmic approach to T-cell disorders is presented in Figures 15.1 and 15.2 (Chapter 15). The major phenotypic characteristics of mature T-cell neoplasms are presented in Table 16.2.

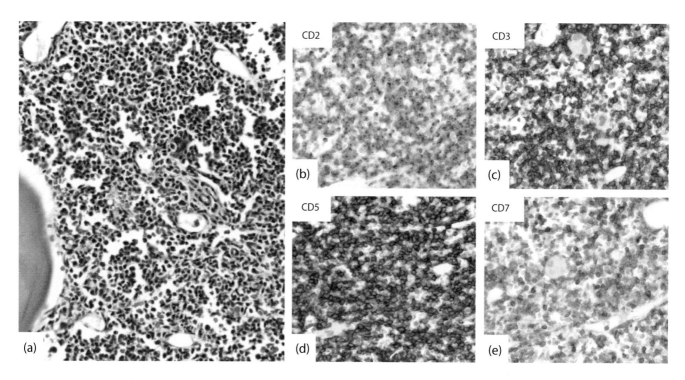

FIGURE 16.2   T-prolymphocytic leukemia (T-PLL) – bone marrow. Core biopsy shows prominent lymphocytosis of predominantly small lymphocytes (a) with positive expression of all four T-cell antigens (b–e). The expression of CD2 and CD7 (a, e) is slightly dimmer than the expression of CD3 and CD5 (c, d).

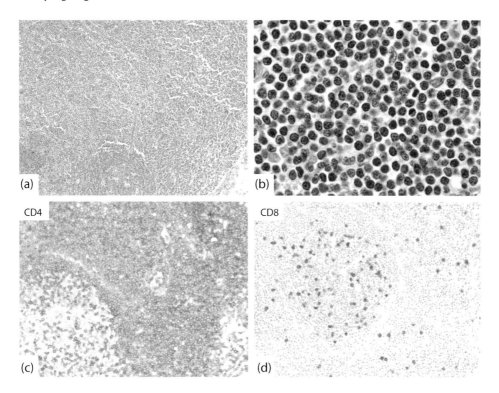

FIGURE 16.3 T-prolymphocytic leukemia (T-PLL) – lymph node. (a) Low magnification shows diffuse lymphoid infiltrate sparing of the follicle. (b) High magnification shows predominance of small, mature-appearing lymphocytes. Neoplastic cells show CD4 restriction (c and d).

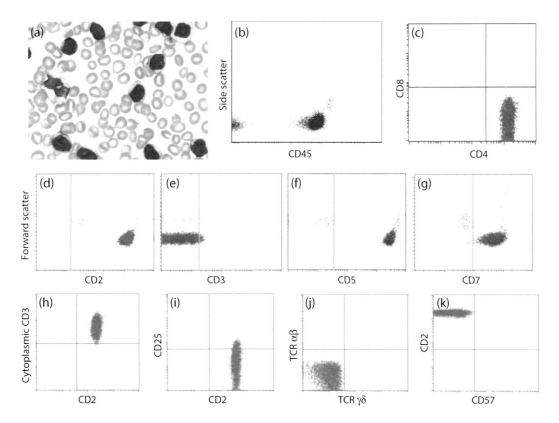

FIGURE 16.4 T-PLL – flow cytometry. (a) Peripheral blood film with marked lymphocytosis. (b–k) Flow cytometry analysis of blood shows predominance of lymphocytes (red dots). Note the paucity of granulocytes and monocytes. Lymphocytes display CD4 subset restriction (c) and bright expression of CD2 (d), lack of surface CD3 (e), bright CD5 (f), and positive CD7 (g). Cytoplasmic CD3 is positive (h). Neoplastic lymphocytes do not co-express CD25 (i), TCR alpha/beta, TCR gamma/delta (j) or CD57 (k).

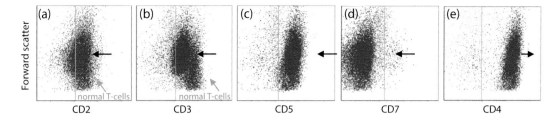

FIGURE 16.5 T-PLL – flow cytometry. Lymphomatous cells (black arrow) show increased forward scatter (a–e; compare to residual normal T-cells), positive CD2 (a), positive (dim) CD3 (b), positive CD5 (c), negative CD7 (d), and positive CD4 (e).

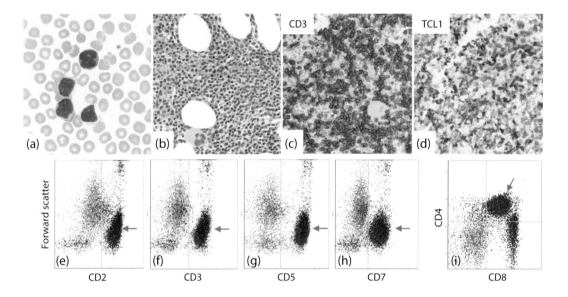

FIGURE 16.6 T-PLL with positive expression of all pan T-cell antigens. (a) Blood film shows atypical lymphoid cells with nucleoli. (b–d) BM shows prominent lymphoid infiltrate (b) expressing CD3 (c), and TCL1 (d). (e–i) Flow cytometry shows lymphoid cells (red dots, arrow) with normal expression of all pan T-cell antigens (e–h) and dual CD4/CD8 positivity (i).

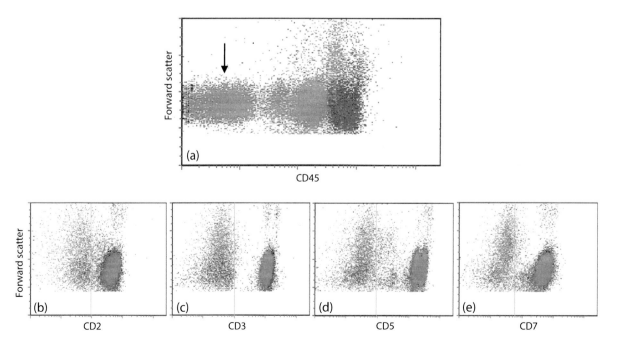

FIGURE 16.7 T-PLL with aberrant (partial) expression of CD45 (a) and normal expression of T-cell antigens (CD2, CD3, CD5, and CD7; b–e) [green dots represent T-PLL; red dots represent benign B- and T-cells; gray dots represent granulocytes; arrows indicates CD45-negative cells].

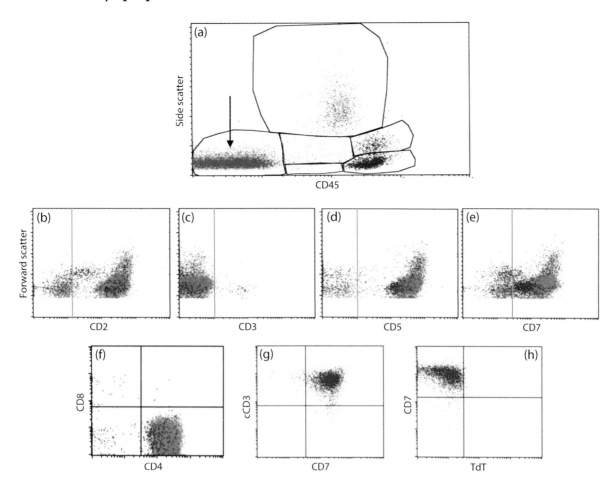

FIGURE 16.8 CD45-negative T-PLL – flow cytometry. T-PLL cells are negative for CD45 (a), surface CD3 (c), CD8 (f), and TdT (h); they express CD2 (b), CD5 (d), CD7 (e), CD8 (f), and cytoplasmic CD3 (g).

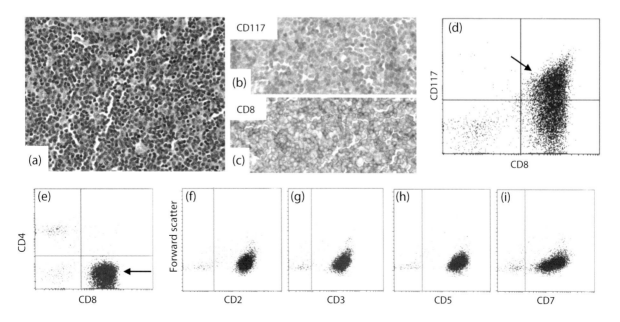

FIGURE 16.9 Lymph node involved by T-PLL with aberrant expression of CD117. (a) Histology: diffuse small lymphocytic infiltrate. (b–c) Immunohistochemistry. (d–i) Flow cytometry. Lymphomatous cells show aberrant expression of CD117 (b, immunohistochemistry; d, flow cytometry) and are CD4⁻/CD8⁺ (c, immunohistochemistry; e, flow cytometry). Leukemic cells show normal expression of all pan T-cell antigens (CD2, CD3, CD5, CD7; f–i).

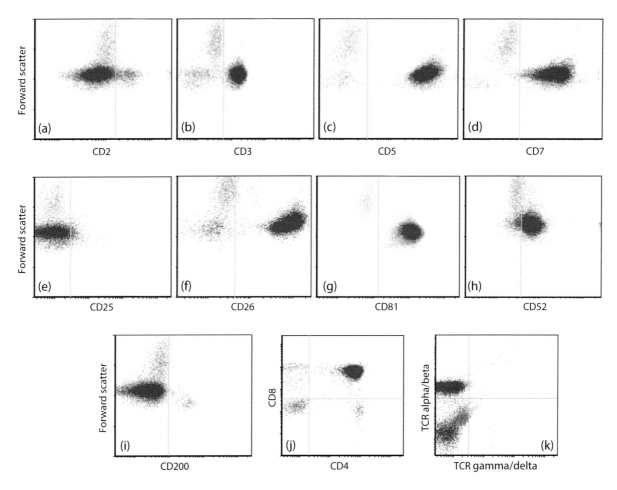

FIGURE 16.10 T-PLL – flow cytometry. Leukemic cells (red dots) display the following phenotype: CD2⁻ (a), CD3⁺ (b), CD5⁺ (c), CD7⁺ (d), CD25⁻ (e), CD26⁺ (f), CD81⁺ (g), CD52⁺ (h), CD200⁻ (i), dual CD4/CD8⁺ (j), and TCR alpha/beta⁺ (k).

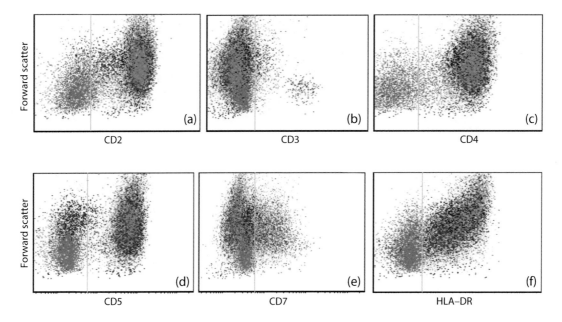

FIGURE 16.11 T-PLL with aberrant loss of CD3 and positive HLA-DR – flow cytometry analysis. 74-year-old man with WBC of 64 × 10⁹/L. Leukemic T-cells (orange dots) show the following phenotype: CD2⁺ (a), CD3⁻ (b, rare benign T-cells are positive – red dots), CD4⁺ (c), CD5⁺ (d), CD7⁻ (e, only rare leukemic cells are positive), and HLA-DR⁺ (f).

TABLE 16.1: Immunophenotypic Profile of T-PLL ($n = 63$ Cases)

All T-cell antigens positive (CD2, CD3, CD5, and CD7)	73%[a]
(All T-cell antigens normally expressed, moderate or bright)	(52%)
(At least one antigen with aberrant expression, dim, partial, or variable)	(19%)
One T-cell antigen negative	23%
Two T-cell antigens negative	6%
≥3 T-cell antigens negative	0
CD2+	95%
CD3+	91%[b]
CD5+	97%
CD7+	86%
CD4+	61%
CD8+	23%
CD4+/CD8+	14%
CD4−/CD8−	5%
CD10+	0
CD11c+	3%
CD45−	9%
CD56+	6%
CD117+	15%[c]
HLA-DR+	2%

[a] Among 33 cases with normal expression of all 4 pan T-cell antigens, 2 cases were CD45−, 7 cases were CD117+, and 5 cases were dual CD4/CD8+.

[b] Surface CD3.

[c] Expression of CD117 (dim or partial) was restricted to CD8+ cases.

Differential diagnosis of T-PLL includes (Figure 16.14):

- Reactive lymphocytosis
- Splenic B-cell lymphoma with prominent nucleoli (SBLPN)
- Chronic lymphocytic leukemia (CLL)
- Adult T-cell lymphoma/leukemia (ATLL)
- Splenic marginal zone lymphoma (SMZL)
- Sézary's syndrome (SS)
- Hairy cell leukemia (HCL)
- Hairy cell leukemia variant (HCL-v)
- B-cell lymphomas in leukemic phase
- Peripheral T-cell lymphomas (PTCLs) in leukemic phase
- T-large granular lymphocyte leukemia (T-LGLL)
- Chronic lymphoproliferative disorder of NK-cells (CLPD-NK)
- T-cell acute lymphoblastic leukemia (T-ALL)
- B-cell acute lymphoblastic leukemia (B-ALL)
- Acute myeloid leukemia (AML)
- Blastic plasmacytoid dendritic cell neoplasm (BPDCN)
- Plasma cell leukemia (PCL)

Benign processes (reactive T-cell lymphocytosis). Reactive T-cell lymphocytosis is seen commonly in blood samples due to transient proliferation of T-cells in acute viral infections, especially Epstein-Barr virus (EBV) and cytomegalovirus (CMV), some medications, post-vaccination, in autoimmune disorders or induced by stress (trauma, myocardial infarct, and cerebrovascular accidents). Relative T-cell lymphocytosis is observed in severe neutropenia. Benign T-cell lymphocytosis is also observed in patients with thymoma. Some of reactive processes (most often due to EBV infection, CMV or HIV) may show expansion of CD8+

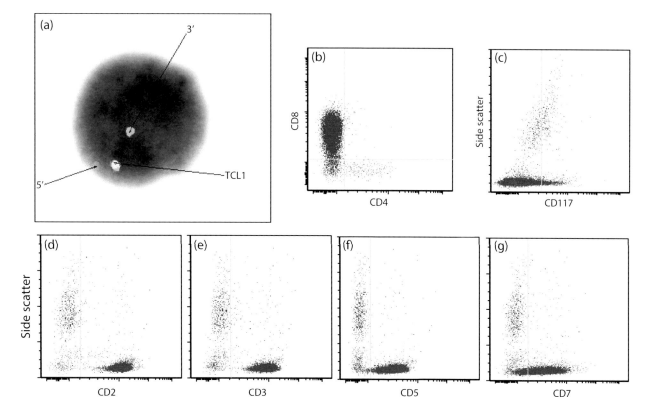

FIGURE 16.12 T-PLL. FISH analysis confirmed the rearrangement of *TCL1* gene (a). Flow cytometry shows CD8 restriction (b), dim CD117 on minute subset (c), and positive expression of all T-cell antigens (d–g) with CD7 being slightly dimmer.

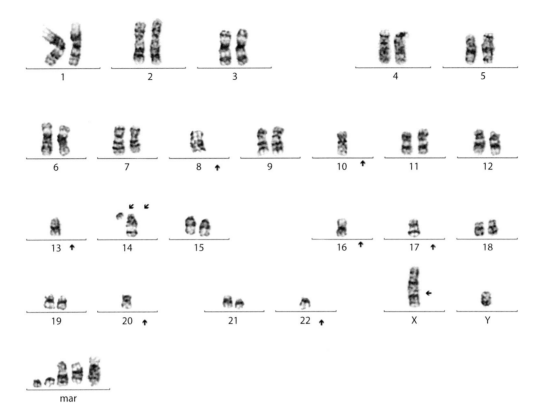

FIGURE 16.13 T-PLL with an abnormal male karyotype positive for translocation t(X;14)(q28;q11.2). Cytogenetic analysis shows an abnormal hypodiploid clone (3 out of 20 cells) characterized by a reciprocal translocation between chromosomes Xq28 and 14q11.2, loss of one copy of chromosomes 8, 10, 13, 16, 17, 20, and 22, addition of material of unknown origin to 14q24, and the presence of 4–6 marker chromosomes. Seventeen normal cells were found during the course of analysis. Translocation t(X;14) is associated with TCR alpha/delta (14q11.2) and *MTCP1* (Xq28) gene rearrangement, which leads to overexpression of *MTCP1*.

T-cells and subtle phenotypic atypia including variably increased forward scatter, dim CD5 expression and/or loss of CD7 expression. These phenotypic features in conjunction with presence of splenomegaly and/or immune-mediated anemia or thrombocytopenia in some patients with viral infections can make the differential diagnosis between reactive process and T-PLL difficult if based solely on FC findings. T-PLL would be more likely if there is CD4 restriction or dual CD4/CD8 positivity, significant and progressing lymphocytosis, and prominent splenomegaly (with or without adenopathy and hepatomegaly). Reactive processes are transient and usually show mixture of B-cells and T-cells including both T-LGL cells (CD3+/CD8+/CD57+) and NK-cells (CD3−/CD56+). Cytologically, reactive lymphocytes in viral infections differ from prolymphocytes with a range of morphologic features, some with immunoblast-like morphology with high nuclear-cytoplasmic ratios and deeply basophilic cytoplasm and other with less condensed chromatin and abundant, pale blue cytoplasm that may appear to "hug" adjacent red blood cells (Downey type II cells). T-PLL occurs usually in elderly patients (men > women) and is characterized by prominent, progressing lymphocytosis in blood (often >100 × 10⁹/L), clonal T-cell gene rearrangement, frequent chromosome 14 abnormalities, prominent splenomegaly with or without hepatomegaly and adenopathy, and characteristic cytologic features on blood smear.

CLL/SLL. Subset of T-PLL presents with lymphocytosis composed of small, mature lymphocytes reminiscent of CLL, and subset of CLL shows increased number of prolymphocytes or

cytologic atypia imitating T-cell process. FC analysis helps in the differential diagnosis. CLL/SLL is positive for B-cell antigens (CD19, CD20), surface light chain immunoglobulins, CD5, CD23, and HLA-DR. Occasional CLL cases may show an aberrant expression of T-cell markers, including CD2, CD4, CD7, or CD8. But CLL is always negative for surface and cytoplasmic CD3.

SBLPN and other mature B-cell lymphomas/leukemias. B-cell lymphomas with blood involvement are distinguished form T-PLL by expression of B-cell antigens (CD19, CD20, CD22, CD79), surface immunoglobulins and HLA-DR. Additional markers seen in mature B-cell disorders include expression of CD10 in follicular lymphoma (FL), Burkitt lymphoma (BL), majority of high grade B-cell lymphomas with *MYC* and *BCL2* rearrangement (HGBL-R), and subset of diffuse large B-cell lymphoma (DLBCL), CD11c, CD25, CD123, and CD103 in HCL, CD103 in HCL-v, and CD5 and CD81 in mantle cell lymphoma (MCL). The majority of cases with B-cell phenotype and marked lymphocytosis with "prolymphocytic" cytomorphology represent leukemic MCL or prolymphocytic transformation of low grade B-cell lymphomas. T-PLL can easily be distinguished from SBLPN by immunophenotyping. SBLPN is positive for B-cell markers (CD19, CD20, CD22, and CD79a), surface immunoglobulins, and HLA-DR (subset of cases may be CD5+ and/or CD23+). Leukemic MCL is confirmed by FISH studies for *CCND1* rearrangement.

ATLL and SS. ATLL (acute variant) and SS may show similar to T-PLL clinical and laboratory features (marked lymphocytosis, skin and lymph node involvement, atypical cytomorphology

TABLE 16.2: Classification of Mature T-Cell Neoplasms

Category	Major Characteristics	Phenotype
T-cell prolymphocytic leukemia (T-PLL)	Marked lymphocytosis; hepatosplenomegaly, lymphadenopathy; inv14q	CD2+, CD3+, CD5+, CD7+
T-cell large granular lymphocytic leukemia (T-LGL leukemia)	Neutropenia; indolent clinical course	CD3+, CD8+, CD57+
Aggressive NK-cell leukemia	Fever, hemophagocytic syndrome	CD2+, CD3–, CD56+
Adult T-cell leukemia/lymphoma (ATLL)	Associated with HTLV-1; blood and lymph node involvement	CD2+, CD3±, CD5+, CD7–, CD25+
Extranodal NK/T-cell lymphoma, nasal type (ENKTL)	Angiodestructive growth pattern	CD2+, CD56+, EBER+
Enteropathy-associated T-cell lymphoma (EATL)	May be associated with celiac disease	CD2+, CD3+, CD5–, CD7–, CD8+ or CD4/CD8–, CD103+
Hepatosplenic T-cell lymphoma (HSTL)	Hepatosplenomegaly	CD2+, CD3+, CD5–, CD7±, TCRγδ+, CD56±
Subcutaneous panniculitis-like T-cell lymphoma (SPTCL)	Subcutaneous nodules	CD8+, CD56–, TCRαβ+
Mycosis fungoides (MF)	Indolent clinical course	CD2+, CD3+, CD5±, CD7–, CD4+/CD8–
Sézary syndrome (SS)	Erythroderma; lymphadenopathy; T-cells with cerebriform nuclei in blood, skin, and lymph nodes	CD2+, CD3+, CD5+/–, CD7–, CD4+/CD8–
Primary cutaneous anaplastic large cell lymphoma		CD30+, ALK–
Lymphomatoid papulosis (LyP)	Chronic, recurrent, and self-healing skin lesions	CD30+
Primary cutaneous γδ T-cell lymphoma		CD2+, CD3+, CD5–, CD7±, CD56+, EBER–
Peripheral T-cell lymphoma, not otherwise specified (PTCL, NOS)	Nodal and extranodal disease	CD2+, CD3+, CD5+, CD7±, may be CD30+
Nodal TFH cell lymphoma, angioimmunoblastic-type (AITL)	Generalized adenopathy; polyclonal hypergammaglobulinemia, hepatosplenomegaly, polytypic plasma cells in blood	CD4+, CD2+, CD3±, CD5+, CD7±, often CD10+
Anaplastic large cell lymphoma (ALCL); ALK+	Nodal and extranodal disease; favorable prognosis compared to ALK– ALCL	CD30+, ALK+;
Anaplastic large cell lymphoma (ALCL); ALK–	Advanced stage disease; morphology similar to ALK+ ALCL; poorer prognosis than in ALK+ ALCL	CD30+, ALK–

of lymphocytes). ATLL often presents with hypercalcemia and lytic bone lesions. The leukemic cells in SS and ATLL are CD4+ and have more pronounced variations in size and shape of nuclei. Both Sézary cells of SS and "flower cells" of ATLL show prominent nuclear irregularities, usually with clumped chromatin without prominent nucleoli. In addition, both SS and ATLL may also show eosinophilia in addition to lymphocytosis (eosinophilia is not a typical feature in T-PLL). In contrast to T-PLL, ATLL always displays an abnormal expression of pan-T antigens (loss of CD7 and less often loss of CD3). CD2 and CD5 are positive in majority of ATLL cases. ATLL are CD25+ and CD26–, while T-PLL are most often CD25– and CD26+. Clinical and laboratory data are helpful in the differential diagnosis, hypercalcemia, lytic bone lesions, skin rash with papulonodular skin lesion and positive HTLV-1 in ATLL or erythroderma involving almost all skin surface area and history of MF in SS.

PTCL. PTCL rarely involves blood and is characterized by more pleomorphic T-cells composed of medium-sized to large cells which display aberrant expression of pan-T antigens in more than 90% of cases. In most cases, blood involvement in PTCL is a manifestation of disease progression, and usually there is a history of adenopathy and/or prior diagnosis of PTCL. Hepatosplenic T-cell lymphoma (HSTL) shows characteristic intrasinusoidal BM involvement and less pronounced lymphocytosis.

BPDCN. Most patients present with skin tumors with frequent progression to leukemic blood (and BM) involvement. Tumor cells are intermediate to large with blastic cytomorphology. They are positive for CD4, CD56, CD43, CD123, and often TdT and are negative for CD3, CD5, and MPO. They may show aberrant expression of CD2, CD7, and/or CD33.

T-LGLL and CLPD-NK. Two main variants of LGL proliferations can be recognized: T-LGLL and CLPD-NK. Both are characterized by lymphoid cells with prominent cytoplasmic azurophilic granules. T-LGLL shows persistent (>6 months) lymphocytosis in blood (≥2 × 10⁹/L) with frequent involvement of BM, liver, and spleen. Most cases have indolent clinical course with neutropenia. T-LGLL may be associated with red cell aplasia, hypergammaglobulinemia, and rheumatoid arthritis. Leukemic cells are most often CD8+, CD2+, CD3+, and CD57+ (subset of cases may also show expression of CD16 and/or CD56). CLPD-NK is less common than T-LGLL and is characterized by persistent (>6 months) increase in NK cells in blood (≥2 × 10⁹/L) and chronic, non-progressive clinical course. Patients with CLPD-NK are most often asymptomatic. Some patients have anemia and/or neutropenia. Lymphadenopathy, organomegaly or skin involvements are infrequent. NK-cells are typically CD2+, CD3–, CD5–, CD7+, CD16+, and CD56+ (only rare cases are CD57+).

T-ALL. Both cytologic features and presence of either dual CD4/CD8 positivity or dual CD4CD8 negativity in T-PLL overlap

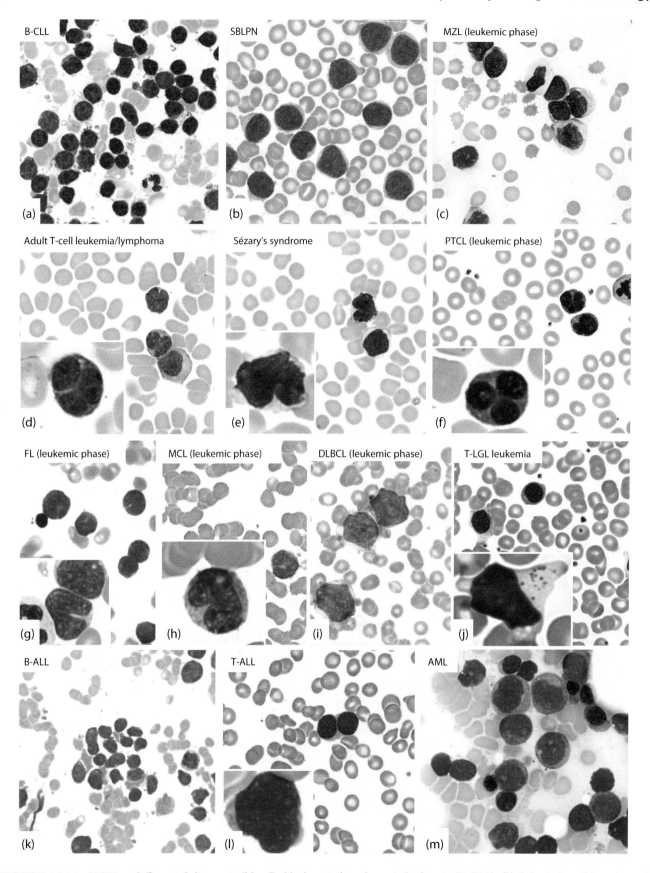

FIGURE 16.14 T-PLL – differential diagnosis (blood): (a) chronic lymphocytic leukemia (B-CLL); (b) Splenic B-cell lymphoma/leukemia with prominent nucleoli (SBLPN); (c) marginal zone lymphoma (MZL); (d) adult T-cell lymphoma/leukemia (ATLL); (e) Sézary's syndrome; (f) peripheral T-cell lymphoma, not otherwise specified (PTCL, NOS); (g) leukemic phase of follicular lymphoma (FL), (h) mantle cell lymphoma (MCL); (i) leukemic phase of DLBCL; (j) T-LGL leukemia; (k) B-ALL; (l) T-ALL; and (m) acute myeloid leukemia (AML).

with T-ALL. T-ALL is distinguished phenotypically by expression of one or more of blastic markers (TdT, CD34, and/or CD1a), moderate to bright expression of CD7 and frequent lack of surface CD3. Majority of T-ALL cases show abnormal chromosomal studies with numerous structural and numeric abnormalities.

B-ALL. B-ALL is positive for CD19, CD79a, HLA-DR, CD34, and TdT, often shows bright CD10.

AML. Cytologic features of T-PLL in conjunction with occasional expression of CD117 may require differential diagnosis from AML. AMLs show expression of pan-myeloid antigens (CD13, CD33), MPO, CD117 and often CD34 and HLA-DR, and most often lack pan-T antigens, except for occasional aberrant expression of CD7 and less often CD5.

Adult T-cell lymphoma/leukemia (ATLL)

ATLL phenotype by FC: CD2$^{+/-}$, CD3$^{+/-}$, CD4$^+$ (rarely CD4/CD8$^+$), CD5$^+$, CD7$^{-/rarely+}$, CD8$^-$, CD25$^+$, CD26$^-$, CD45$^+$, CD56$^-$, CD57$^-$, CCR4$^+$

Introduction
ATLL is an aggressive T-cell malignancy associated with human T-cell leukemia virus type 1 (HTLV1) infection, characterized by marked diversity in clinical manifestations and presence of highly pleomorphic lymphoid cells [1, 15–19]. Tumor cells have prominent nuclear irregularities, often referred to as *cloverleaf* or *flower* cells (seen mostly in acute subtype and only rarely in smoldering or chronic subtypes). ATLL affects adults with leukemic or subleukemic presentation, cutaneous involvement, lymphadenopathy, and/or organomegaly. Hypercalcemia is present in up to 50% of patients and may results in renal failure. Patients are at increased risk for bacterial and viral infections.

Clinical variants. Several clinical variants of ATLL are recognized (Shimoyama classification with 2019 update) [1, 15, 17, 20]:

- Chronic
- Smoldering
- Acute
- Lymphomatous
- Extranodal primary cutaneous

The acute (60% of cases) and lymphomatous (20%) are the most common variants and extranodal primary cutaneous variant is least common. A borderline state between healthy carriers of HTLV1 and ATLL has been named pre-ATLL. Pre-ATLL can resolve or progress into one of the variants of ATLL. The acute type generally presents with lymphocytosis, elevated LDH, hypercalcemia, hepatosplenomegaly, adenopathy, lytic bone lesions, eosinophilia, and frequent involvement of skin. It may involve the BM. The lymphomatous type of ATLL is characterized by prominent adenopathy and often shows other features seen in leukemic form (hepatosplenomegaly, bone and skin lesions, and visceral organ involvement), but without blood involvement. The chronic type presents with mild absolute lymphocytosis (≥4 × 10^9/L) lymphadenopathy and skin involvement but without CNS, bone, gastrointestinal tract, or body cavities involvement. Absolute lymphocytosis ≥4 × 10^9/L of immunophenotypically abnormal lymphocytes (with T-lymphocytes ≥3.5 × 10^9/L) is required for the diagnosis [15, 17]. The smoldering subtype presents with ≥5% abnormal lymphocytes in blood, skin, and/or lung lesions but without absolute lymphocytes, adenopathy, and involvement liver, spleen CNS, gastrointestinal tract, or body cavities. The extranodal primary cutaneous variant has been recently added as a new subtype of ATLL. It is characterized by extensive skin involvement at the time of diagnosis without leukemic presentation or other organ involvement [15].

Prognosis. Chronic and smoldering variants are clinically indolent, whereas acute and lymphomatous variants show a highly aggressive clinical behavior and extremely poor prognosis (median survival <1 year), due to chemoresistance and severe immunosuppression, large tumor burden with multiorgan failure, hypercalcemia, and frequent infections [20–24]. The 4-year survival rate is 66% for the smoldering type, 27% for the chronic type, and 5%–6% for the lymphomatous and acute types [25, 26]. Indolent variants of ATLL can progress to aggressive variants, occasionally referred to as "crisis variants" [19]. On the other hand, spontaneous regression can be observed in sporadic cases [25, 26].

Morphology
Blood. Blood findings vary depending on the stage, gradually progressing from carrier to smoldering, chronic and acute-type leukemia.

Lymphocytes in ATLL display following cytologic features:

- "Flower" ("clover") cells: Intermediate to occasionally large cells with convoluted nuclear contours (flower-petal-like nuclear lobes) without prominent nucleoli and basophilic cytoplasm with or without vacuolation.
- Sézary's cells: Intermediate to occasionally large cells with prominent hyperconvoluted nuclei with cerebriform-like nuclear lobation, condensed chromatin without visible nucleoli, and with abundant, irregularly shaped, and basophilic cytoplasm with occasional vacuoles.
- Immunoblastic cells: Large, transformed lymphocytes with high nuclear-cytoplasmic ratios, prominent often central nucleolus, condensed chromatin, and deeply basophilic cytoplasm.
- Prolymphocytes: Intermediate cells with round to oval central nuclei (without overtly irregular contours) with condensed chromatin with minimally coarse chromatin clumps along margins, prominent single round bluish nucleolus, and moderate amount of basophilic cytoplasm.
- Anaplastic cells: Large often multinucleated cells with prominent pleomorphism, irregular nuclei with hyperchromasia with or without multilobation, several nucleoli, and abundant often irregular cytoplasm. Some of the anaplastic cells may resemble Hodgkin or Reed-Sternberg cells.
- Large lymphocytes: Large cells with round or irregular (pleomorphic) hyperchromatic nuclei with coarse chromatin, several small nucleoli, and abundant pale bluish transparent cytoplasm with occasional vacuoles.
- Small lymphocytes: Small mature appearing lymphocytes with round dense nucleus with clumped chromatin without nucleoli, with thin rim of scant cytoplasm.

The cytomorphologic features varies and depends on the variant of ATLL. In smoldering and chronic variant cytologic atypia is minimal with only occasional "flower" cells, whereas acute and lymphomatous variants show marked atypia with numerous "flower" cells. On blood film the leukemic cells are medium

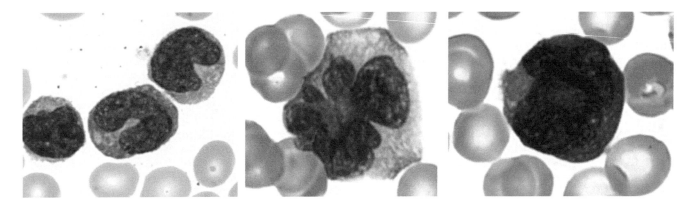

FIGURE 16.15 Adult T-cell leukemia/lymphoma (ATLL). Typical medium to large neoplastic cells with prominent nuclear pleomorphism ("flower cells").

sized to large with prominent nuclear contour irregularities, condensed chromatin, and basophilic cytoplasm (Figure 16.15). Many cells with polylobated nuclei are present with flower-like nuclear configuration giving the description of "flower cells" or "clover leaf". Nucleoli are either small or absent. Cytologic variants, reported in patients with ATLL include large cells, immunoblastic, anaplastic, prolymphocytic-like, and Sézary-like. At least 5% of circulating abnormal T-cells is required for the diagnosis of ATLL in patients without histologically proven lymphoma [20].

Bone marrow biopsy. BM may be involved in the acute variant of ATLL. BM infiltrate is usually subtle (even in patients with prominent lymphocytosis), interstitial and patchy and may be accompanied by fibrosis. Rare cases show mixed interstitial and focally paratrabecular infiltrate or diffuse BM involvement. Eosinophilia is often present. Number of osteoblasts and osteoclasts is often increased, accompanying bone resorption.

Lymph nodes. Lymph nodes are involved in chronic, acute, and lymphomatous variants of ATLL. Smoldering and extranodal primary cutaneous variants do not involve lymph nodes. In the lymphomatous variant, the neoplastic infiltrate may be diffuse (Figure 16.16) or paracortical with dilated sinuses (Figure 16.17). Similarly to other T-cell lymphomas, scattered eosinophils are often seen.

Patterns of lymph node changes in ATLL [19, 27, 28]:

• Anaplastic cell type
• Pleomorphic cell type

• Angioimmunoblastic T-cell lymphoma (AITL)-like type
• Hodgkin lymphoma-like type
• Lymphadenitis-like type
• Marginal zone lymphoma (MZL)-like type

Pleomorphic pattern may be further subdivided into small cell type and medium/large cell type. In pleomorphic small cell type, lymphoid cells are the size of normal blood lymphocytes with only minimal nuclear irregularities. In pleomorphic medium/large cell type, which is most the most characteristic pattern for ATLL, intermediate to large tumor cells show prominent nuclear contour irregularities, bizarre nuclei, and occasional Reed-Sternberg-like cells. Anaplastic large cell type shows monotonous infiltrate of large cells with prominent nucleoli and occasional Reed-Sternberg-like cells. In Hodgkin-like type, the infiltrate is composed of small to medium-sized lymphocytes with clusters of giant cells with multilobated nuclei resembling Reed-Sternberg cells and Hodgkin cells. The latter express CD30 and/or CD15 [27]. The AITL-like type of ATLL is rare and show pleomorphic infiltrate with inflammatory cells, including plasma cells and eosinophils, and clusters of medium to large cells with clear cytoplasm, as seen typically in AITL [27, 28]. Although the lymph node architecture in ATLL is usually effaced without follicle, rare cases may show an unusual MZL-like pattern of involvement.

Skin. Skin is frequently involved (up to 50% of patients) and it may be the first manifestation of the disease. Histologic

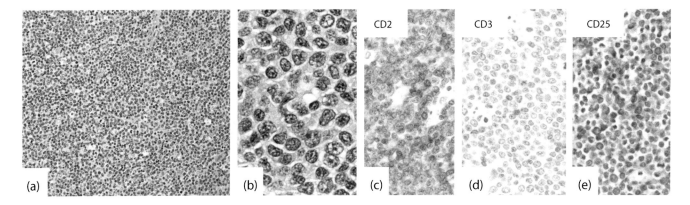

FIGURE 16.16 ATLL – lymph node. Diffuse infiltrate (a) of small to medium-sized lymphocytes with nuclear irregularities (b). Neoplastic T-cells are CD2+ (c), CD3− (d), and CD25+ (e).

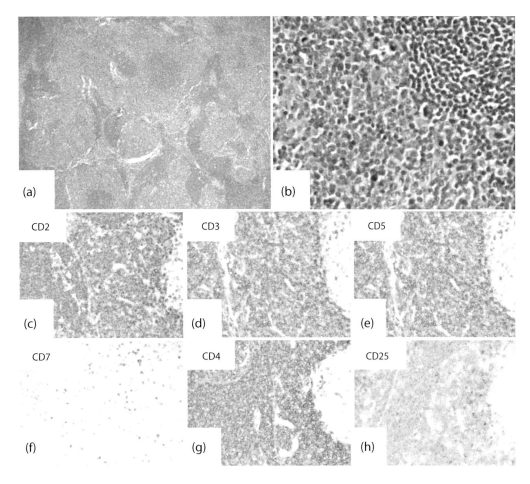

FIGURE 16.17 ATLL – lymph node with paracortical/perifollicular pattern of involvement by ATLL cells (a–b; H&E section at low and high magnification). Neoplastic cells are positive for CD2 (c), CD3 (d), and CD5 (e), do not express CD7 (f), and express CD4 (g) and CD25 (h).

manifestation of ATLL in skin is polymorphous and depending on the type of skin eruption [29].

Miyashiro et al. described three patterns characteristic of ATLL [29]:

- Superficial banded dermal infiltrate with epidermotropism
- Diffuse dermal infiltrate
- Nodular dermal infiltrate

Histomorphology usually resembles MF and less often anaplastic large cell lymphoma (ALCL) [30]. In a series reported by Bittencourt et al., MF-like pattern was found in 19 cases and ALCL-like pattern in two cases. Epidermotropism with Pautrier-type microabscesses, are frequently present. There is often perivascular pattern. Lymphoid cells are accompanied by plasma cells and eosinophils. Many cases show predominantly large cell diffuse lymphoid infiltrate. A variant of ATLL was proposed recently occurring in skin, extranodal primary cutaneous (tumoral) ATLL without leukemic blood involvement, lymph node, and other lesions [15, 31–33].

Other sites. Other sites which may be involved by neoplastic cells of ATLL include liver, skin, gastrointestinal tract, and head and neck [27, 34]. Extranodal adult T-cell leukemia/lymphoma (ATLL) of the head and neck is a rare disease. In a series reported by Miyagi, tumors involved the parotid gland, sinonasal tract, masseter muscle, mandible, and skull. Histopathology includes diffuse pleomorphic-type (with angiocentric features), Hodgkin-like and anaplastic large cell-type. Localized extranodal ATLL of the head and neck may exhibit indolent clinical behaviors [34].

Immunophenotype
ATLL cells are positive for CD4, CD5, CD25, HLA-DR, CCR4 and in most cases also for MUM1, CD2, and CD3 (Figures 16.18 and 16.19). The expression of CD3 is usually dimmer than in normal T-cells. Approximately one third of cases is negative for both TCRαβ and TCRγδ, and the remaining cases express TCRαβ. ATLL is usually negative for CD7 and does not express NK-cell associated antigens (CD16, CD56, and CD57), CD10, CD11b, CD11c, TIA1, granzyme PD1, and CXCL13. Subset of cases (~10%) may be dual CD4/CD8+ and rare cases are CD8+. The large, transformed cells within ATLL infiltrate may be positive for CD30 and cytotoxic molecules. Subset of cells in acute form of ATLL show positive CD30 expression (often variable, ranging from negative to dim to moderate; Figure 15.4; Chapter 15). Rare cases of ATLL may display aberrant expression of CD20 [35, 36]. Similar to cutaneous T-cell lymphomas involving blood (MF/SS), CD26 is often negative in ATLL [37, 38]. The expression of chemokine receptors, CCR4 and CCR7 by ATLL cells correlates with skin and nodal involvement [39, 40]. Kagdi et al. showed prognostic significant of CCR7 expression in ATLL [41]. All patients with aggressive ATLL

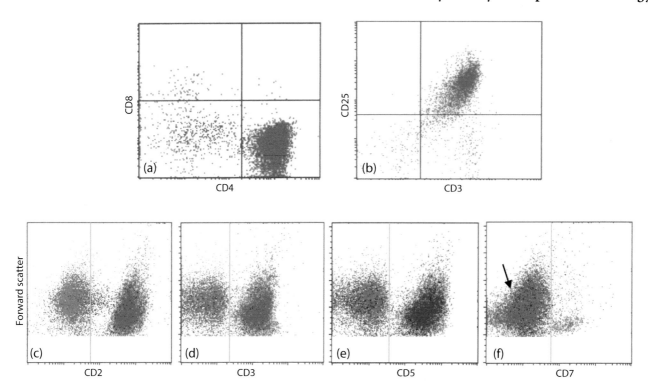

FIGURE 16.18   ATLL – flow cytometry of the bone marrow (a–b, without granulocytes; c–f, with granulocytes). ATLL cells show CD4 subset restriction (a) and CD25 expression (b). CD2 (c), CD3 (d), and CD5 (e) are positive, and CD7 is negative (f).

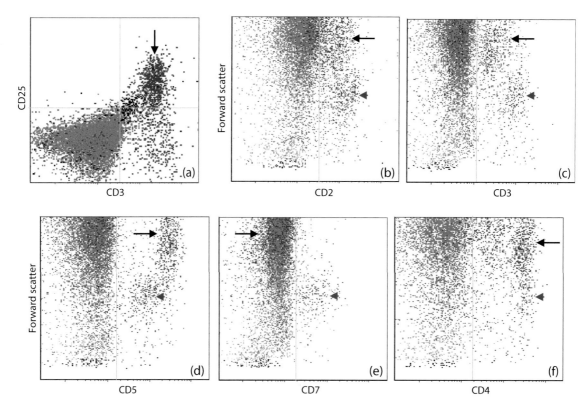

FIGURE 16.19   ATLL – flow cytometry of the bone marrow. Leukemic cells (black arrow) are CD3+ and CD25+ (a). They show high forward scatter (FSC; b-f; black arrows) similar to FSC of granulocytes (black dots). Normal (benign) T–cells (red arrowhead; b–f) show low FSC. The expression of CD2 is moderate (b), comparable to normal T-cells, the expression of CD3 is dim (c), the expression of CD5 is bright (d), and CD7 is negative (e). CD4 is positive (f).

had a CCR7+ (≥30%), whereas 92% with indolent ATLL and 100% non-ATLL had a CCR7− [41]. Immune T-cell activation associated with chronic viral infections, including asymptomatic carriage of HTLV-1, leads to upregulation of CD25 and downregulation of CD127 on T cells, two of the interleukin receptors [41].

Differential diagnosis of ATLL
Blood
Differential diagnosis of ATLL in blood includes (Table 16.2):

- SS
- T-PLL
- T-LGLL
- ALCL in leukemic phase
- PTCL in leukemic phase
- T-ALL
- B-cell lymphoproliferations
- PCL

Based on the presence of atypical circulating lymphocytes in blood, differential diagnosis includes other B- and T-cell lymphoproliferations (both mature and immature). B-cell lymphoproliferations, such a B-CLL, SBLPN, FL, and MCL can be distinguished by FC immunophenotyping. Based on the T-cell phenotype displaying by leukemic cells, diagnostic considerations include T-PLL, SS, T-lymphoblastic leukemia, and other T-cell lymphomas in leukemic phase. Flower cells and hypercalcemia help to exclude PTCL in leukemic phase, which is rare. CD25 is inconsistently and variably expressed in other T-cell lymphomas (including SS), in contrast to uniform and strong expression in ATLL. T-LGLL is positive for CD16, CD56, and/or CD57 and is usually CD8+. Rare PCLs may display flower-like nuclear cytomorphology. FC analysis of blood and testing for HTLV1 is important to confirm the diagnosis of ATLL and excludes its mimics.

Lymph nodes
Differential diagnosis of ATLL in lymph nodes includes:

- Peripheral T-cell lymphoma, not otherwise specified (PTCL, NOS)
- MF
- classic Hodgkin lymphoma (cHL)
- ALCL
- AITL
- T-PLL
- T-cell acute lymphoblastic leukemia/lymphoma (T-ALL/LBL)
- DLBCL
- MZL

ATLL often presents histomorphologic features that mimic other lymphomas, especially cHL. In the lymph node, considerations include HTLV1-associated adenopathy and involvement by PTCL, AITL, MF, T-PLL, T-ALL/LBL, DLBCL, cHL, MZL, AITL, and ALCL. ALCL can be distinguished by strong and uniform expression of CD30 (and ALK in cases of ALK+ ALCL). In contrast to majority of HL, large (transformed) CD30+ cells also express T-cell markers. B-cell lymphomas are distinguished by immunophenotyping. Correlation with clinical history, HTLV1 testing, serum calcium levels and blood smear may be helpful to differentiate lymph node involvement by ATLL from other T-cell lymphoproliferations.

Skin
The differential diagnosis of ATLL in skin includes:

- MF
- Primary cutaneous ALCL (C-ALCL)
- Other T-cell lymphomas

Cutaneous lesions of ATLL are variable and may resemble those of MF, with mostly an indolent course, but some are associated with a poor prognosis. T-PLL in the skin shows either lymphoid infiltrate around blood vessels and appendages, diffuse infiltrate replacing dermis without epidermotropism, or a diffuse subcutaneous infiltrate. ATLL should be distinguished from cutaneous T-cell lymphomas, including MF, and PTCL, especially in endemic areas, by HTLV1 serology.

T-large granular lymphocyte leukemia (T-LGLL)

T-LGLL phenotype by FC: CD2+/rarely−, CD3+/rarely−, CD8+ (rarely CD4+, CD4/CD8−, or CD4/CD8+), CD5+/−, CD7−/+, CD25−, CD26−/+, CD16−/+, CD45+, CD56−/+, CD57+/rarely−, CD81+, CD200−, TCRαβ+ (rarely TCRγδ+)

Introduction
T-LGLL is characterized by persistent (>6 months) lymphocytosis in blood (≥2 × 10⁹/L) and lymphoid cells with abundant cytoplasm and azurophilic (MPO-negative) granules [1, 42–44]. Two main variants of LGL proliferations can be recognized: T-cell LGLL and CLPD-NK, which account for more than 85% and 10% of cases, respectively. Another rare variant of LGL proliferation is called aggressive NK-cell leukemia (ANKL), which is associated with EBV infection and poor prognosis. Rare cases with mixed-phenotype (T-LGLL/CLPD-NK phenotype or αβ/γδ phenotype) have been reported [45].

T-LGLL involves blood, BM, liver, and spleen. Most cases of T-LGLL occur in elderly patients with a median age of ~65 years at diagnosis, have indolent clinical course and severe neutropenia with or without anemia. T-LGLL may be associated with red cell aplasia, hypergammaglobulinemia and rheumatoid arthritis. Other disorders associated with T-LGLL include autoimmune disease (15%–40%), autoimmune cytopenia (5%–10%), B-cell neoplasms (5%–7%), MDS (<4%), solid or hematopoietic neoplasms (<10%), vasculitis (3%), and chronic inflammatory bowel disease (4%). Patients are asymptomatic (28%) or experience fatigue (60%), B-symptoms (12%), recurrent infections (15%), and mouth ulcers [46, 47]. Neutropenia is reported in 85% of patients while severe neutropenia (<0.5 × 10⁹/L) is seen in 50% [48]. Anemia and thrombocytopenia are less common, and seen in approximately 50% and 20% of patients, respectively. Splenomegaly is common, whereas lymphadenopathy is rare. T-LGLL is usually an indolent and non-progressive disorder and it has been suggested that it is at the end of a spectrum which ranges from a reactive/transient disorder, *via* a chronic lymphocytosis to clinically malignant disease requiring intensive therapy [46, 47, 49, 50].

Morphology
T-LGLL in blood or BM aspirate shows mature lymphocytes with small nuclei and abundant cytoplasm with characteristic

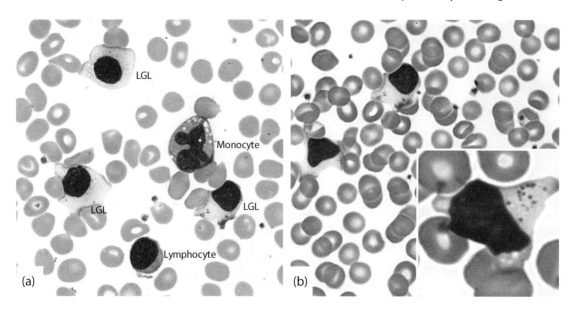

FIGURE 16.20 T-LGL leukemia. Peripheral blood films (a–b) show several LGLs with prominent cytoplasmic granules. Compare with monocytes and normal small lymphocytes (a).

azurophilic granules (Figure 16.20). Number of T-LGL cells >2 × 10⁹/L is compatible with the diagnosis (typically, reactive lymphocytosis has values <5 × 10⁹/L and T-LGLL >5 × 10⁹/L) [1]. In the BM T-LGLs most often display subtle interstitial infiltrate (Figure 16.21) present in approximately 70% of cases [51]. Spleen may be involved, and similarly to BM, the infiltrate is often subtle requiring immunohistochemistry or molecular studies to confirm the involvement.

Immunophenotype

Flow cytometry (FC) analysis. Clonal LGL proliferations are assumed to be derived from normal LGL cells, which comprise 10%–15% of mononuclear cells in blood. T-LGLL has cytotoxic T-cell phenotype (Figures 16.22–16.24), with CD2 (98%), CD3 (100%), CD8 (74%), and TCRαβ expression. CD11b and CD11c are expressed in 15% and 48%, respectively. Of the NK-cell associated markers, CD57 is most frequently expressed (96%), whereas CD16 (Figure 16.25) or CD56 are present in approximately 1/3 cases (Table 16.3). Rare cases may be CD4⁺/CD8⁺ (8%) CD4⁺ (10%; Figure 16.26) or CD4⁻/CD8⁻ (8%; TCRγδ⁺ variant

is discussed below). T-LGLLs generally lack dual CD16/CD56 co-expression, a feature more typical for NK-cell proliferations (co-expression of both markers is seen in 2% of T-LGLL and 53% of CLPD-NK). Presence of all T-cell antigens is seen in 53% but only ~6% of T-LGLLs show normal expression of all pan-T cell antigens. Majority of cases have either lack of one antigen (CD5 or CD7) or aberrant (e.g., dim or partial) expression of one or two markers (most often CD5 and/or CD7). Patients with CD4⁺ T-LGLLs with or without CD8 expression almost never have cytopenias, splenomegaly or autoimmune phenomena [52, 53]. In a series of eight CD4⁺ cases reported by Olteanu et al., none had a history of rheumatoid arthritis, lymphadenopathy or hepatosplenomegaly; all cases showed moderate or bright CD56, seven cases expressed CD57, and four were partially positive for CD8 [54]. Abnormal levels of expression of two or more T-cell antigens were seen in all cases. Subset of T-LGLL may be positive for CD26 and its expression correlate with more aggressive clinical behavior [55].

TCRγδ⁺ LGL leukemia. A minor subgroup of T-LGLL expresses TCRγδ (Figure 16.27). They show predominantly CD4⁻/CD8⁺

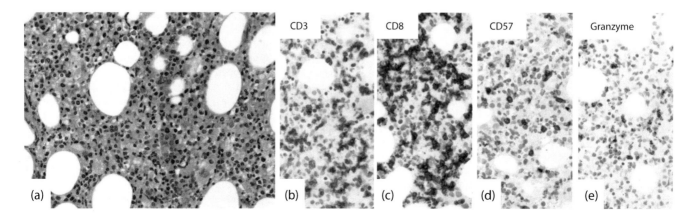

FIGURE 16.21 T-LGL leukemia – bone marrow. (a) T-LGL shows interstitial bone marrow involvement. Leukemic cells express CD3 (b), CD8 (c), CD57 (d), and granzyme B (e).

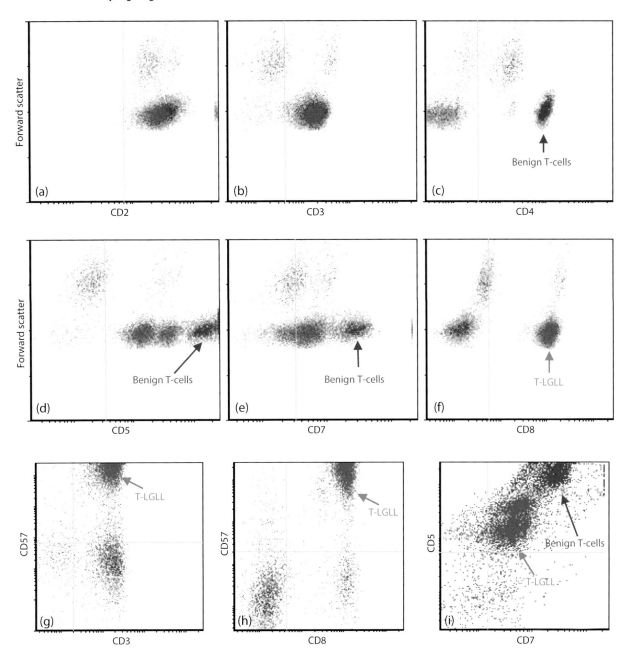

FIGURE 16.22 T-LGLL (blood). Leukemic T-cells (magenta dots) display the following phenotype: CD2+ (a), CD3+ (b), CD4- (c), CD5+ (d, dim expression), CD7+ (f, dim expression), CD8+ (g), and CD57+ (h–i). Note dimmer expression of both CD5 and CD7 when compared to normal T-cells (j) [dot plots a–f, open gate, dot plots g–i, lymphocyte gate].

phenotype (65%) or CD4−/CD8− phenotype (35%), are positive for surface CD3 and variably positive for CD16 (45%), CD56 (45%), and CD57 (86%) [56, 57]. Co-expression of CD56 and CD57 is seen in 43% of patients, while 41% of cases show the CD16/CD57 phenotype. CD2, CD5, CD7, and CD11c are observed in 100%, 86%, 93%, and 83%, respectively [56]. The most common phenotype (57%) of TCRγδ+ T-LGLLs is CD3+/CD8+/CD57+. TCRγδ+ T-lymphocytes in blood, TCRγδ+ thymocytes, as well as TCRγδ+ T-ALL and HSTLs are most often CD4−/CD8−. In the series reported by Sandberg et al., the most common clinical manifestations associated with TCRγδ T-LGLL were chronic cytopenias (neutropenia in 48%, anemia in 23%, thrombocytopenia in 9%, and pancytopenia in 2%), and splenomegaly (18%), as well as multiple autoimmune

(34%) and hematological (14%) disorders [56]. In a series reported by Bourgault-Rouxel et al., the clinical findings of TCRγδ+ T-LGL were similar to T-LGL with ab phenotype [57]. Similar to most TCRαβ+ T-LGL cases, most TCRγδ+ T-LGLLs have an indolent clinical course. In series reported by Bourgault-Rouxel et al., the overall survival at 3 years was 85% [57].

Genetic features

Cytogenetic information on T-LGL is limited. Individual cases with inv(7)(p15q22), inv(14)(q11q32), del(6q), del(1)(p32), t(11;12) (q12;q11), t(3;5)(p26;q13), and t(8;14)(q24;q32) were reported [58–62]. The most common gain-of-function mutations identified in T-LGLL are on *STAT3* and *STAT5b* genes [1, 63].

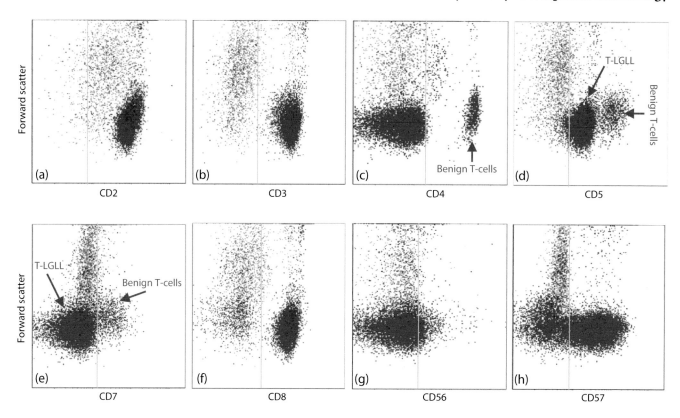

FIGURE 16.23 T-LGLL – FC analysis. Neoplastic cells have the following phenotype: CD2⁺ (a, red dots), CD3⁺ (b), CD4⁻ (c), CD5⁺ (d, dim expression), CD7⁻ (e), CD8⁺ (f), CD56⁻ (g), and CD57⁺ (h).

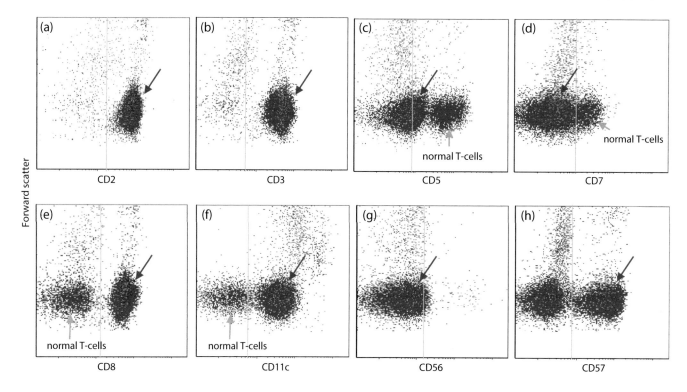

FIGURE 16.24 T-LGLL – flow cytometry. Leukemic cells (red arrow) are positive for CD2 (a), CD3 (b), and CD5 (c; dim expression), negative for CD7 (d), positive for CD8 (e), positive for CD11c (f), negative for CD56 (g), and positive for CD57 (h).

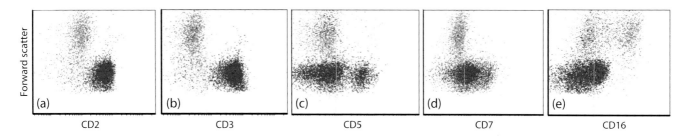

FIGURE 16.25 T-LGLL – FC analysis. Leukemic cells are positive for CD2 (a) and CD3 (b), show negative to partially dim CD5 (c), dim CD7 expression (d), and dim CD16 expression (e).

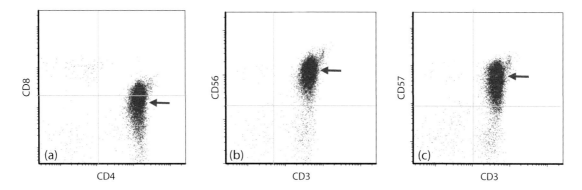

FIGURE 16.26 T-LGLL with CD4 expression. FC analysis shows CD4+ T-LGL cells (a), co-expression CD3 with CD56 (b) and CD57 (c).

TABLE 16.3: Phenotype of T-LGLL (*n* = 106) and CLPD-NK (*n* = 35)

	T-LGLL	CLPD-NK
CD45+	100%	100%
All 4 T-cell antigens+	53%	0
One T-cell antigen−	33%	0
Two T-cell antigens−	11%	91%
Three T-cell antigens−	1%	9%
Four T-cell antigens−	0	0
CD2+	98%	100%
CD3+	100%	3%
CD5+	75%	0
CD7+	66%	88%
CD4+	10%	0
CD8+	74%	32%
CD4+/CD8+	8%	0
CD4/CD8−	8%	56%
CD11b+	15%	62%
CD11c+	48%	79%
CD16+	25%	79%
CD56+	33%	65%
CD57+	96%	65%
CD16+/CD56+/CD57+	1%	29%
CD16+/CD56+/CD57−	1%	24%
CD16−/CD56+/CD57+	30%	18%
CD16+/CD56−/CD57+	23%	18%
CD16+/CD56−/CD57−	1%	9%
CD16−/CD56+/CD57−	2%	3%
CD16−/CD56−/CD57+	43%	9%

Chronic lymphoproliferative disorder of NK-cells (CLPD-NK)

CLPD-NK phenotype by FC: CD2+, CD3−, CD5−, CD7+/rarely−, CD4−/CD8− (rarely CD8+), CD25−, CD26−, CD16+/rarely−, CD45+, CD56+/−, CD57+/−, CD81+, CD200−, TCRαβ−, TCRγδ−

CLPD-NK is less common than T-LGLL and is characterized by persistent (>6 months) increase in NK cells in blood (≥2 × 10^9/L) and chronic, non-progressive clinical course. It is difficult to distinguish between reactive and neoplastic conditions. A transient increase in circulating NK cells may be seen in many conditions such as autoimmune disorders or viral infections. Patients with CLPD-NK cells are most often asymptomatic but may have a gradual increase in circulating large granular lymphocytes (LGLs). NK-LGL leukemia differs clinically from T-LGLL by lack of association with rheumatoid arthritis. Some patients have anemia and/or neutropenia. Lymphadenopathy, organomegaly or skin involvements are infrequent. CLPD-NK cells may occur in association with other medical conditions such as solid and hematologic tumors, vasculitis, splenectomy, neuropathy, and autoimmune disorders.

Morphology. Morphologic features are similar to T-LGLL.

Immunophenotype. The phenotypic hallmark of CLPD-NK is lack of surface CD3 and CD5 expression and positive expression of CD2 and CD7 (Figures 16.28 and 16.29). Cytoplasmic CD3 is often positive. They are dual CD4/CD8-negative (64%) or CD8+ (26%). In contrast to T-LGLLs, CLPD-NK more often shows expression of CD16 (79%) and CD56 (65%), with 35% of cases co-expressing those two antigens. CD57 is present in 65% with 29%

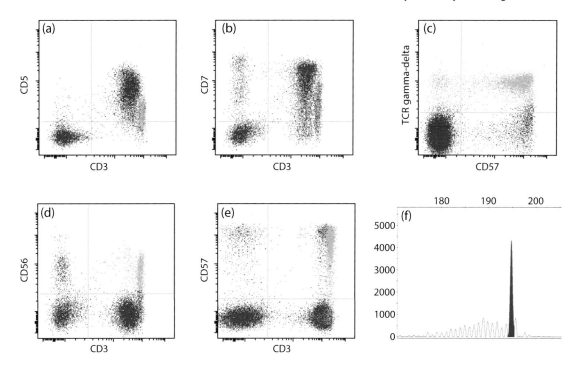

FIGURE 16.27 Early T-LGLL with gamma-delta phenotype (peripheral blood). Gamma-delta⁺ T-cells (green dots) are characterized by bright CD3 expression (a–b), negative to dim CD5 (a), variable CD7 (b), positive gamma-delta (c), and positive CD56 (d), and CD57 (c, e). PCR testing confirmed the clonality of T-cells (f).

of cases co-expressing all NK-cell markers (CD16, CD56, and CD57; Figure 16.30). CLPD-NKs are often positive for CD11b, CD11c, and CD38. There are no rearrangements of the immunoglobulins and TCR genes, as expected for NK cells. Karyotype is normal in most cases. Clinical course is indolent over prolonged period. Disease progression with increasing lymphocytosis and worsening of cytopenias is observed in some cases.

Differential diagnosis of T-LGLL and CLPD-NK

Chronic reactive proliferations of both TCRαβ⁺ and TCRγδ⁺ T-LGL- and NK-cells are seen in various clinical conditions [64, 65]. In these cases, lymphocytosis is often <5 × 10⁹/L while in T-LGLL the lymphocytosis is often >5 × 10⁹/L. Differential diagnosis includes transient and chronic T-cell or NK-cell lymphocytosis in patients with viral infections, autoimmune disorders,

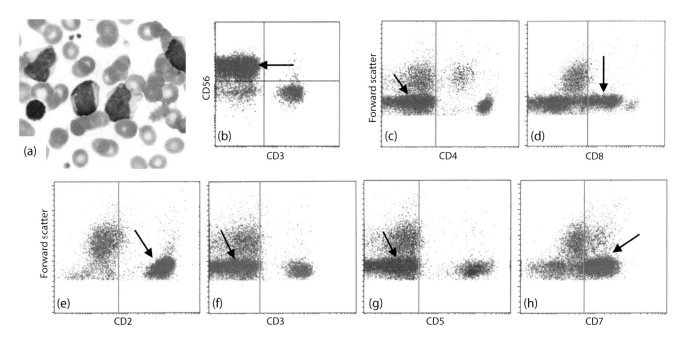

FIGURE 16.28 CLPD-NK – flow cytometry. Atypical lymphocytes (a) are positive for CD56 (b), negative for CD4 and CD8 (c–d). Characteristically, NK-LGL cells are positive for CD2 and CD7 and lack the expression of CD3 and CD5 (e–h).

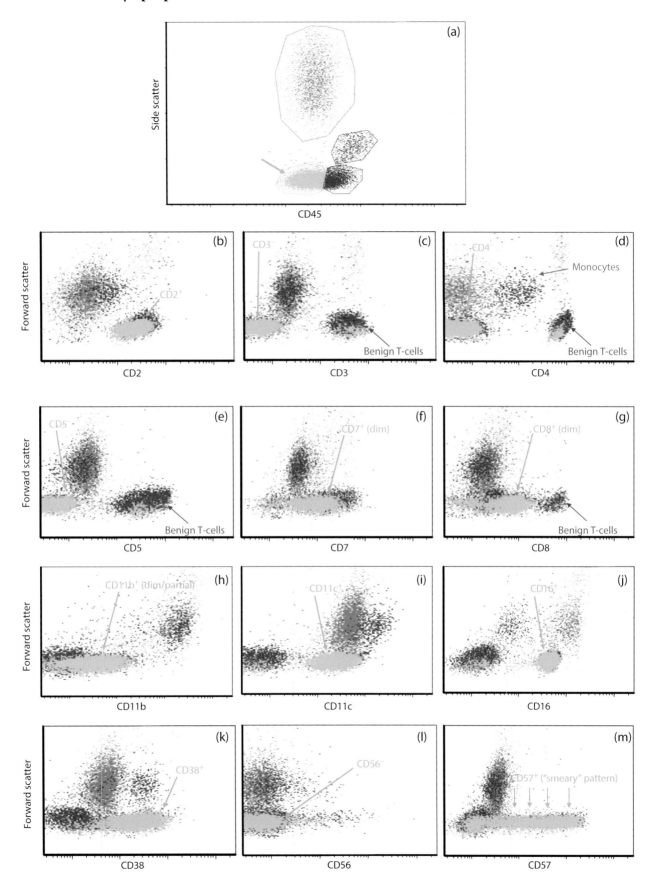

FIGURE 16.29 CLPD-NK – FC analysis (blood). Leukemic NK-cells show dimmer expression of CD45 (a, green dots)) when compared to normal lymphocytes (red dots). Leukemic NK-cells show the following phenotype: CD2$^+$ (b), CD3$^-$ (c), CD4$^-$ (d), CD5$^-$ (e), CD7 dimly$^+$ (f), CD8 dimly$^+$ (g), CD11b dimly$^+$ (h), CD11c$^+$ (i), CD16$^+$ (j), CD38$^+$ (k), CD56$^-$ (l), and CD57 variably$^+$ (m).

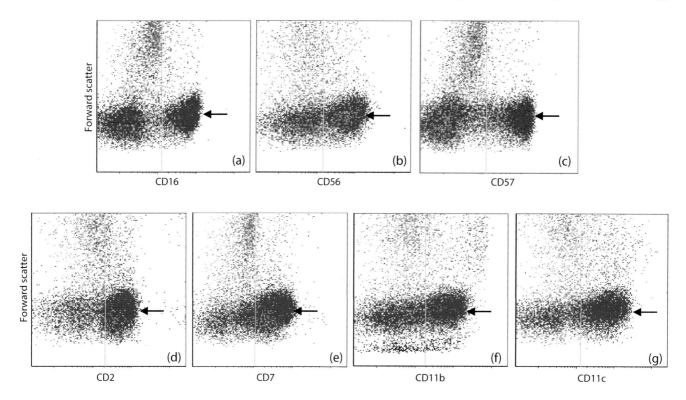

FIGURE 16.30 Chronic NK cell lymphocytosis – bone marrow. NK-cells (arrow) show triple-positive phenotype (CD16⁺, CD56⁺, CD57⁺; a–c), and positive expression of CD2 (d), CD7 (e), CD11b (f), and CD11c (g).

patients with HCL or CLL, after chemotherapy or after organ transplantation (e.g., allogeneic BM transplant). Expansion of T-LGL cells is also observed in some patients with CML [66]. Differential diagnosis includes also T-cell clones of uncertain significance (T-CUS), which can be detected in patients with other malignancies and less often in healthy subjects [67] The T-CUS can be CD4⁻/CD8⁺ (78%), CD4⁻/CD8⁻ (12%), CD4⁺/CD8⁺ (9%), or CD4⁺/CD8⁻ (2%), with phenotypic features similar to T-LGLL, but with brighter CD2 and CD7 and dimmer CD3 expression [67]. In patients with LGL count in blood <0.5 × 10⁹/L without B-symptoms, cytopenias, infections, rheumatoid arthritis and/or splenomegaly and negative TCR gene rearrangement, diagnosis of T-LGLL is unlikely (they should be followed with FC analysis in 6 months). CD4⁺ T-LGLL mimicking SS has been reported [68].

Apart from relatively indolent chronic NK-cell lymphoproliferative disorder, NK cell neoplasms include extranodal nasal type NK cell lymphoma (ENKTL) and aggressive NK cell leukemia [69–71]. ENKTL may involve the BM, but leukemic blood involvement is rare. ANKL differs from chronic NK-cell lymphocytosis by clinical data (fever and constitutional symptoms) and association with EBV infection [70–72]. FC analysis show the phenotype similar to extranodal NK-cell lymphoma and chronic NK-cell lymphoproliferative disorder, except for increased forward scatter, often negative CD7 and CD57 and frequent expression of CD16 and CD11b [73]. Rare cases with CD8 expression have been reported. BM or blood in certain hematopoietic (e.g., CMML) or non-hematopoietic neoplasms or after treatment may show increased number of immature NK-cells with CD117 expression (Figure 16.31).

Peripheral T-cell lymphoma, not otherwise specified (PTCL, NOS)

PTCL phenotype by FC: CD2⁺/⁻, CD3⁺/⁻, CD4⁺/⁻, CD5⁺/⁻, CD7⁻/⁺, CD8⁻/⁺, CD10⁻, CD30⁻/rarely⁺, CD38⁺, CD45⁺, CD56⁻/rarely⁺

Introduction

PTCL, NOS, is a heterogeneous group of tumors with variable clinical features, histology, genetic alteration, response to treatment and prognosis. It is a mature T-cell lymphoma which does not fulfill morphologic, phenotypic or genetic criteria for any distinctive mature T-cell lymphoma category, hence the designation "not otherwise specified" [1, 74–77]. PTCL, although most common category of peripheral T-LPDs (it accounts for approximately 30% of PTCLs in Western countries) accounts for less than 5%–20% of all non-Hodgkin lymphomas. PTCL occurs at any age, usually in older patients with the median age of 60 years. It occurs often as a nodal disease, but any other site, including blood, BM, bone, omentum, skin, CNS, soft tissues, gastrointestinal tract, spleen, liver, and lung may be involved, often concurrently with lymph node involvement.

Prognosis. Despite aggressive therapy, the prognosis is poor [78–80], with more than half of the patients dying of their disease [81]. The estimated overall survival is 41%–49% at 5 years [82–84]. The International Prognostic Index (IPI) is a significant prognostic factor for both progression-free and overall survival [83, 85–87].

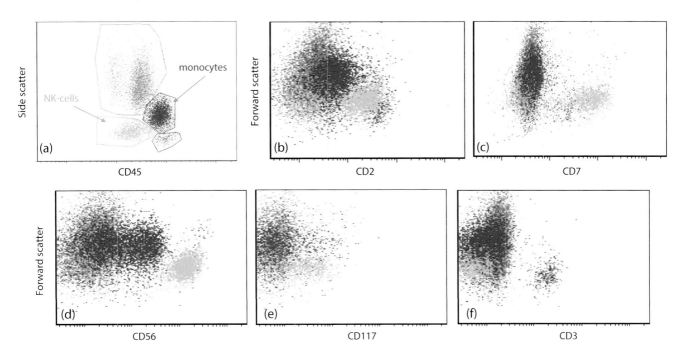

FIGURE 16.31 Immature NK-cells with CD117 expression. FC analysis of blood in patient with CMML after therapy. Monocytes (blue dots) have bright expression of CD45 (a) and immature NK-cells (a, green dots) show dimmer CD45 expression. NK-cells are positive for CD2 (b), CD7 (c), CD56 (d, bright expression), and CD117 (e, dim expression). Surface CD3 is negative (f).

Besides IPI, systemic symptoms and BM infiltration have been found to correlate with prognosis [86]. BM is involved in 20%–40% of PTCL and appears to worsen the prognosis [81, 84].

Morphology

Lymph nodes. Most cases of PTCL show complete effacement of lymph node architecture, but subset of cases shows characteristic expansion of perifollicular or paracortical area (T-zone pattern). The cellular composition of PTCL is very heterogeneous with variable cells' size and cytomorphology, but medium-sized to large cells predominate. Nuclei are irregular and pleomorphic with unevenly distributed coarse chromatin and nucleoli. Cells with prominent nuclear irregularities, including cerebriform-like cells, clear cells, signet-ring-like cells, multinucleated Reed-Sternberg-like cells, or blastoid cells with prominent nucleoli and mitotic figures are often present within otherwise very pleomorphic infiltrate. Lymphomatous cells are usually accompanied by inflammatory infiltrate of small lymphocytes, histiocytes, plasma cells, clusters of epithelioid histiocytes (which may form granulomas), and characteristically, eosinophils. Rare cases of PTCL are composed of rather small to medium-sized lymphocytes, which otherwise display cytologic atypia in the form of prominent variation is the shape of nuclei (with many cells showing highly irregular nuclear contours) and one or more prominent nucleoli.

Morphologic variants of PTCL, NOS include:

- PTCL with diffuse pattern: histologic examination shows diffuse infiltration with effacement of the normal lymph node architecture (Figure 16.32).
- Lennert's lymphoma (lymphoepithelioid variant of PTCL): a rare variant of PTCL with numerous aggregates of epithelioid histiocytic cells is designated as Lennert's lymphoma. Similar pattern is retained in the BM. Lennert's lymphoma is more often CD8+ when compared to other variants of PTCL.
- PTCL with T-zone pattern (T-zone lymphoma): neoplastic infiltrate limited to expanded paracortical area (Figure 16.33).
- PTCL with clear cytoplasm and/or signet-ring cell features: clusters of clear cells are more typical for AITL.
- PTCL with Hodgkin-like and/or Reed-Sternberg-like cells: neoplastic infiltrate with scattered large multilobated Reed-Sternberg-like or Hodgkin-like cells with macronucleoli. In contrast to cHL, large tumor cells are CD45+ and show expression of one of pan-T-cell makers with or without CD30.
- PTCL with fibrosis creating nodular pattern: neoplastic infiltrate is accompanied by bands of fibrosis which create pseudo-nodular pattern.
- PTCL with angioimmunoblastic lymphoma-like features: PTCL with increased vessels (high endothelial venules) and proliferation of follicular dendritic cells (FDCs), but not as prominent as seen in AITL. In contrast to AITL, neoplastic T-cells do not display follicular T-helper cell phenotype (FTH).

Prior follicular variant of PTCL it is now classified under the separate category of nodal PTCLs of T-follicular helper cell origin, which includes AITL, follicular T-cell lymphoma (FTCL), and nodal peripheral T-cell lymphoma with T-follicular helper cell phenotype (PTCL-TFH) [1, 88].

Extranodal sites. PTCLs may occur in extranodal sites, including spleen, gastrointestinal tract, liver, skin, and soft tissues. The morphologic and immunophenotypic features are heterogeneous, and PTCL is diagnosed only in the absence of characteristic features for specific T-cell lymphoma category, especially MF, enteropathy-associated T-cell lymphoma (EATL),

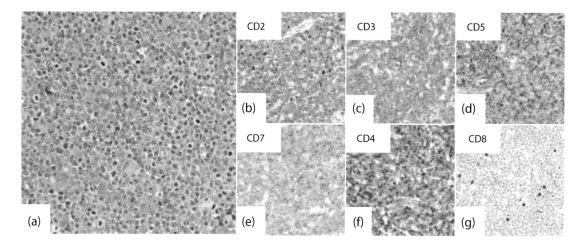

FIGURE 16.32 PTCL, NOS. Diffuse lymph node involvement by medium-sized to large cells with irregular nuclei and nucleoli (a). Tumor cells are positive for all pan-T-cell markers (CD2, CD3, CD5, and CD7, b–e) with CD7 being dimly expressed. They are CD4⁺ (f) and CD8⁻ (g).

monomorphic epitheliotropic intestinal T-cell lymphoma (MEITL), ATLL, subcutaneous panniculitis-like T-cell lymphoma (SPTCL), or HSTL.

   Bone marrow and blood. BM is quite often involved in patients with PTCL, and advanced disease may also be associated with leukemic blood involvement. On H&E sections of the

core biopsy, the pattern of involvement varies, and may be nodular, interstitial, and diffuse, but often is mixed [89]. Rare cases of intrasinusoidal pattern have also been reported [89]. FC is often helpful in identifying atypical T-cell population in BM or blood. PTCL with BM involvement have a similar aggressive course and poor survival compared to DLBCL with BM involvement [90].

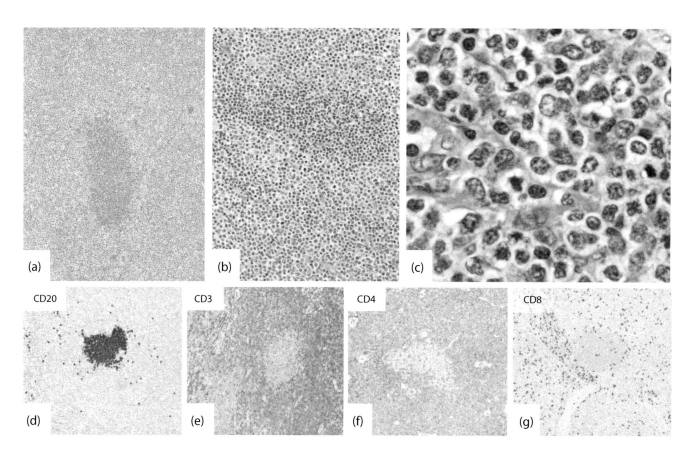

FIGURE 16.33 PTCL. (a–b) Interfollicular pattern of involvement (T-zone variant). (c) High magnification shows pleomorphic lymphomatous cells with irregular nuclear outlines. CD20 staining shows preserved B-cell areas (d). Neoplastic cells are positive for CD3 (e) and CD4 (f) Only rare CD8⁺ small T-cells are present (g).

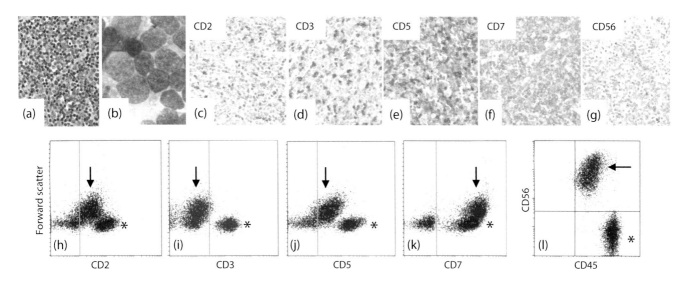

FIGURE 16.34 PTCL – comparison of immunohistochemistry and flow cytometry. (a) Tissue section shows diffuse lymphoid infiltrate. (b) Touch smear shows medium-sized lymphoid cells with inconspicuous nucleoli. Immunohistochemistry (c–g) and flow cytometry (h–l) shows the following phenotype of neoplastic cells: CD2$^+$ (dim; a, h), CD3$^-$ (d, i), CD5$^+$ (e, j), CD7$^+$ (f, k), and CD56$^+$ (g, l).

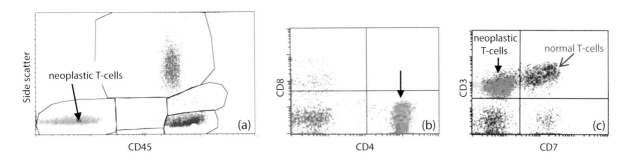

FIGURE 16.35 Leukemic blood involvement by PTCL – flow cytometry analysis. Tumor cell display aberrant lack of CD45 (a; orange dots), CD4 restriction (b; arrow), positive, although slightly dimmer CD3 (c; orange dots) and loss of CD7 (c; orange dots). Normal T-cells (red dots) are positive for both CD3 and CD7 (c).

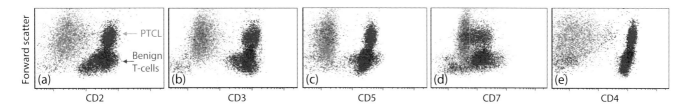

FIGURE 16.36 PTCL – FC analysis of lymph node. Lymphoma cells show (blue dots) shows positive expression of all pan-T-cell antigens (a–d). Only high forward scatter and CD4 restriction (e) allows for identification of abnormal T-cell population.

Immunophenotype

Immunohistochemistry. PTCL are positive for CD45, pan-T-cell antigens (CD2, CD3, CD5, and CD7), CD4 (less often CD8) and in subset of cases CD30 and cytotoxic proteins (granzyme B, TIA1, and/or perforin). The expression of T-cell markers is often aberrant, most commonly CD5 and/or CD7, but CD2 or CD3 may also be either dim or missing. Unusual cases may show co-expression of CD30 and CD15, or aberrant expression of CD56. Figure 16.34 shows immunohistochemistry and FC data of PTC with aberrant expression of CD2, loss of CD3, and positive CD56. The

expression of CD30 is usually dimmer in PTCL than in ALCL but in rare cases may be similarly strong.

Flow cytometry (FC). The expression of CD45 in PTCL is usually bright positive (~96%) but some cases show either dim (~10%) or negative (~4%) CD45 (Figure 16.35). In 23% of cases, all T-cell markers are positive, including 8% cases which do not reveal any loss or diminution of pan-T antigens expression (Figures 16.36 and 16.37). Majority of PTCLs show increased forward scatter and prominent phenotypic atypia (Figures 16.38–16.41). Among pan-T antigens, CD7 is most frequently lost (52%), followed by

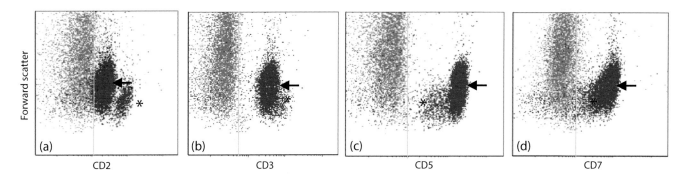

FIGURE 16.37 PTCL – flow cytometry. Lymphomatous cells (arrow) show positive expression of all T-cell markers. The expression of CD2 (a) is dim, CD3 is moderate (b), CD5 is bright (c), and CD7 is moderate (d). Forward scatter is increased when compared to benign T-cells (*).

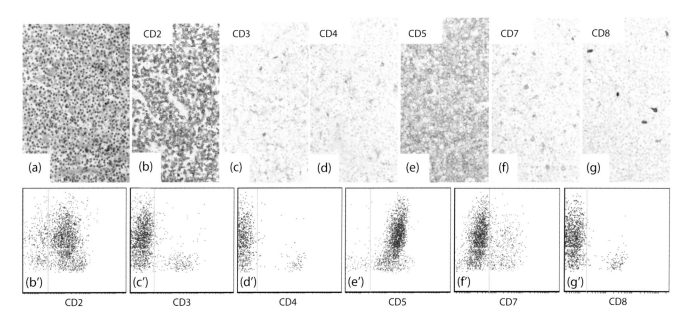

FIGURE 16.38 PTCL with clear cell cytoplasm (a) and prominent phenotypic atypia. Immunohistochemistry (b–g) and flow cytometry (b′–g′, blue dots) show positive CD2 and CD5 only and lack of CD3, CD7, CD4, and CD8.

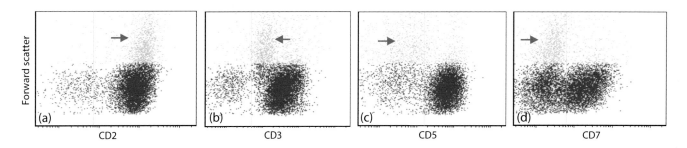

FIGURE 16.39 PTCL (lymph node from 34-year man) with prominent phenotypic atypia. Neoplastic cells (blue dots, arrow) shows increased forward scatter), positive CD2 (a), dim CD3 (b), and negative CD5 and CD7 (c–d). Benign T-cells (red dots) show normal expression of T-cell markers.

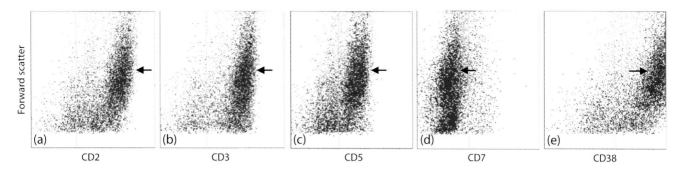

FIGURE 16.40   PTCL – flow cytometry (lymph node). Lymphomatous cells (arrow) show high forward scatter (a–e), positive CD2 (a), CD3 (b), and CD5 (c), negative CD7 (d), and bright expression of CD38 (e).

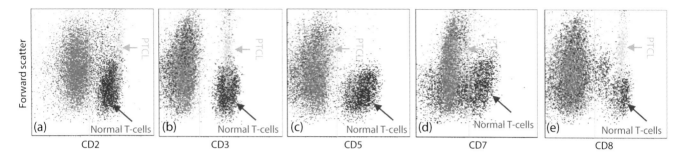

FIGURE 16.41   PTCL – flow cytometry. Blood with predominance of granulocytes (gray dots), benign T-cells (red dots) and minor population of atypical T-cells. Despite minimal involvement by PTCL, lymphomatous cells (blue dots) are easily identifiable by FC based on increased FSC (a–e), brighter CD2 expression when compared to normal T-cells (a), negative CD5 (c) and CD7 (d), and CD8 restriction (e).

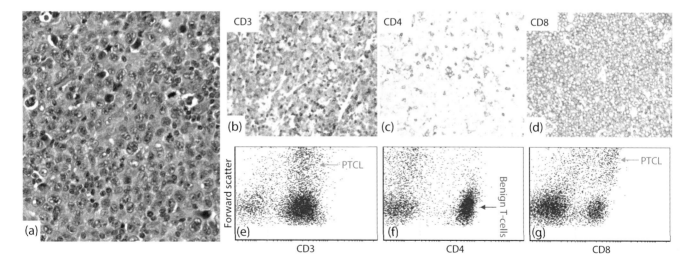

FIGURE 16.42   PTCL with CD8 expression (lymph node). (a) Histology shows highly atypical pleomorphic large cell infiltrate with numerous mitoses. Immunohistochemistry (b–d) and flow cytometry (e–g) shows positive CD3 (b, e), negative CD4 (c, f), and positive CD8 (d, g).

loss of CD3 (35%) and CD5 (16%). CD2 is negative in only 10% of cases. Dim expression of CD2, CD3, CD5, and CD7 is noted in ~4%, ~12%, ~18%, and ~9% cases, respectively. CD4$^+$ lymphomas predominate (61%), dual negative expression of CD4/CD8 is observed on significant proportions of tumors (26%) and occasional cases are either CD8$^+$ (9%; Figure 16.42) or CD4/CD8$^+$ (4%). Of additional markers, CD11c, CD15, CD25, CD30, CD56, CD57,

CD117, EMA, and HLA-DR may be occasionally expressed (CD10 expression is typical for AITL and FTCL). The summary of phenotype of PTCL is presented in Table 16.4.

Genetic features

Specific chromosomal translocations are unknown in PTCL. Lepretre et al. reported cytogenetic findings in 71 untreated

TABLE 16.4: Phenotype of PTCL (*n* = 111)

CD45+	96%
All four T-cell antigens positive (normal expression)	23% (8%)
One T-cell antigen−	48%
Two T-cell antigens−	23%
Three T-cell antigens−	6%
All four T-cell antigens−	0
CD2+	90%
CD3+	65%
CD5+	84%
CD7+	48%
CD4+	61%
CD8+	9%
CD4+/CD8+	4%
CD4−/CD8−	26%
CD56+	12%
CD57+	10
CD10+	0

patients with PTCL: 57 patients (80.3%) had abnormal clones, whereas 9 karyotypes (12.7%) showed only normal metaphases; 5 karyotypes (7%) could not be analyzed [91]. Recurrent numerical chromosomal abnormalities included +3 (21%), +5 (15.7%), +7 (15.5%), +21 (14%), −13 (14%), +8 (12.2%), +19 (12.2%), −10 (10.5%), and −Y (9% of male patients) and chromosomes involved in structural rearrangements included chromosome 6 (31.5%), mainly due to 6q deletions (19.2%), 1q (22.8%), 7q (22.8%), 9p (19.4%), 9q (19.2%), 4q (19.2%), 3q (19.2%), 2p (17.5%), 1p (17.5%), and 14q (17%) (trisomies 3 and 5 mainly correlated with AITL, while isochromosome 7q, associated with trisomy 8, was present in two cases of hepatosplenic gd T-cell lymphoma) [91].

Differential diagnosis of PTCL

The distinction from other (specific) peripheral T-cell disorders is based on clinical, morphologic, phenotypic, and genetic data, but is not always clear, especially at the time of initial diagnosis. The main entities from which PTCL has to be differentiated include nodal involvement by T-PLL, lymphomatous variant of ATLL, ALCL, AITL, nodal PTCL with TFH phenotype and reactive T-cell infiltrates in benign processes (such as Kikuchi lymphadenitis) or accompanying B-cell lymphomas (e.g., T-cell/histiocyte-rich large B-cell lymphoma; THRLBCL), cHL, or non-hematopoietic. Algorithmic approach to T-cell lymphomas is presented in Figure 15.1 (Chapter 15) and algorithmic approach to lymph node with atypical T-cell infiltrate is presented in Figure 15.2 (Chapter 15). Figure 16.43 presents histologic differential diagnosis of PTCL involving lymph nodes.

Differential diagnosis of PTCL includes:

- Reactive lymphoid hyperplasia
- Kikuchi disease
- Dermatopathic lymphadenitis
- Granulomatous lymphadenitis
- AITL
- ALCL
- MF and SS
- ATLL
- EATL
- MEITL

- HSTL
- T-PLL
- BPDCN
- T-ALL/LBL
- Extranodal NK/T-cell lymphoma, nasal type (ENKTL)

Reactive processes

Reactive processes with paracortical and/or interfollicular pattern may display some cytologic and/or phenotypic atypia and require differential diagnosis with PTCL. These reactive processes include viral infections, drug-induced lymphadenopathies, postvaccination adenopathy, dermatopathic lymphadenitis, and Kikuchi disease (necrotizing lymphohistiocytic lymphadenitis). Kikuchi lymphadenopathy (Kikuchi-Fujimoto disease/lymphadenitis) is a benign, self-limited disease often confused with B- and especially T-cell lymphomas due effacement of lymph node architecture (at least partial) and scattered atypical lymphocytes with immunoblastic features. The lymph node shows reactive germinal centers and focal areas of necrosis (necrosis may be subtle is early stages, when only occasional apoptotic cells are present within histiocytic aggregates) [92–94]. The histiocytic cells with engulfed cellular debris have abundant cytoplasm and crescentic nuclei (C-shaped forms), a characteristic feature of Kikuchi lymphadenopathy. The infiltrate is composed of pleomorphic population of small, intermediate to large lymphocytes (predominantly T-cells, especially in areas of necrosis; CD8+ T-cells are more abundant than CD4+), histiocytes (CD68+, CD163+, and CD4+) and plasmacytoid dendritic cells (CD123+, CD68+, and CD303+). Scattered weakly CD30+ immunoblasts may be present (they are of T-cell lineage, usually CD8+). Characteristically, there are no neutrophils and only rare plasma cells may be seen. Karyorrhectic debris are present in the necrotic areas and may be prominent. Based on the cellular composition, some authors distinguish several variants of Kikuchi lymphadenopathy: lymphohistiocytic, phagocytic, necrotic, and foamy cell type [95]. Lymphadenopathy in Kikuchi-Fujimoto disease may be accompanied by similar changes in the skin. Similar pattern to Kikuchi lymphadenopathy may be seen in systemic lupus erythematosus (SLE). SLE adenopathy differs by the presence of numerous plasma cells, hematoxylin bodies, and degenerated nuclear material in the blood walls (Azzopardi phenomenon). FC analysis of Kikuchi lymphadenopathy shows reactive pattern with polytypic B-cells, minor subset of CD10+ B-cells, and many small T-cells with normal expression of pan T-cell antigens. The characteristic FC feature of Kikuchi lymphadenopathy is CD38 expression by the majority of CD19+ small B cells, IgD+ B cells lacking surface IgM and decreased expression of CD57 by both CD4+ and CD8+ T-cells [96].

AITL

Typical AITL can be differentiated from PTCL by prominent arborizing high endothelial venules, expanded FDC meshwork outside the follicles, clusters of atypical cells with clear cytoplasm, especially around vessels, expression of CD10 and/or BCL6, expression of PD1 and CXCL13, more prominent inflammatory background and scattered EBV-infected (EBER+) cells. FC analysis often show rather characteristic for AITL pattern, including CD10 expression, variably increased forward scatter, and presence of population of CD4+ T-cells with negative to dim CD3 expression. WHO classification requires expression of at least two of TFH cell markers (CXCL13, CD10, PD1, ICOS, BCL6, or CD200) for the diagnosis of AITL and other T-cell lymphomas with TFH phenotype (FTCL and PTCL-TFH).

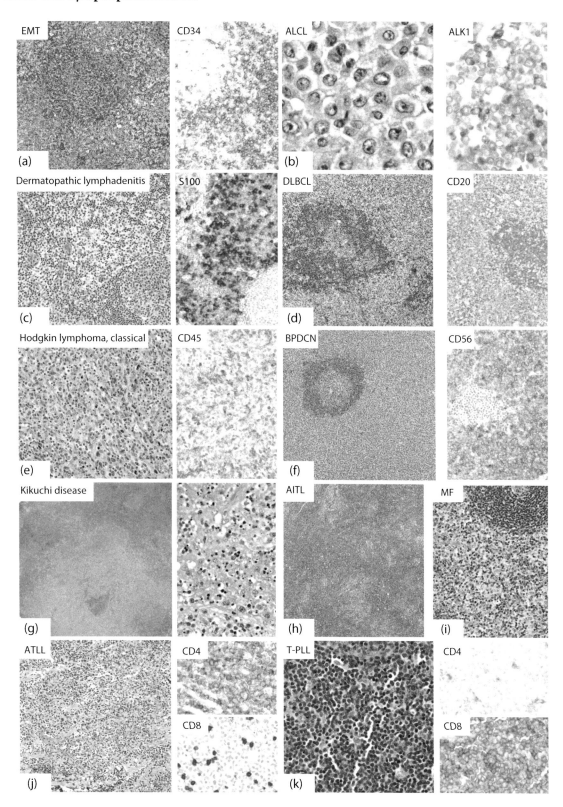

FIGURE 16.43 PTCL – differential diagnosis (lymph node). (a) Extramedullary myeloid tumor (EMT). Lack of pan-T antigens and positivity for CD34 and pan-myeloid antigens (MPO, muramidase, CD68) excludes PTCL. (b) Anaplastic large cell lymphoma (ALCL). (c) Dermatopathic lymphadenitis. It is characterized by the presence pigmented cells and clusters of atypical S100⁺ interdigitating reticulum cells. (d) DLBCL with unusual interfollicular distribution. (e) Hodgkin lymphoma (HL, classical). Neoplastic cells in HL are negative for CD45, pan-T cell markers and CD4/CD8. (f) Blastic plasmacytoid dendritic cell neoplasm (BPDCN). (g) Kikuchi disease. Prominent histiocytic infiltrate with necrosis and karyorrhectic nuclear debris without neutrophils. (h) Nodal TFH cell lymphoma, angioimmunoblastic-type (AITL). (i) Mycosis fungoides (MF) involving the lymph node. (j) Adult T-cell lymphoma/leukemia (ATLL). (k) T-cell prolymphocytic leukemia (T-PLL).

ALCL

ALK+ ALCL occurs more often in younger patients whereas PTCL is more common in older patients. The malignant cells in ALCL are more uniformly atypical and "anaplastic", forming cohesive, often intrasinusoidal clusters. By immunostaining, ALK+ ALCL can be easily distinguished from PTCL by positive expression of ALK protein. The differential diagnosis of ALK− ALCL from CD30+ PTCL is more problematic. Molecular genetic profiling studies suggest that ALK− ALCL has distinct profile from both ALK+ ALCL and PTCL. Presence of single lymph node with ALK−/CD30+ neoplastic lymphoid infiltrate should raise the possibility of ALK− ALLC, PTCL with CD30 expression, ATLL, MF and nodal dissemination of other forms of ALK− ALCL, such as primary C-ALCL or breast implant associated ALCLs [74]. Patients with ALK− ALCL are usually older than those affected by ALK+ ALCL. The WHO classification recognizes ALK− ALCL, but the morphologic and immunophenotypic distinction between CD30+ PTCL and ALK− ALCL is somewhat subjective and not always reliable. The staining with CD30 is stronger and more homogenous in ALCL, with typical membranous and Golgi pattern, whereas in CD30+ PTCL is weaker and heterogeneous. ALCL differs also by more pronounced phenotype atypia (aberrant expression of T-cell markers), including so-called null-cell type cases (CD2−, CD3−, CD5−, and CD7−), and more frequent expression of EMA and cytotoxic proteins.

MF/SS

Early stages of MF involving the lymph node show paracortical expansion with dermatopathic changes. In advanced involvement, the lymph node is replaced by sheets of atypical medium sized to large cells with highly irregular nuclei. Both morphologic and immunophenotypic features may be indistinguishable from PTCL, especially in transformed cases of MF with predominance of large cells. History of MF, presence of skin lesions and/or Sézary's cells in the blood help to exclude PTCL. T-cells in MF are positive for CD4 and usually express CD2, CD3, and CD5, while CD7 and cytotoxic proteins are frequently negative. Cases with large cell transformation show often CD30 expression. Apart from transformed MF, increased number of atypical CD30+ T-cells in lymph node may be seen in other cutaneous processes, such as lymphomatoid papulosis (LyP) or primary cutaneous anaplastic large cell lymphoma (C-ALCL).

ATLL

Lymph nodes are often involved in both chronic, acute, and lymphomatous variants, blood is involved in chronic and acute variants, BM is involved in acute variant (and less often in chronic and lymphomatous forms) and skin can be involved in all variants of ATLL. The cytologic and histologic features of ATLL vary depending on the type of disease. In chronic variant cytologic atypia may be minimal, but in lymphomatous or acute variants, cytologic features are very pleomorphic including characteristic "flower" cells with multilobulated nuclei, large anaplastic cells or multinucleated cells resembling Reed-Sternberg cells, often accompanied by eosinophils and occasionally plasma cells. In skin, the pattern of dermal infiltrate in ATLL is variable, including superficial banded dermal infiltrate with epidermotropism, diffuse, or nodular infiltrate [29]. In lymph nodes, there is paracortical expansion with atypical CD4+ T-cell infiltrate, which may mimic Hodgkin lymphoma, AITL, ALCL, or PTCL. In BM the infiltrates are either focal, interstitial or prominent, diffuse. Phenotypically, ATLLs are CD4+ and CD7− and show strong expression of CD25. CD5 is positive in most cases, and the

expression of CD3 is often positive. Cases with increased large cells may show CD30 expression. Correlation with HTLV1 status helps to differentiate between PTCL and ATLL.

EATL

EATL occurs in the gastrointestinal tract, where PTCLs may occur. The immunophenotypic and morphologic features are highly variable, similarly to nodal PTCL. Patients with EATL often have history of celiac disease. In EATL tumor cells are often positive for CD2, CD3, and CD7, express CD103, and are negative for CD5. Majority of cases are dual CD4/CD8 negative, but some tumors may express CD8.

MEITL

In MEITL tumor cells are positive for CD3, CD8, and CD56.

HSTL

HSTL involves hepatic sinusoids and splenic red pulp. In the lymph nodes and BM, HSTL displays intrasinusoidal pattern. Tumor cells are positive pan-T-cell antigens, except for CD5 which is usually absent. There is often aberrant dim or negative expression of CD7. HSTLs are either CD4−/CD8− (majority) or CD4−/CD8+ (minority). TIA1, a cytotoxic granule-associated marker, is often positive, and CD56 may be expressed. EBV/EBER is most often negative. HSTL is characterized by presence of isochromosome 7.

T-PLL

T-PLL is characterized by prominent lymphocytosis and splenomegaly. The involvement of the lymph node is usually paracortical with preserved follicles but may be diffuse with total effacement of lymph node architecture. The diagnosis of T-PLL is made most often based on blood findings. When analyzed by FC T-PLLs often show positive expression of all four pan-T cell markers (CD2, CD3, CD5, and CD7) whereas PTCLs frequently show aberrant expression of one or more pan-T-cell markers. T-PLL show strong expression of TCL1. PTCL may involve blood, but this occurs most often at the advanced stages of the disease. Characteristic for T-PLL inv(14)(q11;q32.1) or t(14;14)(q11;q32.1) leading to rearrangement of *TCL1* gene (detectable by FISH) is not seen in PTCL.

BPDCN

BPDCN involves skin and frequently disseminates to blood and/or BM. BPDCN is positive for CD4, CD43, CD45, CD56, and CD123, but often shows also strong expression of CD2 and CD7. Subset of BPDCNs may be positive for TdT. It can be distinguished from PTCL by immature cytologic features, lack of CD3 and CD5 expression, and positive CD56, CD123, and HLA-DR. PTCL are most often HLA-DR− and are rarely CD56+.

T-ALL/LBL

T-ALL cells are usually positive for CD34, TdT, and/or CD1a. In addition, they are most often either CD4/CD8+ or CD4/CD8−, whereas the majority of PTCL cases are CD4+ or less often CD8+. When analyzed by FC, T-ALL often show dimmer CD45 expression, lack of surface CD3 expression, strong FC analysis may also be helpful, often showing lack of the expression of surface CD3, dimmer CD45 expression and strong expression of CD7 in T-ALL.

Follicular variant of PTCL

FTCL is a T-cell lymphoma with a follicular growth pattern derived from T follicular helper cells (TFHs). FTCLs show overlapping cytomorphologic and immunophenotypic features with AITL (e.g., neoplastic clear cells, presence of B immunoblasts, EBV⁺ cells, expression of CD10, BCL6, PD1, SAP, CCR5, and CXCL13) suggesting a possible relationship [97–99]. A few patients with FTCL can relapse as AITL and vice versa. In a series of PTCL with follicular pattern reported by Huang et al., neoplastic cells were medium-sized with clear cytoplasm and were CD4⁺ in 89%, CD10⁺ in 72%, BCL6⁺ in 74%, and CXCL13⁺ in 85% [97]. The main difference between FTC and AITL is the diffuse growth pattern of AITL with expanded FDC meshwork surrounding blood vessels, hyperplastic arborizing high endothelial venules and the polymorphic background [100]. Apart from AITL and FTCL, TFH-derived neoplasms include PTCL-TFH and primary cutaneous CD4⁺ small/medium T-cell lymphoma. Because of nodular architecture, FTCL needs to be differentiated from NLPHL, lymphocyte-rich cHL, FL, and some MZLs. The FTCL may mimic cHL, especially lymphocyte rich variant. Moroch et al. described five cases of FTCL originally diagnosed as HL [100]. All those cases showed scattered large polylobated cells with cytologic and immunophenotypic features typical for Reed-Sternberg cells, including expression of CD15, CD30, and EBV (EBER). Extensive immunophenotyping with demonstration of atypical cells expressing TFH-associated markers (CD10, SAP, BCL6, PD-1, CCR5, and CXCL13) helps to differentiate T-cell lymphomas with TFH phenotype from PTCL, NOS. According to WHO classification, cases are qualified as a TFH lymphoma if there is positive expression of at least two, or ideally three TFH immunophenotypic markers [1].

Nodal TFH cell lymphoma, angioimmunoblastic-type (AITL)

AITL phenotype by FC: CD2⁺/⁻, CD3⁻/⁺, CD4⁺, CD5⁺/⁻, CD7⁺/⁻, CD8⁻, CD10⁺/rarely⁻, CD30⁻/rare cells⁺, CD45⁺, CD56⁻, CD81⁺, CD200⁺/rarely⁻

Introduction

Current WHO classification divides nodal T-follicular helper (TFH) cell lymphomas into three subtype: nodal TFH cell lymphoma, angioimmunoblastic-type (AITL; previously named angioimmunoblastic T-cell lymphoma), nodal TFH cell lymphoma, follicular type (FTCL) and nodal TFH cell lymphoma, NOS (PTCL-TFH). AITL is an uncommon but aggressive nodal, mature T-cell lymphoma characterized by systemic symptoms, polyclonal hypergammaglobulinemia and generalized lymphadenopathy with a polymorphous lymphoid infiltrate and increased vascularity [1, 75, 77, 101–105]. AITL affects elderly adults in their 6th and 7th decade (median age ranges from 59 to 65 years) [106, 107]. The expression of the chemokine CXCL13 by the neoplastic cells in conjunction with gene-expression profile suggest that AITL mostly likely derives from TFHs a finding that explains many of its pathological and clinical features [108–111]. Common clinical symptoms include subacute or acute systemic illness, fever, weight loss, adenopathy, skin rash, arthritis, and edema with pleural and/or peritoneal effusions. Generalized adenopathy is present in 90% of cases, constitutional symptoms (B symptoms) in 77% of cases, spleen enlargement in 51%–79%, hepatomegaly in 50%, skin manifestations in 45%–50% pruritus, pleuritis (22%–37%), arthralgia or arthritis (17%), ear, nose, and throat involvement (14%); central or peripheral neurologic manifestations (10%), and ascites (5%–25%) [101, 112–114]. Most patients present with advanced disease at diagnosis with BM involvement seen in

60%–70%. The other abnormalities include: elevated LDH (50%–80%), inflammatory syndrome (67%), hypergammaglobulinemia (50%–80%), anemia (51%–88%), lymphopenia (20%–52%), hypereosinophilia (35%–50%), auto- or dysimmune manifestations (30%), autoimmune hemolytic anemia (19%), thrombocytopenic purpura (7%), and vasculitis (12%) [112, 114]. One of rare immunologic abnormalities observed in AITL is exuberant polyclonal plasmacytosis in blood mimicking PCL.

Morphology

Lymph nodes. In typical cases histology shows variable degrees of effacement of the lymph node architecture (often with capsular and perinodal infiltration) by polymorphous infiltrate composed of small reactive lymphocytes, histiocytes or epithelioid cells, immunoblasts, eosinophils, plasma cells, and clusters of atypical small to medium-sized T-cells (Figures 16.44–16.46). The atypical cells have a tendency for clustering or have prominent perivascular distribution. There is characteristic irregular proliferation of FDCs, best visualized by CD21, CD23, and/or CD35) and increased vascularity due to marked proliferation of high endothelial venules, many of which show thickened or hyalinized PAS⁺ walls [115–117]. The meshwork of FDC surrounds the vessels and may have the characteristic for AITL appearance of "burn out" germinal centers [118]. B-cells are sparse and pushed toward the periphery of the lymph node, and in most cases, there are no germinal centers. Large B-cells with immunoblastic features are scattered individually throughout the lymph node. Neoplastic T-cell infiltrate is usually polymorphic composed predominantly of small to medium-sized cells with occasional large, highly atypical cells. The latter may resemble Reed-Sternberg cells. Typical neoplastic cells have round, oval or slightly irregular nuclei and abundant, clear cytoplasm with distinct cell membranes. In less typical cases, the neoplastic cells are small with minimal atypia without characteristic clear cytoplasm.

Based on the presence of hyperplastic follicles, regressed follicles or absence of follicles, AITL can be subdivided morphologically into three categories [1, 74, 115–117]:

- Pattern I (AITL with hyperplastic follicles; Figure 16.46): The lymph node has mostly preserved architecture and contains hyperplastic follicles with poorly developed mantles merging with paracortex expanded by a polymorphous infiltrate that often comprises inconspicuous neoplastic cells, which tend to distribute around the follicles [114, 119].
- Pattern II (AITL with depleted follicles): Occasional depleted follicles are present. In pattern I and II, FDC are normal or only minimally increased.
- Pattern III (AITL without follicles): Classic type of AITL with complete effacement of the lymph node architecture.

Other variants of AITL include:

- Clear cell-rich variant: AITL with numerous neoplastic cells with clear cytoplasm.
- Epithelioid variant: AITL with many histiocytes with occasional granulomatous pattern resembling Lennert's lymphoma.
- B-cell-rich variant: It contains high proportion of large B-cells (>25%), which are usually (but not always) infected by EBV. In cases with very prominent large B-cell component, the diagnosis of EBV⁺ DLBCL may be rendered. This complication occurs most commonly during the evolution of the disease.

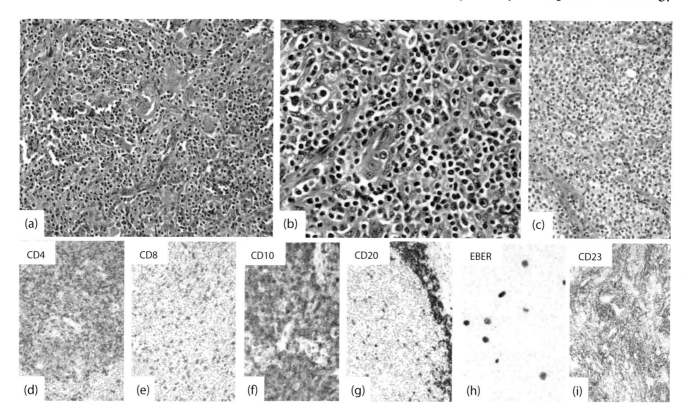

FIGURE 16.44 AITL. (a) Low power shows effacement of the architecture by a polymorphous lympho-vascular infiltrate. (b) Higher magnification shows the mixture of small and medium-sized lymphocytes, plasma cells, eosinophils, and blood vessels. (c) Another area shows clusters of atypical lymphocytes with clear cytoplasm. (d) CD4+ T-cells predominate. (e) Only rare CD8+ T-cell are present. (f) T-cells display aberrant expression of CD10. (g) B-cells are sparse and tend to accumulate at the periphery of the lymph node. (h) Scattered B-immunoblasts are expressing EBER. (i) Staining for CD23 highlights the expansion of follicular dendritic cells.

- Plasma cell-rich variant: AITL with high proportion of polytypic plasma cells. Occasional cases of AITL may even show marked polytypic plasmacytosis in blood (mimicking PCL). Rare cases of cutaneous T-cell lymphomas of TFH origin (including cutaneous CD4+ small/medium T-LPD and AITL) with monoclonal plasma cells have been reported. In contrast to cutaneous MZLs, the plasma cells do not form prominent sheets.
- Small cell variant: AITL composed of predominantly small lymphoid cells with scant cytoplasm.

Bone marrow (BM). Although the general adenopathy is the main presenting sign, many patients have evidence of extranodal involvement at the time of diagnosis. The most frequent extranodal sites include BM, spleen, skin, and lungs. BM involved by AITL shows either large interstitial lymphoid aggregates, interstitial, paratrabecular (Figure 16.47), diffuse or mixed pattern. Often the BM involvement is subtle. The infiltrate shows mixed population of small, medium-sized, and occasional large lymphocytes with cytologic and immunophenotypic features similar to lymph nodes with AITL. The background which may be focally myxoid shows eosinophils, plasma cells, and histiocytes, increased reticulin fibers and small blood vessels. Reactive plasmacytosis is frequently observed in patients with AITL (~60%), more often in cases with than without BM involvement by AITL [120]. In some cases, plasmacytosis is very prominent, raising the differential diagnosis of plasma cell myeloma (PCM). Other reactive changes include erythroid hyperplasia, eosinophilia,

myelofibrosis, or hemophagocytosis. In series reported by Cho et al., BM involvement was observed in 70% of cases, most often in the form of nodular (57%) infiltrate [120]. Remaining cases shows either focal or interstitial infiltrate. Blood vessel proliferation is observed in ~40% and clear cells in ~35% [120]. In contrast to strong CD3 and CD5 expression, staining with CD2 is often weak. Almost half of the cases show mixed infiltration by neoplastic T cells and reactive B-cells. Aberrant expression of CD10 is seen in 50% and BCL6 in ~60% [120].

Skin. In the skin the infiltrate may be subtle with non-specific mild perivascular accumulation of lymphocytes to (less often) an overt and diffuse infiltrate. In most cases, eosinophils, vascular proliferation and large immunoblasts are not obvious. EBV+ cells are only rarely demonstrated in skin lesions.

Blood. Occasional cases of AITL present at initial diagnosis with marked blood plasmacytosis mimicking PCL. FC of blood confirms in those cases benign (polytypic) character of plasma cells (Figure 16.48).

Immunophenotype

Immunohistochemistry. AITL is a neoplasm derived from TFHs, and as such, neoplastic T-cells express several markers characteristic of, although not entirely specific to, TFH: CXCL13, CD10, PD1, ICOS, BCL6, or CD200 [110, 121–124]. CD10 and CXCL13 are considered most specific and PD1 and ICOS most sensitive to identify TFH phenotype [121]. Immunophenotyping reveals predominance of T-cells with both CD4+ and CD8+ T-lymphocytes (neoplastic CD4+ T-cells usually predominate). Tumor cells

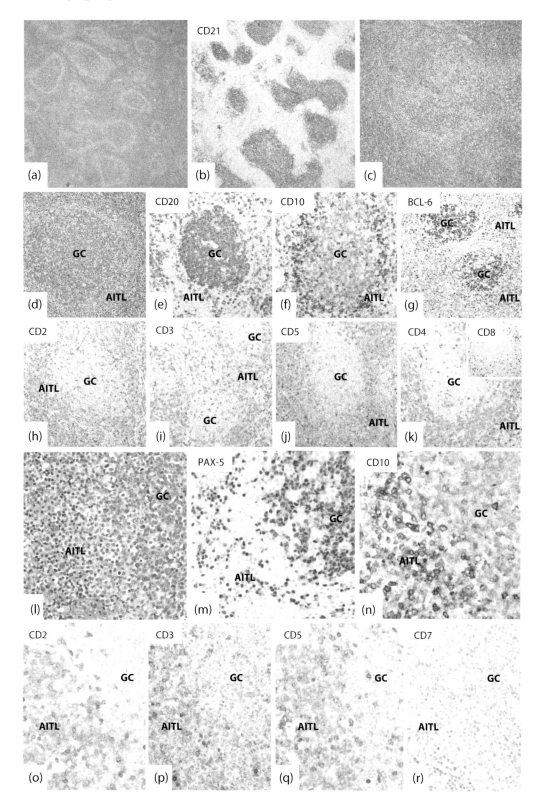

FIGURE 16.45 AITL. (a) Low magnification of the lymph node shows preserved architecture with secondary follicles surrounded by rim of clear cells. (b) Immunostaining with CD21 shows rather cohesive follicular dendritic meshwork, which does not expand into interfollicular area. (c) Intermediate magnification shows reactive germinal center surrounded by neoplastic cells with clear cytoplasm. (d–k) Immunostaining of the area depicted in d, shows residual germinal center positive for CD20 (e), CD10 (f), and BCL6 (g) surrounded by neoplastic T-cells (AITL), which express CD10 (f), BCL6 (g), CD2 (h), CD3 (i), CD5 (j), and CD4 (k; *inset*: CD8 staining for comparison). (l–r) High magnification focusing on the border of germinal center shows two distinct populations: benign B-cells (l; germinal center, GC) and lymphomatous cells with clear cytoplasm (l; AITL). Timor cells are negative for PAX5 (m) and positive for CD10 (n; note brighter expression compared to B-cells), CD2 (o), CD3 (p), and CD5 (q). CD7 is not expressed (r).

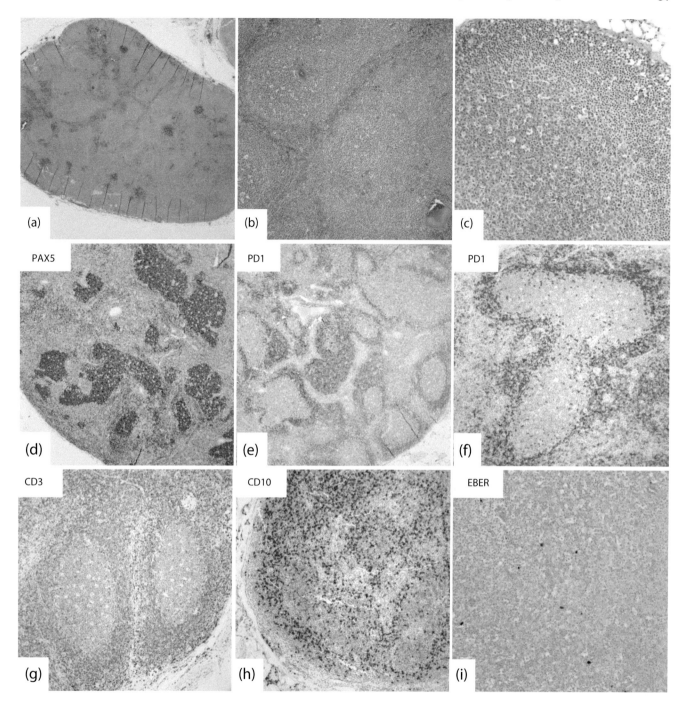

FIGURE 16.46 Perifollicular AITL with reactive germinal centers. The histologic section shows lymph node with numerous reactive germinal centers (a–c). The reactive B-cell follicles are positive for PAX5 (d). Neoplastic T-cell population is identified by immunostaining with PD1 (e–f, low and intermediate magnification), CD3 (g) and CD10 (h). Note dimmer expression of CD3 by neoplastic T-cells (immediately around the follicles) when compared to reactive T-cells in the background (g). The expression of CD10 is stronger among AITL cells than in germinal center cells (h). Scattered EBV-infected cells are noted by EBER (ISH) staining (i).

usually display aberrant expression of pan-T markers, most often loss of CD3 and/or CD7, but occasional tumors show expression of all pan T-cell markers (CD2, CD3, CD5, and CD7; Figure 16.49). The expression of T-markers may be much dimmer than in residual small (benign) T-cells. Majority of cases (80%) display co-expression of CD10 by neoplastic T-cells (Figures 16.44–16.46), but CD10 expression is often heterogeneous and the number of CD10+ T-cells in individual tumor may vary [106, 115, 116, 125].

Attygalle et al. reported CD10 expression in 89% of AITL [116]. BCL6 is expressed by T-cells in approximately one-third of cases. Both neoplastic T-cells and activated B-cells may express CD30. The presence of scattered CD30+ cells, often with irregular nuclei and prominent nucleoli (Reed-Sternberg-like cells) should not be confused with classic HL. Staining with CD21 or CD23 shows expansion of FDC meshwork in majority of cases. The majority of cases (regardless of the stage of the disease) contain EBV+ B-cells

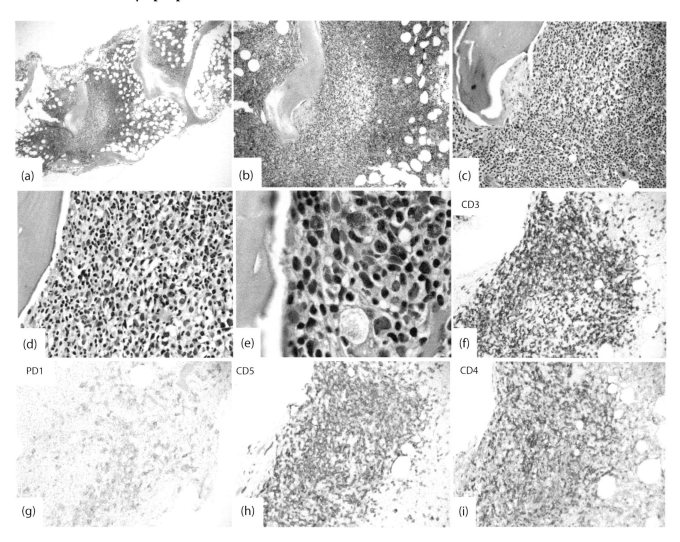

FIGURE 16.47 AITL – paratrabecular BM involvement. (a–e) Histology. Prominent paratrabecular involvement of BM by polymorphic lymphoid infiltrate of small to medium to large cells mixed with eosinophils. (f–I) Immunohistochemistry. Lymphomatous cells are positive for CD3 (f), PD1 (g), CD5 (h), and CD4 (I).

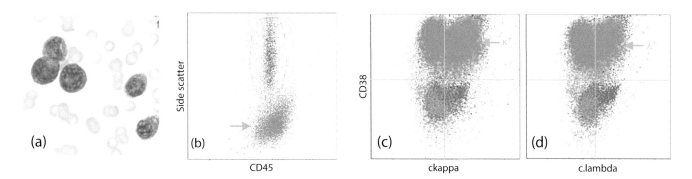

FIGURE 16.48 Blood with marked polytypic plasmacytosis in young patient with history of AITL. (a) Blood smear shows highly atypical plasma cells with occasional immature features. (b–d) Flow cytometry shows plasma cells with low side scatter and positive CD45 (b) and bright CD38 (c–d). Analysis of cytoplasmic light chains shows polytypic pattern with both kappa (c) and lambda (d) expression.

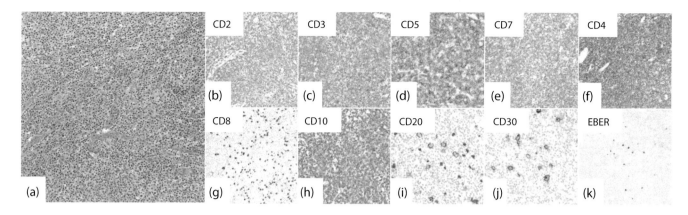

FIGURE 16.49 AITL – immunohistochemistry. Histology show typical features of AITL (a). Lymphomatous cells express all pan T-cell markers (CD2, CD3, CD5, and CD7; b–e), are CD4⁺/CD8⁻ (f–g) and show aberrant expression of CD10 (h). Scattered B-cells (CD20⁺; i), CD30⁺ cells (j), and EBV-infected cells (k) are noted.

[126]. CXCL13, a chemokine involved in B-cell migration into germinal centers, characteristic for follicular helper T cells, is expressed by majority of AITL [110]. Other markers for germinal center T cells, such as SAP and PD1 are also positive in most cases of AITL [124, 127].

Flow cytometry (FC). FC analysis reveals atypical T-cell population in majority of AITL, including cases with predominance of reactive component (Figures 16.50–16.54). The neoplastic T-cells are CD4⁺ and often show dim or negative expression of one or more of the pan-cell antigens, increased (often variable or "smeary") forward scatter and partial CD10 positivity. Subset of cells may be positive for CD71 (dim). Rare CD30⁺ cells are also often present. In some cases, the phenotypic atypia is easily identifiable (e.g., loss of surface CD3, CD5, and/or CD7), but immunophenotypic changes in the expression of pan-T-cell antigens may be subtle and abnormal population is identified through variable but increased forward scatter and CD4 restriction (Figure 16.53). CD56 expression (often partial) may be present in AITL by FC analysis. Presence of CD3⁻/dimCD4⁺ T-cell

population helps to identify AITL by FC analysis [75]. Loghavi et al. reported less frequent expression of CD10 in AITL involving BM or blood when compared to lymph nodes, and more frequent loss of surface CD3 expression by AITL cells in blood and BM than in lymph nodes [128].

Genetic features

Chromosomal abnormalities can be identified in ~62% of AITL. The most common chromosomal changes reported in AITL include trisomy 3, trisomy 5, and additional copy of chromosome X, +18, +19, and −7 [91, 112, 129, 130]. Majority of cases are positive for clonal *TCR* gene rearrangement, and subset of cases (~10%–30%) shows also clonal rearrangement of the immunoglobulin gene [118, 131–133]. Gene-expression profiling of AITL has demonstrated overexpression of several genes characteristic of follicular helper T cells and vascular endothelial growth factor-A [109, 134]. The molecular profile of genes mutated in AITL resembles myeloid diseases, including mutations in epigenetic modifiers (*TET2*, *IDH2*, and *DNMT3A*) [135]. *TET2* mutations are seen

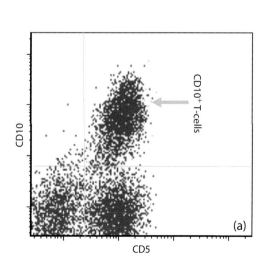

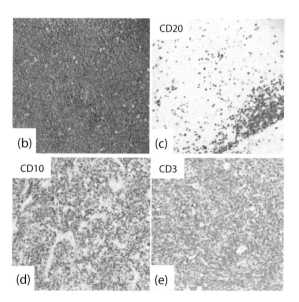

FIGURE 16.50 AITL with strong CD10 expression by both flow cytometry and IHC. (a) FC analysis shows significant T-cell population showing CD5 and CD10 co-expression (arrows). (b) Histology. (c–e) Immunohistochemistry. Only rare CD20⁺ B-cells are present, mostly in the subcapsular area (c). T-cells show aberrant expression of CD10 (d–e).

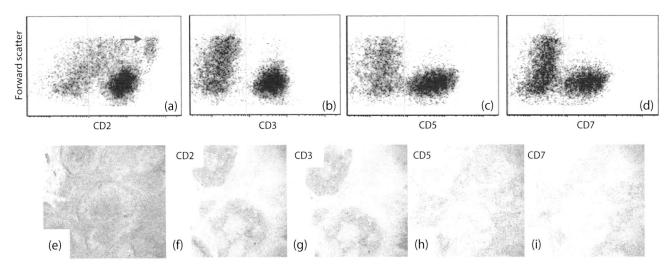

FIGURE 16.51 AITL (perifollicular pattern) – flow cytometry. (a–d) FC analysis shows predominance of small T-cells with normal expression of T-cell antigens. Only minor subset of T-cells with high forward scatter (arrow) show positive CD2 expression (a) and lack of surface CD3 (b), CD5 (c), and CD7 (d). (e) Histology shows atypical clusters of clear cells around lymphoid follicles. (f–j). Immunohistochemistry. Neoplastic T-cells are positive for CD2 (f), CD3 (g), and negative for CD5 (h) and CD7 (I).

in 80%, *RHOA* mutations in 50%–70%, *DNMT3A* mutations in 20%–40%, and *IDH2* mutations in 20%–30%. Other mutations include *TP53, JAK2,* and *STAT3* [135, 136].

Differential diagnosis of AITL
Differential diagnosis of AITL includes [74, 97, 100, 116, 117, 137–139]:

- Reactive lymphoid hyperplasia (e.g., HIV-associated or EBV-associated, drug reactions)
- Reactive lymph node with progressive transformation of germinal centers (PTGCs)
- Rosai-Dorfman disease

- PTCL, NOS
- FTCL
- Nodal TFH cell lymphoma, NOS (PTCL-TFH)
- ATLL
- MZL

Differential diagnosis of AITL based on TFH phenotype includes:

- Nodal TFH cell lymphoma, follicular-type FTCL
- Nodal TFH cell lymphoma, NOS (PTCL-TFH)
- FL
- DLBCL, subset
- Other CD10+ B-cell lymphomas

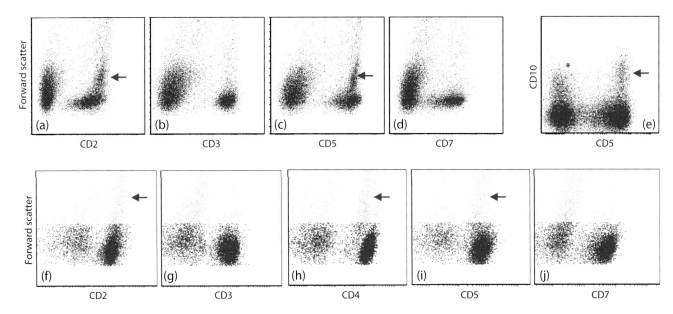

FIGURE 16.52 AITL – FC analysis (two cases). (a–e). Case #1. AITL cells have increased forward scatter. They are positive for CD2 (a, arrow), negative for CD3 (b), positive for CD5 (c, arrow), negative for CD7 (d), and positive for CD10 (e, arrow; benign germinal center cells are CD5− and CD10+, *). (f–k) Case #2. AITL cells (blue dots) have increased forward scatter. They are positive for CD2 (f, arrow), negative for CD3 (g), positive for CD4 (h, arrow), positive for CD5 (i, arrow), and negative for CD7 (j).

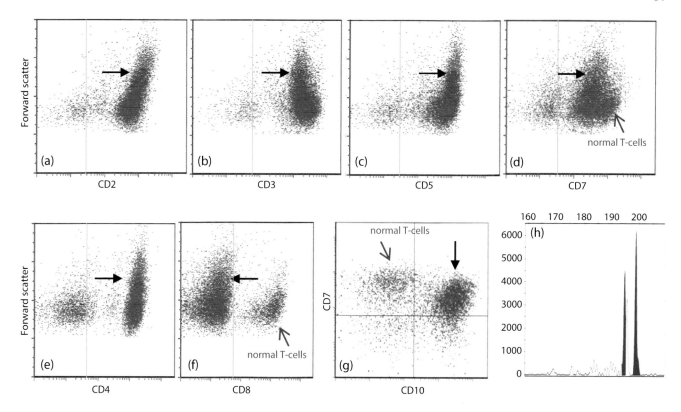

FIGURE 16.53 AITL. Neoplastic T-cells (black arrow) show partially increased forward scatter and subtle changes in the expression of pan-T-cell antigens, including minimally dimmer expression of CD3 (b) and CD7 (d). Other changes typical for AITL are easily identifiable, such as CD4 restriction (e) and aberrant expression of CD10 (g). Molecular testing confirmed T-cell clonality (PCR; h).

Differential diagnosis of AITL based on presence of circulating plasma cells:

- Reactive plasmacytosis in blood
- PCL

Reactive processes

Early AITL may show preserved reactive germinal centers with mostly interfollicular distribution of neoplastic cells, and therefore it may be difficult to differentiate from reactive processes (especially those accompanying autoimmune conditions) Identification of clusters of atypical lymphoid cells with clear cytoplasm and aberrant phenotype, presence of a prominent arborizing vascular network of high endothelial venules and proliferation of the FDCs helps to establish the diagnosis of AITL. Correlation with molecular testing for T-cell clonality may be needed in difficult cases.

Cook et al. reported the presence of rare benign CD10+ T-cells in reactive lymph nodes and B-cell disorders and therefore the identification of minute population of CD10+ T-cells should not be considered an indication of AITL [140, 141]. PD1 staining is a highly sensitive marker in the diagnosis of PTCLs: increased extrafollicular PD1+ cells are seen in 93% (76/82) of AITL, 62% (16/26) of PTCL, and 11% (2/18) of anaplastic-lymphoma-kinase (ALK)-negative ALCL [142]. The majority of reactive lymphadenopathies including cat-scratch disease, Kikuchi lymphadenitis, Castleman's disease, and reactive follicular hyperplasia show no PD1 staining outside follicles. The reactive processes with increased extrafollicular PD1+ cells in a pattern similar to AITL

and PTCL, include PTGCs, viral lymphadenitis (EBV and human immunodeficiency virus), and Rosai-Dorfman disease [142].

Lymph node in infectious mononucleosis shows follicular hyperplasia, which is absent in typical AITL (lymphoid follicles are present in early AITL, type I). Reactive processes lack atypical T-cells with clear cytoplasm expressing CD10 or BCL6, an arborizing vascular proliferation and atypical expansion of FDC meshwork. Many viral infections are characterized by increased proportion of CD8+ T-cells, rather than CD4+ T-cells typical for AITL. Most of the reactive conditions do not have clonal rearrangement of *TCR* gene.

ATLL

ATLL may occasionally show AITL-like pattern in the involved lymph nodes [28]. Positive HTLV1 status confirms the diagnosis of ATLL. Prominent lymphocytosis with "flower cells" on blood film, hypercalcemia and elevated LDH are characteristic for acute variant of ATLL, which also may show adenopathy, hepatosplenomegaly, and skin involvement. Lymphomatous variant of ATLL lacks lymphocytosis and typically presents with prominent adenopathy, but often also involves skin, liver, and spleen. Mild adenopathy is also seen in chronic variant, but both smoldering ATLL and primary cutaneous ATLL present without lymph node involvement.

PTCL

Patients with PTCL do not have hypergammaglobulinemia, typically present in AITL. In contrast to AITL, PTCL shows usually more monomorphic T-cell infiltrate with or without clear cells. The tumor cells are negative for TFH markers and they lack EBV+ B-cells, expanded meshwork of FDCs and prominent

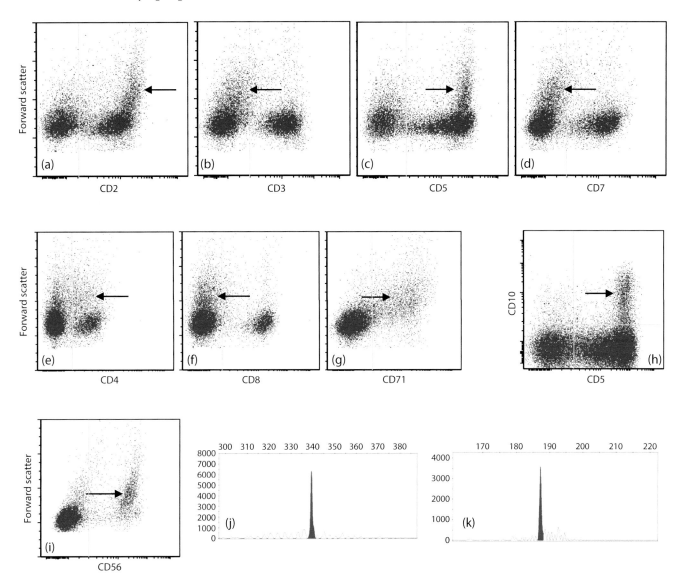

FIGURE 16.54 AITL – flow cytometry. Neoplastic T-cells show increased forward scatter (a–g; arrow), positive CD2 (a) and CD5 (c), negative CD3 (b) and CD7 (d), dimly positive CD4 (e), negative CD8 (f), positive CD71 (g), positive CD10 (h), and positive CD56 (i). Molecular testing (PCR) revealed clonal rearrangement of both IGH (j) and TCR (k).

vascular proliferation [115–117]. If there is increased vascularity in PTCL, it is most often mild [117]. The lymph node architecture in PTCL is effaced without too many residual B-cells (except for PTCL with T-zone pattern). In contrast to frequent expression of CD10 in AITL (89%), Attygalle et al. did not observe CD10 positivity in PTCL or ALCL [116]. EBER+ immunoblasts, so typical for AITL may be seen in PTCL as well [126].

PTCL-TFH
Nodal TFH cell lymphomas are defined by expression of at least 2 TFH markers (CD10, BCL6, CXCL13, PD1 (CD279), ICOS, SAP, CCR5, c-MAF, and CD200) in addition to CD4 expression. They include AITL, FTCL and nodal TFH cell lymphoma, NOS (PTCL-TFH). AITL cases were more likely than PTCL-TFH cases to contain expanded CD21+ FDC meshworks, clear cell cytology and polymorphous inflammatory background [143]. In contrast to FTCL the infiltrate is diffuse or less often T-zone-like. Lack of prominent polymorphic inflammatory background, vascular

proliferation and expansion of FDC meshwork differentiate this lymphoma from AITL, but the difference may be subtle, and it is suggested that PTCL-TFH may actually represent a tumor cell-rich variant of AITL [1, 144].

FTCL
TFH cells are considered as the normal counterpart of AITL, but TFH phenotype is not entirely specific for AITL because similar features are seen in rare variant of TFH cell lymphoma with nodular pattern (follicular-type; FTCL) and has also been reported in primary cutaneous CD4+ small to medium-sized pleomorphic T-cell lymphoma [145]. FTCL is a recently recognized rare variant of TFH cell lymphoma and nodular architecture [97–100, 146–151]. Because of overlapping phenotypic features between AITL and FTCL, close relationship between those two lymphomas has been suggested. However, presence of recurrent translocation t(5;9)(q23;q22) described in ~20% of FTCL [97, 152], but not in AITL, may suggest that at least a subset

of FTCL is distinct from AITL [100]. Clinical features of FTCL and AITL overlap. Morphologically, FTCL differs from AITL by lack of extrafollicular proliferation of FDCs and proliferation of high endothelial venules typical for AITL. Morphologically FTCL resembles either FL or PTGCs.

B-cell lymphomas

Based on positive CD10 expression by AITL, presence of increased (activated) large B-cells in some cases of AITL or histologic features mimicking MZL or FL with reversed pattern, differential diagnosis of AITL also includes B-cell lymphomas. Those are differentiated from AITL by FC by showing clonal B-cell population often mixed with reactive T-cells without aberrant phenotype.

Anaplastic large cell lymphoma (ALCL)

ALCL phenotype by FC: high forward scatter, CD2[+/rarely−], CD3[+/−], CD4[+] or less often CD8[+] (rare tumors are either CD4/8− or CD4/CD8[+]), CD5[+/−], CD7[−/rarely+], CD10−, CD25[+/−], CD26[+/rarely−], CD30[+], CD43[+], CD45[+], CD56[−/rarely+]

Introduction

ALCL is a T-cell lymphoma composed of large pleomorphic cells, which have irregular kidney-shaped nuclei ("hallmark cells") and are positive for CD30, and in majority of cases ALK (anaplastic lymphoma kinase protein). In current WHO classification, ALCL is divided into ALK[+] and ALK[−] type [1]. ALCL involves lymph nodes and extranodal sites, including skin, soft tissues, liver, lung, and bone and less often CNS and gastrointestinal tract. ALCL occurs at any age including children. ALK[+] ALCL occurs most commonly in the first three decades of life, is more common in men, presents as aggressive stage III to IV disease with systemic symptoms, have frequently extranodal involvement and has good response to chemotherapy [153–158]. ALK[−] ALCL occurs

in older patients (peak incidence in 6th decade), with a lower male predominance and less advanced stage, but with frequent involvement of skin, gastrointestinal tract and liver and but lower frequency of BM involvement [158]. A separate variant of ALK[−] ALCL in adults occurs in patients with breast implants [159–161].

Prognosis. The prognosis of ALK[+] ALCL is favorable, except for cases with blood involvement, which are aggressive. ALCL without ALK expression occurs in older patients with similar distribution in male and female patients is associated with poor prognosis, and lower incidence of stage III to IV disease and extranodal involvement. Supervised analysis with microarray gene-expression profiling, showed that ALK[+] ALCL and ALK[−] ALCL have different gene-expression profiles, further confirming that they are different entities [162]. Among the most significantly differentially expressed genes between ALK[+] and ALK[−] samples, Lamant et al. found *BCL6, PTPN12, CEBPB,* and *SERPINA1* genes to be overexpressed in ALK[+] ALCL [162]. It is therefore suggested that ALK[−] lymphomas with anaplastic features may represent a variant of CD30[+] PTCL.

Morphology

Lymph nodes. ALK[+] ALCL shows a wide range of morphological spectrum including common, lymphohistiocytic, small cell, giant cell, monomorphic, and Hodgkin-like variants [147, 156, 162–171].

Five morphological variants of AKL[+] ALCL have been described:

- Classic (common)
- Lymphohistiocytic
- Monomorphic
- Small cell
- Hodgkin-like
- Composite

The classic (common) variant of ALCL (Figure 16.55) comprises the majority of cases of ALCL (60%) [155, 163]. Typical cases show

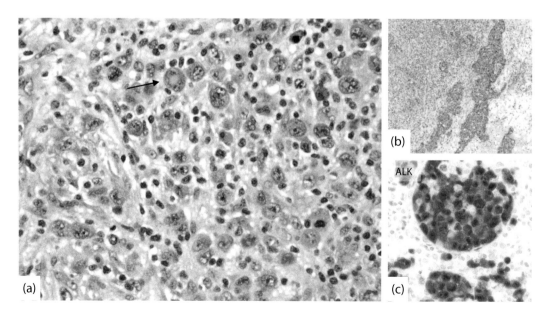

FIGURE 16.55 Anaplastic large cell lymphoma (ALCL) – common variant. (a) Pleomorphic large cell lymphoid infiltrate. Many nuclei are irregular with a horseshoe shape, so-called hallmark cells (arrow). (b) Low power shows focal intrasinusoidal distribution of tumor cells. (c) Intrasinusoidal clusters of tumor cells show strong nuclear and cytoplasmic expression of ALK.

large neoplastic cells with characteristic horseshoe or kidney-shaped nuclei ("hallmark cells"), prominent nucleoli, eosinophilic region near the nucleus, and abundant cytoplasm. The lympho-histiocytic variant is characterized by a mixture of tumor cells, which are usually smaller than in the common variant and a large number of histiocytes [172]. The monomorphic variant contains a diffuse infiltrate of large monomorphic cells with predominantly round nuclei and prominent nucleoli, resembling immunoblastic lymphoma. The small cell variant has a predominance of small to medium-sized lymphocytes with scattered large hallmark cells. Expression of ALK put this variant into ALCL category, despite small cell size and lack of overt anaplastic features. The Hodgkin-like variant is seen rarely (<5%) and is characterized by morphologic features similar to nodular sclerosis subtype of cHL. Subset

of ALK+ ALCL shows infiltrate composed of more than one histomorphologic variant (15%) [171]. The pattern of lymph node involvement may be diffuse, perifollicular/T-zone or focal with characteristic intrasinusoidal distribution of tumor cells, mimicking metastatic tumor. Some of the tumor cells have prominent invagination of the nuclear membrane creating "doughnut" like cells, whereas other cells resemble Reed-Sternberg cells. Giant-cell variant of ALCL shows large cells with irregular often bizarre nuclei. Rare ALCL may show prominent spindle cells in a myxoid stroma [108]. Histologic features of ALK− ALCL are similar to ALK+ tumors.

Extranodal sites. ALCL often involves extranodal sites (Figure 16.56), including cerebrospinal fluid (CSF), liver, skin, spleen, lungs, testes, and bone/BM, body cavities and soft tissues

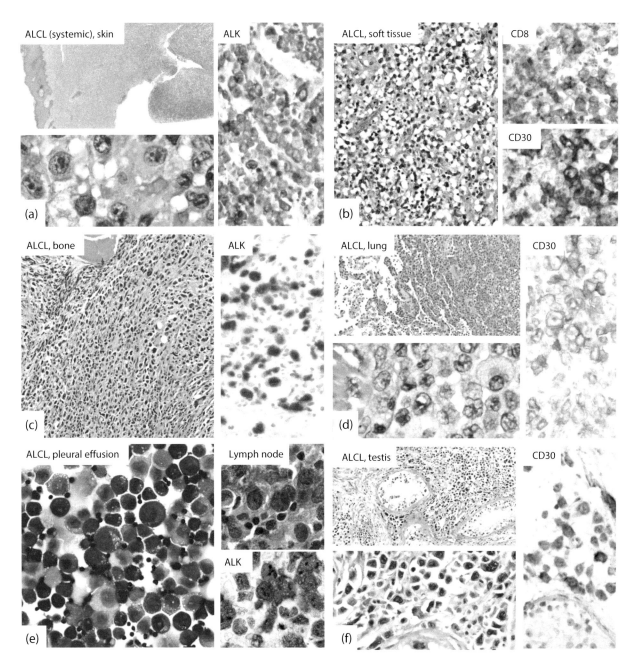

FIGURE 16.56 Extranodal ALK+ ALCL. (a) Skin. (b) Soft tissue. (c) Bone. (d) Lung. (e) Pleural effusion with concurrent involvement of the lymph node. (f) Testis.

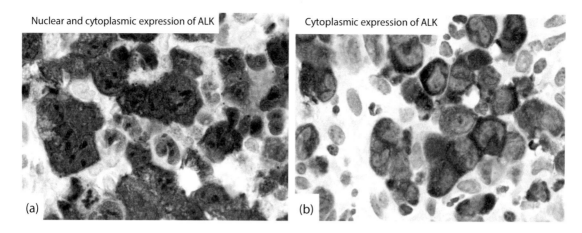

FIGURE 16.57   ALCL – two patterns of ALK expression: (a) nuclear, nucleolar, and cytoplasmic staining; (b) cytoplasmic staining.

[167, 173–178]. ALCL is rarely associated with leukemic blood involvement, and those cases may show extensive extranodal disease [175]. Most cases involving blood belong to the small cell category of ALCL [167, 168, 175].

Bone marrow. ALCL show either diffuse, nodular, interstitial, or rarely intrasinusoidal pattern of BM involvement. Interstitial pattern is seen more often in ALK⁺ tumors and nodular pattern more often in ALK⁻ tumors [179]. Tumor cells are strongly positive for CD30, CD43s, and usually some of the pan-T-cell markers. Immunohistochemical staining for CD30 and/or ALK is especially useful in identification of BM involvement by small cell variant of ALCL.

Immunophenotype

Immunohistochemistry. The ALK expression in ALCL may be nuclear, nucleolar, and cytoplasmic (Figure 16.57). The t(2;5) is associated with nuclear/nucleolar and cytoplasmic staining, whereas ALCL with variant translocations, other than t(2;5) show cytoplasmic staining. The neoplastic cells are positive for CD30 with strong membrane staining and perinuclear Golgi accentuation (Figure 16.58). The expression of CD30 may be less prominent in small cell variant of ALCL. Majority of cases are positive

for CD45, CD43, and EMA. Pan-T antigens are often aberrantly expressed (only about 10% of ALCL are positive for all four pan-T antigens). CD7 is most frequently absent and CD2 is least frequently absent. Subset of ALCL may be negative for all four pan-T antigens ("null cell type"). Majority of cases are CD4⁺ (~70%), but CD8⁺, CD4⁺/8⁺, or CD4⁻/8⁻ cases do occur. ALCLs are predominantly TCRab⁺ (~70%), and remaining cases do not express TCR. A subset of ALCL may be CD56⁺. MUM1, a plasma cell marker, may be positive. Patients with CD56⁺ ALCL have much poorer prognosis than those with CD56⁻ tumors in both the ALK⁺ and ALK⁻ subgroups [180]. Subset of cases displays aberrant lack of CD45 expression. PAX5 is negative in ALCL. Rare cases of ALCL may display aberrant expression of CD15. Most ALCLs are positive for cytotoxic markers (TIA1, granzyme B, perforin) as well as EMA and clusterin. Cytotoxic protein expression (TIA1, granzyme B, or perforin) is slightly more pronounced in ALK⁺ compared to ALK⁻ tumors.

Flow cytometry. FC may show cluster of cells with high forward scatter as well as increased side scatter, which put tumor cells in "monocytic" or "granulocytic" regions on CD45 versus side scatter display (as with other high-grade lymphomas, FC often underestimate the number of tumor cells due to selective

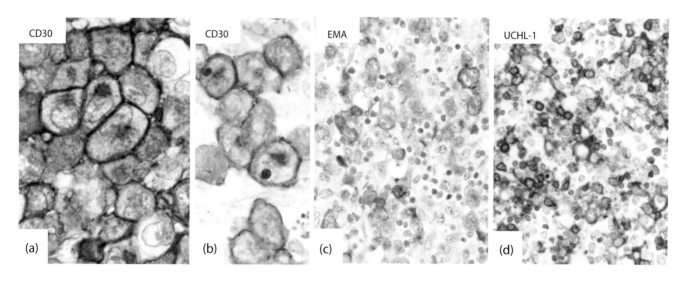

FIGURE 16.58   ALCL – immunohistochemistry. Neoplastic cells are positive for CD30 (a–b, strong membranous and Golgi-area staining), EMA (c), and UCHL-1 (d).

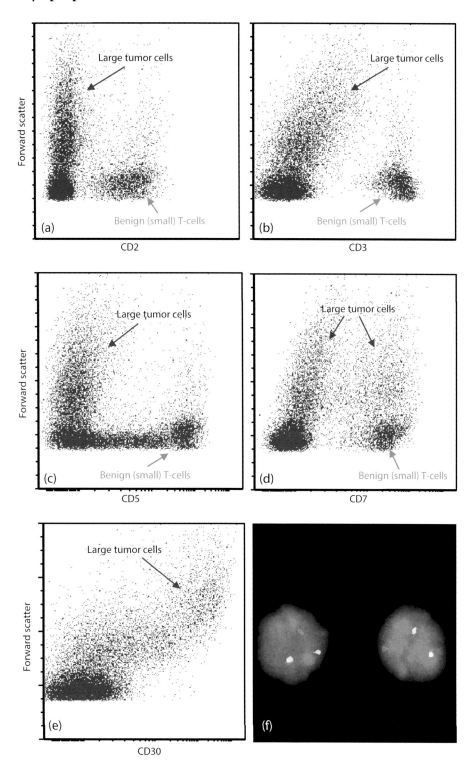

FIGURE 16.59 ALCL – flow cytometry. ALCL (cervical lymph node from 12-year-old boy) shows negative expression of T-cell antigens (a–c), except for partial CD7 expression (d). CD30 is strongly positive (e). FISH analysis showed *ALK* rearrangement (f; break-apart probe).

loss of tumor cells). The neoplastic cells often display aberrant phenotype, easily identifiable by FC data (Figures 16.59 and 16.60; Table 16.5). Most cases show aberrant expression of T-cell markers with loss of surface CD3, CD5, or TCR. In a FC series of 19 cases reported by Juco et al., the neoplastic cells expressed CD45, HLA-DR, and CD30 in all cases, CD2 in 71%, CD3 in 32%, CD4 in 63%, CD5 in 26%, CD7 in 32%, CD8 in 21%, and CD25 in 88% [181]. In a series reported by Kesler et al. (29 cases), CD4 was expressed most commonly (80%), followed by CD2 (72%), CD3 (40%), and CD5 and CD7 (32% each); CD45 was expressed in 23 of 25 cases and CD13 in 7 of 9 cases [182]. FC is helpful in identifying cases with leukemic blood involvement

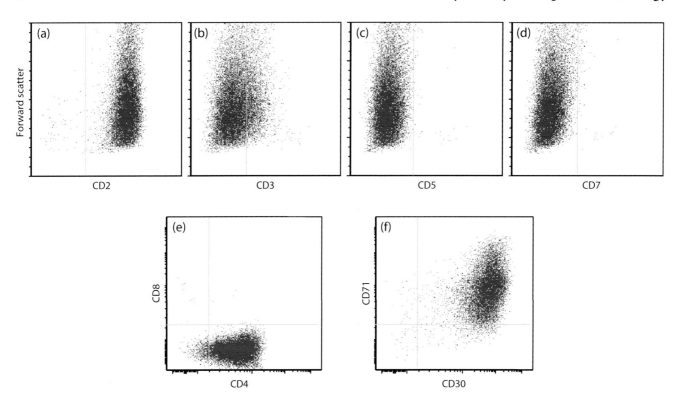

FIGURE 16.60 ALCL – flow cytometry. Lymphomatous cells are positive for CD2 (a), CD4 (e), CD30 (f), and CD71 (f). CD3 (b), CD5 (c), and CD7 (d) are negative.

(Figure 16.61), BM involvement (Figure 16.62), body cavities (effusions; Figure 16.63), or CSF. In blood or BM analysis, the sensitivity of FC approaches that of molecular testing for *NPM-ALK* (PCR) [183, 184].

Genetic features
ALK+ and ALK− ALCL differ in terms of genomic profiles [185]. The most common losses affect 17p13.3-p12 (25%), in which *TP53* gene is located, 6q21 (17%), the region containing *PRDM1* and *ATG5*, 13q32.3-q33.3, and 16q23.2 (16%) [185]. More than 20% of

TABLE 16.5: Phenotype of ALCL (*n* = 33)

CD45+	**97%**
All four T-cell antigens positive (normal expression)	9% (9%)
One T-cell antigen−	15%
Two T-cell antigens−	27%
Three T-cell antigens−	30%
All four T-cell antigens−	18%
CD2+	67%
CD3+	30%
CD5+	42%
CD7+	27%
CD4+	70%
CD8+	18%
CD4+/CD8+	3%
CD4−/CD8−	9%
CD56+	12%
CD57+	0
CD10+	0

ALCL show gains f different regions of the long arm of chromosome 1 and 16% cases show gains of 8q24.22. In ALK− ALCL, 52% show *PRDM1* inactivation and/or loss of 17p (52%), and remaining 48% are negative for those changes, and in ALK+ ALCL, 45% show genetic aberrations (in addition to *ALK*) and the remaining 55% are without additional genetic changes [185]. Subset of ALCL carry the t(2;5)(p23;q35) [166]. The t(2;5) disrupts the nucleophosmin (*NPM*) gene at 5q35 and the anaplastic lymphoma kinase (*ALK*) gene at 2p23, generating a novel *NPM-ALK* fusion gene. *ALK* (CD246) belongs to the insulin receptor superfamily with a role in both neural development and oncogenesis. *NPM-ALK* fusion leads to a chimeric mRNA molecule and a unique 80-kDa NPM-ALK fusion protein referred to as p80 [186]. The t(2;5)(p23;q35) and variant translocations involving 2p23 result in overexpression of ALK protein, which can be detected by routine immunohistochemistry [187–191]. ALCL with *NPM-ALK* fusion shows strong nuclear, nucleolar, and cytoplasmic ALK staining. Several cytogenetic and molecular studies have demonstrated that chromosomal aberrations other than the t(2;5) (p23;q35) may give rise to *ALK* fusion in ALCL. These alternative partners to *NPM* gene include *TPM3* (nonmuscle tropomyosin) associated with t(1;2)(q21;p23), *TFG* (*TRK*-fused gene) associated with t(2;3)(p23;q21), *CLTC* (clathrin heavy chain gene) associated with t(2;17)(p23;q23) and *MSN* (moesin) [188, 190, 192]. Contrary to the nuclear and cytoplasmic distribution of the NPM-ALK protein, variant ALK fusion proteins show a variable subcellular localization, for example in ALC with t(1;2) [*TPM3-ALK*], ALK expression is restricted to cytoplasm with strong membrane staining [188, 193]. ALK identification by immunostaining on routine tissue section (immunohistochemistry) or *ALK* FISH with break-apart probes are most commonly applied to identify ALK+ ALCL.

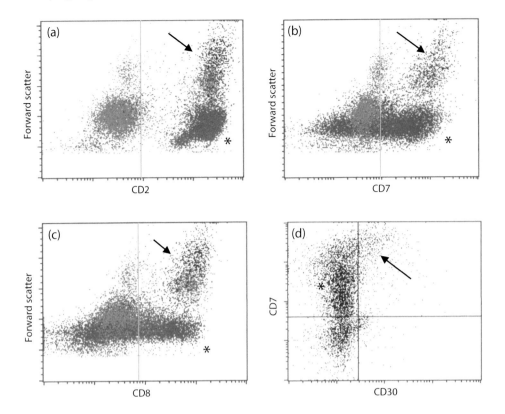

FIGURE 16.61 ALCL – leukemic phase (blood involvement). Flow cytometry of blood shows population of large cells (increased forward scatter; arrows) expressing CD2 (a), CD7 (b), CD8 (c), and CD30 (d), Benign small T-cells (*) are positive for CD2, CD7, CD8, and negative for CD30.

Differential diagnosis

Differential diagnosis of ALCL depends on the location of the tumor and includes large cell hematolymphoid and non-hematopoietic tumors, especially, DLBCL, classical Hodgkin lymphoma (HL), PTCL, NOS, "gray zone" lymphoma (large B-cell lymphoma with features intermediate between cHL and DLBCL), and some non-hematopoietic tumors (carcinoma, melanoma, or sarcoma), as shown in Figure 16.64. Positive ALK expression excludes most tumors, except ALK+ DLBCL and occasional ALK+ non-hematopoietic tumors. Non-hematolymphoid tumors expressing ALK include subset of breast carcinomas, of lung carcinomas, rhabdomyosarcoma (alveolar), neuroblastoma, and inflammatory myofibroblastic tumor. Neither CD30 nor ALK is absolutely specific for ALCL and the diagnostic significance of the expression of these proteins must be carefully assessed in combination with other phenotypic, morphological, clinical, and even genetic information.

Differential diagnosis of ALCL (ALK+ and ALK−) based on morphology:

- cHL
- DLBCL, especially with anaplastic features
- Intravascular large B-cell lymphoma (IVLBCL)
- Primary effusion lymphoma (PEL), especially solid organ variant
- DLBCL with ALK expression
- Primary mediastinal B-cell lymphoma (PMBL)
- PTCL, NOS
- Mediastinal grey zone lymphoma
- EATL

- Primary cutaneous CD30+ T-cell lymphoproliferations
- Non-hematopoietic tumors (carcinoma, sarcoma, and melanoma)
- Breast implant-associated ALCL
- Atypical reactive hyperplasia (e.g., EBV lymphadenitis)

Differential diagnosis of ALCL (ALK+ and ALK−) based on CD30 expression:

- cHL
- DLBCL, especially with anaplastic features
- PMBL
- PTCL, NOS
- Mediastinal grey zone lymphoma
- Primary cutaneous CD30+ T-cell lymphoproliferations, transformed MF
- EATL
- Breast implant-associated ALCL
- ATLL

Reactive processes

Occasional cases of reactive lymph node hyperplasia (especially atypical processes accompanying viral infections) may contain increased number of large (activated) B-cells in the paracortex which are CD30+; immunostaining with B- and T-cell markers, EBV/EBER and careful analysis of cytomorphologic and histologic (architectural) features helps to exclude ALCL and classical HL.

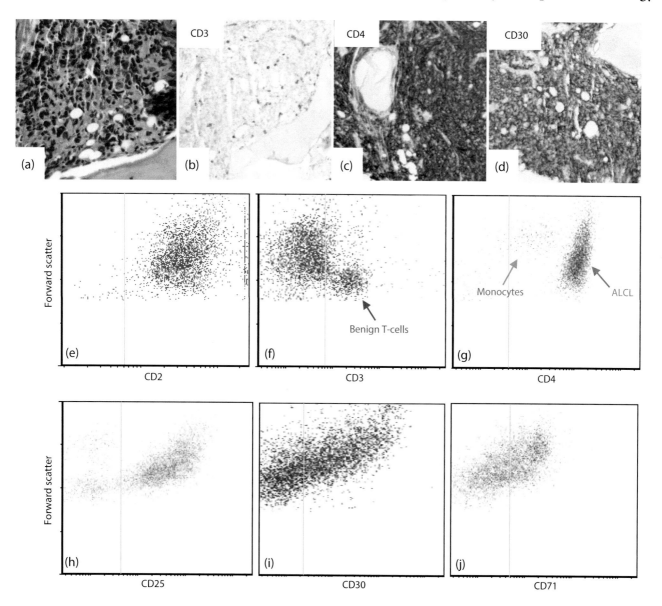

FIGURE 16.62 ALCL with extensive BM involvement. Histology of the core biopsy (a) shows diffuse infiltrate of large atypical lymphoid cells. (b–d) Immunohistochemistry analysis shows lack of CD3 expression (b) and positive CD4 (c), and CD30 (d). (e–j) Flow cytometry shows lymphomatous cells (magenta dots) positive for CD2 (e), negative for CD3 (f), and positive for CD4 (g), CD25 (h), CD30 (i), and partially CD71 (j).

Primary cutaneous CD30⁺ T-cell lymphoproliferations

Primary cutaneous CD30⁺ lymphomas, including primary C-ALCL and LyP, show strong expression of CD30 with membranous and Golgi pattern. The majority of C-ALCL are ALK⁻ by immunohistochemistry. Very rare cases may show cytoplasmic ALK expression associated with variant *ALK* rearrangement [other than t(2;5)], but occasional cases with cytoplasmic and nuclear ALK staining have also been reported (more often in pediatric population) [194–197]. Regardless of classical or variant *ALK* translocation, FISH "break-apart" probe for *ALK* gene can identify *ALK* rearrangement in those cases. Very often, correlation with clinical presentation is crucial to differentiate between systemic ALCL involving skin, LyP and C-ALCL. Correlation with clinical data (history, skin status) is necessary

to differentiate lymphatic drainage from C-ALCL or LyP and systemic ALCL. Both secondary lymph node involvement form cutaneous CD30⁺ tumors and systemic ALCL may show subcapsular and sinusoidal infiltration [197]. Approximately 5%–10% of LyP cases may involve lymph nodes [198]. CD30 expression is seen also in majority of transformed MF cases. Those cases often have history of MF. Histologically, transformed MF shows sheets of large atypical lymphoid cells expressing T-cell markers and CD30, with some cases showing epidermotropism (in contrast to MF, transformed cases rarely show Pautrier microabscesses).

Breast implant-associated anaplastic large cell lymphoma

This is a rare variant of ALK⁻ ALCL arising in association with a breast implant [1, 159, 160, 199]. Tumor cells (similar in

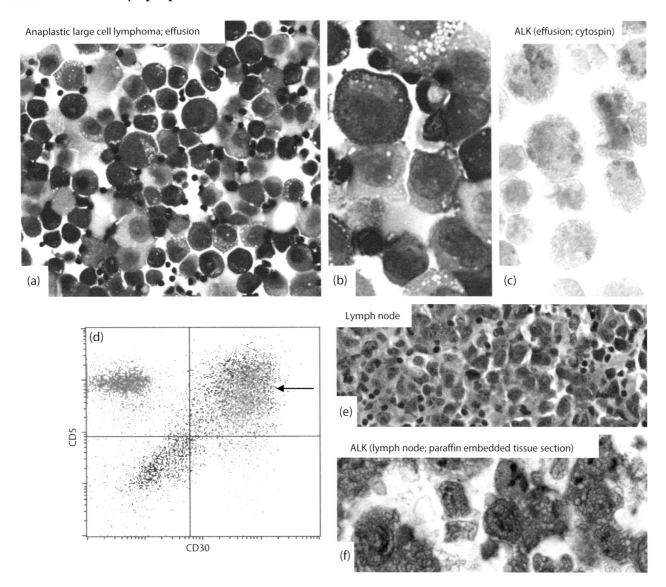

FIGURE 16.63 Pleural effusion – ALCL. (a) Cytospin preparation shows numerous malignant cells with large nuclei, dense cytoplasm with occasional vacuoles. (b) High magnification shows detailed cytologic features. (c) Immunohistochemical staining with ALK (effusion). (d) Flow cytometry shows T-cells co-expressing CD30 (arrow). (e) Histologic section of the lymph node from the same patients shows diffuse large cell infiltrate. (f) Tumor cells show nuclear, nucleolar, and cytoplasmic staining with ALK.

appearance to other variants of ALCL) infiltrate the capsule surrounding breast implant (Figure 16.65). They are positive for CD30 and pan-T-cell antigens (ALK is negative). In contrast to other ALK⁻ ALCL, the prognosis is favorable after excision alone.

Aggressive NK-cell leukemia (ANKL)

ANKL phenotype by FC: CD2⁺, s.CD3⁻, c.CD3⁺, CD4⁻, CD5⁻, CD7⁺/⁻, CD8⁻, CD16⁺, CD56⁺, CD57⁻

Introduction

ANKL is a very rare, systemic neoplastic proliferation of mature NK-cells with an aggressive fulminant clinical course and median survival of less than 2 months [1, 70, 200–206]. ANKL usually

develops de novo in young adults with no gender preference. Patients with ANKL typically present acutely with fever, B symptoms, hemophagocytic lymphohistiocytosis (HLH), raised LGH levels and disseminated intravascular coagulopathy (DIC) [201, 202]. Hepatosplenomegaly with or without lymphadenopathy can be the predominant presentation. Common sites of involvement include BM, blood, lymph nodes, liver, and spleen. Less common sites of involvement include skin, soft tissue, lungs, and omentum.

Morphology
Blood. The leukemic cells are larger than normal LGLs. Some cells may resemble LGL cells with pale cytoplasm with azurophilic granules and nuclei with open chromatin and inconspicuous nucleoli, but subset of cells show more prominent atypia including large nucleoli.

Lymph node and extranodal sites. The neoplastic cells of ANKL have variable morphological features ranging from

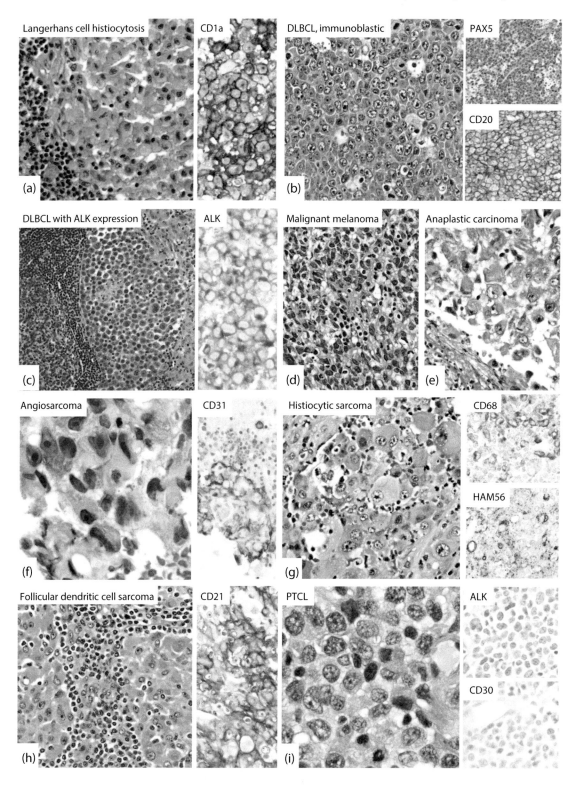

FIGURE 16.64 ALCL – differential diagnosis. (a) Langerhans cell histiocytosis. Tumor cells have abundant cytoplasm, characteristic nuclear features (grooves) and are positive for CD1a and S100. (b) DLBCL, immunoblastic variant. It may resemble monomorphic subtype of ALCL, but is expresses B-cell markers, including CD20 and PAX5. (c) Large B-cell lymphoma with cytoplasmic ALK expression. This unusual variant of DLBCL is negative for CD20 and expresses CD138, IgA and ALK (cytoplasmic). (d) Malignant melanoma. (e) Anaplastic large cell carcinoma. (f) Angiosarcoma. Tumor cells express vascular markers and are negative for ALK. (g) Histiocytic sarcoma. The neoplastic cells lack reactivity with pan-T antigens, B-cell markers and show variable staining with CD68 (and other histiocytic markers) and CD15. With the use of immunostaining and FISH/molecular tests, majority of those tumors are now diagnosed as ALCL. (h) Follicular dendritic cell sarcoma. Tumor cells are positive for CD21. (i) Peripheral T-cell lymphoma, not otherwise specified (PTCL, NOS). CD30 expression is variable, but ALK-1 is negative. *(Continued)*

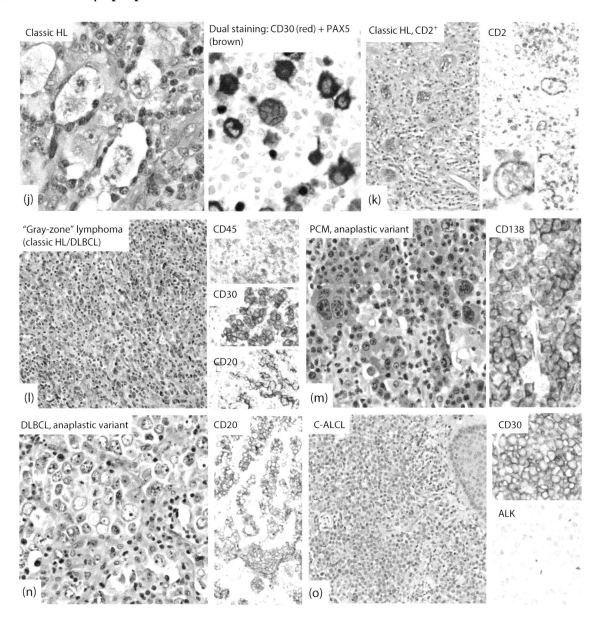

FIGURE 16.64 *(Continued)* (j-k) Classic HL. (l) Mediastinal grey zone lymphoma. (m) Anaplastic variant of plasma cell myeloma (PCM). (n) DLBCL with anaplastic features. (o) Primary cutaneous ALCL (C-ALCL).

monotonous medium-sized cells with round to irregular nuclei, and ample cytoplasm containing azurophilic granules to medium- or large-sized cells with prominent nuclear pleomorphism. The involvement of lymph nodes, liver, and spleen can be focal and subtle, intrasinusoidal or extensive with diffuse effacement of the architecture, angiodestruction, and geographical necrosis. Histiocytes with hemophagocytosis can be present. Areas of necrosis with or without angioinvasion are commonly seen.

Bone marrow*.* BM involvement is often subtle, focal, and interstitial, with some cases showing more pronounced diffuse involvement. Some cases show prominent involvement with necrosis (Figure 16.66) and accompanying HLH.

Immunophenotype
Neoplastic cells are positive for CD2 (cytoplasmic), CD3, CD7, CD16 (majority of cases), FASL, CD56, EBV (EBER), and cytotoxic proteins (granzyme B, TIA1, and perforin). Surface CD3

and CD5 are negative, CD57 is usually negative and TCR genes show a germline configuration.

Differential diagnosis of ANKL
The differential diagnosis of ANKL includes T-LGL leukemia, chronic indolent NK-cell lymphoproliferative disorder, extranodal T/NK-cell lymphoma, nasal type (ENKTL) and systemic EBV⁺ T-cell lymphoma of childhood (STCLC). T-LGL leukemia occurs in adults and elderly patients and is frequently associated with severe neutropenia, autoimmune disorders (especially rheumatoid arthritis), and follows an indolent usually not progressive course. Phenotypically, T-LGL leukemia is most often surface CD3⁺, CD8⁺, and CD57⁺ with variable expression of CD16 (CD56 is usually negative but may be co-expressed with CD57). Chronic indolent NK-cell lymphoproliferative disorder is an indolent, non-progressive disorder of mature NK-cells which morphologically resembles T-LGLL but differs from it by less common association with

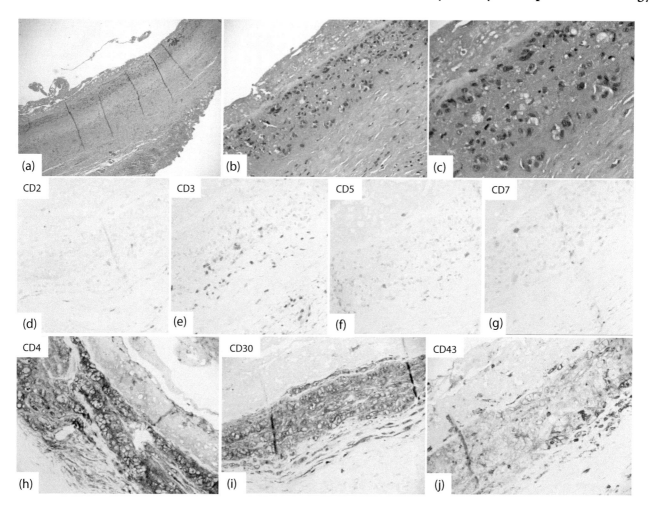

FIGURE 16.65   Breast-implant associated ALCL. (a–c) Section of the capsule surrounding breast implant showing large cell infiltrate (low, intermediate, and high magnification). (d–j) Immunohistochemistry. Anaplastic lymphoma cells show null cell phenotype (CD2⁻, CD3⁻, CD5⁻, and CD7⁻; d-g). They are positive for CD4 (h), CD30 (i), and CD43 (j).

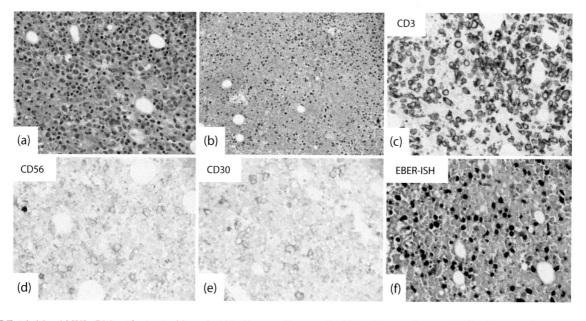

FIGURE 16.66   ANKL. BM with atypical lymphoid infiltrate of large cells (a) and areas of necrosis (b). Tumor cells are positive for CD3 (c), CD56 (d), CD30 (e, focal expression), and EBV (f, EBER-ISH).

neutropenia or rheumatoid arthritis and by phenotype showing expression of CD2, CD7, CD16, and CD56 with lack of surface CD3 and CD5. STCLC affect children, while ANKL occurs more often in adults. ENKTL has similar phenotype to ANKL but is most often limited to involvement of the upper aerodigestive tract.

Extranodal NK/T-cell lymphoma, nasal type (ENKTL)

ENKTL phenotype by FC: CD2⁺, s.CD3⁻, c.CD3⁺, CD4⁻, CD5⁻, CD7⁺/⁻, CD8⁻/rare cases⁺, CD16⁻, CD25⁻/⁺, CD30⁻/⁺, CD56⁺, CD57⁻

Introduction
ENKTL, previously known as lethal midline granuloma or angiocentric T-cell lymphoma, is a distinct clinico-pathological entity associated with EBV infection, cytotoxic phenotype and vascular destruction with accompanying necrosis [1, 207]. ENKTL has a predilection for the nasal cavity (midface) and the upper aerodigestive tract including the nasopharynx, paranasal sinuses, oropharynx, orbital walls, and palate (where it often presents as an ulcerative lesion) and may extends to local lymph nodes and in

some cases can also develop outside of the nasopharynx, including skin, lymph nodes, soft tissue, gastrointestinal tract, breast, spleen, testis, lung, and upper respiratory tract [1, 200, 208–227]. Regional lymph node involvement can be seen in a minority of patients. Most cases are genuine NK-cell neoplasms but a very small proportion of them show a cytotoxic T-cell phenotype [71].

The clinical presentation varies, depending on the site of involvement. ENKTL is usually diagnosed in adults with a wide age range and median age in the 5th decade (46 years) and a male predominance. Systemic dissemination is often late and common metastatic sites include skin, gastrointestinal tract, and genital organs [71, 223]. Many patients have lymphadenopathy [224]. Nasal lesions usually present with nasal obstruction or a mid-facial destructive tumor. Systemic symptoms are common and include fever, malaise, and weight loss. The prognosis is generally poor except for occasional solitary nasal NK-cell lymphomas. Early stage disease may respond to radiotherapy alone, however late stage disease does not respond well to any available therapies. The median overall survival is better in nasal compared with the extra-nasal cases [223].

Morphology
The neoplastic infiltrate is diffuse and may be composed of small, medium-sized, large, or mixed small and large lymphocytes (Figure 16.67). Tumors composed of medium-sized lymphocytes

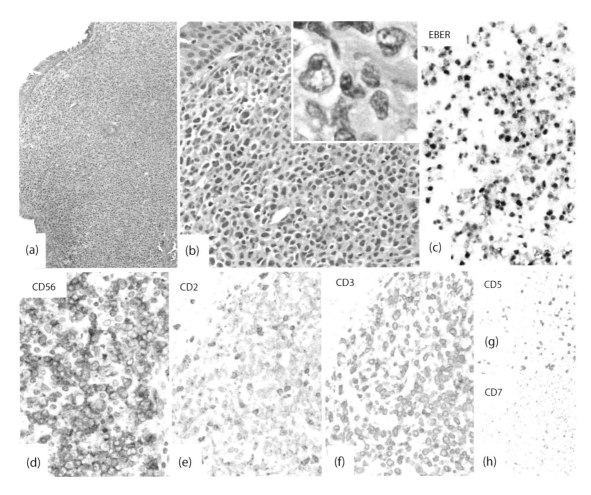

FIGURE 16.67 Extranodal NK/T-cell lymphoma, nasal type – nasopharynx. (a–b) Diffuse lymphoid infiltrate within nasal mucosa (*inset*: pleomorphic lymphoid cells). Lymphomatous cells are positive for EBER (c), CD56 (d), and T-cell antigens CD2 and CD3 (e–f), and do not express CD5 and CD7 (g–h).

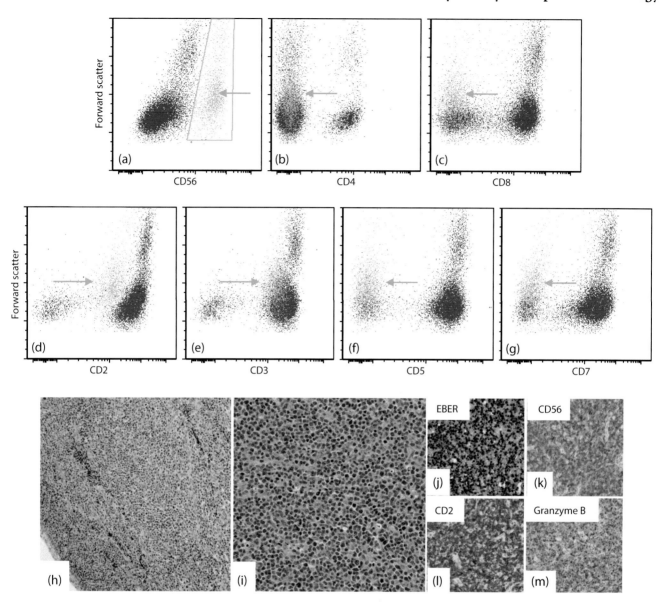

FIGURE 16.68 ENKTL composed of medium-sized cells (nasal cavity). Flow cytometry analysis (a–g) shows predominance of reactive small T-cells (red dots) and minor population of atypical cells (green dots) with slightly increased forward scatter, positive CD56 (a), negative CD4 (b), negative CD8 (c), positive CD2 (d), positive CD3 (e), negative CD5 (f), and negative CD7 (g). Histologic section shows diffuse infiltrate of medium sized cells (h–i), expressing EBV/EBER (j), CD56 (k), CD2 (l), and granzyme B (m).

or mixed small and large cells predominate [224]. Neoplastic cells have irregular and hyperchromatic nuclei and pale to clear cytoplasm. Inflammatory cells (eosinophils, histiocytes, plasma cells, and rare granulocytes) are often present, and histiocytes may show hemophagocytosis. A characteristic feature of ENKTL is its angiocentric growth pattern (vascular invasion), which may lead to angiodestruction and prominent zonal necrosis with abundant karyorrhectic debris. Admixture of inflammatory background including small lymphocytes, histiocytes, plasma cells, and eosinophils is often seen.

Immunophenotype

The neoplastic cells express some T-cell associated antigens, most commonly CD2 and cytoplasmic CD3, cytotoxic markers, and CD56 (Figures 16.68 and 16.69). Most cases display typical NK-cell phenotype: CD2+, surface CD3−, cytoplasmic CD3+,

CD5−, CD7+/−, CD4−, CD8−, TCRαβ−, TCRγδ− CD16−, CD56+, and CD57−. In contrast to benign NK-cells which are CD2+ and CD7+, the expression of CD7 in ENKTL is variable. Cytotoxic granule-associated antigens including granzyme B, perforin, and TIA1 (T-cell-restricted intracellular antigen-1) are usually positive. Subset of cases is positive for CD8, HLA-DR, CD25 (20%–40%), CD30 (30%–40%), and S100. Rare cases of ENKTL with typical histomorphology are CD56− and CD8+. The cases with predominance of large lymphocytes do not pose a diagnostic dilemma, but cases with predominance of small to medium-sized lymphocytes may be difficult to interpret due to prominent reactive component. One clue to the correct diagnosis of ENKTL is the presence of necrosis. Careful evaluation of phenotypic markers under high magnification in those cases usually shows cells with an aberrant phenotype: positive expression of EBV (EBER) and CD56, lack of CD5, and dual CD4/CD8-negativity. All cases

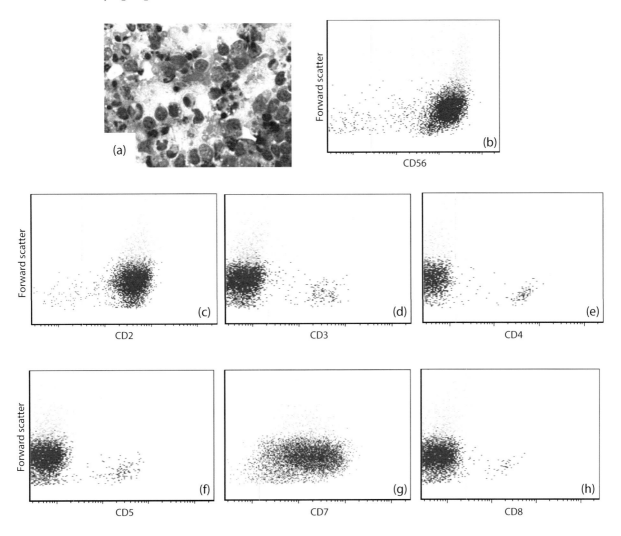

FIGURE 16.69   ENKTL, right nasal mass from 28-year-old man (FC analysis). (a) Touch smear shows highly atypical large neoplastic cells with irregular nuclei, basophilic cytoplasmic and "dirty" background. (b–h) Flow cytometry shows strong CD56 expression (b), positive CD2 (c), negative CD3 (d), CD4 (e) and CD5 (f), positive CD7 (g), and negative CD8.

are EBV+ (with all of lymphoma cells being positive). FC analysis shows atypical T/NK-cells with increased forward scatter, positive CD56, negative CD4 and CD8, and aberrant expression of pan-T-cell antigens.

Genetic features

Chromosomal abnormalities are commonly found in ENKTL, the aberrations involving chromosome 6q being most frequent. Other non-random abnormalities include +X, i(1q), i(7q), +8, del(13q), del(17p), i(17q), and 11q23 rearrangement [228, 229]. CGH of ENKTL showed gain of 2q, and loss of 6q16.1-q27, 11q22.3-q23.3, 5p14.1-p14.3, 5q34-q35.3, 1p36.23-p36.33, 2p16.1-p16.3, 4q12, and 4q31.3-q32.1 [72].

Differential diagnosis of ENKTL

Differential diagnosis of ENKTL (Figure 16.70) includes [207, 211, 212, 218, 230–236]:

- Reactive inflammatory lesions, Kikuchi lymphadenitis
- PCM
- Plasmablastic lymphoma (PBL)
- DLBCL

- EBV+ DLBCL
- Lymphomatoid granulomatosis (LyG)
- PTCL, NOS
- NK-cell enteropathy
- Malignant melanoma
- Nasopharyngeal carcinoma
- Extramedullary myeloid tumor (EMT)
- BPDCN
- T-LGL leukemia (T-LGL leukemia)
- HSTL
- SPTCL
- Primary cutaneous γδ T-cell lymphoma (PGD-TCL)
- Chronic indolent NK-cell lymphoproliferative disorder (CLPD-NK)
- ANKL

Differential diagnosis of ENKTL based on CD56 expression includes:

- CD56+ AML (especially acute monoblastic leukemia),
- BPDCN
- Extranodal DLBCL with CD56 expression

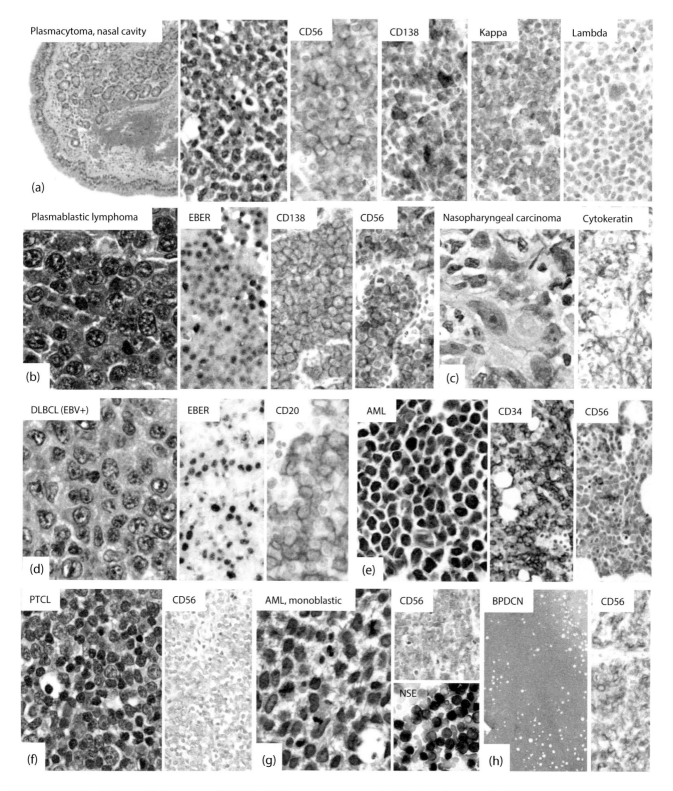

FIGURE 16.70 Differential diagnosis of ENKTL. (a) Plasmacytoma. Atypical diffuse plasma cell infiltrate within nasal cavity may suggest NK-cell lymphoma. Expression of light chain immunoglobulins and negative expression of EBER helps in diagnosis of plasma cell neoplasm. (b) Plasmablastic lymphoma. Positive expression of EBER and CD56 is common for both plasmablastic lymphoma and NK-cell lymphoma. Lack of angiocentrism and lack of expression of pan-T antigens (e.g., CD2) and cytotoxic granule associated proteins (granzyme B, TIA1) distinguish these two neoplasms. (c) Poorly differentiated nasopharyngeal carcinoma. Pleomorphic infiltrate with expression of EBV in nasopharyngeal carcinoma may be confused with nasal NK-cell lymphoma. Expression of cytokeratin establishes the correct diagnosis. (d) DLBCL: EBV-associated DLBCL (e.g., in immunocompromised or elderly patients) may be mistaken for nasal NK-cell lymphoma. (e) AML with CD56 expression. (f) Peripheral T-cell lymphoma, not otherwise specified (PTCL, NOS) with CD56 expression. (g) Acute monoblastic leukemia. (h) Blastic plasmacytoid dendritic cell neoplasm (BPDCN).

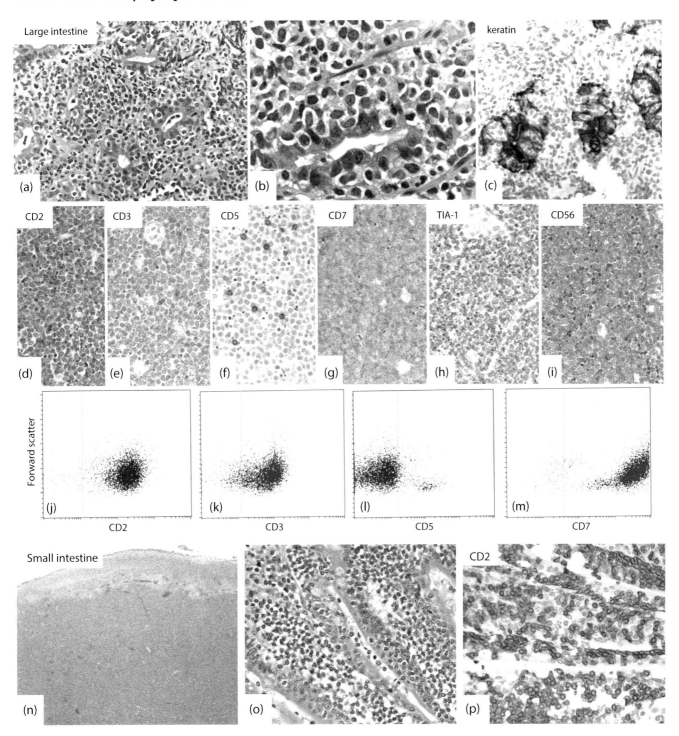

FIGURE 16.78 MEITL with involvement of large intestine (a–m) and small intestine (n–p). Neoplastic cells display prominent tropism to epithelium (a–b; o). Cytokeratin staining (c) shows prominent intraepithelial lymphocytosis. The tumor cells are small to medium in size with pale cytoplasm (a–b; o). They are positive for CD2 (d and p, immunohistochemistry; j, flow cytometry), CD3 (dim; e and k), CD7 (bright; g and m), TIA1 (h) and CD56 (i); they are negative for CD5 (f and l).

infiltration of colonic crypt epithelium or surface epithelium by lymphoid cells, although subtle lymphoepithelial lesions may be observed in some cases. The infiltrates are composed of predominantly small to medium-sized, monotonous lymphoid cells with slightly irregular nuclei, mature nuclear chromatin, inconspicuous nucleoli, and scant pale cytoplasm. Occasional eosinophils or histiocytes are intermixed with the lymphoid cells. Some cases

may show presence of lymphoid follicles and/or granulomas, mimicking Crohn's disease.

Immunophenotype

Lymphomatous cells have the following phenotype: CD2+, CD3+, CD5+/-, CD7+/-, CD30-, CD56-, EBER-, TIA-1+/-, and granzyme B- [261]. The pan-T-cell markers CD2, CD3, CD5, and CD7 are

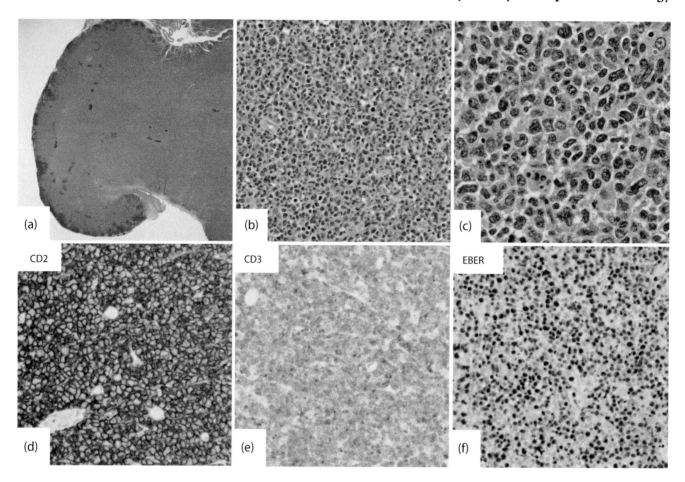

FIGURE 16.79 ENKTL – small intestine. Large polypoid mass (a) shows highly atypical and diffuse lymphoid infiltrate (b–c). Tumor cells are positive for CD2 (d), CD3 (e; weak expression) and EBV (f; EBER-ISH); CD5 and CD7 were negative (not shown).

generally positive, but loss of CD5 or CD7 is seen is some cases. All cases show TCRβ (Beta-F1) positive phenotype. There is usually no expression of CD30, CD56, or CD103, although CD103 has been reported [266, 270, 271]. The majority of cases (~60%) are CD4+, with the remaining cases being CD8+ or rarely CD4−/CD8− or CD4+/CD8+. CD8+ lesions express TIA-1, but granzyme B is negative in most cases. Ki-67 index is low (<10%).

Differential diagnosis of indolent T-LPD
The differential diagnosis includes EATL, MEIT, PTCL (NOS), inflammatory bowel disease (Crohn disease), and celiac sprue, and careful integration of the endoscopic, histologic, and immunophenotypic features is necessary to make the correct diagnosis (Table 16.6).

EATL
EATL most commonly presents with extensive mucosal ulcerations and deep infiltration of the bowel wall. Frequently, there is multifocal involvement as well as infiltration of adjacent abdominal structures and associated ascites. In contrast, indolent T-LPD usually presents as 1 or more shallow mucosal ulcers with associated erythema or as multiple small polyps. Colonic lesions can be confluent, giving the endoscopic appearance of inflammatory bowel disease. Histologically, these lesions are nondestructive, involving mostly the lamina propria and muscularis mucosae, and are composed predominantly of small, mature-appearing lymphoid cells. In contrast, EATL is usually a

large and destructive lesion composed of medium- to large-sized pleomorphic cells with prominent nucleoli. In EATL, the intestinal mucosa adjacent to the main tumor mass frequently shows evidence of enteropathy, whereas none of our T-LPD patients had a history of celiac disease or showed histologic evidence of enteropathy. The immunophenotype of EATL can overlap with that of indolent T-LPD. However, the macroscopic appearance of the lesions, the morphology, and destructive nature of the infiltrates as well as the associated enteropathy should all point toward a diagnosis of EATL.

MEIT
In MEIT the cells are monotonous and small to medium in size, and lesions are also infiltrative and highly destructive. Importantly, MEIT is characterized by florid infiltration of the intestinal crypt epithelium and adjacent intestinal mucosa by lymphoma cells, whereas indolent T-LPD shows little or no involvement of the crypt or surface epithelium. MEIT has a characteristic immunophenotype, with the tumor cells being positive for CD3, CD8, CD56, and often TCR-G, but negative for CD4. In contrast, indolent T-LPD is negative for CD56.

Inflammatory bowel disease (IBD)
Indolent T-LPD have some morphologic features, such as crypt distortion, that superficially mimic the changes seen in ulcerative colitis, careful examination reveals no other diagnostic features such as cryptitis, crypt abscesses, reduced intraepithelial mucin,

basal plasmacytosis, submucosal fibrosis, hypertrophic muscularis mucosae, and Paneth cell hyperplasia. Presence of reactive follicles and/or granulomas in some cases of indolent T-LPD may mimic Crohn's disease (indolent T-LPD lacks other well-defined morphologic characteristics of Crohn's disease, such as transmural non-necrotizing granulomatous infiltrate without ulceration affecting discontinuously entire gastrointestinal tract from esophagus to anus).

Mycosis fungoides (MF)

MF phenotype by FC: CD2$^{+/-}$, CD3$^+$, CD4$^+$, CD5$^+$, CD7$^{-/rarely+}$, CD8$^-$, CD10$^-$, CD25$^{-/+}$, CD26$^-$, CD30$^-$

Introduction
MF is the most common type of cutaneous T-cell lymphoma, characterized clinically by indolent course and morphologically by atypical lymphocytes with irregular (cerebriform) nuclei and their clustering within epithelium (epidermotropism, including Pautrier microabscesses) [1, 272, 273]. MF accounts for almost 50% of all primary lymphomas involving the skin [147]. It typically affects older adults (median age at diagnosis 50–60 years), but may occur in children and adolescent [273, 274]. MF is limited to the skin, with erythematous patches, plaques, and less frequently tumors. Occasional lesions may be atrophic and dyspigmented (hyperpigmented or hypopigmented) in a variant termed poikilodermatous MF. MF most often affects areas infrequently exposed to sunlight (i.e., trunk). After an initial indolent and protracted course, MF usually progresses to generalized erythroderma and involvement of blood, lymph nodes, liver, and spleen (SS). BM involvement is rare. The course of MF is indolent except when complicated by transformation to large cell lymphoma [275, 276].

Morphology
Skin. The MF is an indolent disease developing slowly over several years, and its definite diagnosis, particularly in early (patch/plaque) stage is difficult due to non-specific clinical and pathologic features overlapping with those of reactive dermatoses such as eczema or parapsoriasis. The correct diagnosis of MF relies on clinical presentation, histopathology with immunophenotyping and often gene rearrangement testing for T-cell clonality. The early stages of MF are difficult to diagnose based solely on morphologic features. It is not uncommon for the diagnosis of MF to remain elusive for many years, often requiring observation and repeated biopsies, with an average time to diagnosis of 3–6 years [277, 278].

The morphologic pattern depends on the stage of the disease. In early skin involvement there is a patchy lymphoid infiltrate in the upper dermis with epidermotropism (Figure 16.80), scattered

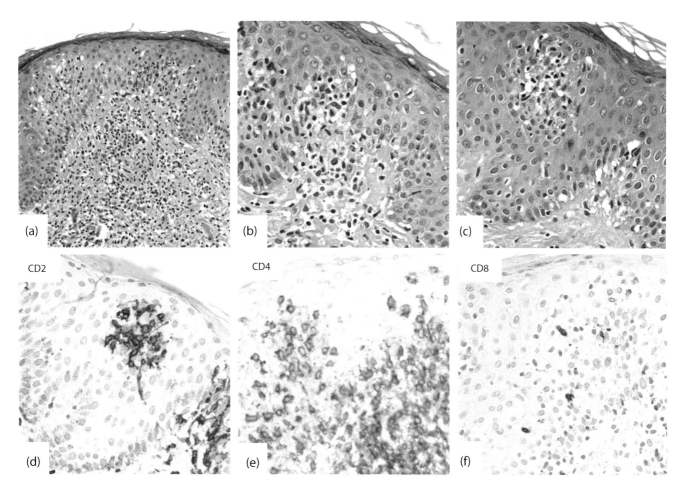

FIGURE 16.80 MF (early stage) showing prominent epidermotropism (a–c) with characteristic accumulation of lymphomatous cells within epidermis (c). Tumor cells are positive CD2 (d) and CD4 (e) and negative CD8 (f).

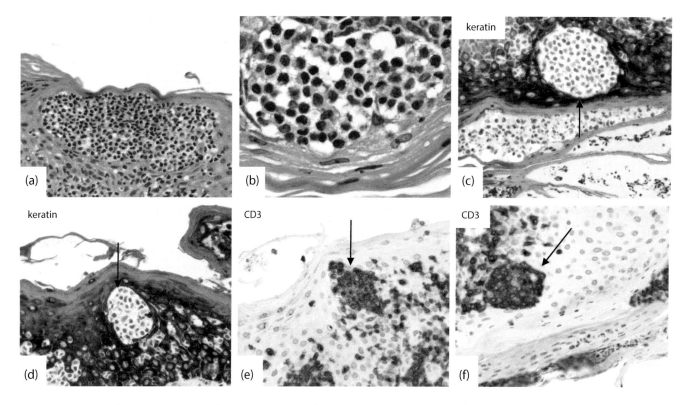

FIGURE 16.81 MF – Pautrier microabscesses (a–b) Histology sections show prominent lymphoid aggregated within epidermis (a, low magnification; b, high magnification of different area). (c–f) Immunostaining with cytokeratin (c–d) and CD3 (e–f) helps to visualize lymphoid aggregates in the epidermis.

histiocytes and single cell exocytosis, or less commonly aggregates of atypical lymphocytes within the epidermis (Pautrier microabscesses; Figure 16.81). The lymphoid cells are small to medium-sized and often have irregular, extremely convoluted or cerebriform (indented) hyperchromatic nuclei. Pautrier microabscesses consisting of aggregates of neoplastic T-cells and epidermal dendritic cells (Langerhans cells) are fairly specific but are present only in subset of patients and may be seen occasionally in other disorders. Occasional large lymphocytes may be also present, as well as reactive small lymphocytes and eosinophils. Eosinophils are sparse in early patch-stage disease but may be more prominent in plaque and tumor-stage disease.

Lymph nodes. The involvement of the lymph node by neoplastic T-cell infiltrate can be assessed by histologic examination, especially when combined with immunophenotyping. However, early lymph node involvement may be difficult for morphologic assessment especially differentiating it from reactive dermatopathic changes. Lymph nodes show variable histologic patterns depending on the stage of the disease. Cases without lymph node involvement (category I) often show dermatopathic changes and paracortical hyperplasia. Scattered rare, atypical lymphocytes may be present. In early involvement (category II), there is a paracortical expansion with focal/partial effacement of the architecture and sheets of atypical lymphocytes with irregular nuclear contours. Increased number of atypical cells is often seen in the subcapsular region. In cases with massive involvement (category III) there is complete replacement of lymph node architecture by a diffuse atypical lymphoid infiltrate (Figure 16.82). Correlation with FC analysis of the fresh lymph node sample is often helpful in diagnosis of involvement by MF by identifying aberrant phenotype of T-cells.

Histologic transformation (HT)
Diagnosis of large cell transformation (HT) in MF relies of clinical history and pathological-immunophenotypic findings. Disease is usually classified as transformed if biopsy showed large cells (≥4 times the size of a small lymphocyte) in more than 25% of the infiltrate or if they formed microscopic nodules [279–281]. The transformed lymphocytes are usually large with blastoid appearance, cerebriform nuclei and prominent nucleoli. Highly atypical anaplastic or Reed-Sternberg-like cells may be present. HT has been associated with expression of CD30 in approximately 40% of cases [282]. The HT is more common in patients with tumors and with more advances clinical stage of the disease. Some studies showed the presence of usually small, but variable numbers of CD30+ cells in nontransformed MF [283]. Figure 16.83 shows MF with large cell HT.

MF variants
MF variants include folliculotropic MF, pagetoid reticulosis (Figure 16.84), granulomatous slack skin, mucosal MF, and poikilodermatous.

Immunophenotype
The neoplastic cells in MF typically express CD4, TCRαβ, CD45RO, and pan T-cell markers. Aberrant phenotype (loss of one or more pan T-cell antigens, usually CD7, and less often CD2, CD3, or CD5) may be observed and helps in differentiating MF from reactive T-cell infiltrates [284–286]. The aberrant loss of CD7 can be seen also in reactive conditions, and therefore CD7 should be negative in more than 90% to be considered suggestive for MF (for CD2, CD3, and CD5, the threshold is lower, at 50%) [287]. Cytotoxic protein markers and CD30 are most often

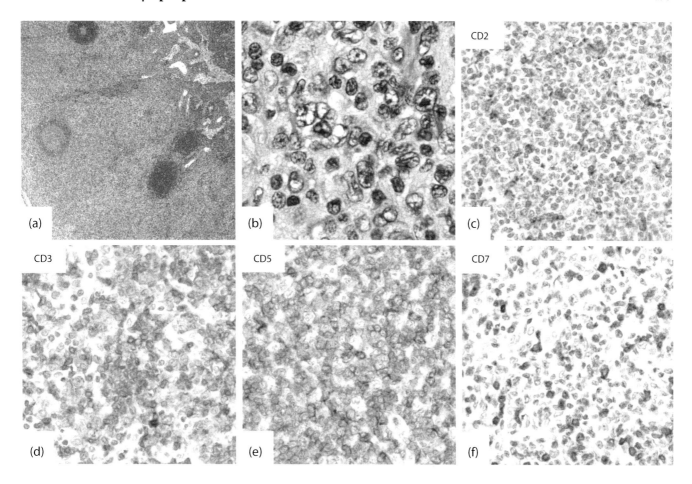

FIGURE 16.82 MF – lymph node involvement. (a) Low magnification shows prominent paracortical/interfollicular infiltrate. (b) High magnification shows medium-sized to large lymphoid cells with nuclear pleomorphism and nucleoli. Neoplastic cells show lack of CD2 (c), positive CD3 (d) and CD5 (e), and lack of CD7 expression (f).

negative [288]. The expression of TIA1 or granzyme B is seen more often in tumors showing blastic transformation. The subtle immunophenotypic differences in the expression of pan-T cell markers among dermal and epidermal lymphocytes are helpful in the diagnosis of early MF epidermal/dermal discordance of CD2, CD3, CD5, or CD7 expression [289]. In rare cases of otherwise classical MF, a CD4$^-$/CD8$^+$ mature T-cell phenotype may be seen [284, 290–292]. Such cases have the same clinical behavior and prognosis and should not be considered separately. CD8$^+$ MF occurs more often in children. Figure 16.85 presents the phenotypic feature of MF involving the lymph node.

Genetics

Chromosomal abnormalities, mostly complex, are seen in about 50% of patients with mycosis fungoides/Sézary's syndrome (MF/SS), but recurrent rearrangements are rare. PCR analysis of *TCR* gene rearrangements can demonstrate the clonality in up to 99% of cases [293–296]. The application of multiplex PCR with heteroduplex analysis is associated with a high specificity and sensitivity for cutaneous T-cell lymphoma diagnosis [297] and is very helpful in differential diagnosis between lymphoma and benign inflammatory disease. The percentage of clonality in benign conditions is low: Ponti et al. reported clonal T-cell population only in 2.3% of inflammatory changes [297]. The frequency with which a T-cell clone is detected in lymph

increases with extent of skin involvement, overall clinical stage and with abnormal histomorphology.

Differential diagnosis of MF
Differential diagnosis of MF in the skin

Differential diagnosis of MF includes reactive skin disorders with lymphoid infiltrate (benign eczematous skin lesions), primary and secondary B- and T-cell lymphomas and nonhematopoietic tumors with prominent reactive lymphoid infiltrate. Reactive conditions that may mimic MF include drug-induced reversible lymphoid hyperplasia, persistent nodular arthropod bite reactions, secondary syphilis, lymphomatoid dermatitis, nodular scabies, chronic actinic dermatitis, fungal infections, lymphomatoid lichenoid keratosis, pigmented *purpuric dermatitis*, lupus, inflamed vitiligo, HIV-related dermatitis, psoriasis, and regressed malignant melanoma [277]. Drugs implicated in the skin lesions that may resemble MF include phenytoin, carbamazepine, sodium valproate, gemcitabine, gold, and clonidine patch [298]. Their discontinuation leads to clearing of the skin lesions. Reactive lesions show dense lymphoid infiltrate with small lymphocytes, plasma cells, eosinophils, and histiocytes.

The following characteristics favor the diagnosis of MF over reactive conditions [273, 287, 299–301]:

- Superficial lymphoid infiltrate
- Lack of ulceration

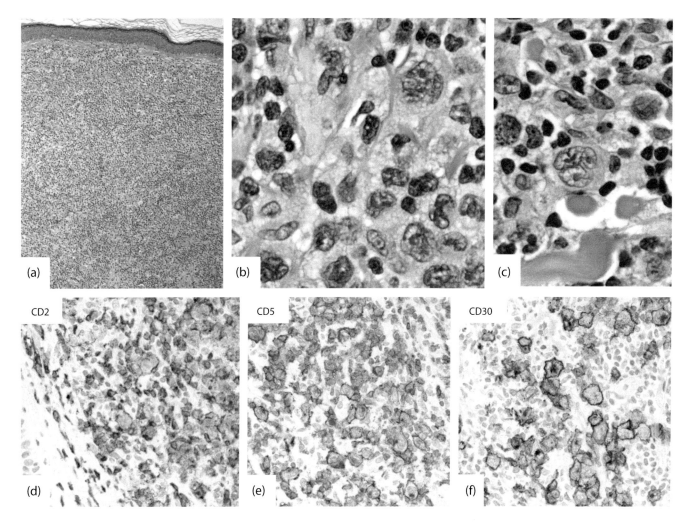

FIGURE 16.83 Large cell transformation of MF. Dense lymphoid infiltrate involving dermis (a), composed of pleomorphic cells with numerous large anaplastic lymphocytes (b–c). Neoplastic cells are positive for CD2 (d), CD5 (e), and CD30 (f).

- Epidermotropism without spongiosis (intercellular edema)
- Superficial dermal sclerosis
- Cytologic atypia (defined as cells with enlarged, hyperchromatic nuclei and irregular or cerebriform or hyperconvoluted nuclei)
- Aberrant T-cell antigen expression (lack of CD2, CD3, and/ or CD5 in ≥50% of T-cells; lack of CD7 in ≥90% of T-cells)
- Presence of lymphocytes with extremely convoluted nuclei (cerebriform cells) within epidermis
- Clusters of cells within epithelium (Pautrier's microabscesses)
- Haloed lymphocytes
- Exocytosis
- Epidermal lymphocytes larger than dermal lymphocytes
- Lymphocytes aligned within basal layer of epidermis
- T-cell antigen loss confined to epidermis (discordant phenotype of T-cells within epidermis and those in dermis)
- Clonal TCR gene rearrangement

MF needs to be differentiated from other cutaneous T-cell lymphomas (the major phenotypic characteristics of cutaneous T-cell lymphomas are presented in Table 16.7). Very prominent epidermotropism should raise the possibility of pagetoid reticulosis, cutaneous γδ T-cell lymphoma, LyP (type D) and primary cutaneous aggressive epidermotropic CD8⁺ T-cell lymphoma (CD8⁺

AECTCL). On the other hand, epidermotropism may be absent in early MF, tumor-stage MF or in folliculotropic MF. Among LyP cases, LyP type B can display histomorphology similar to MF, and type D LyP similar to pagetoid reticulosis. Since MF often displays aberrant loss of CD7 (CD2⁺, CD3⁺, CD5⁺, CD7⁻), presence of CD7 and lack of CD2 would favor the diagnosis of other T-cell lymphomas, especially cutaneous aggressive epidermotropic CD8⁺ T-cell lymphoma. Differential diagnosis of transformed MF, which may be CD30⁺ includes C-ALCL, systemic ALCL, LyP and PTCL. LyP with *DUSP-IRF4* rearrangement (6p25.3) displays large cells in the dermis and small lymphocytes in the epidermis mimicking MF with large cell transformation. LyP is characterized by recurrent self-healing papules and nodules. Subset of C-ALCL has *IRF4-DUSP22* rearrangement, which can be detected by FISH in ~26% [302, 303].

Differential diagnosis of MF in lymph nodes

The diagnosis of MF in the lymph node may be difficult, especially at the early stages. Differential diagnosis includes dermatopathic lymphadenitis [304] and other reactive conditions, B-cell lymphoma (especially DLBCL), T-cell lymphoproliferations, cHL, and EMT. Dermatopathic lymphadenitis shows characteristic increase of the Langerhans cells in paracortical area and scattered macrophages with pigment. Early stages of MF involving

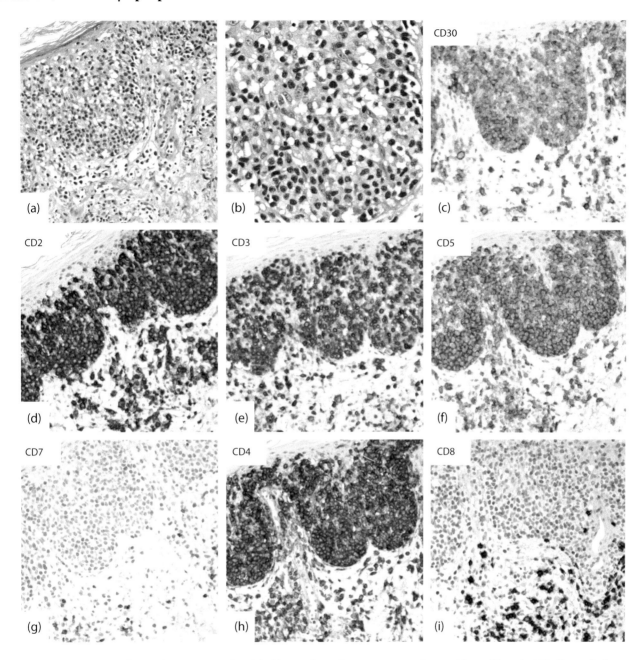

FIGURE 16.84 Pagetoid reticulosis variant of MF. (a–b) Histology shows prominent intraepidermal lymphoid infiltrate (a, low magnification; b, high magnification). Tumor cells show the following phenotype: CD30+ (c), CD2+ (d), CD3+ (e), CD5+ (f, CD7− (g), CD4+ (h), and CD8− (i).

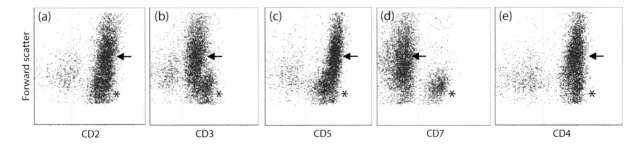

FIGURE 16.85 Mycosis fungoides (MF) involving the lymph node. Lymphomatous cells (arrow) display increased forward scatter (FSC; a–e), positive CD2 (a), positive (dim) CD3 (b), positive CD5 (c), negative CD7 (d), and positive CD4 (e). Residual (benign) T-cells (*) show normal expression of T-cell antigens and low FSC.

TABLE 16.7: Differential Diagnosis of Cutaneous T-Cell Lymphomas

	MF/SS	LyP	C-ALCL	SPTCL	PTCL	ATLL	CD4+ C-PTCLPD	CD8+ C-ATCL
CD2	+	+/−	+/−	+/−	+/−	+/(−)	+	+/−
CD3	+	+/−	+/−	+/−	+/−	+/(−)	+	+
CD4/CD8	CD4	CD4*	CD4>CD8	CD8	CD4 or CD8	CD4	CD4	CD8
CD5	+/(−)	+/−	+/−	+/−	+/−	+	+	+/−
CD7	−/(+)	−/(+)	−/(+)	+/−	−/+	−	+	+/−
CD10	−	−	−	−	−	−	−	−
CD25	−/(+)	+	−	−	−/+	+	−	−
CD30	−/(+)	+	+	−	+/−	+	−	−
Cytology	Sézary cells	Reed-Sternberg-like or immunoblast-like cells	Hallmark cells	Large pleomorphic cells	Pleomorphic cells	Cells with irregular nuclei (flower-like)		
Histology	Epidermotropism	Wedge-shaped infiltrate	Large cell diffuse infiltrate	Rimming of fat cells by tumor cells		Similar to MF or C-ALCL	Nodular or diffuse infiltrate with folliculotropism	Monomorphic diffuse infiltrate

Abbreviations: MF, mycosis fungoides; SS, Sézary's syndrome; LyP, lymphomatoid papulosis; SPTCL, subcutaneous panniculitis-like T-cell lymphoma; ATLL, adult T-cell leukemia/lymphoma; PTCL, peripheral T-cell lymphoma; CD4+ C-PTCLPD, primary cutaneous CD4+ small/medium pleomorphic T-cell lymphoproliferative disorder; CD8+ C-ATCL, primary cutaneous acral CD8+ T-cell lymphoma.

Notes: +, positive; (+), rarely positive; −, negative; (−) rarely negative; *, rare cases CD8+.

the lymph node are usually limited to subcapsular and interfollicular (paracortical) areas and may be inconspicuous on H&E examination, and therefore, difficult to differentiate from reactive conditions. Clusters of lymphocytes with pleomorphic, atypical nuclei and phenotypic abnormalities (e.g., lack of the expression of one or more of pan-T-cell antigen) help to diagnose early MF involvement. Molecular testing for T-cell clonality is often needed for final diagnosis, however. Advanced stages with diffuse infiltrate of highly atypical medium-sized to large cells, often with multilobated nuclei (Reed-Sternberg-like), do not create a diagnostic problem, but need to be differentiated from other T-cell lymphomas, especially PTCL, ATLL, lymphomatous type, and ALCL. Blastic appearance of tumor cells in subset of cases in conjunction with paracortical distribution may raise the suspicion of EMT on routine histologic examination. DLBCL, cHL, and EMT are distinguished by immunophenotypic studies.

Sézary's syndrome (SS)

SS phenotype by FC: CD2+/−, CD3+, CD4+, CD5+, CD7−/rarely+, CD8−, CD10−, CD25−/+, CD26−, CD30−/+

Introduction

SS (Figures 16.86 and 16.87) is a rare leukemic type and aggressive erythrodermic type of cutaneous T-cell lymphoma with poor prognosis. It is defined historically by the triad of erythroderma (now defined as affecting >80% of body surface area), generalized lymphadenopathy, and the presence of neoplastic T-cells (Sézary's cells) in skin, lymph nodes, and peripheral blood (≥5%) [1, 272]. SS is considered by some authors to be an erythrodermic leukemic variant of MF but is classified separately in the new WHO classification of cutaneous lymphomas. Some patients with MF develop erythroderma, leading to a

disorder termed erythrodermic MF, which may be difficult to distinguish clinically from SS. Only patients with true SS will have a substantial leukemic T-cell burden in the blood [305, 306]. The criteria recommended for the diagnosis of SS (apart from demonstration of clonally related neoplastic T-cells in skin and blood), include either an absolute Sézary's cell count of >1000 cells/μL, an expanded CD4+ T-cell population resulting in CD4/CD8 ratio >10, loss of CD7 (CD4+/CD7− ≥30%); or loss of CD26 (CD4+/CD26− ≥40%) WHO, EORTC [272]. It remains practically incurable, with a median survival of 2–3 years [307]. The prognostic factors in multivariate analysis are age at diagnosis, interval before diagnosis and presence of EBV genome in keratinocytes [307]. Univariate analysis revealed LDH level as a prognostic indicator. Fast evolution of the disease, increased level of LDH and increased level of serum b_2-microglobulin are associated with poor prognosis in MF/SS [308]. Chromosomal abnormalities occur in 43% of patients [309], usually involving chromosomes 1, 6, 10, 14, and 17. Most patients die of opportunistic infections that are due to immunosuppression.

Staging

Blood stages of MF/SS were defined by the European Organization of Research and Treatment of Cancer (EORTC) Cutaneous Task Force Committee. Stage B0 is defined as ≤5% MF/SS cells among circulating lymphocytes and an absolute count of CD4+/CD26− or CD4+/CD7− cells of <250 events/μL, stage B1 as >5% MF/SS cells and ≥250 to <1000 CD4+/CD26− or CD4+/CD7− events/μL, and stage B2 as ≥1000 MF/SS cells or CD4+/CD26− or CD4+/CD7− events/μL [310].

Morphology

SS is characterized by the presence of atypical lymphocytes with irregular convoluted nuclei. The neoplastic cells have a peculiar skin-homing tendency due to the presence of the cutaneous lymphocyte antigen and chemokine receptor CCR4 and CCR10 [311–313]. In the skin biopsy, the infiltrate may be similar to MF,

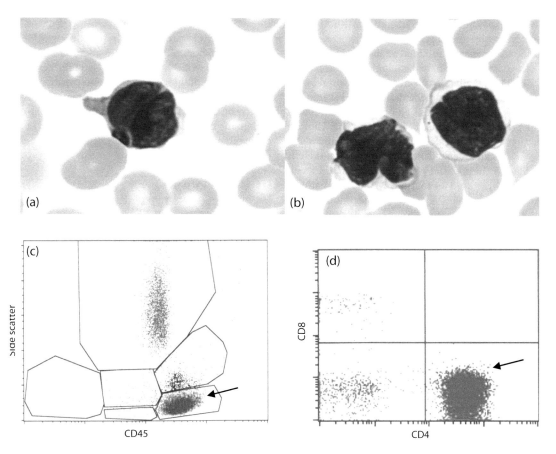

FIGURE 16.86 Sézary's syndrome. Blood smear with atypical lymphocytes (a–b). Flow cytometry (c–d) shows lymphocyte with predominance of CD4⁺ cells.

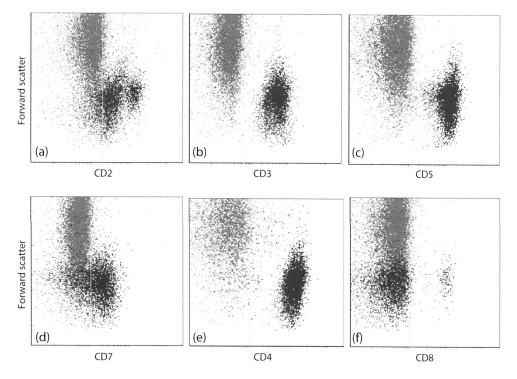

FIGURE 16.87 Sézary's syndrome (blood) – flow cytometry. Neoplastic T-cells (blue dots) are positive for CD2 (a), CD3 (b), CD5 (c), CD7 (d), and CD4 (e) and are negative for CD8 (f). The expression of CD2 is dim (a; compare with benign T-cells – red dots) and expression of CD5 is brighter than in normal T-cells (c).

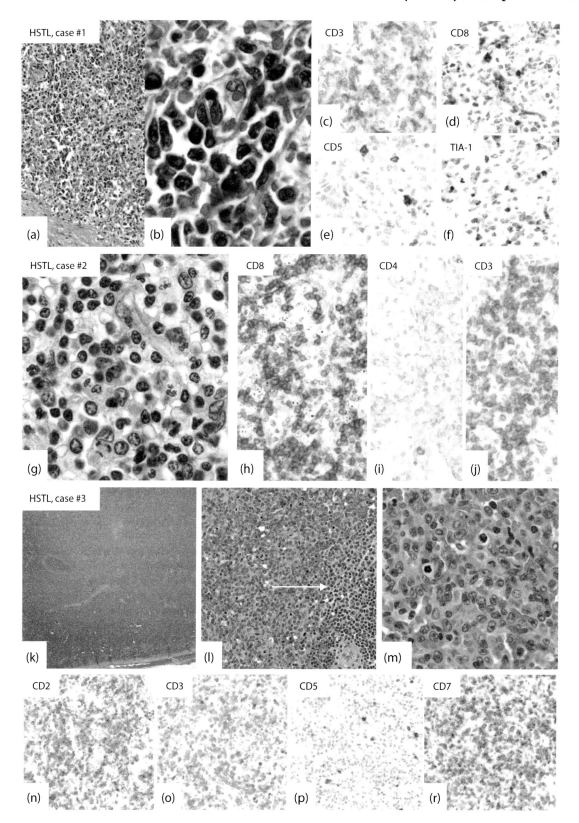

FIGURE 16.89 Spleen – HSTL. (a–f) Case #1: (a) low magnification shows clusters of atypical lymphoid cells; (b) high magnification shows intrasinusoidal distribution of neoplastic cells; (c–f) immunohistochemistry shows positive CD3 (c), negative CD8 (d), negative CD5 (e), and positive TIA-1 (f). (g–j) Case #2: (g) atypical lymphoid infiltrate; (h–j) immunohistochemistry shows positive CD8 (h), negative CD4 (i), and positive CD3 (j). (k–r) Case #3. HSTL in 17 y/o male patient. Low magnification (k) shows expanded red pulp with diffuse atypical lymphoid infiltrate. Tumor cells are larger when compared to residual germinal center cells (l, arrow points to benign lymphocytes). High magnification (m) shows large atypical cells with irregular nuclei, nucleoli and pale cytoplasm. Mitotic figures are easily identifiable. Lymphomatous cells are positive for CD2 (n) and CD3 (o), negative for CD5 (p), and positive for CD7 (ı).

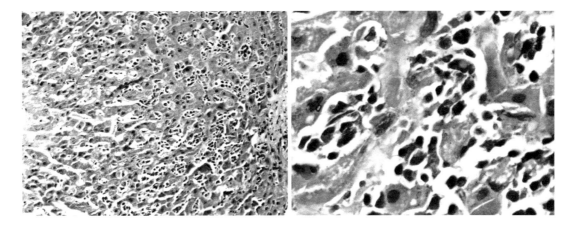

FIGURE 16.90 Liver – HSTL. Atypical, mostly intrasinusoidal infiltrate of medium-sized cells.

Chronic active EBV infection of T- and NK-cell type, systemic form

Current WHO classification includes chronic active EBV infection of T- and NK-cell type, systemic form as category of EBV⁺ T/NK-cell lymphoproliferative disease of childhood [147]. As name implies, the disease is systemic, involving liver, spleen, lymph nodes, BM, and skin. It has strong racial predisposition to Asia, but has also been reported in Latin America [1]. Morphologically, white pulp is atrophic with lymphoid infiltrate involving predominantly the sinuses. There is usually no cytologic or phenotypic atypia except for some scattered immunoblasts, but areas of necrosis may be present.

T-cell neoplasms

T-LGL leukemia. T-LGL leukemia is most often diagnosed by FC analysis of blood with confirmatory PCR testing for T-cell clonality. It is characterized by indolent clinical course, often with infections and may sometimes splenomegaly. The leukemic cells show characteristic azurophilic granules in the cytoplasm (lymphocytes in HSTL do not have cytoplasmic granules). Phenotypically, T-LGL leukemias are CD8⁺ or dual CD4/CD8⁻, CD57⁺ and often CD16 and/or CD56 positive. Distinguishing HSTL from T-LGL leukemia with γδ phenotype may be difficult without morphologic analysis of spleen [338]. T-LGL leukemia differs from HSPT by often positive CD5 and CD57 and negative granzyme B and perforin

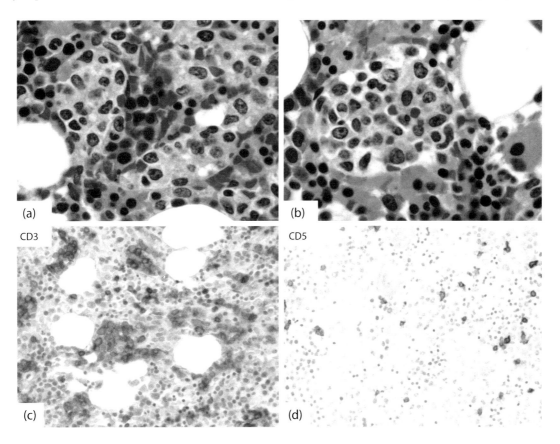

FIGURE 16.91 Bone marrow with typical intrasinusoidal involvement by HSTL. (a–b) Histology (BM core biopsy). (c–d) Immunohistochemistry. Tumor cells express CD3 (c) and are negative for CD5 (d).

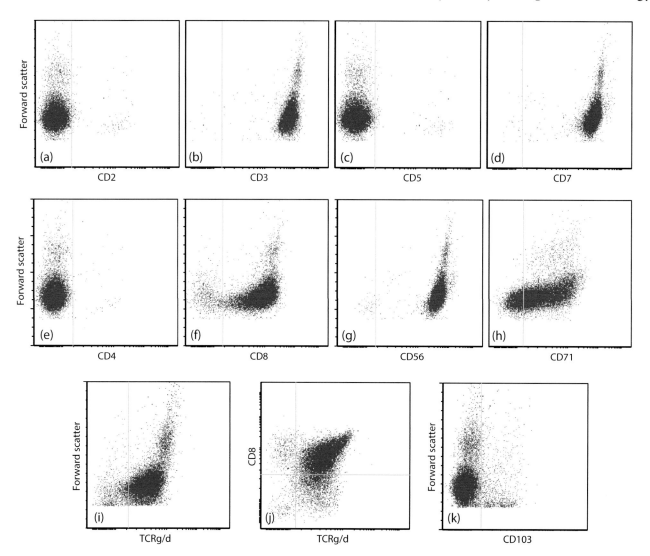

FIGURE 16.92   HSTL – flow cytometry analysis. Lymphomatous T-cells show the following phenotype: CD2⁻ (a), CD3⁺ (b), CD5⁻ (c), CD7⁺ (d), CD4⁻ (e), CD8⁺ (f), CD56⁺ (g), CD71⁺ (h, partial), TCRγδ⁺ (i–j), and CD103⁻ (k).

(opposite pattern is seen in HSTL). The spleen shows mostly pre-served architecture with subtle T-cell infiltrate in the red pulp. Focal T-cell aggregates and intrasinusoidal T-cells may be present (intrasinusoidal infiltrate is much less conspicuous than in HSTL). Occasional cases show reactive plasmacytosis around the blood vessels. Massive splenomegaly, BM sinusoidal involvement and lack of azurophilic granules would favor the diagnosis of HSTL [338].

Aggressive NK-cell leukemia. ANKL may have a clinical presen-tation similar to HSTL. Cytologically, neoplastic cells are medium to large with azurophilic cytoplasmic granules. Phenotypically it expresses CD2, NK-cell markers (CD56), cytotoxic granules and often EBV, and is negative for CD5, surface CD3 (by FC analysis and both CD4 and CD8).

PTCL. PTCL usually involves lymph node, although extranodal involvement is quite common. PTCLs in most cases lack intravas-cular distribution. The morphology and phenotype are similar to PTCL in lymph nodes. Majority of splenic PTCL are composed of αβ T-cells which are either CD4⁺ or CD8⁺ and display aberrant expression of T-cell antigens (most often CD7).

T-PLL. High WBC, hepatosplenomegaly red pulp infiltrate, often show typical prolymphocytic cytomorphology and are

positive for inv14q or t(14;14)(q11;q32). Most pan-T-cell mark-ers are positive, and many tumors are TCL1⁺. The expression of CD45 may be partially negative. Subset of CD8⁺ cases often shows CD117 expression.

T-ALL. Leukemic presentation, involvement of spleen, liver, and BM and occurrence in young patients (more often males) are common for both T-ALL and HSTL. T-ALL differ from HSTL but dimmer expression of CD45, lack of surface CD3, bright expres-sion of CD7 and positive expression of one or more blastic mark-ers (CD34, TdT), and occasionally CD1a. Subset of T-ALL cases is dual CD4/CD8⁺.

References

1. Swerdlow, S.H., et al., ed. *WHO classification of tumors of haema-topoietic and lymphoid tissues.* 2016, IARC: Lyon.
2. Laribi, K., et al., *Advances in the understanding and manage-ment of T-cell prolymphocytic leukemia.* Oncotarget, 2017. **8**(61): p. 104664–86.
3. Catovsky, D., E. Matutes, and V. Brito-Babapulle, *Is T-cell CLL a disease entity?* Br J Haematol, 1996. **94**(3). p. 580.

4. Frater, J.L., *T-cell prolymphocytic leukemia: review of an entity and its differential diagnostic considerations.* Int J Lab Hematol, 2020. **42 Suppl 1**: p. 90–8.

5. Matutes, E., *T-cell prolymphocytic leukemia.* Cancer Control, 1998. **5**(1): p. 19–24.

6. Dearden, C.E., *T-cell prolymphocytic leukemia.* Clin Lymphoma Myeloma, 2009. **9 Suppl 3**: p. S239–43.

7. Graham, R.L., B. Cooper, and J.R. Krause, *T-cell prolymphocytic leukemia.* Proc (Bayl Univ Med Cent), 2013. **26**(1): p. 19–21.

8. Matutes, E., et al., *Clinical and laboratory features of 78 cases of T-prolymphocytic leukemia.* Blood, 1991. **78**(12): p. 3269–74.

9. Dearden, C., *How I treat prolymphocytic leukemia.* Blood, 2012. **120**(3): p. 538–51.

10. Garand, R., et al., *Indolent course as a relatively frequent presentation in T-prolymphocytic leukaemia. Groupe Francais d'Hematologie Cellulaire.* Br J Haematol, 1998. **103**(2): p. 488–94.

11. Pawson, R., et al., *Absence of HTLV-I/II in T-prolymphocytic leukaemia.* Br J Haematol, 1998. **102**(3): p. 872–3.

12. Ravandi, F. and S. O'Brien, *Chronic lymphoid leukemias other than chronic lymphocytic leukemia: diagnosis and treatment.* Mayo Clin Proc, 2005. **80**(12): p. 1660–74.

13. Bartlett, N.L. and D.L. Longo, *T-small lymphocyte disorders.* Semin Hematol, 1999. **36**(2): p. 164–70.

14. Costa, D., et al., *High levels of chromosomal imbalances in typical and small-cell variants of T-cell prolymphocytic leukemia.* Cancer Genet Cytogenet, 2003. **147**(1): p. 36–43.

15. Cook, L.B., et al., *Revised adult T-cell leukemia-lymphoma international consensus meeting report.* J Clin Oncol, 2019. **37**(8): p. 677–87.

16. Tsukasaki, K., et al., *Diagnostic approaches and established treatments for adult T cell leukemia lymphoma.* Front Microbiol, 2020. **11**: p. 1207.

17. Adkins, B.D., et al., *Updates in lymph node and skin pathology of adult T-cell leukemia/lymphoma, biomarkers, and beyond.* Semin Diagn Pathol, 2020. **37**(1): p. 1–10.

18. Bazarbachi, A., et al., *How I treat adult T-cell leukemia/lymphoma.* Blood, 2011. **118**(7): p. 1736–45.

19. Jaffe, E.S., et al., *The pathologic spectrum of adult T-cell leukemia/lymphoma in the United States. Human T-cell leukemia/lymphoma virus-associated lymphoid malignancies.* Am J Surg Pathol, 1984. **8**(4): p. 263–75.

20. Shimoyama, M., *Diagnostic criteria and classification of clinical subtypes of adult T-cell leukaemia-lymphoma. A report from the Lymphoma Study Group (1984–87).* Br J Haematol, 1991. **79**(3): p. 428–37.

21. Takatsuki, K., et al., *Clinical diversity in adult T-cell leukemia-lymphoma.* Cancer Res, 1985. **45**(9 Suppl): p. 4644s–5s.

22. Kawano, F., et al., *Variation in the clinical courses of adult T-cell leukemia.* Cancer, 1985. **55**(4): p. 851–6.

23. Bazarbachi, A., et al., *New therapeutic approaches for adult T-cell leukaemia.* Lancet Oncol, 2004. **5**(11): p. 664–72.

24. Yamaguchi, K. and T. Watanabe, *Human T lymphotropic virus type-I and adult T-cell leukemia in Japan.* Int J Hematol, 2002. **76 Suppl 2**: p. 240–5.

25. Shimoyama, M., *Treatment of patients with adult T-cell leukemia-lymphoma: an overview.*, in Advances in adult T-cell leukemia and HTLV-1 research., K. Takatsuki, Hinuma, Y., Yoshida, M., Editor. 1992, Japan Scientific Societies Press: Tokyo. p. 43–6.

26. Shimoyama, M., *Chemotherapy of ATL.*, in Adult T-cell leukemia., K. Takatsuki, Editor. 1994, Oxford University Press: London. p. 221–36.

27. Ohshima, K., *Pathological features of diseases associated with human T-cell leukemia virus type I.* Cancer Sci, 2007. **98**(6): p. 772–8.

28. Karube, K., et al., *Adult T-cell lymphoma/leukemia with angioimmunoblastic T-cell lymphoma-like features: report of 11 cases.* Am J Surg Pathol, 2007. **31**(2): p. 216–23.

29. Miyashiro, D. and J.A. Sanches, *Cutaneous manifestations of adult T-cell leukemia/lymphoma.* Semin Diagn Pathol, 2020. **37**(2): p. 81–91.

30. Bittencourt, A.L., et al., *Adult T-cell leukemia/lymphoma (ATL) presenting in the skin: clinical, histological and immunohistochemical features of 52 cases.* Acta Oncol, 2009. **48**(4): p. 598–604.

31. Takasaki, Y., et al., *Long-term study of indolent adult T-cell leukemia-lymphoma.* Blood, 2010. **115**(22): p. 4337–43.

32. Tsukasaki, K., et al., *Definition, prognostic factors, treatment, and response criteria of adult T-cell leukemia-lymphoma: a proposal from an international consensus meeting.* J Clin Oncol, 2009. **27**(3): p. 453–9.

33. Kataoka, K., et al., *Integrated molecular analysis of adult T cell leukemia/lymphoma.* Nat Genet, 2015. **47**(11): p. 1304–15.

34. Miyagi, T., et al., *Extranodal adult T-cell leukemia/lymphoma of the head and neck: a clinicopathological study of nine cases and a review of the literature.* Leuk Lymphoma, 2009. **50**(2): p. 187–95.

35. Buckner, C.L., et al., *CD20 positive T-cell lymphoma/leukemia: a rare entity with potential diagnostic pitfalls.* Ann Clin Lab Sci, 2007. **37**(3): p. 263–7.

36. Kawano, R., D. Niino, and K. Ohshima, *Six cases of CD20-positive adult T-cell leukemia.* J Clin Exp Hematop, 2016. **56**(2): p. 119–25.

37. Jones, D., et al., *Absence of CD26 expression is a useful marker for diagnosis of T-cell lymphoma in peripheral blood.* Am J Clin Pathol, 2001. **115**(6): p. 885–92.

38. Kelemen, K., et al., *The usefulness of CD26 in flow cytometric analysis of peripheral blood in Sézary syndrome.* Am J Clin Pathol, 2008. **129**(1): p. 146–56.

39. Hasegawa, H., et al., *Increased chemokine receptor CCR7/EBI1 expression enhances the infiltration of lymphoid organs by adult T-cell leukemia cells.* Blood, 2000. **95**(1): p. 30–8.

40. Yoshie, O., *Expression of CCR4 in adult T-cell leukemia.* Leuk Lymphoma, 2005. **46**(2): p. 185–90.

41. Kagdi, H.H., et al., *Risk stratification of adult T-cell leukemia/lymphoma using immunophenotyping.* Cancer Med, 2017. **6**(1): p. 298–309.

42. Zambello, R., et al., *Are T-LGL leukemia and NK-chronic lymphoproliferative disorder really two distinct diseases?* Transl Med UniSa, 2014. **8**: p. 4–11.

43. Yabe, M., et al., *Clinicopathologic, immunophenotypic, cytogenetic, and molecular features of gammadelta T-cell large granular lymphocytic leukemia: an analysis of 14 patients suggests biologic differences with alphabeta T-cell large granular lymphocytic leukemia. [corrected].* Am J Clin Pathol, 2015. **144**(4): p. 607–19.

44. Lamy, T. and T.P. Loughran, Jr., *How I treat LGL leukemia.* Blood, 2011. **117**(10): p. 2764–74.

45. Neff, J.L., et al., *Mixed-phenotype large granular lymphocytic leukemia: a rare subtype in the large granular lymphocytic leukemia spectrum.* Hum Pathol, 2018. **81**: p. 96–104.

46. Dhodapkar, M.V., et al., *Clinical spectrum of clonal proliferations of T-large granular lymphocytes: a T-cell clonopathy of undetermined significance?* Blood, 1994. **84**(5): p. 1620–7.

47. Lamy, T. and T.P. Loughran, Jr., *Clinical features of large granular lymphocyte leukemia.* Semin Hematol, 2003. **40**(3): p. 185–95.

48. Loughran, T.P., Jr., *Clonal diseases of large granular lymphocytes.* Blood, 1993. **82**(1): p. 1–14.

49. van Oostveen, J.W., et al., *Polyclonal expansion of T-cell receptor-gamma delta⁺ T lymphocytes associated with neutropenia and thrombocytopenia.* Leukemia, 1992. **6**(5): p. 410–8.

50. Langerak, A.W., Y. Sandberg, and J.J. van Dongen, *Spectrum of T-large granular lymphocyte lymphoproliferations: ranging from expanded activated effector T cells to T-cell leukaemia.* Br J Haematol, 2003. **123**(3): p. 561–2.

51. Morice, W.G., et al., *Distinct bone marrow findings in T-cell granular lymphocytic leukemia revealed by paraffin section immunoperoxidase stains for CD8, TIA-1, and granzyme B.* Blood, 2002. **99**(1): p. 268–74.

52. Garrido, P., et al., *Monoclonal TCR-Vbeta13.1⁺/CD4⁺/NKa⁺/CD8⁻/⁺dim T-LGL lymphocytosis: evidence for an antigen-driven chronic T-cell stimulation origin.* Blood, 2007. **109**(11): p. 4890–8.

53. Lima, M., et al., *TCRalphabeta+/CD4+ large granular lymphocytosis: a new clonal T-cell lymphoproliferative disorder.* Am J Pathol, 2003. **163**(2): p. 763–71.

54. Olteanu, H., et al., *Laboratory findings in CD4(+) large granular lymphocytoses.* Int J Lab Hematol, 2010. **32**(1 Pt 1): p. e9–e16.

55. Dang, N.H., et al., *T-large granular lymphocyte lymphoproliferative disorder: expression of CD26 as a marker of clinically aggressive disease and characterization of marrow inhibition.* Br J Haematol, 2003. **121**(6): p. 857–65.

56. Sandberg, Y., et al., *TCRgammadelta+ large granular lymphocyte leukemias reflect the spectrum of normal antigen-selected TCRgammadelta+ T-cells.* Leukemia, 2006. **20**(3): p. 505–13.

57. Bourgault-Rouxel, A.S., et al., *Clinical spectrum of gammadelta+ T cell LGL leukemia: analysis of 20 cases.* Leuk Res, 2008. **32**(1): p. 45–8.

58. Wong, K.F., et al., *Chromosomal abnormalities in T-cell large granular lymphocyte leukaemia: report of two cases and review of the literature.* Br J Haematol, 2002. **116**(3): p. 598–600.

59. Man, C., et al., *Deletion 6q as a recurrent chromosomal aberration in T-cell large granular lymphocyte leukemia.* Cancer Genet Cytogenet, 2002. **139**(1): p. 71–4.

60. Salido, M., et al., *New t(11;12)(q12;q11) characterized by RxFISH in a patient with T-cell large granular lymphocyte leukemia.* Cancer Genet Cytogenet, 2001. **125**(1): p. 70–3.

61. Brito-Babapulle, V., et al., *A t(8;14)(q24;q32) in a T-lymphoma/leukemia of CD8+ large granular lymphocytes.* Leukemia, 1987. **1**(12): p. 789–94.

62. Schmidt, H.H., et al., *Translocation (3;5)(p26;q13) in a patient with chronic T-cell lymphoproliferative disorder.* Cancer Genet Cytogenet, 1998. **104**(2): p. 82–5.

63. Teramo, A., et al., *Insights into genetic landscape of large granular lymphocyte leukemia.* Front Oncol, 2020. **10**: p. 152.

64. Rose, M.G. and N. Berliner, *T-cell large granular lymphocyte leukemia and related disorders.* Oncologist, 2004. **9**(3): p. 247–58.

65. McClanahan, J., P.I. Fukushima, and M. Stetler-Stevenson, *Increased peripheral blood gamma delta T-cells in patients with lymphoid neoplasia: a diagnostic dilemma in flow cytometry.* Cytometry, 1999. **38**(6): p. 280–5.

66. Kreutzman, A., et al., *Mono/oligoclonal T and NK cells are common in chronic myeloid leukemia patients at diagnosis and expand during dasatinib therapy.* Blood, 2010. **116**(5): p. 772–82.

67. Shi, M., et al., *T-cell clones of uncertain significance are highly prevalent and show close resemblance to T-cell large granular lymphocytic leukemia. Implications for laboratory diagnostics.* Mod Pathol, 2020. **33**(10): p. 2046–57.

68. Zhang, L., M. Van den Bergh, and L. Sokol, *CD4-positive T-cell large granular lymphocytosis mimicking Sézary syndrome in a patient with mycosis fungoides.* Cancer Control, 2017. **24**(2): p. 207–12.

69. Chang, S.T., et al., *The spectrum of T-cell and natural killer/T-cell neoplasms with leukaemic presentation in a single institution in Taiwan.* Int J Lab Hematol, 2012. **34**(4): p. 422–6.

70. Suzuki, R., *NK/T-cell lymphomas: pathobiology, prognosis and treatment paradigm.* Curr Oncol Rep, 2012. **14**(5): p. 395–402.

71. Kwong, Y.L., *Natural killer-cell malignancies: diagnosis and treatment.* Leukemia, 2005. **19**(12): p. 2186–94.

72. Nakashima, Y., et al., *Genome-wide array-based comparative genomic hybridization of natural killer cell lymphoma/leukemia: different genomic alteration patterns of aggressive NK-cell leukemia and extranodal Nk/T-cell lymphoma, nasal type.* Genes Chromosomes Cancer, 2005. **44**(3): p. 247–55.

73. Jiang, N.G., et al., *Flow cytometric immunophenotyping is of great value to diagnosis of natural killer cell neoplasms involving bone marrow and peripheral blood.* Ann Hematol, 2013. **92**(1): p. 89–96.

74. de Leval, L., *Approach to nodal-based T-cell lymphomas.* Pathology, 2020. **52**(1): p. 78–99.

75. Alikhan, M., et al., *Peripheral T-cell lymphomas of follicular helper T-cell type frequently display an aberrant CD3(-/dim)CD4(+) population by flow cytometry: an important clue to the diagnosis of a Hodgkin lymphoma mimic.* Mod Pathol, 2016. **29**(10): p. 1173–82.

76. Vega, F. and L.J. Medeiros, *A suggested immunohistochemical algorithm for the classification of T-cell lymphomas involving lymph nodes.* Hum Pathol, 2020. **102**: p. 104–16.

77. Jaffe, E.S., *The 2008 WHO classification of lymphomas: implications for clinical practice and translational research.* Hematology Am Soc Hematol Educ Program, 2009: p. 523–31.

78. Savage, K.J., *Peripheral T-cell lymphomas.* Blood Rev, 2007. **21**(4): p. 201–16.

79. Horwitz, S.M., *Novel therapies and role of transplant in the treatment of peripheral T-cell lymphomas.* Hematology Am Soc Hematol Educ Program, 2008: p. 289–96.

80. Horwitz, S.M., *Management of peripheral T-cell non-Hodgkin's lymphoma.* Curr Opin Oncol, 2007. **19**(5): p. 438–43.

81. Ascani, S., et al., *Peripheral T-cell lymphomas. Clinico-pathologic study of 168 cases diagnosed according to the R.E.A.L. Classification.* Ann Oncol, 1997. **8**(6): p. 583–92.

82. Arrowsmith, E.R., et al., *Peripheral T-cell lymphomas: clinical features and prognostic factors of 92 cases defined by the revised European American lymphoma classification.* Leuk Lymphoma, 2003. **44**(2): p. 241–9.

83. Gisselbrecht, C., et al., *Prognostic significance of T-cell phenotype in aggressive non-Hodgkin's lymphomas. Groupe d'Etudes des Lymphomes de l'Adulte (GELA).* Blood, 1998. **92**(1): p. 76–82.

84. Gallamini, A., et al., *Peripheral T-cell lymphoma unspecified (PTCL-U): a new prognostic model from a retrospective multicentric clinical study.* Blood, 2004. **103**(7): p. 2474–9.

85. Kim, K., et al., *Clinical features of peripheral T-cell lymphomas in 78 patients diagnosed according to the Revised European-American lymphoma (REAL) classification.* Eur J Cancer, 2002. **38**(1): p. 75–81.

86. Lopez-Guillermo, A., et al., *Peripheral T-cell lymphomas: initial features, natural history, and prognostic factors in a series of 174 patients diagnosed according to the R.E.A.L. Classification.* Ann Oncol, 1998. **9**(8): p. 849–55.

87. Ansell, S.M., et al., *Predictive capacity of the International Prognostic Factor Index in patients with peripheral T-cell lymphoma.* J Clin Oncol, 1997. **15**(6): p. 2296–301.

88. Swerdlow, S.H., et al., *The 2016 revision of the World Health Organization classification of lymphoid neoplasms.* Blood, 2016. **127**(20): p. 2375–90.

89. Dogan, A. and W.G. Morice, *Bone marrow histopathology in peripheral T-cell lymphomas.* Br J Haematol, 2004. **127**(2): p. 140–54.

90. Yi, S., et al., *The significance of bone marrow involvement in aggressive lymphomas: a retrospective comparison of clinical outcomes between peripheral T cell lymphoma and diffuse large B cell lymphoma in China.* Acta Haematol, 2010. **124**(4): p. 239–44.

91. Lepretre, S., et al., *Chromosome abnormalities in peripheral T-cell lymphoma.* Cancer Genet Cytogenet, 2000. **117**(1): p. 71–9.

92. Pileri, S., et al., *Histiocytic necrotizing lymphadenitis without granulocytic infiltration.* Virchows Arch A Pathol Anat Histol, 1982. **395**(3): p. 257–71.

93. Felgar, R.E., et al., *Histiocytic necrotizing lymphadenitis (Kikuchi's disease): in situ end-labeling, immunohistochemical, and serologic evidence supporting cytotoxic lymphocyte-mediated apoptotic cell death.* Mod Pathol, 1997. **10**(3): p. 231–41.

94. Menasce, L.P., et al., *Histiocytic necrotizing lymphadenitis (Kikuchi-Fujimoto disease): continuing diagnostic difficulties.* Histopathology, 1998. **33**(3): p. 248–54.

95. Tsang, W.Y., J.K. Chan, and C.S. Ng, *Kikuchi's lymphadenitis. A morphologic analysis of 75 cases with special reference to unusual features.* Am J Surg Pathol, 1994. **18**(3): p. 219–31.

96. Scott, G.D., et al., *Histology-independent signature distinguishes Kikuchi-Fujimoto disease/systemic lupus erythematosus-associated lymphadenitis from benign and malignant lymphadenopathies.* Am J Clin Pathol, 2020. **154**(2): p. 215–24.

97. Huang, Y., et al., *Peripheral T-cell lymphomas with a follicular growth pattern are derived from follicular helper T cells (TFH) and may show overlapping features with angioimmunoblastic T-cell lymphomas.* Am J Surg Pathol, 2009. **33**(5): p. 682–90.

98. Agostinelli, C., et al., *Peripheral T cell lymphomas with follicular T helper phenotype: a new basket or a distinct entity? Revising Karl Lennert's personal archive.* Histopathology, 2011. **59**(4): p. 679–91.

99. Laurent, C., N. Fazilleau, and P. Brousset, *A novel subset of T-helper cells: follicular T-helper cells and their markers.* Haematologica, 2010. **95**(3): p. 356–8.

100. Moroch, J., et al., *Follicular peripheral T-cell lymphoma expands the spectrum of classical Hodgkin lymphoma mimics.* Am J Surg Pathol, 2012. **36**(11): p. 1636–46.

101. Patsouris, E., H. Noel, and K. Lennert, *Angioimmunoblastic lymphadenopathy–type of T-cell lymphoma with a high content of epithelioid cells. Histopathology and comparison with lymphoepithelioid cell lymphoma.* Am J Surg Pathol, 1989. **13**(4): p. 262–75.

102. Ferry, J.A., *Angioimmunoblastic T-cell lymphoma.* Adv Anat Pathol, 2002. **9**(5): p. 273–9.

103. Dunleavy, K., *Angioimmunoblastic T-cell lymphoma (AILT): a unique clinical and pathobiological entity.* Onkologie, 2008. **31**(10): p. 509–10.

104. Nakamura, S., et al., *Angioimmunoblastic T-cell lymphoma (angioimmunoblastic lymphadenopathy with dysproteinemia [AILD]-type T-cell lymphoma) followed by Hodgkin's disease associated with Epstein-Barr virus.* Pathol Int, 1995. **45**(12): p. 958–64.

105. Jaffe, E.S., *Angioimmunoblastic T-cell lymphoma: new insights, but the clinical challenge remains.* Ann Oncol, 1995. **6**(7): p. 631–2.

106. Mourad, N., et al., *Clinical, biologic, and pathologic features in 157 patients with angioimmunoblastic T-cell lymphoma treated within the Groupe d'Etude des Lymphomes de l'Adulte (GELA) trials.* Blood, 2008. **111**(9): p. 4463–70.

107. Vose, J., J. Armitage, and D. Weisenburger, *International peripheral T-cell and natural killer/T-cell lymphoma study: pathology findings and clinical outcomes.* J Clin Oncol, 2008. **26**(25): p. 4124–30.

108. Jaffe, E.S., *Pathobiology of peripheral T-cell lymphomas.* Hematology Am Soc Hematol Educ Program, 2006: p. 317–22.

109. Dunleavy, K., W.H. Wilson, and E.S. Jaffe, *Angioimmunoblastic T cell lymphoma: pathobiological insights and clinical implications.* Curr Opin Hematol, 2007. **14**(4): p. 348–53.

110. Dupuis, J., et al., *Expression of CXCL13 by neoplastic cells in angioimmunoblastic T-cell lymphoma (AITL): a new diagnostic marker providing evidence that AITL derives from follicular helper T cells.* Am J Surg Pathol, 2006. **30**(4): p. 490–4.

111. Grogg, K.L., et al., *Angioimmunoblastic T-cell lymphoma: a neoplasm of germinal-center T-helper cells?* Blood, 2005. **106**(4): p. 1501–2.

112. Lachenal, F., et al., *Angioimmunoblastic T-cell lymphoma: clinical and laboratory features at diagnosis in 77 patients.* Medicine (Baltimore), 2007. **86**(5): p. 282–92.

113. Siegert, W., et al., *Angioimmunoblastic lymphadenopathy (AILD)-type T-cell lymphoma: prognostic impact of clinical observations and laboratory findings at presentation. The Kiel Lymphoma Study Group.* Ann Oncol, 1995. **6**(7): p. 659–64.

114. de Leval, L., C. Gisselbrecht, and P. Gaulard, *Advances in the understanding and management of angioimmunoblastic T-cell lymphoma.* Br J Haematol, 2009. **148**(5): p. 673–89.

115. Attygalle, A., et al., *Neoplastic T cells in angioimmunoblastic T-cell lymphoma express CD10.* Blood, 2002. **99**(2): p. 627–33.

116. Attygalle, A.D., et al., *Distinguishing angioimmunoblastic T-cell lymphoma from peripheral T-cell lymphoma, unspecified, using morphology, immunophenotype and molecular genetics.* Histopathology, 2007. **50**(4): p. 498–508.

117. Attygalle, A.D., et al., *Histologic evolution of angioimmunoblastic T-cell lymphoma in consecutive biopsies: clinical correlation and insights into natural history and disease progression.* Am J Surg Pathol, 2007. **31**(7): p. 1077–88.

118. Feller, A.C., et al., *Clonal gene rearrangement patterns correlate with immunophenotype and clinical parameters in patients with angioimmunoblastic lymphadenopathy.* Am J Pathol, 1988. **133**(3): p. 549–56.

119. Ree, H.J., et al., *Angioimmunoblastic lymphoma (AILD-type T-cell lymphoma) with hyperplastic germinal centers.* Am J Surg Pathol, 1998. **22**(6): p. 643–55.

120. Cho, Y.U., et al., *Distinct features of angioimmunoblastic T-cell lymphoma with bone marrow involvement.* Am J Clin Pathol, 2009. **131**(5): p. 640–6.

121. Gaulard, P. and L. de Leval, *Follicular helper T cells: implications in neoplastic hematopathology.* Semin Diagn Pathol, 2011. **28**(3): p. 202–13.

122. Dorfman, D.M., et al., *Programmed death-1 (PD-1) is a marker of germinal center-associated T cells and angioimmunoblastic T-cell lymphoma.* Am J Surg Pathol, 2006. **30**(7): p. 802–10.

123. Krenacs, L., et al., *Phenotype of neoplastic cells in angioimmunoblastic T-cell lymphoma is consistent with activated follicular B helper T cells.* Blood, 2006. **108**(3): p. 1110–1.

124. Roncador, G., et al., *Expression of two markers of germinal center T cells (SAP and PD-1) in angioimmunoblastic T-cell lymphoma.* Haematologica, 2007. **92**(8): p. 1059–66.

125. Karube, K., et al., *Usefulness of flow cytometry for differential diagnosis of precursor and peripheral T-cell and NK-cell lymphomas: analysis of 490 cases.* Pathol Int, 2008. **58**(2): p. 89–97.

126. Tan, B.T., R.A. Warnke, and D.A. Arber, *The frequency of B- and T-cell gene rearrangements and Epstein-Barr virus in T-cell lymphomas: a comparison between angioimmunoblastic T-cell lymphoma and peripheral T-cell lymphoma, unspecified with and without associated B-cell proliferations.* J Mol Diagn, 2006. **8**(4): p. 466–75; quiz 527.

127. Rodriguez-Justo, M., et al., *Angioimmunoblastic T-cell lymphoma with hyperplastic germinal centres: a neoplasia with origin in the outer zone of the germinal centre? Clinicopathological and immunohistochemical study of 10 cases with follicular T-cell markers.* Mod Pathol, 2009. **22**(6): p. 753–61.

128. Loghavi, S., et al., *Immunophenotypic and diagnostic characterization of angioimmunoblastic T-cell lymphoma by advanced flow cytometric technology.* Leuk Lymphoma, 2016: p. 1–9.

129. Schlegelberger, B., et al., *Detection of aberrant clones in nearly all cases of angioimmunoblastic lymphadenopathy with dysproteinemia-type T-cell lymphoma by combined interphase and metaphase cytogenetics.* Blood, 1994. **84**(8): p. 2640–8.

130. Kaneko, Y., et al., *Characteristic karyotypic pattern in T-cell lymphoproliferative disorders with reactive "angioimmunoblastic lymphadenopathy with dysproteinemia-type" features.* Blood, 1988. **72**(2): p. 413–21.

131. O'Connor, N.T., et al., *Evidence for monoclonal T lymphocyte proliferation in angioimmunoblastic lymphadenopathy.* J Clin Pathol, 1986. **39**(11): p. 1229–32.

132. Weiss, L.M., et al., *Clonal T-cell populations in angioimmunoblastic lymphadenopathy and angioimmunoblastic lymphadenopathy-like lymphoma.* Am J Pathol, 1986. **122**(3): p. 392–7.

133. Lipford, E.H., et al., *Clonality of angioimmunoblastic lymphadenopathy and implications for its evolution to malignant lymphoma.* J Clin Invest, 1987. **79**(2): p. 637–42.

134. de Leval, L., et al., *The gene expression profile of nodal peripheral T-cell lymphoma demonstrates a molecular link between angioimmunoblastic T-cell lymphoma (AITL) and follicular helper T (TFH) cells.* Blood, 2007. **109**(11): p. 4952–63.

135. Odejide, O., et al., *A targeted mutational landscape of angioimmunoblastic T-cell lymphoma.* Blood, 2014. **123**(9): p. 1293–6.

136. Chiba, S. and M. Sakata-Yanagimoto, *Advances in understanding of angioimmunoblastic T-cell lymphoma.* Leukemia, 2020. **34**(10): p. 2592–606.

137. Quintanilla-Martinez, L., et al., *Peripheral T-cell lymphoma with Reed-Sternberg-like cells of B-cell phenotype and genotype associated with Epstein-Barr virus infection.* Am J Surg Pathol, 1999. **23**(10): p. 1233–40.

138. Nakamura, N., et al., *Peripheral T-cell lymphoma other than angioimmunoblastic T-cell lymphoma (AILD), with follicular dendritic cells proliferation and infection of B immunoblasts with Epstein Barr virus.* Fukushima J Med Sci, 1999. **45**(1): p. 45–51.

139. Frizzera, G., Y. Kaneko, and M. Sakurai, *Angioimmunoblastic lymphadenopathy and related disorders: a retrospective look in search of definitions.* Leukemia, 1989. **3**(1): p. 1–5.

140. Cook, J.R., F.E. Craig, and S.H. Swerdlow, *Benign CD10-positive T cells in reactive lymphoid proliferations and B-cell lymphomas.* Mod Pathol, 2003. **16**(9): p. 879–85.

141. Stacchini, A., et al., *The usefulness of flow cytometric CD10 detection in the differential diagnosis of peripheral T-cell lymphomas.* Am J Clin Pathol, 2007. **128**(5): p. 854–64.

142. Krishnan, C., et al., *PD-1 expression in T-cell lymphomas and reactive lymphoid entities: potential overlap in staining patterns between lymphoma and viral lymphadenitis.* Am J Surg Pathol, 2010. **34**(2): p. 178–89.

143. Basha, B.M., et al., *Application of a 5 marker panel to the routine diagnosis of peripheral T-cell lymphoma with T-follicular helper phenotype.* Am J Surg Pathol, 2019. **43**(9): p. 1282–90.

144. Attygalle, A.D., et al., *Peripheral T-cell and NK-cell lymphomas and their mimics; taking a step forward – report on the lymphoma workshop of the XVIth meeting of the European Association for Haematopathology and the Society for Hematopathology.* Histopathology, 2014. **64**(2): p. 171–99.

145. Rodriguez Pinilla, S.M., et al., *Primary cutaneous CD4+ small/medium-sized pleomorphic T-cell lymphoma expresses follicular T-cell markers.* Am J Surg Pathol, 2009. **33**(1): p. 81–90.

146. Bacon, C.M., et al., *Peripheral T-cell lymphoma with a follicular growth pattern: derivation from follicular helper T cells and relationship to angioimmunoblastic T-cell lymphoma.* Br J Haematol, 2008. **143**(3): p. 439–41.

147. Swerdlow, S.H., Campo, E., Harris, N. L., Jaffe, E. S., Pileri, S. A., Stein, H., et al., ed. WHO classification of tumors of haematopoietic and lymphoid tissues. 2008, IARC: Lyon.

148. de Leval, L., et al., *Peripheral T-cell lymphoma with follicular involvement and a CD4+/bcl-6+ phenotype.* Am J Surg Pathol, 2001. **25**(3): p. 395–400.

149. Qubaja, M., et al., *Nodal follicular helper T-cell lymphoma may present with different patterns. A case report.* Hum Pathol, 2009. **40**(2): p. 264–9.

150. Rudiger, T., et al., *Peripheral T-cell lymphoma with distinct perifollicular growth pattern: a distinct subtype of T-cell lymphoma?* Am J Surg Pathol, 2000. **24**(1): p. 117–22.

151. Marafioti, T., et al., *The inducible T-cell co-stimulator molecule is expressed on subsets of T cells and is a new marker of lymphomas of T follicular helper cell-derivation.* Haematologica, 2010. **95**(3): p. 432–9.

152. Streubel, B., et al., *Novel t(5;9)(q33;q22) fuses ITK to SYK in unspecified peripheral T-cell lymphoma.* Leukemia, 2006. **20**(2): p. 313–8.

153. Shiota, M. and S. Mori, *Anaplastic large cell lymphomas expressing the novel chimeric protein p80NPM/ALK: a distinct clinicopathologic entity.* Leukemia, 1997. **11 Suppl 3**: p. 538–40.

154. Gascoyne, R.D., et al., *Prognostic significance of anaplastic lymphoma kinase (ALK) protein expression in adults with anaplastic large cell lymphoma.* Blood, 1999. **93**(11): p. 3913–21.

155. Benharroch, D., et al., *ALK-positive lymphoma: a single disease with a broad spectrum of morphology.* Blood, 1998. **91**(6): p. 2076–84.

156. Pileri, S.A., et al., *Anaplastic large cell lymphoma: a concept reviewed.* Adv Clin Path, 1998. **2**(4): p. 285–96.

157. Falini, B., et al., *ALK+ lymphoma: clinico-pathological findings and outcome.* Blood, 1999. **93**(8): p. 2697–706.

158. Inghirami, G. and S.A. Pileri, *Anaplastic large-cell lymphoma.* Semin Diagn Pathol, 2011. **28**(3): p. 190–201.

159. Adrada, B.E., et al., *Breast implant-associated anaplastic large cell lymphoma: sensitivity, specificity, and findings of imaging studies in 44 patients.* Breast Cancer Res Treat, 2014. **147**(1): p. 1–14.

160. Miranda, R.N., et al., *Breast implant-associated anaplastic large-cell lymphoma: long-term follow-up of 60 patients.* J Clin Oncol, 2014. **32**(2): p. 114–20.

161. Lechner, M.G., et al., *Survival signals and targets for therapy in breast implant-associated ALK–anaplastic large cell lymphoma.* Clin Cancer Res, 2012. **18**(17): p. 4549–59.

162. Lamant, L., et al., *Gene-expression profiling of systemic anaplastic large-cell lymphoma reveals differences based on ALK status and two distinct morphologic ALK+ subtypes.* Blood, 2007. **109**(5): p. 2156–64.

163. Falini, B., et al., *ALK expression defines a distinct group of T/null lymphomas ("ALK lymphomas") with a wide morphological spectrum.* Am J Pathol, 1998. **153**(3): p. 875–86.

164. Pileri, S.A., et al., *Anaplastic large cell lymphoma: update of findings.* Leuk Lymphoma, 1995. **18**(1–2): p. 17–25.

165. Ott, G., et al., *A lymphohistiocytic variant of anaplastic large cell lymphoma with demonstration of the t(2;5)(p23;q35) chromosome translocation.* Br J Haematol, 1998. **100**(1): p. 187–90.

166. Stein, H., et al., *CD30(+) anaplastic large cell lymphoma: a review of its histopathologic, genetic, and clinical features.* Blood, 2000. **96**(12): p. 3681–95.

167. Bayle, C., et al., *Leukaemic presentation of small cell variant anaplastic large cell lymphoma: report of four cases.* Br J Haematol, 1999. **104**(4): p. 680–8.

168. Kinney, M.C., et al., *A small-cell-predominant variant of primary Ki-1 (CD30)+ T-cell lymphoma.* Am J Surg Pathol, 1993. **17**(9): p. 859–68.

169. Chan, J.K., R. Buchanan, and C.D. Fletcher, *Sarcomatoid variant of anaplastic large-cell Ki-1 lymphoma.* Am J Surg Pathol, 1990. **14**(10): p. 983–8.

170. Zinzani, P.L., et al., *Anaplastic large cell lymphoma Hodgkin's-like: a randomized trial of ABVD versus MACOP-B with and without radiation therapy.* Blood, 1998. **92**(3): p. 790–4.

171. Ferreri, A.J., et al., *Anaplastic large cell lymphoma, ALK-positive.* Crit Rev Oncol Hematol, 2012. **83**(2): p. 293–302.

172. Pileri, S.A., et al., *Frequent expression of the NPM-ALK chimeric fusion protein in anaplastic large-cell lymphoma, lymphohistiocytic type.* Am J Pathol, 1997. **150**(4): p. 1207–11.

173. Burke, A.P., J.A. Andriko, and R. Virmani, *Anaplastic large cell lymphoma (CD 30+), T-phenotype, in the heart of an HIV-positive man.* Cardiovasc Pathol, 2000. **9**(1): p. 49–52.

174. Chan, A.C., et al., *Anaplastic large cell lymphoma presenting as a pleural effusion and mimicking primary effusion lymphoma. A report of 2 cases.* Acta Cytol, 2003. **47**(5): p. 809–16.

175. Grewal, J.S., et al., *Highly aggressive ALK-positive anaplastic large cell lymphoma with a leukemic phase and multi-organ involvement: a report of three cases and a review of the literature.* Ann Hematol, 2007. **86**(7): p. 499–508.

176. Kadin, M.E. and C. Carpenter, *Systemic and primary cutaneous anaplastic large cell lymphomas.* Semin Hematol, 2003. **40**(3): p. 244–56.

177. Nakamura, S., et al., *Rapidly growing primary gastric CD30 (Ki-1)-positive anaplastic large cell lymphoma.* Dig Dis Sci, 1998. **43**(2): p. 300–5.

178. Villamor, N., et al., *Anaplastic large-cell lymphoma with rapid evolution to leukemic phase.* Ann Hematol, 1999. **78**(10): p. 478–82.

179. Park, S.H., et al., *Immunohistopathological features of anaplastic large-cell lymphoma according to anaplastic lymphoma kinase expression and bone marrow involvement pattern.* Histopathology, 2013. **63**(1): p. 13–8.

180. Suzuki, R., et al., *Prognostic significance of CD56 expression for ALK-positive and ALK-negative anaplastic large-cell lymphoma of T/null cell phenotype.* Blood, 2000. **96**(9): p. 2993–3000.

181. Juco, J., J.T. Holden et al., *Immunophenotypic analysis of anaplastic large cell lymphoma by flow cytometry.* Am J Clin Pathol, 2003. **119**: p. 205–12.

182. Kesler, M.V., et al., *Anaplastic large cell lymphoma: a flow cytometric analysis of 29 cases.* Am J Clin Pathol, 2007. **128**(2): p. 314–22.

183. Damm-Welk, C., et al., *Prognostic significance of circulating tumor cells in bone marrow or peripheral blood as detected by qualitative and quantitative PCR in pediatric NPM-ALK-positive anaplastic large-cell lymphoma.* Blood, 2007. **110**(2): p. 670–7.

184. Damm-Welk, C., et al., *Flow cytometric detection of circulating tumour cells in nucleophosmin/anaplastic lymphoma kinase-positive anaplastic large cell lymphoma: comparison with quantitative polymerase chain reaction.* Br J Haematol, 2007. **138**(4): p. 459–66.

185. Boi, M., et al., *PRDM1/BLIMP1 is commonly inactivated in anaplastic large T-cell lymphoma.* Blood, 2013. **122**(15): p. 2683–93.

186. Morris, S.W., et al., *Fusion of a kinase gene, ALK, to a nucleolar protein gene, NPM, in non-Hodgkin's lymphoma.* Science, 1994. **263**(5151): p. 1281–4.

187. Falini, B., *Anaplastic large cell lymphoma: pathological, molecular and clinical features.* Br J Haematol, 2001. **114**(4): p. 741–60.

188. Lamant, L., et al., *A new fusion gene TPM3-ALK in anaplastic large cell lymphoma created by a (1;2)(q25;p23) translocation.* Blood, 1999. **93**(9): p. 3088–95.

189. Lamant, L., et al., *High incidence of the t(2;5)(p23;q35) translocation in anaplastic large cell lymphoma and its lack of detection in Hodgkin's disease. Comparison of cytogenetic analysis, reverse transcriptase-polymerase chain reaction, and P-80 immunostaining.* Blood, 1996. **87**(1): p. 284–91.

190. Ma, Z., et al., *Inv(2)(p23q35) in anaplastic large-cell lymphoma induces constitutive anaplastic lymphoma kinase (ALK) tyrosine kinase activation by fusion to ATIC, an enzyme involved in purine nucleotide biosynthesis.* Blood, 2000. **95**(6): p. 2144–9.

191. Falini, B., et al., *Lymphomas expressing ALK fusion protein(s) other than NPM-ALK.* Blood, 1999. **94**(10): p. 3509–15.

192. Hernandez, L., et al., *TRK-fused gene (TFG) is a new partner of ALK in anaplastic large cell lymphoma producing two structurally different TFG-ALK translocations.* Blood, 1999. **94**(9): p. 3265–8.

193. Mason, D.Y., et al., *Nucleolar localization of the nucleophosmin-anaplastic lymphoma kinase is not required for malignant transformation.* Cancer Res, 1998. **58**(5): p. 1057–62.

194. Kadin, M.E., et al., *Primary cutaneous ALCL with phosphorylated/activated cytoplasmic ALK and novel phenotype: EMA/MUC1+, cutaneous lymphocyte antigen negative.* Am J Surg Pathol, 2008. **32**(9): p. 1421–6.

195. Su, L.D., et al., *The t(2;5)-associated p80 NPM/ALK fusion protein in nodal and cutaneous CD30+ lymphoproliferative disorders.* J Cutan Pathol, 1997. **24**(10): p. 597–603.

196. Song, S.X., et al., *Mycosis fungoides: report of the 2011 society for hematopathology/European association for haematopathology workshop.* Am J Clin Pathol, 2013. **139**(4): p. 466–90.

197. Quintanilla-Martinez, L., et al., *Non-mycosis fungoides cutaneous T-cell lymphomas: report of the 2011 society for hematopathology/European association for haematopathology workshop.* Am J Clin Pathol, 2013. **139**(4): p. 491–514.

198. Bekkenk, M.W., et al., *Primary and secondary cutaneous CD30(+) lymphoproliferative disorders: a report from the Dutch Cutaneous Lymphoma Group on the long-term follow-up data of 219 patients and guidelines for diagnosis and treatment.* Blood, 2000. **95**(12): p. 3653–61.

199. Irshaid, L. and M.L. Xu, *ALCL by any other name: the many facets of anaplastic large cell lymphoma.* Pathology, 2020. **52**(1): p. 100–10.

200. Chan, J.K., *Natural killer cell neoplasms.* Anat Pathol, 1998. **3**: p. 77–145.

201. Song, S.Y., et al., *Aggressive natural killer cell leukemia: clinical features and treatment outcome.* Haematologica, 2002. **87**(12): p. 1343–5.

202. Suzuki, R., et al., *Aggressive natural killer-cell leukemia revisited: large granular lymphocyte leukemia of cytotoxic NK cells.* Leukemia, 2004. **18**(4): p. 763–70.

203. Li, C., et al., *Abnormal immunophenotype provides a key diagnostic marker: a report of 29 cases of de novo aggressive natural killer cell leukemia.* Transl Res, 2014. **163**(6): p. 565–77.

204. Ryder, J., et al., *Aggressive natural killer cell leukemia: report of a Chinese series and review of the literature.* Int J Hematol, 2007. **85**(1): p. 18–25.

205. Zhang, Q., et al., *Six cases of aggressive natural killer-cell leukemia in a Chinese population.* Int J Clin Exp Pathol, 2014. **7**(6): p. 3423–31.

206. Montes-Mojarro, I.A., et al., *Epstein-Barr virus positive T and NK-cell lymphoproliferations: morphological features and differential diagnosis.* Semin Diagn Pathol, 2020. **37**(1): p. 32–46.

207. Hue, S.S., et al., *Epstein-Barr virus-associated T- and NK-cell lymphoproliferative diseases: an update and diagnostic approach.* Pathology, 2020. **52**(1): p. 111–27.

208. Chiang, A.K., et al., *Nasal T/natural killer (NK)-cell lymphomas are derived from Epstein-Barr virus-infected cytotoxic lymphocytes of both NK- and T-cell lineage.* Int J Cancer, 1997. **73**(3): p. 332–8.

209. Kwong, Y.L., et al., *CD56+ NK lymphomas: clinicopathological features and prognosis.* Br J Haematol, 1997. **97**(4): p. 821–9.

210. Cheung, M.M., J.K. Chan, and K.F. Wong, *Natural killer cell neoplasms: a distinctive group of highly aggressive lymphomas/leukemias.* Semin Hematol, 2003. **40**(3): p. 221–32.

211. Cuadra-Garcia, I., et al., *Sinonasal lymphoma: a clinicopathologic analysis of 58 cases from the Massachusetts General Hospital.* Am J Surg Pathol, 1999. **23**(11): p. 1356–69.

212. Gaal, K., et al., *Sinonasal NK/T-cell lymphomas in the United States.* Am J Surg Pathol, 2000. **24**(11): p. 1511–7.

213. Jaffe, E.S., *Classification of natural killer (NK) cell and NK-like T-cell malignancies.* Blood, 1996. **87**(4): p. 1207–10.

214. Jaffe, E.S., et al., *Extranodal peripheral T-cell and NK-cell neoplasms.* Am J Clin Pathol, 1999. **111**(1 Suppl 1): p. S46–55.

215. Jaffe, E.S., L. Krenacs, and M. Raffeld, *Classification of cytotoxic T-cell and natural killer cell lymphomas.* Semin Hematol, 2003. **40**(3): p. 175–84.

216. Natkunam, Y., et al., *Aggressive cutaneous NK and NK-like T-cell lymphomas: clinicopathologic, immunohistochemical, and molecular analyses of 12 cases.* Am J Surg Pathol, 1999. **23**(5): p. 571–81.

217. Oshimi, K., *NK cell lymphoma.* Int J Hematol, 2002. **76 Suppl 2**: p. 118–21.

218. Ratech, H., et al., *A clinicopathologic study of malignant lymphomas of the nose, paranasal sinuses, and hard palate, including cases of lethal midline granuloma.* Cancer, 1989. **64**(12): p. 2525–31.

219. Siu, L.L., J.K. Chan, and Y.L. Kwong, *Natural killer cell malignancies: clinicopathologic and molecular features.* Histol Histopathol, 2002. **17**(2): p. 539–54.

220. Weiss, L.M., D.A. Arber, and J.G. Strickler, *Nasal T-cell lymphoma.* Ann Oncol, 1994. 5 **Suppl 1**: p. 39–42.

221. Al-Hakeem, D.A., et al., *Extranodal NK/T-cell lymphoma, nasal type.* Oral Oncol, 2007. **43**(1): p. 4–14.

222. Liang, R., *Advances in the management and monitoring of extranodal NK/T-cell lymphoma, nasal type.* Br J Haematol, 2009. **147**(1): p. 13–21.

223. Au, W.Y., et al., *Clinical differences between nasal and extranasal natural killer/T-cell lymphoma: a study of 136 cases from the International Peripheral T-Cell Lymphoma Project.* Blood, 2009. **113**(17): p. 3931–7.

224. Li, S., et al., *Extranodal NK/T-cell lymphoma, nasal type: a report of 73 cases at MD Anderson Cancer Center.* Am J Surg Pathol, 2013. **37**(1): p. 14–23.

225. Lee, J., et al., *Extranodal natural killer T-cell lymphoma, nasal-type: a prognostic model from a retrospective multicenter study.* J Clin Oncol, 2006. **24**(4): p. 612–8.

226. Wu, X., et al., *A clinical study of 115 patients with extranodal natural killer/T-cell lymphoma, nasal type.* Clin Oncol (R Coll Radiol), 2008. **20**(8): p. 619–25.

227. Huang, Y., et al., *De novo testicular extranodal NK/T-cell lymphoma: a clinicopathologic study of 21 cases with review of additional 18 cases in the literature.* Am J Surg Pathol, 2019. **43**(4): p. 549–58.

228. Wong, K.F., J.K. Chan, and Y.L. Kwong, *Identification of del(6)(q21q25) as a recurring chromosomal abnormality in putative NK cell lymphoma/leukaemia.* Br J Haematol, 1997. **98**(4): p. 922–6.

229. Wong, K.F., Y.M. Zhang, and J.K. Chan, *Cytogenetic abnormalities in natural killer cell lymphoma/leukaemia–is there a consistent pattern?* Leuk Lymphoma, 1999. **34**(3–4): p. 241–50.

230. Chan, J.K., et al., *Most nasal/nasopharyngeal lymphomas are peripheral T-cell neoplasms.* Am J Surg Pathol, 1987. **11**(6): p. 418–29.

231. Chan, J.K. and C.S. Ng, *Malignant lymphoma, natural killer cells and hemophagocytic syndrome.* Pathology, 1989. **21**(2): p. 154–5.

232. Chen, S.H., et al., *Primary sinonasal non-Hodgkin's lymphoma masquerading as chronic rhinosinusitis: an issue of routine histopathological examination.* J Laryngol Otol, 2003. **117**(5): p. 404–7.

233. Cheung, M.M., et al., *Primary non-Hodgkin's lymphoma of the nose and nasopharynx: clinical features, tumor immunophenotype, and treatment outcome in 113 patients.* J Clin Oncol, 1998. **16**(1): p. 70–7.

234. Ferry, J.A., et al., *Nasal lymphoma. A clinicopathologic study with immunophenotypic and genotypic analysis.* Am J Surg Pathol, 1991. **15**(3): p. 268–79.

235. Liu, Q., et al., *Nasal CD56 positive small round cell tumors. Differential diagnosis of hematological, neurogenic, and myogenic neoplasms.* Virchows Arch, 2001. **438**(3): p. 271–9.

236. Mansoor, A., et al., *NK-cell enteropathy: a benign NK-cell lymphoproliferative disease mimicking intestinal lymphoma: clinicopathologic features and follow-up in a unique case series.* Blood, 2011. **117**(5): p. 1447–52.

237. Ashton-Key, M., et al., *Molecular analysis of T-cell clonality in ulcerative jejunitis and enteropathy-associated T-cell lymphoma.* Am J Pathol, 1997. **151**(2): p. 493–8.

238. de Bruin, P.C., et al., *Enteropathy-associated T-cell lymphomas have a cytotoxic T-cell phenotype.* Histopathology, 1997. **31**(4): p. 313–7.

239. Baumgartner, A.K., et al., *High frequency of genetic aberrations in enteropathy-type T-cell lymphoma.* Lab Invest, 2003. **83**(10): p. 1509–16.

240. Isaacson, P.G., *Relation between cryptic intestinal lymphoma and refractory sprue.* Lancet, 2000. **356**(9225): p. 178–9.

241. Murray, A., et al., *Study of the immunohistochemistry and T cell clonality of enteropathy-associated T cell lymphoma.* Am J Pathol, 1995. **146**(2): p. 509–19.

242. Pricolo, V.E., et al., *Gastrointestinal malignancies in patients with celiac sprue.* Am J Surg, 1998. **176**(4): p. 344–7.

243. Chott, A., et al., *Classification of intestinal T-cell neoplasms and their differential diagnosis.* Am J Clin Pathol, 1999. **111**(1 Suppl 1): p. S68–74.

244. Zettl, A., et al., *Enteropathy-type T-cell lymphoma.* Am J Clin Pathol, 2007. **127**(5): p. 701–6.

245. Delabie, J., et al., *Enteropathy-associated T-cell lymphoma: clinical and histological findings from the International Peripheral T-Cell Lymphoma Project.* Blood, 2011. **118**(1): p. 148–55.

246. Chan, J.K., et al., *Type II enteropathy-associated T-cell lymphoma: a distinct aggressive lymphoma with frequent gammadelta T-cell receptor expression.* Am J Surg Pathol, 2011. **35**(10): p. 1557–69.

247. van Vliet, C. and D.V. Spagnolo, *T- and NK-cell lymphoproliferative disorders of the gastrointestinal tract: review and update.* Pathology, 2020. **52**(1): p. 128–41.

248. Isaacson, P.G. and M.Q. Du, *Gastrointestinal lymphoma: where morphology meets molecular biology.* J Pathol, 2005. **205**(2): p. 255–74.

249. Soderquist, C.R. and G. Bhagat, *Gastrointestinal T- and NK-cell lymphomas and indolent lymphoproliferative disorders.* Semin Diagn Pathol, 2020. **37**(1): p. 11–23.

250. Malamut, G., et al., *Enteropathy associated T cell lymphoma in celiac disease: a large retrospective study.* Dig Liver Dis, 2013. **45**(5): p. 377–84.

251. Moffitt, A.B., et al., *Enteropathy-associated T cell lymphoma subtypes are characterized by loss of function of SETD2.* J Exp Med, 2017. **214**(5): p. 1371–86.

252. Verkarre, V., et al., *Recurrent partial trisomy 1q22-q44 in clonal intraepithelial lymphocytes in refractory celiac sprue.* Gastroenterology, 2003. **125**(1): p. 40–6.

253. Deleeuw, R.J., et al., *Whole-genome analysis and HLA genotyping of enteropathy-type T-cell lymphoma reveals 2 distinct lymphoma subtypes.* Gastroenterology, 2007. **132**(5): p. 1902–11.

254. Zettl, A., et al., *Chromosomal gains at 9q characterize enteropathy-type T-cell lymphoma.* Am J Pathol, 2002. **161**(5): p. 1635–45.

255. Nicolae, A., et al., *Mutations in the JAK/STAT and RAS signaling pathways are common in intestinal T-cell lymphomas.* Leukemia, 2016. **30**(11): p. 2245–7.

256. Roberti, A., et al., *Type II enteropathy-associated T-cell lymphoma features a unique genomic profile with highly recurrent SETD2 alterations.* Nat Commun, 2016. **7**: p. 12602.

257. Mosnier, J.F., et al., *Lymphocytic and collagenous colitis: an immunohistochemical study.* Am J Gastroenterol, 1996. **91**(4): p. 709–13.

258. Goranzon, C., et al., *Immunohistochemical characterization of lymphocytes in microscopic colitis.* J Crohns Colitis, 2013. **7**(10): p. e434–42.

259. Tan, S.Y., et al., *Type II EATL (epitheliotropic intestinal T-cell lymphoma): a neoplasm of intra-epithelial T-cells with predominant CD8alphaalpha phenotype.* Leukemia, 2013. **27**(8): p. 1688–96.

260. Soderquist, C.R., et al., *Genetic and phenotypic characterization of indolent T-cell lymphoproliferative disorders of the gastrointestinal tract.* Haematologica, 2020. **105**(7): p. 1895–906.

261. Perry, A.M., et al., *Indolent T-cell lymphoproliferative disease of the gastrointestinal tract.* Blood, 2013. **122**(22): p. 3599–606.

262. Zivny, J., et al., *CD4+ T-cell lymphoproliferative disorder of the gut clinically mimicking celiac sprue.* Dig Dis Sci, 2004. **49**(4): p. 551–5.

263. Svrcek, M., et al., *Small intestinal CD4+ T-cell lymphoma: a rare distinctive clinicopathological entity associated with prolonged survival.* Virchows Arch, 2007. **451**(6): p. 1091–3.

264. Margolskee, E., et al., *Indolent small intestinal CD4+ T-cell lymphoma is a distinct entity with unique biologic and clinical features.* PLoS One, 2013. **8**(7): p. e68343.

265. Leventaki, V., et al., *Indolent peripheral T-cell lymphoma involving the gastrointestinal tract.* Hum Pathol, 2014. **45**(2): p. 421–6.

266. Malamut, G., et al., *Small intestinal CD4+ T-cell lymphoma is a heterogenous entity with common pathology features.* Clin Gastroenterol Hepatol, 2014. **12**(4): p. 599–608.e1.

267. Sena Teixeira Mendes, L., et al., *CD4-positive small T-cell lymphoma of the intestine presenting with severe bile-acid malabsorption: a supportive symptom control approach.* Br J Haematol, 2014. **167**(2): p. 265–9.

268. Sharma, A., et al., *Recurrent STAT3-JAK2 fusions in indolent T-cell lymphoproliferative disorder of the gastrointestinal tract.* Blood, 2018. **131**(20): p. 2262–6.

269. Perry, A.M., et al., *Disease progression in a patient with indolent T-cell lymphoproliferative disease of the gastrointestinal tract.* Int J Surg Pathol, 2019. **27**(1): p. 102–7.

270. Hirakawa, K., et al., *Primary gastrointestinal T-cell lymphoma resembling multiple lymphomatous polyposis.* Gastroenterology, 1996. **111**(3): p. 778–82.

271. Matnani, R., et al., *Indolent T- and NK-cell lymphoproliferative disorders of the gastrointestinal tract: a review and update.* Hematol Oncol, 2017. **35**(1): p. 3–16.

272. Willemze, R., et al., *The 2018 update of the WHO-EORTC classification for primary cutaneous lymphomas.* Blood, 2019. **133**(16): p. 1703–14.

273. Willemze, R., et al., *WHO-EORTC classification for cutaneous lymphomas.* Blood, 2005. **105**(10): p. 3768–85.

274. van Doorn, R., et al., *Mycosis fungoides: disease evolution and prognosis of 309 Dutch patients.* Arch Dermatol, 2000. **136**(4): p. 504–10.

275. Benner, M.F., et al., *Prognostic factors in transformed mycosis fungoides: a retrospective analysis of 100 cases.* Blood, 2012. **119**(7): p. 1643–9.

276. Cerroni, L., et al., *Clinicopathologic and immunologic features associated with transformation of mycosis fungoides to large-cell lymphoma.* Am J Surg Pathol, 1992. **16**(6): p. 543–52.

277. Reddy, K. and J. Bhawan, *Histologic mimickers of mycosis fungoides: a review.* J Cutan Pathol, 2007. **34**(7): p. 519–25.

278. Kim, Y.H., et al., *Long-term outcome of 525 patients with mycosis fungoides and Sézary syndrome: clinical prognostic factors and risk for disease progression.* Arch Dermatol, 2003. **139**(7): p. 857–66.

279. Diamandidou, E., et al., *Transformation of mycosis fungoides/Sézary syndrome: clinical characteristics and prognosis.* Blood, 1998. **92**(4): p. 1150–9.

280. Salhany, K.E., et al., *Transformation of cutaneous T cell lymphoma to large cell lymphoma. A clinicopathologic and immunologic study.* Am J Pathol, 1988. **132**(2): p. 265–77.

281. Vergier, B., et al., *Transformation of mycosis fungoides: clinicopathological and prognostic features of 45 cases. French Study Group of Cutaneous Lymphomas.* Blood, 2000. **95**(7): p. 2212–8.

282. Arulogun, S.O., et al., *Long-term outcomes of patients with advanced-stage cutaneous T-cell lymphoma and large cell transformation.* Blood, 2008. **112**(8): p. 3082–7.

283. Edinger, J.T., et al., *CD30 expression and proliferative fraction in nontransformed mycosis fungoides.* Am J Surg Pathol, 2009. **33**(12): p. 1860–8.

284. Massone, C., et al., *The prognosis of early mycosis fungoides is not influenced by phenotype and T-cell clonality.* Br J Dermatol, 2008. **159**(4): p. 881–6.

285. Ralfkiaer, E., *Immunohistological markers for the diagnosis of cutaneous lymphomas.* Semin Diagn Pathol, 1991. **8**(2): p. 62–72.

286. Ralfkiaer, E., et al., *Immunophenotypic studies in cutaneous T-cell lymphomas: clinical implications.* Br J Dermatol, 1993. **129**(6): p. 655–9.

287. Pimpinelli, N., et al., *Defining early mycosis fungoides.* J Am Acad Dermatol, 2005. **53**(6): p. 1053–63.

288. Vermeer, M.H., et al., *Expression of cytotoxic proteins by neoplastic T cells in mycosis fungoides increases with progression from plaque stage to tumor stage disease.* Am J Pathol, 1999. **154**(4): p. 1203–10.

289. Smith, B.D. and L.D. Wilson, *Cutaneous lymphoma.* Curr Probl Cancer, 2008. **32**(2): p. 43–87.

290. Berti, E., et al., *Primary cutaneous CD8-positive epidermotropic cytotoxic T cell lymphomas. A distinct clinicopathological entity with an aggressive clinical behavior.* Am J Pathol, 1999. **155**(2): p. 483–92.

291. Agnarsson, B.A., E.C. Vonderheid, and M.E. Kadin, *Cutaneous T cell lymphoma with suppressor/cytotoxic (CD8) phenotype: identification of rapidly progressive and chronic subtypes.* J Am Acad Dermatol, 1990. **22**(4): p. 569–77.

292. Whittam, L.R., et al., *CD8-positive juvenile onset mycosis fungoides: an immunohistochemical and genotypic analysis of six cases.* Br J Dermatol, 2000. **143**(6): p. 1199–204.

293. Bruggemann, M., et al., *Powerful strategy for polymerase chain reaction-based clonality assessment in T-cell malignancies Report of the BIOMED-2 Concerted Action BHM4 CT98-3936.* Leukemia, 2007. **21**(2): p. 215–21.

294. Wood, G.S., et al., *Detection of clonal T-cell receptor gamma gene rearrangements in early mycosis fungoides/Sézary syndrome by polymerase chain reaction and denaturing gradient gel electrophoresis (PCR/DGGE).* J Invest Dermatol, 1994. **103**(1): p. 34–41.

295. Trainor, K.J., et al., *Gene rearrangement in B- and T-lymphoproliferative disease detected by the polymerase chain reaction.* Blood, 1991. **78**(1): p. 192–6.

296. Bottaro, M., et al., *Heteroduplex analysis of T-cell receptor gamma gene rearrangements for diagnosis and monitoring of cutaneous T-cell lymphomas.* Blood, 1994. **83**(11): p. 3271–8.

297. Ponti, R., et al., *T-cell receptor gamma gene rearrangement by multiplex polymerase chain reaction/heteroduplex analysis in patients with cutaneous T-cell lymphoma (mycosis fungoides/Sézary syndrome) and benign inflammatory disease: correlation with clinical, histological and immunophenotypical findings.* Br J Dermatol, 2005. **153**(3): p. 565–73.

298. Horn, T.a.K.H., *Cutaneous toxicities of drugs.*, in Lever's histopathology of the skin, D. Elder, Elenitsas, R., Johnson, BL., Murphy, GF., Editor. 2005, Lippincott Williams and WIlkins: New York. p. 331.

299. Wilcox, R.A., *Cutaneous T-cell lymphoma: 2011 update on diagnosis, risk-stratification, and management.* Am J Hematol, 2011. **86**(11): p. 928–48.

300. Guitart, J. and C. Magro, *Cutaneous T-cell lymphoid dyscrasia: a unifying term for idiopathic chronic dermatoses with persistent T-cell clones.* Arch Dermatol, 2007. **143**(7): p. 921–32.

301. Zinzani, P.L., A.J. Ferreri, and L. Cerroni, *Mycosis fungoides.* Crit Rev Oncol Hematol, 2008. **65**(2): p. 172–82.

302. Pham-Ledard, A., et al., *IRF4 gene rearrangements define a subgroup of CD30-positive cutaneous T-cell lymphoma: a study of 54 cases.* J Invest Dermatol, 2010. **130**(3): p. 816–25.

303. Wada, D.A., et al., *Specificity of IRF4 translocations for primary cutaneous anaplastic large cell lymphoma: a multicenter study of 204 skin biopsies.* Mod Pathol, 2011. **24**(4): p. 596–605.

304. Winter, L.K., J.H. Spiegel, and T. King, *Dermatopathic lymphadenitis of the head and neck.* J Cutan Pathol, 2007. **34**(2): p. 195–7.

305. Vonderheid, E.C., et al., *Update on erythrodermic cutaneous T-cell lymphoma: report of the International Society for Cutaneous Lymphomas.* J Am Acad Dermatol, 2002. **46**(1): p. 95–106.

306. Vonderheid, E.C., J. Pena, and P. Nowell, *Sézary cell counts in erythrodermic cutaneous T-cell lymphoma: implications for prognosis and staging.* Leuk Lymphoma, 2006. **47**(9): p. 1841–56.

307. Foulc, P., J.M. N'Guyen, and B. Dreno, *Prognostic factors in Sézary syndrome: a study of 28 patients.* Br J Dermatol, 2003. **149**(6): p. 1152–8.

308. Marti, R.M., et al., *Sézary syndrome and related variants of classic cutaneous T-cell lymphoma. A descriptive and prognostic clinicopathologic study of 29 cases.* Leuk Lymphoma, 2003. **44**(1): p. 59–69.

309. Mao, X., et al., *Molecular cytogenetic characterization of Sézary syndrome.* Genes Chromosomes Cancer, 2003. **36**(3): p. 250–60.

310. Scarisbrick, J.J., et al., *Blood classification and blood response criteria in mycosis fungoides and Sézary syndrome using flow cytometry: recommendations from the EORTC cutaneous lymphoma task force.* Eur J Cancer, 2018. **93**: p. 47–56.

311. Picker, L.J., et al., *Differential expression of homing-associated adhesion molecules by T cell subsets in man.* J Immunol, 1990. **145**(10): p. 3247–55.

312. Notohamiprodjo, M., et al., *CCR10 is expressed in cutaneous T-cell lymphoma.* Int J Cancer, 2005. **115**(4): p. 641–7.

313. Sokolowska-Wojdylo, M., et al., *Circulating clonal CLA(+) and CD4(+) T cells in Sézary syndrome express the skin-homing chemokine receptors CCR4 and CCR10 as well as the lymph node-homing chemokine receptor CCR7.* Br J Dermatol, 2005. **152**(2): p. 258–64.

314. Sentis, H.J., R. Willemze, and E. Scheffer, *Histopathologic studies in Sézary syndrome and erythrodermic mycosis fungoides: a comparison with benign forms of erythroderma.* J Am Acad Dermatol, 1986. **15**(6): p. 1217–26.

315. Trotter, M.J., et al., *Cutaneous histopathology of Sézary syndrome: a study of 41 cases with a proven circulating T-cell clone.* J Cutan Pathol, 1997. **24**(5): p. 286–91.

316. Sibaud, V., et al., *Bone marrow histopathologic and molecular staging in epidermotropic T-cell lymphomas.* Am J Clin Pathol, 2003. **119**(3): p. 414–23.

317. Scheffer, E., et al., *Lymph node histopathology in mycosis fungoides and Sézary's syndrome.* Curr Probl Dermatol, 1990. **19**: p. 105–13.

318. Scheffer, E., et al., *A histologic study of lymph nodes from patients with the Sézary syndrome.* Cancer, 1986. **57**(12): p. 2375–80.

319. Novelli, M., et al., *Blood flow cytometry in Sézary syndrome: new insights on prognostic relevance and immunophenotypic changes during follow-up.* Am J Clin Pathol, 2015. **143**(1): p. 57–69.

320. Klemke, C.D., et al., *The diagnosis of Sézary syndrome on peripheral blood by flow cytometry requires the use of multiple markers.* Br J Dermatol, 2008. **159**(4): p. 871–80.

321. Lyapichev, K.A., et al., *Determination of immunophenotypic aberrancies provides better assessment of peripheral blood involvement by mycosis fungoides/Sézary syndrome than quantification of CD26$^-$ or CD7$^-$ CD4$^+$ T-cells.* Cytometry B Clin Cytom, 2021. **100**(2): p. 183–91.

322. Horna, P., et al., *Quantitative flow cytometric identification of aberrant T cell clusters in erythrodermic cutaneous T cell lymphoma. Implications for staging and prognosis.* J Clin Pathol, 2014. **67**(5): p. 431–6.

323. Horna, P., et al., *Flow cytometric evaluation of peripheral blood for suspected Sézary syndrome or mycosis fungoides: international guidelines for assay characteristics.* Cytometry B Clin Cytom, 2021. **100**(2): p. 142–55.

324. Cetinozman, F., et al., *Differential expression of programmed death-1 (PD-1) in Sézary syndrome and mycosis fungoides.* Arch Dermatol, 2012. **148**(12): p. 1379–85.

325. Cetinozman, F., P.M. Jansen, and R. Willemze, *Expression of programmed death-1 in primary cutaneous CD4-positive small/medium-sized pleomorphic T-cell lymphoma, cutaneous pseudo-T-cell lymphoma, and other types of cutaneous T-cell lymphoma.* Am J Surg Pathol, 2012. **36**(1): p. 109–16.

326. Hurabielle, C., et al., *Eruption of lymphocyte recovery with atypical lymphocytes mimicking a primary cutaneous T-cell lymphoma: a series of 12 patients.* Hum Pathol, 2018. **71**: p. 100–8.

327. Illingworth, A., et al., *International guidelines for the flow cytometric evaluation of peripheral blood for suspected Sézary syndrome or mycosis fungoides: assay development/optimization, validation, and ongoing quality monitors.* Cytometry B Clin Cytom, 2021. **100**(2): p. 156–82.

328. Ferreri, A.J., S. Govi, and S.A. Pileri, *Hepatosplenic gamma-delta T-cell lymphoma.* Crit Rev Oncol Hematol, 2012. **83**(2): p. 283–92.

329. Belhadj, K., et al., *Hepatosplenic gammadelta T-cell lymphoma is a rare clinicopathologic entity with poor outcome: report on a series of 21 patients.* Blood, 2003. **102**(13): p. 4261–9.

330. Cooke, C.B., et al., *Hepatosplenic T-cell lymphoma: a distinct clinicopathologic entity of cytotoxic gamma delta T-cell origin.* Blood, 1996. **88**(11): p. 4265–74.

331. Farcet, J.P., et al., *Hepatosplenic T-cell lymphoma: sinusal/sinusoidal localization of malignant cells expressing the T-cell receptor gamma delta.* Blood, 1990. **75**(11): p. 2213–9.

332. Vega, F., L.J. Medeiros, and P. Gaulard, *Hepatosplenic and other gammadelta T-cell lymphomas.* Am J Clin Pathol, 2007. **127**(6): p. 869–80.

333. Wong, K.F., et al., *Hepatosplenic gamma delta T-cell lymphoma. A distinctive aggressive lymphoma type.* Am J Surg Pathol, 1995. **19**(6): p. 718–26.

334. Yamaguchi, M., *Hepatosplenic gammadelta T-cell lymphoma: difficulty in diagnosis.* Intern Med, 2004. **43**(2): p. 83–4.

335. Kumar, S., C. Lawlor, and E.S. Jaffe, *Hepatosplenic T-cell lymphoma of alphabeta lineage.* Am J Surg Pathol, 2001. **25**(7): p. 970–1.

336. Lai, R., et al., *Hepatosplenic T-cell lymphoma of alphabeta lineage in a 16-year-old boy presenting with hemolytic anemia and thrombocytopenia.* Am J Surg Pathol, 2000. **24**(3): p. 459–63.

337. Macon, W.R., et al., *Hepatosplenic alphabeta T-cell lymphomas: a report of 14 cases and comparison with hepatosplenic gammadelta T-cell lymphomas.* Am J Surg Pathol, 2001. **25**(3): p. 285–96.

338. Yabe, M., et al., *Distinguishing between hepatosplenic T-cell lymphoma and gammadelta T-cell large granular lymphocytic leukemia: a clinicopathologic, immunophenotypic, and molecular analysis.* Am J Surg Pathol, 2017. **41**(1): p. 82–93.

339. McKinney, M., et al., *The genetic basis of hepatosplenic T-cell lymphoma.* Cancer Discov, 2017. **7**(4): p. 369–79.

340. Tamaska, J., et al., *Hepatosplenic gammadelta T-cell lymphoma with ring chromosome 7, an isochromosome 7q equivalent clonal chromosomal aberration.* Virchows Arch, 2006. **449**(4): p. 479–83.

341. Suarez, F., et al., *Hepatosplenic alphabeta T-cell lymphoma: an unusual case with clinical, histologic, and cytogenetic features of gammadelta hepatosplenic T-cell lymphoma.* Am J Surg Pathol, 2000. **24**(7): p. 1027–32.

342. Gorczyca, W., et al., *An approach to diagnosis of T-cell lymphoproliferative disorders by flow cytometry.* Cytometry, 2002. **50**(3): p. 177–90.

343. Gorczyca, W., *Differential diagnosis of T-cell lymphoproliferative disorders by flow cytometry multicolor immunophenotyping. correlation with morphology.* Methods Cell Biol, 2004. **75**: p. 595–621.

344. Wlodarska, I., et al., *Fluorescence in situ hybridization study of chromosome 7 aberrations in hepatosplenic T-cell lymphoma: isochromosome 7q as a common abnormality accumulating in forms with features of cytologic progression.* Genes Chromosomes Cancer, 2002. **33**(3): p. 243–51.

345. Alonsozana, E.L., et al., *Isochromosome 7q: the primary cytogenetic abnormality in hepatosplenic gammadelta T cell lymphoma.* Leukemia, 1997. **11**(8): p. 1367–72.

346. Francois, A., et al., *Hepatosplenic gamma/delta T-cell lymphoma: a report of two cases in immunocompromised patients, associated with isochromosome 7q.* Am J Surg Pathol, 1997. **21**(7): p. 781–90.

347. Steurer, M., et al., *Hepatosplenic gammadelta-T-cell lymphoma with leukemic course after renal transplantation.* Hum Pathol, 2002. **33**(2): p. 253–8.

17

B-CELL ACUTE LYMPHOBLASTIC LEUKEMIA/LYMPHOMA

B-ALL phenotype by flow cytometry: CD10$^{+(bright)/rarely-}$, CD13$^{-/rarely+}$, CD19^{+}, CD20$^{-/rarely+}$, CD22^{+}, CD33$^{-/rarely+}$, CD34$^{+/rarely-}$, CD38$^{+(bright)}$, CD45$^{-/+dim}$, CD56^{-}, CD71$^{-/+dim}$, CD79a^{+}, CD81^{+dim}, CD123$^{+/-}$, CD200$^{+/-}$, HLA-DR^{+}, MPO^{-}, TdT$^{+/rarely-}$

Introduction

B-cell acute lymphoblastic leukemia/lymphoma (B-ALL/LBL) is a lymphoproliferative disorder of immature B-cells with blastic morphology and specific phenotype (CD10$^{+/-}$, CD19^{+}, CD20^{-}, CD22$^{+/-}$, cCD79a^{+}, CD34^{+}, TdT^{+}, and CD45$^{+/-}$) [1–6]. Several clinical, phenotypic, and genetic features define prognosis in B-ALL. The total WBC count at the time of diagnosis is the single most powerful clinical predictor of remission induction and duration, and long-term survival for all age groups [7–9]. Patients with high WBC counts often have extramedullary disease at diagnosis and are at high risk for relapse in central nervous system (CNS) and testes. Age at diagnosis, certain chromosomal changes, immunophenotype, and persistence of leukemia after induction therapy comprise other important prognostic parameters [10–12]. B-ALL have been historically divided into pro-B-ALL (early-pre-B-ALL; TdT^{+}/CD19^{+}/CD10^{-}), common ALL (CD10^{+} or CALLA^{+}), pre-B-ALL (CD10$^{+/-}$; cytoplasmic IgM^{+}), and mature B-ALL (surface IgM^{+}). Majority of mature B-ALL, which are characterized by medium-sized to large blasts with round hyperchromatic nuclei, one or more nucleoli and basophilic cytoplasm with prominent vacuoles, expression of surface immunoglobulins and higher incidence of CNS involvement are now classified as Burkitt lymphoma (BL) in leukemic phase. Common and pre-B ALL are often positive for t(9;22)/BCR-ABL (30%–50%). The pro-B-ALLs show t(4;11)(q34;q11)/ALL1-AF4. In a series by Cimino et al., adult patients with pro-B-ALL had the ALL1/AF4 fusion transcript, originating from the t(4;11) translocation in 36.4%, and the t(9;22)/BCR/ABL in 9% [13]. B-ALL with t(9;22) often display aberrant expression of pan-myeloid antigens (CD33 or less often CD13). Adult patients with early-pre-B-ALL and t(4;11) or t(9;22) have poor prognosis and the absence of both of these translocations correlates with a significantly better clinical outcome after intensive chemotherapy treatment [13]. CD10-negative pre-B-ALL has been identified as a high risk subgroup of adult ALL associated with a high frequency of MLL aberrations and worse prognosis [14]. Pro-B and/or t(4;11)$^{+}$ ALL is associated with worse prognosis but responds well to high dose cytarabine therapy and stem cell transplantation.

WHO classification (2016) divides B-ALL into following categories [1]:

- B-lymphoblastic leukemia/lymphoma, not otherwise specified (B-ALL, NOS)
- B-lymphoblastic leukemia/lymphoma with recurrent genetic abnormalities:

- B-ALL with t(9;22)(q34;q11.2) [BCR-ABL1]
- B-ALL with t(v;11q23), KMT2A (MLL) rearranged
- B-ALL with t(12;21)(p13;q22) [ETV6-RUNX1]
- B-ALL with high hyperdiploidy
- B-ALL with hypodiploidy
- B-ALL with t(5;14)(q31;q32) [IL3-IGH]
- B-ALL with t(1;19)(q23;p13.3) [TCF3-PBX1]
- B-ALL, BCR-ABL1-like features
- B-ALL with iAMP21

Morphology

Cytomorphology. Lymphoblasts are generally small to medium-sized with little variation in their shape and size, increased nuclear-cytoplasmic ratio, finely dispersed nuclear chromatin, inconspicuous nucleoli, and occasionally vacuolated cytoplasm (Figure 17.1). Occasional cases show less monotonous appearing blasts with larger and more irregular nuclei or blasts with basophilic cytoplasm and prominent cytoplasmic vacuoles. The latter is often seen in B-ALL with t(1;19). Some of the blasts may show unevenly distributed cytoplasm creating cytoplasmic pseudopods, termed "hand-mirror" cells (similar features are seen in T-lymphoblastic leukemia and some less differentiated acute myeloid leukemias, AMLs). Occasional cases may show blasts with some cytoplasmic granules (usually seen only on minor subset of blasts). Historically, lymphoblasts (L) were divided into three cytological categories: L1 (small blasts with round to oval nuclei, scanty cytoplasm, coarse chromatin, inconspicuous nucleolus), L2 (medium-sized to large blasts with often irregular nuclei, more abundant cytoplasm, fine, open chromatin, and enlarged nucleolus), and L3 (medium-sized to large blasts with abundant basophilic cytoplasm with many vacuoles, hyperchromatic nuclei, and one or more prominent nucleoli). Presence of L3 blasts is mostly limited to BL in leukemic phase.

Bone marrow. The bone marrow (BM) shows a diffuse and monotonous infiltrate of cells with immature vesicular chromatin, inconspicuous nucleoli, and scanty cytoplasm (Figure 17.2). Based on current WHO recommendation, the diagnosis of B-ALL should be avoided when there are <20% blasts in BM (many treatment protocols require ≥25% marrow blasts to define leukemia, but in contrast to AML, there is no agreed upon lower limit for the proportion of blasts required for the diagnosis of B-ALL).

Lymph nodes. Involvement of the lymph nodes shows either diffuse (Figure 17.3) or paracortical infiltrate of monotonous, medium-sized cells with round to oval nuclei with open chromatin, small nucleoli). Some cases show prominent "starry-sky" pattern. Lymph node capsule and fibrous trabeculae (septae) are often infiltrated, but sinuses are often intact.

Immunophenotyping

Immunohistochemistry
Immunohistochemistry staining of BM shows expression of CD10, CD19, CD22, CD79a, Fli-1, CD34, PAX5, TdT, CD43, and CD45 (Figures 17.2 and 17.3). Subset of cases may be CD45^{-}.

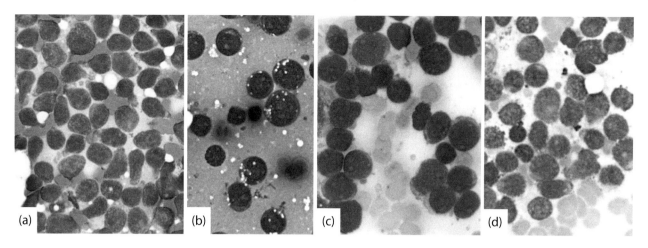

FIGURE 17.1   B-lymphoblastic leukemia – cytology. BM aspirate smears from four B-ALL cases (a–d) show lymphoblasts with increased nuclear-cytoplasmic ratio, scanty cytoplasm, nucleoli, and occasional cytoplasmic vacuoles (Wright-Giemsa, ×1000).

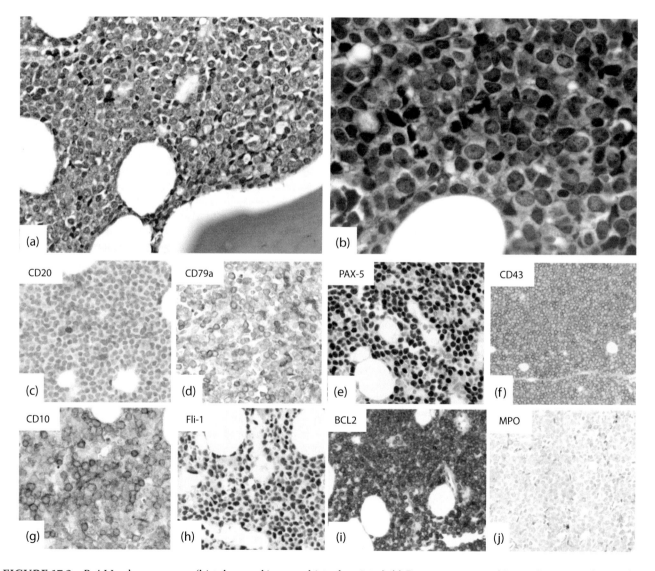

FIGURE 17.2   B-ALL – bone marrow (histology and immunohistochemistry). (a) Bone marrow core biopsy shows complete replacement of marrow elements by lymphoblasts. (b) Higher magnification shows rather monomorphic blasts with scanty cytoplasm, evenly distributed chromatin and nucleoli. (c–j) Immunohistochemistry: blasts are negative for CD20 (c), and positive for CD79a (d), PAX-5 (e), CD43 (f), CD10 (g), Fli-1 (h), and BCL2 (i). MPO is not expressed (j).

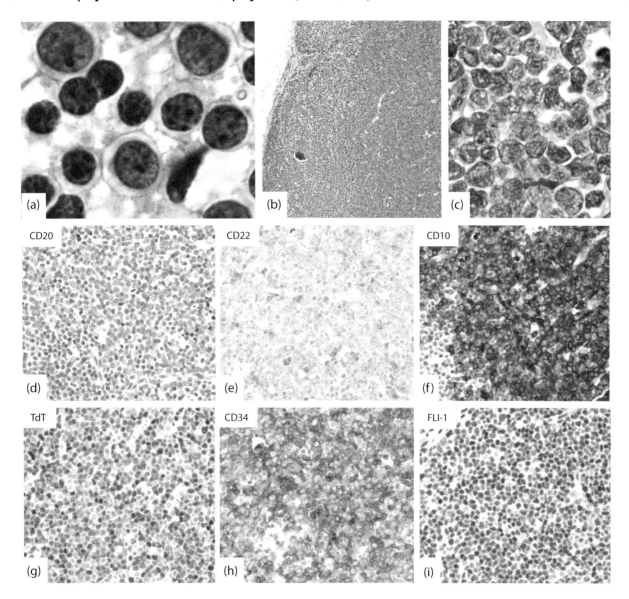

FIGURE 17.3 Precursor B-cell lymphoblastic lymphoma – lymph node. (a) Touch smear shows blasts with round regular nuclei and few inconspicuous nucleoli. (b–c) Histology section of the lymph node shows sheets of lymphoblasts (low and high magnification). Residual small lymphocytes are also noted (left side). (d–i) Immunohistochemistry. Blasts are negative for CD20 (d) and are positive for CD22 (e), CD10 (f), TdT (g), CD34 (h), and Fli-1 (i).

Proliferation fraction (Ki-67 labeling) is moderate to high. Most cases do not express CD20 and only very rare cases express BCL6, which differentiate B-ALL from BL (BCL6 expression, if present, is weak in B-ALL, while in BL both CD20 and BCL6 are strongly positive).

Flow cytometry
Phenotypic categories of B-ALL
B-ALL can be subdivided into following categories (stages of maturation):

- Pro-B-ALL (B-I, early-pre-B-ALL): CD10−, CD19+, TdT+, CD45+dim
- Common ALL: CD10+ (B-II, common B, CALLA+), CD19+, CD34+, TdT+
- Pre-B-ALL (B-III, pre-B): CD10+(dim)/−; cytoplasmic (c) IgM+; CD34+/−, TdT+/−, CD45+moderate

- Mature B-ALL (B-IV, mature B): surface IgM+, CD34− (maybe positive), TdT− (maybe positive)
- Philadelphia chromosome+ B-ALL: bright CD10+, CD11b+/−, CD13+ (dim)/−, CD15+/−, CD19+, CD20− (rarely dimly+), CD22+, CD25+, CD33+dim (maybe negative), CD34+/− (maybe partial), CD38+/−, CD45+(dim)/−, CD66c+, and TdT+/−
- B-ALL with *MLL* alterations: CD10− (rare cases maybe partially positive), CD15+/−, CD19+, CD22+, CD33+/−, CD34+, CD65s+/−, and TdT+/− [occasional cases may show mature B-cell phenotype with clonal surface light chains, blastic morphology and lack of CD10, CD20, CD34, and TdT]

The immunophenotype of B-ALL
B-cell maturation is presented in Figure 2.8 in Chapter 2 and phenotypic criteria for identification of B-lymphoblasts are presented in Chapter 6. On flow cytometry (FC) analysis (Figures 17.4–17.9) B-lymphoblasts lack the expression of surface light chain

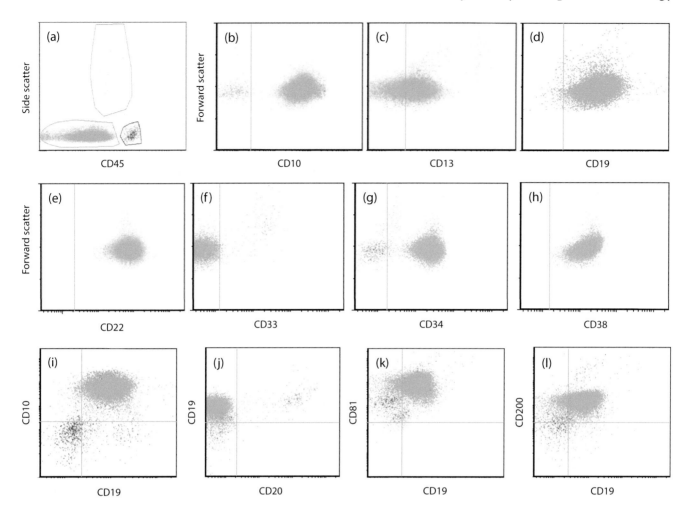

FIGURE 17.4 B-ALL – flow cytometry (bone marrow from 5-year-old patient). Blasts (green dots) have the following phenotype: CD45-/dim+ (a), CD10+ (bright; b), CD13+ (dim/partial; c), CD19+ (d), CD22+ (e), CD33− (f), CD34+ (g), and CD38+ (h). Note typical for B-ALL bright expression of CD10 (i) and negative CD20 (j). Majority of B-ALL are positive for CD81 (k). The expression of CD200 varies, ranging from positive (l) to negative.

immunoglobulins, are most often positive for CD10, CD19, CD22, CD34, CD38, CD79a, CD81, HLA-DR, and TdT, negative or dimly positive for CD45 (the expression maybe partial), negative or less often dimly positive for CD20, and may show aberrant expression of pan-myeloid markers (CD11b, CD13, CD15, or CD33; Figures 17.8 and 17.9). MPO staining is negative in B-ALL (except for minor subset of blasts). Presence of myeloid

antigens is associated with worse prognosis and often with Philadelphia chromosome (*BCR-ABL1* fusion), balanced t(12;17) or extra *ETV6-RUNX1*+ fusion. There is no significant correlation between CD11b expression and most of the initial laboratory, cytogenetic, and diagnostic parameters in B-ALL. CD11b positivity was reported to show a 5-fold increased risk of minimal residual disease (MRD) after induction therapy (day 33). In the

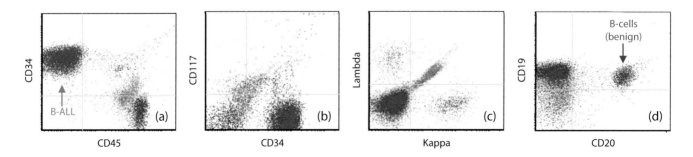

FIGURE 17.5 Identification of B-lymphoblasts by flow cytometry. B-lymphoblasts (magenta dots) are negative for CD45 (a), positive for CD34 (a–b), negative for CD117 (b), negative for surface light chain immunoglobulins (c), positive for CD19 (d), and negative for CD20 (d).

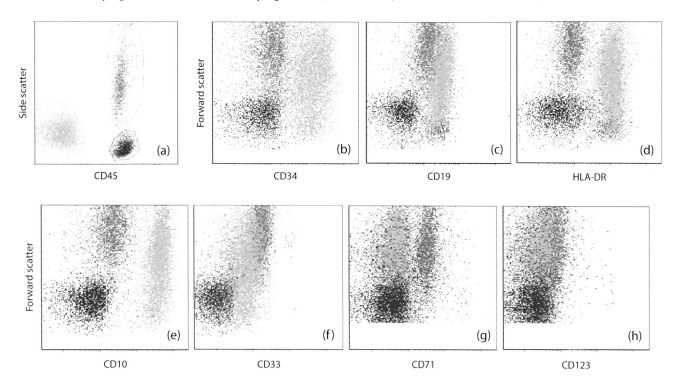

FIGURE 17.6 B-ALL – flow cytometry. Blasts (green dots) show low side scatter (a), negative CD45 expression (a) and increased forward scatter (b–h). They are positive for CD34 (b), CD19 (c), HLA-DR (d), CD10 (e), and CD33 (f), whereas CD71 (g) and CD123 (h) are negative. Note very bright CD10 expression (e; much brighter when compared to neutrophils represented by gray dots).

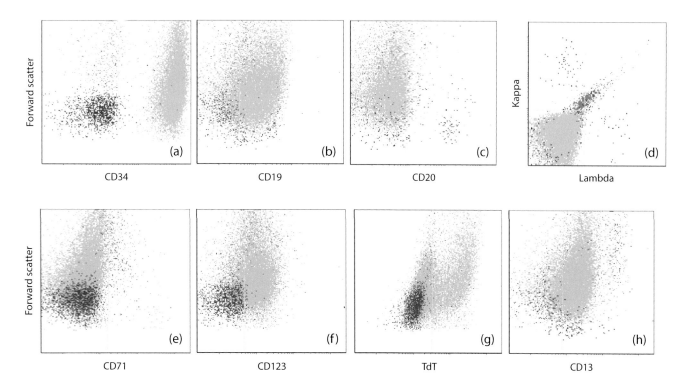

FIGURE 17.7 B-ALL – flow cytometry. Blasts (green dots) show bright expression of CD34 (a), positive CD19 (b), negative CD20 (c), negative surface light chain immunoglobulins (d), negative CD71 (e), positive CD123 (f), positive TdT (g), and positive CD13 (h).

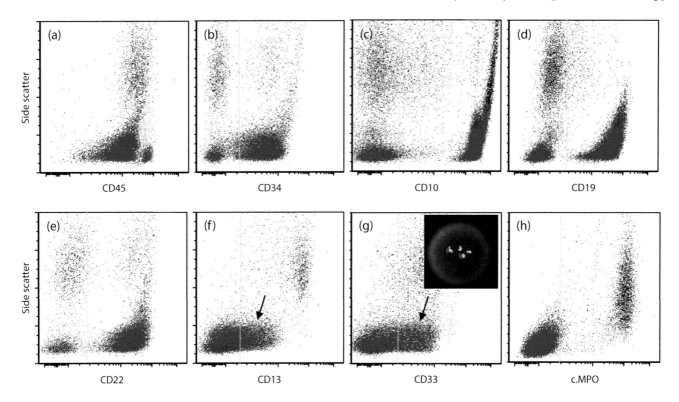

FIGURE 17.8 B-ALL with aberrant expression of pan-myeloid antigens – flow cytometry. B-lymphoblasts (blue dots) are positive for CD45 (a), CD34 (b), CD10 (c; bright expression), CD19 (d; bright expression), CD22 (e), and partially for both CD13 (f; arrow) and CD33 (g; arrow). Negative cytoplasmic MPO excludes mixed phenotype acute leukemia (MPAL). FISH (g; inset) shows several copies of BCR-ABL fusion; (*ASS1*-aqua, *ABL1*-orange, *BCR*-green).

multivariate analysis CD11b expression is an independent prognostic factor compared with other clinically relevant parameters at diagnosis. Most cases show moderate CD19, but occasional cases have been reported with reduced level of CD19. The expression of CD10 is most often bright, which is helpful in differential diagnosis from mature CD10+ B-cell neoplasms (which usually show dim or moderate expression). The expression of CD38 is either dim or moderate. The expression of CD71 varies in B-ALL with ~30%–50% of cases being positive (most often with dim or partial expression). AMLs are positive for CD71 in 70%–80% with acute erythroid leukemia showing very bright expression, while other leukemias are usually dimly positive. The expression of CD81 is usually dim and CD200 may be either positive or negative. Subset of B-ALL may display expression of CD123 (Figure 17.10). Minor subset of B-ALL cases is negative for CD34 (~29%) or TdT (~15%), and very rare cases (~5%) lack both TdT and CD34. Very rare cases show aberrant expression of CD56. Surface light chain immunoglobulins expression can be seen in ~5%. Pediatric B-ALL with CD56 and CD200 expression have worse prognosis [15]. Immunophenotypic prolife of B-ALL is presented in Table 17.1.

CD20 and CD45 expression. CD20 expression was reported to be associated with adverse prognosis in adult *BCR-ABL1*-negative ALL [16]. In univariate analysis, fluorescence intensity of CD45 and CD20 is significantly associated with event-free survival, whereas other phenotypic markers showed no significant correlation with outcome. Patients whose blasts were greater than the 75th percentile of intensity for CD45 fared significantly worse than those with lower-density CD45, and those whose blasts were greater than the 25th percentile of intensity for CD20 had a poorer event-free survival. The intensity of both

CD45 and CD20 is independently correlated with outcome [17]. There was no significant correlation between intensity of expression of either antigen and traditional clinical risk factors, ploidy, or t(9;22) or t(1;19). In multivariate analysis, both CD45 intensity greater than the 75th percentile and CD20 intensity greater than the 25th percentile were significantly correlated with poor outcome independently of previously reported poor prognostic factors including National Cancer Institute (NCI) risk group, ploidy, trisomies of 4 and 10, and adverse translocations including t(1;19), t(9;22), and t(4;11). CD20 expression has adverse prognostic significance in ALL, in both Philadelphia− and Philadelphia+ cases, but its significance is limited mostly to younger patients [16, 18]. The introduction of rituximab into frontline therapy for patients with Philadelphia−/CD20+ ALL appears to improve the outcome. The presence of CD34+/CD38−/CD58− blasts at diagnosis identifies a group of patients with higher risk. Figure 17.11 shows B-ALL with unusual CD20 and CD45 expression and Figure 17.12 shows early B-ALL with moderate CD45 expression.

Aberrant phenotype of B-ALL blasts. B-ALL shows often aberrant expression of antigens, which can be divided into (1) aberrant expression of antigens associated with immature B-cells (hematogone-associated antigens), including CD10, CD19, CD20, CD22, CD34, CD38, CD45, and TdT, or (2) aberrant expression of non B-cell markers (lineage "infidelity"), including either myeloid associated antigens (CD11b, CD13, CD14, CD15, and/or CD33) or T- and NK-cell antigens (e.g., CD4, CD5, CD7, CD56). Identification of abnormal phenotype of blasts by FC (leukemia-associated phenotype; LAP) is important to diagnose B-ALL and to identify measurable (minimal) residual disease (MRD; see below). The phenotypic aberrancies include discordant expression of CD34 and TdT, asynchronous co-expression

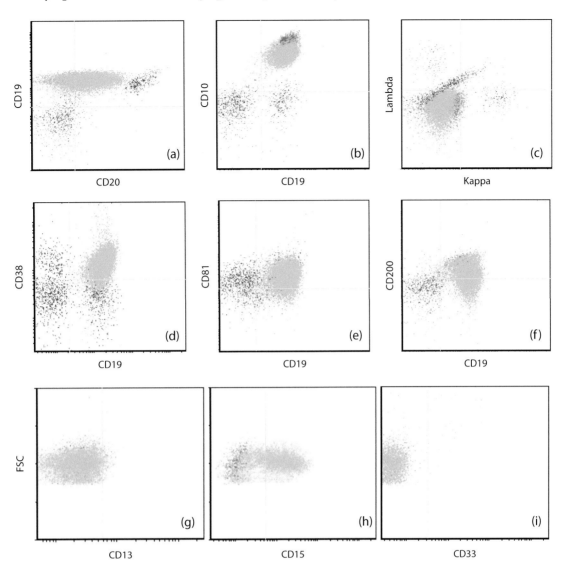

FIGURE 17.9 B-ALL with aberrant expression of CD15. B-lymphoblasts (green dots) show positive CD19 (a, b), partially dim CD20 (a), bright CD10 (b), negative surface light chain immunoglobulins (c), moderate CD38 (d), dim CD81 (e), and dim (partial) CD200 (f). Among myeloid antigens, CD13 is negative (g), CD15 is dimly positive (h), and CD33 is negative (i).

of CD34 (or TdT) and CD20, increased (bright) expression of CD10 and CD22, lack of CD34 and/or TdT expression, lack or only partial expression of CD45, aberrant expression of myeloid markers (CD11b, CD13, CD15, CD33), and negative or abnormally dim CD38 expression. In a series published by Seegmiller et al., co-expression of CD20 and CD34 was seen in ~30%, negative or very dim CD45 in 66%, overexpression of CD10 in 60%, negative or dim CD38 in 58%, negative or very dim CD45 in 66% [3]. The expression of at least one myeloid antigen was seen in 86% (including 28.5% of cases with one antigen, 39% with two antigens, 13% with three antigens, 4.5% with four antigens, and 1.5% with five myeloid antigens) with the most frequently expressed antigen being CD13 (54.5%) followed by CD33 (43%), CD15 (36%), and CD11b (20%) [3]. Expression of T-cell antigens is observed in 9% of cases, the most common antigen being CD4 (other antigens include CD2, CD5, and CD7) and aberrant expression of CD56 is seen in ~5% [3]. Aberrant CD56 expression is seen more often in pediatric population. CD123 expression is seen often in hyperdiploid cases and CRLF2 in B-ALL with *CRLF2* rearrangement.

Surface light chain immunoglobulins (kappa and lambda) expression in B-ALL

Surface light chain restriction is a feature of mature B-cell malignancies but rarely (~5%) can be seen in B-ALL often associated with *MLL* or BCR-ABL1 rearrangements (Figure 6.8 in Chapter 6). Negative or very dim expression of CD45, presence of myeloid antigens (CD13 or CD33), lack or dim and partial CD20 expression, and positive expression of CD34 and/or TdT help to identify B-ALL with clonal surface kappa or lambda expression. False positive expression of kappa or lambda due to spectral overlap of bright CD10 expression conjugated with PE-Cy7 which "spills over" to PE-conjugated surface immunoglobulin detector channel should be excluded.

B-ALL without expression of CD34 and TdT

Rare B-ALL cases (~4%) lack both CD34 and TdT by FC analysis, making the diagnosis of precursor B-cell neoplasm difficult without correlation with cytology and additional (often) extensive) immunophenotypic markers. Blastic cytology, lack or partially dim expression of CD45, lack of surface light chain

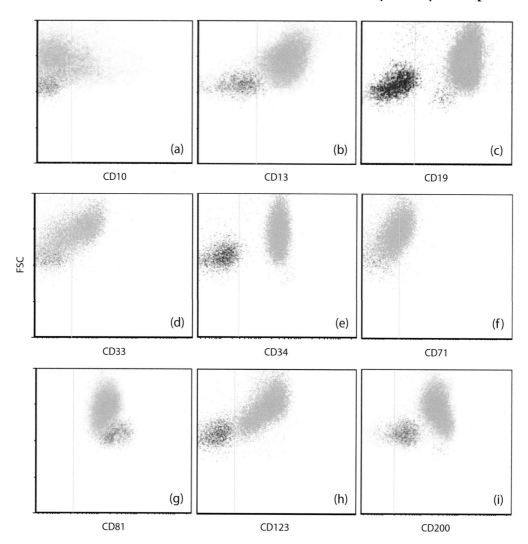

FIGURE 17.10 B-ALL with mostly negative CD10 (a), aberrant expression of CD13 (b), moderate CD19 (c), aberrant expression of CD33 (d), positive CD34 (e), negative to partially dim CD71 (f), dim CD81 (g), positive CD123 (h), and moderate CD200 (i).

TABLE 17.1: Immunophenotypic Profile of B-ALL ($n = 116$)

Marker	Frequency	Comments
CD10+	87%	Majority showed bright expression (62% of total cases) while 3.5% showed partial and 20% moderate expression
CD13+	8%	Only 3.5% showed dual CD13/CD33 positivity
CD19+	100%	
CD20+	30%	Including 7% of total cases with dim, 12% with moderate, 5% with variable (smeary), and 4% with partial expression
CD33+	33%	Mostly dim expression
CD34+	71%	Including 3.5% with partial expression; ~80% (of total cases) showed both TdT and CD34 expression, ~15% showed TdT expression without CD34, and 6% showed CD34 expression without TdT
CD45+	80%	Including 11% with partial expression; expression of CD45 was either dim or moderate
CD45−	22%	
CD56+	2%	
HLA-DR+	99%	
TdT+	85%	Including 3.5% with partial expression
CD34−/TdT−	~5%	Pre-B phenotype
κ or λ expression	4.6%	The expression of surface light chain immunoglobulins may be dim to moderate

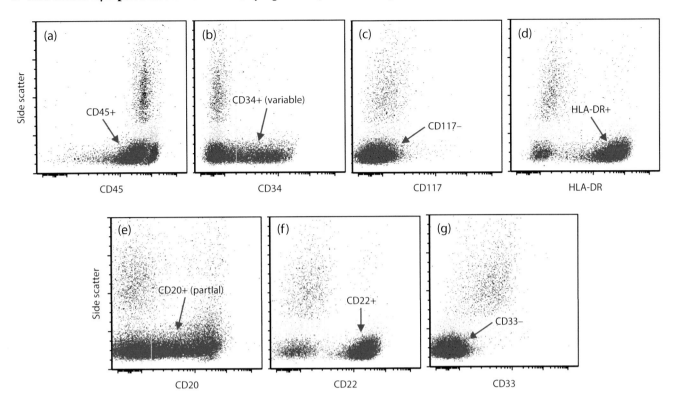

FIGURE 17.11 B-ALL – flow cytometry. B-lymphoblasts (blue dots) are positive for CD45 (a), CD34 (b; variable expression), HLA-DR (d), CD20 (e; variable and partial expression), and CD22 (f). CD117 (c) and CD33 (g) are not expressed.

immunoglobulins and CD20, very bright expression of CD10 and co-expression of myeloid antigens by B-cells helps to diagnose B-ALL in those rare cases. In rare cases, concurrent (pretreatment) FC analysis of blood and BM samples may show discrepant results of CD34 and/or TdT expression.

MPO expression in B-ALL. Some ALL categories may express myeloid antigens, yet usually with a weaker intensity then in AML. CD13 and CD33 are the myeloid antigens most often expressed on the most immature B-ALL as well as the most immature T-ALL [19]. B-ALL cases are often homogeneous in their immunophenotypic characteristics. The issue of MPO-only positive B-ALL (cases where the general immunophenotype of blasts is consistent with B-ALL but a fraction of blasts appears to be MPO+) is of uncertain clinical significance [20–22]. In a study by Oberley

et al., this group of B-ALL had an increased rate of relapse and a worse event-free survival than the patients with B-ALL who did not express MPO [21]. In majority of these cases, MPO cannot be detected by cytochemistry and/or IHC. Most probably, cases with only a single blast population should not be considered mixed phenotype acute leukemia (MPAL) if weak MPO expression by FC is the only evidence of myeloid differentiation [1, 20]. The proportion of MPO positive cells is controversial, but a 3% cutoff is the level retained in cytochemistry. Published MPO positivity thresholds are 10% for FC and 3% for cytochemistry. Identifying the MPO expression by FC is not completely equal to assessing the enzymatic activity, but the suggested threshold in FC ranges between 10% and 28% [23–25]. It is recommended to use benign lymphocytes as an internal negative control with blasts

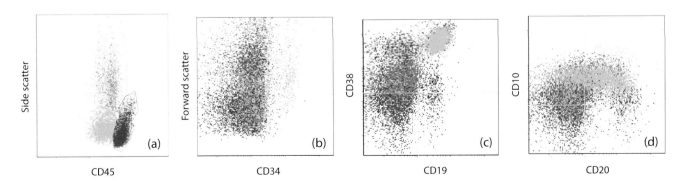

FIGURE 17.12 Early (emerging) B-ALL – blood (WBC = 18k/μL). Blasts (green dots) show moderate CD45 expression (a), mostly negative CD34 (b; only minor population of blasts is positive), bright CD38 (c), moderate CD19 (c), positive CD10 (d), and variable expression of CD20 ranging from negative to moderate (d).

positivity for MPO defined by fluorescence greater than upper limit of fluorescence of normal lymphocytes [24]. McGinnis et al. suggested that B-ALL can be considered MPO⁺ with ≥20% blasts in the MPO positive region, while cases <20% MPO⁺ blasts to be considered MPO⁻ [24]. In study by Guy et al., a 13% threshold was found to be relevant using an isotype control as background-reference (sensitivity 95%, specificity 91%) while using residual normal lymphocytes as an alternative reference a threshold of 28% yielded improved 97% sensitivity and 96% specificity [25].

B-lymphoblasts versus mature B-cell neoplasms. Subset of mature B-cell lymphoproliferative disorders [most often follicular lymphoma (FL), chronic lymphocytic leukemia (CLL), diffuse large B-cell lymphoma (DLBCL), hairy cell leukemia (HCL), high grade B-cell lymphoma with *MYC* and *BCL2* rearrangement (HGBL-R, double hit lymphoma) or transformed large B-cell neoplasms from low grade B-cell lymphomas] may lack surface light chain immunoglobulin expression and may have dim or moderate expression of CD45, mimicking precursor lesions. Positive CD20, lack of very bright CD10, and lack of blastic markers (TdT/ CD34) indicate mature disorder. Lack of CD45 is characteristic for plasma cell myeloma (PCM) and high-grade B-cell lymphomas with plasmablastic features (e.g., plasmablastic lymphoma, PBL). Similar to B-ALL, PBLs are negative for surface and cytoplasmic immunoglobulins. Strong expression of MUM1 and CD138, lack of TdT and CD34, and positive EBV/EBER expression excludes B-ALL and indicates PBL. PCM is recognized by cytomorphology and positive expression of cytoplasmic light chain immunoglobulins. B-cell lymphomas, including FL and SLL/CLL may undergo transformation to B-ALL or to B-cell lymphomas with phenotypic features overlapping between mature and immature neoplasms.

B-lymphoblasts versus maturing B-cell precursors (hematogones). Maturing B-cell precursors (hematogones) can be identified by FC in majority of samples from BM (~1% of marrow elements). Their number decreases with age but may be increased in regenerating marrow from patients after chemotherapy or stem cell transplantation, in some neoplasms, autoimmune disorders (ITP), iron deficiency or infections. Majority of patients with MDS and myeloproliferative neoplasms (MPN) show lack of hematogones or significant decrease in their number (more pronounced in MPN than in MDS). The identification of hematogones is important in FC monitoring B-ALL patients after treatment to exclude MRD.

The phenotypic differential diagnosis between hematogones and B-ALL is presented in Chapter 6 (Figures 6.8–6.12). The phenotype of hematogones is variable depending on the stage of differentiation (Figures 17.13 and 17.14). Very early B-cell lymphoid progenitors are TdT⁺/CD24⁺ and lack CD19 expression [26, 27]. Hematogones show progressively maturing patterns of antigen expression, which can be divided into three distinct stages: stage I, II, and III hematogones [28, 29]. The most immature hematogones (stage I hematogones) are positive for TdT, CD10 (bright), CD19, CD34, CD38, CD58, CD200, and entirely negative for CD20. As hematogones mature, they lose CD34 and TdT expression and become less bright for CD10 and CD200. Stage II hematogones are positive for CD10 (dimmer than stage I), CD19, CD38, and cytoplasmic IgM and do not express CD34, CD58, and TdT, and stage III hematogones differ from stage II by acquiring dim (often variable) expression of CD20 and surface immunoglobulin light chains. At stage III hematogones, progressive acquisition of CD20 expression is associated with progressive loss of CD10 expression. The expression of CD45 varies with progressive

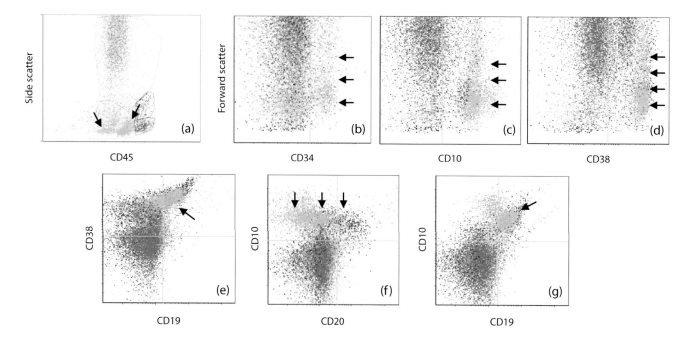

FIGURE 17.13 Flow cytometry features of hematogones. On the CD45 versus side scatter (SCC; a) hematogones show two distinct populations, one with dim CD45 and one with moderate CD45 expression (arrows). Subset of hematogones is positive for CD34 (b). Forward scatter (FSC) is characteristically variable (b–d; arrows) ranging from low to high, with majority of hematogones display low FSC. Hematogones are positive for CD10 (c, f–g) and CD38 (d–e), with CD10 being dimmer than in B-ALL and CD38 being brighter than in B-ALL. The expression of CD20 (f) is variable, ranging from negative (majority of hematogones) to dimly positive (minor subset).

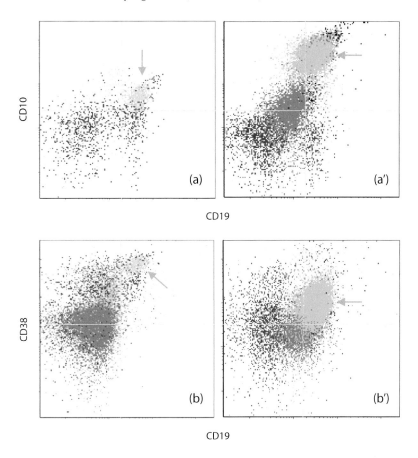

FIGURE 17.14 Comparison of the expression of CD10 and CD38 versus CD19 in hematogones (a, b) and B-ALL (a′, b′). Hematogones (a–b; blue dots) and B-ALL (a′–b′; green dots) are CD19+, CD10+, and CD38+, but deferrer in the intensity of staining: CD10 is much brighter in B-ALL and CD38 is dimmer in B-ALL, when compared to hematogones.

increase in the intensity of CD45 expression as hematogones progress from stage I to stage III. Hematogone express CD22 and bright CD38 throughout all stages of maturation. The transition to mature B-lymphocytes occurs with the loss of CD10, decreased CD38, and increased CD22.

Generally, hematogones show very low side scatter (SSC) by FC, variable forward scatter, with majority of hematogones having low forward scatter and subset showing increased but variable ("smeary") forward scatter, and variable (heterogeneous) expression of CD20, CD34, and CD45. A subset of hematogones with dim CD45 is usually CD34+ and a subset of hematogones with moderate CD45 is CD34−. The marrow with increased number of hematogones show spectrum of B-cell maturation with small proportion of very immature, CD19+/CD22+/CD200+/CD20−/TdT+/CD34+ B-cells (I hematogones) and predominant population of more mature stage II hematogones (CD10+/CD200+dim/TdT−/CD34+/−/surface immunoglobulins− CD20−). Stage II hematogones usually predominate (~65%) [28, 30]. Hematogones are negative for myeloid antigens (CD13, CD33) and usually lack CD123.

B-lymphoblasts are characterized by higher SSC, usually slightly higher, but more cohesive forward scatter and form a more cohesive cluster of cells on FC dot plot displays when compared to hematogones (Figure 17.15). In contrast to B-lymphoblasts, hematogones show usually at least two distinct populations (stage I and stage II), and even for stage II hematogones the expression of many markers is variable ("smeary"). This continuous fashion of antigen expression, most easily identifiable with CD10, CD20, and CD45 antigens, reflects changes in the level of antigen expression at different stages of B-cell maturation and is most helpful FC feature in differentiating hematogones form B-ALL. Hematogones differ from B-ALL by discordant expression of CD34 and CD123 [31]. Less mature hematogones (dim CD45+) express CD34 and lack CD123 expression, whereas the more mature hematogones (moderate CD45+) lack CD34 but always express CD123. In contrast with this discordant pattern of CD34 and CD123 expression in hematogones, blasts in majority of B-ALL (91%) show concordant expression of the two antigens: 80% (36 of 45) cases expressed both antigens, whereas 11% (5 of 45) expressed neither. In contrast to B-ALL hematogones do not display antigens from an inappropriate cell lineage (e.g., pan-myeloid markers CD13, CD15, and/or CD33). The expression of CD10 and CD38 is much brighter in B-ALL than in hematogones (subset of B-ALL may be CD10−). The expression of TdT in hematogones is downregulated (from negative to dim), as opposed to B-ALL blasts, which are strongly TdT+ (subset of B-ALL cases may be TdT−). Many B-ALL cases are either negative or dimly positive for CD45, whereas majority of hematogones (stage II) show moderate CD45. B-ALL are positive for CD58, whereas this antigen is only positive in early stages of B-cell maturation as the majority of hematogones are CD58− [32]. CD38 and CD81 expression is brighter in hematogones and CD200 expression is much brighter in B-ALL than stage II hematogones, but the difference in CD200 between B-ALL and early hematogones is not that significant. Figure 6.11

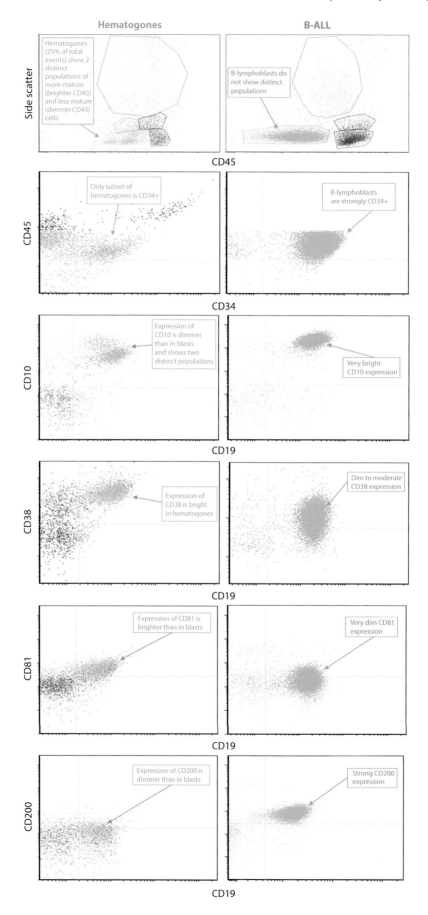

FIGURE 17.15 Comparison of FC pattern of hematogones (blue dots, left column) and B-ALL (green dots, right column).

in Chapter 6 compares hematogones with measurable (minimal) residual B-ALL. Don et al. proposed recently an algorithmic approach to differentiate between hematogones and B-ALL by using CD58 and CD81 antigens showing significant difference in mean fluorescent intensity (MFI) for CD81 and CD58 when comparing hematogones and B-ALL populations: B-ALL cases had a mean (SD) MFI of 24.6 (27.5; range, 2–125) for CD81 and 135.6 (72.6; range, 48–328) for CD58, while hematogones cases had a mean (SD) MFI of 70.2 (19.2; range, 42–123) for CD81 and 38.8 (9.4; range, 23–58) for CD58 [33]. Tembhare et al. reported significant difference in intensity of expression of CD24, CD44, CD73, CD86, and CD200 between B-ALL and early and late hematogones [34]. In that study, MFIs in early hematogones (stage I), late hematogones (stage II), and B-ALL cases were 48.65, 55.15, and 29.35 for CD24, 0.34, 0.29, and 0.595 for CD44, 0.25, 0.365, and 2.85 for CD73, 0.26, 0.26, and 0.65 for CD86 and 3.63, 1.68, and 5.33 for CD200, respectively [34]. Saumell et al. reported the distinct pattern of expression of LILRB1 (leukocyte immunoglobulin-like receptor B1; CD85j) in hematogones and neoplastic B-lymphoblasts, which might be useful in analysis of MRD of B-ALL after treatment [35]. LILRB1 expression is higher on CD34$^+$/CD10$^{bright+}$ stage 1 hematogones, which is downregulated to a dim level of expression on CD34$^-$/CD10$^{moderate+}$ stage 2 hematogones and then upregulated to a moderate level of expression on CD10^{dim+}/CD20$^+$ stage 3 hematogones [35]. In B-ALL the expression of LILRB1 is homogeneous and brighter when compared to hematogones.

Genetic features

Numerous structural and numerical chromosomal aberrations have been identified in B-ALL, many of which are associated with specific disease characteristic and patient outcome. Approximately 75% of childhood ALL cases harbor recurring chromosomal or genetic aberrations detectable by karyotyping, FISH, or molecular techniques. Many of the aberrations are used to diagnose and classify B-ALL (see above). They can be broadly divided into chromosomal translocations and numerical changes (hyper- or hypodiploidy). The common changes in pediatric B-ALL include hyperdiploidy, t(12;21)/*ETV6-RUNX1*, t(1;19)/*TCF3-PBX1*, t(9;22)/*BCR-ABL1*, and rearrangement of *MLL* at 11q23. Approximately 20%–30% of adult ALLs and 5% of pediatric ALLs are positive for *BCR-ABL1* (Philadelphia chromosome). In addition to *BCR*, six other genes have been reported to form rearrangements with *ABL1*: *ETV6* at 12p13, *RCD1* at 1q24, *SFPQ* at 1p34, *ZMIZ1* at 10q22.3, *NUP214* at 9q34.13, *FOXP1* at 3p12, *SNX2* at 5p23 and *EML1* at 14q32. Several chromosomal abnormalities have been associated with favorable outcome: high hyperdiploidy, trisomies of chromosomes 4 and 10, and t(12;21)/*ETV6-RUNX1*. In contrast, hypodiploidy (≤45 chromosomes), t(17;19) (encoding TCF3-HLF fusion), and KMT2A fusions are each associated with adverse outcome. In addition, *BCR-ABL1* fusions are associated with adverse outcome and determine of using therapeutic regimens containing a tyrosine kinase inhibitor (TKI). A subset of *BCR-ABL1*$^-$ B-ALL patients harbors gene expression profile similar to *BCR-ABL1*$^+$ B-ALL, which led to recognition of a provisional subtype of *BCR-ABL1*-like ALL: *ABL1*, *ABL2*, *CLF2*, *CSF1R*, *JAK2*, *NTRK3*, *PDGFR*β, and *TYK2* [36, 37]. High hyperdiploidy, *ETV6-RUNX1*, and *TCF3-PBX1* are less common in adult ALL. In relapsed pediatric ALL, deletion of *IKZF1* and alteration of *TP53* identify patients with significantly inferior outcome [38]. Genes implicated in treatment resistance include *CDKN2A/B* and *IKZF1* [39].

Measurable (minimal) residual disease (MRD) in B-ALL

Introduction

The most common cause of treatment failure in pediatric ALL is relapse, occurring in 15%–20% of patients [40]. The detection of MRD in childhood and adult ALL is an independent risk parameter in both de novo and relapsed ALL and in patients undergoing stem cell transplantation [6, 41–45]. In childhood ALL, MRD is an independent prognostic factor allowing for risk stratification [46, 47]. Early elimination of leukemic cells is a favorable prognostic indicator. The absence of MRD at the end of induction therapy is considered the main favorable outcome predictor [6, 48–50]. The most widely applied MRD assays in ALL are flow cytometric identification of leukemia immunophenotypes (Figures 17.16 and 17.17) and PCR analysis of immunoglobulin gene rearrangement or fusion transcripts. The prerequisite for analysis of immunoglobulin gene rearrangement is the molecular characterization of leukemia-specific immunoglobulin gene rearrangement for each individual patient. Among fusion transcript as targets for MRD detection in ALL, *BCR-ABL1* and *MLL* have the broadest clinical use. MRD evaluation by FC achieves a sensitivity of 10^{-3} to 10^{-4}, which is lower than the sensitivity achieved by RQ-PCR. By measuring MRD on days 33 and 78 by RQ-PCR, Conter et al. showed that patient with standard risk (42%) had estimated 5-year event-free survival at 92.3%, those with intermediate risk (52%) at 77.6% and those with high risk (6%) at 50.1% [48]. Analysis of disease-free survival rates for MRD$^+$ and MRD$^-$ patients shows that MRD positivity is associated with increased relapses (being most significant at 3–5 months post-induction and beyond). The association of MRD test results and disease-free survival better predicts the outcome than other standard parameters and is therefore important in determining managements of individual patients [51, 52].

Flow cytometry analysis of MRD in B-ALL

FC analysis has broad applicability, since most of ALL blasts have identifiable leukemia-associated immunophenotype (LAIP) at diagnosis [6, 34, 53–62]. LAIP can be identified in ~95% of B-ALL cases [50, 54, 57]. The major advantages of FC analysis of MRD in B-ALL are the speed of obtaining results, wide availability of FC analysis, and relative simplicity. The limitations include inadequate number of cells for analysis, difficulties in separating leukemic cells from normal marrow precursors and change of antigenic profile of leukemic cells after therapy.

LAIP can be divided into the following categories:

a. asynchronous antigen expression (presence of mature myeloid markers such as surface light chain immunoglobulin or CD20 on CD34$^+$ and/or TdT$^+$ blasts
b. lineage infidelity or cross-lineage expression, e.g., expression of myeloid markers (CD11b, CD13, CD15, CD33, CD56, CD65) by lymphoblasts
c. lack of antigen expression (e.g., lack of HLA-DR, CD34, CD38, CD45) by lymphoblasts
d. underexpression of individual marker(s) e.g., very dim or partial antigen expression (CD19, CD22, CD34, CD38, CD45, CD81, HLA-DR, TdT)
e. overexpression of antigen(s) (e.g., very bright expression of CD34, CD10, CD38, CD49f, CD58, CD123)

MRD assessment by FC has many advantages including high sensitivity, fast turnaround time, and lower cost [59]. The proposed

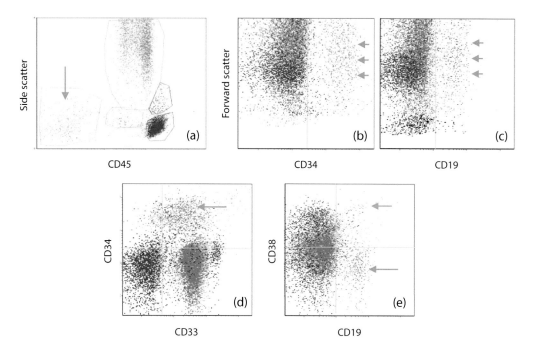

FIGURE 17.16   B-ALL – measurable (minimal) residual disease. B-lymphoblasts (orange dots, orange arrows) are negative for CD45 (a) and positive for CD34 (b), CD19 (c), and CD33 (d). Rare hematogones are also noted; they show bright expression of CD38 (e; blue dots, blue arrow).

FC panels to analyze MRD in ALL include variable combination of the following antibodies: CD10, CD13, CD19, CD20, c.CD22, CD24, CD33, CD34, CD38, CD44, CD45, CD58, CD66b, CD73, c.CD79b, CD81, CD86, CD99, CD123, CD200, CRLF2, HLA-DR, IgM, kappa, lambda, and TdT [34, 59–64]. Basso et al. published MRD analysis results by FC on day 15 of treatment of 830 patient who underwent the same therapeutic protocol and have identified three risk groups: standard (42%), intermediate (47%), and high (11%), which showed increasing relapse incidences in 5 years (7.5%, 17.5%, and 47.2%) [65]. The finding of TdT+ cells or cells with aberrant phenotype in a RBC-free cerebrospinal fluid (CSF) sample with a negative cytomorphology is highly predictive for impending CNS relapse [66, 67].

Differential diagnosis of B-ALL

Differential diagnosis of B-ALL/LBL includes malignant lymphomas, AML (especially minimally differentiated or AML without maturation), MPAL, T-lymphoblastic lymphoma/leukemia, acute

undifferentiated leukemia (AUL), hematogones, and metastatic small blue-cell tumors (Figure 17.18).

Differential diagnosis of B-ALL includes:

* BL
* High grade B-cell lymphoma with *MYC* and *BCL2*, rearrangement (HGBL-R)
* DLBCL
* FL and histologic transformation of FL to high grade lymphoma
* Mantle cell lymphoma (MCL, blastoid variant)
* Peripheral T-cell lymphoproliferations
* PCM
* PBL
* TdT+ blastic B-cell neoplasm with *BCL2* and/or *MYC* rearrangements
* AML
* MPAL
* AUL

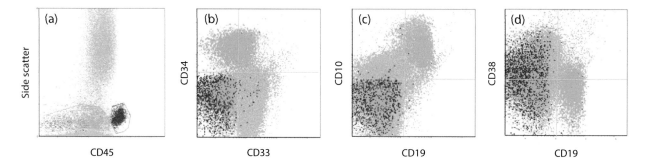

FIGURE 17.17   B-ALL – measurable (minimal) residual disease. B-lymphoblasts (green dots) show dim to moderate CD45 expression (a), positive CD34 (b), partial CD33 expression (b), bright CD10 expression (c), positive CD19 (c–d), and negative to partially dim CD38 expression (d) [flow data represent higher number of events collected when compared to standard flow cytometry analysis].

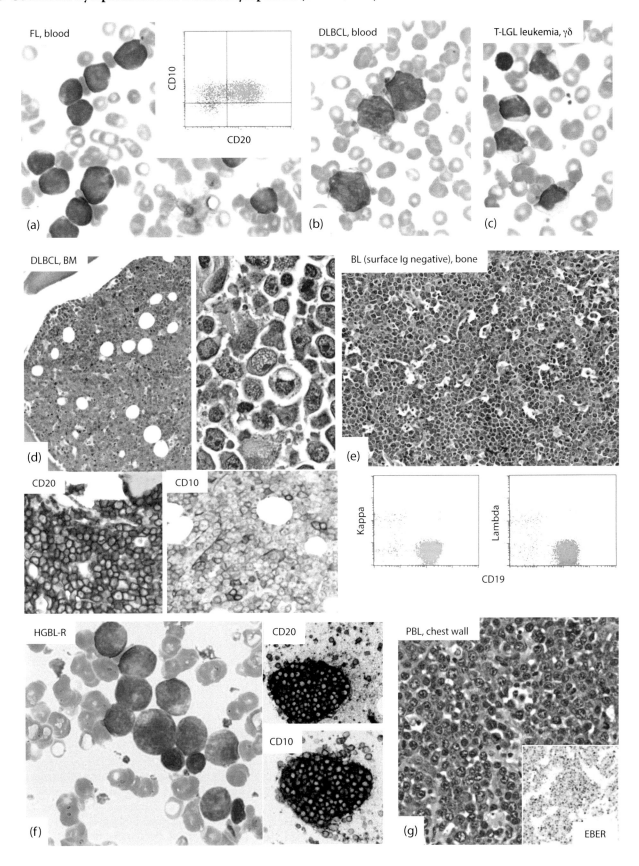

FIGURE 17.18 B-ALL – differential diagnosis. (a) Follicular lymphoma (leukemic phase in the peripheral blood). (b) DLBCL involving blood. (c) T-LGL leukemia (gamma/delta). (d) DLBCL involving BM. (e) Burkitt lymphoma (surface immunoglobulin negative). (f) High grade lymphoma with MYC and BCL2 rearrangement (HGBL-R; double hit lymphoma, BM aspirate and clot section). (g) Plasmablastic lymphoma (chest wall). *(Continued)*

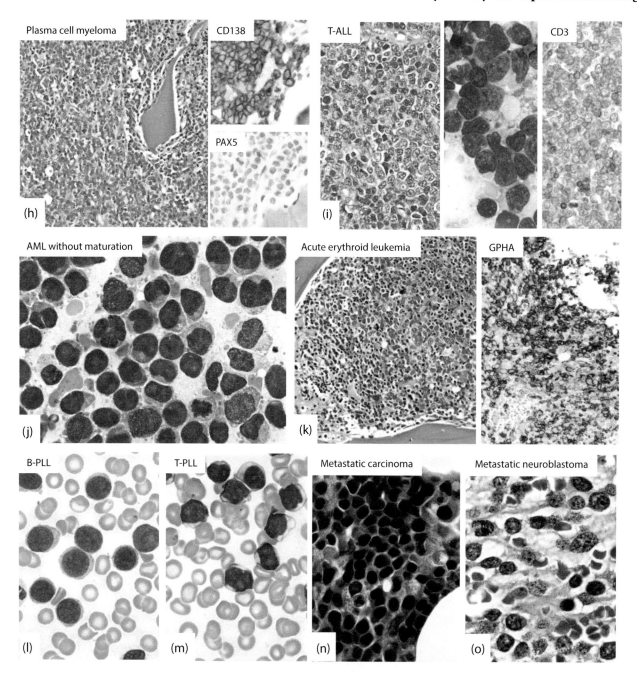

FIGURE 17.18 *(Continued)* B-ALL – differential diagnosis. (h) Plasma cell myeloma (PCM). (i) T-ALL. (j) AML. (k) Acute erythroid leukemia. (l) B-PLL. (m) T-PLL. (n) Metastatic small cell carcinoma. (o) Metastatic neuroblastoma.

- T-cell prolymphocytic leukemia (T-PLL)
- T-cell lymphoblastic leukemia/lymphoma (T-ALL/LBL)
- Metastatic carcinoma/small blue cell tumors
- Hematogones

B-cell lymphomas

B-cell lymphomas including the leukemic phase of FL, DLBCL, BL, HGBL-R, and immunoblastic lymphoma are differentiated from B-ALL/LBL by expression of surface light chain immunoglobulins, CD20 and lack of blastic markers (TdT and CD34). Blastic mantle cell leukemia is positive for B-cell markers and CD5 (as well as *CCND1* rearrangement). B-cell lymphomas of follicle center cell origin show bright expression of CD45, moderate to bright CD20 and moderate to bright expression of surface immunoglobulins (kappa or lambda) by FC. CD10 is usually either dimly or moderately expressed, not as bright as in CD10+ B-ALLs. Subset of FL (and DLBCLs with CD10 expression) may lack surface light chain immunoglobulins (Figure 17.19) but differ from B-ALL by intensity of CD20, CD45, and CD10 expression, as well as lack of blastic markers. In some cases, the final subclassification must be based on cytogenetic/FISH and/or molecular tests (e.g., *MYC*, *BCL6*). HGBL-R is differentiated from B-ALL by presence of *MYC* and *BCL2* (and/or *BCL6*) rearrangement and lack of blastic markers (see also below). BL lacks TdT or CD34 expression and is positive for *MYC* rearrangement. The summary of phenotypic markers used in differential diagnosis of large cell (high-grade) B-cell lymphomas, and B-ALL is presented in Table 12.2 in Chapter 12.

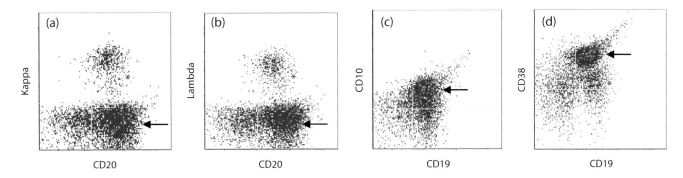

FIGURE 17.19 Follicular lymphoma without expression of surface light chain immunoglobulins. Lymphomatous cells (arrow) are positive for CD20 (a–b), CD19 (c–d), CD10 (c), and CD38 (d). Surface light chain immunoglobulins are negative (a–b; residual benign B-cells marked with (*) show normal expression of kappa and lambda). Note slightly brighter expression of CD20 by lymphomatous cells when compared to polytypic B-cells. In contrast to typical B-ALL, follicular lymphomas show dimmer expression of CD10 and CD38 and strong (homogeneous) expression of CD20.

Double/triple hit B-cell lymphomas with TdT expression (B-ALL with MYC and BCL2 rearrangement; high-grade TdT+ blastic B-cell lymphoma/leukemia)

High grade B-cell lymphomas with *BCL2* and *MYC* rearrangements (HGBL-R; Figure 17.20), also known as "double-hit" lymphomas (DHL), are rare neoplasms characterized by highly aggressive clinical behavior, complex karyotypes, and a spectrum of pathologic features overlapping with BL, DLBCL, and B-lymphoblastic lymphoma/leukemia (B-ALL/LBL). Rare high grade B-cell lymphomas with rearrangement of *MYC* and *BCL2* (and/or *BCL6*), so called double or triple hit lymphomas express TdT, and based on current WHO recommendation those cases are classified as B-cell acute lymphoblastic lymphoma/leukemia, although some authors suggest to use term high-grade TdT+ blastic B-cell lymphoma/leukemia, as lack of other features of immaturity, presence of monotypic surface immunoglobulin by FC, partial BCL6 expression and double/triple-hit genetics indicate a mature B-cell lymphoma [1, 68, 69].

Patients with double hit B-ALL most often present with large abdominal and/or retroperitoneal masses and diffuse BM replacement by sheets of blasts [2, 70]. Blasts are medium to large and may show prominent cytoplasmic vacuoles especially in double hit cases. Tumor cells are positive for TdT, CD10, CD19, negative or partially positive for CD34, negative or partially dimly positive for CD20 and negative for surface immunoglobulins [2]. Some of these neoplasms may represent transformation of prior low-grade lymphoma (e.g., FL). In some of these neoplasms FC may show a mature B-cell lymphoma component and BM core biopsy may show peri- to paratrabecular infiltrate of small cells in addition to "blasts" [2]. De novo B-ALL with *BCL2* rearrangement [t(14;18) (q32;q21)] has also been reported [2, 71–76]. These tumors may be indistinguishable morphologically and immunophenotypically from FL with lymphoblastic transformation.

Double-hit events are extremely rare in B-ALL, especially in pediatric patients or young adults. In adult population they often represent progression from FL [2, 75, 77, 78]. *MYC* rearrangement is rarely observed in B-ALL/LBL in the absence of the t(14;18) [*IGH/BCL2* rearrangement]. Since 1980, only 13 cases of B-ALL/LBL with isolated *MYC* rearrangement were reported [79–85]. Like other B-ALL/LBLs, most of the cases occur in pediatric patients and only three cases were reported in adults. In a study of 5280 cases of pediatric ALL, only five (<0.1%) with isolated

MYC rearrangement were identified [79]. Geyer et al. published a series of seven patients with TdT+ B-lymphoblastic transformation of FL [75]. In that series, the authors raise the possibility that patients presenting with de novo double-hit B-LBL may have a pre-existing low-grade FL masked by the higher-grade process. TdT positivity was reported in subset of patients with DHL or THL by Moench et al. [86]. One of the cases was positive for TdT but expressed monotypic surface light chain, bright CD45 and CD20, and had a centroblastic morphology, favoring a mature neoplasm, one case showed blastic morphology but mature FC immunophenotype and two cases represented transformation of FL. Ok et al. reported several variants of TdT+ B-cell lymphomas with double or triple hit: (1) de novo double or triple hit high grade B-cell lymphoma with TdT expression, (2) FL transformed to transformed to DHL with TdT expression, and (3) initial relapse of FL to TdT– aggressive B-cell lymphoma, followed by relapses in which the neoplasm acquired TdT expression [68, 69].

FC immunophenotypic analysis shows an immature B-cell immunophenotype (CD10+, CD19+, TdT+, surface Ig–) and immunohistochemistry shows high expression of MYC and BCL2. In three B-ALL cases described by Li et al., flow cytometric analysis showed dim CD45, positive CD10, CD19, TdT, and dim to absent CD20 (one of the cases showed lambda chain restriction) [87]. In a series by Moench et al., FC dim CD45, absence of CD20 or surface light chain, or expression of TdT suggesting of immature phenotype. All patients show complex karyotypes associated with 8q24 abnormalities in the form of t(8;9)(q24;p13) or t(8;14) (q24;q32) and t(14;18)(q32;q21) [69, 88]. B-ALL cases with MYC rearrangement appear to represent a distinct biological phenomenon, in which a *MYC* translocation may be acquired at an immature stage of differentiation, in which the tumor cells still express TDT and lack a mature B-cell phenotype. Figure 17.21 shows high-grade TdT+ blastic B-cell lymphoma/leukemia with *MYC* and *BCL2* rearrangement.

Peripheral (mature) T-cell disorders

Mature T-cell lymphoproliferations involving blood or BM are distinguished by T-cell phenotype and negative TdT and CD34 expression.

T-lymphoblastic leukemia/lymphoma

T-ALL/LBL is positive for cytoplasmic (and less often surface) CD3, often shows bright CD7 expression and lacks CD19, CD22, or CD79a expression. Subset of T-ALL may be CD10+.

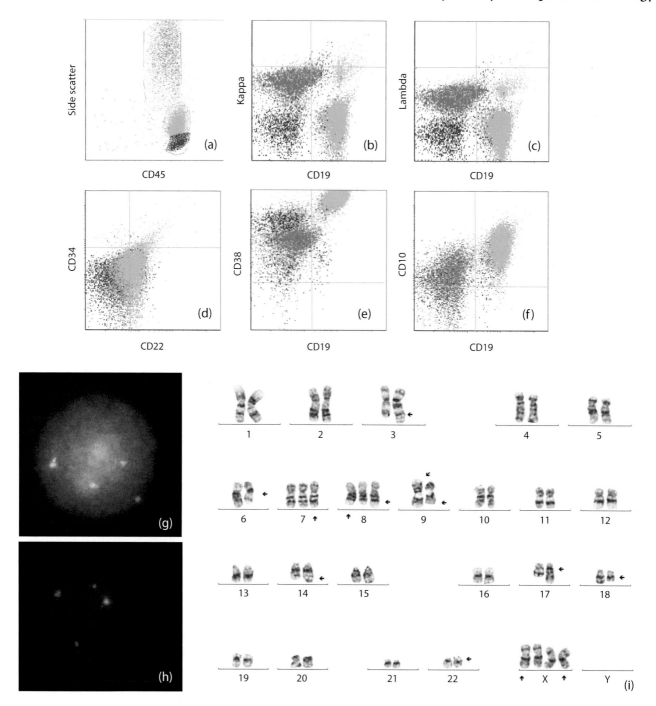

FIGURE 17.20 High grade B-cell lymphoma (CD10⁺) with rearrangement of *BCL2* and *MYC* and complex karyotype. B-cells (green dots) show bright CD45 (a), lack of surface light chain immunoglobulins (b–c), negative CD34 (c), bright CD38 (d), and positive CD10 (e). FISH studies show *BCL2* (g) and *MYC* (h) rearrangement. Metaphase cytogenetics shows complex karyotype (i): 50,XX,+X,+X,add(3) (q12),der(4)t(1;4)(q12;q31.1), t(6;17)(p10;q10),+7, +8, t(8;22)(q24.1;q11.2), add(9)(p22), add(9)(q22), t(14;18)(q32;q21.3)[5]/50,sl,-add(3) (q12), +der(3)ins(3;?)(q12;q12),-der(4)t(1;4)(q12;q31.1),+4[3]/46,XX[12].

B- or T-cell prolymphocytic leukemia

Prolymphocytic leukemias (both of B- and T-cell origin) are distinguished by lack of TdT, CD10, and CD34 expression.

Plasma cell myeloma (PCM)

B-ALL and PCM share lack of CD45, CD20, and surface light chain immunoglobulin expression. PCMs lack TdT, HLA-DR, CD10, CD19, and CD34 expression and are positive for CD138,

and cytoplasmic light and heavy chain immunoglobulins and often CD56 and CD117.

Acute myeloid leukemia (AML)

AML are differentiated by expression of CD117, pan-myeloid antigens (CD13, CD33), MPO and lack of B-cell antigens (in most cases). However, a subset of B-ALL/LBL (especially with BCR-ABL1 fusion) may express CD13 and/or CD33, and a subset of

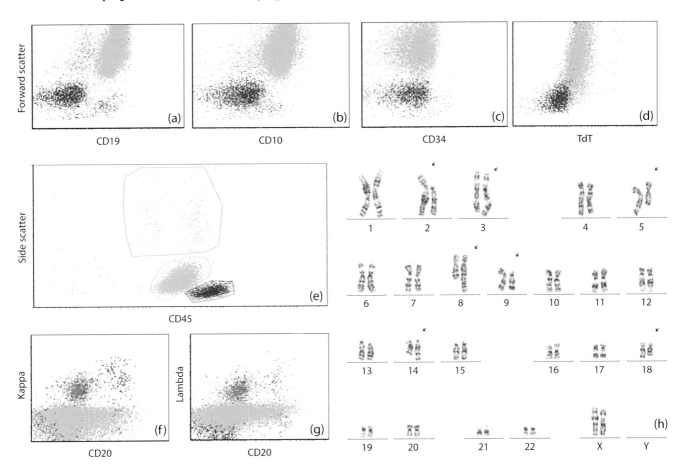

FIGURE 17.21 High-grade TdT⁺ blastic B-cell lymphoma/leukemia with *MYC* and *BCL2* rearrangement. Neoplastic B-cells (green dots) are positive for CD19 (a) and CD10 (b), negative for CD34 (c), dimly positive for TdT (d) and show moderate expression of CD45 and slightly increased side scatter placing them in "blastic" region on CD45 versus side scatter display (e). CD20 is partially positive (dim) without expression of surface light chain immunoglobulins (f–g). Metaphase cytogenetics (h) shows an abnormal female karyotype positive for translocation t(2;8)(p11;q24) and translocation t(14;18)(q32;q21). The translocation t(14;18) identified in this specimen is associated with BCL2-IGH gene rearrangement and is a characteristic finding in follicular lymphoma and diffuse large B-cell lymphoma of follicular center cell origin. Translocation between 8q24.2 (where the MYC gene is located) and 2p11.2 (where the Immunoglobulin Kappa gene is located) has been reported mostly in Burkitt lymphoma, diffuse large B-cell lymphoma, and also in other B-cell lymphomas.

AML, usually with t(8;21) may express CD19, CD79a, and CD56. Acute erythroid leukemia is strongly positive for CD71 and often expresses glycophorin A (GPHA, CD235a) and/or hemoglobin A, lacks B-cell markers and CD10.

Mixed phenotype acute leukemia (MPAL)

MPAL (biphenotypic acute leukemia) is a very rare disease [20, 89–91]. MPAL cases are often characterized by the presence of several subset of blasts, morphologically and/or immunophenotypically. Two pattern of antigen expression are associated with MPAL: co-expression of antigens classically associated with different lineages on the same cells (biphenotypic acute leukemia; BAL) or co-occurrence in the same sample of two or more blast populations from different lineages (bilineal leukemia). Current WHO classification replaced previous scoring system proposed by the European Group for the immunological classification of Leukemias [1]. In the new WHO classification of leukemias, only markers considered most lineage-specific have been retained for lineage assignment [1]. The B-lineage is confirmed by strong expression of CD19 and positive at least one of the following

markers: cytoplasmic CD22, cytoplasmic CD79a or CD10. If the expression of CD19 is dim, two those additional markers are needed for B-lineage assignment. T-lineage is confirmed by either surface or cytoplasmic CD3 expression. Myeloid lineage is confirmed by positive myeloperoxidase (MPO) staining. If MPO is negative, MPAL can be diagnosed if blasts show strong expression of other myeloid markers such as CD117, CD33, and/or CD13. A clear differentiation toward the monocytic lineage (CD11c, CD14, CD64, or lysozyme) on a subpopulation of blasts may also define MPAL in the absence of MPO expression. MPAL co-expresses myeloid (or monocytic) markers with B- or T-cell lineage specific marker. It is often positive for CD34, TdT, and HLA-DR.

In large series of 100 patients with MPAL published by Matutes et al., morphology was consistent with acute lymphoblastic leukemia in 43% and AML in 42% (remaining 15% of patients had inconclusive cytomorphology); the phenotype was either B + myeloid (59%), T + myeloid (35%), B + T (4%), or B + T + myeloid (trilineage; 2%) and cytogenetics showed t(9;22) (20%), 11q23 *MLL* rearrangement (8%), complex changes (32%) or normal karyotype (13%), with age, presence of *BCR-ABL1* fusion and

AML therapy being the predictors of poor outcome [89]. MPAL shows by frequent *WT1* mutations (18%) and *BCR-ABL1* translocations (30%) [90]. In the same series, TdT was positive in 89%, HLA-DR (human leukocyte antigen-D-related) in 92% and D34 in 74%. Among cases with myeloid differentiation, MPO was expressed in at least 5% of blasts in 98% of cases and in >20% of blasts in 76% of the cases. In B-myeloid cases, CD19 was positive in 93% and was always associated with the expression of CD10, cytoplasmic CD22 and/or cytoplasmic CD79a. Figures 26.2–26.5 in Chapter 26 show examples of MPAL.

Metastatic tumors

Metastatic tumors with blastoid morphology are distinguished by FC and immunohistochemical analysis:

Metastatic carcinoma: CD45⁻, CD56⁺/⁻, CD117⁻/⁺, CD38⁻/⁺, keratin⁺

Rhabdomyosarcomas: CD45⁻, CD56⁺, CD90⁺, CD117⁺/⁻, myogenin⁺

Neuroblastoma: CD45⁻, CD56⁺, CD2⁺, CD81⁺

Primitive neuroectodermal tumors/Ewing sarcoma: CD45⁻, CD271⁺, CD99⁺

Hematogones

See FC immunophenotyping of B-ALL, above.

References

1. Swerdlow, S.H., et al., ed. *WHO classification of tumors of haematopoietic and lymphoid tissues.* 2016, IARC: Lyon.
2. Loghavi, S., J.L. Kutok, and J.L. Jorgensen, *B-acute lymphoblastic leukemia/lymphoblastic lymphoma.* Am J Clin Pathol, 2015. **144**(3): p. 393–410.
3. Seegmiller, A.C., et al., *Characterization of immunophenotypic aberrancies in 200 cases of B acute lymphoblastic leukemia.* Am J Clin Pathol, 2009. **132**(6): p. 940–9.
4. Pui, C.H., M.V. Relling, and J.R. Downing, *Acute lymphoblastic leukemia.* N Engl J Med, 2004. **350**(15): p. 1535–48.
5. Onciu, M., *Acute lymphoblastic leukemia.* Hematol Oncol Clin North Am, 2009. **23**(4): p. 655–74.
6. Borowitz, M.J., et al., *Clinical significance of minimal residual disease in childhood acute lymphoblastic leukemia and its relationship to other prognostic factors: a Children's Oncology Group study.* Blood, 2008. **111**(12): p. 5477–85.
7. Greaves, M.F., et al., *Immunologically defined subclasses of acute lymphoblastic leukaemia in children: their relationship to presentation features and prognosis.* Br J Haematol, 1981. **48**(2): p. 179–97.
8. Baccarani, M., et al., *Adolescent and adult acute lymphoblastic leukemia: prognostic features and outcome of therapy. A study of 293 patients.* Blood, 1982. **60**(3): p. 677–84.
9. Amadori, S., et al., *Long-term survival in adolescent and adult acute lymphoblastic leukemia.* Cancer, 1983. **52**(1): p. 30–4.
10. Pui, C.H., D. Campana, and W.E. Evans, *Childhood acute lymphoblastic leukaemia–current status and future perspectives.* Lancet Oncol, 2001. **2**(10): p. 597–607.
11. Gustafsson, G. and A. Kreuger, *Sex and other prognostic factors in acute lymphoblastic leukemia in childhood.* Am J Pediatr Hematol Oncol, 1983. **5**(3): p. 243–50.
12. Miller, D.R., et al., *Prognostic factors and therapy in acute lymphoblastic leukemia of childhood: CCG-141. A report from childrens cancer study group.* Cancer, 1983. **51**(6): p. 1041–9.
13. Cimino, G., et al., *Clinico-biologic features and treatment outcome of adult pro-B-ALL patients enrolled in the GIMEMA 0496 study: absence of the ALL1/AF4 and of the BCR/ABL fusion genes correlates with a significantly better clinical outcome.* Blood, 2003. **102**(6): p. 2014–20.
14. Gleissner, B., et al., *CD10⁻ pre-B acute lymphoblastic leukemia (ALL) is a distinct high-risk subgroup of adult ALL associated with a high frequency of MLL aberrations: results of the German Multicenter Trials for Adult ALL (GMALL).* Blood, 2005. **106**(13): p. 4054–6.
15. Aref, S., et al., *Prognostic impact of CD200 and CD56 expression in pediatric B-cell acute lymphoblastic leukemia patients.* Pediatr Hematol Oncol, 2017. **34**(5): p. 275–85.
16. Maury, S., et al., *Adverse prognostic significance of CD20 expression in adults with Philadelphia chromosome-negative B-cell precursor acute lymphoblastic leukemia.* Haematologica, 2010. **95**(2): p. 324–8.
17. Borowitz, M.J., et al., *Prognostic significance of fluorescence intensity of surface marker expression in childhood B-precursor acute lymphoblastic leukemia. A Pediatric Oncology Group Study.* Blood, 1997. **89**(11): p. 3960–6.
18. Thomas, D.A., et al., *Prognostic significance of CD20 expression in adults with de novo precursor B-lineage acute lymphoblastic leukemia.* Blood, 2009. **113**(25): p. 6330–7.
19. Bene, M.C., et al., *Proposals for the immunological classification of acute leukemias. European Group for the Immunological Characterization of Leukemias (EGIL).* Leukemia, 1995. **9**(10): p. 1783–6.
20. Porwit, A. and M.C. Bene, *Multiparameter flow cytometry applications in the diagnosis of mixed phenotype acute leukemia.* Cytometry B Clin Cytom, 2019. **96**(3): p. 183–94.
21. Oberley, M.J., et al., *Clinical significance of isolated myeloperoxidase expression in pediatric B-lymphoblastic leukemia.* Am J Clin Pathol, 2017. **147**(4): p. 374–81.
22. Raikar, S.S., et al., *Isolated myeloperoxidase expression in pediatric B/myeloid mixed phenotype acute leukemia is linked with better survival.* Blood, 2018. **131**(5): p. 573–7.
23. van den Ancker, W., et al., *A threshold of 10% for myeloperoxidase by flow cytometry is valid to classify acute leukemia of ambiguous and myeloid origin.* Cytometry B Clin Cytom, 2013. **84**(2): p. 114–8.
24. McGinnis, E., et al., *Clinical and laboratory features associated with myeloperoxidase expression in pediatric B-lymphoblastic leukemia.* Cytometry B Clin Cytom, 2021. **100**(4): p. 446–53.
25. Guy, J., et al., *Flow cytometry thresholds of myeloperoxidase detection to discriminate between acute lymphoblastic or myeloblastic leukaemia.* Br J Haematol, 2013. **161**(4): p. 551–5.
26. Israel, E., et al., *Expression of CD24 on CD19⁻ CD79a⁺ early B-cell progenitors in human bone marrow.* Cell Immunol, 2005. **236**(1–2): p. 171–8.
27. Dworzak, M.N., et al., *Four-color flow cytometric investigation of terminal deoxynucleotidyl transferase-positive lymphoid precursors in pediatric bone marrow: CD79a expression precedes CD19 in early B-cell ontogeny.* Blood, 1998. **92**(9): p. 3203–9.
28. Carulli, G., et al., *Multiparameter flow cytometry to detect hematogones and to assess B-lymphocyte clonality in bone marrow samples from patients with non-Hodgkin lymphomas.* Hematol Rep, 2014. **6**(2): p. 5381.
29. Sedek, L., et al., *The immunophenotypes of blast cells in B-cell precursor acute lymphoblastic leukemia: how different are they from their normal counterparts?* Cytometry B Clin Cytom, 2014. **86**(5): p. 329–39.
30. Rimsza, L.M., et al., *Benign hematogone-rich lymphoid proliferations can be distinguished from B-lineage acute lymphoblastic leukemia by integration of morphology, immunophenotype, adhesion molecule expression, and architectural features.* Am J Clin Pathol, 2000. **114**(1): p. 66–75.
31. Hassanein, N.M., et al., *Distinct expression patterns of CD123 and CD34 on normal bone marrow B-cell precursors ("hematogones") and B lymphoblastic leukemia blasts.* Am J Clin Pathol, 2009. **132**(4): p. 573–80.
32. Lee, R.V., R.C. Braylan, and L.M. Rimsza, *CD58 expression decreases as nonmalignant B cells mature in bone marrow and is frequently overexpressed in adult and pediatric precursor B-cell acute lymphoblastic leukemia.* Am J Clin Pathol, 2005. **123**(1): p. 119–24.

33. Don, M.D., et al., *Improved recognition of hematogones from precursor B-lymphoblastic leukemia by a single tube flow cytometric analysis.* Am J Clin Pathol, 2020. **153**(6): p. 790–8.

34. Tembhare, P.R., et al., *Evaluation of new markers for minimal residual disease monitoring in B-cell precursor acute lymphoblastic leukemia: CD73 and CD86 are the most relevant new markers to increase the efficacy of MRD 2016; 00B: 000–000.* Cytometry B Clin Cytom, 2018. **94**(1): p. 100–11.

35. Saumell Tutusaus, S., et al., *LILRB1: a novel diagnostic B-cell marker to distinguish neoplastic B lymphoblasts from hematogones.* Am J Clin Pathol, 2021. **156**(6): p. 941–9.

36. Mullighan, C.G., et al., *BCR-ABL1 lymphoblastic leukaemia is characterized by the deletion of Ikaros.* Nature, 2008. **453**(7191): p. 110–4.

37. Roberts, K.G., et al., *Targetable kinase-activating lesions in Ph-like acute lymphoblastic leukemia.* N Engl J Med, 2014. **371**(11): p. 1005–15.

38. Krentz, S., et al., *Prognostic value of genetic alterations in children with first bone marrow relapse of childhood B-cell precursor acute lymphoblastic leukemia.* Leukemia, 2012. **27**(2): p. 295–304.

39. Yang, J.J., et al., *Genome-wide copy number profiling reveals molecular evolution from diagnosis to relapse in childhood acute lymphoblastic leukemia.* Blood, 2008. **112**(10): p. 4178–83.

40. Locatelli, F., et al., *How I treat relapsed childhood acute lymphoblastic leukemia.* Blood, 2012. **120**(14): p. 2807–16.

41. Bruggemann, M., T. Raff, and M. Kneba, *Has MRD monitoring superseded other prognostic factors in adult ALL?* Blood, 2012. **120**(23): p. 4470–81.

42. Bassan, R., et al., *Improved risk classification for risk-specific therapy based on the molecular study of minimal residual disease (MRD) in adult acute lymphoblastic leukemia (ALL).* Blood, 2009. **113**(18): p. 4153–62.

43. Cave, H., et al., *Clinical significance of minimal residual disease in childhood acute lymphoblastic leukemia. European Organization for Research and Treatment of Cancer–Childhood Leukemia Cooperative Group.* N Engl J Med, 1998. **339**(9): p. 591–8.

44. Coustan-Smith, E., et al., *Prognostic importance of measuring early clearance of leukemic cells by flow cytometry in childhood acute lymphoblastic leukemia.* Blood, 2002. **100**(1): p. 52–8.

45. Lee, S., et al., *Minimal residual disease-based role of imatinib as a first-line interim therapy prior to allogeneic stem cell transplantation in Philadelphia chromosome-positive acute lymphoblastic leukemia.* Blood, 2003. **102**(8): p. 3068–70.

46. Foroni, L., et al., *Investigation of minimal residual disease in childhood and adult acute lymphoblastic leukaemia by molecular analysis.* Br J Haematol, 1999. **105**(1): p. 7–24.

47. Bruggemann, M., et al., *Significance of minimal residual disease in lymphoid malignancies.* Acta Haematol, 2004. **112**(1–2): p. 111–9.

48. Conter, V., et al., *Molecular response to treatment redefines all prognostic factors in children and adolescents with B-cell precursor acute lymphoblastic leukemia: results in 3184 patients of the AIEOP-BFM ALL 2000 study.* Blood, 2010. **115**(16): p. 3206–14.

49. Stow, P., et al., *Clinical significance of low levels of minimal residual disease at the end of remission induction therapy in childhood acute lymphoblastic leukemia.* Blood, 2010. **115**(23): p. 4657–63.

50. Gaipa, G., et al., *Detection of minimal residual disease in pediatric acute lymphoblastic leukemia.* Cytometry B Clin Cytom, 2013. **84**(6): p. 359–69.

51. Foroni, L. and A.V. Hoffbrand, *Molecular analysis of minimal residual disease in adult acute lymphoblastic leukaemia.* Best Pract Res Clin Haematol, 2002. **15**(1): p. 71–90.

52. Gruhn, B., et al., *Minimal residual disease after intensive induction therapy in childhood acute lymphoblastic leukemia predicts outcome.* Leukemia, 1998. **12**(5): p. 675–81.

53. Basso, G., et al., *Flow cytometric immunophenotyping of acute lymphoblastic leukemia: is the time ready for consensus the guidelines?* J Biol Regul Homeost Agents, 2002. **16**(4): p. 257–8.

54. Campana, D., *Status of minimal residual disease testing in childhood haematological malignancies.* Br J Haematol, 2008. **143**(4): p. 481–9.

55. Dworzak, M.N., et al., *Prognostic significance and modalities of flow cytometric minimal residual disease detection in childhood acute lymphoblastic leukemia.* Blood, 2002. **99**(6): p. 1952–8.

56. Spinelli, O., et al., *Prognostic significance and treatment implications of minimal residual disease studies in Philadelphia-negative adult acute lymphoblastic leukemia.* Mediterr J Hematol Infect Dis, 2014. **6**(1): p. e2014062.

57. Campana, D., *Minimal residual disease monitoring in childhood acute lymphoblastic leukemia.* Curr Opin Hematol, 2012. **19**(4): p. 313–8.

58. Irving, J., et al., *Establishment and validation of a standard protocol for the detection of minimal residual disease in B lineage childhood acute lymphoblastic leukemia by flow cytometry in a multi-center setting.* Haematologica, 2009. **94**(6): p. 870–4.

59. Wood, B.L., *Flow cytometric monitoring of residual disease in acute leukemia.* Methods Mol Biol, 2013. **999**: p. 123–36.

60. Ravandi, F., et al., *Minimal residual disease assessed by multi-parameter flow cytometry is highly prognostic in adult patients with acute lymphoblastic leukaemia.* Br J Haematol, 2016. **172**(3): p. 392–400.

61. Dworzak, M.N., et al., *AIEOP-BFM consensus guidelines 2016 for flow cytometric immunophenotyping of Pediatric acute lymphoblastic leukemia.* Cytometry B Clin Cytom, 2018. **94**(1): p. 82–93.

62. Cherian, S., et al., *A novel flow cytometric assay for detection of residual disease in patients with B-lymphoblastic leukemia/lymphoma post anti-CD19 therapy.* Cytometry B Clin Cytom, 2018. **94**(1): p. 112–20.

63. van Dongen, J.J., et al., *EuroFlow antibody panels for standardized n-dimensional flow cytometric immunophenotyping of normal, reactive and malignant leukocytes.* Leukemia, 2012. **26**(9): p. 1908–75.

64. Coustan-Smith, E., et al., *New markers for minimal residual disease detection in acute lymphoblastic leukemia.* Blood, 2011. **117**(23): p. 6267–76.

65. Basso, G., et al., *Risk of relapse of childhood acute lymphoblastic leukemia is predicted by flow cytometric measurement of residual disease on day 15 bone marrow.* J Clin Oncol, 2009. **27**(31): p. 5168–74.

66. Hooijkaas, H., et al., *Terminal deoxynucleotidyl transferase (TdT)-positive cells in cerebrospinal fluid and development of overt CNS leukemia: a 5-year follow-up study in 113 children with a TdT-positive leukemia or non-Hodgkin's lymphoma.* Blood, 1989. **74**(1): p. 416–22.

67. Subira, D., et al., *Flow cytometry and the study of central nervous disease in patients with acute leukaemia.* Br J Haematol, 2001. **112**(2): p. 381–4.

68. Ok, C.Y. and L.J. Medeiros, *High-grade B-cell lymphoma: a term re-purposed in the revised WHO classification.* Pathology, 2020. **52**(1): p. 68–77.

69. Ok, C.Y., et al., *High-grade B-cell lymphomas with TdT expression: a diagnostic and classification dilemma.* Mod Pathol, 2019. **32**(1): p. 48–58.

70. Agbay, R.L., et al., *High-grade transformation of low-grade B-cell lymphoma: pathology and molecular pathogenesis.* Am J Surg Pathol, 2016. **40**(1): p. e1–e16.

71. Mufti, G.J., et al., *Common ALL with pre-B-cell features showing (8;14) and (14;18) chromosome translocations.* Blood, 1983. **62**(5): p. 1142–6.

72. Carli, M.G., et al., *Lymphoblastic lymphoma with primary splenic involvement and the classic 14;18 translocation.* Cancer Genet Cytogenet, 1991. **57**(1): p. 47–51.

73. Kramer, M.H., et al., *De novo acute B-cell leukemia with translocation t(14;18): an entity with a poor prognosis.* Leukemia, 1991. **5**(6): p. 473–8.

74. Nacheva, E., et al., *C-MYC translocations in de novo B-cell lineage acute leukemias with t(14;18)(cell lines Karpas 231 and 353).* Blood, 1993. **82**(1): p. 231–40.

75. Geyer, J.T., et al., *Lymphoblastic transformation of follicular lymphoma: a clinicopathologic and molecular analysis of 7 patients.* Hum Pathol, 2015. **46**(2): p. 260–71.

76. Subramaniyam, S., et al., *De novo B lymphoblastic leukemia/ lymphoma in an adult with t(14;18)(q32;q21) and c-MYC gene rearrangement involving 10p13.* Leuk Lymphoma, 2011. **52**(11): p. 2195–9.

77. Kobrin, C., et al., *Molecular analysis of light-chain switch and acute lymphoblastic leukemia transformation in two follicular lymphomas: implications for lymphomagenesis.* Leuk Lymphoma, 2006. **47**(8): p. 1523–34.

78. de Jong, D., et al., *Activation of the c-myc oncogene in a precursor-B-cell blast crisis of follicular lymphoma, presenting as composite lymphoma.* N Engl J Med, 1988. **318**(21): p. 1373–8.

79. Navid, F., et al., *Acute lymphoblastic leukemia with the (8;14) (q24;q32) translocation and FAB L3 morphology associated with a B-precursor immunophenotype: the Pediatric Oncology Group experience.* Leukemia, 1999. **13**(1): p. 135–41.

80. Komrokji, R., et al., *Burkitt's leukemia with precursor B-cell immunophenotype and atypical morphology (atypical Burkitt's leukemia/lymphoma): case report and review of literature.* Leuk Res, 2003. **27**(6): p. 561–6.

81. Meznarich, J., et al., *Pediatric B-cell lymphoma with lymphoblastic morphology, TdT expression, MYC rearrangement, and features overlapping with Burkitt lymphoma.* Pediatr Blood Cancer, 2016. **63**(5): p. 938–40.

82. Hassan, R., et al., *Burkitt lymphoma/leukaemia transformed from a precursor B cell: clinical and molecular aspects.* Eur J Haematol, 2008. **80**(3): p. 265–70.

83. Gupta, A.A., et al., *Occurrence of t(8;22)(q24.1;q11.2) involving the MYC locus in a case of pediatric acute lymphoblastic leukemia with a precursor B cell immunophenotype.* J Pediatr Hematol Oncol, 2004. **26**(8): p. 532–4.

84. Higa, B., et al., *Precursor B-cell acute lymphoblastic leukaemia with FAB L3 (i.e., Burkitt's leukaemia/lymphoma) morphology and co-expression of monoclonal surface light chains and TdT: report of a unique case and review of the literature.* Pathology, 2009. **41**(5): p. 495–8.

85. Slavutsky, I., et al., *Variant (8;22) translocation in lymphoblastic lymphoma.* Leuk Lymphoma, 1996. **21**(1–2): p. 169–72.

86. Moench, L., et al., *Double- and triple-hit lymphomas can present with features suggestive of immaturity, including TdT expression, and create diagnostic challenges.* Leuk Lymphoma, 2016. **57**(11): p. 2626–35.

87. Li, Y., et al., *B lymphoblastic leukemia/lymphoma with Burkitt-like morphology and IGH/MYC rearrangement: report of 3 cases in adult patients.* Am J Surg Pathol, 2018. **42**(2): p. 269–76.

88. Liu, W., et al., *De novo MYC and BCL2 double-hit B-cell precursor acute lymphoblastic leukemia (BCP-ALL) in pediatric and young adult patients associated with poor prognosis.* Pediatr Hematol Oncol, 2015. **32**(8): p. 535–47.

89. Matutes, E., et al., *Mixed-phenotype acute leukemia: clinical and laboratory features and outcome in 100 patients defined according to the WHO 2008 classification.* Blood, 2011. **117**(11): p. 3163–71.

90. Heesch, S., et al., *Acute leukemias of ambiguous lineage in adults: molecular and clinical characterization.* Ann Hematol, 2013. **92**(6): p. 747–58.

91. Bene, M.C. and A. Porwit, *Acute leukemias of ambiguous lineage.* Semin Diagn Pathol, 2012. **29**(1): p. 12–8.

18

T-CELL ACUTE LYMPHOBLASTIC LEUKEMIA/LYMPHOMA

T-ALL phenotype by flow cytometry (FC): CD1a$^{-/+}$, CD2$^+$, surface CD3$^{-/rare\ cases+}$, cytoplasmic CD3$^+$, CD4$^-$/CD8$^-$ or CD4$^+$/CD8$^+$, CD5$^{+/-}$, CD7$^+$, CD10$^{-/+}$, CD13$^{-/rarely+}$, CD15$^{-/rarely+}$, CD33$^{-/rarely+}$, CD34$^{+/-}$, CD38$^+$, CD56$^{-/rare\ cases+}$, CD71$^{-/+}$, CD79a$^{-/rarely+}$, CD117$^-$, CD123$^-$, HLA-DR$^-$, MPO$^-$, TdT$^{+/rarely-}$

Introduction

T-cell lymphoblastic leukemia (T-ALL) is a neoplasm of immature T-cell precursors (T-lymphoblasts), which accounts for approximately 20%–25% of patients with ALL (15% of childhood and 25% of adult ALL) [1–8]. T-ALL has clinical, immunologic, cytogenetic, and molecular features that are distinct from those with B-ALL. T-ALL is closely related to precursor T-cell lymphoblastic lymphoma but differs in clinical presentation and site of relapse: T-lymphoblastic lymphoma usually presents as a mediastinal mass or lymphadenopathy whereas T-ALL patients present with predominantly bone marrow (BM) and blood disease. T-ALL occurs more often in male than female patients (at ratio ~6:1) and involves BM and blood, mediastinum and less commonly lymph nodes, skin, gonads, and central nervous system (CNS). Mediastinal involvement and adenopathy are more common in younger patients than in patients older than 60 years. Patients with <25% of BM involvement are classified as T-LBL while patients with ≥25% BM blasts are diagnosed with T-ALL [1]. With intensive chemotherapy, cure rates for T-ALL approach 80%.

Morphology

Cytomorphology

Morphologically, T-lymphoblasts are similar to B-lymphoblasts. They are medium-sized with scanty, often eccentric cytoplasm which occasionally creates a "mirror-hand" appearance. The nuclei show finely dispersed chromatin and several nucleoli, which may be prominent or inconspicuous, depending on the degree of differentiation (Figure 18.1).

Histomorphology

T-ALL regardless of the site of involvement shows replacement by normal elements by a diffuse monotonous infiltrate of medium-sized cells, often with a "starry-sky" pattern (Figures 18.2 and 18.3). Occasional cases may display interfollicular involvement of the lymph node (Figure 18.4).

Flow cytometry

Identification of T-lymphoblasts by flow cytometry

Identification of T-lymphoblasts by FC is presented in detail in Chapter 6. T-lymphoblasts (Figure 18.5) are characterized by low side scatter (SSC), dim or moderate (not bright) CD45, lack of surface CD3, positive cytoplasmic CD3 (c.CD3), moderate to bright CD7, positive CD10 expression, and presence of one or more of

blastic markers (CD1a, TdT, and/or CD34). In contrast to benign T-cells, majority of T-ALL are dual CD4/CD8$^-$ or dual CD4/CD8$^+$. Given the lack of surface CD3 in the majority of T-ALL, staining for cytoplasmic CD3 is required to confirm T-lineage.

Maturation stages

The earliest marker of T-cell lineage is CD7, but it is not specific as it may be positive in acute myeloid leukemias (AMLs) or blastic plasmacytoid dendritic cell neoplasm (BPDCN). CD3 is most specific T-cell marker, especially surface CD3 (cytoplasmic CD3 appears earlier in T-cell differentiation but is less specific). The distinction between different immunological maturation stages (pro-T-ALL, pre-T-ALL, cortical T-ALL, and medullary T-ALL) is not always possible. Presence of surface CD3 (s.CD3) and either CD4 or CD8 expression favors medullary (mature) T-ALL, expression of CD1a is more typical for cortical T-ALL, and presence of HLA-DR or myeloid markers and dual CD4/CD8 negativity points toward pro-T-ALL [9, 10]. Pro-T-ALL (early T-cell precursor, ETP) are often positive for myeloid antigens (CD13, CD33), negative for CD1a, negative CD5 (it may be dimly$^+$), dual CD4/CD8$^-$, and positive for CD7, c.CD3, CD34, and HLA-DR. ETPs represent immature progenitors that have recently immigrated from the BM to the thymus and apart from T-lymphoid potential may also differentiate into NK-cell, dendritic cell, or myeloid cell. Pre-T-ALL is either dual CD4/CD8$^-$ or CD4/CD8$^+$, may be positive for pan-myeloid markers (CD13, CD33, CD65s), is often CD10$^+$ and TdT$^+$, and may express CD79a. CD1a is negative. Cortical T-ALL are strongly positive for CD1a, are most often dual CD4/CD8$^+$ and CD10$^+$, rarely show CD34 expression and are usually negative for CD13 or CD33. Medullary (mature) T-ALL is most often either CD4 or CD8 positive and shows surface CD3 expression.

The phenotypic stages of T-cell development can be divided into [11]:

- Pro-T (T-I): CD7$^+$, s.CD3$^-$, c.CD3$^+$, CD1a$^-$, CD34$^{+/-}$, CD2$^-$, CD5$^-$, CD4$^-$/CD8$^-$;
- Pre-T (T-II): CD2$^+$ and/or CD5$^+$, s.CD3$^-$, c.CD3$^+$, CD7$^+$, CD1a$^-$, CD34$^{+/-}$, CD4$^-$/CD8$^-$ or CD4$^+$/CD8$^+$), TdT$^+$
- Cortical T (T-III): CD1a$^+$, s.CD3$^{+/-}$, c.CD3$^+$, CD2$^+$, CD5$^+$, CD1a$^+$, CD34$^-$, CD4$^+$/CD8$^+$, TdT$^+$;
- Mature (medullary) T cells (T-IV): CD4$^+$ or CD8$^+$, CD2$^+$, CD5$^+$, CD7$^+$, s.CD3$^+$, c.CD3$^+$, CD1a$^-$, CD34$^-$.

Based on the expression of CD1a and surface CD3 (s.CD3), WHO recognizes the following categories of T-ALL:

- Early T-ALL (CD1a$^-$, s.CD3$^-$)
- Thymic T-ALL (CD1a$^+$, s.CD3$^-$)
- Mature T-ALL (CD1a$^-$, s.CD3$^+$)

The flow cytometric profile of T-ALL

The phenotypic profile of T-ALL is presented in Table 18.1. CD45 expression is often dim to moderate but may be bright similarly to mature (peripheral) T-cell lymphomas. Almost all cases of T-ALL display aberrant expression of T markers (either loss, diminished or partial expression), with CD7 being most often positive (98%)

DOI: 10.1201/9781003197935-18

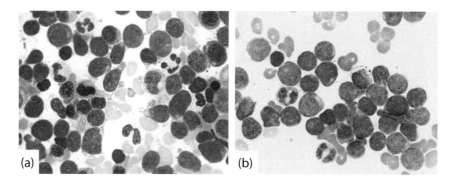

FIGURE 18.1   T-lymphoblastic leukemia/lymphoma (T-ALL/LBL) – cytology (a–b, two cases). Bone marrow aspirate with numerous blasts with delicate chromatin, round eccentric nuclei with nucleoli, and occasional "hand-mirror" appearance.

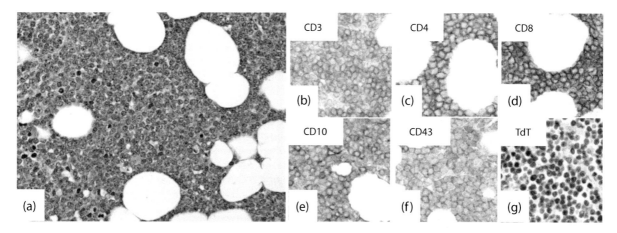

FIGURE 18.2   Precursor T-cell acute lymphoblastic leukemia (T-ALL) – bone marrow. (a) Histology shows replacement of the bone marrow by blasts. (b–g) Immunohistochemistry shows expression of CD3 (b), CD4 (c), CD8 (d), CD10 (e), CD43 (f), and TdT (g).

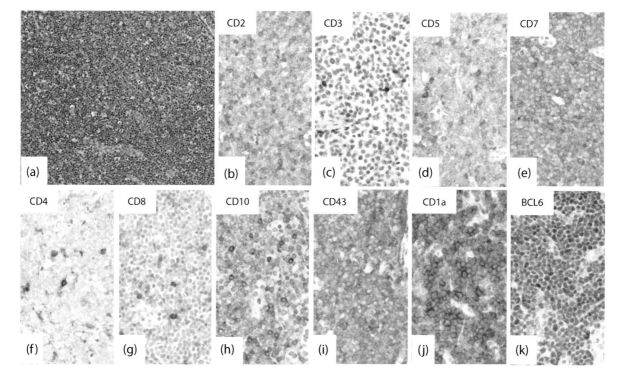

FIGURE 18.3   T-LBL – lymph node. (a) Histologic section shows monotonous lymphoid infiltrate with blastic appearance. (b–k) Immunohistochemistry. T-lymphoblasts have the following phenotype: CD2+ (b), CD3− (c), CD5+ (d), CD7+ (e), CD4− (f), CD8− (g), CD10+ (h), CD43+ (i), CD1a+ (j), and BCL6+ (k).

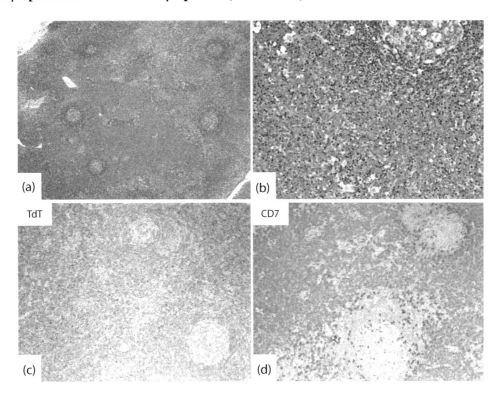

FIGURE 18.4 T-LBL with T-zone pattern (paracortical, interfollicular lymph node involvement; a–b). Blasts are positive for TdT (c) and CD7 (e).

and surface CD3 being most often negative (75%). The expression of CD2 and CD5 is seen 72% and 88% of cases, respectively. Only ~20% of cases show positive expression of all T-cell markers (Figure 18.6). In those cases, T-ALL is identified by either dual CD4/CD8 positivity or negativity, and presence of CD34, TdT, CD10, and/or CD1a expression. Among blastic markers, TdT is most often expressed (86%) followed by CD34 (36%) and CD1a (33%). Among T-cell antigens, CD7 is most often positive (~98%) usually with bright expression and surface CD3 is usually absent (Figures 18.7 and 18.8), reflecting T-cell maturation. CD7 is expressed at initial stages of T-cell development, followed by CD2 and then by CD5. The subtype of T-ALL, an ETP acute lymphoblastic leukemia (ETP-ALL), is positive for CD2, cytoplasmic CD3, and CD7 but lacks CD5 expression. The staining for cytoplasmic CD3 is positive, confirming T-lineage. Figure 18.9 shows a T-ALL case with lack of CD7 expression. Most T-ALL cases are either dual CD4/CD8− (~53%; Figure 18.10) or dual CD4/CD8+ (~36%; Figure 18.11), and only rare cases are either CD4+ (Figure 18.12) or CD8+. Occasional cases may show only partial expression of CD4 and CD8. All T-ALL cases are positive for CD38. A subset of T-ALL is positive for CD10 (37%), CD56 (~16%), CD1a (~32%), and myeloid antigens (CD13 in 7% and CD33 in 12%; Figure 18.13). CD1a expression (cortical T-cell phenotype) is associated with better prognosis. HLA-DR is usually negative, but rare cases, especially less differentiated leukemias may be positive (Figure 18.14). Expression of myeloid antigens (CD13, CD33) or CD79a can be seen in subset of cases [12–14]. CD71 may be positive in half of the cases. Myeloid antigens in T-ALL may suggest the presence of Philadelphia chromosome (*BCR-ABL1* fusion). T-ALLs most often lack TCR expression (as expected from negative s.CD3), about one-third of cases are TCRαβ+, and only rare cases TCRγδ+ (Figure 18.15). T-lymphoblasts in the lymph nodes

(or other organs) can easily be recognized by increased forward scatter, lack of CD4 and CD8 (or dual positivity), and aberrant expression of T-cell markers. Rare T-ALL cases may be of NK-cell origin with expression of CD16, CD56, and/or CD57 (CD2+/−, CD3−, CD5−, and CD7+/−). Status of CD135 and CD117 was suggested to predict the *FLT3*, *IL-7R*, and *TLX3* mutations in pediatric T-ALL (CD135high+ and CD117intermediate/high+ with *FLT3*, CD117low+ with *IL-7R* and CD135high+ with *TLX3*) [15].

Adult T-ALL

In a series of adult T-ALL patients reported by Marks et al., CD13 was expressed in 51%, CD33 in 30%, CD65 in 4%, and CD15 in 12%. 31% of patients expressed CD1a and lack CD13, 46% were CD1a−/CD13+, 7% co-expressed CD1a and CD13 and remaining 16% of patients were negative for both antigens [7]. T-ALL patients with positive CD1a and lack of CD13 have better survival than CD1a−/CD13+ patients [7]. In the same study, patients expressing CD2 rarely had complex karyotype. Significantly fewer CD13+ than CD13− patients survive 5 years, whereas CD33 does not add to this inferior outcome. CD13, and particularly CD13/CD33 dual positivity is often associated with a CD34+, triple CD3/CD4/CD8 negative, immature phenotype.

Pediatric T-ALL

In a series of pediatric T-LBL, the vast majority of cases were positive for CD45 (99.3%), TdT (90%), CD2 (66.7%), cytoplasmic and/or surface CD3 (84% and 46%, respectively), CD5 (95%) and CD7 (96.5%) [16]. Most cases were also positive for CD1a (66.7%), CD43 (86%), and CD10 (57%). CD34 was positive in 20%, CD13 in 7%, CD33 in 13%, and CD30 in 3.2%. Dual CD4 and CD8 expression was noted in 71% and lack of both CD4 and CD8 in 16.7%. CD79a was present in 5.2%.

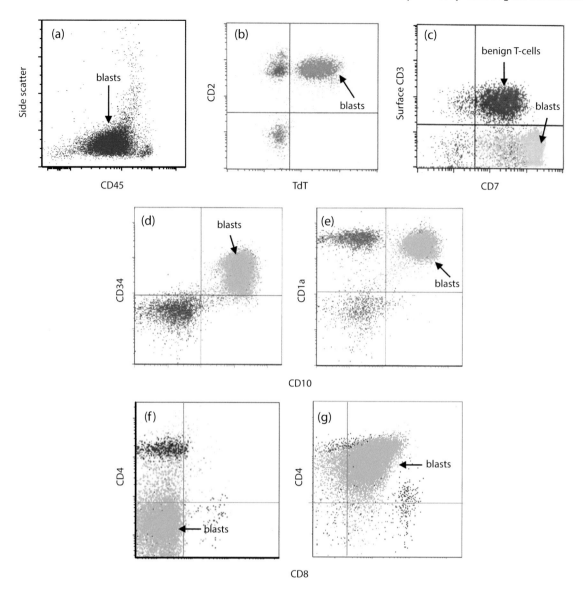

FIGURE 18.5 Identification of T-lymphoblasts by flow cytometry: T-lymphoblasts can be identified by moderate CD45 expression (a), positive TdT (b), lack of surface CD3 expression (c), positive CD34 (d), positive CD10 (d–e), positive CD1a (e), and by either dual CD4/CD8 negativity (f) or dual CD4/CD8 positivity (g).

Early T-cell precursor T-ALL (ETP-ALL)

The phenotype and differential diagnosis of ETP-ALL is discussed at the end of this chapter.

Differential diagnosis of T-ALL

Based on morphology, differential diagnosis includes hematopoietic and non-hematopoietic neoplasms with blastic (blastoid) appearance, and based on the immunophenotype, differential diagnosis includes neoplasms, which are positive for T-cell markers and/or blastic markers (TdT, CD34, CD1a):

- Indolent T-lymphoblastic proliferation
- B-cell lymphoblastic leukemia/lymphoma (B-ALL)
- Poorly differentiated (non-hematopoietic) small blue cell tumors
- Peripheral (mature/post-thymic) T cell lymphoproliferative disorders

- Diffuse large B-cell lymphoma (DLBCL)
- T-cell prolymphocytic leukemias (T-PLL)
- High grade B-cell lymphomas with "blastoid" or plasmablastic features: Burkitt lymphoma (BL), high grade B-cell lymphoma with rearrangement of MYC and BCL2 (HGBL-R), plasmablastic lymphoma (PBL), blastoid variant of mantle cell lymphoma (MCL)
- AML and extramedullary myeloid tumor (EMT)
- BPDCN
- Mixed phenotype acute leukemia (MPAL)
- Acute undifferentiated leukemia (AUL)
- Thymoma and thymic hyperplasia

Indolent T-lymphoblastic proliferation

Few cases of indolent T-lymphoblastic proliferations have been reported [4, 17–19]. They show predilection for involvement of the oropharynx/nasopharynx, a long-term clinical course with frequent recurrences but no evidence of systemic dissemination, association

TABLE 18.1: Phenotype of T-ALL ($n = 118$ Cases)

CD45+	98%
All four T-cell antigens positive	22%
(Normal expression)	(8%)
(Positive but aberrant expression)	(92%)
One T-cell antigen⁻	53%
Two T-cell antigens⁻	19%
Three T-cell antigens⁻	5%
Four T-cell antigens⁻	0
CD2+	72%
s.CD3+	25%
CD5+	88%
CD7+	98%
CD4+	8%
CD8+	3%
CD4+/CD8+	36%
CD4⁻/CD8⁻	53%
CD56+	16%
CD10+	37%
CD117+	11%
HLA-DR+	3%
TdT+	86%
CD34+	36%
CD1a+	33%
CD1a⁻/TdT+/CD34⁻	36%
CD1a⁻/TdT⁻/CD34+	5%
CD1a+/TdT⁻/CD34⁻	3%
CD1a+/TdT+/CD34+	8%
CD1a⁻/TdT⁻/CD34⁻	1%
CD13+	7%
CD33+	12%
CD13+/CD33+	3%

with Castleman disease, various types of carcinoma, follicular dendritic tumors, and angioimmunoblastic T-cell lymphoma (AITL). Morphologically and phenotypically they are characterized by focal collection of T-lymphoblasts with a cortical T-cell immunophenotype (CD4+, CD8+, CD1a+, and TdT+) [4]. It is negative for CD34 and there is no monoclonal T-cell population by PCR.

B-lymphoblastic leukemia/lymphoma (B-ALL)

B-ALLs are positive for CD19, CD10, HLA-DR, CD34, TdT, CD22, and CD79a and negative for T-cell markers.

Poorly differentiated small blue cell tumors

Small blue cell tumors resemble morphologically T-ALL. Immunohistochemistry staining helps in differential diagnosis. Small cell carcinomas are positive for cytokeratin, CD56, thyroid transcription factor 1 (TTF1), and Ki-67. Ewing sarcomas (and related tumors) are positive for CD99, FLI1, caveolin1, Leu7, chromogranin, neuron-specific enolase (NSE), and synaptophysin. Rhabdomyosarcomas are positive for muscle-specific markers, including MyoD1, myogenin, desmin, and muscle-specific actin. Neuroblastomas are positive for NSE and chromogranin A, and desmoplastic small round cell tumors are positive for keratins, epithelial membrane antigen (EMA), desmin, and often neuron specific enolase. FC may also play a role in subclassification of small blue cell tumors as shown by Ferreira-Facio et al. [20]. Based on their study, FC in neuroblastomas showed a uniform population of CD45⁻, CD56+, CD90+, CD58+, CD9+, CD81hi, and GD2+ tumors cells with heterogeneous expression of CD57⁻/+ and CD58+/++. Rhabdomyosarcoma showed a specific phenotype with MYOD1 and myogenin expression, lack of CD45 and CD57, and positive CD56 and CD90 [20]. Germ cell tumors presented with positive expression of CD56, CD10, NG2, and lack of CD45 and CD38 [20].

Thymoma and thymic hyperplasia

Flow cytometric characteristics of thymocytes (from thymoma or thymic hyperplasia):

Forward scatter shows two distinct populations (larger and smaller cells), CD1a+, CD2+(variable), surface CD3+(subset; variable), cytoplasmic CD3+, CD4+/CD8+, CD5+(variable), CD7+(variable), CD10+(subset), CD13⁻, CD15⁻, CD33⁻, CD34+(subset), CD38+, CD56⁻, CD71+(subset), CD81+(variable), CD117⁻, CD123⁻, HLA-DR⁻, MPO⁻, TdT+(subset)

FC shows very characteristic pattern in thymoma or thymic hyperplasia with variable surface CD3 expression, partially positive CD10, positive CD2 and CD5, and dual CD4/CD8 positivity. Less mature thymocytes are positive for CD10 and negative for surface CD3 and more mature cells show negative CD10 and smeary (heterogeneous) surface CD3 (see also Chapter 6 for more details). The diagnosis of thymoma or thymic hyperplasia can easily be confirmed by histologic and immunostaining analysis by showing immature (TdT+/CD4+/CD8+/CD1a+) T-cells mixed with variable proportion of cytokeratin+ cells. Figure 18.16 compares flow cytometric features of thymoma with T-lymphoblasts.

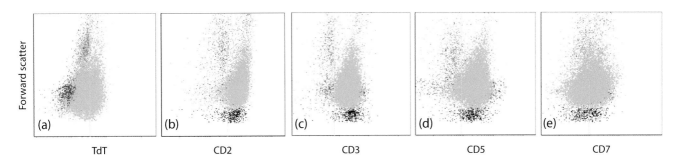

FIGURE 18.6 T-ALL with positive expression of all pan-T-cell antigens. Blasts (green dots) show dim expression of TdT (a), positive CD3 (b), positive surface CD3 (c), positive CD5 (d), and dimly positive CD7 (e).

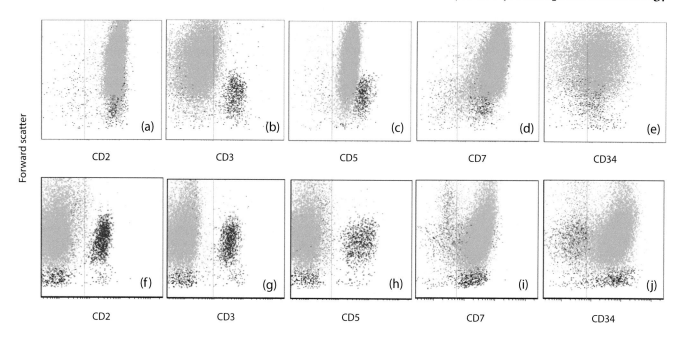

FIGURE 18.7 T-lymphoblastic lymphoma (lymph node) – flow cytometry (two cases). Case #1 (a–e): blasts show increased forward scatter and the following phenotype: CD2⁺, CD3⁻, CD5⁺, CD7⁺, and CD34⁺. Case #2: (f–j): blasts show loss of all T-cell antigens (f–h) except for CD7 (i). CD34 is positive (j).

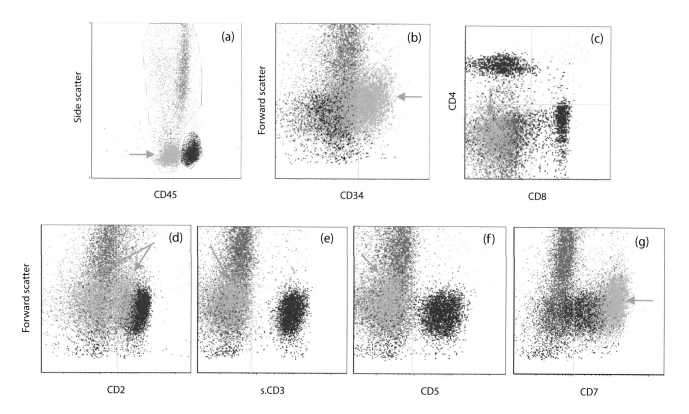

FIGURE 18.8 Partial blood involvement by T-ALL. Blasts (green dots, arrow) show moderate expression of CD45 (a), low side scatter (a), positive CD34 (b), negative CD4 and CD8 (c), low forward scatter (d–g), partial expression of CD2 (d), negative surface CD3 (e), negative CD5 (f) and bright expression of CD7 (g). Normal (benign) T-cells (red dots) show bright CD45 (a), either CD4 or CD8 expression (c), and moderate expression of T-cell markers (d–g).

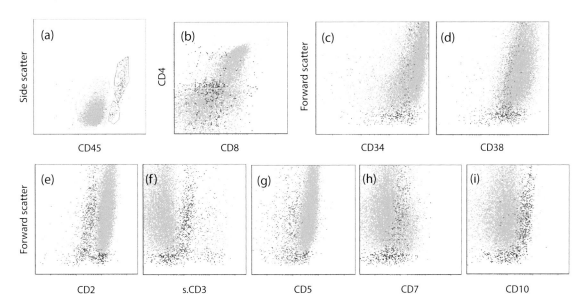

FIGURE 18.9 T-ALL/LBL – lymph node. Flow cytometry analysis shows T-lymphoblasts (green dots) with partial expression of CD4 and CD8, negative CD3 and lack of CD7 on majority of blasts. The forward scatter is increased and variable. The lymphoblasts have the following phenotype: CD45+ (a; moderate expression), CD4/CD8+/− (b; partial positive expression), CD34+ (c), CD38+ (d; bright expression), CD2+ (e), surface CD3− (f), CD5+ (g), CD7− (h; minor subset dimly+), and CD10 (i; dim expression).

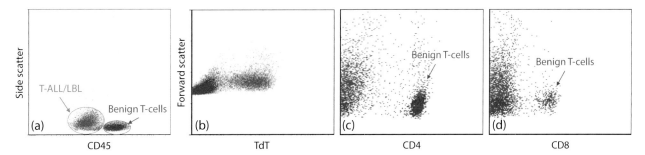

FIGURE 18.10 Precursor T-cell lymphoblastic lymphoma of the mediastinum from 4-year-old boy. Blasts (magenta dots) show dim to moderate CD45 (a), positive TdT (b) and dual CD4/CD8 negativity (c).

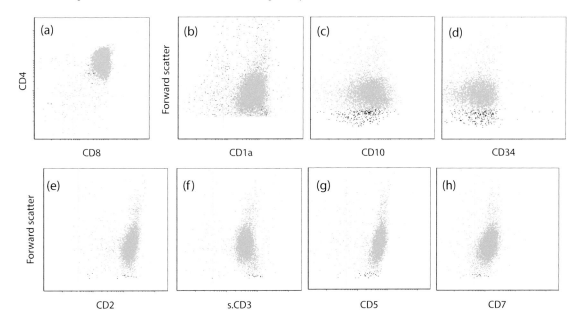

FIGURE 18.11 Precursor T-cell lymphoblastic lymphoma of the mediastinum – flow cytometry. Blasts show "cortical" T-cell phenotype with positive expression of all T-cell markers (including surface CD3): dual CD4/CD8+ (a), CD1a+ (b), CD10+ (c), CD34− (d), CD2+ (e), CD3+ (f), CD5+ (g), and CD7+ (h).

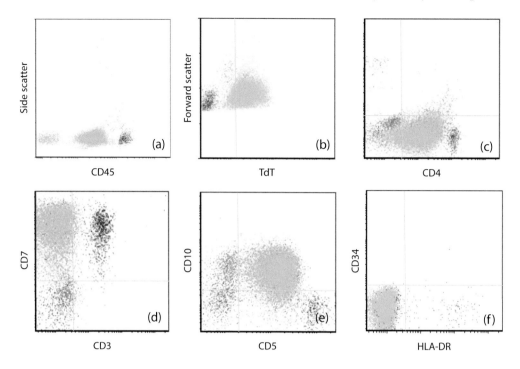

FIGURE 18.12 T-ALL with CD4 expression. Blasts (blue dots) are positive for CD45 (a), TdT (b), CD4 (c), CD7 (d), CD5 (e), and CD10 (e). They are negative for surface CD3 (d), CD34 (f), and HLA-DR (f).

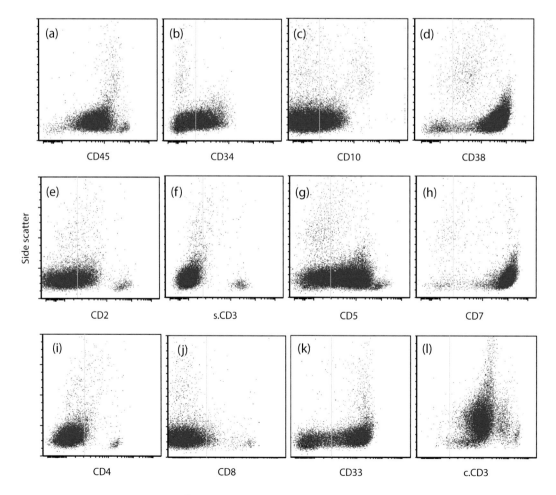

FIGURE 18.13 T-ALL/LBL - bone marrow. Flow cytometry analysis shows predominance of T-lymphoblasts (blue dots) with the following phenotype: CD45+ (a), CD34+ (b; partial expression), CD10+ (c; partial expression), CD38+ (d; strong expression), CD2+ (e; partial expression), surface CD3− (f), CD5+ (g), CD7+ (h; bright expression), CD4− (i), CD8− (j), CD33+ (k), and cytoplasmic CD3+ (l).

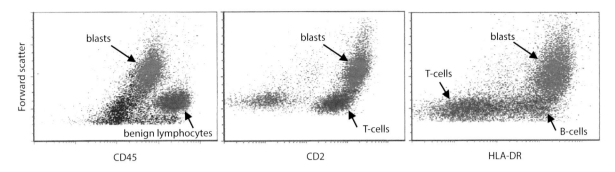

FIGURE 18.14   T-ALL/LBL with positive HLA-DR.

Peripheral T-cell lymphoproliferations

In contrast to T-ALL, mature (peripheral) T-cell lymphoproliferations are usually either CD4+ or CD8+ and do not express blastic markers (TdT, CD34, CD1a). CD10 expression is not specific for T-ALL as it can be seen in AITL and other T-cell lymphoproliferations of T-follicular helper (TFH) origin. Differential diagnosis between T-ALL and peripheral T-cell lymphoproliferations is presented in Chapter 6.

B-cell lymphoproliferations with "blastoid" appearance

Occasional B-cell lymphoproliferations may resemble morphologically T-ALL/LBL or express T-cell antigens (including CD2, CD3, CD5, or CD7). Presence of clonal expression of surface light chain immunoglobulins by FC and/or presence of B-cell markers by both FC and immunohistochemistry helps in establishing the correct diagnosis. PBL, which are usually CD45− and CD20−, often show phenotype similar to plasma cell myeloma and EBER-ISH positivity. Blastoid variant of MCL is positive for CD20, CD5, BCL1 (cyclin D1), and SOX11, and does not express TdT or CD34. Subset of MCLs may be CD10+. HGBL-R shows strong expression of B-cell markers, is usually positive for both CD10 and BCL2, and lacks T-cell antigen expression.

Acute myeloid leukemia

The phenotype of AMLs (EMTs) may overlap with T-ALL. T-cell markers (CD2, CD5, and most often CD7) are often aberrantly expressed in AML and CD2 and CD4 are often positive in acute monoblastic leukemia. On the other hand, myeloid antigens may be positive in T-ALL (usually CD13 or CD33. ETP acute lymphoblastic leukemia (ETP-ALL) may show positive CD117. Minimally differentiated AML with CD7 expression may be especially difficult to differentiate from T-ALL with aberrant expression of CD13 or CD33, as it has <3% of blasts expressing myeloperoxidase (MPO). Presence of surface or cytoplasmic CD3 expression and lack of MPO expression favor the diagnosis of T-ALL. If blasts are negative for surface CD3 but show strong expression of CD7 and additional T-cell marker(s) (e.g., CD2 or CD5), staining for cytoplasmic CD3 should be added to confirm (or exclude) T-ALL or MPAL (T/myeloid).

Mixed phenotype acute leukemia (T/myeloid; T-ALL/AML)

MPAL cases are often characterized by the presence of several subset of blasts, morphologically and/or immunophenotypically. Two pattern of antigen expression are associated with MPAL: co-expression of antigens classically associated with different lineages on the same cells (biphenotypic leukemia) or co-occurrence in the same sample of two or more blast populations from different lineages (bilineal leukemia). T-lineage is confirmed by either surface or cytoplasmic CD3 expression. Myeloid lineage is confirmed by positive MPO staining. If MPO is negative, MPAL can be diagnosed if blasts show strong expression of other myeloid markers such as CD117, CD33, and/or CD13 or monocytic

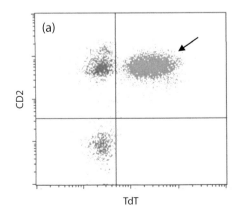

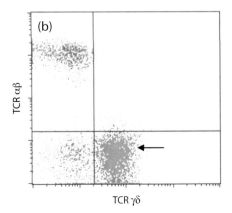

FIGURE 18.15   Precursor T-lymphoblastic lymphoma with TCRγδ phenotype. Lymphoblasts are positive for CD2 (a), TdT (a), and TCRγδ (b).

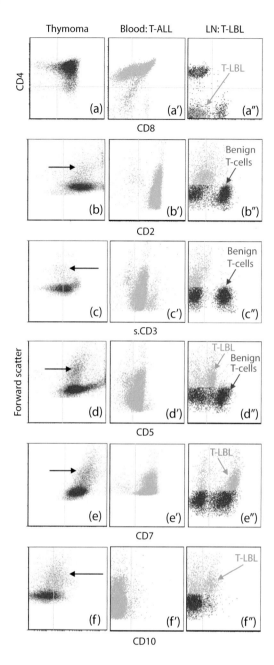

FIGURE 18.16 Comparison of flow cytometry patterns of thymocytes (immature T-cells from thymoma; left column) with T-lymphoblasts (middle and right columns). Thymocytes are dual CD4/CD8 positive (a) and show positive expression of all pan-T-cell markers (b–e). Based on forward scatter properties (b–f), two distinct populations are easily identifiable: more mature cells with low forward scatter and less mature cells with high forward scatter (arrow). More mature cells with low forward scatter show variable (mostly positive) expression of surface CD3 while less mature cells with high forward scatter are mostly surface CD3⁻ (c, arrow) and show dim expression of CD10 (f, arrow). T-lymphoblasts are either dual CD4/CD8⁺ (a′) or dual CD4/CD8⁻ (a″) and are homogeneous on forward scatter analysis (b′/b″ to f′/f″). Most T-ALL cases are surface CD3⁻, but minor subset may be surface CD3⁺ (c′). The expression of pan T-cell markers is often aberrant (either dim or negative) and subset of cases may be CD10⁺ (f″). A case of T-lymphoblastic lymphoma (a″–f″) from lymph node shows many residual (benign) T-cells with normal expression of CD4, CD8 and pan-T-cell antigens.

differentiation with expression of non-specific esterase (NSE), CD11c, CD14, CD64, or lysozyme. Cases with only a single blast population should not be considered MPAL if weak MPO expression by FC is the only evidence of myeloid differentiation [1, 21]. The proportion of MPO positive cells is controversial but a 3% cutoff is the level retained in cytochemistry. Identifying the MPO expression by FC is not completely equal to assessing the enzymatic activity, but the suggested threshold in FC is 10% or 13% [22].

Blastic plasmacytoid dendritic cell neoplasm
BPDCN is positive for CD4, CD56, and CD123 and often expresses CD7 and may be positive for CD2 and TdT. It differs from T-ALL by positive HLA-DR and lack of CD3 expression.

Acute undifferentiated leukemia
AUL is characterized phenotypically by presence of blastic markers and lack of any lineage specific markers. It is negative for CD3.

Early T-cell precursor T-ALL (ETP-ALL)

ETP-ALL phenotype by FC: CD1a⁻, CD2⁺, surface CD3⁻, cytoplasmic CD3⁺, CD4⁻/CD8⁻ CD5⁻/dim+(<75%), CD7⁺, CD10⁻/⁺, CD13⁺, CD15⁻/rarely+, CD33⁺, CD34⁺/⁻, CD38⁺, CD56⁻/rare cases+, CD65⁺, CD71⁻/⁺, CD79a⁻/rarely+, CD117⁻/⁺, CD123⁻, HLA-DR⁻, MPO⁻, TdT⁺/rarely⁻

A subset of T-ALL shows the phenotype similar to ETPs of the thymus. The normal ETP, or double negative 1 (DN1) thymocyte retains the ability to differentiate into cells of both the T-cell and myeloid, but not B-cell, lineages. ETP-ALL is characterized by the absence of CD1a and CD8 expression, absent or dim CD5 (<75% of blasts), and expression of one or more myeloid or stem cell markers (CD11b, CD13, CD33, CD34, CD65, CD117, and/or HLA-DR) in at least 25% of the lymphoblasts [2]. Inukai et al. devised a scoring system based on the expression of six markers (Table 18.2). Figures 18.17–18.19 show examples of ETP-ALL.

ETP-ALL has genetic profile distinct from non-ETP T-ALL and more similar to myeloid leukemias or mixed-phenotype acute leukemia (MPAL; T-ALL/AML) [23–25]. It is associated with worse prognosis, poor response to therapy, with

TABLE 18.2: Inukai Scoring System for ETP-ALL Based on 11 Markers (ETP-ALL Diagnosis Requires >6 Points)

Score (points)	−2	−1	+1	+2
CD2⁺		≥75%	<20%	
CD3⁺		≥75%	<20%	
CD4⁺		≥75%	<20%	
CD5⁺	≥75%			<75%
CD8⁺	≥5%			<5%
CD10⁺		≥75%	<20%	
CD13⁺			≥25%	≥75%
CD33⁺			≥25%	≥75%
CD34⁺			≥25%	≥75%
CD56⁺			≥20%	
HLA-DR⁺			≥25%	≥75%

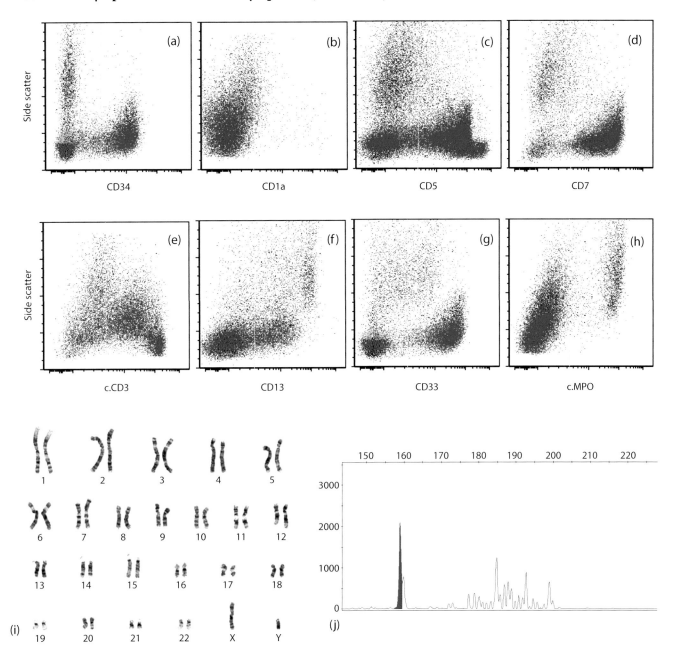

FIGURE 18.17 ETP-ALL. (a–h) Flow cytometry shows blasts (blue dots) with positive CD34 (a), negative CD1a (b), positive CD5 (c; <75%), positive CD7 (d), positive cytoplasmic CD3 (e), partially positive CD13 (f), positive CD33 (g), and negative MPO (h). (i) Karyotype is normal by metaphase cytogenetics. (j) PCR testing confirmed T-cell clonality.

much higher rates of MRD and relapse at 10 years [2]. In T-lymphoblastic lymphoma cases reported by Patel et al., ETP-ALL accounted for approximately 14% [16]. Neumann et al. have shown early T-cell phenotype in 32% of adult T-ALL cases [26]. The outcome of adults with ETP-ALL was poor with an overall survival of only 35% at 10 years, comparable to the inferior outcome of early T-ALL with 38%.

The molecular characterization of adult ETP-ALL revealed overexpression of stem cell-related genes (*BAALC, IGFBP7, MN1, WT1*). *FLT3* mutations, rare in the overall cohort of T-ALL, were very frequent and nearly exclusively found in ETP-ALL [26]. *FLT3* mutated ETP-ALL is often CD2+, CD5−, CD13+, and CD33−, has low rate of TCR rearrangement, lack of

NOTCH1 mutations and aberrant expression of *IGFBP7, WT1*, and *GATA3* [27]. Whole-genome sequencing of 12 ETP-ALL cases performed by Zhang et al., showed activating mutations in genes regulating cytokine receptor and *RAS* signaling (67% of cases; *NRAS, KRAS, FLT3, IL7R, JAK3, JAK1, SH2B3*, and *BRAF*), inactivating lesions disrupting hematopoietic development (58%; *GATA3, ETV6, RUNX1, IKZF1*, and *EP300*) and histone-modifying genes (48%; *EZH2, EED, SUZ12, SETD2*, and *EP300*) [23]. The mutational spectrum is similar to myeloid tumors, and moreover, the global transcriptional profile of ETP-ALL is similar to that of normal myeloid hematopoietic stem cells and AML. These findings suggest that addition of myeloid-directed therapies might improve

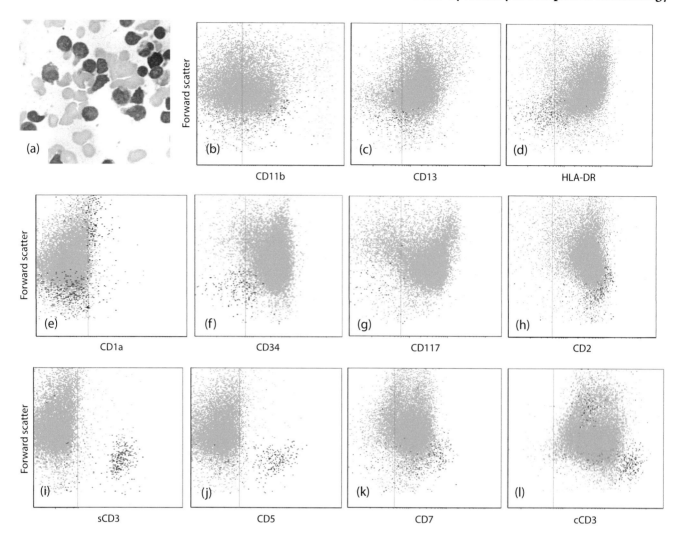

FIGURE 18.18 ETP-ALL (flow cytometry from BM). (a) Aspirate smear shows lymphoblasts with hand-mirror appearance. Blasts display typical phenotype for ETP-ALL: CD11b$^+$, CD13$^+$, HLA-DR$^+$, CD1a$^-$, CD34$^+$, CD117$^+$, CD2$^+$, surface CD3$^-$, CD5$^-$, CD7$^+$, and cytoplasmic CD3$^+$.

the poor outcome of ETP-ALL [23]. Implementation of *FLT3* inhibitors in addition to early allogeneic stem cell transplantation may be considered in ETP-ALL.

Differential diagnosis of ETP-ALL

The main differential diagnosis of ETP-ALL includes MPAL (T-ALL/AML), AUL, T-ALL with aberrant expression of myeloid

antigens (CD13 and/or CD33), acute megakaryoblastic leukemia, and minimally differentiated AML (Table 18.3). The current WHO classification considers expression of MPO or at least two monocytic markers (CD11c, CD14, CD64, or lysozyme) as proof of myeloid lineage and surface or cytoplasmic CD3 expression as T cell lineage. Although in current WHO classification ETP-ALL is classified as a subtype of T-ALL due to the expression of CD3,

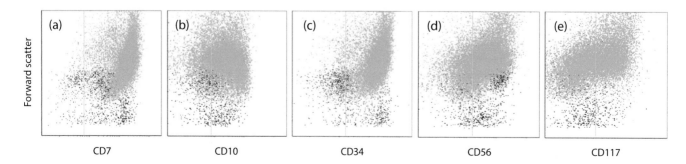

FIGURE 18.19 T-ALL/LBL with expression of CD56 and CD117. Blasts (green dots) are positive for CD7 (a), CD10 (b), CD34 (c), CD56 (d), and partially CD117 (e).

TABLE 18.3: Differential Diagnosis of ETP-ALL

	ETP-ALL	T-ALL	MPAL (T-ALL/AML)	AUL
CD1a	−	+/−	−	−
CD2	−/(+)	+/−	+/−	−
Cytoplasmic CD3	+	+	+	−
CD4	−	a	−/+	−
CD5	−/(+)weak<75%	+/−	+/−	−
CD7	+	+/(−)	+/−	−
CD8	−	a	−	−
CD10	−/(+)	−/+	−	−
CD11b	+/(−)	−	−	−
CD13	+/−	−/+	+/(−)	−
CD33	+/−	−/+	+/(−)	−
CD34	+	+/−	+	+
CD38	+	+	+/−	+
CD56	−/(+)	−/(+)	−/(+)	−
CD117	+/(−)	−	+/(−)	−
HLA-DR	−/(+)	−/(+)	+/−	+
MPOb	−	−	+(>10%)b	−

Abbreviations: ETP-ALL, early T-cell precursor acute lymphoblastic leukemia; T-ALL, T-cell acute lymphoblastic leukemia (not including ETP-ALL); MPAL, mixed phenotype acute leukemia; AML, acute myeloid leukemia; AUL, acute undifferentiated leukemia; MPO, myeloperoxidase (by flow cytometry).

Notes: +, positive (+), rarely positive; −, negative; (−) rarely negative.

a Either dual CD4/CD8+ or dual CD4/CD8−.

b MPO positivity is 3% by cytochemistry and 10% by flow cytometry.

Gutierrez et al. proposed to use the term acute myeloid/T-lymphoblastic leukemia (AMTL), defined as acute leukemias that fit the diagnostic criteria of ETP-ALL or of T/myeloid MPALs, together with AMLs with clonal TCR gene rearrangements and evidence of T-lymphoid differentiation (CD3, CD7, CD2, or CD4 expression) [28]. Leukemias with positive megakaryoblastic markers (CD41 and CD61) are excluded from this group and are classified as acute megakaryoblastic leukemia. In the series by Gutierrez et al., CD34, CD117, CD13/CD33, and CD11b had similar frequency distributions in both ETP-ALL and MPAL (T-ALL/AML), whereas CD2 and HLA-DR were more frequent in the MPAL group [28]. Cytoplasmic CD3 was present in more than 30% of blast cells, and MPO was found in more than 20% in MPAL (T-ALL/AML) [28]. Four cases in that series had Inukai scores that would classify them as ETP-ALL but were classified as MPAL (T-ALL/AML) based on strong MPO expression and/or myelomonocyte differentiation. Gutierrez et al. demonstrated that ETP-ALL and MPAL (T-ALL/AML), irrespective of phenotypic similarities or differences, have *NOTCH1* mutations, which was a good predictor of response to treatment and was associated with significantly better overall survival [28]. ETP-ALL is differentiated from typical T-ALL by applying diagnostic criteria devised by Coustan-Smith et al. or scoring system published by Inukai et al. [2, 8].

References

1. Swerdlow, S.H., et al., ed. *WHO classification of tumors of haematopoietic and lymphoid tissues.* 2016, IARC: Lyon.
2. Coustan-Smith, E., et al., *Early T-cell precursor leukaemia: a subtype of very high-risk acute lymphoblastic leukaemia.* Lancet Oncol, 2009. **10**(2): p. 147–56.
3. Teachey, D.T. and D. O'Connor, *How I treat newly diagnosed T-cell acute lymphoblastic leukemia and T-cell lymphoblastic lymphoma in children.* Blood, 2020. **135**(3): p. 159–66.
4. You, M.J., L.J. Medeiros, and E.D. Hsi, *T-lymphoblastic leukemia/lymphoma.* Am J Clin Pathol, 2015. **144**(3): p. 411–22.
5. Onciu, M., *Acute lymphoblastic leukemia.* Hematol Oncol Clin North Am, 2009. **23**(4): p. 655–74.
6. Belver, L. and A. Ferrando, *The genetics and mechanisms of T cell acute lymphoblastic leukaemia.* Nat Rev Cancer, 2016. **16**(8): p. 494–507.
7. Marks, D.I., et al., *T-cell acute lymphoblastic leukemia in adults: clinical features, immunophenotype, cytogenetics, and outcome from the large randomized prospective trial (UKALL XII/ECOG 2993).* Blood, 2009. **114**(25): p. 5136–45.
8. Inukai, T., et al., *Clinical significance of early T-cell precursor acute lymphoblastic leukaemia: results of the Tokyo Children's Cancer Study Group Study L99-15.* Br J Haematol, 2012. **156**(3): p. 358–65.
9. Lewis, R.E., et al., *The immunophenotype of pre-TALL/LBL revisited.* Exp Mol Pathol, 2006. **81**(2): p. 162–5.
10. Oschlies, I., et al., *Diagnosis and immunophenotype of 188 pediatric lymphoblastic lymphomas treated within a randomized prospective trial: experiences and preliminary recommendations from the European childhood lymphoma pathology panel.* Am J Surg Pathol, 2011. **35**(6): p. 836–44.
11. Bene, M.C., et al., *Proposals for the immunological classification of acute leukemias. European Group for the Immunological Characterization of Leukemias (EGIL).* Leukemia, 1995. **9**(10): p. 1783–6.
12. Pilozzi, E., et al., *Co-expression of CD79a (JCB117) and CD3 by lymphoblastic lymphoma.* J Pathol, 1998. **186**(2): p. 140–3.
13. Khalidi, H.S., et al., *Acute lymphoblastic leukemia. Survey of immunophenotype, French-American-British classification, frequency of myeloid antigen expression, and karyotypic abnormalities in 210 pediatric and adult cases.* Am J Clin Pathol, 1999. **111**(4): p. 467–76.
14. Uckun, F.M., et al., *Clinical features and treatment outcome of children with myeloid antigen positive acute lymphoblastic leukemia: a report from the Children's Cancer Group.* Blood, 1997. **90**(1): p. 28–35.
15. Noronha, E.P., et al., *Immunophenotyping with CD135 and CD117 predicts the FLT3, IL-7R and TLX3 gene mutations in childhood T-cell acute leukemia.* Blood Cells Mol Dis, 2016. **57**: p. 74–80.
16. Patel, J.L., et al., *The immunophenotype of T-lymphoblastic lymphoma in children and adolescents: a Children's Oncology Group report.* Br J Haematol, 2012. **159**(4): p. 454–61.
17. Ohgami, R.S., et al., *Indolent T-lymphoblastic proliferation (iT-LBP): a review of clinical and pathologic features and distinction from malignant T-lymphoblastic lymphoma.* Adv Anat Pathol, 2013. **20**(3): p. 137–40.
18. Strauchen, J.A., *Indolent T-lymphoblastic proliferation: report of a case with an 11-year history and association with myasthenia gravis.* Am J Surg Pathol, 2001. **25**(3): p. 411–5.
19. Ohgami, R.S., et al., *TdT+ T-lymphoblastic populations are increased in Castleman disease, in Castleman disease in association with follicular dendritic cell tumors, and in angioimmunoblastic T-cell lymphoma.* Am J Surg Pathol, 2012. **36**(11): p. 1619–28.
20. Ferreira-Facio, C.S., et al., *Contribution of multiparameter flow cytometry immunophenotyping to the diagnostic screening and classification of pediatric cancer.* PLoS One, 2013. **8**(3): p. e55534.
21. Porwit, A. and M.C. Bene, *Multiparameter flow cytometry applications in the diagnosis of mixed phenotype acute leukemia.* Cytometry B Clin Cytom, 2019. **96**(3): p. 183–94.
22. van den Ancker, W., et al., *A threshold of 10% for myeloperoxidase by flow cytometry is valid to classify acute leukemia of ambiguous and myeloid origin.* Cytometry B Clin Cytom, 2013. **84**(2): p. 114–8.
23. Zhang, J., et al., *The genetic basis of early T-cell precursor acute lymphoblastic leukaemia.* Nature, 2012. **481**(7380): p. 157–63.

24. Liu, Y., et al., *The genomic landscape of pediatric and young adult T-lineage acute lymphoblastic leukemia.* Nat Genet, 2017. **49**(8): p. 1211–8.

25. Alexander, T.B., et al., *The genetic basis and cell of origin of mixed phenotype acute leukaemia.* Nature, 2018. **562**(7727): p. 373–9.

26. Neumann, M., et al., *Clinical and molecular characterization of early T-cell precursor leukemia: a high-risk subgroup in adult T-ALL with a high frequency of FLT3 mutations.* Blood Cancer J, 2012. **2**(1): p. e55.

27. Neumann, M., et al., *FLT3 mutations in early T-cell precursor ALL characterize a stem cell like leukemia and imply the clinical use of tyrosine kinase inhibitors.* PLoS One, 2013. **8**(1): p. e53190.

28. Gutierrez, A. and A. Kentsis, *Acute myeloid/T-lymphoblastic leukaemia (AMTL): a distinct category of acute leukaemias with common pathogenesis in need of improved therapy.* Br J Haematol, 2018. **180**(6): p. 919–24.

19

MYELODYSPLASTIC NEOPLASMS

Introduction

Myelodysplastic neoplasm (MDS) is a group of heterogeneous clonal hematopoietic stem cell disorders characterized clinically and morphologically by ineffective hematopoiesis and dyspoiesis leading to cytopenia(s) (which often result in transfusion-dependent anemia and/or increased infections or hemorrhage) and risk of progression to acute leukemia [1–20]. MDS may be proceeded by clonal hematopoiesis of indeterminate potential (CHIP), idiopathic cytopenia of unknown significance (ICUS), clonal cytopenia of unknown significance (CCUS), age-related clonal hematopoiesis (ARCH), idiopathic dysplasia of unknown significance (IDUS), or clonal hematopoiesis with oncogenic potential (CHOP) [7, 10, 14, 21–26].

Definition of idiopathic cytopenia of unknown significance (ICUS)

Persistent cytopenia of any degree in one or more major blood cell lineages (erythrocytes, neutrophils, or platelets), in patients not meeting the minimal diagnostic criteria for MDS, chronic myelomonocytic leukemia (CMML), or myeloproliferative neoplasm (MPN) and the cytopenic state cannot be explained by any other (hematologic or non-hematologic) etiology. The clinical course of ICUS is variable, but may be followed by CMML, MDS, AML, systemic mastocytosis (SM), or even lymphoma. Initial investigations required to establish the diagnosis of ICUS include: detailed clinical history (toxins, drugs, mutagenic events, etc.), clinical evaluation with radiologic imaging, differential blood count and complete serum chemistry, bone marrow (BM) histology with immunohistochemistry, BM smear including iron staining, flow cytometry (FC), chromosomal analysis (cytogenetics/FISH), exclusion of viral infections (hepatitis C virus [HCV], parvovirus, human immunodeficiency virus [HIV], cytomegalovirus [CMV], Epstein-Barr virus [EBV], other), and molecular tests (e.g., to exclude T-cell large granular lymphocyte [T-LGL] leukemia in patients with neutropenia).

Definition of idiopathic dysplasia of unknown significance (IDUS)

IDUS is diagnosed when BM or blood analysis shows significant dysplasia (e.g., macrocytosis/megaloblastoid changes, dysmegakaryopoiesis, hypogranulated neutrophils, pseudo-Pelger-Huët cells) without accompanying cytopenia and without fulfilling the criterial for diagnosis of MDS, CMML, or MPN. Presence of molecular abnormalities (somatic mutations) in patients with IDUS (but without any other evidence of MDS or CMML), changes the diagnosis from IDUS to CHIP. Although IDUS is rare, patients need to be followed, as they may progress to frank myeloid malignancy.

Definition of clonal hematopoiesis of indeterminate potential (CHIP)

The diagnosis of CHIP is based on the presence of at least one somatic mutation that is relevant clinically and is otherwise found in MDS (or other myeloid neoplasms), the absence of significant cytopenia, and the exclusion of MDS and of all other WHO-defined hematopoietic neoplasms or recognized clonal entity, such as monoclonal B-lymphocytosis (MBL) or paroxysmal nocturnal hemoglobinuria (PNH) [10, 21, 27–30]. The most common mutations found in CHIP are *DNMT3A*, *TET2*, and *ASHL1* (*TP53*, *JAK2*, and *SF3B1* are less frequent) [14, 27]. A clone size, or variant allele fraction (VAF), of at least 2% has been used in the literature as a defined cutoff, although smaller clones can be detected using deeper sequencing techniques. The variant allele frequency in CHIP may remain stable or increase over many years without being associated with clinical evidence of hematologic malignancy [14, 24, 31]. Presence of CHIP is associated with slightly increased risk of developing a hematologic malignancy (MDS or other myeloid neoplasms). The rate of development of overt neoplasia in patients with CHIP, as currently defined, is 0.5%–1% per year. Mutations in *TP53*, *JAK2*, *SF3B1*, *SRSF2*, and *U2AF1* have been linked with a higher risk of developing AML.

Definition of clonal cytopenia of unknown significance (CCUS)

In patients with CCUS, cytopenia and clonal abnormalities can be detected, but no dysplasia is seen and no other features (criteria) sufficient to diagnose MDS or another clonal BM neoplasm are found [10]. The differential diagnosis between MDS, early CMML and CCUS may be difficult (especially in cases when subtle dysplasia is present but is limited to <10% of marrow cells). Follow-up morphologic and genetic BM analysis is those cases is recommended.

Definition of age-related clonal hematopoiesis (ARCH)

ARCH is defined as the gradual, clonal expansion of hematopoietic stem and progenitor cells (HSPC) carrying specific, disruptive, and recurrent genetic variants, in individuals without clear diagnosis of hematological malignancies [7, 24–26]. Detectable somatic mutations are rare in persons younger than 40 years of age but rise appreciably in frequency with age. Among persons 70–79 years of age, 80–89 years of age, and 90–108 years of age, clonal mutations are observed in 9.5%, 11.7%, and 18.4%, respectively [24]. The majority of the variants occur in three genes: *DNMT3A*, *TET2*, and *ASXL1*.

WHO classification of MDS (Table 19.1):

- MDS with low blasts (MDS-LB)
- MDS with low blasts and SF3B1 mutation (MDS-SF3B1; MDS with ring sideroblasts)
- MDS with low blast and isolated 5q deletion (MDS-5q)
- MDS with increased blasts (MDS-IB-1 with5-9% blasts in BM or 2-4% in blood; MDS-IB-2 with 10-19% blasts in BM or 5-19% in blood or Auer rods)
- MDS hypoplastic (MDS-h)
- MDS with biallelic TP53 inactivation (MDS-biTP53)

TABLE 19.1: MDS Classification

	Blood[a]	BM
MDS-LB	Cytopenia(s)	<5% blasts
	Blasts <2%	<15% ring sideroblasts[b]
MDS-SF3B1	Cytopenia(s)	≥15% ringed sideroblasts[b]
	Blasts <2%	<5% blasts
MDS-IB-1	Cytopenia(s); 2%–4% blasts; no Auer rods;	Single lineage/multilineage dysplasia
		5%–9% blasts; no Auer rods
MDS-IB-2	Cytopenia(s); 5%–19% blasts;	Single lineage/multilineage dysplasia
	Auer rods±	10%–19% blasts; Auer rods±
MDS-5q	Anemia, leukopenia and/or thrombocytopenia; blasts <2%	<5% blasts; no Auer rods; isolated del(5q)
MDS-h	-	<25% BM cellularity (age adjusted)

Abbreviations: MDS, myelodysplastic neoplasm; LB, low blasts; IB, increased blasts; MDS-h, MDS, hypoplastic

[a] <1 × 10⁹/L monocytes.

[b] Ring sideroblasts counted as percentage of erythroid precursors, only ≥5% ring sideroblasts is required if SF3BP1⁺

MDS and other myeloid neoplasms, such as acute myeloid leukemia (AML), MPN, and mixed MDS/MPNs including CMML developing after exposure to chemo- or radiation therapy are classified as therapy-related myeloid neoplasm (tMDS/tAML/tMPN). Apart from MDS, dysplastic changes are also typical for mixed MDS/MPN neoplasms, such as CMML characterized by presence of absolute monocytosis, MDS/MPN with neutrophilia, characterized by prominent neutrophilia or mixed myelodysplastic syndrome/MPN with SF3B1 and thrombocytosis (MDS/MPN-SF3B1-T) characterized by presence of leukocytosis and thrombocytosis (see differential diagnosis below).

Minimal diagnostic criteria

The diagnosis of MDS is suspected based on the presence of unexplained cytopenia(s). Recently, minimal diagnostic criteria for MDS have been proposed by introducing MDS prerequisite-type criteria (both must be fulfilled), MDS-related criteria (one of these must be fulfilled), and several co-criteria [1, 15, 22, 32, 33].

Diagnosis of MDS require:

1. persistent cytopenia(s) without another reversible cause, such as nutritional deficiency or the effect of drug and
2. extensive dysplasia (>10% of marrow cells in at least one lineage), karyotypic evidence of clonality with typical MDS-associated changes, such as deletion 5q or monosomy 7 (excluding nonspecific changes such as trisomy 8, loss of Y, isolated del(20q), or trisomy 15) and/or increased blasts (<20%).

Supplemental co-criteria for the diagnosis of MDS include:

1. abnormal findings on histologic or immunohistochemical studies of marrow biopsy that can be consistent with MDS, such as abnormally localized immature precursors, clusters of CD34⁺ blasts, or >10% dysplastic micromegakaryocytes detected by immunohistochemistry with CD61
2. abnormal immunophenotype by FC with multiple MDS-associated abnormalities
3. evidence of a clonal population of myeloid cells by molecular genetic testing.

Morphology

Blood

Blood, apart from anemia, which is the most common findings in MDS, may show neutropenia and/or thrombocytopenia. Red blood cells are most often macrocytic but may be normocytic (microcytic anemia is unusual for MDS). The MDS-SF3B1 is usually associated with MCV values above 100 fL. The red cells often display aniso-poikilocytosis and may show basophilic stippling. Poikilocytosis includes dacrocytes (tear-drop shaped cells), acanthocytes (spur-like cells), and oval macrocytes. Granulocytes are often hypogranular and hypolobated. Hypolobated granulocytes are reminiscent of inborn Pelger-Huët anomaly and therefore are called pseudo-Pelger cells. Platelets may also display atypia (including giant forms) when examined on oil magnification. Blasts, nucleated red blood cells, basophils, and micromegakaryocytes may be present. Presence of 2%–4% blasts in blood is diagnostic for MDS-IB-1 (even in the number of blasts in the BM is <5%) and 5%–19% for MDS-IB-2. Based on WHO classification, presence of Auer rods is diagnostic for MDS-IB-2, even if the number of blasts in blood is <5%.

Bone marrow aspirate

The presence of dysplasia is necessary for the diagnosis of MDS. At least 10% of all cells of a given hematopoietic lineage must be dysplastic to allow for the diagnosis of MDS. Dysplasia in red cell lineage (dyserythropoiesis) is characterized by nuclear and cytoplasmic abnormalities. Increased numbers of blasts, the presence of ring sideroblasts, micromegakaryocytes, and pseudo-Pelger-Huët cells correlate most strongly with the presence of clonal cytogenetic abnormalities in MDS. Dyserythropoiesis (Figure 19.1) includes nuclear budding, macronormoblasts, megaloblastoid changes, binuclearity, multinuclearity (three or more nuclei), internuclear bridging, cytoplasmic bridging, karyorrhexis, basophilic stippling (presence in the cytoplasm of multiple basophilic inclusions), nuclear fragment(s), cytoplasmic vacuolization, incomplete hemoglobinization (areas of empty cytoplasm), ring sideroblasts, mitotic figures, and prominent nucleoli. Dysgranulopoiesis (Figure 19.2) include increased blasts, Auer rods, pseudo Pelger-Huët anomaly, abnormal nuclear shape, nuclear extrusions, nuclear hypolobation, hypersegmentation, and hypogranulation. Dysmegakaryopoiesis (Figure 19.3) includes micromegakaryocytes, small binucleated megakaryocytes, hyperchromatic nuclei,

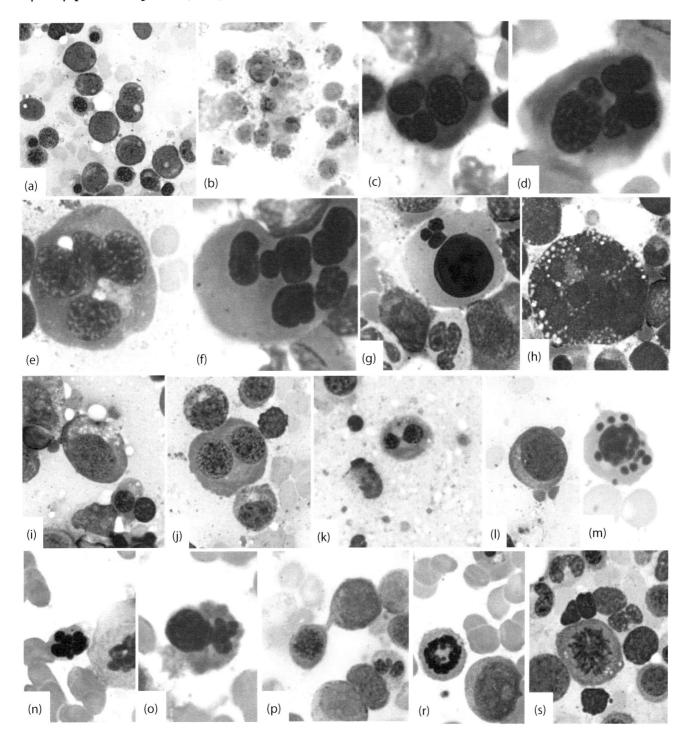

FIGURE 19.1 Dyserythropoiesis: megaloblastoid changes (a), ring sideroblasts (b, iron staining), multinucleation (c–f), giant erythroblasts with detached nuclear fragments (f), (c–h), cytoplasmic vacuoles (h–i), binucleation (j), internuclear bridging (k), cytoplasmic blebs (l), prominent nucleoli (l, r), nuclear disintegration/karyorrhexis (m–o), intercytoplasmic bridging (p), and mitotic figures (r–s).

hypolobulated/monolobulated megakaryocytes, and megakaryocytes with multiple widely separated nuclei.

Histomorphology

The cytomorphologic findings are complemented by histologic features, which include increased marrow cellularity, increased number of megakaryocytes, megakaryocytic atypia, abnormal localization of immature precursors (ALIP), decreased M:E ratio due to erythroid hyperplasia and/or increased reticulin fibrosis. In majority of patients with MDS the BM is hypercellular, but BM may be hypocellular in minor subset of patients (~10%) in so-called hypocellular variant of MDS (MDS-h). Other histologic features seen in MDS include accentuated paratrabecular immaturity, variable size of erythroid cell clusters and increased (scattered) mast cells. Ring sideroblasts may be visible in clot sections stained for iron. Histologic analysis is also helpful to exclude other disorders

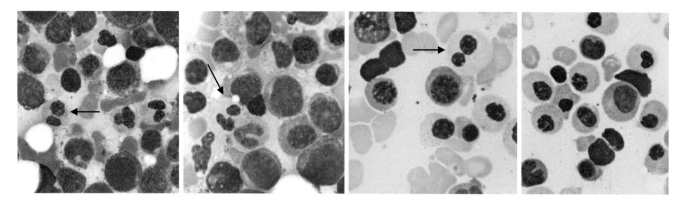

FIGURE 19.2 Dysgranulopoiesis. Atypical granulocytes with hypolobated nuclei, pelgeroid features (arrows), increased size and hypogranular cytoplasm are present.

(both hematopoietic and non-hematopoietic) which present with cytopenia(s) and to separate MDS from aplastic anemia (AA).

Immunohistochemistry

The immunohistochemistry staining of BM in patients with MDS provides additional information, which may be very helpful in the diagnosis of MDS, mostly to exclude other neoplasms, which can be associated with cytopenia(s), and to access the number and phenotype of blasts. Immunostaining with CD34 and CD117 helps to determine the number and distribution of blasts and the immunostaining with myeloperoxidase (MPO), GPHA (glycophorin A; CD235a), CD71, E-cadherin, CD68, HLA-DR, CD45, CD61, and muramidase helps to evaluate the myeloid to erythroid (M:E) ratio, erythroid maturation, monocytes, and number and distribution of megakaryocytes (Figure 19.4). Erythroid precursors are positive for both GPHA, E-cadherin and/or CD71. Immature erythroid cells are also often positive for EMA and CD117. CD117, apart from being positive on myeloblasts and subset of immature erythroid cells, stains mast cells, promyelocytes, and plasma cells. Aberrant expression of CD34 is often observed on dysplastic megakaryocytes.

Flow cytometry

FC provide useful information in management of patients with MDS and it is recommended that FC immunophenotypic findings be incorporated in the integrated BM report which should also include peripheral blood counts, a description of BM aspirate and trephine morphology with any relevant immunohistochemistry, and the complete conventional karyotype and FISH data, as well as mutational status, if available [7, 8, 34–53]. FC is especially useful in cases in which morphology did not reveal increased blasts or ring sideroblasts, cytogenetics studies showed normal karyotype and molecular testing (next generation sequencing, NGS) did not reveal any mutations. Apart from identifying dysgranulopoiesis, FC analysis allows also to rule out other causes of cytopenia(s), such as acute leukemia, hairy cell leukemia (HCL), plasma cell myeloma (PCM), or extensive involvement of BM by lymphomas or mature B-cell or T-cell leukemias (e.g., chronic lymphocytic leukemia, adult T-cell lymphoma/leukemia, T-cell prolymphocytic leukemia). FC analysis of blood may also identify T-cell large granular lymphocyte leukemia (T-LGLL) responsible for neutropenia.

The routine FC does not include the evaluation of red cell precursors for features of dyserythropoiesis as they are mostly lysed together with red blood cells during sample preparation, and therefore typical FC analysis in MDS concentrates on the phenotype of maturing myeloid cells and monocytes, and on the phenotype and number of blasts and B-cell progenitors. However, since most of the MDS cases are characterized by erythroid hyperplasia with dyserythropoiesis, analysis of erythroid precursors in properly lysed sample has been shown to add value to FC applications in patients with MDS [50, 54–57]. FC is not used for analysis of dysmegakaryopoiesis, as megakaryocytes are too scanty to be harvested for analysis.

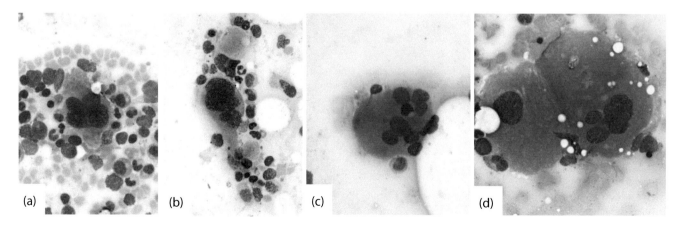

(a)   (b)   (c)   (d)

FIGURE 19.3 Megakaryocytic atypia. (a–d) Atypical megakaryocytes with hyperlobulated or hypolobated nuclei.

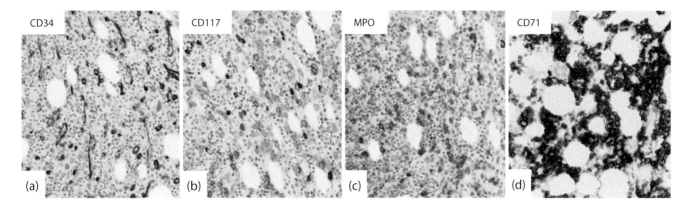

FIGURE 19.4 MDS – immunohistochemistry. The staining with CD34 (a) and CD117 (b) shows increased number of blasts indicating MDS-EB (even when excluding plasma cells and mast cells, it is evident that subset of blasts is negative for CD34). Aberrant phenotype of blasts is often seen in MDS cases. Myeloblasts are positive for MPO (c). The staining with CD71 (d) shows erythroid hyperplasia with leftward shift (compare with MPO).

The abnormalities which can be identified by FC in patients with MDS include:

- Decreased side scatter (SSC) of neutrophils/maturing myeloid precursors
- The aberrant phenotype of neutrophils/maturing myeloid precursors (aberrant expression of individual markers, including CD10, CD11b, CD13, CD14, CD15, CD16, CD33, CD45, CD56, CD64, CD66, CD117, and/or HLA-DR)
- Asynchronous shift to the left by neutrophils/maturing myeloid cells and abnormal maturation pattern (aberrant relationship between CD11b versus CD13, CD11b versus HLA-DR, CD11b versus CD16, CD15 versus CD10, and/or CD13 versus CD16)
- Presence of CD34, CD117, CD133, and/or HLA-DR on neutrophils/maturing myeloid precursors
- Aberrant phenotype of monocytes (abnormal expression of CD2, CD5, CD7, CD11b, CD11c, CD13, CD14, CD15, CD16, CD33, CD34, CD36, CD45, CD56, CD117, CD133, and/or HLA-DR)
- Altered maturation pattern on monocytes (aberrant relationship between HLA-DR and CD11b, CD14 and CD36, CD13, and CD33)
- Increased number of myeloblasts
- Aberrant phenotype of myeloblasts (abnormal expression of CD2, CD5, CD7, CD11b, CD13, CD15, CD19, CD33, CD45, CD56, CD65, HLA-DR, and TdT)
- Asynchronous expression of blastic markers on myeloblasts (CD34, CD117, and CD133)
- Decreased number or complete lack of B-cell progenitors (hematogones)
- Increased or decreased number of monocytes (compared to lymphocytes)
- Increased SSC of monocytes
- Decreased myeloid versus lymphoid ratio (<1)
- Increased number of CD45$^-$ and/or CD45^{dim+} nucleated erythroid precursors
- Aberrant expression of CD71 and GPHA on nucleated erythroid precursors
- Presence of a minute PHN clone (in the analysis of blood samples)

Decreased SSC

Decreased granularity of maturing myeloid cells, one of the most important features of dysgranulopoiesis observed in MDS, can be identified by FC as decreased SSC. The SSC of maturing neutrophils should be expressed as a ratio relative to that obtained for lymphocytes as an internal control (with ≤6 being positive). In rare cases the SSC may be so low that dysplastic granulocytes appear in "blastic" gate on SSC versus CD45 display (Figure 19.5). In majority of cases the decrease of SSC is subtle or partial. Evaluation of "blastic" markers (CD34 and CD117) and markers associated with maturation (CD10, CD11b, CD15, CD16, and CD65) helps to distinguish granulocytes/maturing myeloid precursors with low SSC from blasts and monocytes.

Aberrant expression of myeloid, monocytic, and/or lymphoid markers on maturing myeloid precursors

Figure 19.6 shows antigen expression during normal myeloid maturation. Any deviation from normal maturation pattern identified by FC, although not specific, may be associated with dysgranulopoiesis and is helpful in establishing the diagnosis of MDS. All FC features may be present on a subset of cells or involve entire population. Single antigenic abnormality is less specific for MDS than accumulation of several abnormalities. The intensity of aberrant expression is also variable, but often correlates with the degree of myelodysplasia. Low grade MDS tends to have less obvious changes, whereas high grade MDS (MDS-IB) shows more pronounced changes.

During normal maturation, increasing expression of CD11b and CD16 is seen in final stages of maturation with neutrophils showing brightest expression. The expression of CD13 is high in blasts, decreases during transition from promyelocytes to myelocytes, and starts to increase again as the cells progress from bands to segmented forms. CD10 and CD16 are expressed by mature granulocytic cells and the expression of CD11b starts to appear in late myelocytes and is highest in bands and neutrophils. Comparing CD13 versus CD16 expression in normal BM shows transition from CD13$^+$/CD16$^-$ promyelocytes, to CD13$^{+(dim)}$/CD16$^-$ immature myeloid cells to finally CD13$^+$/CD16$^+$ neutrophils. In MDS, this pattern is often lost. MDS patients may show also asynchronous pattern of expression of CD16 versus CD11b. The phenotypic abnormalities identified in MDS include aberrant

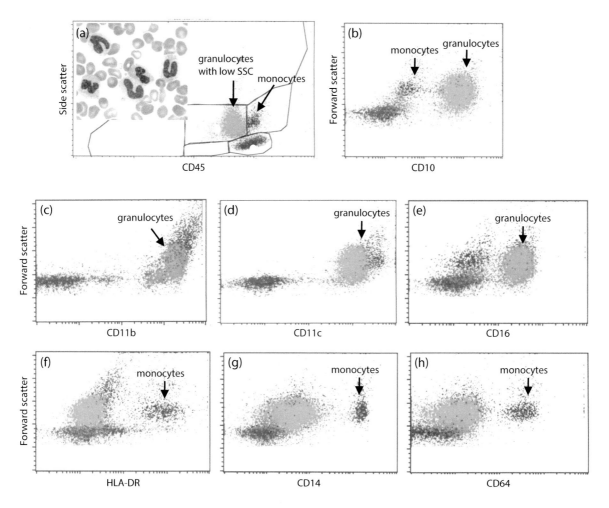

FIGURE 19.5 MDS. Granulocytes (green dots) display low side scatter (a), which may mimic blasts on CD45 versus side scatter display (a) or monocytic cells due to their expression of CD11b (c) and CD11c (d). Dysplastic granulocytes differ phenotypically from blasts by lack of CD34 and CD117 expression and from monocytic cells by strong CD10 (b) and CD16 (e) expression and lack of HLA-DR (f), CD14 (g), and CD64 (h) expression. Cytologic evaluation (a; *inset*) confirmed dysplastic (agranular) granulocytes.

expression of CD10, CD11b, CD13, CD14, CD15, CD16, CD33, CD45, CD56, CD64, and HLA-DR in granulocytic series and aberrant expression of CD2, CD5, CD7, CD11b, CD11c, CD13, CD14, CD15, CD16, CD33, CD36, CD45, CD56, and HLA-DR by monocytes. Figures 19.7–19.11 show FC features seen in MDS. The most common phenotypic abnormalities of granulocytes in MDS include loss or decreased expression of CD10, CD11b, CD16, and aberrant (positive) expression of CD56 or HLA-DR. Bowen and Davis reported consistently normal pattern of CD11b and CD16 expression in the granulocytic series in healthy individuals, but in MDS patients there was an increased percentage of granulocytic cells with low CD16 or both low CD16 and low CD11b [58]. Chang et al. reported significantly lower percentage of CD10+ mature granulocytes in patients with MDS than in controls [59]. Maturing myeloid cells in MDS may display dim CD15 without a concomitant shift to the left by CD11b, CD13, CD16, and HLA-DR (asynchronous maturation) [39]. In a series reported by Stetler-Stevenson et al., the most common myelomonocytic abnormalities detected by FC in MDS were granulocytic hypogranulation (84%), abnormal CD13/CD16 (78%) or CD11b/CD16 (70%) patterns, and CD64 negativity (66%) [34]. Wells et al. reported that the most common FC abnormalities in MDS patients were the

presence of abnormal myeloblasts (62%), abnormal relationship between CD13 and CD16 in maturing myeloid cells and monocytes (23%), asynchronous shift to the left (23%), and the presence of CD56 on maturing myeloid cells (16%) and monocytes (17%) [39]. In monocytes, the most frequent immunophenotypic abnormalities include abnormal intensity of CD13, CD14, CD36, CD33, or CD64, abnormal pattern of CD11b versus HLA-DR, presence of CD56 and expression of CD2, CD7, or CD19 [34, 38, 39, 60–62]. Presence of increased number of monocytes with aberrant phenotype should prompt the differential diagnosis between MDS with increased monocytes and CMML. Neutrophils with diminished or absent CD10 expression, abnormal CD10 pattern and CD10/15 ratios are associated with dysplasia. Vikentiou et al. showed that analyzing CD16/MPO/lactoferrin expression can differentiate between lower- and higher-risk MDS patients [63]. In series reported by Loosdrecht et al., 14/50 patients had single immunophenotypic abnormality and 32/50 patients had multiple abnormalities with abnormal relations between CD11b, CD13, CD15, and CD16 being most common [60]. Myeloid neoplasms with monosomy 7 typically demonstrate multiple immunophenotypic abnormalities on myeloid blasts and maturing myelomonocytic cells. Increased CD14 expression on maturing granulocytic

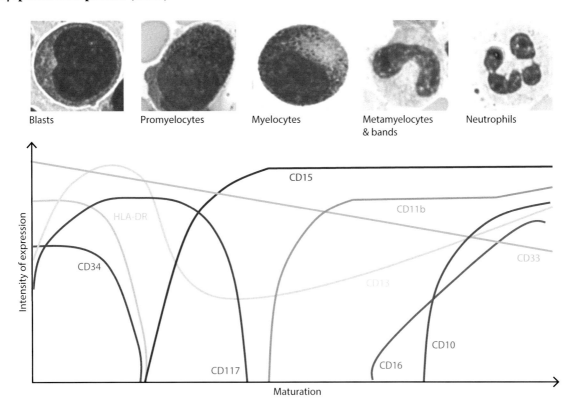

FIGURE 19.6   Antigen expression during myeloid maturation.

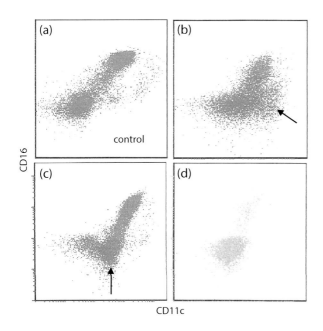

FIGURE 19.7   Abnormal CD11c/CD16 pattern in MDS. Panel a shows CD11c/CD16 pattern in normal bone marrow. Note two distinct populations, one negative and the other positive for CD11c and CD16 with only few cells in between. In MDS (b–d), the distinction between those two populations is less visible (b, c). Panel b shows up-regulation of CD11c on CD16-negative cells (arrow), panel c shows down-regulation of CD16 and up-regulation of CD11c on subset of cells (arrow, compare with a), and panel d shows marked down-regulation of both markers.

cells is characteristically seen in myeloid neoplasms with monosomy 7 [64]. This abnormality was significantly more frequent in myeloid neoplasms with monosomy 7 than in those with del(7q). Rare cases of MDS may show aberrant expression of CD117 on maturing myeloid precursors (Figure 19.12).

Aberrant phenotype of neutrophils/maturing myeloid precursors can be incorporated into scoring systems, as proposed by Ogata et al. and Barreau et al., allowing for more sensitive and specific FC diagnosis of MDS-related cytopenias [46, 65–67]. In a series by Barreau et al., neutrophils/maturing myeloid precursors were analyzed for maturations pathways and mean fluorescence intensity for each marker (CD10, CD11b, CD13, CD14, CD16, CD33, CD34, CD45, CD56, and CD64) and compared to the reference maturation database using the maturation tool of the Infinicyt software [65]. Parameters that were outside the threshold defined by the mean ±2SD (standard deviation) of the reference database were considered to be aberrant. "Diff score" was calculated by the sum of absolute values of SD outside the threshold of all markers ($n = 10$) at all stages of granulocytic and monocytic maturation. The "Diff score" was significantly greater in patients with MDS than in patients without MDS. Only 6 of the 93 non-MDS patients in that report had high (false positive) "Diff score" suggestive of MDS (among those six patients, the cytopenia(s) were in fact related to B12 deficiency, autoimmune disorders, chronic alcohol intake, and iron deficiency) [65].

Increased blasts

MDS patients show increased proportions of the more immature immunophenotypic compartments (CD33+/CD16−; CD45+/CD16−; CD13+/CD16−) of myeloid cells and decreased proportions of mature granulocytes (CD33+/CD16+bright; CD45+/CD16+bright; CD13+/CD16+bright) [68]. Myeloblasts are increased in MDS

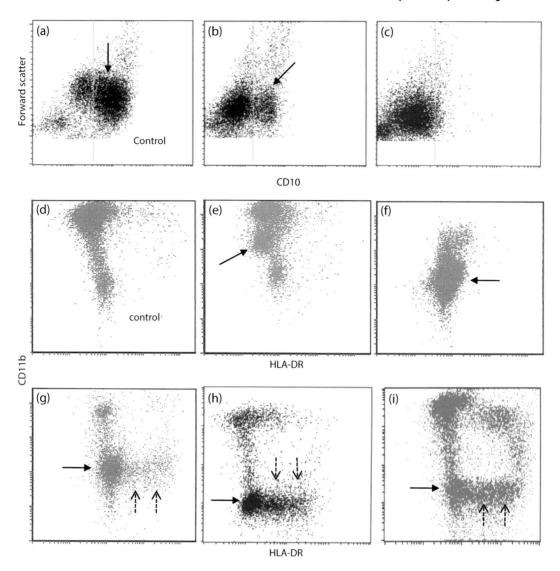

FIGURE 19.8   MDS – flow cytometry (dysgranulopoiesis). MDS – flow cytometry (dysgranulopoiesis). (a–c) CD10 expression. (a) Normal (control) sample with positive CD10 expression (arrow). (b) MDS with partial loss of CD10 expression; only minute subset of granulocytes (arrow) is CD10⁺. (c) MDS with complete lack of CD10 expression by granulocytes. (d–i) Aberrant expression of CD11b and HLA-DR by granulocytes. (d) Normal (control) sample with variable but mostly bright expression of CD11b and negative HLA-DR. Panels e through i show gradual increase in the severity of phenotypic atypia associated with MDS. e shows distinct subset of granulocytes with subtle down-regulation of CD11b (arrow), whereas f shows majority of granulocytes being negative CD11b (arrow). In g and h, apart from prominent down-regulation of CD11b (arrow), subset of granulocytes shows also aberrant expression of HLA-DR (dashed arrows). Panel i shows prominent down regulation of CD11b (arrow) and up-regulation of HLA-DR (dashed arrows), creating characteristic "window" pattern.

(Figures 19.13–19.15), regardless of the morphologic subtype of MDS, but number of CD34⁺/CD10⁺ B-cell precursors (hematogones) and CD34⁺ plasmacytoid dendritic cell precursors is decreased. Loosdrecht et al. reported the median percentage of myeloid progenitor cells of 2.4% in MDS patients compared to 1.2% in normal BM samples [50, 60, 61]. Identification of patients with MDS-IB is one of the most straightforward features offered by FC in evaluation of MDS. Based on number of blasts, MDS-IB is further subdivided into MDS-IB-1 with 5%–9% blasts in BM or 2%–4% blasts in blood, and MDS-IB-2 with 10% 19% of blasts

in BM or 5%–19% blasts in blood. It is suggested that the cut-off level for blasts in FC analysis is 3% rather than 5% used in by cytomorphology [39, 46, 50, 60, 61, 69]. Circulating CD34⁺ blasts >10/μL predict MDS leukemic evolution independently of WHO categories [70].

Since myeloblasts may be negative for CD34, and cells other than myeloblasts (mast cells, plasma cells, immature erythroid cells) may express CD117, the enumeration of blasts in MDS should include CD34, CD117, HLA-DR, CD11b, and CD45 (blasts being defined as CD34⁺⁻, CD117⁺⁻, CD11b⁻,

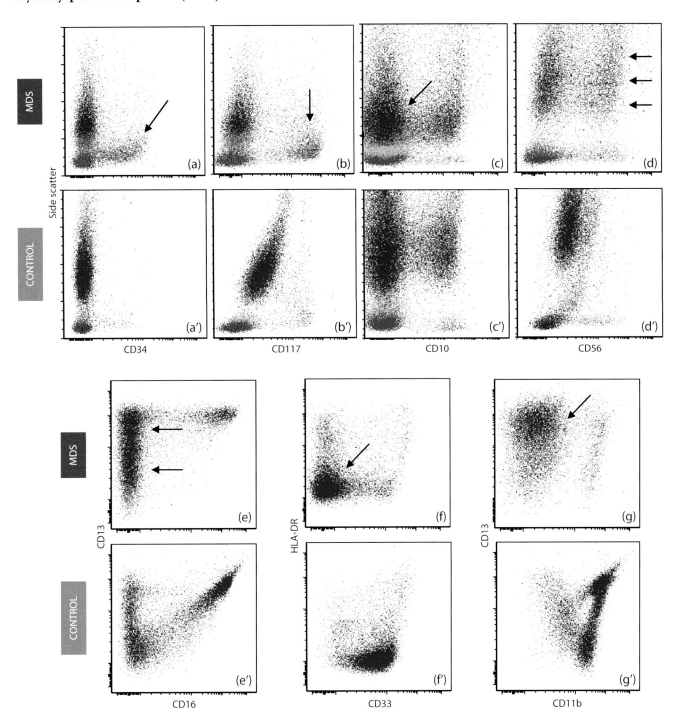

FIGURE 19.9 MDS – flow cytometry. Flow cytometry analysis (different MDS cases) shows increased blasts (a–b; compare with control samples in a′ and b′), decreased side scatter and down-regulation of CD10 (c; compare with control on c′), and normal side scatter and aberrant expression of CD56 (d; compare with control on d′). Gating on granulocytes/maturing myeloid precursors (e–g) shows down-regulation of CD16 (e), CD33 (f) and down-regulation of CD11b (g). Control (benign) bone marrow samples are shown in a′–d′ and e′–g′.

CD45[+(dim to moderate)], HLA-DR[+], and SSC[low]). The FC count of blasts based on CD34 expression underestimates the number of blasts, whereas the strategy based on the CD34[+] and/or CD117[+] and CD45[+(dim to moderate)] phenotype overestimates the blast number [71]. The study by Huang et al. showed that ratio of CD34[+] and/or CD117[+]/HLA-DR[+] cells to the number of total events shows the highest degree of correlation with morphological blast count [71]. This criterion includes the measurement of CD34[+] blasts, CD34[−]/CD117[+/−]/HLA-DR[+] neutrophils, and erythroid-committed precursors as well as early CD117[low]/HLA-DR[high] monocytic and dendritic cell precursors [69, 72, 73].

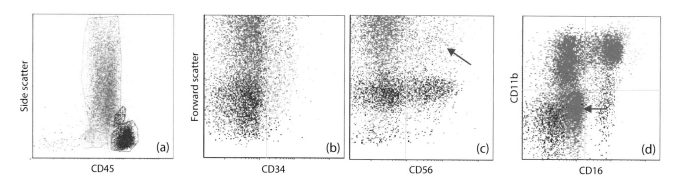

FIGURE 19.10   Low grade MDS (MDS-SLD) – flow cytometry. Granulocytes (grey dots) show minimally decreased side scatter and normal expression of CD45 (a). CD34 staining shows rare blasts (b; green dots). Occasional granulocytes show aberrant expression of CD56 (c; arrow). The analysis of CD11b and CD16 shows decreased expression of both markers (d; arrow).

Aberrant phenotype of blasts

The abnormal antigen expression by blasts in MDS (Figure 19.16) is similar to changes occurring in AMLs (leukemia associated immunophenotype; LAIP). The aberrant phenotypic changes of blasts observed in patients with MDS include overexpression of CD34, CD117, and CD38, discordant expression of CD34 and CD117, dim, partial or negative CD34, dim CD38 and negative or dim CD45, abnormal expression of CD4, positive CD11b, CD15, and/or CD65, lack, partial or aberrantly dim expression of CD13, CD33, and HLA-DR, and cross-lineage expression of CD2, CD5, CD7, CD19, CD56, and/or TdT [36, 37, 39, 42, 60, 69, 74–77]. Analyzing the expression of CD13 versus HLA-DR on CD34+ blasts in normal BM shows usually heterogeneous staining with several distinct populations of blasts. This heterogeneity is often lost in MDS. Some MDS patients display decreased expression of CD45 on blasts [39, 75]. Aberrant phenotype of blasts in MDS patients (e.g., CD7 and/or TdT) correlates with poor prognosis [36, 60, 78]. Loosdrecht et al. demonstrated that

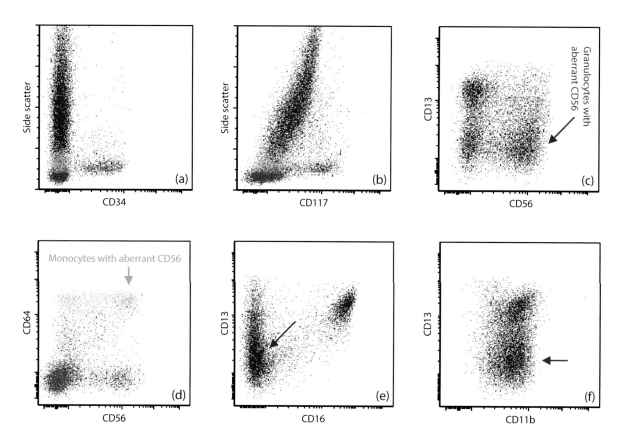

FIGURE 19.11   MDS-IB – flow cytometry. Blasts expressing CD34 and CD117 are increased (a–b; blue dots). In addition, granulocytes and monocytes display aberrant expression of CD56 (c–d; arrow). Significant subset of granulocytes shows also down-regulation of CD13 and CD16 (e–f).

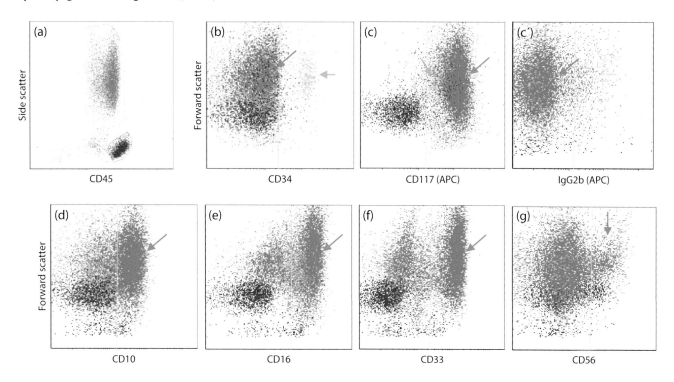

FIGURE 19.12 MDS-EIB – flow cytometry. CD45 versus side scatter (a) shows slightly increased blasts (green dots) and normal expression of CD45 by granulocytes/maturing myeloid precursors (gray dots). The side scatter of granulocytes appears normal (a). Blasts are positive for CD34 and CD117 (b–c; green arrow). Granulocytes (gray arrow) are negative for CD34 (b) and display aberrant expression of CD117 (c; compare with isotypic control on c′) and show normal expression of CD10 (d), CD16 (e), and CD33 (f). Minor subset of granulocytes shows aberrant expression of CD56 (g). Bright CD45 (instead of moderate) and strong expression of both CD10 and CD16 confirms that CD117 is aberrantly expressed by granulocytes and excludes promyelocytes.

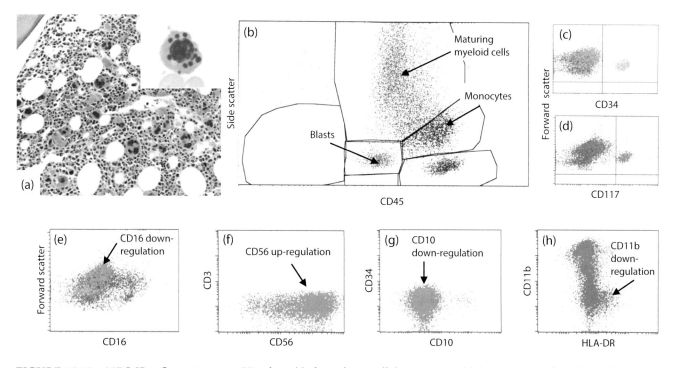

FIGURE 19.13 MDS-IB – flow cytometry. Histology (a) shows hypercellular marrow with increased number of megakaryocytes which display atypical cytomorphology (*Inset*: red cell precursor with prominent dyserythropoiesis as seen on aspirate smear). Flow cytometry (b–h) shows mixed population of myeloid cells, monocytes, lymphocytes, and blasts. Granulocytes do not display decreased side scatter (b) but show down-regulation of CD16 (e), CD10 (g), and CD11b (h), and up-regulation of CD56 (f). Blasts (b; green dots) are increased in number. They express CD34 (c) and CD117 (d).

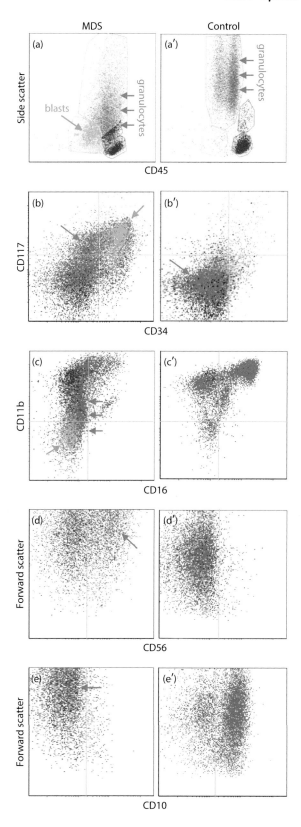

FIGURE 19.14 MDS-IB – flow cytometry. Blasts (green arrow) are increased (a). They are positive for CD34 and CD117 (b). Granulocytes display markedly decreased side scatter (a; gray arrows), partial (aberrant) expression of Cd117 (b; gray arrow), decreased expression of CD11b and CD16 (c; gray arrow), aberrant expression of CD56 (d; arrow) and completely negative CD10 (e, arrow). The right column (a′–e′) shows benign bone marrow for comparison.

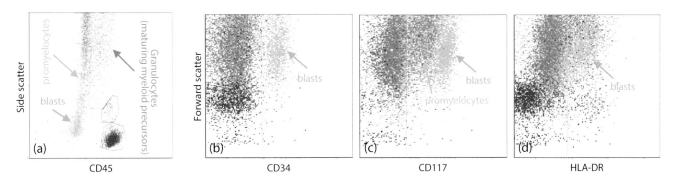

FIGURE 19.15 MDS-IB with prominent leftward shift with increased blasts (green dots) and promyelocytes (orange dots). Blasts show low side scatter and dim CD45 (a), positive CD34 (b), positive CD117 (c) and positive HLA_DR (d). Promyelocytes show high side scatter (a), negative CD34 (b), positive CD117 (c), and negative HLA-DR (d). Granulocytes (gray dots) show decreased CD45 expression (a) indicating leftward shift and negative CD34, CD117, and HLA-DR (b–d).

patient with MDS with single lineage dysplasia (as defined by WHO classification) with expression of lineage infidelity markers on myeloblasts (e.g., CD5, CD7, and/or CD56) had an adverse clinical outcome [50, 60, 61]. MDS cases with aberrant phenotype of blasts often display abnormal karyotype by cytogenetic and/or FISH studies.

Aberrant phenotype of monocytes
Normal monocytes are positive for CD4, CD11b (moderate), CD11c (bright), CD13, CD14 (bright), CD33 (bright), CD38, CD45 (bright), CD64 (bright), and HLA-DR (moderate to bright). In MDS, monocytes may be decreased, normal, or increased in number. They are usually mature with normal pattern of expression of

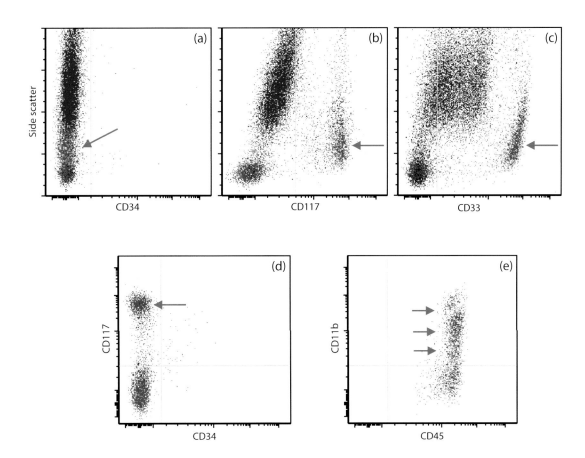

FIGURE 19.16 MDS – flow cytometry. BM analysis by flow cytometry shows increased blasts (blue dots; arrow) with aberrant phenotype: negative CD34 (a, d), positive CD117 (b, d) and partial expression of CD11b (e). The 2 lower panels shows only mononuclear gate (without granulocytes).

CD14 versus CD64. Some cases display variable or partial expression of CD14 (complete loss of CD14 is rare in MDS). Similar to CD14, also CD11b may be aberrantly expressed with either dim or variable ("smeary") pattern. Rare cases of MDS display unusually bright CD11b. The most common phenotypic abnormality in MDS (although not specific) is the aberrant expression of CD56 (the expression may be partial or variable). Other abnormalities seen in MDS include reduced expression of CD13 and/or CD33, reduced or lost expression of HLA-DR, decreased expression of CD45, strong expression of CD2, presence of CD23 or rarely partial expression of blastic markers (CD34, CD117).

Decreased lymphoid progenitors (hematogones)

Patients with MDS usually have decreased number of hematogones [36, 46, 60, 79], but normal or even increased number of hematogones may be seen in MDS, more often in MDS-IB. Hematogones have very low SSC and can be visualized on CD45 versus SSC display. The most immature hematogones (stage 1) express CD34, TdT, CD10, and usually CD19 and CD22. The detailed phenotypic characteristics of hematogones are presented in Chapters 5 and 40. Ogata et al. recommend quantitation of stage I CD10[+]/CD34[+] hematogones as a percentage of all CD34[+] cells in the BM [46].

Dyserythropoiesis

Della Porta et al. developed a quantitative FC approach to identify sideroblastic anemia by analyzing the expression of CD71, CD105, cytosolic H-ferritin, cytosolic L-ferritin, and mitochondrial ferritin in erythroblasts [80]. Compared with pathologic and healthy controls, MDS patients had higher expression of cytosolic H-ferritin and CD105, and lower expression of CD71 [80]. Mitochondrial ferritin was specifically detected in MDS-RS, and there was a close relationship between its expression and Prussian blue staining. This FC approach provided an accurate quantitative evaluation of erythroid dysplasia and allowed a reliable diagnosis of sideroblastic anemia [80]. The FC RED score was developed as a whole BM FC protocol using the nuclear dye CyTRAK orange to gate nucleated cells without lysing red blood cells. The RED score is based on the evaluation of dyserythropoiesis with CD71 and CD36 coefficient of variation values and hemoglobin levels according to gender. It ranges from 0 to 7, with a RED score ≥3 predicting MDS with a sensitivity of 77.5% and a specificity of 90% [57, 81]. Westers et al. showed that analysis of expression of CD36 and CD71 (expressed as coefficient of variation), in combination with CD71 fluorescence intensity and the percentage of CD117[+] erythroid progenitors provided the best discrimination between MDSs and non-clonal cytopenias (specificity 90%; 95% confidence interval: 84%–94%) [55]. Relative expression of CD105 was either increased or decreased in MDS and therefore, CD105 expression did not discriminate between MDS and controls in that series [55].

Presence of minute PNH clone

Identification of minute PNH clone in the granulocytic (Figure 19.17), red blood cell and/or monocytic populations have been reported in association with AA and MDS [82].

Flow cytometry scoring systems in MDS

Ogata et al. have proposed a widely accepted and tested combination of four parameters to evaluate MDS by FC [36, 46, 66, 67, 83]:

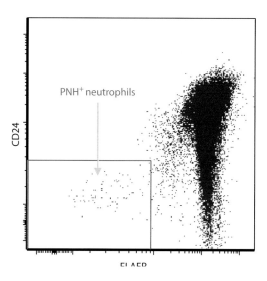

FIGURE 19.17 "Minute PNH+ granulocytic population."

- The percentage of CD34[+] myeloid progenitor cells within CD45[+] population [1 point if ≥2%)
- The frequency of hematogones within CD34[+] compartment [1 point if <5%]
- CD45 expression on myeloid progenitors relative to CD45 expression on lymphocytes [1 point if the ratio of mean fluorescence intensity (MFI) of CD45 on lymphocytes/MFI of CD45 on gated CD34[+] myeloblasts ≤4 or ≥7.5]
- The evaluation of neutrophils granularity by orthogonal SSC compared to SSC of benign lymphocytes [1 point if ratio of SSC peak channel on total granulocytic cells (CD10[+] and CD10[−])/SSC peak channel of lymphocytes ≤6]

Based on Ogata score, MDS is indicated if the sum of the abnormal parameters is ≥2 [84]. Several other groups have published FC scoring methods and guidelines for MDS diagnosis based on the detection of immunophenotypic abnormalities during maturation of granulocytes, monocytes and lymphocytes [8, 39, 47, 50, 52, 57, 61, 65, 67, 68, 84–88]. Barreau et al. demonstrated that the scoring of abnormal expression patterns on both granulocytic and monocytic cell populations ("Diff score") added to the Ogata score is a simple multiparameter flow cytometric tool allowing reproducible MDS diagnosis [65]. Chu et al. proposed another scoring system based on antigen expression in neutrophils and monocytes [89]. European LeukemiaNet Working Group proposed the integrated flow cytometry score (iFC) based on the adopted Wells scoring system which includes Ogata score and aberrant phenotype of neutrophils and monocytes and aberrant antigen expression of blasts [39, 52, 60, 61]. Table 19.2 lists FC parameters used in the MDS scoring systems.

FC results based on iFC [52]:

- A: FC results show no sign of MDS
- B: FC results show signs of MDS, If FC results are contradictory with other diagnostic parameters, it is recommended to repeat the BM analysis after appropriate clinical interval
- C: FC results may fit MDS. These results should always be interpreted in the context of other diagnostic parameters. Calculation of iFC is presented in Table 19.3.

TABLE 19.2: FC Parameters Used in Scoring Systems for the Diagnosis of MDS

Blasts	Neutrophils/Maturing Myeloid Cells	Monocytes
Increased number (>3%)	Decreased SSC	Decreased or increased SSC
Abnormal SSC	Decreased myeloid to lymphoid ratio	Increased or decreased number when compared to lymphocytes
Positive expression of CD11b	Abnormal CD11b versus CD13 pattern	Abnormal expression of CD13
Abnormal expression of CD13	Abnormal CD13 versus CD16 pattern	Abnormal expression of CD14
Positive expression of CD15	Abnormal expression of CD15	Abnormal expression of CD33
Abnormal expression of CD33	Abnormal expression of CD33	Abnormal expression of CD36
Abnormal expression of CD34	Positive expression of CD34	Abnormal expression of CD45
Abnormal expression of CD45	Positive expression of HLA-DR	Abnormal expression of HLA-DR
Abnormal expression of CD117	Overexpression of CD56	Positive expression of CD34
Positive "lineage infidelity" (presence of CD5, CD7, CD19, or CD56)	Positive "lineage infidelity" (presence of CD5, CD7, CD19)	Positive "lineage infidelity" (presence of CD5, CD7, CD19)
Abnormal expression of HLA-DR	Asynchronous shift to the left	Overexpression of CD56

TABLE 19.3: Calculation of iFC MDS Scoring by Flow Cytometry

iFC Score	A	A/B[a]	A/B[a]	A/B[a]	B/C[a]	B/C[a]	C	C
FC score (Ogata)	<2	<2	<2	≥2	≥2	≥2	<2	≥2
Aberrant phenotype of blasts	–	–	+	–	–	+	+	+
Aberrant phenotype of neutrophils[b] or monocytes[c]	–	+	–	–	+	–	+	+

Source: After van de Loosdrecht et al. (2013).

[a] Choice for "A" or "B" depends on the kind and number of aberrancies that are noted by FC (see Table 19.2).

[b] Low SSC or ≥2 other abnormalities.

[c] CD56 positivity of ≥2 other abnormalities.

The score, adopted from Wells et al. is calculated as below [61]:

- 0: no FC abnormalities
- 1 point: Single abnormality in either neutrophils/maturing myeloid cells or monocytes
- 2 points: Single abnormality in both neutrophils/maturing myeloid cells or monocytes, 2 or 3 abnormalities in either neutrophils/maturing myeloid cells or monocytes or expression of CD34 or lineage infidelity markers on either neutrophils/maturing myeloid cells or monocytes
- 3 points: 4 or more abnormalities in either neutrophils/maturing myeloid cells or monocytes
- 4 points: 2 or 3 abnormalities in both neutrophils/maturing myeloid cells or monocytes
- 1 additional point for decreased myeloid/lymphoid ratio (<1), normal percentage of myeloid blasts (<5%) with flow cytometric abnormalities
- 2 additional points for increased percentage of abnormal myeloid blasts (5%–10%)
- 3 additional points for increased percentage of abnormal myeloid blasts (11%–20%)
- 4 additional points for blasts >20% (those cases are classified as AML based on current WHO classification).

Davydova et al. compared Ogata, Wells, and iFC scores and confirmed the usefulness of scoring systems in the diagnosis of MDS [53]. In their series, the frequency of Ogata score ≥2 was higher in all variants of MDS compared with control, except for MDS-LB, in which Ogata score ≥2 was obtained only in 50% of cases. In the same report, the median Wells score was higher in the MDS group compared to the score in control group. The highest Wells score was found in MDS-IB-2 [53]. Relatively high Wells scores (4 and 5) were found in 18.1% patients in control group (five patients with PNH, three with AA two patients each with vitamin B12 deficiency and lymphomas, and three patients with autoimmune disorders) [53].The iFC score frequency of A, B, and C in the entire MDS cohort was 12.75%, 8.89%, and 78.45%, respectively. The B score was noted in four patients with PNH, two cases of each, AA, and lymphoma, and one case of B12 deficiency. The score C was found in one case of each PNH and B12 deficiency [53]. The overall sensitivity and specificity values reported by Davydova et al. were 77.5% and 90.4% for the Ogata score, 79.4% and 81.9% for Wells score, and 87.3% and 87.6% for the iFC score [53].

Genetic features

Cytogenetics/FISH

None of the morphologic findings is specific for MDS, as they may be seen in nutritional deficiency, viral infections, medications (toxic therapy or Neupogen therapy), or congenital or acquired marrow failure syndromes. Therefore, current WHO classification defined specific criteria for the diagnosis of MDS, including finding of ≥10% dysplastic cells in a least one hematopoietic lineage, an abnormal karyotype (exclusive of certain nonspecific changes such as –Y), or an increase in myeloblasts (5%–19%) [1]. Recurring chromosomal abnormalities occur in 40%–70% of patients with primary MDS and in 95% of therapy-related MDS (tMDS), and are strong and independent prognostic indicators [12, 15, 90–99]. Presence of −Y, +8, or del(20q) as a sole abnormality does not allow for a definite diagnosis of MDS in the absence of morphological criteria or other criteria. Other abnormalities, such as −7/del(7q), −5/del(5q), i(17q)/t(17q), −13/del(13q), del(11q), del(12p), del(9q) in the presence of a refractory cytopenia but no morphologic evidence of dysplasia, are considered diagnostic for MDS.

Molecular testing

Somatic point mutations are common in MDS and are associated with specific clinical features. More than 40 different recurrent gene mutations have been associated with MDS. Mutated genes can be grouped into several functional pathways, including messenger RNA splicing, DNA methylation, chromatin modification (remodeling), transcription factors, DNA repair, and signal transduction. Although no single mutation is detectable in more than 25%–30% of patients, almost all patients with MDS defined by WHO criteria will have at least one of these somatic mutations detectable. The most commonly mutated genes in MDS include *TET2* (20%–30%), *SF3B1* (20%–30%), *ASXL1* (14%–22%), *SFRS2* (15%), *DNMT3A* (10%), *EZH2* (6%–10%), *U2AF1* (5%–10%), ZRSR2 (5%–10%), *TP53* (10%), *STAG2* (5%–7%), *IDH1/2* (5%), *RUNX1* (6%–12%), *BCOR* (5%), *NRAS* (5%), and *CBL* (5%) [11, 12, 100]. *JAK2* is rare in MDS (1%–5%) and usually occurs in MPN or mixed MDS/MPN such as MDS/MPN with SF3B1 mutation and thrombocytosis (MDS/MPN-SF3B1-T). Whole genome sequencing studies showed that the most frequent recurrent mutations in MDS affect the spliceosome machinery (40%–45%). The strongest genotype-phenotype correlation exists between mutations of *SF3B1* and the sideroblastic phenotype, which is caused by iron accumulation in erythroblast mitochondria. *SF3B1* mutations are found in 60%–80% of patients with MDS-SF3B1 and MDS/MPN-SF3B1-T [101–103]. Except for *SF3B1*, *DNMT3A*, *JAK2*, an *MPL* mutations, the majority of common mutations occur more frequently in higher-risk MDS [11].

Differential diagnosis of MDS

General considerations in differential diagnosis of MDS

The diagnosis of MDS is complex and requires correlation between multiple technologies including morphology, cytogenetics, immunophenotyping, molecular tests, and routine laboratory tests. Although the diagnosis is straightforward in cases

with profound dyspoiesis in one or more of the myeloid lineages and/or increased number of blasts, it is often challenging, especially in early stages of the disease. Differential diagnosis is also difficult in hypocellular and fibrotic variants of MDS, which need to be differentiated from AA and primary myelofibrosis (PMF), respectively. MDS is associated with anemia, thrombocytopenia, leukopenia, bi-cytopenia, or pancytopenia, and therefore differential diagnosis includes numerous conditions with unexplained cytopenias(s). Major considerations include iron deficiency anemia, anemia of chronic disease, hemolytic anemia, B12/folate deficiency, ITP, chronic infectious diseases, marrow damage due to exposure to toxins (e.g., arsenic, lead, ethanol, chloramphenicol, anti-tuberculosis drugs, antineoplastic drugs), viral infections (e.g., parvovirus, HIV; Figure 19.18), AIDS, thymoma, congenital dyserythropoietic anemia, acute leukemias (especially aleukemic leukemia), hypersplenism, chronic MPNs (especially PMF), AA, and infiltrative marrow processes (e.g., metastatic tumors, HCL and other B- and T-lymphoproliferations, Hodgkin lymphoma, Gaucher disease, and multiple myeloma). Certain lymphomas, e.g., angioimmunoblastic T-cell lymphoma (AITL) often present with anemia and/or other cytopenias. When parvovirus infection is considered, viral DNA testing is recommended for patients in aplastic crisis and for those who are immunocompromised.

The presence of dysplastic features (morphology and/or FC immunophenotyping) does not per se is diagnostic of MDS. Parvovirus B19 infection in HIV patients may be associated with erythroblastopenia with parvovirus infected giant megaloblastoid erythroblasts (Figure 19.18). Dysmaturation may be seen in healthy individuals and in conditions other than MDS, e.g., B12/folate deficiency, essential elements deficiency, certain drugs (e.g., cotrimoxazole), treatment with granulocyte colony stimulating factors (Figure 19.19), exposure to heavy metals (especially arsenic), therapeutic drugs (Figure 19.20) and toxins, PNH (Figure 19.21), viral infections, immunologic disorders, and hereditary conditions (e.g., congenital dyserythropoietic anemia). Antibiotic cotrimoxazole causes prominent neutrophilic nuclear hypolobation similar to changes seen in MDS. Identification of ALIP is not specific for MDS, as it can be seen in reactive conditions with increased blasts (e.g., BM regeneration after treatment of toxic insult), after treatment with Neupogen or in MPNs. Dyspoietic features are present (by definition) in CMML and MDS/MPN with neutrophilia, both representing mixed MDS/MPN neoplasms. Correlation with CBC data, blood smear, BM morphology, and immunophenotyping helps to diagnose CMML

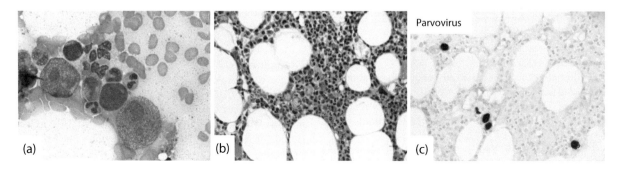

(a)   (b)   (c) Parvovirus

FIGURE 19.18 BM with parvovirus infection. (a) Aspirate smear with highly "dysplastic" erythroid precursors with typical viral inclusions. (b–c) BM core biopsy shows rare erythroid precursors infected by parvovirus (c, immunohistochemistry).

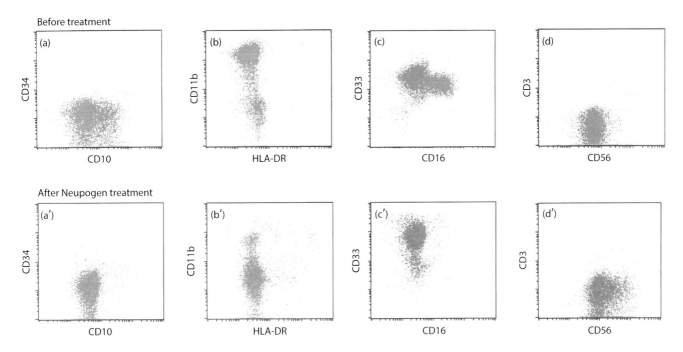

FIGURE 19.19 Dysmaturation associated with growth factor treatment (G-CSG; Neupogen). Patient with chronic renal failure and recent onset of pancytopenia with significant reduction in the expression of CD10 (a, a'), CD11b (b, b'), and CD16 (c, c') and aberrant expression of CD56 (d, d') one month after Neupogen (filgrastim) treatment (upper panels, before treatment; lower panels, after treatment).

Differential diagnosis of pancytopenia:

- MDS
- AML ("aleukemic")
- Acute promyelocytic leukemia (APL)
- Acute erythroid leukemia (AEL, pure erythroid leukemia)
- PMF
- SM
- HCL
- T-LGL leukemia
- PNH
- Hemophagocytic lymphohistiocytosis (HLH)
- Metastatic tumor/other bone marrow infiltrative process
- AA, congenital or acquired
- Gelatinous transformation of bone marrow
- Hypersplenism
- Toxic marrow damage (therapy, toxins, radiation)
- Infections (sepsis, malaria, viruses, other)

Morphologic differential diagnosis of MDS (Figure 19.22) includes:

- Dysplasia not associated with MDS
- Sideroblastic anemia
- IDUS
- Acute myeloid leukemia with myelodysplasia-related changes (AML-MRC)
- MPNs
- CMML

- MDS/MPN with neutrophilia
- MDS/MPN with SF3B1 mutation and thrombocytosis (MDS/MPN-SF3B1-T)
- Some B- and T-cell lymphomas
- SM
- AML
- Acute lymphoblastic leukemia (ALL)
- AEL (pure erythroid leukemia)
- Acute panmyelosis with myelofibrosis (APMF)

Differential diagnosis of dysgranulopoiesis identified by flow cytometry
Low side scatter of granulocytes
Abnormal granulocytes with low SSC must be differentiated from other cells with moderate CD45 and low SSC including blasts, monocytes, hypogranular variant of APL, and large cell lymphomas.

Phenotypic atypia of granulocytes
Many of the immunophenotypic abnormalities observed in patients with MDS are not specific and can be observed in reactive (benign) BM or blood samples, e.g., in post-chemotherapy marrow regeneration, viral infections, marrow involvement by lymphoma and treatment with growth factors (granulocyte colony-stimulating factor; G-CSF). MDS changes observed by FC may be similar to other myeloid disorders, especially MPNs or mixed MDS/MPN such as CMML. Presence of prominent neutrophilia with eosinophilia, basophilia, and lymphopenia helps to differentiate CML from MDS. Essential thrombocythemia

548   **Flow Cytometry in Neoplastic Hematology**

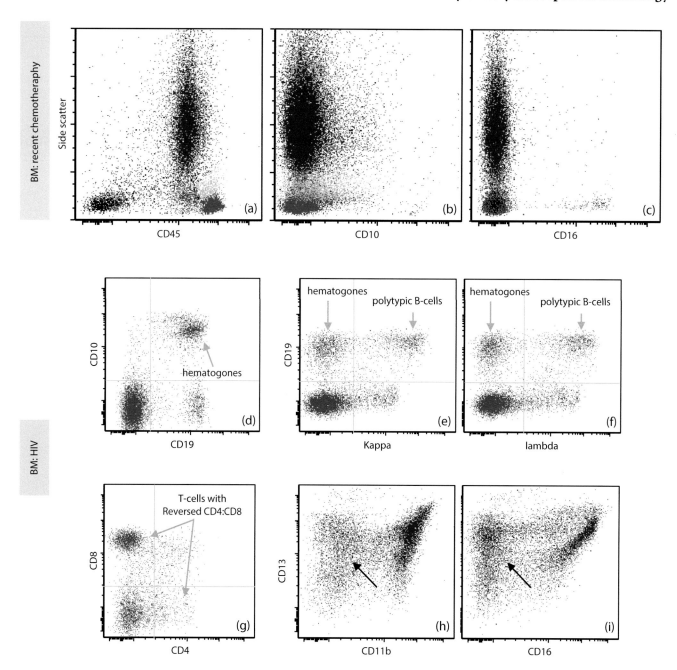

FIGURE 19.20 (a–c) Transient dyspoietic features and leftward shift following recent chemotherapy (for lymphoma). Granulocytes (purple dots) show down-regulation of CD45 (a), CD10 (b), and CD16 (c). (d–i) BM analysis from patient with HIV: increased hematogones (d); non-specific adsorption of surface immunoglobulins on B-cells (e–f; it is difficult to separate kappa+ from lambda+ B-cells); T-cells with reversed CD4:CD8 ratio (g); and subtle phenotypic atypia of maturing myeloid precursors (h–i; arrow).

(ET) or MPNs in early stages of the disease often yield normal FC results, but differentiating MDS from some of the MPNs, especially early (pre-fibrotic) phase of PMF is often not possible by FC analysis. Regenerating marrow may display marked myeloid shift, indicated by the predominance of granulocytes with low SSC and low-to-negative expression of CD10, CD11b, and CD16 and relatively bright CD33. CD56 may be aberrantly expressed on subset of granulocytes and/or monocytes in reactive conditions, including regenerating marrow, infections, and treatment with

G-CSF. The G-CSF treated marrow display increased immature cells, dyssynchronous expression of CD13 and CD16 among the maturing granulocytes, decreased SSC of maturing myeloid cells and increased CD45 expression on the immature granulocytes [104]. Maturing myeloid cells with prominent down-regulation of CD10 and CD16 need to be differentiated form neoplastic promyelocytes. Aberrant lack of expression of CD14 by monocytes is seen in PNH patients. Patients with viral infections, especially HIV often display aberrant pattern of myeloid

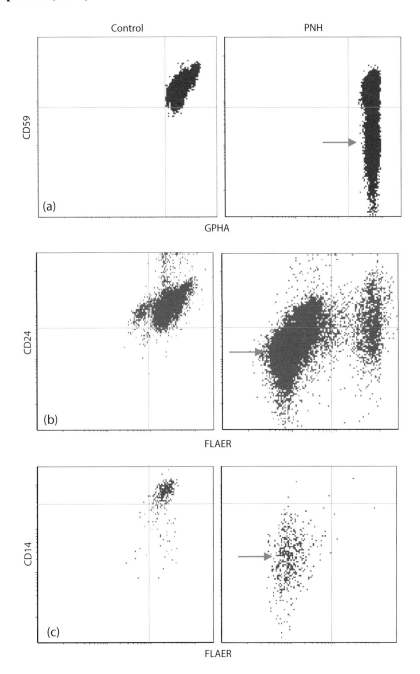

FIGURE 19.21 PNH – FC analysis. PNH clones (arrow) detected by FC show down-regulation of CD59 on red blood cells (a), down-regulation of CD24 and FLAER on neutrophils (b) and down-regulation of CD14 and FLAER on monocytes (c).

maturation. Other FC features associated with HIV in the BM samples include lack polytypic plasmacytosis, increased hematogones, T-cells with reversed CD4:CD8 ratio and non-specific adsorption of surface immunoglobulins on polyclonal B-cells.

Increased blasts

Increased number of myeloblasts may be seen in other processes, such as chronic MPNs (accelerated phase), MDS/MPN (e.g., CMML, MDS/MPN with neutrophilia), regenerating marrow or residual AML.

Aberrant phenotype of blasts

Aberrant phenotype of blasts can be observed in regenerating marrow or after treatment with growth factors, in AML (see Chapters 5 and 24), in CMML (Chapter 20) and MPNs (Chapter 21).

Aberrant phenotype of monocytes

Aberrant phenotype of monocytes can be observed in CMML (see Chapter 20), acute monocytic leukemia (see Chapter 22), MPNs (see Chapter 21), and in certain reactive conditions.

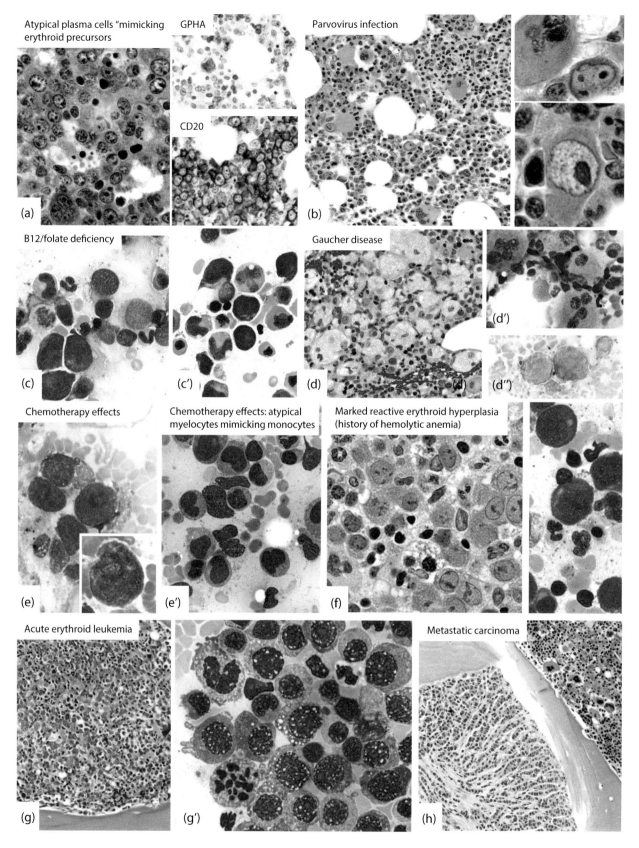

FIGURE 19.22 MDS – differential diagnosis (part 1). (a) MM. Atypical plasma cells mimic dysplastic red cell precursors (GPHA staining is negative; CD20 staining is positive). (b) Parvovirus infection. (c) B12/folate deficiency. (d) Gaucher disease (d, core biopsy; d′ aspirate smear stained with W-G; d″, aspirate smear with iron staining). (e) Post-treatment dyspoiesis (atypical myeloid precursor mimicking promyelocytes). (f) Reactive erythroid hyperplasia associated with hemolysis. (g) Acute erythroid leukemia (AEL). (h) Metastatic carcinoma. (*Continued*)

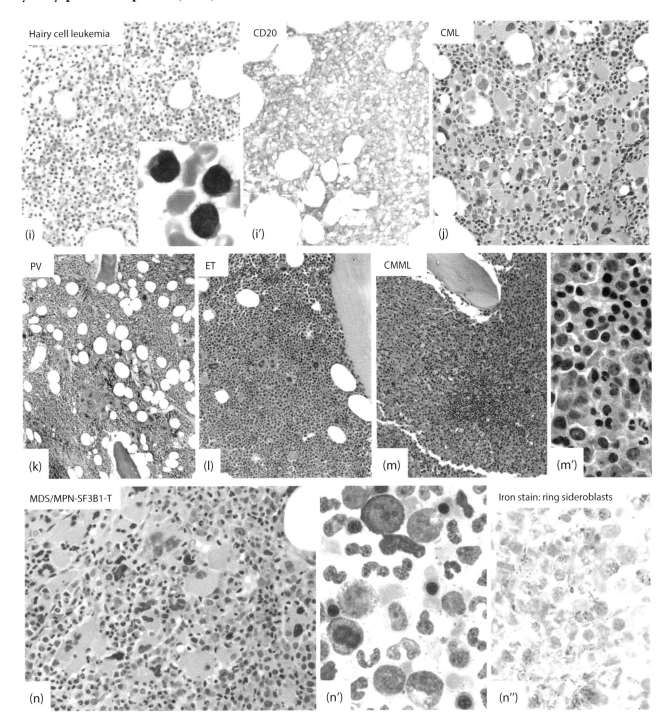

FIGURE 19.22 (*Continued*) MDS – differential diagnosis (part 2). (i) HCL. (j–n) Myeloproliferative neoplasms: CML (j), PV (k), ET (l), CMML (m), and mixed myelodysplastic/myeloproliferative neoplasm – MDS/MPN-SF3B1-T (n).

Lack of hematogones

Decreased percentage or complete lack of progenitor B-cells may be seen in elderly patients and in patient with immunodeficiency. MPNs, including CML, show decreased or complete lack of hematogones, often more prominent than in MDS.

References

1. Swerdlow, S.H., et al., ed. *WHO classification of tumors of haematopoietic and lymphoid tissues*. 2016, IARC: Lyon.

2. Bono, E., et al., *Clinical, histopathological and molecular characterization of hypoplastic myelodysplastic syndrome*. Leukemia, 2019. **33**(10): p. 2495–505.

3. Schanz, J., et al., *Coalesced multicentric analysis of 2,351 patients with myelodysplastic syndromes indicates an underestimation of poor-risk cytogenetics of myelodysplastic syndromes in the international prognostic scoring system*. J Clin Oncol, 2011. **29**(15): p. 1963–70.

4. Heim, S., *Cytogenetic findings in primary and secondary MDS*. Leuk Res, 1992. **16**(1): p. 43–6.

5. Taylor, J., W. Xiao, and O. Abdel-Wahab, *Diagnosis and classification of hematologic malignancies on the basis of genetics*. Blood, 2017. **130**(4): p. 410–23.

6. Mufti, G.J., et al., *Diagnosis and classification of myelodysplastic syndrome: International Working Group on Morphology of myelodysplastic syndrome (IWGM-MDS) consensus proposals for the definition and enumeration of myeloblasts and ring sideroblasts.* Haematologica, 2008. **93**(11): p. 1712–7.

7. Mufti, G.J., et al., *Diagnostic algorithm for lower-risk myelodysplastic syndromes.* Leukemia, 2018. **32**(8): p. 1679–96.

8. Takeuchi, A., et al., *Diagnostic value of flow cytometry standardized using the European LeukemiaNet for myelodysplastic syndrome.* Acta Haematol, 2020. **143**(2): p. 140–5.

9. Graubert, T. and M.J. Walter, *Genetics of myelodysplastic syndromes: new insights.* Hematology Am Soc Hematol Educ Program, 2011. **2011**: p. 543–9.

10. Valent, P., *ICUS, IDUS, CHIP and CCUS: diagnostic criteria, separation from MDS and clinical implications.* Pathobiology, 2019. **86**(1): p. 30–38.

11. Haferlach, T., et al., *Landscape of genetic lesions in 944 patients with myelodysplastic syndromes.* Leukemia, 2013. **28**(2): p. 241–7.

12. Della Porta, M.G., et al., *Minimal morphological criteria for defining bone marrow dysplasia: a basis for clinical implementation of WHO classification of myelodysplastic syndromes.* Leukemia, 2015. **29**(1): p. 66–75.

13. Pellagatti, A. and J. Boultwood, *The molecular pathogenesis of the myelodysplastic syndromes.* Eur J Haematol, 2015. **95**(1): p. 3–15.

14. Caponetti, G.C. and A. Bagg, *Mutations in myelodysplastic syndromes: Core abnormalities and CHIPping away at the edges.* Int J Lab Hematol, 2020. **42**(6): p. 671–84.

15. Zhou, J., A. Orazi, and M.B. Czader, *Myelodysplastic syndromes.* Semin Diagn Pathol, 2011. **28**(4): p. 258–72.

16. Orazi, A. and M.B. Czader, *Myelodysplastic syndromes.* Am J Clin Pathol, 2009. **132**(2): p. 290–305.

17. Garcia-Manero, G., *Myelodysplastic syndromes: 2012 update on diagnosis, risk-stratification, and management.* Am J Hematol, 2012. **87**(7): p. 692–701.

18. Gangat, N., M.M. Patnaik, and A. Tefferi, *Myelodysplastic syndromes: contemporary review and how we treat.* Am J Hematol, 2016. **91**(1): p. 76–89.

19. Stetler-Stevenson, M. and C.M. Yuan, *Myelodysplastic syndromes: the role of flow cytometry in diagnosis and prognosis.* Int J Lab Hematol, 2009. **31**(5): p. 479–83.

20. Valent, P. and R. Wieser, *Update on genetic and molecular markers associated with myelodysplastic syndromes.* Leuk Lymphoma, 2009. **50**(3): p. 341–8.

21. Valent, P., et al., *Proposed diagnostic criteria for classical CMML, CMML variants and pre-CMML conditions.* Haematologica, 2019. **104**(10): p. 1935–49.

22. Valent, P., et al., *Proposed minimal diagnostic criteria for myelodysplastic syndromes (MDS) and potential pre-MDS conditions.* Oncotarget, 2017. **8**(43): p. 73483–500.

23. Wimazal, F., et al., *Idiopathic cytopenia of undetermined significance (ICUS) versus low risk MDS: the diagnostic interface.* Leuk Res, 2007. **31**(11): p. 1461–8.

24. Jaiswal, S., et al., *Age-related clonal hematopoiesis associated with adverse outcomes.* N Engl J Med, 2014. **371**(26): p. 2488–98.

25. Shlush, L.I., *Age-related clonal hematopoiesis.* Blood, 2018. **131**(5): p. 496–504.

26. Xie, M., et al., *Age-related mutations associated with clonal hematopoietic expansion and malignancies.* Nat Med, 2014. **20**(12): p. 1472–8.

27. Steensma, D.P., et al., *Clonal hematopoiesis of indeterminate potential and its distinction from myelodysplastic syndromes.* Blood, 2015. **126**(1): p. 9–16.

28. Genovese, G., et al., *Clonal hematopoiesis and blood-cancer risk inferred from blood DNA sequence.* N Engl J Med, 2014. **371**(26): p. 2477–87.

29. Heuser, M., F. Thol, and A. Ganser, *Clonal hematopoiesis of indeterminate potential.* Dtsch Arztebl Int, 2016. **113**(18): p. 317–22.

30. Link, D.C. and M.J. Walter, *'CHIP'ping away at clonal hematopoiesis.* Leukemia, 2016. **30**(8): p. 1633–5.

31. Young, A.L., et al., *Clonal haematopoiesis harbouring AML-associated mutations is ubiquitous in healthy adults.* Nat Commun, 2016. **7**: p. 12484.

32. Valent, P., et al., *Idiopathic cytopenia of undetermined significance (ICUS) and idiopathic dysplasia of uncertain significance (IDUS), and their distinction from low risk MDS.* Leuk Res, 2012. **36**(1): p. 1–5.

33. Valent, P. and H.P. Horny, *Minimal diagnostic criteria for myelodysplastic syndromes and separation from ICUS and IDUS: update and open questions.* Eur J Clin Invest, 2009. **39**(7): p. 548–53.

34. Stetler-Stevenson, M., et al., *Diagnostic utility of flow cytometric immunophenotyping in myelodysplastic syndrome.* Blood, 2001. **98**(4): p. 979–87.

35. Maynadie, M., et al., *Immunophenotypic clustering of myelodysplastic syndromes.* Blood, 2002. **100**(7): p. 2349–56.

36. Ogata, K., et al., *Clinical significance of phenotypic features of blasts in patients with myelodysplastic syndrome.* Blood, 2002. **100**(12): p. 3887–96.

37. Del Canizo, M.C., et al., *Immunophenotypic analysis of myelodysplastic syndromes.* Haematologica, 2003. **88**(4): p. 402–7.

38. Benesch, M., et al., *Flow cytometry for diagnosis and assessment of prognosis in patients with myelodysplastic syndromes.* Hematology, 2004. **9**(3): p. 171–7.

39. Wells, D.A., et al., *Myeloid and monocytic dyspoiesis as determined by flow cytometric scoring in myelodysplastic syndrome correlates with the IPSS and with outcome after hematopoietic stem cell transplantation.* Blood, 2003. **102**(1): p. 394–403.

40. Wood, B.L., *Myeloid malignancies: myelodysplastic syndromes, myeloproliferative disorders, and acute myeloid leukemia.* Clin Lab Med, 2007. **27**(3): p. 551–75, vii.

41. Wood, B.L., et al., *2006 Bethesda International Consensus recommendations on the immunophenotypic analysis of hematolymphoid neoplasia by flow cytometry: optimal reagents and reporting for the flow cytometric diagnosis of hematopoietic neoplasia.* Cytometry B Clin Cytom, 2007. **72 Suppl 1**: p. S14–22.

42. Kussick, S.J., et al., *Four-color flow cytometry shows strong concordance with bone marrow morphology and cytogenetics in the evaluation for myelodysplasia.* Am J Clin Pathol, 2005. **124**(2): p. 170–81.

43. Cherian, S., et al., *Flow-cytometric analysis of peripheral blood neutrophils: a simple, objective, independent and potentially clinically useful assay to facilitate the diagnosis of myelodysplastic syndromes.* Am J Hematol, 2005. **79**(3): p. 243–5.

44. Truong, F., et al., *The utility of flow cytometric immunophenotyping in cytopenic patients with a non-diagnostic bone marrow: a prospective study.* Leuk Res, 2009. **33**(8): p. 1039–46.

45. Loken, M.R., et al., *Flow cytometry in myelodysplastic syndromes: report from a working conference.* Leuk Res, 2008. **32**(1): p. 5–17.

46. Ogata, K., *Diagnostic flow cytometry for low-grade myelodysplastic syndromes.* Hematol Oncol, 2008. **26**(4): p. 193–8.

47. Satoh, C., et al., *Flow cytometric parameters with little interexaminer variability for diagnosing low-grade myelodysplastic syndromes.* Leuk Res, 2008. **32**(5): p. 699–707.

48. Wells, D.A. and K. Ogata, *On flow cytometry in myelodysplastic syndromes, with caveats.* Leuk Res, 2008. **32**(2): p. 209–10.

49. Lorand-Metze, I., et al., *Detection of hematopoietic maturation abnormalities by flow cytometry in myelodysplastic syndromes and its utility for the differential diagnosis with non-clonal disorders.* Leuk Res, 2007. **31**(2): p. 147–55.

50. van de Loosdrecht, A.A., et al., *Standardization of flow cytometry in myelodysplastic syndromes: report from the first European LeukemiaNet working conference on flow cytometry in myelodysplastic syndromes.* Haematologica, 2009. **94**(8): p. 1124–34.

51. Cremers, E.M., et al., *Multiparameter flow cytometry is instrumental to distinguish myelodysplastic syndromes from non-neoplastic cytopenias.* Eur J Cancer, 2015. **54**: p. 49–56.

52. van de Loosdrecht, A.A. and T.M. Westers, *Cutting edge: flow cytometry in myelodysplastic syndromes.* J Natl Compr Canc Netw, 2013. **11**(7): p. 892–902.

53. Davydova, Y.O., et al., *Diagnostic significance of flow cytometry scales in diagnostics of myelodysplastic syndromes.* Cytometry B Clin Cytom, 2021. **100**(3): p. 312–21.

54. Westers, T.M., et al., *Standardization of flow cytometry in myelodysplastic syndromes: a report from an international consortium and the European LeukemiaNet Working Group.* Leukemia, 2012. **26**(7): p. 1730–41.

55. Westers, T.M., et al., *Immunophenotypic analysis of erythroid dysplasia in myelodysplastic syndromes. A report from the IMDSFlow working group.* Haematologica, 2017. **102**(2): p. 308–19.

56. Cremers, E.M., et al., *Implementation of erythroid lineage analysis by flow cytometry in diagnostic models for myelodysplastic syndromes.* Haematologica, 2017. **102**(2): p. 320–6.

57. Mathis, S., et al., *Flow cytometric detection of dyserythropoiesis: a sensitive and powerful diagnostic tool for myelodysplastic syndromes.* Leukemia, 2013. **27**(10): p. 1981–7.

58. Bowen, K.L., B.H Davis, *Abnormal pattern of expression of CD16 (FcR-III) and CD11b (CRIII) antigens by developing neutrophils in the bone marrow of patients with myelodysplastic syndrome.* Lab Hematol, 1997. **3**: p. 292–8.

59. Chang, C.C. and R.P. Cleveland, *Decreased CD10-positive mature granulocytes in bone marrow from patients with myelodysplastic syndrome.* Arch Pathol Lab Med, 2000. **124**(8): p. 1152–6.

60. van de Loosdrecht, A.A., T.M. Westers, and G.J. Ossenkoppele, *Flowcytometry in myelodysplastic syndromes: towards a new paradigm in diagnosis and prognostication?* Leuk Res, 2008. **32**(2): p. 205–7.

61. van de Loosdrecht, A.A., et al., *Identification of distinct prognostic subgroups in low- and intermediate-1-risk myelodysplastic syndromes by flow cytometry.* Blood, 2008. **111**(3): p. 1067–77.

62. Stachurski, D., et al., *Flow cytometric analysis of myelomonocytic cells by a pattern recognition approach is sensitive and specific in diagnosing myelodysplastic syndrome and related marrow diseases: emphasis on a global evaluation and recognition of diagnostic pitfalls.* Leuk Res, 2008. **32**(2): p. 215–24.

63. Vikentiou, M., et al., *Distinct neutrophil subpopulations phenotype by flow cytometry in myelodysplastic syndromes.* Leuk Lymphoma, 2009. **50**(3): p. 401–9.

64. Chen, X., B.L. Wood, and S. Cherian, *Immunophenotypic features of myeloid neoplasms associated with chromosome 7 abnormalities.* Cytometry B Clin Cytom, 2019. **96**(4): p. 300–9.

65. Barreau, S., et al., *Phenotypic landscape of granulocytes and monocytes by multiparametric flow cytometry: a prospective study of a 1-tube panel strategy for diagnosis and prognosis of patients with MDS.* Cytometry B Clin Cytom, 2020. **98**(3): p. 226–37.

66. Ogata, K., et al., *Diagnostic application of flow cytometric characteristics of CD34+ cells in low-grade myelodysplastic syndromes.* Blood, 2006. **108**(3): p. 1037–44.

67. Ogata, K., et al., *Diagnostic utility of flow cytometry in low-grade myelodysplastic syndromes: a prospective validation study.* Haematologica, 2009. **94**(8): p. 1066–74.

68. Malcovati, L., et al., *Flow cytometry evaluation of erythroid and myeloid dysplasia in patients with myelodysplastic syndrome.* Leukemia, 2005. **19**(5): p. 776–83.

69. Matarraz, S., et al., *The immunophenotype of different immature, myeloid and B-cell lineage-committed CD34+ hematopoietic cells allows discrimination between normal/reactive and myelodysplastic syndrome precursors.* Leukemia, 2008. **22**(6): p. 1175–83.

70. Cesana, C., et al., *Prognostic value of circulating CD34+ cells in myelodysplastic syndromes.* Leuk Res, 2008. **32**(11): p. 1715–23.

71. Huang, M., et al., *Correlation between bone marrow blasts counts with flow cytometry and morphological analysis in myelodysplastic syndromes.* Ann Lab Med, 2017. **37**(5): p. 450–3.

72. Orfao, A., et al., *Immunophenotyping of acute leukemias and myelodysplastic syndromes.* Cytometry A, 2004. **58**(1): p. 62–71.

73. Matarraz, S., et al., *Bone marrow cells from myelodysplastic syndromes show altered immunophenotypic profiles that may contribute to the diagnosis and prognostic stratification of the disease: a pilot study on a series of 56 patients.* Cytometry B Clin Cytom, 2010. **78**(3): p. 154–68.

74. Arroyo, J.L., et al., *Impact of immunophenotype on prognosis of patients with myelodysplastic syndromes. Its value in patients without karyotypic abnormalities.* Hematol J, 2004. **5**(3): p. 227–33.

75. Pirruccello, S.J., K.H. Young, and P. Aoun, *Myeloblast phenotypic changes in myelodysplasia. CD34 and CD117 expression abnormalities are common.* Am J Clin Pathol, 2006. **125**(6): p. 884–94.

76. Monreal, M.B., et al., *Increased immature hematopoietic progenitor cells CD34+/CD38dim in myelodysplasia.* Cytometry B Clin Cytom, 2006. **70**(2): p. 63–70.

77. Jilani, I., et al., *Differences in CD33 intensity between various myeloid neoplasms.* Am J Clin Pathol, 2002. **118**: p. 560–6.

78. Font, P., et al., *Evaluation of CD7 and terminal deoxynucleotidyl transferase (TdT) expression in CD34+ myeloblasts from patients with myelodysplastic syndrome.* Leuk Res, 2006. **30**(8): p. 957–63.

79. Sternberg, A., et al., *Evidence for reduced B-cell progenitors in early (low-risk) myelodysplastic syndrome.* Blood, 2005. **106**(9): p. 2982–91.

80. Della Porta, M.G., et al., *Flow cytometry evaluation of erythroid dysplasia in patients with myelodysplastic syndrome.* Leukemia, 2006. **20**(4): p. 549–55.

81. Park, S., et al., *Dyserythropoiesis evaluated by the RED score and hepcidin:ferritin ratio predicts response to erythropoietin in lower-risk myelodysplastic syndromes.* Haematologica, 2019. **104**(3): p. 497–504.

82. Wang, H., et al., *Clinical significance of a minor population of paroxysmal nocturnal hemoglobinuria-type cells in bone marrow failure syndrome.* Blood, 2002. **100**(12): p. 3897–902.

83. Ogata, S., K. Okumura, and H. Taguchi, *A simple and rapid method for the detection of poly(ADP-ribose) by flow cytometry.* Biosci Biotechnol Biochem, 2000. **64**(3): p. 510–5.

84. Della Porta, M.G., et al., *Multicenter validation of a reproducible flow cytometric score for the diagnosis of low-grade myelodysplastic syndromes: results of a European LeukemiaNET study.* Haematologica, 2012. **97**(8): p. 1209–17.

85. Porwit, A., et al., *Revisiting guidelines for integration of flow cytometry results in the WHO classification of myelodysplastic syndromes-proposal from the International/European LeukemiaNet Working Group for Flow Cytometry in MDS.* Leukemia, 2014. **28**(9): p. 1793–8.

86. Porwit, A., *Is there a role for flow cytometry in the evaluation of patients with myelodysplastic syndromes?* Curr Hematol Malig Rep, 2015. **10**(3): p. 309–17.

87. Bento, L.C., et al., *The use of flow cytometry in myelodysplastic syndromes: a review.* Front Oncol, 2017. **7**: p. 270.

88. Alhan, C., et al., *Application of flow cytometry for myelodysplastic syndromes: pitfalls and technical considerations.* Cytometry B Clin Cytom, 2016. **90**(4): p. 358–67.

89. Chu, S.C., et al., *Flow cytometric scoring system as a diagnostic and prognostic tool in myelodysplastic syndromes.* Leuk Res, 2011. **35**(7): p. 868–73.

90. Fenaux, P., *Myelodysplastic syndromes.* Hematol Cell Ther, 1996. **38**(5): p. 363–80.

91. Fenaux, P., P. Morel, and J.L. Lai, *Cytogenetics of myelodysplastic syndromes.* Semin Hematol, 1996. **33**(2): p. 127–38.

92. Morel, P., et al., *Prognostic factors in myelodysplastic syndromes: critical analysis of the impact of age and gender and failure to identify a very-low-risk group using standard mortality ratio techniques.* Br J Haematol, 1996. **94**(1): p. 116–9.

93. Schiffer, C.A., et al., *Prognostic impact of cytogenetic abnormalities in patients with de novo acute nonlymphocytic leukemia.* Blood, 1989. **73**(1): p. 263–70.

94. Berger, R., et al., *Prognostic significance of chromosomal abnormalities in acute nonlymphocytic leukemia: a study of 343 patients.* Cancer Genet Cytogenet, 1987. **28**(2): p. 293–9.

95. Greenberg, P., et al., *International scoring system for evaluating prognosis in myelodysplastic syndromes.* Blood, 1997. **89**(6): p. 2079–88.

96. Bernasconi, P., et al., *World Health Organization classification in combination with cytogenetic markers improves the prognostic stratification of patients with de novo primary myelodysplastic syndromes.* Br J Haematol, 2007. **137**(3): p. 193–205.

97. Bernasconi, P., et al., *Incidence and prognostic significance of karyotype abnormalities in de novo primary myelodysplastic syndromes: a study on 331 patients from a single institution.* Leukemia, 2005. **19**(8): p. 1424–31.

98. Olney, H.J. and M.M. Le Beau, *Evaluation of recurring cytogenetic abnormalities in the treatment of myelodysplastic syndromes.* Leuk Res, 2007. **31**(4): p. 427–34.

99. Cazzola, M., M.G. Della Porta, and L. Malcovati, *The genetic basis of myelodysplasia and its clinical relevance.* Blood, 2013. **122**(25): p. 4021–34.

100. Hou, H.A., et al., *Incorporation of mutations in five genes in the revised International Prognostic Scoring System can improve risk stratification in the patients with myelodysplastic syndrome.* Blood Cancer J, 2018. **8**(4): p. 39.

101. Visconte, V., et al., *SF3B1 haploinsufficiency leads to formation of ring sideroblasts in myelodysplastic syndromes.* Blood, 2012. **120**(16): p. 3173–86.

102. Visconte, V., et al., *SF3B1, a splicing factor is frequently mutated in refractory anemia with ring sideroblasts.* Leukemia, 2012. **26**(3): p. 542–5.

103. Papaemmanuil, E., et al., *Somatic SF3B1 mutation in myelodysplasia with ring sideroblasts.* N Engl J Med, 2011. **365**(15): p. 1384–95.

104. Kussick, S.J. and B.L. Wood, *Using 4-color flow cytometry to identify abnormal myeloid populations.* Arch Pathol Lab Med, 2003. **127**(9): p. 1140–7.

20

MIXED MYELODYSPLASTIC-MYELOPROLIFERATIVE NEOPLASMS

Chronic myelomonocytic leukemia

Introduction

Chronic myelomonocytic leukemia (CMML) is a clonal hematopoietic malignancy characterized by a persistent peripheral blood monocytosis $\geq 0.5 \times 10^9$/L with overlapping features of both myeloproliferative neoplasm (MPN) and a myelodysplastic neoplasm (MDS) [1–12]. Myelodysplastic component includes dysplasia, and myeloproliferative component includes leukocytosis and splenomegaly. Median age at diagnosis of CMML varies between 65 and 75 years and there is 2:1 male predominance [13, 14]. CMML is stratified into myelodysplastic variant (white blood cell count <13 × 10^9/L) and myeloproliferative variant (white blood cell count ≥13 × 10^9/L). Some patients present with skin lesions due to leukemia cutis. Similar to blastic phase (crisis) of chronic myeloid leukemia (CML), some patients with CMML may directly present in the blastic phase (acute myeloid leukemia, AML). Algorithmic approach to monocytosis and CMML is presented in Figure 20.1.

CMML is defined by WHO criteria [1]:

1. persistent absolute ($\geq 0.5 \times 10^9$/L) and relative (≥ 10%) monocytosis in the blood (with absolute monocytosis (>0.5–<1 × 10^9/L diagnosis requires presence of clonal cytogenetic or molecular abnormality and dysplasia)
2. <20% blasts in blood and bone marrow (BM) – blast count includes myeloblasts, monoblasts, and promonocytes
3. not meeting diagnostic criteria of CML or other MPNs
4. not meeting diagnostic criteria of myeloid/lymphoid neoplasms with tyrosine kinase fusions
5. Supporting criteria: (1) dysplasia in at least one lineage (in at least 10% of cells); (2) acquired clonal cytogenetic or molecular abnormality; (3) abnormal partitioning of blood monocytes (>94% classical monocytes with positive CD14 and negative CD16)
6. Requirements for diagnosis: criteria 1-4 must be present in all cases; if monocytosis is >1 × 10^9/L, one or more supporting criteria must be met; if monocytosis is <1 × 10^9/L, supporting criteria 1 and 2 must be met.

MPN such as CML (*BCR-ABL1*⁺), PV, and PMF, or other mixed MDS/MPNs such as MDS/MPN with neutrophilia may show absolute monocytosis (monocytes ≥1 × 10^9/L), but the monocytes do not exceed 10% of leukocytes [15–17]. MDS patients may show occasional monocytosis (even absolute), but monocytosis is neither chronic nor persistent as in CMML. CMML may occur in patients with mastocytosis and D816V *KIT* mutation, other myeloid or lymphoid neoplasms or as a therapy-related myeloid neoplasm (tCMML) following cytotoxic therapy [18–20]. Systemic mastocytosis (SM) with concurrent CMML represents a variant of SM with an associated hematologic neoplasm (SM-AHN). In some of patients with CMML and other neoplasms, the CMML clone is dominant, and the additional sub-clone is smaller in size and usually not relevant clinically, even if these smaller clones express certain driver mutations, such as *KIT* D816V or

a rearranged *PDGFRA* or *PDGFRB*. Rarely a *BCR-ABL1*⁺ CML may develop as an additional small-sized (sub)clone in patient with CMML. Cases with monocytosis, ring sideroblasts (>15%) and thrombocytosis (≥450 × 10^9/L) are diagnosed as mixed MDS/MPN with SF3B1 mutation and thrombocytosis (MDS/MPN-SF3B1-T). The presence of additional (chronic) myeloid, mast cell, or lymphoid neoplasms does not exclude the diagnosis of concurrent CMML, provided that the diagnostic WHO criteria for CMML are fulfilled [1, 10]. However, before making the diagnosis of CMML, other neoplasms should be excluded based on current WHO criteria including *BCR-ABL1*⁺ CML, MPN with *PDGFRA*, *PDGFRB*, *FGFR1* or *PCM1-JAK2*, *JAK2*⁺ PV, PMF, or ET with *JAK2*, *MPL*, or *CALR* mutation, AML with inv(16)/t(16;16), MDS/MPN with neutrophilia, or *CRSF3*⁺ chronic neutrophilic leukemia (CNL). Both the classic form of CMML and the special variants of CMML should be divided into primary (de novo) and secondary CMML (sCMML).

The sCMML includes patients who:

- received chemotherapy and/or radiation therapy in the past (therapy related CMML, tCMML), or
- have a history of a preceding MDS, MPN, or another indolent myeloid or mast cell neoplasm prior to the CMML diagnosis.

Similar to other myeloid neoplasms (MDS, MPN, AML), CMML may be proceeded by clonal hematopoiesis of indeterminate potential (CHIP), clonal cytopenia of unknown significance (CCUS), age-related clonal hematopoiesis (ARCH), idiopathic dysplasia of unknown significance (IDUS), or clonal hematopoiesis with oncogenic potential (CHOP) [10, 21–23]. ICUS is characterized by persistent cytopenia of any degree in one or more major blood cell lineages (erythrocytes, neutrophils, or platelets), in patients not meeting the minimal diagnostic criteria for CMML (or MDS, MPN) and the cytopenic state cannot be explained by any other (hematologic or non-hematologic) etiology. The clinical course of ICUS is variable, but may be followed by CMML, MDS, AML, SM, or even lymphoma. IDUS is diagnosed when BM or blood analysis shows significant dysplasia (e.g., macrocytosis, hypogranulated neutrophils, pseudo-Pelger cells) without accompanying cytopenia and without fulfilling the criterial for diagnosis of CMML, MDS, or MPN. Presence of molecular changes in patients with IDUS (but without any other evidence of MDS or CMML), changes the diagnosis to CHIP. The diagnosis of CHIP is based on the presence of at least one somatic mutation that is relevant clinically and is otherwise found in MDS (or other myeloid neoplasms), the absence of persistent cytopenia, and the exclusion of MDS and of all other hematopoietic neoplasms (and other clonal disorders) as underlying conditions [10, 21]. In patients with CCUS, cytopenia and clonal abnormalities can be detected, but no dysplasia is seen and no other features (criteria) sufficient to diagnose MDS or another clonal BM neoplasm are found [21]. The differential diagnosis between MDS, early CMML and CCUS may be difficult (especially in cases when subtle dysplasia

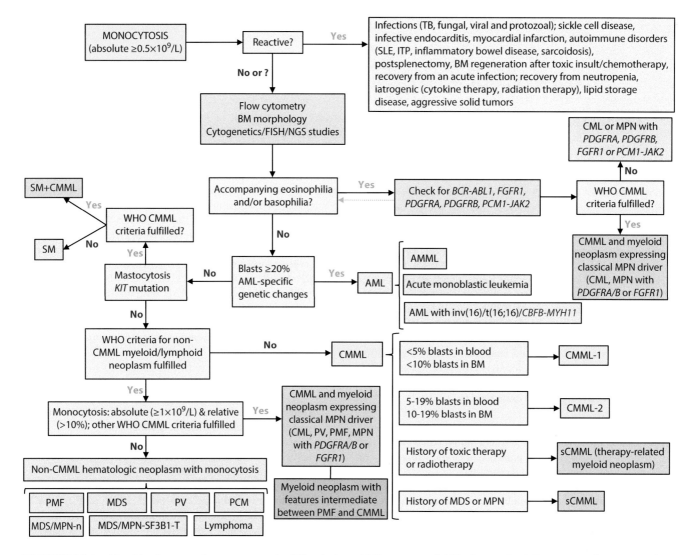

FIGURE 20.1 Algorithmic approach to monocytosis. *Abbreviations*: AML, acute myeloid leukemia; AMML, acute myelomonocytic leukemia; MDS/MPN-n, MDS/MPN with neutrophilia; CML, chronic myeloid leukemia; CMML, chronic myelomonocytic leukemia; sCMML, secondary CMML; TB, tuberculosis; PMF, primary myelofibrosis; PV, polycythemia vera; MDS; myelodysplastic syndrome; PCM, plasma cell myeloma; MPN, myeloproliferative neoplasm; MDS/MPN-RS-T, MDS/MPN with ring sideroblasts and thrombocytosis; SM, systemic mastocytosis; SLE, systemic lupus erythematosus; ITP, immune thrombocytopenic purpura; NGS, next gene sequencing.

is present but is limited to <10% of marrow cells). Follow-up morphologic and genetic BM analysis is those cases is recommended.

Minimal diagnostic criteria

Recently, minimal diagnostic criteria for classical CMML and its variants, as well as pre-CMML criteria were proposed by Valent et al. [10].

Minimal diagnostic criterial of classical CMML [the diagnosis of CMML can be established when all prerequisite criteria (A) and either morphologic dysplasia (B) or one or more of the co-criteria (C) are fulfilled]:

A. *Prerequisite criterial (all must be fulfilled):*
   - Persistent (3 months) peripheral blood monocytosis $\geq 1 \times 10^9$/L and relative monocytosis of $\geq 10\%$ of circulating blood leukocytes
   - Exclusion of *BCR-ABL1*+ leukemia, classical MPN, and all other BM neoplasms that could serve as a primary source of chronic persistent monocytosis

   - Blast cell count <20% in blood and BM smears and exclusion of all other histopathological, morphologic, molecular, and cytogenetic features that count as evidence for the presence of AML, such as Auer rods, overt AML by histology or immunohistochemistry, presence of AML-specific diagnostic cytogenetic and/or molecular markers, such as inv16, t(8;21), or t(15;17)

B. *Morphologic criterion = Dysplasia:*
   - Dysplasia in at least 10% of all cells in one of the three lineages in the BM smear: erythroid, neutrophilic, megakaryocytic

C. *Co-criteria (for patients fulfilling A but not B, and otherwise show typical clinical features of CMML such as splenomegaly):*
   - Typical chromosome abnormalities by conventional karyotyping or FISH [+8, −7/del(7q), −Y, complex karyotype, −20/del(20q), +21, TET2 deletions, NT1 deletions, ETV6 deletions]

- Abnormal findings in histologic and/or immunohisto-chemical studies of BM biopsy sections supporting the diagnosis of CMML (leukemic infiltration of CD14+ monocytes and exclusion of AML)
- Abnormal immunophenotype of BM and blood cells by flow cytometry (FC), with multiple CMML-associated phenotypic aberrancies indicating the presence of an abnormal/dysplastic population of monocytic and other myeloid cells (utilizing a cutoff value of >94% MO1 monocytes, phenotyping can identify CMML cases with sensitivity of >90% and a specificity of >5%, and the decrease in MO3 monocytes is even as diagnostic as the increase in MO1 cells) [7, 24, 25]
- Evidence of clonal population of myeloid cells determined by molecular (sequencing) studies revealing CMML-related mutations (genes that are often mutated in the CMML/MDS context include, among other, *TET2*, *SRSF2*, *ASXL1*, and *SETBP1*. Minimal allele burden proposed to count as co-criterion: ≥10%)

Grading

Based on the number of blasts, CMML is divided into two categories (Table 20.1): CMML-0 (<2% blasts in blood, <5% blasts in BM), CMML-1 (2%–4% blasts in blood, 5%–9% blasts in BM), and CMML-2 (5%–19% blasts in blood and 10%–19% blasts in BM). Depending on the leukocyte count, CMML can be divided into a "dysplastic" variant (leukocyte count ≤13×10⁹/L) and a "proliferative" variant (leukocyte count>13 × 10⁹/L). The resulting grading system defines six distinct CMML variants with variable clinical outcome [26]. In patients who progress from CMML-1 to CMML-2 the CMML-status must be reconfirmed with all diagnostic approaches, including BM histology and immunohistochemistry, molecular studies, and FC in order to exclude AML (especially in cases with proliferative CMML-2).

Special variants of CMML

The special variants of CMML form a heterogeneous group of neoplasms comprising distinct clinical and biological entities [10]:

Oligomonocytic CMML

Former cases diagnosed as oligomonocytic CMML are not classified as CMML: the threshold for absolute monocytosis was lowered to 0.5 × 10⁹/L. To enhance diagnosis accuracy, when absolute monocytosis is <1 × 10⁹/L, detection of dysplasia in at least one lineage and clonal genetic abnormality is required for diagnosis.

Systemic mastocytosis (SM) with concomitant CMML (SM-CMML)

WHO criteria for SM are fulfilled. In most patients, CMML monocytes exhibit *KIT* D816V mutation.

CMML with a concomitant myeloid neoplasm expressing a classical MPN-driver, such as JAK2 V617F, BCR-ABL1 or rearranged PDGFRA/B or FGFR1.

WHO criteria for classical MPN such as CML, PMF, or a myeloid neoplasm with rearranged *PDGFRA/B* are fulfilled in addition to the criteria of CMML

CMML with expression of a molecular MPN-driver

Molecular drivers of classical MPN such as *JAK2* V617F or rearranged *PDGFRA/B* are found but diagnostic criterial for such MPN are not fulfilled (only criterial for CMML are met).

CMML with a concomitant lymphoid/ lymphoproliferative neoplasm

WHO criteria for a lymphoid neoplasm are met (e.g., Hodgkin lymphoma, CLL, MGUS, plasma cell myeloma, or B-cell lymphoma) in addition to CMML.

CMML with ring sideroblasts (CMML-RS)

Presence of absolute monocytosis in blood and >15% ring sideroblasts in BM is an unusual finding. Those cases are diagnosed as CMML-RS. CMML-RS has a clinical course close to that of classical MDS-RS and markedly better prognosis than classical CMML.

CMML with eosinophilia

CMML with eosinophilia is diagnosed when all criteria for CMML are met and there is also prominent eosinophilia (≥1.5 × 10⁹/L). All cases with CMML and eosinophilia should be tested for *PDGFRA*, *PDGFRB*, *FGFR1*, and *PCM1-JAK2*.

Therapy-related CMML (tCMML)

Therapy-related mycloid neoplasm in the form of CMML represents a CMML following chemotherapy or radiotherapy. sCMML develops in patients with a prior history of MDS or MPN.

Morphology
Cytology (blood)
Neoplastic cells in patients with CMML include blasts and monocytes at different stages of maturation:

- Myeloblasts are smaller than monocytes, have round or oval nucleus with fine chromatin, nucleolus, and basophilic cytoplasm with occasional granules.

TABLE 20.1: CMML Grading

Grading-based Variants	Diagnostic Features/Criteria
CMML-1	<10% blasts in BM smears and <5% blasts in blood[a]
Dysplastic CMML-1	Blood leukocytes ≤13 × 10⁹/L
Proliferative CMML-1	Blood leukocytes >13 × 10⁹/L
CMML-2	10%–19% blasts in BM smears and 5%–19% blasts in blood[a]
Dysplastic CMML-2	Blood leukocytes ≤13 × 10⁹/L
Proliferative CMML-2	Blood leukocytes >13 × 10⁹/L

[a] When blast cell count obtained from BM smears and those obtained from blood differ and do not fit into one distinct grade of CMML (e.g., BM blasts 4% and blood blasts 6%) grading should be based on the higher blast cell percentage.

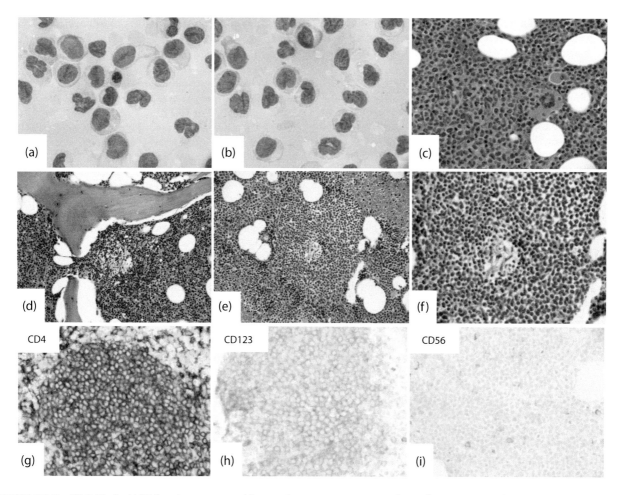

FIGURE 20.2 CMML. (a–b) BM aspirate smear with prominent monocytosis with cytologic atypia and only occasional immature monocytes. (c) BM core biopsy shows hypercellular marrow with monocytosis and megakaryocytic atypia. (d–i) Aggregates of plasmacytoid dendritic cells with ≥10 cells/aggregate. Core biopsy (d) shows paratrabecular cluster of plasmacytoid dendritic cells (low magnification). Clot section (e–f, H&E, low and higher magnification; g–I, immunohistochemistry) shows cluster of plasmacytoid dendritic cells which are positive for CD4 (g) and CD123 (h), and negative for CD56 (i).

- Monoblasts have round or oval nucleus with delicate, finely dispersed (lace-like) chromatin, prominent nucleolus, and basophilic cytoplasm with absent to rare azurophilic granules. It is larger than mature monocyte.
- Promonocytes are larger than mature monocytes, have convoluted (indented or folded) nucleus with delicate immature chromatin, visible nucleoli, and variable basophilic cytoplasm with occasional granules. Promonocytes differ from monoblasts by their nuclear shape.
- Mature monocyte has irregular (convoluted) nucleus with condensed chromatin without nucleolus, and gray to pink cytoplasm with occasional vacuoles or granules (atypical monocytes differ from mature monocytes by slightly smaller size, inconspicuous to prominent nucleolus, prominent nuclear shape irregularities, and more condensed chromatin).

Monocytes at different stages of maturation are positive for the nonspecific esterases (NSEs; alpha-naphthyl acetate, and alpha-naphthyl butyrate) and most often negative for myeloperoxidase (MPO). Blood smear shows leukocytosis with monocytosis (≥1 × 10^9/L; on average ~8 × 10^9/L). Monocytes comprise >10% of the leukocytes. There is no prominent eosinophilia or basophilia. Some cases may show normal or even decreased leukocyte count. Monocytes are mostly mature without significant atypia (Figures 20.2 and 20.3), but atypical monocytes with granulation, nuclear lobation or convolutions, grayish cytoplasm, or even immature monocytes may be present [27]. Some cells may display an unusual chromatin condensation pattern. Similar to MDS, neutrophils may display Pelgeroid changes and hypogranulation. Dysgranulopoiesis is more prominent in cases with lower white blood cells count (dysplastic CMM), when compared to proliferative variant of CMML. Monocytosis is often accompanied by anemia and/or thrombocytopenia. Some patients have monocytosis and neutrophilia, prompting the differential diagnosis of CML and aCML. Immature cells (blasts and promonocytes) account for <20% of the leukocytes.

Bone marrow

The BM aspirate smear shows increased number of mature monocytes, often with cytologic atypia. Immature cells (myeloblasts, monoblasts, and promonocytes comprise <20% of marrow nucleated cells). The BM in CMML is hypercellular (usually 80%–90%)

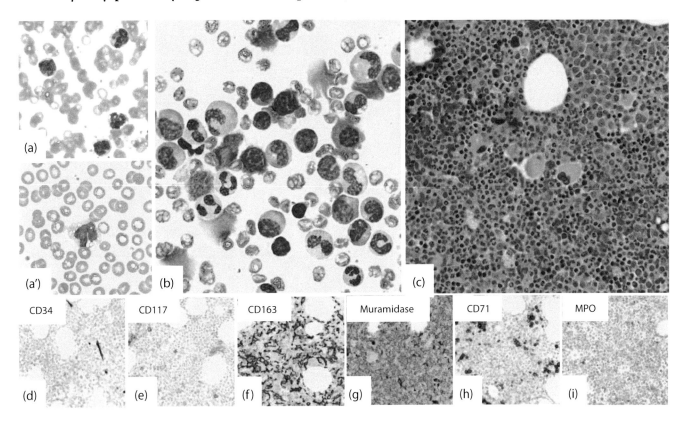

FIGURE 20.3 CMML – morphology and immunohistochemistry. Blood smear (a, a′) shows atypical, but mostly mature-appearing monocytes. BM aspirate smear (b) shows maturing myeloid and erythroid precursors with increased monocytic cells. BM histology (c) shows markedly hypercellular marrow with trilineage maturation, atypical megakaryocytes, and increased monocytes (best visualized with immunohistochemistry stainings; d–i). Blasts are not increased (d–e). Staining with CD163 (f) shows only scattered positive cells, but muramidase staining is strongly positive (g). Only rare erythroid precursors are noted (h). Some of the neoplastic monocytes display dim staining with MPO (i).

with prominent monocytosis, myeloid hyperplasia, megakaryocytic atypia, and dysgranulopoiesis and/or dyserythropoiesis (Figures 20.2–20.4). Only rare cases of CMML have been reported to show normocellular or even hypocellular BM. The myeloid to lymphoid ratio (M:E ratio) is increased. Majority of cases show clusters or nodules of myelomonocytic cells with relatively abundant finely granular cytoplasm, indented nuclei, and fine chromatin. Immunostaining with monocytic markers may help to identify monocytes and their precursors in BM. ALIP (at least three clusters of myeloid precursors) are often seen, especially in CMML-2. Blasts and promonocytes may be seen, but <20% of total white blood cells. In most cases, blasts and promonocytes account for fewer than 5% of blood leukocytes and fewer than 10% of the nucleated marrow cells. Higher number of blasts (plus promonocytes) may indicate transformation into AML. Subset of cases shows nodules of plasmacytoid dendritic cells which are CD4+ and CD123+ and usually CD56− (Figure 20.2)

Dysplastic changes involving at least one lineage are present, most often in the form of dysgranulopoiesis, but dyserythropoiesis (megaloblastoid changes, abnormal nuclear contours, and rarely ring sideroblasts) and megakaryocytic atypia may also be prominent (including hypolobated forms and micromegakaryocytes). Number of megakaryocytes varies but is usually normal or mildly increased. Reticulin fibrosis is often seen, usually focal and is more pronounced in CMML-2. Subset of cases shows mild lymphocytosis and plasmacytosis. If myelodysplasia is minimal,

CMML can still be diagnosed if an acquired cytogenetic or FISH abnormality is demonstrated or monocytosis has persisted for >3 months (and all other causes have been excluded). Staining with non-specific esterase (NSE) and MPO helps to differentiate between promonocytes, monocytes, and dyspoietic granulocytic precursors. NSE stains the cytoplasm of mature monocytes and can help differentiate promonocytes from monocytes. The sum of promonocytes and monocytes can be counted as "monocytic" cells for purposes of classification. The ratio of monocytes, granulocytes, and erythroid precursors varies.

Immunohistochemistry

The immunohistochemical evaluation of the BM core (or clot) sections (including CD34, CD117, monocytic markers, myeloid markers, and erythroid markers) is often helpful in patients suspected of having CMML (Figure 20.5). Staining with CD34 and CD117 (in addition to differential count on good quality BM aspirate smear) helps in differentiate between CMML-1 (blasts <10%), and CMML-2 (blasts 10%–19%), and acute myelomonocytic leukemia (AMML) (blasts and blasts equivalents ≥20%). Monocytic cells are strongly positive for muramidase, express CD68 and are often positive for CD163. MPO is most often negative. Muramidase (lysozyme) is often strongly positive. Neoplastic monocytes are often positive for CD56 (the staining by immunohistochemistry may be weak in decalcified core biopsy samples). Erythroid precursors can be visualized by GPHA, CD71, E-cadherin, and hemoglobin A. They are

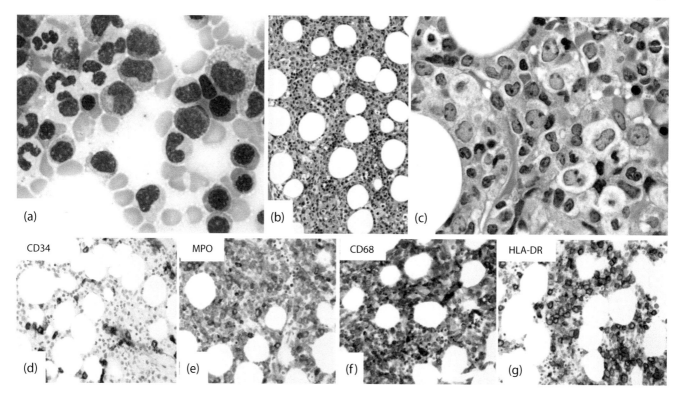

FIGURE 20.4   CMML. (a) BM aspirate with maturing myeloid cells and increased monocytes. (b–c) BM core biopsy is hypercellular marrow with prominent monocytosis. Immunohistochemical staining (d–g) demonstrates slightly increased blasts (d; CD34 staining), and predominance of cells positive for MPO (e), CD68 (f), and HLA-DR (g).

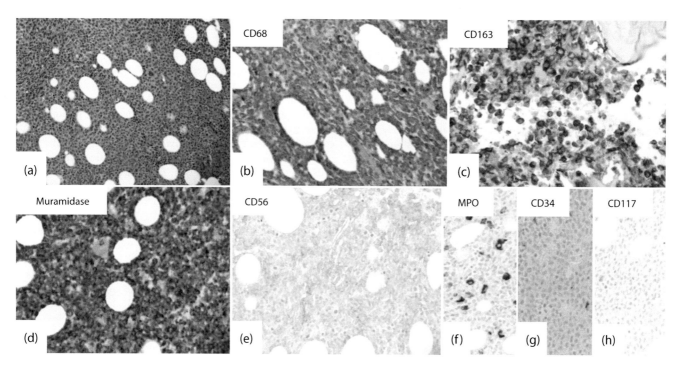

FIGURE 20.5   CMML – immunohistochemistry. (a) BM shows prominent involvement by CMML. Neoplastic monocytes are mature with strong expression of CD68 (b), CD163 (c), and muramidase (d), and weakly positive for CD56 (e). MPO (f), CD34 (g), and CD117 (h) are negative.

usually decreased in number and leftward shifted (CD71 or e-cadherin staining is more pronounced than GPHA). The CD68 staining helps to identify monocytic cells (phagocytic histiocytes show diffuse dense cytoplasmic staining, often vacuolated, dendritic histiocytes show long dendritic processes, monocytes have dark, coarse cytoplasmic granules, and promonocytes show fine cytoplasmic granules). The percentage of CD68+ cells is increased (it is higher in CMML-2) [28]. Interstitially located CD68+ cells had coarser and more easily identifiable granules (monocytes), whereas cells positive within myelomonocytic aggregates had fainter and finer granules (promonocytes) [28]. The staining with CD34 and CD117 shows increased number of immature cells in CMML-2. BM in CMML may show increased number of plasmacytoid dendritic cells expressing CD4, CD43, CD68, CD123, granzyme B, and rarely CD56.

Flow cytometry (FC)
Phenotype of monocytes
The percentage of monocytes assessed by FC ranges from 5% to 65% with average of 20%. The neoplastic monocytes in CMML have the phenotype of mature monocytes with bright expression of CD11b, CD11c, CD13, CD14, CD15, CD33, CD45, and CD64 (Figures 20.6–20.9; Table 20.2). A majority of cases express

HLA-DR (~77%), CD56 (~73%), and CD4 (~83%), and subset of cases is positive for CD2 (~48%), CD7 (~8%), CD10 (~17%), CD16 (~31%), and CD23 (~23%). Aberrant expression of CD14 (negative, variable, or partial expression) is seen in ~15% of cases. The aberrant phenotype of monocytes, including moderate (not bright) CD45 (6.3%), aberrant HLA-DR (partial, dim or variable; 12.6%), positive CD56 (72.9%), positive CD7 (8.3%), positive CD10 (16.7%), positive CD16 (31.3%), positive CD23 (22.9%), dim or variable CD64 (8.4%), dim or variable CD13 (20.9%), variable CD11b (4.2%), and/or partial or variable expression of CD14 (12.5%) is observed in majority of CMML cases (93.7%). Monocytes in CMML do not express blasts markers (CD34, CD117, CD133). Most cases exhibit aberrant expression of more than one antigen. Although many of the phenotypic abnormalities of monocytes present in CMML may be also seen in reactive monocytes, the changes observed in benign conditions are usually much less pronounced and involve minor population of monocytes. Low levels of CD56 expression (dim expression on <25% of monocytes) is reported in about half control cases [25, 29]. In majority of CMML cases the pattern of CD45 versus side scatter (SSC) is similar to normal monocytes (bright CD45 and low to mildly increased SSC).

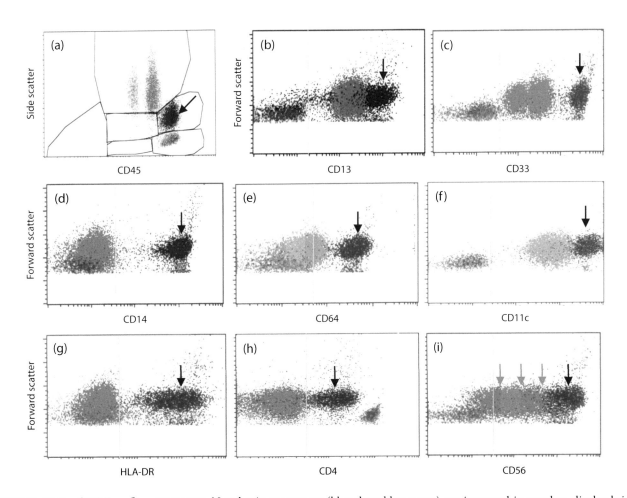

FIGURE 20.6 CMML – flow cytometry. Neoplastic monocytes (blue dots; blue arrow) are increased in number, display bright expression of CD45 (a), and have the phenotype similar to benign monocytes [with bright CD13 (b), bright CD33 (c), bright CD14 (d), bright CD64 (e), bright CD11c (f), positive HLA-DR (g), and positive CD4 (h)] with the exception of aberrant expression of CD56 (i). Granulocytes (gray dots; gray arrows) show aberrant expression of CD56 (i).

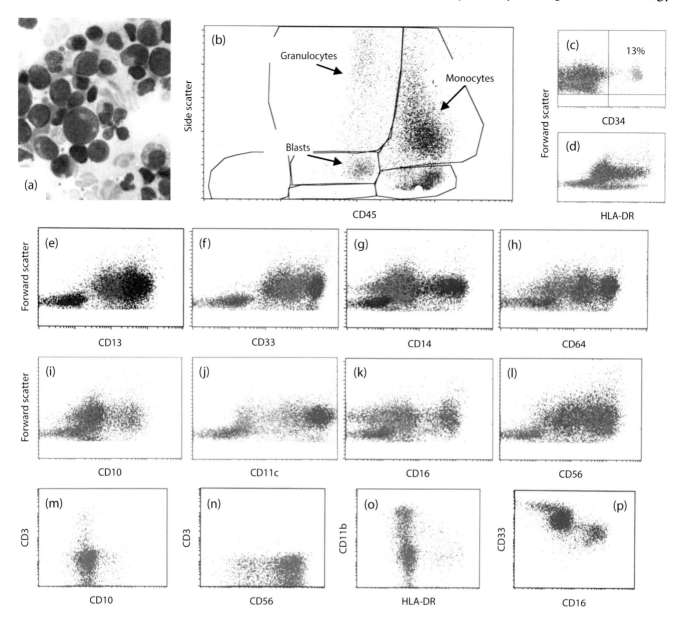

FIGURE 20.7   CMML – flow cytometry. BM aspirate (a) shows increased number of atypical monocytes. Flow cytometry (b–p) shows increased number of blasts (b–c; green dots) and monocytes (blue dots). Neoplastic monocytes are positive for CD13 (e), CD33 (f), CD14 (g), CD64 (h), and CD11c (j), and display aberrant expression of CD10 (i), CD16 (k), and CD56 (l). Granulocytes (b; gray dots) display aberrant expression of CD10 (m), CD56 (n), CD11b (o), and CD16 (p).

Monocyte subsets

Human blood monocytes can be classified into three distinct populations (Figure 20.10), classical CD16−/CD14bright+ mono-cytes (classical monocytes, MO1), intermediate CD16+/CD14bright+ monocytes (MO2), and non-classical CD16+/CD14dim+/− mono-cytes (MO3), with different gene expression profiles, chemokine receptor expression and phagocytic activities (Table 20.3) [3, 30, 31]. The MO1 constitute the major monocyte population (85%) in healthy conditions. The proportion of CD16+/CD14dim non-classical monocytes increases in various inflammatory condi-tions, and in malignancies including plasma cell myeloma [32] and AML [33]. In contrast to healthy persons or patients with reactive monocytosis, CMML patients demonstrate an increase in the fraction of CD14+/CD16− cells (classical monocytes, MO1;

Figure 20.11) and decreased fraction of "intermediate" monocytes (CD14+/CD16+, MO2) and "non-classical" monocytes (CD14dim+/−/ CD16+, MO3) [3]. Similar distribution of classical, intermediate, and non-classical monocytes as in CMML is observed in oligo-monocytic CMML [34].

Myeloblasts

The number of CD34+ blasts in the BM ranges from 0.2% to 12% (determined by FC analysis), with the median percentage of 1.25% (average, 3.1%; SD, 3.7). Shen et al. reported similar number of blasts (range from 0.02% to 12.6%; median 4.0%) [25]. Number of circulating blasts is higher in CMML-2 (median 1%) when compared to CMML-1 (median 0.5%) [35]. Similar to MDS, blasts in CMML often display aberrant phenotype,

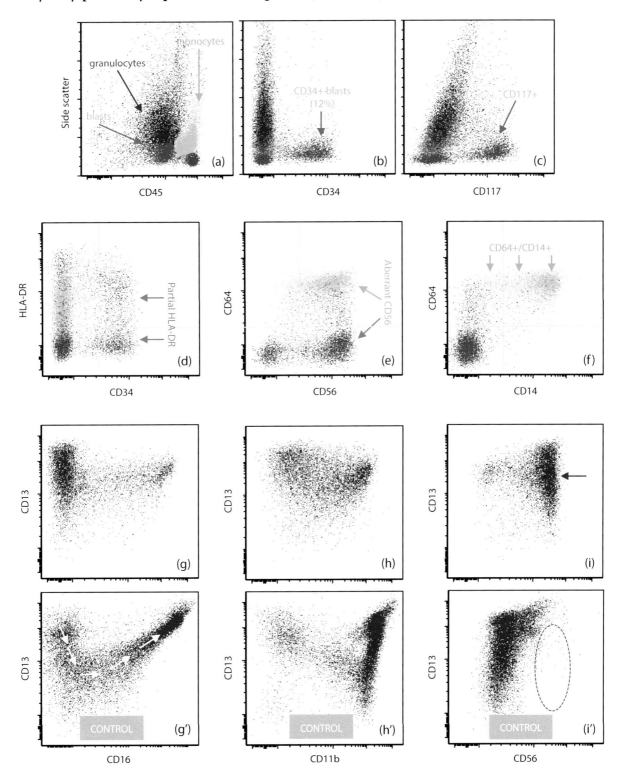

FIGURE 20.8 CMML – flow cytometry. Flow cytometric analysis of the BM shows increased monocytes (a; green dots), decreased side scatter of granulocytes (a; purple dots) and increased blasts (a; blue dots). Blasts are positive for CD34 (b) and CD117 (c) and display aberrant expression of CDHLA-DR (d; variable and partially negative) and CD56 (e; blue dots). Monocytes (green dots) are positive for HLA-DR (d) and show aberrant (positive) expression of CD56 (e). The majority of monocytes are positive for both CD64 and CD14 (f), but minor population of monocytes show variable expression of CD14 with some cells being negative. Gating on granulocytes only (g–i) shows abnormal phenotype indicating dyspoiesis, in the form of down-regulation of CD16 (g), aberrant pattern of CD13 versus CD11b (h) and prominent up-regulation of CD56 (i; arrow). Panels g′ to i′ represent normal control to better visualize phenotypic atypia of granulocytes (show in g–i).

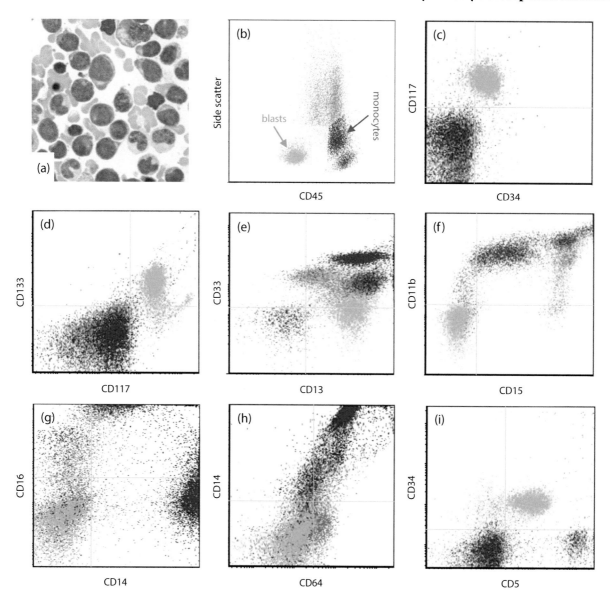

FIGURE 20.9 CMML 2 – flow cytometry. Aspirate smear shows myeloid leftward shift with blasts and monocytes (a). Flow cytometry (b–i) shows mixed population of blasts (green dots), monocytes (blue dots), neutrophils/maturing myeloid precursors (grey dots) and lymphocytes (red dots). Blasts are positive for CD45 (b), CD34 (c), CD117 (c–d), CD133 (d), CD13 (e) and show aberrant expression of CD33 (negative to dim; e) and CD5 (positive; i). Monocytes are positive for CD45 (b), CD13 and CD33 (e), CD11b and CD15 (f), CD14 and CD64 (g–h). Majority of monocytes are CD16⁻ (g).

including increased intensity of expression of CD117, CD123, CD33, and CD34, and/or presence of lymphoid lineage markers (CD19, CD7, CD56, CD2, or CD5) [25]. Aberrant phenotype of blasts was present in all CMML cases reported by Feng et al. compared to 16.7% of patients with reactive monocytosis [35].

In CMML, 94.1% cases showed ≥2 phenotypic abnormalities on blasts and 91% had ≥3 phenotypic abnormalities. The most common blast aberrancies identified in CMML included brighter expression of CD13, CD34, and CD117, and altered pattern of CD45/SSC [35].

TABLE 20.2: **Phenotypic Classification of Monocytes Based on CD14 and CD16 Expression, and Distribution of Monocyte-Subsets in CMML and Controls**

Monocytes Subset	Defining Phenotype	Frequency		
		CMML	MDS or MPN	Reactive BM
Classical (MO1)	CD14^bright+/CD16⁻	≥94%	70%–97%	<94%
Intermediate (MO2)	CD14^bright+/CD16⁺	<20%	5%–20%	5%–15%
Non-classical (MO3)	CD14^dim+/CD16⁺	<5%	5%–10%	5%–20%

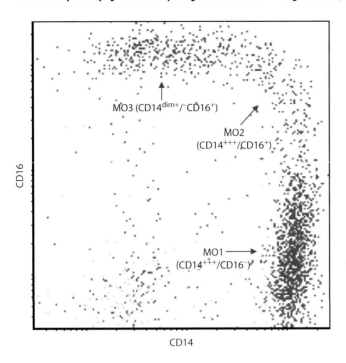

FIGURE 20.10 Classification of monocytes based on CD14 and CD16 expression.

Additional FC features

Additional FC features helpful in identifying CMML and excluding reactive monocytosis include circulating blasts (<20%), higher percentage of myeloblasts (<20% blasts), promonocytes and monocytes, lack or decreased number of hematogones, and/or

TABLE 20.3: Immunophenotypic Profile of CMML (*n* = 49)

	Frequency	Comments
CD2	49%	Including 29% dim, 8% subset, and 4% moderate expression
CD4	83%	Dim to moderate expression
CD7	8%	
CD10	16%	Includes 1 case positive on subset
CD11b	100%	Bright expression
CD11c	100%	Bright expression
CD13	96%	Includes 2 cases with dim expression on subset of cells
CD14	96%[a]	Includes 2 cases positive on subset; most often bright expression (only 1 case showed variable expression
CD16	30%	Mostly dim and/or partial expression (only 3 cases showed moderate expression)
CD23	22%	Includes 4 cases positive on subset
CD33	100%	Bright expression
CD34	0	1 case showed dim expression on minute population
CD45	100%	Bright expression
CD56	73%	
CD64	98%[a]	Usually bright expression
CD117	0	
HLA-DR	77%	Moderate to bright expression

[a] One case was negative for both CD14 and CD64 (CD11b and CD11c were positive).

phenotypic atypia of granulocytes (CD56 expression, decreased SSC, abnormal maturation pattern of CD11b/CD13/CD16, and decreased expression of CD10, CD11b, CD13, and/or CD16). In a series of CMML cases reported by Feng et al., granulocyte aberrancies were present in 91.2% CMML patient and only in 8.3% of patients with reactive monocytosis [35]. 20% or more blasts in blood or BM indicate AML.

Genetic features

No specific cytogenetic abnormalities are reported in patients with CMML. Clonal chromosomal changes are present in 20%–40%, with +8, −7/del(7q), and 12p rearrangements, complex karyotype, trisomy 21, isochromosome 17, deletion 5q, and deletion 20q being most common [27, 36–42]. Oo et al. reported therapy-related CMML with monosomy 7 and t(12;17)(p13;q11.2) [20]. Presence of specific MPN driver rearrangement such as *BCR-ABL1*, *PCM1-JAK2*, *FGFR1*, *PDGFRA*, or *PDGFRB* excludes CMML based on current WHO criteria, but a minor group of myeloid neoplasms may fulfill WHO criteria for both CMML and MPN and are classified as CMML with a concomitant myeloid neoplasm expressing a classical MPN-driver. CMML with mastocytosis and *KIT* mutation is classified as SM associated with other (non-mast cell) hematopoietic neoplasms (SM-AHN; SM-CMML).

CMML is associated with mutations in genes that encode epigenetic modifiers (*TET2*, *ASXL1*, *EZH2*), regulators of mRNA splicing (*SRSF2 SF3B1*, ZRSF2), cytokine signaling (*NRAS*, *KRAS*, *CBL*, *JAK2*), transcription factors (*RUNX1*), and mediators of DNA damage response (*TP53*, *PHF6*). Mutations in *TET2* are present in ~55%–60%, *SRSF2* in ~50%, *ASXL1* in ~40%, *RAS* mutation in ~10%–30%, *DNMT3A* in ~5%, *JAK2* mutations in ~8%–10%, and *SETBP1* mutations in ~18% of CMML [2, 4, 27, 43–50]. The association of *SRSF2* and *TET2* mutations may be highly specific for CMML [51]. Very rare cases of CMML with *NPM1* mutations have been reported (~5%) [52, 53]. Compared with CMML without *NPM1* mutations, CMML patients with *NPM1* mutation present with more severe anemia, higher BM monocyte percentage (Figure 20.12), an increased tendency for AML progression and an inferior overall survival. Oligomonocytic CMML share molecular profile with over CMML except for the presence of a lower percentage of *RAS* pathway mutations [34].

Mutations in *DNMT3A*, *TET2*, and *ASXL1* can be also present in hematologically normal adults, representing either age related clonal hematopoiesis (ARCH) or CHIP. Both ARCH and CHIP have been associated with aging and increased incidence of hematological malignancies, including CMML (as well as cardiovascular diseases).

Differential diagnosis of CMML

Differential diagnosis of CMML includes:

- Reactive monocytosis
- CML (*BCR-ABL1*[+])
- MDS/MPN-n (MDS/MPN with neutrophilia)
- MPNs with *PDGFRA*, *PDGFRB*, or *FGFR1* rearrangement
- PMF with monocytosis
- PV with monocytosis
- ET with monocytosis
- MDS with monocytosis
- Juvenile myelomonocytic leukemia (JMML)
- CNL
- AMML

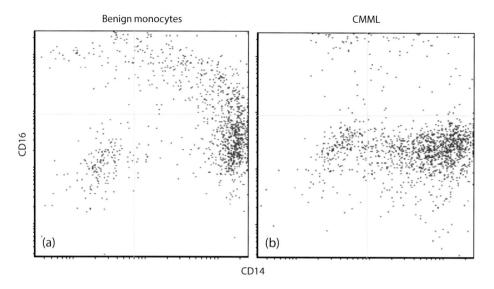

FIGURE 20.11   Comparison of distribution of classical CD16$^-$/CD14$^{bright+}$ monocytes (MO1), intermediate CD16$^+$/CD14$^{bright+}$ monocytes (MO2) and non-classical CD16$^+$/CD14^{dim+} monocytes (MO3) in normal BM (a) and in CMML (b). Note the predominance of MO1 monocytes in CMML (b).

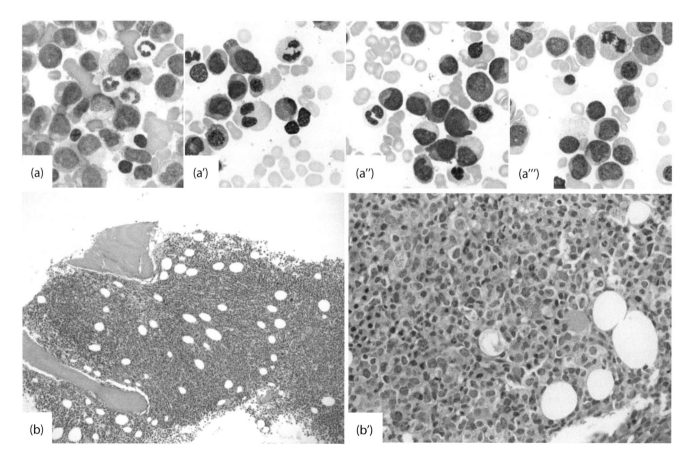

FIGURE 20.12   CMML with *NPM1* mutation. (a) Aspirate smear showing predominance of atypical monocytes, dysgranulopoiesis, and dyserythropoiesis (blasts and blasts equivalents are <20%). BM core biopsy (b, low and intermediate magnification) shows hypercellular marrow with increased monocytes, mild eosinophilia but without significantly increased blasts.

- AML with inv(16)/t(16;16)/*CBFB* rearrangement
- Acute monocytic (monoblastic) leukemia
- SM with monocytosis
- Plasma cell leukemia
- Diffuse large B-cell lymphoma (DLBCL) in leukemia phase

Reactive monocytosis

Algorithmic approach to monocytosis and CMML is presented in Figure 20.1. Reactive monocytosis occurs in patients with chronic infections and autoimmune processes, following toxic therapies and in post-trauma patients. Infectious etiology includes tuberculosis, fungal infections, infective endocarditis, viral infections, congenital syphilis, and protozoal infections. Recovery from acute infections or the BM regeneration after cytotoxic therapy is often associated with transient monocytosis. Connective tissue disorders associated with monocytosis include systemic lupus erythematous (SLE), inflammatory bowel disease, immune thrombocytopenia, and sarcoidosis. Other disorders which may be associated with monocytosis include lipid storage diseases, sickle cell disease, postsplenectomy, and chronic stress.

Reactive monocytes usually do not display overtly aberrant phenotype (Figure 20.13), but minor population of monocytes may show some atypia, most often in the form of expression of CD16 or CD56, or decreased expression of CD11b, CD13, CD14, CD15, CD45, and/or HLA-DR. Alteration of 1 antigen was reported in 55% of the reactive monocytosis, but abnormal expression of 2 or more antigens in only 15% of the cases [29]. Peripheral blood from healthy individuals shows a minor CD56+ monocytic population (0%–16%–3.5%; mean ± SD, 1.3% ± 1%) [54]. Since dim or partial CD2 expression if often seen on benign monocytes, I do not consider the CD2 evaluation helpful in differentiating CMML from reactive monocytosis. In blood, reactive monocytes rarely show decreased (moderate) or partially negative expression of CD14, but benign BM samples often show very minor population of CD14- monocytes (usually less than 10%). In contrast to healthy persons or patients with reactive monocytosis, CMML patients demonstrate an increase in the fraction of CD14+/CD16- cells (classical monocytes, MO1) and decreased fraction of "intermediate" monocytes (CD14+/CD16+, MO2) and "non-classical" monocytes (CD14low/CD16+, MO3) [3, 55–58]. An increase in the CD14bright+/CD16- (MO1) classical monocyte fraction ≥94% of the total monocytes was proposed to rapidly and efficiently distinguish CMML and oligomonocytic CMML from reactive monocytosis with specificity of 88.2%–95.1% and sensitivity of 90.6%–93.8% [3, 34, 58]. The 94% threshold was subsequently validated in two other studies [31, 59].

Pophali et al. reported a sub-optimal sensitivity of using a cut-off value of >94% for MO1 classical monocytes and <1.13% for MO3 non-classical monocytes in differential diagnosis between CMML and other reactive process [56]. They also reported CML with monocytosis that had a MO1 fraction of >94%. Using the visual interactive stochastic neighbor embedding (viSNE) FC method, Thomas et al. defined monocytes by incorporating all cell surface markers simultaneously and found that although classical monocytes were defined with high purity using CD14 and CD16, intermediate and nonclassical monocytes defined using CD14 and CD16 alone are frequently contaminated, with average intermediate and nonclassical monocyte purity of approximately 86.0% and 87.2%, respectively [55]. To improve the monocyte purity, they devised a new gating scheme that takes advantage of the shared coexpression of cell surface markers on each subset concluding that addition of CCR2, CD36, HLA-DR, and CD11c to CD14/CD16 analysis help with better discrimination of the three monocyte populations [55].

Chronic myeloid leukemia (BCR-ABL1+)

CML is characterized morphologically by prominent leukocytosis with blood smear showing predominance of granulocytes at different stages of maturation, basophilia, eosinophilia and scattered blasts and nucleated erythroid precursors. CML shows also increased number of monocytes, which on occasional may be prominent (Figure 20.14). In most cases, however, granulocytes predominate, and monocytes usually do not exceed 10% of cells in differential count. In contrast to CML, CMML does not contain pseudo-Gaucher like cells and is not associated with prominent basophilia. The diagnosis of CML is confirmed by presence of Philadelphia chromosome [t(9;22)] or the *BCR-ABL1* fusion.

Myeloproliferative neoplasms with PDGFRA, PDGFRB, or FGFR1

Presence of leukocytosis with eosinophilia in the absence of *BCR-ABL1* transcripts may indicate MPNs with *PDGFRA* or *PDGFRB* rearrangement, a rare neoplasm characterized by marked eosinophilia. CMML cases with prominent eosinophilia may mimic those myeloid neoplasms with specific genetic changes. If WHO criteria are both for both CMML and MPN with specific driver mutation, a diagnosis of CMML with a concomitant myeloid neoplasm expressing a classical MPN-driver, such as *JAK2 V617F*, *BCR-ABL1* or rearranged *PDGFRA/B* or *FGFR1*. If the criteria for MPN are not met, the case is diagnosed as CMML with expression of a molecular MPN-driver.

Primary myelofibrosis (PMF) with monocytosis

Presence of reticulin fibrosis is not specific for PMF and can be seen in other myeloid neoplasms, including CMML, and presence of monocytosis is not specific for CMML and can be seen in other myeloid neoplasms, such as MDS, PV, or PMF. Monocytosis in PMF patients can be seen at presentation, or appears later, especially during disease progression (often with appearance of dysplasia). Other features overlapping in CMML and PMF are presence of leukocytosis, splenomegaly (in CMML, splenomegaly is usually associated with infiltration of spleen by leukemic CMML cells) and/or *JAK2* mutation. Megakaryocytes in PMF are highly atypical with many immature, cloud-like, large, hypersegmented, and hyperchromatic forms often with prominent megakaryocytic clustering (>15 cells). Megakaryocytes in CMML are more often either normal or show dysplastic features more typical for MDS, such as megakaryocytes with hypolobated or abnormally lobated nuclei. The dysplastic variant of CMML usually shows erythroid hyperplasia with dyserythropoiesis, while PMF is most often characterized by increased M:E ratio due to granulocytic proliferation and erythroid hypoplasia. Presence of MPN-associated "driver" mutations (*JAK2*, *MPL*, or *CALR*) favors the diagnosis of PMF with monocytosis [1]. Those mutations, however, are not specific for PMF, as they may be present in CMML. PMF may also acquire secondary mutations, such as *TET2*, *DNMT3A*, *EZH2*, *ASXL1*, *SRSF2*, and *U2AF1*, which occur also commonly in CMML. In comparison to PMF with monocytosis, patients with CMML are older, have lower platelet count, higher BM blasts, presence of micromegakaryocytes or hypolobated forms and dysplasia in other lineages, higher frequency of *TET2* mutations and lower *JAK2* allelic burden. The neoplasms with overlapping features between PMF with monocytosis and

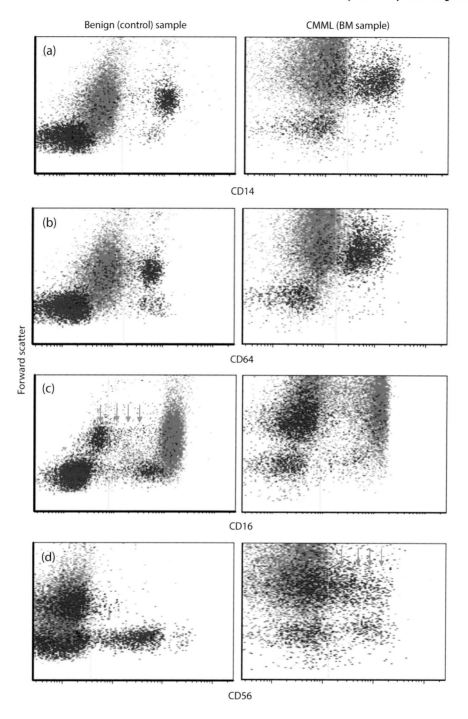

FIGURE 20.13   Comparison of benign monocytes (left column) with CMML (right column). Neoplastic monocytes in CMML show bright expression of CD14 (a) and CD64 (b), negative CD16 (c), and partially positive CD56 (d).

CMML with marrow fibrosis may represent either "gray-zone" neoplasm (hybrid between PMF and CMML) or unusual PMF with monocytosis, dysplasia, and CMML-like mutations [1, 17, 60–62].

MDS/MPN with neutrophilia (MDS/MPN-n)
In contrast to CMML, MDS/MPN-n shows admixture of pro-myelocytes, myelocytes, and metamyelocytes which comprise

at least 10% of leukocytes. All three BM lineages may display dyspoiesis. Staining of the BM aspirate with NSE may be helpful to identify monocytes and differentiate CMML from MDS/MPN-n. Despite monocytosis in MDS/MPN-n, neutrophilia is still a predominant feature. Patients with significant neutrophilia but displaying monocytosis fulfilling the WHO criteria are diagnosed with CMML rather than MDS/MPN-n [27].

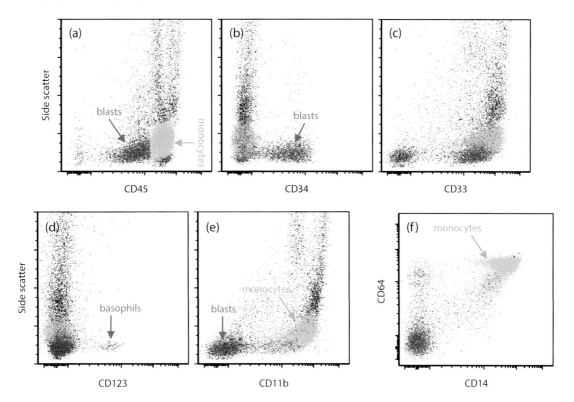

FIGURE 20.14 CML (*BCR-ABL1+*) with increased blasts and monocytes (blood). In rare cases of CML, flow cytometric analysis of peripheral blood may mimic CMML. FC analysis of blood shows blasts (blue dots) with moderate CD45 (a), positive CD34 (b) and positive CD13 (c) and numerous monocytes (green dots) with bright CD45 (a), bright CD13 (c), negative CD123 (d), bright CD11b (e), and bright CD14 (f). Cytogenetic and FISH testing for *BCR-ABL1* (Philadelphia chromosome) is crucial in the differential diagnosis.

Myelodysplastic neoplasms (MDS)

CMML and MDS show some overlapping features, as CMML is associated with dysplastic changes and MDS may be associated with monocytosis (occasionally seen only in BM). In addition, characteristic (albeit not specific) mutation of TET2 and SRSF2) may be also seen in MDS. Monocytosis in MDS is usually not chronic or persistent. If dysplastic features are accompanied by absolute and persistent monocytosis, a diagnosis of CMML can be rendered, keeping in mind that there is a significant clinical, morphologic, and immunophenotypic overlap between MDS and CMML and some cases of MDS may represent an early stage of CMML. MDS often is characterized by erythroid hyperplasia, whereas in CMML the M:E ratio is typically increased with normal or decreased erythropoiesis. Patients with MDS may progress into CMML [63–65]. Some MDS cases may show persistent nodular BM lesions composed of immature monocytes [66]. Monocytic leukemoid reaction in a patient with MDS has also been reported [67]. Rare cases of CMML show >15% ring sideroblasts in BM.

Acute myelomonocytic leukemia (AMML)

AMML has at least 20% myeloblasts or blast equivalents (e.g., promonocytes). In CMML the number of blasts and promonocytes is <20%. Monocytes in AMML usually display less prominent phenotypic atypia by FC analysis when compared to both CMML and acute monocytic leukemia. Occasionally, due to presence of prominent trilineage dyspoiesis and leftward shift of myeloid cells, erythroid precursors and monocytes, differential diagnosis between CMML-2 and emerging AMML may be very difficult. Careful cytologic analysis of good quality BM aspirate

smear with differential count of at least 500 cells, FC analysis and immunohistochemical analysis of BM core biopsy are helpful in reaching the correct diagnosis.

Acute myeloid leukemia with inv(16)/t(16;16)

AML with inv(16)/t(16;16) often presents with increased monocytes and abnormal eosinophils. It differs from CMML presence of inv(16)/t(16;16) by cytogenetic/FSH studies (corresponding to *CBFB-MYH11* fusion) and ≥20% blasts (or blasts equivalents such as monoblasts or promonocytes).

Acute monoblastic leukemia

Acute monoblastic leukemia differs from CMML by presence of immature monocytes (promonocytes and monoblasts) with prominent cytologic and phenotypic atypia and at much higher number than in CMML (Figure 20.15). Monoblasts is characterized by fine chromatin, round nuclei, nucleolus and pale basophilic cytoplasm, whereas promonocytes have irregular, often folded nuclei, prominent nucleoli, and paler cytoplasm. Frequently monocytes display aberrant expression of CD14 (either partial or complete loss or variable expression) and positive CD56. In addition, poorly differentiated cases may be positive for CD34 and/or CD117. Aberrant expression of HLA-DR (negative or dim), CD10 (positive), CD33 (negative or dim), and CD11b (variable or dim) is also seen more often in acute monoblastic leukemia than in CMML.

Polycythemia vera (PV) with monocytosis

Monocytosis can occur in patients with PV (~20%) and is associated with poor outcome. PV is diagnosed with sustained erythrocytosis with red blood cells >25% above mean normal predicted

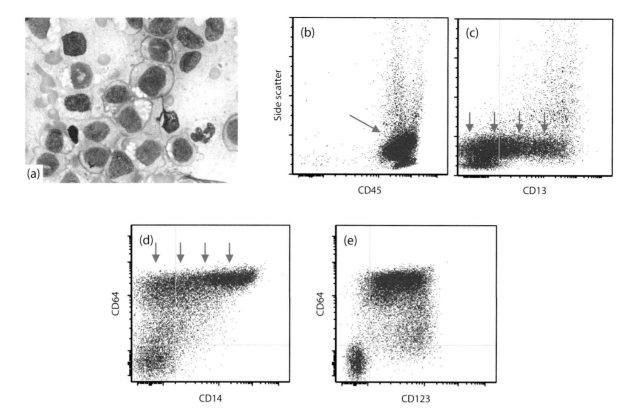

FIGURE 20.15 Acute monoblastic leukemia is characterized by immature and atypical monocytic cells (a) composed of promono-cytes and monoblasts. When analyzed by flow cytometry the monocytes comprise the predominate population (b; blue dots, arrow) and frequently show very aberrant phenotype, such as partially negative CD13 (c), heterogeneous ("smeary") expression of CD14 (d) and positive CD123 (e).

value and hemoglobin >16.5g/dL (men) or >16.0g/dL (women), and/or hematocrit >49% in men and >48% in women.

B-cell lymphoproliferations

DLBCL, Burkitt lymphoma (BL), and high-grade B-cell lympho-mas, as well as unusual "blastoid" variants of hairy cell leukemia or mantle cell lymphoma may resemble cytologically immature monocytic cells. FC immunophenotyping helps to distinguish between monoblasts and B-cell neoplasms (see Figure 22.28 in Chapter 22).

Juvenile myelomonocytic leukemia

JMML is MPN of early childhood (a median age of years) with a varied clinical presentation that may include failure to thrive, malaise, fever, bleeding, pallor, lymphadenopathy, skin rash, and hepatosplenomegaly [1, 68–75]. It has aggressive clinical course and poor prognosis. Patients with JMML lack of *BCR-ABL1*, and usually show leukocytosis with monocytosis, circulating granu-locytic precursors and red cell precursors, increased hemo-globin F and clonal chromosomal abnormalities. Monocytes display dysplastic features. An absolute monocyte count >1 × 10^9/L is required for the diagnosis. The percentage of blasts in blood averages 2% and rarely exceeds 20% [73]. BM is hypercel-lular due to myelomonocytic proliferation. Megakaryocytes are often decreased in number. Dyspoietic features are present but are usually subtle. Karyotype is normal in majority of cases, while monosomy 7 is seen in 25% and other abnormalities in 10% [73]. Monocytosis in BM is less pronounced than in blood. The

hallmark of JMML is hypersensitivity of marrow progenitors to granulocyte-monocyte colony stimulating factor in vitro result-ing from mutations in components of the RAS-signaling pathway [75]. Current standard of care for patient with JMML is allogeneic hematopoietic stem-cell transplant [74].

MDS/MPN with SF3B1 mutation and thrombocytosis

Introduction
The presence of anemia, ring sideroblasts and thrombocytosis is classified under current WHO system as MDS/MPN with SF3B1 mutation and thrombocytosis (MDS/MPN-SF3B1-T) [1, 76, 77]. Patients with MDS/MPN-SF3B1-T have features of MDS with SF3B1 mutation (MDS-SF3B1) with additional presence of persis-tent thrombocytosis [76, 77].

The diagnostic criteria for MDS/MPN-SF3B1-T include:

- Anemia associated with erythroid lineage dysplasia with or without multilineage dysplasia
- ≥15% ring sideroblasts (even if *SF3B1* mutation is detected)
- <1% blasts in blood and <5% blasts in the BM
- Persistent thrombocytosis with platelet count ≥450 × 10^9/L
- Presence of a *SF3B1* mutation or, in the absence of *SF3B1* mutation, no history of recent cytotoxic or growth factor therapy [a diagnosis of MDS/MPN-SF3B1-T is strongly supported by the presence of *SF3B1* mutation together with a mutation in *JAK2* V617F, *CALR*, or *MPL* genes]

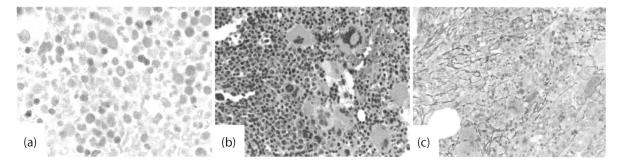

FIGURE 20.16 MDS/MPN-RS-T. Aspirate smear shows many ring sideroblasts (a). BM core biopsy shows hypercellular marrow with megakaryocytic atypia (b) and mild reticulin fibrosis (c).

- Lack of *BCR-ABL1* fusion gene, no rearrangement of *PDGFRA*, *PDGFRB*, or *FGFR1*; or *PCM1-JAK2*; no (3;3) (q21;q26), inv(3)(q21q26), or del(5q) [in a case which otherwise fulfills the diagnostic criteria for MDS with isolated del(5q) – no or minimal absolute basophilia; basophils usually <2% of leukocytes]
- No preceding history of MPN, MDS (except MDS-RS), or other type of MDS/MPN

Morphology

Patients with MDS/MPN-SF3B1-T present with some signs of ET, including a marked thrombocytosis, hypercellular marrow, and increased megakaryocytes, but also have ≥15% ring sideroblasts (Figures 20.16 and 20.17), a feature usually associated with MDS. Ring sideroblasts are defined as erythroid precursors with abnormal perinuclear mitochondrial iron accumulation (≥5 sideroblastic granules covering ≥⅓ of the nuclear circumference) visualized

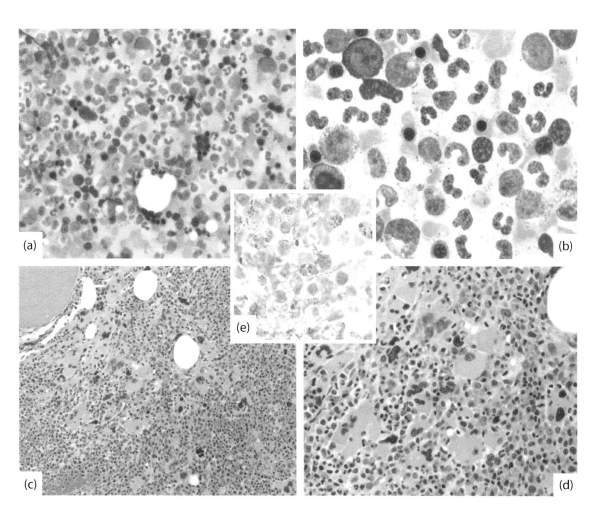

FIGURE 20.17 MDS/MPN-SF3B1-T shows features of myelodysplastic syndrome (such as MDS-RS) overlapping with a MPN (such as ET or PMF). BM aspirate (a–b) and core biopsy (c–d) show hypercellular marrow with trilineage dyspoiesis. There is marked megakaryocytosis with atypia and clustering. An iron stain on fresh aspirate (e) shows >15% ringed sideroblasts.

TABLE 20.4: Differential Diagnosis of Mixed MDS/MPNs

		CMML	MDS/MPN-n	MDS/MPN-SF3B1-T
Persistent ≥0.5 × 10⁹/L and relative monocytosis of ≥10% of blood leukocytes		+	−	−
Persistent thrombocytosis ≥450 × 10⁹/L		−	−	+
Leukocytosis ≥13 × 10⁹/L		+/−	+	+/−
Dysplasia involving ≥1 myeloid lineage		+	+[a]	+[a]
Ring sideroblasts (≥15%)		−/(+)	−	+
Mutations	ASXL1	+$^{40\%}$/−	−/+$^{25\%}$	−/+$^{10\%}$
	JAK2	−/+$^{10\%}$	−/(+)$^{4\%}$	+$^{50-60\%}$/−
	MPL	−	−	−/+$^{10-20\%}$
	CBL	−/+$^{8\%}$	−/+$^{10-20\%}$	−/(+)$^{2\%}$
	CSF3R	−/(+)$^{4\%}$	−/(+)$^{<10\%b}$	−
	SF3B1	−/(+)$^{5\%}$	−/(+)	+$^{80-90\%}$/(−)
	TET2	+$^{60\%}$/−	−/+$^{30\%}$	−/+$^{10-25\%}$
	DNMT3A	−/(+)$^{5\%}$	−/(+)	−/+$^{15\%}$
	SRSF2	+$^{50\%}$/−	−	−/(+)$^{7\%}$
	SETBP1	−/+$^{10-20\%}$	−/+$^{25-30\%}$	−/(+)$^{10\%}$
BCR-ABL1 fusion		−	−	−

Notes: +, positive; −, negative; (+), rarely positive; (−), rarely negative.

[a] MDS/MPN-n is characterized by marked dysgranulopoiesis (dysplasia in other lineages is less pronounced) and MDS/MPN-SF3B1-T usually shows prominent dyserythropoiesis and less pronounced dysgranulopoiesis than in MDS/MPN-n.

[b] If CSF3R is positive, chronic neutrophilic leukemia is more likely.

by Prussian blue staining (Perls reaction). In contrast to MDS with ring sideroblasts which is defined by either ≥15% ring sideroblasts or ≥5% ring sideroblasts if *SF3B1* mutation is present, MDS/MPN-SF3B1-T requires ≥15% ring sideroblasts regardless of the mutational status.

Blood. There are no circulating blasts (<1%). Red blood cells often show hypochromia with anisocytosis. Thrombocytosis is always present (≥450 × 10⁹/L). Some cases may show mild leukocytosis.

BM. Being an overlap syndrome, MDS/MPN-SF3B1-Ts displays morphologic features typical for MDS and/or non-CML MPNs. The M:E ratio is usually decreased due to erythroid hyperplasia. Dyserythropoiesis may be accompanied by dysgranulopoiesis. Megakaryocytes are increased and atypical, showing cytologic atypia comparable to either ET or PMF. Reticulin fibrosis (at least focal) is often present.

Genetic features
Genes mutations in MDS/MPN-SF3B1-T include: *SF3B1* (~85%–90%), *JAK2* (~33%–60%), *TET2* (~10%–25%), *ASHXL1* (~15%–29%), *DNMT3A* (~15%), *SETBP1* (~13%), *SRSF2* (~7%), *EZH2* (~7%), *U2AF1* (~5%), *IDH2* (~4%), *ZRSR2* (~3%), *MPL* (~3%), and *CBL* (~2%) [77–79]. Presence of *SETBP1* or *ASXL1* mutations is associated with poor survival.

Differential diagnosis of MDS/MPN-SF3B1-T

Differential diagnosis of MDS/MPN-SF3B1-T includes:

- MDS-SF3B1
- CMML with ring sideroblasts
- PMF and early primary myelofibrosis (prePMF)
- ET
- Acquired disorders associated with ring sideroblasts (copper deficiency, lead poisoning, zinc toxicity, alcoholism)
- Drug induced sideroblastic anemia
- Hereditary sideroblastic anemia

- Unclassifiable MDS/MPN (MDS/MPN-U)

Table 20.4 shows major factors in differential diagnosis between CMML, MDS/MPN-n, and MDS/MPN-SF3B1-T.

PMF and prePMF
MDS/MPN-SF3B1-T may show reticulin fibrosis which in conjunction with prominent megakaryocytic atypia raise the possibility of non-CML MPN, including PMF. PMF usually shows increased M:E ratio due to myeloid hyperplasia and lack of significant dyserythropoiesis, although rare cases of PMF may show ring sideroblasts (PMF-RS), which together of thrombocytosis observed in some PMFS require differential diagnosis from MDS/MPN-SF3B1-T. Blood smears form PMF show often leukoerythroblastosis, rarely observed in MDS/MPN-SF3B1-T. The most typical histomorphologic features of PMF includes megakaryocytic hyperplasia with marked atypia and clustering (>7 cells), often around bone trabeculae or sinuses, and intrasinusoidal hematopoiesis. Those features are rarely observed in MDS/MPN-SF3B1-T. On the molecular level, *JAK2* mutation is common in both neoplasms, whereas presence of SF3B1 mutation together with JAK2, CALR, or MPL mutation strongly support the diagnosis of MDS/MPN-SF3B1-T [1]. Splenomegaly is seen in majority of patients with PMF and is only rarely observed in MDS/MPN-SF3B1-T.

ET
ET differs from MDS/MPN-SF3B1-T by lack of prominent dyserythropoiesis and ring sideroblasts.

Disorders associated with ring sideroblasts
MDS-SF3B1. MDS-SF3B1 and MDS/MPN-SF3B1-T share many morphologic, genetic, and clinical features except for presence of persistent thrombocytosis typical for the latter.

CMML with ring sideroblasts. CMML with ring sideroblasts fulfills all criteria diagnostic for CMML (see above) in addition to being positive for ring sideroblasts. CMML with ring sideroblasts differs from MDS/MPN-RS-T by lack of thrombocytosis and presence of absolute monocytosis.

PMF with ring sideroblasts. See preceding text.

Secondary (non-clonal) disorders associated with ring sideroblasts, anemia with/without myelodysplasia. Alcoholism, lead poisoning, zinc toxicity, and copper or pyridoxine deficiency may lead to anemia with ring sideroblasts (with or without features of myelodysplasia in BM). Especially copper deficiency should be excluded, as it can mimic MDS.

Drug-induced sideroblastic anemia. Drugs associated with ring sideroblasts include isoniazid, chloramphenicol, linezolid, and penicillamine.

Hereditary sideroblastic anemia. The hereditary disorders with ring sideroblasts include X-linked sideroblastic anemia (with *ALAS2* mutations or with ataxia), *SLC25A38*-related sideroblasts anemia, *GLRX5*-related sideroblastic anemia, Kearns Sayre syndrome, Pearson marrow-pancreas syndrome, thiamine-responsive megaloblastic anemia syndrome and myopathy, lactic acidosis, and sideroblastic anemia [80].

MDS/MPN-U. MDS/MPN-U shows features typical for either MDS or MPN, which do not fulfill the WHO criteria for any specific category. MDS/MPN-U may show increased number of ring sideroblasts.

MDS/MPN with neutrophilia (MDS/MPN-n)

Introduction

MDS/MPN-n is a rare mixed MDS/MPN neoplasm formerly classified as atypical CML (aCML) [1, 81–86]. The median overall survival is ~14 months and cumulative incidence of AML transformation after 1 year is ~12%. It is characterized by overlap of myeloproliferative and myelodysplastic features, including leukocytosis with leftward-shifted granulocytic series, dysgranulopoiesis, dysmegakaryopoiesis, and dyserythropoiesis, but without basophilia and monocytosis [27, 81, 83, 87–90]. It usually affects older adults. There is no *BCR-ABL1* fusion or Philadelphia chromosome, which differentiates it from CML. Patients present with anemia and/or thrombocytopenia, high white blood cell count, splenomegaly and often hepatomegaly.

Diagnostic criteria

Diagnostic criterial for MDS/MPN-n include:

- Persistent leukocytosis $\geq 13 \times 10^9$/L due to neutrophilia
- Immature myeloid precursors $\geq 10\%$ of leukocytes
- Marked dysgranulopoiesis
- Absence of *BCR-ABL1, PDGFRA, PDGFRB, FGFR1,* or *PCM1-JAK2*
- Absent or minimal monocytosis (<10% of leukocytes)
- Absent or minimal basophilia (often <2%)
- Hypercellular BM with granulocytic hyperplasia and dysgranulopoiesis (with or without dyserythropoiesis and dysmegakaryopoiesis)
- WHO criteria for PMF, PV, or ET are not met

Morphology

Granulocytic precursors (promyelocytes, myelocytes, and metamyelocytes) comprise $\geq 10\%$, basophils <2% and monocytes <10% of WBC. Granulocytic cells display dysgranulopoietic features,

most often in the form of acquired Pelger-Huët abnormality, clumped nuclear chromatin, bizarrely hypersegmented nuclei, binucleated cells, hypogranularity, and/or abnormal cytoplasmic hypergranularity (Figure 20.18). In a series reported by Wang et al., marked dysgranulopoiesis ($\geq 50\%$ of granulocytes) was seen in 52% MDS/MPN-n (aCML) patients, and the remaining 48% had 10% to 49% dysgranulopoiesis. In a series reported by Xubo et al., the percentage of blasts, nucleated erythrocytes, monocytes, eosinophils and basophils was 2.45% (±2), 7.8% (±2.9), 1.3% (±1.2), 1.5% (±1.6), and 1.2% (±1), respectively [89]. Megakaryocytes often show atypia in the form of non-lobulated nuclei. Red cell precursors often show dyserythropoiesis.

The BM biopsy is hypercellular due to granulocytic hyperplasia (M:E ratio is usually >10:1). Blasts are increased (<20%) and some cases may display abnormal localization of immature precursors (ALIP). Number of megakaryocytes varies; they often display atypia including hypolobated or non-lobulated nuclei and/or micromegakaryocytes. Moderate reticulin fibrosis (1 to 2/4) is present in majority of cases. There is no eosinophilia, basophilia, monocytosis, lymphocytosis, plasmacytosis, or myelomonocytic clusters.

Genetic features

Patient with MDS/MPN-n have higher frequency of chromosomal changes than those with CMML. Cytogenetic abnormalities have been reported in up to 80% of patients, including +8, +13, del(20q), del5(q), i(17q), and del(20q). Occasional cases of MDS/MPN-n with t(5;12)(q33;p13), t(6;8)(p22;q22), del(12p), del(15q), −7, or t(4;22)(q12;q11.2) were reported [27, 89]. Unusual fusion of *BCR-JAK2* from ins(22;9)(q11;p13p24) has been reported in MDS/MPN-n [91]. 24%–1% patients with MDS/MPN-n have *SETBP1* mutations [86, 92]. Those patients have higher WBC counts and worse prognosis. In contrast to CNL which is often *CSF3R+*, the *CSF3R* mutation status is not as clear in MDS/MPN-n. Maxson et al. and Gotlib et al. reported frequent *CSF3R* mutations in MDS/MPN-n (approx. 40%), whereas Pardanani et al. and Wang et al. showed that *CSF3R* mutations were mostly absent in MDS/MPN-n [84, 85, 90, 93]. It is suggested that presence of *CSF3R* mutation in a patient with predominantly neutrophilic MPN should be considered diagnostic for CNL [90, 94]. Mutations typical for MPN (*JAK2, CALR, MPL,* and *CSF3R*) are either absent or infrequent in MDS/MPN-n, and their detection should prompt the differential diagnosis of CNL, PMF, or MPN unclassifiable (MPN-U). SETBP1 mutations have been noted in up to 32% of MDS/MPN-n [43].

Differential diagnosis of MDS/MPN-n

Differential diagnosis of MDS/MPN-n includes:

- CML
- CMML
- MDS
- CNL
- Myelodysplastic/MPN, unclassifiable
- PMF

CML (BCR-ABL1+)

CML differs from MDS/MPN-n by presence of *BCR-ABL1* fusion. Basophilia, thrombocytosis, hypolobated micromegakaryocytes and lack of Pelgeroid features favor the diagnosis of CML. CML with unusual or cryptic ("masked") *BCR-ABL1* rearrangements such as atypical *BCR-ABL1* transcripts (e.g., e8/a2 or e6a2) or variant translocation such as t(8;10;21)(q22;q24;q22) or t(6;9)

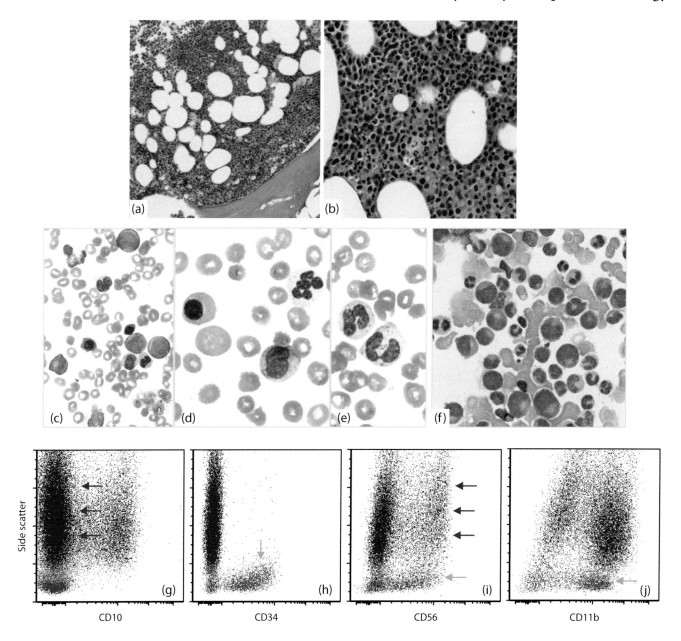

FIGURE 20.18 MDS/MPN-n. Patient underwent BM biopsy due to marked leukocytosis (90 × 10⁹/L). H&E section from the BM core biopsy (a–b) shows hypercellular marrow with myeloid hyperplasia and leftward shift. Blood smear (c–e) shows leukoerythroblastosis. BM aspirate (f) shows myeloid hyperplasia with leftward shift without basophilia or hypolobated micromegakaryocytes. Flow cytometry analysis (g–j) shows increased myeloid to lymphoid ratio due to myeloid hyperplasia (granulocytes are represented by purple dots), aberrant expression of CD10 on majority of granulocytes (g), increased blasts (h; blue dots), aberrant expression of CD56 on subset of granulocytes and subset of blasts (i), and aberrant expression of CD11b on majority of blasts (j; blue dots).

(p21;q34.1) should be excluded when diagnosing MDS/MPN-n. A novel multiplex PCR methodology offer improved detection of typical and atypical *BCR-ABL1* fusion transcripts [95].

CMML

Monocytosis is the hallmark of CMML (by definition monocytes are >1 × 10⁹/L). Presence of persistent monocytosis is diagnostic of CMML and does not favor MDS/MPN-n. The absolute monocytes count in MDS/MPN-n may be increased but in contrast to CMML the relative count is <10%.

MDS

In contrast to MDS, which is characterized by BM failure (leading to cytopenia or often pancytopenia), MDS/MPN-n shows both dysplastic as well as proliferative features leading to neutrophilia and dysgranulopoiesis. Multilineage dysplasia may be also present in MDS/MPN-n, an overlapping feature with MDS with multilineage dysplasia (MDS-MLD). In contrast to MDS/MPN-n, MDS patients do not present with prominent neutrophilia. Dysgranulopoiesis manifested as abnormal nuclear hypersegmentation is not typically seen in MDS.

CNL

CNL is a very rare type of leukemia characterized by a proliferation mainly of mature neutrophils, elevated neutrophil-alkaline phosphatase activity, splenomegaly, and lack of the Philadelphia chromosome. CNL is associated with *CSF3R* mutations, whereas MDS/MPN-n often shows *SETBP1* mutations (25%–32%) and is only rarely positive for *CSFR3* mutation.

Myelodysplastic/myeloproliferative disease, unclassifiable (MDS/MPN-U)

MDS/MPN-U is a diagnosis of exclusion and is restricted to cases of mixed myelodysplastic/myeloproliferative disorders which do not fulfill the criteria for the diagnosis of CMML, MDS/MPN-n, and JMML, without prior history of any specific myeloid disorder. One or more of the myeloid lineages proliferates (as seen in chronic myeloproliferative disease), whereas the other lineages show dyspoiesis with ineffective proliferation (as seen in MDS).

References

1. Swerdlow, S.H., et al., ed. *WHO classification of tumors of haematopoietic and lymphoid tissues.* 2016, IARC: Lyon.
2. Patnaik, M.M., et al., *ASXL1 and SETBP1 mutations and their prognostic contribution in chronic myelomonocytic leukemia: a two-center study of 466 patients.* Leukemia, 2014. **28**(11): p. 2206–12.
3. Selimoglu-Buet, D., et al., *Characteristic repartition of monocyte subsets as a diagnostic signature of chronic myelomonocytic leukemia.* Blood, 2015. **125**(23): p. 3618–26.
4. Patnaik, M.M. and A. Tefferi, *Chronic myelomonocytic leukemia: 2018 update on diagnosis, risk stratification and management.* Am J Hematol, 2018. **93**(6): p. 824–40.
5. Ouyang, Y., et al., *Clinical significance of CSF3R, SRSF2 and SETBP1 mutations in chronic neutrophilic leukemia and chronic myelomonocytic leukemia.* Oncotarget, 2017. **8**(13): p. 20834–41.
6. Itzykson, R., et al., *Clonal architecture of chronic myelomonocytic leukemias.* Blood, 2013. **121**(12): p. 2186–98.
7. Harrington, A.M., et al., *Immunophenotypes of chronic myelomonocytic leukemia (CMML) subtypes by flow cytometry: a comparison of CMML-1 vs CMML-2, myeloproliferative vs dysplastic, de novo vs therapy-related, and CMML-specific cytogenetic risk subtypes.* Am J Clin Pathol, 2016. **146**(2): p. 170–81.
8. Elena, C., et al., *Integrating clinical features and genetic lesions in the risk assessment of patients with chronic myelomonocytic leukemia.* Blood, 2016. **128**(10): p. 1408–17.
9. Onida, F., *Models of prognostication in chronic myelomonocytic leukemia.* Curr Hematol Malig Rep, 2017. **12**(6): p. 513–21.
10. Valent, P., et al., *Proposed diagnostic criteria for classical CMML, CMML variants and pre-CMML conditions.* Haematologica, 2019. **104**(10): p. 1935–49.
11. Elmariah, H. and A.E. DeZern, *Chronic myelomonocytic leukemia: 2018 update to prognosis and treatment.* Curr Hematol Malig Rep, 2019. **14**(3): p. 154–63.
12. Thomopoulos, T.P., et al., *Chronic myelomonocytic leukemia – a review.* Expert Rev Hematol, 2021. **14**(1): p. 59–77.
13. Beran, M., *Chronic myelomonocytic leukemia.* Cancer Treat Res, 2008. **142**: p. 107–32.
14. Beran, M., et al., *Prognostic factors and risk assessment in chronic myelomonocytic leukemia: validation study of the M.D. Anderson Prognostic Scoring System.* Leuk Lymphoma, 2007. **48**(6): p. 1150–60.
15. Barraco, D., et al., *Monocytosis in polycythemia vera: clinical and molecular correlates.* Am J Hematol, 2017. **92**(7): p. 640–5.
16. Hu, Z., et al., *Utility of JAK2 V617F allelic burden in distinguishing chronic myelomonocytic leukemia from primary myelofibrosis with monocytosis.* Hum Pathol, 2019. **85**: p. 290–8.
17. Chapman, J., et al., *Myeloid neoplasms with features intermediate between primary myelofibrosis and chronic myelomonocytic leukemia.* Mod Pathol, 2018. **31**(3): p. 429–41.
18. Sotlar, K., et al., *Detection of c-kit mutation Asp 816 to Val in microdissected bone marrow infiltrates in a case of systemic mastocytosis associated with chronic myelomonocytic leukaemia.* Mol Pathol, 2000. **53**(4): p. 188–93.
19. Ahmed, F., et al., *Therapy related CMML: a case report and review of the literature.* Int J Hematol, 2009. **89**(5): p. 699–703.
20. Oo, T.H. and L. Kenney, *Therapy-related chronic myelomonocytic leukemia with unique chromosomal abnormalities: monosomy 7 and t(12;17)(p13;q11.2).* Am J Hematol, 2007. **82**(3): p. 248–9.
21. Valent, P., *ICUS, IDUS, CHIP and CCUS: diagnostic criteria, separation from MDS and clinical implications.* Pathobiology, 2019. **86**(1): p. 30–38.
22. Valent, P., et al., *Proposed minimal diagnostic criteria for myelodysplastic syndromes (MDS) and potential pre-MDS conditions.* Oncotarget, 2017. **8**(43): p. 73483–500.
23. Wimazal, F., et al., *Idiopathic cytopenia of undetermined significance (ICUS) versus low risk MDS: the diagnostic interface.* Leuk Res, 2007. **31**(11): p. 1461–8.
24. Lacronique-Gazaille, C., et al., *A simple method for detection of major phenotypic abnormalities in myelodysplastic syndromes: expression of CD56 in CMML.* Haematologica, 2007. **92**(6): p. 859–60.
25. Shen, Q., et al., *Flow cytometry immunophenotypic findings in chronic myelomonocytic leukemia and its utility in monitoring treatment response.* Eur J Haematol, 2015. **95**(2): p. 168–76.
26. Schuler, E., et al., *Refined medullary blast and white blood cell count based classification of chronic myelomonocytic leukemias.* Leuk Res, 2014. **38**(12): p. 1413–9.
27. Muramatsu, H., H. Makishima, and J.P. Maciejewski, *Chronic myelomonocytic leukemia and atypical chronic myeloid leukemia: novel pathogenetic lesions.* Semin Oncol, 2012. **39**(1): p. 67–73.
28. Ngo, N.T., I.A. Lampert, and K.N. Naresh, *Bone marrow trephine morphology and immunohistochemical findings in chronic myelomonocytic leukaemia.* Br J Haematol, 2008. **141**(6): p. 771–81.
29. Xu, Y., et al., *Flow cytometric analysis of monocytes as a tool for distinguishing chronic myelomonocytic leukemia from reactive monocytosis.* Am J Clin Pathol, 2005. **124**(5): p. 799–806.
30. Ziegler-Heitbrock, L., et al., *Nomenclature of monocytes and dendritic cells in blood.* Blood, 2010. **116**(16): p. e74–80.
31. Patnaik, M.M., et al., *Flow cytometry based monocyte subset analysis accurately distinguishes chronic myelomonocytic leukemia from myeloproliferative neoplasms with associated monocytosis.* Blood Cancer J, 2017. **125**(23): p. 3618–26.
32. Sponaas, A.M., et al., *The proportion of CD16(+)CD14(dim) monocytes increases with tumor cell load in bone marrow of patients with multiple myeloma.* Immun Inflamm Dis, 2015. **3**(2): p. 94–102.
33. Ziegler-Heitbrock, L., *Blood monocytes and their subsets: established features and open questions.* Front Immunol, 2015. **6**: p. 423.
34. Calvo, X., et al., *Oligomonocytic and overt chronic myelomonocytic leukemia show similar clinical, genomic, and immunophenotypic features.* Blood Adv, 2020. **4**(20): p. 5285–96.
35. Feng, R., et al., *Application of immunophenotypic analysis in distinguishing chronic myelomonocytic leukemia from reactive monocytosis.* Cytometry B Clin Cytom, 2018. **94**(6): p. 901–9.
36. Fenaux, P., et al., *Chronic and subacute myelomonocytic leukaemia in the adult: a report of 60 cases with special reference to prognostic factors.* Br J Haematol, 1987. **65**(1): p. 101–6.
37. Fenaux, P., P. Morel, and J.L. Lai, *Cytogenetics of myelodysplastic syndromes.* Semin Hematol, 1996. **33**(2): p. 127–38.
38. Anonymous, *Chronic myelomonocytic leukemia: single entity or heterogeneous disorder? A prospective multicenter study of 100 patients. Groupe Francais de Cytogenetique Hematologique.* Cancer Genet Cytogenet, 1991. **55**(1): p. 57–65.
39. Germing, U., et al., *Problems in the classification of CMML–dysplastic versus proliferative type.* Leuk Res, 1998. **22**(10): p. 871–8.

ET or PMF with non-mutated *JAK2* or *MPL*, *CALR* mutations are reported in 67% of those with ET and 88% of those with PMF [29]. Patients with mutated *CALR* have lower risk of thrombosis and longer overall survival than patients with mutated *JAK2* [29].

CSFR3. *CSFR3* mutations are strongly associated with CNL.

JAK2. Molecular genetic analysis for the detection of the $JAK2^{V617F}$ (exon 14) mutation, as well as mutations within *JAK2* exon 12 and *MPL* exon 10, is part of routine diagnostic workup for patient suspected to have MPN. The Janus family of cytosolic tyrosine kinases (JAK) plays an essential role in development and normal hematopoiesis [30]. *JAK2*, encoded on chromosome 9p24, plays a central role in non-protein tyrosine kinase receptor signaling pathways, which could explain its involvement in malignancies of different hematologic lineages [30, 31]. The fusion of *TEL* to *JAK2* has been reported in acute leukemia and BP of CML. Novel *JAK2* somatic mutation (a G-C to T-a transversion, at nucleotide 1849 of exon 14, resulting in the substitution of valine to phenyloalanine at codon 617; *JAK2* V617F) has been implicated in pathogenesis of non-CML classic MPN [32–35]. $JAK2^{V617F}$ mutation is observed in majority of patients with PV (≥95%) and in ~50% (49%–57%) patients with ET and ~50% (44%–55%) of patients with PMF [32–38]. *JAK2* is mutated in approximately half of the cases of mixed MDS/MPN with ringed sideroblasts and marked thrombocytosis (MDS/MPN-RS-T) but is uncommon in other myeloid disorders such as MDS, AML, or CMML. Scott et al., identified four somatic gain-of-function mutations affecting *JAK2* exon 12 in 10 V617F-negative patients who presented with an isolated erythrocytosis, distinctive bone marrow (BM) morphology, and several also had reduced serum erythropoietin levels (three of the exon 12 mutations included a substitution of leucine for lysine at position 539 of *JAK2*) [39]. Most patients with PV carrying an exon 12 mutation had isolated erythrocytosis at clinical onset, unlike patients with $JAK2^{V617F}$-positive PV, most of whom had also elevations in white blood cell and/or platelet counts [40]. In contrast to $JAK2^{V617F}$, exon 12 mutations are not associated with ET and PMF, although *JAK2* exon 12 PV may progress to a secondary myelofibrosis.

MPL. Recently, two mutations in the thrombopoietin receptor (c-*MPL*) have been found in patients with MPNs: W515L and W515K [41–43]. These mutations have been evident in patients with ET and PMF but not in PV [44]. $MPL^{W515L/K}$ and $JAK2^{V617F}$ may occur concurrently, suggesting that these alleles may have functional complementation in myeloproliferative disease [41, 42]. Multiple molecular abnormalities are involved in the pathogenesis of the MPNs and aberrant *MPL* expression may be a common denominator of aberrant signaling in both the $JAK2^{V617F}$-positive and $JAK2^{V617F}$-negative MPNs [45].

PDGFRA. Platelet-derived growth factor receptor α (*PDGFRA*; chromosome 4q12) and β (*PDGFRB*; chromosome 5q31-q32) are involved in mutations occurring in chronic MPNs. Activating *PDGFRA* mutations due to *FIP1L1/PDGFRA* fusion has been described in subset of patients with SM associated with eosinophilia and hypereosinophilic syndrome/CEL (HES/CEL) [46–49]. *FIP1L1/PDGFRA* fusion results from karyotypically occult interstitial deletion of part of chromosome 4, del(4)(q12). *PDGFRA* mutations can be identified by FISH or RT-PCR (*CHIC2* deletion can serve as a surrogate marker for *FIP1L1/PDGFRA* fusion) [46].

Morphology
Blood

MPNs are most often associated with cytosis (thrombocytosis, neutrophilia, eosinophilia, basophilia, and/or erythrocytosis). Platelets in ET show anisocytosis ranging from small to giant forms. Thrombocytosis is often present in CML, early phases of both PV and PMF, and in mixed MPN/myelodysplastic syndrome (MDS) with ring sideroblasts and thrombocytosis (MPN/MDS-RS-T). Algorithmic approach to thrombocytosis is presented in Figure 21.2. Myelofibrosis can present with anemia, thrombocytopenia, and/or leukoerythroblastosis (presence of immature cells of both the myeloid and erythroid lineages). Apart from PMF, leukoerythroblastosis is seen in other MPNs in fibrotic stage, MDS/MPN-RS-T, acute myeloid leukemia (AML), especially AML with myelodysplasia-related changes (MDS-MRC) and reticulin fibrosis, infiltrative process in BM (metastatic carcinoma, lymphoma, Hodgkin lymphoma, plasma cell myeloma [PCM], CLL, mastocytosis, amyloidosis, granulomas, etc.) and in some infections. Neutrophilia is typical for CML and CNL but can be present in other MPNs, including PMF or PV. Algorithmic approach to neutrophilia is presented in Figure 21.3. PV is characterized by erythrocytosis, but often presents also with neutrophilia and/or thrombocytosis. Algorithmic approach to diagnosis of PV is presented in Figure 21.4, and algorithmic approach to eosinophilia is presented in Figure 21.5.

Bone marrow

Morphology plays central role is diagnosis and classification of MPNs and constitute some of WHO defined major criteria for a diagnosis. Although there is a significant overlap in morphologic features between various MPNs, especially in early and late stages of disease, many of the morphologic characteristics in conjunction with mutation screening help to establish a definite diagnosis of specific type of MPN. Generally, MPNs are characterized by hyperplasia of at least one of BM main lineages (granulocytic, erythroid and/or megakaryocytic) leading to increased production of granulocytes (most typical for CML), platelets (a major feature of ET), and red cells (a major feature of PV). Both PMF and PV show panmyelosis, that is, proliferation of all three lineages, while ET is usually associated with megakaryocytic hyperplasia only. PMF is characterized by BM fibrosis, cytopenia(s), and splenomegaly. Typical morphologic features of MPN are presented in Figure 21.6. BM aspirate is often hypercellular with increased megakaryocytes. BM cellularity and proportion of different lineages is best evaluated on the core biopsy. BM cellularity decreases with age; on average the expected (normal) cellularity corresponds to 100 minus patient age (e.g., 50-year-old person show 50% BM cellularity, whereas 70-year-old person shows cellularity of 30). The age-adjusted BM cellularity is usually increased with either panmyelosis or hyperplasia of one or two myeloid lineages. Myeloid hyperplasia may be accompanied by a leftward shift and accentuated paratrabecular myeloid immaturity. Megakaryocytes are increased and display atypia and often clustering. Megakaryocytic clustering generally correlates with an increase in reticulin fibers. Hypolobated micromegakaryocytes are more typical for CML, giant and bizarre forms of megakaryocytes with bulbous or balloon-shaped nuclei are typical for PMF, giant hyperlobulated megakaryocytes occur in ET, and PV shows pleomorphic megakaryocytes with cytologic atypia and variable size. Reticulin fibers are variably increased. Fibrosis is most pronounced in PMF and in the late (fibrotic) stage of other MPNs but can be mild and focal in early PMF (pre-PMF). ET usually does not show reticulin fibrosis, while PV may show mild and focal increase in reticulin fibers. Sinuses may be dilated with intravascular hematopoiesis and accompanying extramedullary hematopoiesis (as seen often in PMF). BM fibrosis may also accompany CML, mastocytosis, and less often PV.

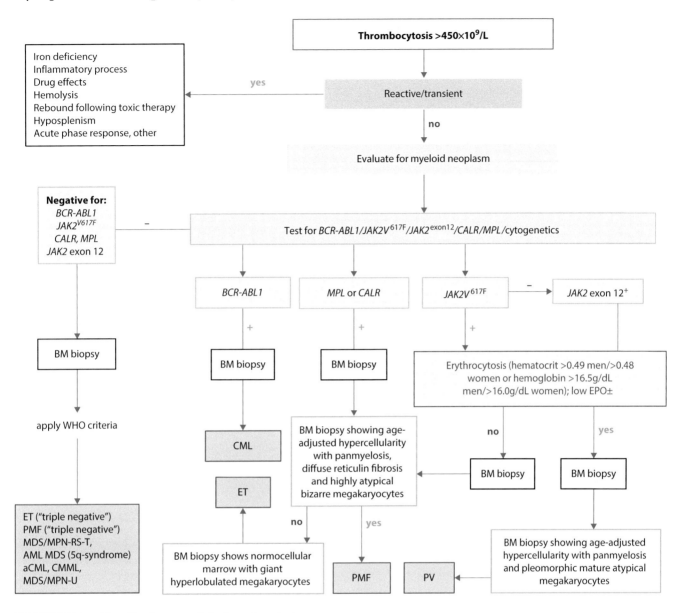

FIGURE 21.2 Algorithmic approach to thrombocytosis.

Flow cytometry

Characterization of normal BM cells (maturation pattern) and peripheral blood cells by flow cytometry (FC; Figure 21.7) is well established and allows for the distinction between normal and abnormal patterns, which proves useful not only for the diagnosis of acute leukemia but also allows for the analysis of myelodysplasia and MPN [50–66]. FC abnormalities are more frequently observed in cases with substantial myelofibrosis and are more frequent in cases with ≥5% BM blasts and/or circulating blasts [66]. Hematopoietic progenitors are positive for CD34, CD133, CD117, and HLA-DR. Neutrophilic maturation from blasts through promyelocytes, myelocytes, metamyelocytes, bands, and neutrophils is characterized by the loss of CD34 and HLA-DR expression at promyelocytic stage, loss CD117 expression, and the acquisition of CD11b and CD11c expression at myelocytic stage and acquisition of CD10 expression by neutrophils [67]. Myeloblasts are positive for CD34, CD38, HLA-DR, CD117, CD4, CD13 (dim), and CD33 (CD34 is expressed by all hematopoietic precursors, including early myeloblasts; CD117 expression

appears after CD34). Promyelocytes lose CD34 and HLA-DR, retain CD117 and show positive expression of CD13 and CD33 (bright). They show dim expression of CD4 and start to acquire CD15. At the transition to myelocytes, the expression of CD117 is lost. Myelocytes start to acquire the expression of CD11b and its intensity increases as the cell mature to late myelocytes and metamyelocytes (at the same time, the expression of CD4 disappear). CD33 expression progressively decreases. Metamyelocytes start to express CD10 and CD16 which increases in intensity as the cells progress to mature neutrophils. Segmented forms display bright expression of CD11b, CD11c, CD10, CD16, and CD15. FC analysis also permits identification of different subtypes of stem cells, based on the expression of CD34, CD38, and a panel of myeloid and lymphoid markers.

FC helps to differentiate between lymphocytosis, monocytosis, acute leukemia, and neutrophilia or eosinophilia. FC can determine the number and phenotype of blasts, thus helping to exclude MPN in accelerated or blasts phase. Additionally, there are subtle phenotypic abnormalities displayed by granulocytes

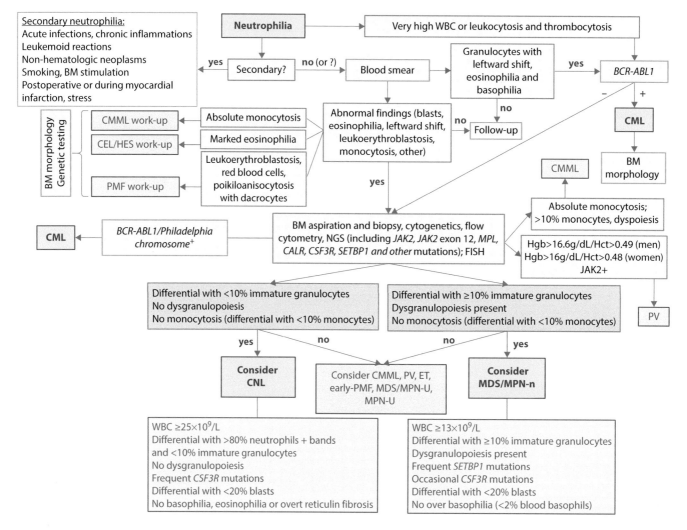

FIGURE 21.3 Algorithmic approach to neutrophilia. *Abbreviations: MDS/MPN-n, MDS/MON with neutrophilia; BM, bone marrow; CEL, chronic eosinophilic leukemia; CML, chronic myeloid leukemia; CNL, chronic neutrophilic leukemia; CMML, chronic myelomonocytic leukemia; ET, essential thrombocythemia; FISH, fluorescence in situ hybridization; HES, hypereosinophilic syndrome; NGS, next generation sequencing; PMF, primary myelofibrosis; PV, polycythemia vera; WBC, white blood cell count.*

and maturing myeloid precursors in the chronic phase (CP) of MPN (among other changes) which might be helpful in the diagnosis. Those include slightly increased number of blasts in BM or presence of circulating blasts in blood, decreased side scatter of granulocytes, aberrant expression of several markers, mainly CD10, CD11b, CD13, CD16, and CD56 by granulocytes/maturing myeloid precursors, circulating CD45-/CD71+/GPHA+ erythroid precursors, presence of basophilia and/or eosinophilia, immunophenotypic atypia of monocytes and abnormal ratio of myeloid cells to lymphocytes (due to granulocytosis and corresponding lymphopenia). Some of the phenotypic features seen in MPN by FC are not specific, as they may be seen in other myeloid neoplasms (e.g., MDS) or reactive processes.

Chronic myeloid leukemia

Introduction

CML, *BCR-ABL1+*, is a clonal stem cell disorder characterized by a formation of *BCR-ABL1* fusion gene as a result of translocation t(9;22)(q34;q11) [Philadelphia chromosome; Ph] leading to

enhanced tyrosine kinase activity and proliferation of myeloid cells at all stages of differentiation [2, 68, 69]. The c-abl protein, a tightly regulated tyrosine kinase, is predominantly present in the nucleus and plays a key role in cell cycle control. In majority of CML cases, the breakpoint in *BCR* is in the major breakpoint cluster region M-BCR (exons 13 or 14 of the BCR gene) to exon 2 of the ABL gene (e13a2 and e14a2) with formation of fusion protein, p210. In occasional cases, the breakpoint occurs in the μ-BCR region (exons 17-20; previously c1-c4) and formation of p230. Breakpoints in the minor breakpoint region, m-BCR (exons 1 of BCR) with exon 2 of ABL gene (e1a2) with the formation of shorter fusion protein, p190 occur rarely in CML and most frequently associated with Ph+ acute lymphoblastic leukemia (ALL). CML main characteristics include Philadelphia chromosome, leukocytosis with basophilia, hypercellular BM with myeloid hyperplasia, and leftward shift and hypolobated dwarf megakaryocytes (Figure 21.8). Most patients are diagnosed in CP and present with fatigue, night sweats, splenomegaly, weight loss, and anemia or are asymptomatic with leukocytosis (with/without thrombocytosis) identified during routine medical

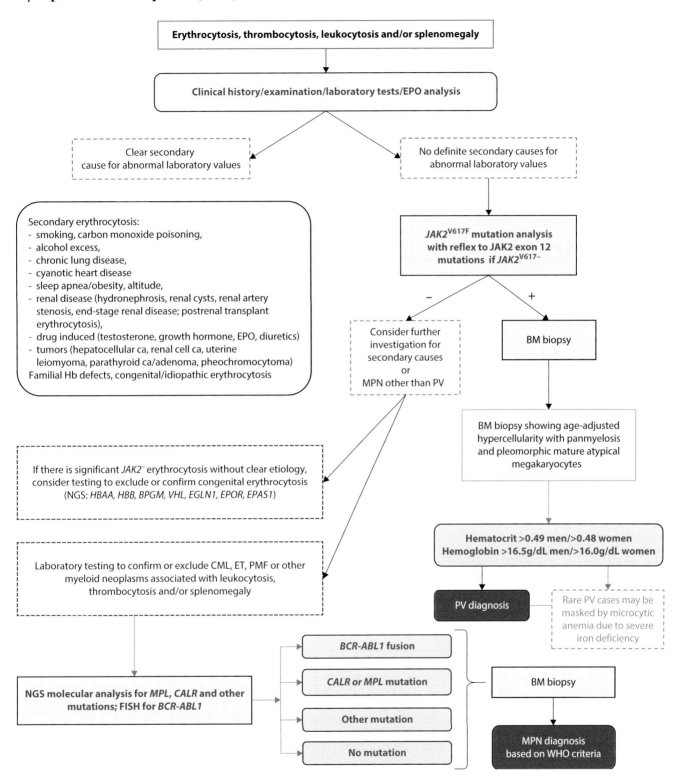

FIGURE 21.4 Algorithm for the diagnosis of PV (PV, polycythemia vera; MPN, myeloproliferative neoplasm, EPO, erythropoietin; BM, bone marrow; NGS, next Gene sequencing).

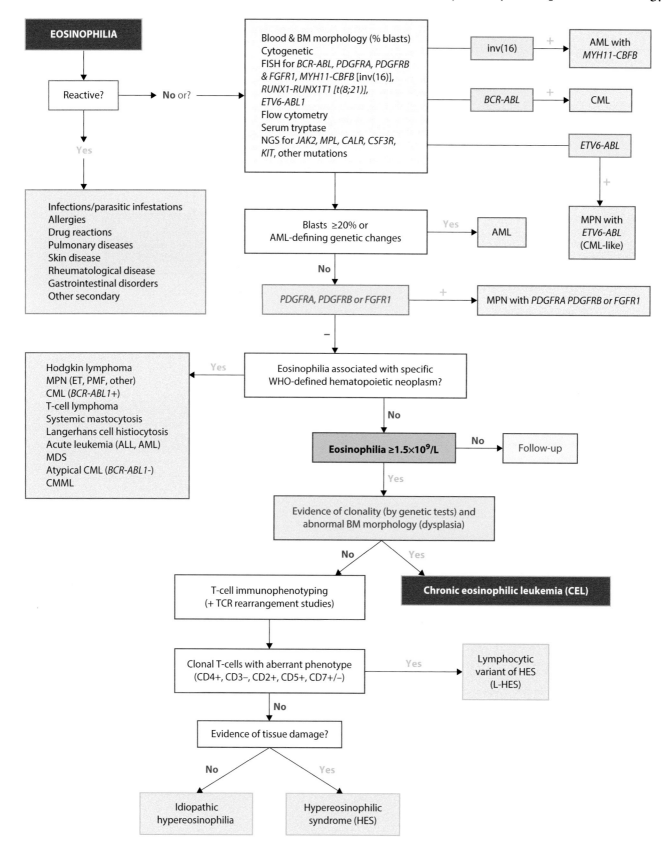

FIGURE 21.5 Algorithmic approach to eosinophilia. CEL is diagnosed with persistent eosinophilia with evidence of clonality by genetics testing and/or increased blasts (*PDGFRA, PDGFRB, FGFR1, BCR-ABL, and MYH11-CBFB* must be negative). HES shows sign of organ damage or involvement; It differs from CEL by lack of clonality and increased blasts. MPN with *FGFR1* may be associated with T-ALL, eosinophilia, and mastocytosis. *Abbreviations: CEL, chronic eosinophilic leukemia; HES, hypereosinophilic syndrome; CML, chronic myeloid leukemia (BCR-ABL+); MPN, myeloproliferative neoplasm; MDS, myelodysplastic syndrome; ALL, acute lymphoblastic leukemia.*

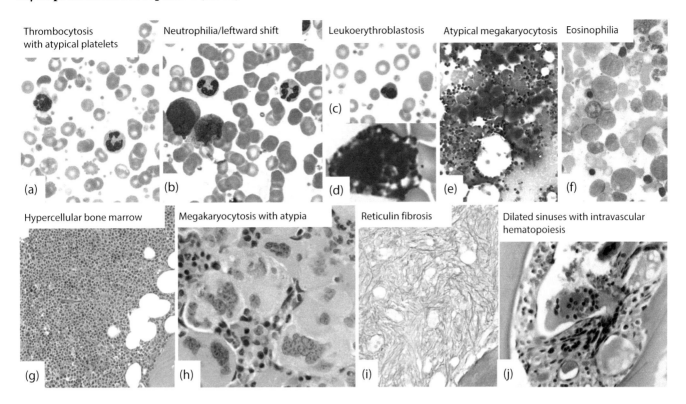

FIGURE 21.6 Myeloproliferative neoplasms (MPN) – general morphologic features: (a) blood film with thrombocytosis; (b) blood film with neutrophilia with leftward shift; (c) blood film with erythroid precursors; (d) basophilia; (e) BM aspirate with prominent megakaryocytosis with atypia; (f) BM aspirate with prominent eosinophilia; (g) BM core biopsy showing hypercellular marrow with myeloid hyperplasia and atypical hypolobated megakaryocytes; (h) BM core biopsy with atypical megakaryocytic clustering; (i) BM core biopsy with prominent reticulin fibrosis; (j) dilated sinuses with intravascular hematopoiesis.

checkup. Rarely, patients are diagnosed in accelerated phase (AP) or blastic phase (as *BCR-ABL1*⁺ AML or ALL). Introduction of the tyrosine kinase inhibitors, such as imatinib mesylate (Gleevec), revolutionized the treatment of CML with complete cytogenetic response (CyR) rate at 70%–90% and 5-year progression-free and overall survival between 80% and 95% [70–72].

Morphology
Blood
In CP of CML, blood shows prominent leukocytosis (with predominance of neutrophils), absolute basophilia and often eosinophilia. Granulocytic cells show a leftward shift with a "non-symmetrical" distribution (myelocytes > metamyelocytes). Although myelocytes predominate among immature cells, promyelocytes and blasts are increased (blasts usually do not exceed 2%). The blasts count between 10% and 19% defines AP and with 20% or more the disease is classified as AML (WHO classification). Platelets are usually increased, although platelet count may be normal or even reduced. Platelets display atypia with anisocytosis and occasional giant form. Monocytes are also increased (absolute monocytosis), but disproportionally to the number of granulocytes (<10% monocytes). Prominent monocytosis is typically seen in association with *BCR-ABL1* fusion at exons 1–2. Erythrocytosis is not seen in CML, but rare circulated red blood cell precursors are present in blood.

Bone marrow aspirate
BM aspirate is hypercellular with an increased M:E ratio due to both myeloid hyperplasia and erythroid hypoplasia (myeloid to erythroid ratio is usually around 10:1 to 30:1). Granulocytic cells show full maturation to segmented forms with a leftward shift and a peak ("myelocyte bulge") in the percentage of myelocytes. Erythroid and granulocytic series do not exhibit overt dyspoiesis. Megakaryocytes may be increased in number and display atypia, most characteristically in the form of smaller cells with centrally located hypolobated nucleus. In CP, blasts do not exceed 5% of the marrow cells. Eosinophils and basophils are increased in number. Scattered sea-blue histiocytes may be present (pseudo-Gaucher cell; storage histiocytes).

Bone marrow histology
Histologic examination of the BM core biopsy reveals a hypercellular marrow with myeloid and often megakaryocytic hyperplasia, myeloid leftward shift without increased number of blasts (CP) or increased blasts (AP). Myeloblasts and promyelocytes often accumulate against the bone trabeculae (accentuated paratrabecular immaturity) and around blood arterioles. Megakaryocytes are increased, usually smaller in size and have hypolobated nuclei. Significantly increased number of atypical megakaryocytes is seen in A megakaryocyte-rich subtype of CML as opposed to a more common granulocytic subtype. Prominent clustering or bizarre, hyperchromatic forms typical for non-CML MPNs, are absent. Except for cases with increased megakaryocytes, reticulin fibrosis is not prominent in CML in CP (prominent fibrosis may develop during the course of the disease and signify the disease progression). Eosinophils, mast cells, and basophils are increased in numbers. Plasma cells are often increased as well. BM vascularity is often increased in CML. Based on histomorphologic

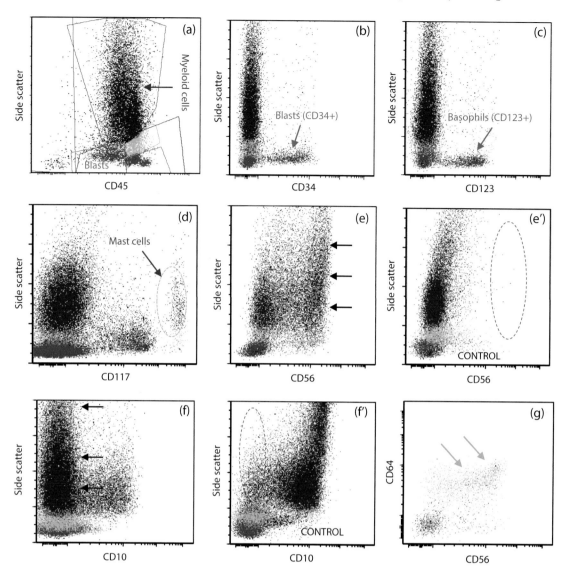

FIGURE 21.7 Myeloproliferative neoplasm (MPN) – flow cytometry. Flow cytometry analysis of blood (a) shows increased granulocytes with leftward shift (decreased CD45 expression) and increased blasts (a–b; blue dots). Basophilia (b) may be prominent as show by CD123 staining (c). Analysis of BM aspirate may show mast cells (d). Granulocytes display aberrant expression of CD56 (e; compare with healthy control shown on e'), decreased side scatter (f) and down-regulation of CD10 (f; compare with healthy control shown on f'). In contrast to CMML, monocytes are not increased but display aberrant phenotype (CD56 expression; g).

features, CML may display three variants: (1) granulocytic variant, (2) the megakaryocyte-rich variant, and (3) myelofibrotic variant [73–75]. The megakaryocyte-rich subtype is associated with increased risk of transformation into myelofibrosis.

Immunophenotype
Immunohistochemistry
Blasts are positive for CD34, CD117, CD33, MPO, and HLA-DR. Promyelocytes are positive for CD117, CD33, and MPO; they do not express CD34 and HLA-DR. The staining with MPO, CD71, and GPHA shows marked predominance of myeloid cells. Megakaryocytes are positive for CD61. In case with increased blasts, immunostaining with TdT, CD34, CD117, myeloid markers, and B- and T-cell markers is helpful to establish the lineage of immature cells and their proportion (e.g., to differentiate between myeloid and lymphoid blast crisis).

Flow cytometry
The analysis of peripheral blood by FC shows characteristic features in CP CML, which allow its distinction from reactive neutrophilia or eosinophilia (Figure 21.9). The most typical phenotypic features suggestive of CML in blood include an increased proportion of granulocytes when compared to other cell types, the presence of a distinct population of blasts, basophilia and phenotypic features of dysmaturation, and/or leftward shift displayed by granulocytes. CML cases show (on average) 1.3% of CD34+ blasts and 2.1% CD117+ precursors (those number in benign control cases range from 0.02% to 0.05%). There is on average 2.4% basophils in CML (Figure 21.10), compared to 0.5% in controls. The features of dysmaturation and leftward shift displayed by granulocytes include decreased granularity (decreased side scatter), aberrant expression of CD56 on subset of cells, and the lack of expression of CD10, CD11b, CD13, and CD16 in a significant

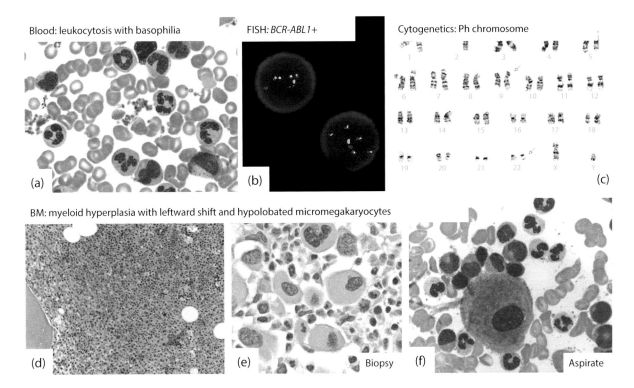

FIGURE 21.8   Major characteristics of CML: blood smear (a) with neutrophilia and leftward shift, FISH (b) and cytogenetic (c) with *BCR-ABL1* rearrangement (Philadelphia chromosome). Bone marrow biopsy (d–e) and aspirate smear (f) showing myeloid hyperplasia and atypical hypolobated dwarf megakaryocytes.

population. Many cases show an aberrant expression of CD56 by monocytes. Reactive neutrophilia, except of an increased proportion of granulocytes does not differ significantly in FC analysis from healthy controls. Rare cases of CML show minor population of circulating immature B-lymphoblasts resembling phenotypically hematogones in the BM or B-ALL (Figures 21.11 and 21.12). These cells are positive for CD22, CD19, and CD10 with variable expression of CD34, and likely represent partially mature B-lymphoid precursors derived from Ph+ stem cells. The flow cytometric features of CML in the BM are more subtle than in blood and include aberrant expression of CD56 by granulocytes and monocytes, increased number of blasts, increased proportion of granulocytes to lymphocytes, decreased granularity (lowered side scatter on granulocytes), abnormal maturation pattern (evaluated by expression of CD10, CD11b, CD13, CD16, and CD56), aberrant phenotype of monocytes, increased basophils, and a loss or significantly decreased number of hematogones (Figure 21.13).

Disease progression

CML may progress from the CP to AP and/or BP. Majority of patients with CML are diagnosed in CP (~80%) [76, 77]. In most untreated patients, there is progressive increase in leukocyte count. In untreated patients, transformation to BP occurs after a median of 3 years. With new treatments (imatinib, other TK inhibitors), the course of CML differs from that observed under prior treatment protocols. The progression is frequently preceded or accompanied by recurring secondary chromosomal abnormalities and oncogene alteration, most often including mutation or deletions of *TP53*, trisomy 8, upregulation of *Rb*, *MYC*, and *RAS* genes, doubling of the Ph chromosome, isochromosome 17 [i(17q)], and less often trisomy 19, trisomy 21, deletion 7, and loss

of the Y chromosome [78–86]. Patients who had a complete CyR or in whom levels of *BCR/ABL* transcripts had fallen by at least 3 log had a significantly lower risk of disease progression than did patients without a complete CyR [87].

Based on WHO classification, AP is suggested if any of the following parameters are present: (1) persistent or increasing leukocytosis (>10 × 10^9/L) and/or persistent of increasing splenomegaly unresponsive to therapy; (2) persistent thrombocytosis (>1000 × 10^9/L) unresponsive to therapy; (3) persistent thrombocytopenia (<100 × 10^9/L) unrelated to therapy; (3) ≥20% basophils in the peripheral blood; (4) 10%–19% myeloblasts in BM or blood; and (5) clonal cytogenetic evolution (the appearance of additional genetic abnormalities that were not present at the time of diagnosis) [88]. Figure 21.14 shows CML in AP.

In WHO classification, BP of CML is defined by (1) ≥20% blasts; or (2) extramedullary blast proliferation. The transformation into acute leukemia may be abrupt or may follow the AP. Occasional cases of CML are detected in blast crisis without a prior diagnosis of CML. Majority of cases shows features of AML, with either granulocytic, monocytic, erythroid, or megakaryocytic differentiation. AML with marked basophilia or acute basophilic leukemia may also complicate CML. The remaining cases (~20%) show lymphoblastic differentiation or bilineage (mixed phenotype) acute leukemia. Extramedullary acute leukemic infiltrate may involve any part of the body, most commonly the skin, spleen, lymph node, and brain. The immunophenotypic features of CML in BP correspond to those of *de novo* acute leukemias and are determined by FC and/or immunohistochemistry and cytochemical staining for non-specific esterase (NSE) and myeloperoxidase (MPO). The median survival of BP is 2–6 months (long-term survival is uncommon) [89–91]. The response

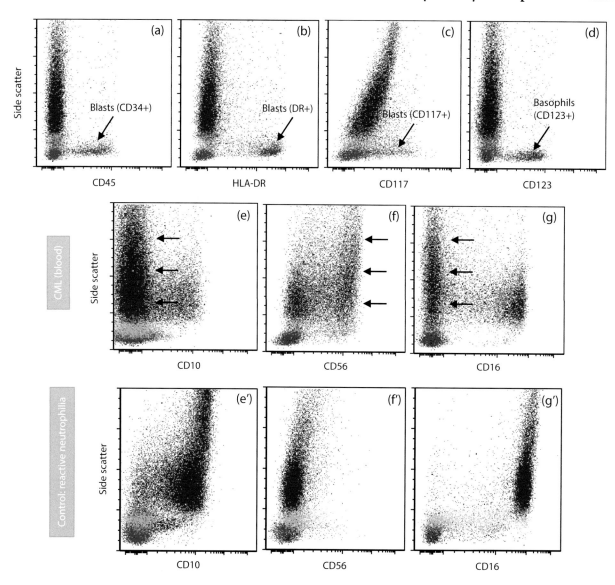

FIGURE 21.9 Flow cytometric features of CML in peripheral blood. The features differentiating CML from reactive neutrophilia include increased blasts expressing CD34, HLA-DR, and CD117 (a–c), increased basophils, expressing CD123 (d), decreased side scatter of granulocytes (e–g), down-regulation of CD10 (e; compare with control shown on e'), up-regulation of CD56 on granulocytes (f; compare with control shown on f') and down-regulation of CD16 on granulocytes (g; compare with control shown on g').

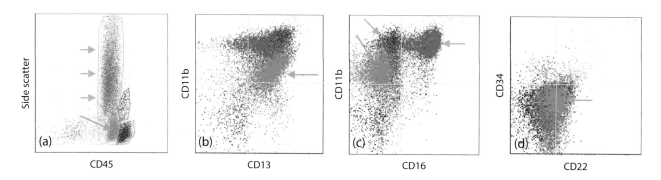

FIGURE 21.10 CML – blood. FC analysis shows increased basophils (a; green dots; green arrow). Granulocytes (gray dots; gray arrows) display moderate CD45 and slightly decreased side scatter (a), bright CD11b (b–c) and CD13 (b), and variable expression of CD16 (majority of granulocytes show bright CD16, but subset is CD16-negative; c). Basophils show slightly brighter expression of CD45 than neutrophils (a), low side scatter (a), moderate CD11b (dimmer than in neutrophils; b-c), bright CD13 (b), negative CD16 (c), and partially dim CD22 (d).

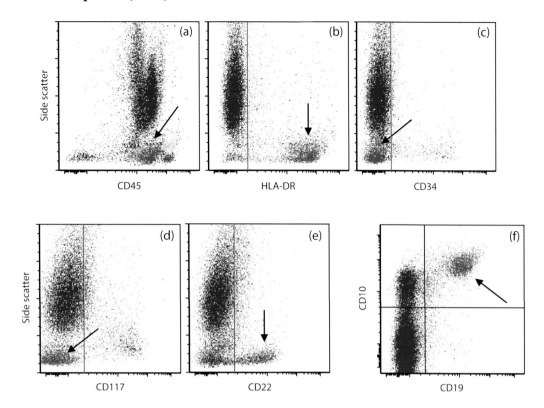

FIGURE 21.11 Flow cytometric features of CML. Rare cases of CML show small but distinct population of circulating immature B-cells ("hematogones-like") with the following phenotype: CD45$^+$ (a), HLA-DR$^+$ (b), CD34$^-$ (c), CD117$^-$ (d), CD22$^+$ (e), CD10$^+$ (f), and CD19$^+$ (f). It is uncertain whether this population represents an emerging B-ALL blast crisis.

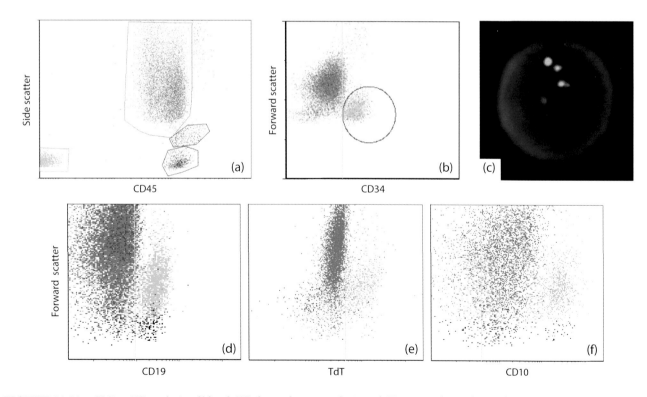

FIGURE 21.12 CML – FC analysis of blood. FC shows down-regulation of CD45 on subset of granulocytes (gray dots), resembling FC from bone marrow sample rather than blood (granulocytes at different stages of maturation), and presence of CD45$^-$ (a) and CD34$^+$ (b) B-lymphoblasts. FISH studies confirmed the diagnosis of CML (*BCR-ABL* rearrangement; c). Immature B-cells are positive for CD19 (d), TdT (e), and CD10 (f).

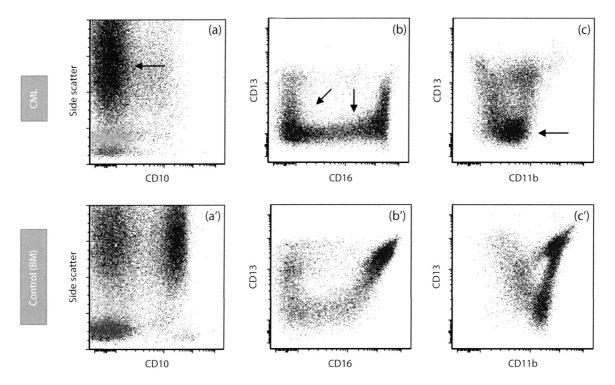

FIGURE 21.13 FC features of CML in the BM aspirate. Granulocytes/maturing myeloid precursors (purple dots) display aberrant pattern of maturation including down-regulation of CD10 (a; compare with control on a'), CD13 versus CD16 (b; compare with control on b') and CD11b versus CD13 (c; compare with control on c').

to high-dose chemotherapy with allogeneic stem cell transplantation is poor [89], due to up-regulation of anti-apoptotic signals and multidrug resistance (MDR). Despite the generally dismal prognosis of CML in BP when compared to *BCR-ABL1*-negative acute leukemia, determination of blast lineage in transformed CML is clinically important. Patients with lymphoblastic transformation have a better response to chemotherapy and longer survival than patients with myeloblastic transformation [92, 93]. Leukocyte alkaline phosphatase (LAP) is reduced in CML patients at diagnosis and the LAP values increase when CML transforms to more advanced disease (AP or BP). Cytogenetic clonal evolution is a known poor prognostic factor in CML. The lack of CyR

at 3 months appears to be a stronger independent poor prognostic factor for survival than clonal evolution for both chronic and AP. Presence of additional *BCR-ABL1* copies suggests disease progression and poor prognosis. The phenotype of blasts in BP of CML is often very abnormal, including lack of CD34 and CD117 expression (see Figure 5.35 in Chapter 5). Figures 21.15 and 21.16 show examples of CML in BP. Figure 21.17 shows an unusual progression of CML. The BM analysis showed typical CML in CP. Concurrent analysis of the inguinal lymph node showed involvement by T-lymphoblastic lymphoma. The leukemic cells in the BM (CML) and lymphomatous cells in the lymph node (T-ALL/LBL) had numerous copies of *BCR-ABL1*.

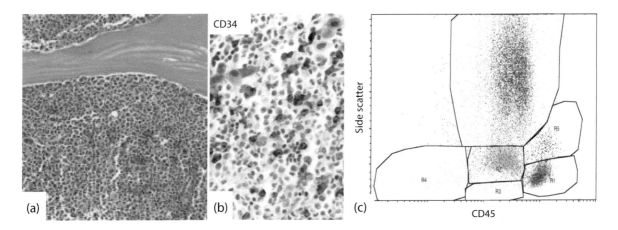

FIGURE 21.14 CML – accelerated phase (AP). The core biopsy shows hypercellular bone marrow (a) with increased blasts on core biopsy (a, histology; b, immunostaining with CD34). Flow cytometry analysis (c) revealed increased blasts (green dots).

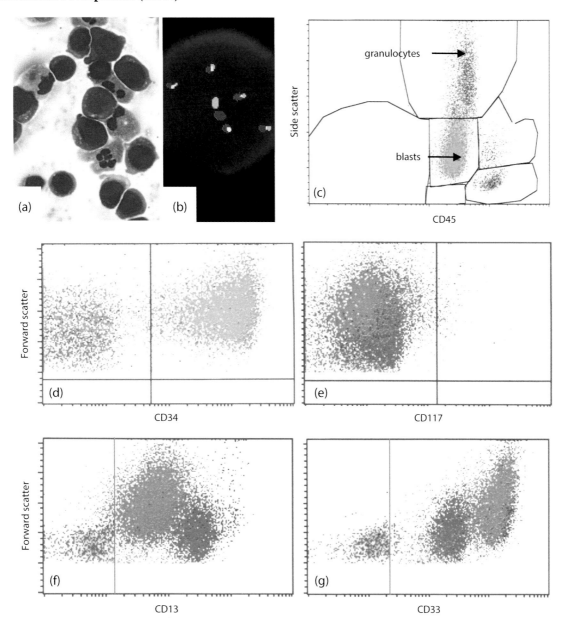

FIGURE 21.15   CML – myeloid blast phase. Aspirate smear (a) shows blasts. FISH studies (b) show increased number of *BCR-ABL1* copies. Flow cytometry (c–g) shows blasts (green dots; Arrow) expressing CD45 (c), CD34 (d), CD13 (f; Dim expression), and CD33 (g; Bright expression). CD117 is negative (e). Residual granulocytes (gray dots) have higher Side scatter (c) and lower forward scatter (d–g) when compared to blasts.

Disease monitoring

Imatinib mesylate can induce complete or nearly complete remission in up to 80% of patients [70, 94–98]. 90% of patients with early-stage (CP) CML and 60% of patients with advances stage CML (BP) achieve hematologic response (HR) to imatinib [70, 99]. The response to treatment is based on the hematologic, cytogenetic, and molecular parameters [72, 94–96, 100–102]. An HR indicates a return of peripheral blood cell counts and BM morphology to normal. CyR can be divided into complete, major, minor, and minimal. Complete cytogenetic response (CCyR) indicates the disappearance of the Philadelphia chromosome (Ph) and major cytogenetic response (MCyR) indicates less than 35% Ph+ cells in BM. Major molecular response is defined as 3 log reduction in *BCR-ABL1* transcript (≤0.1% on the international scale), deeper molecular response is ≤0.01% on the international scale and complete molecular response (CMR) is synonymous with undetectable transcripts by qRT-PCR (RQ-PCR). The preferred initial treatment is daily imatinib or second-generation tyrosine kinase inhibitors [72]. FC features associated with residual or recurrent disease include the presence of circulating blasts with atypical phenotype (Figure 21.18), myeloid dysmaturation, basophilia, or eosinophilia and in the BM presence of increased blasts with phenotypic atypia or aberrant expression of CD56 on myeloid cells.

Differential diagnosis of CML

Differential diagnosis of CML includes

- Reactive neutrophilia (leukemoid reaction, infections, plasma cell neoplasms, treatment (e.g., Neupogen)
- MDS/MPN-n

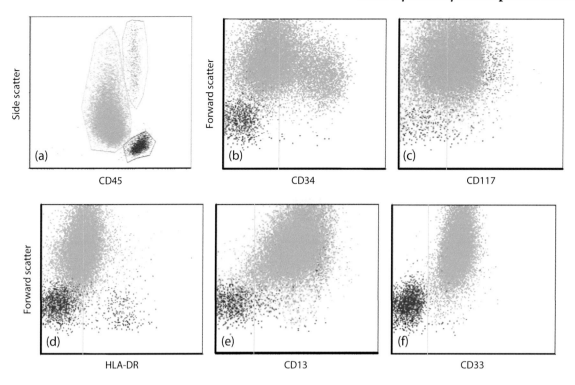

FIGURE 21.16   CML in blast phase. Blasts (green dots) show moderate CD45 (a), partial expression of CD34 (b), dim positive CD117 (c), negative to dim HLA-DR (d), and positive expression of CD13 (e) and CD33 (f).

- Chronic myelomonocytic leukemia (CMML)
- CEL
- CNL
- ET
- PMF
- AML
- PV
- MDS

Reactive neutrophilia

Prominent neutrophilia (leukemoid reaction) is seen in infections and as a paraneoplastic syndrome in patients with malignant tumors (hematopoietic and non-hematopoietic), including PCM, carcinomas of the lung, stomach, and kidney and rarely sarcomas. Leukemoid reaction is characterized by prominent leukocytosis (usually ~40 × 10^9/L) with a significant increase in early neutrophil precursors, toxic granulocytic vacuolation, and Döhle's bodies in the granulocytes. The samples from patients with leukemoid reaction usually do not show basophilia, increased micromegakaryocytes, increased blasts, or reticulin fibrosis [103]. CML patients have reduced LAP index, which is high in leukemoid reaction. Transient prominent neutrophilia with a left shift can be seen in patients receiving corticosteroids.

ET

Morphologically, CML with thrombocytosis differs from ET by granulocytic leftward shift, basophilia, and presence of hypolobated dwarf megakaryocytes. ET typically shows giant hyperlobulated megakaryocytes. The presence of BCR-ABL1 fusion excludes the diagnosis of ET.

PV

PV with associated iron deficiency, which causes normal hemoglobin and hematocrit (Hct) values, can manifest with leukocytosis and thrombocytosis mimicking CML. Leukocytosis, BM fibrosis, and occasionally eosinophilia and basophilia may be seen in some PV, especially as disease progresses. PV differs from CML by prominent megakaryocytic atypia with bizarre hyperchromatic forms, lack of BCR-ABL1 fusion, and presence of JAK2 mutation. Patients with history of PV developing BCR-ABL1$^+$ clones, and vice versa, CML patients with JAK2$^+$ clones have been reported [22, 23, 104].

PMF

Patients with CML may develop significant reticulin fibrosis, which require differentiation from PMF. History of CML and/or positive BCR-ABL1 rearrangement excludes de novo PMF.

MDS/MPN-n

MDS/MPN-n is a variant of mixed myeloproliferative/myelodysplastic neoplasm characterized by neutrophilia, cytologic features of dysplasia in BM and lack of BCR-ABL1 fusion. MDS/MPN-n is not associated with basophilia or thrombocytosis and megakaryocytes show more pronounced atypia not limited only to hypolobated micromegakaryocytes. As in MDS cases, MDS/MPN-n often shows dyserythropoiesis (mostly in the form of megaloblastoid changes) and dysgranulopoiesis (Pelgeroid changes), not typically seen in CML.

CNL

CNL is a rare disease occurring mostly in elderly patients. It is characterized by neutrophilia and splenomegaly. It does not show basophilia, hypolobated micromegakaryocytes, myeloid leftward shift, and most importantly BCR-ABL1 fusion. Neutrophils often show prominent cytoplasmic granules (toxic granulation). CNL is characterized by frequent mutations in receptor of colony stimulating factor 3 (CSF3R). Mutations in CSF3R are highly prevalent in CNL and may support the diagnosis of this disease in the appropriate clinical context. CSF3R mutations have also been reported less commonly in other myeloid disorders including MDS/MPN-n, CMML, and AML.

BONE MARROW

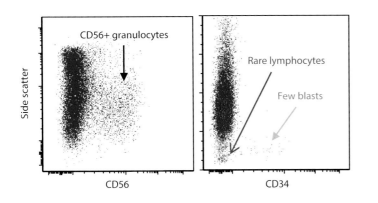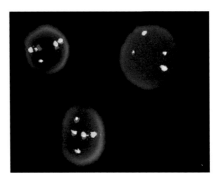

INGUINAL LYMPH NODE

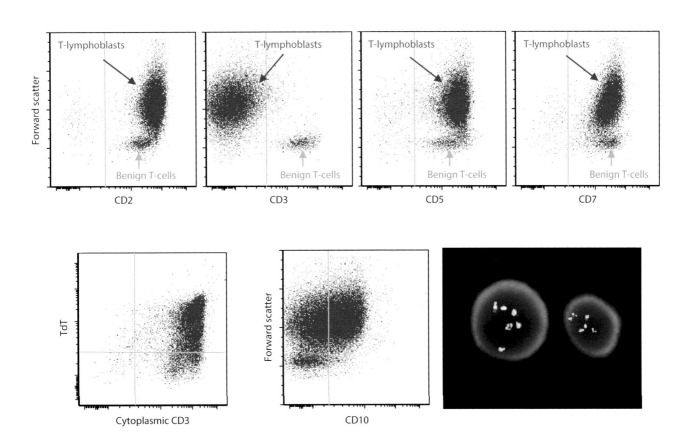

FIGURE 21.17 CML in chronic phase (in the BM) and "localized T-lymphoblastic blast crisis" (inguinal adenopathy with T-lymphoblastic lymphoma diagnosed at the time of CML diagnosis). Patient had no prior history of CML or other malignancy. The morphologic, flow cytometric, and FISH analysis of the BM showed CML in chronic phase with extra copies of *BCR-ABL1*. Concurrent analysis of the lymph node showed involvement by T-lymphoblastic lymphoma with extra copies of *BCR-ABL1*. Lymphomatous cells in the lymph node were positive for CD2, CD5, CD7, cytoplasmic CD3, TdT, and partially CD10. Surface CD3 was not expressed. The flow cytometric analysis of the BM shows marked lymphopenia (no blasts, including T-lymphoblasts have been identified). Granulocytes displayed aberrant expression of CD56 on subset. FISH: aqua, arginosuccinate synthetase 1 gene on 9q34; green, *BCR* gene on chr.22; and red, *ABL1* gene on chromosome 9; yellow signal indicates *BCR-ABL1* fusion.

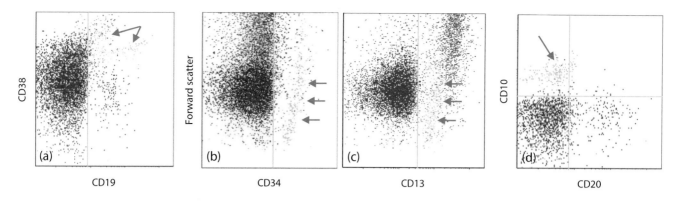

FIGURE 21.18 CML (after treatment) – blood. FC analysis shows a minute population of blasts (blue dots; arrow) with aberrant phenotype: CD19+ (a), CD38+ (a), CD34+ (b), CD13+ (c), CD10+ (d), and CD20− (d). Some of the FC features resemble hematogones (variable forward scatter, CD10 positivity, and CD19 versus CD38 pattern).

Myeloid neoplasm with ETV6

MPN associated with *ABL1-ETV6* fusions are rare. Patients usually show high WBC count with neutrophilia, eosinophilia, and basophilia. BM is hypercellular with myeloid hyperplasia with leftward shift. The clinicopathological features mimic CML, but there is no t(9;22)/*BCR-ABL1* fusion, although some patients respond to tyrosine kinase inhibitors.

Eosinophilia

Apart from CML (*BCR-ABL1+*), eosinophilia may be present in a variety of reactive and malignant disorders (*BCR-ABL1−*), including CEL, HES, and MPNs associated with rearrangement of *PDGFRA*, *PDGFRB*, or *FGFR1*. Eosinophilia may be also seen in peripheral T-cell disorders, classic Hodgkin lymphoma (cHL), SM, and ALL. Molecular testing (including *BCR-ABL1*), BM morphology, and FC immunophenotyping helps to confirm or exclude CML.

MDS

CML, especially in AP, may resemble MDS (MDS with excess blasts). MDS differs by erythroid hyperplasia and corresponding myeloid hypoplasia, lack of leukocytosis (in majority of cases), and lack of *BCR-ABL1* fusion.

CMML

Monocytosis may be present in CML and when prominent may mimic CMML (see Figure 20.14 in Chapter 20). CMML is a mixed myelodysplastic/MPN characterized by presence of absolute monocytosis, dysplasia, and risk of progression to AML. As per the definition, the Philadelphia chromosome and its related *BCR-ABL1* fusion gene are absent in CMML. Somatic mutations identified in CMML patients include *SRSF2*, *TET2*, or *RAS*. The diagnosis of CMML requires both an absolute monocytosis (≥1 × 10⁹/L) and relative monocytosis (≥10% of leukocytes) in the peripheral blood. In CML, the monocytes do not exceed 10%.

AML

AML differs by ≥20% and/or presence of specific chromosomal (molecular changes), such as t(8;21), t(15;17), or inv(16) [2]. Primary *BCR-ABL1+* AML is rare, but *de novo BCR-ABL1+* ALL occurs more frequently, especially in older patients.

Flow cytometric differential diagnosis of CML in blood

Many of the flow cytometric features observed in CML are not unique and therefore based on the FC pattern alone, the

differential diagnosis includes eosinophilia (reactive and neoplastic), MDS, CMML, paroxysmal nocturnal hemoglobinuria (PNH), and classic (non-CML) MPN such as ET, PV, or PMF. [52–56, 59, 61, 63–65, 105–115]. Eosinophils are negative for CD10 and CD16 but show significantly higher side scatter and lower forward scatter when compared to neutrophils. They do not display aberrant expression of CD11b, CD13, or CD56. Many flow cytometric findings in CML overlap with those of MDS. Granulocytes in MDS display low side scatter (decreased granularity), abnormal CD10/CD13/CD16 maturation pattern, and aberrant expression of CD56. MDS is also characterized by an increased number of blasts, a lack of hematogones, and an aberrant phenotype of monocytes. Patients with MDS, however, present with different clinical manifestations, which are easily distinguished from those of CML. In contrast to CML, samples from MDS patients show a decreased proportion of granulocytes, an increased number of CD45-negative events (representing erythroid precursors), and a lack of basophilia (in most cases). The presence of basophilia (>1%) in MDS is rare and is associated with worse prognosis [116]. CMML patients are characterized by absolute monocytosis, with FC analysis showing a predominance of monocytes with aberrant phenotype including CD56 expression and loss or variable expression of CD14 [56, 109, 117, 118]. Granulocytes in ET or PMF display phenotypic abnormalities overlapping with those observed in MDS. [52] Patients with PNH and some rare genetic disorders may display aberrant loss of CD10 and/or CD16 by granulocytes [119]. In some patients, CD16 appears negative as a result of genetic polymorphism of the CD16 molecule [120]. Neutrophil apoptosis is associated with diminished expression of CD16 [121]. Monocytes may be increased in CML cases, and therefore work-up of patients with monocytosis should include testing for *BCR-ABL1*. Similar to CMML, monocytes in CML are mature and often display aberrant expression of CD56 and/or variable expression of CD14. The proportion of granulocytes to monocytes is reversed or significantly reduced in CMML, whereas in CML is usually normal or decreased.

Polycythemia vera

Introduction

PV is an MPN characterized by increased and autonomous production of red cells, and to lesser degree other myeloid cells [2, 37, 122–128]. The abnormal proliferation in PV is caused by a constitutively active JAK-STAT signal transduction pathway, due to unique V617F mutation within exon 14 (~95% of PV) [32, 34, 129] and by different mutation within exon 12 (~4% of PV) of the *JAK2* gene [130, 131].

Two phases of PV can be recognized: (1) polycythemic and (2) post-polycythemic myelofibrosis (post-PV-MF) phase. In the revised WHO classification, the diagnostic threshold for hemoglobin and Hct concentrations required for the diagnosis of PV was lowered to >16.5g/dL and 49% for men and >16g/dL and 48% for women. Based on this lowered threshold, cases designated before pre-polycythemic phase of PV also termed "masked" PV, as well as some of MPN, unclassifiable are now diagnosed as PV (polycythemic phase). The polycythemic phase shows typical clinical and laboratory features of PV. The course of PV is mainly dominated by thrombosis and symptoms related to increased red cell mass (RCM) such as hypertension, headache, and pruritus (due to hyperhistaminemia), dizziness, splenomegaly, hemorrhage, and complications of either thrombosis or hemorrhage. Splenomegaly is most often seen in advanced disease. After a period of stable disease, PV usually progresses to a "spent" (post-polycythemic) phase with cytopenia(s), BM fibrosis, and extramedullary hematopoiesis. In some patients, the PV is complicated by MDS or acute leukemia (BP).

Laboratory and morphologic findings depend on the stage of the disease. In the initial polycythemic stage, the red cell indices are increased: red blood cells >25% above mean normal predicted value and hemoglobin >16.5g/dL (men) or >16.0g/dL (women), and/or Hct >49% in men and >48% in women. Hct has been shown to perform better in identifying patients with a raised RCM than hemoglobin concentration. In rare cases of (masked) PV associated with severe iron deficiency or less often increased splenic sequestration (e.g., in Budd Chiari syndrome), the values of hemoglobin and Hct may be below WHO defined criteria [132, 133]. Increased RCM >25% above mean normal predicted value helps to confirm the diagnosis of PV [2]. Aladağ et al., proposed using red blood cell count as an alternative to red blood cell mass to differentiate between PV with concurrent iron deficiency-induced microcytic anemia and unclassifiable MPN [132]. Since PV is a clonal proliferation of all three BM lineages, pan-myeloproliferative pattern (erythrocytosis with leukocytosis and/or thrombocytosis) is more consistent with PV than isolated erythrocytosis. Thrombosis and bleeding are major causes of morbidity and death in patients with PV. Neutrophilia and rarely basophilia may be present mimicking CML. Subset of cases may be associated with prominent thrombocytosis mimicking ET.

The diagnosis of PV is based on clinical and biological parameters defined by WHO (Table 21.2). In isolated erythrocytosis, secondary causes for polycythemia should be excluded first, including smoking, pulmonary, or cardiac problems, overweight with nocturnal dyspnea, or hepatic and renal tumors. Assessing serum erythropoietin (EPO) level is an excellent discriminatory test, being high in secondary polycythemia (e.g., due to exogenous administration or endogenous overproduction) and in hypoxic conditions, and is typically low in PV, although in the setting of *JAK2* mutation testing the role of EPO utility is limited. An algorithmic approach to the diagnosis of PV is presented in Figure 21.4.

Morphology

Blood shows erythrocytosis and in some cases thrombocytosis, neutrophilia, and/or basophilia. There is no leukoerythroblastosis, except for late, post-PV myelofibrosis phase. The polycythemic stage of PV (Figure 21.19) is characterized by a hypercellular

TABLE 21.2: WHO Criteria for PV (Diagnosis Requires All Three Major Criteria or the First Two Major Criteria and the Minor Criterion)

Major criteria

1. Hemoglobin >16.5 g/dL in men, >16.0 g/dL in women or elevated hematocrit >49% in men, >48% in women or increased red blood mass (>25% above normal)
2. BM biopsy showing age-adjusted hypercellularity with panmyelosis and pleomorphic mature megakaryocytes of variable size
3. Presence of *JAK2* V617F or *JAK2* exon 12 mutation

Minor criterion

Serum erythropoietin levels below the reference range for normal

Major criterion #2 may not be required in patients with sustained absolute erythrocytosis (hemoglobin >18.5g/dL or hematocrit >55.5% for men and hemoglobin >16.5g/dL or hematocrit >49.5% for women) if major criterion #3 and minor criterion are present

BM due to panmyelosis (erythroid, myeloid, and megakaryocytic hyperplasia) [73, 75, 134–138]. The presence of reactive lymphoid aggregates is not unusual for PV. Minute subset of patients may show normocellular and/or slightly hypercellular marrow, a feature more typical for ET. Erythroid precursors are increased with formation of prominent clusters. Granulocytes display slight leftward shift, but there is no increase in number of blasts. Megakaryocytes are increased in number and are dispersed individually or form loose aggregates, often close to bone trabeculae. Megakaryocytes display focally prominent atypia with anisocytosis ranging from small, intermediate to giant forms and hyperlobated nuclei. Bizarre, bulky nuclei with prominent nuclear-cytoplasmic dyssynchrony may be seen but are not as prominent as in PMF. Many normal appearing megakaryocytes are also present, feature that helps to distinguish PV from PMF. Majority of the cases do not display reticulin fibrosis at the initial diagnosis, but focal mild to moderate reticulin fibrosis may be present in early PV as well. Marked fibrosis or collagen deposition is typical for either PMF or late stage of PV. There are no iron particles in the aspirate smear or clot sections in most PV cases.

Postpolycythemic myelofibrosis. The spent phase is characterized by diffuse reticulin fibrosis and marrow hypocellularity with clusters of atypical, often hyperchromatic megakaryocytes (Figure 21.20). The peripheral blood and BM histomorphology findings are similar to PMF. Diagnostic criteria for post-PV-MF, published by Barosi et al., and incorporated into WHO classification are presented in Table 21.3 [2, 139]. The progression to PP-MF is observed in 15% of patients at a median of 10 years (range 2–23) from the diagnosis of PV, and 35% at 15 years [140].

Flow cytometry

FC has limited role in PV. It is used mostly to exclude disease progression to accelerated or BP and to exclude other accompanying hematologic neoplasms (e.g., chronic lymphocytic leukemia, lymphoma, or PCM). Herborg et al., reported that enumeration of circulating human Myeloid Inhibitory C-type Lectin (hMICL)-positive stem cells by FC can discriminate between MPN phenotypes and holds potential for monitoring disease evolution [141]. Maugeri et al., showed that fraction of circulating neutrophils and monocytes that had phagocytosed platelets, as assessed by FC, was significantly higher in patients with PV or ET, independently of hydroxyurea treatment, than in controls [142].

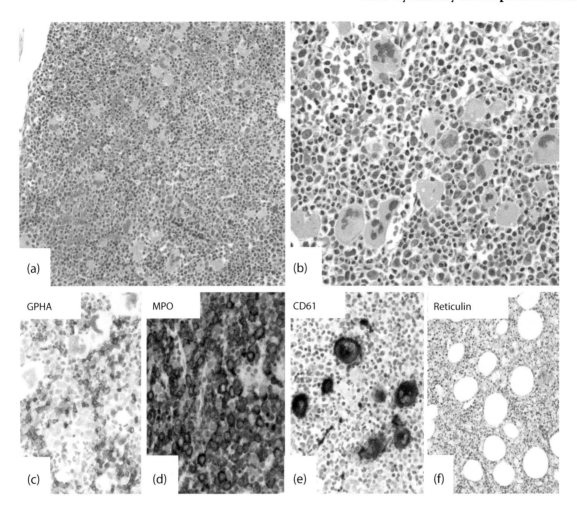

FIGURE 21.19   PV. (A) BM core biopsy shows hypercellular marrow with increased m:E ratio and megakaryocytosis. (b) High magnification displays numerous atypical megakaryocytes including hyperlobulated forms mimicking ET. (c–e) Immunohistochemical staining shows scattered red cell precursors (c), myeloid hyperplasia (d), and megakaryocytosis (E). Reticulin fibrosis is mildly increased (f).

Genetic features

Somatic point mutation of the tyrosine kinase *JAK2* (*JAK2* V617F) located in exon 14 of the gene has been reported in ~98% of PV [32, 34, 35]. Rare patients with PV, which are negative for *JAK2* V617F mutation, harbor the mutation of *JAK2* at exon 12. The *JAK2* exon 12 mutation positive PV is associated with higher hemoglobin levels and lower white cell and platelet count compared to typical *JAK2* V617F+ cases. Chromosomal abnormalities are found in 15%–20% of PV patients at diagnosis. The most common recurring abnormalities include +8, +9, del(20q), and 1q duplications [143–148]. FISH analysis increases the percentage of abnormal cases by 1.5%–6% when compared to conventional cytogenetics [146, 149], but trisomies 8 and 9 and deletions in 13q and 20q are more often detected by classic cytogenetics than FISH [149]. Similar to other chronic MPNs, as disease progresses, chromosomal abnormalities become more frequent [145, 148]. Patients treated with myelosuppressive agents show a significantly greater risk of chromosome abnormalities than did patients who had been phlebotomized [145]. Next gene sequencing studies revealed additional (non-driver) mutations in PV, including *DNMT3A*

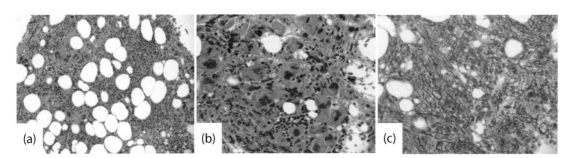

FIGURE 21.20   Post-polycythemia myelofibrosis (PPMF). (a–b) histology (intermediate and high magnification) shows megakaryocytic hyperplasia with marked cytologic atypia. (c) reticulin staining shows grade 3 fibrosis.

TABLE 21.3: WHO Criteria for Post PV Myelofibrosis (PPMF)

Required criteria

1. Documentation of a previous diagnosis of PV
2. BM fibrosis grade 2–3 (0–3 scale) or 3–4 (0–4 scale)

Additional criteria (Two are required)

1. Anemia
2. Leukoerythroblastosis
3. Increasing splenomegaly
4. Two of the following constitutional symptoms: >10% weight loss in 6 months, unexplained fever (>37.5°C)

(3%–15%), *IDH1/2* (<2%), *TET2* (15%–30%), *ASXL1* (5%–10%), *EZH2* (<5%) and *SF3B1* (<6%), *SRSF2* (<5%), *CEBP1* (2%–6%), *KIT* (3%), *TP53* (<5%), and *CBL* (<7%) [6].

Disease progression

Accelerated phase. The presence of ≥10% blasts in blood or BM indicates AP of PV.

   Blasts phase. The presence of ≥20% blasts in blood or BM indicates BP of PV (PV in BP; AML following PV).

The risk of disease transformation into BM fibrosis, myelodysplasia (MDS) or AML increases over time,[145, 150–153]. In a series reported by Fruchtman et al., 2.8% of patients with PV developed MDS/AML[154]. Exposure to P32, busulphan, and pipobroman, but not to hydroxyurea alone, had an independent role in producing an excess risk for progression to AML/MDS compared with treatment with phlebotomy or interferon [155]. Recent studies suggest that patients receiving hydroxyurea as the only cytoreductive therapy do not have increased risk of progression to AML[155–157]. Recent studies have shown that genetic variations in the DNA repair predispose patients with ET and PV [158]. Newer agents, including pegylated interferon alpha-2a, ruxolitinib, and other *JAK2* inhibitors, may replace hydroxyurea in the treatment of PV in the near future. Most of the patients die from thrombosis or hemorrhage, but up to 20% succumb to MDS or AML. Comprehensive analysis of post-PV AML cells identified several mutations involving *IDH1-IDH2, TET2, IKZF, NRAS, TP53,* and *RUNX1* genes. Blasts, even in *JAK2*+ PV cases, have been shown to be *JAK2*− [159].

Differential diagnosis of PV

Differential diagnosis of PV based on erythrocytosis includes

- Hypoxia associated erythrocytosis (lung disease, cardiac disease, high-altitude habitat, renal artery stenosis, intrinsic renal disease, obstructive sleep apnea)
- Ectopic erythropoietin secretion (uterine leiomyoma, hepatocellular carcinoma, cerebellar hemangioblastoma)
- Drug-associated erythrocytosis (exogenous erythropoietin, androgen preparations)
- Inherited erythrocytosis (high oxygen-affinity hemoglobin, erythropoietin receptor mutation, 2,3-biphosphoglycerate mutase deficiency)
- Relative erythrocytosis (e.g., due to dehydration)

Differential diagnosis of PV based on JAK2 mutation includes

- ET ~50%−60%
- PMF ~50%−60%
- CNL, rare cases
- CEL, rare cases

- Mixed myelodysplastic/MPN with ring sideroblasts and thrombocytosis (MDS/MPN-RS-T)
- AML, rare cases

Differential diagnosis of PV based on morphology includes

- PMF
- ET
- CML
- MDS

PMF

PMF differs from PV by the presence of significant reticulin fibrosis and more pronounced and uniform megakaryocytic atypia. In PMF, blood smear shows leukoerythroblastosis with numerous dacrocytes and abnormal platelets. In the prefibrotic stage of PMF, the BM is hypercellular with myeloid hyperplasia and prominent clusters of highly atypical megakaryocytes showing hyperchromatic nuclei, abnormal nuclear lobation often described as cloud-like, bulbous, or balloon-like. The laboratory findings in PV and pre-fibrotic PMF are most helpful in the differential diagnosis between both disorders.

ET

There is significant morphologic overlap between ET and PV, especially in early PV. Transformation of *JAK2*-mutated ET to PV has been reported, while no transformation to PV was observed in CALR-mutated ET patients [160]. The hemoglobin levels ≥16.5g/dL in men and 16.0g/dl in women or a Hct level of 49% in men and 48% in women help to differentiate most cases of *JAK2*-mutated ET from PV. The BM in ET is usually normocellular or only slightly hypercellular, whereas all PV cases display age-adjusted increased hematopoietic cellularity due to panmyelosis (proliferation of all three lineages) [125]. In ET, megakaryocytes are dispersed individually and mostly large (giant) with hyperlobulated (staghorn) nuclei, while PV shows cytologic pleomorphism among megakaryocytes, which vary in size and occasionally may show feature reminiscent of PMF. Reticulin staining is also helpful in differential diagnosis with ET showing no increase in reticulin fibers (<5%) and PV usually showing mild increase in fibrosis (<20%) [125]. JAK2 mutation is seen in 100% of PV cased and in 64% of ET. The presence of *MPL*, CALR, or lack of *JAK2, CALR,* and *MPL* (triple negative status) indicates ET.

CML

CML differs by the presence of hypolobated micromegakaryocytes, basophilia, and predominance of granulocytic hyperplasia. The BM in MDS is hypercellular with erythroid hyperplasia, but clinical presentation and laboratory data are different in MDS (cytopenias) from PV in polycythemic phase (cytoses).

MDS

BM in MDS patients is often hypercellular with erythroid hyperplasia and megakaryocytic atypia, especially presence of small hypolobated megakaryocytes. Hemoglobin and Hct levels are decreased, which differs from increased values in PV.

Essential thrombocythemia

Introduction

ET is a relatively indolent and often asymptomatic clonal MPN that involves predominantly megakaryocytic lineage characterized primarily by a sustained elevation in platelets (≥450 × 10⁹/L),

TABLE 21.4: WHO Criteria for ET (All Four are Required for Diagnosis)

Major criteria:

1. Platelet count ≥450 × 10⁹/L
2. Bone marrow biopsy specimen showing proliferation mainly of the megakaryocytic lineage with increased numbers of enlarged, mature megakaryocytes with hyperlobulated nuclei, no significant increase or left shift of neutrophil granulopoiesis or erythropoiesis; no or very minimal (grade 1) reticulin fibrosis
3. Not meeting WHO criteria for PV, BCR-ABL1⁺ CML, PMF, MDS or other myeloid neoplasm
4. JAK2, CALR, or MPL mutation

Minor criterion:

Presence of a clonal markers or absence of evidence of reactive thrombocytosis

The diagnosis of ET requires that either all major criteria are met, or the first three major criteria plus the minor criterion

megakaryocytosis and minimal to absent BM fibrosis [2, 161–170]. The acquired mutations in the *JAK2, CALR,* and *MPL* genes occur in ~60%, 30%, and 3%–4% of cases, respectively (~12% are triple-negative). Since other MPNs, especially CML, PV and PMF often present with thrombocytosis, morphologic evaluation of the BM plays important role in the diagnosis of ET. Increase and loose clustering of large megakaryocytes with mature cytoplasm and multilobulated staghorn-like nuclei in a normocellular or only slightly hypercellular BM represent major hallmarks of ET [137, 165, 171]. Early (prefibrotic) phase of PMF (pre-PMF) differs by marrow hypercellularity and cohesive clusters of megakaryocytes with often bulbous, bizarre nuclei with maturation defect [172].

Table 21.4 presents current WHO criteria for ET [2]. Generally, ET can be diagnosed in a patients with sustained platelet ≥450 × 10⁹/L with *JAK2*^V617F (or other clonal marker) who do not meet the criteria for the diagnosis of PV, CML, PMF, MDS, and other MPN, and whose biopsy shows atypical large and mature megakaryocytes not accompanying by BM fibrosis (in the absence of clonal marker, there should be no evidence for reactive thrombocytosis). This means that to diagnose ET, one has to exclude *BCR-ABL1* fusion, significant BM reticulin or collagen fibrosis and dyserythropoiesis and dysgranulopoiesis, and to prove the failure of iron replacement therapy to increase the hemoglobin level to PV range in the presence of decreased serum ferritin.

Morphology

The blood shows an increase in number of platelets, which may display atypia and anisocytosis. Leukocytosis, if present, is mild. The BM aspirate is normocellular to slightly hypercellular with increased megakaryocytes, which often cluster within spicules. Megakaryocytes are large and occasionally giant with mature cytoplasm and irregular (hyperlobulated) nuclei (staghorn-like). The biopsy shows normocellular to hypercellular marrow (Figure 21.21) without significant leftward shift of neutrophil granulopoiesis or erythropoiesis. There is megakaryocytic hyperplasia with atypia, but without overt maturation defects (typical for PMF). Megakaryocytes may be seen abnormally close to the bony trabeculae; usually they are in the deep interstitium. In rare cases, reticulin fibers may be focally increased (<25% of the marrow area), but typical ET usually lacks reticulin or collagen fibrosis. The granulocytic series does not show leftward shift.

Flow cytometry

Majority of ET cases do not display abnormalities identifiable by routine FC analysis.

Genetic features

Janus kinase 2 (*JAK2*) mutations constitute the most frequent mutation in ET (60%), followed by *CALR* exon 9 insertions/deletions (25%–32%) and myeloproliferative leukemia virus oncogene (*MPL*) mutations (3%–4%) [16, 29, 160, 165, 173–175]. Remaining ET cases (~12%) are triple-negative (they lack *JAK2, CALR,* and *MPL* mutations). *JAK2, CALR,* and *MPL* mutations are mutually exclusive. ET patients with *CALR* mutation show higher platelets count, lower leukocyte count, lower hemoglobin level, lower risk of thrombosis, and better survival when compared to patients with *JAK2*-mutated ET [29]. Nangalia et al., reported higher platelet count, lower hemoglobin level, and higher incidence of fibrotic transformation in patients with *CALR*⁺ cases, compared to *JAK2* mutated cases [174]. More recent reports did not find significant difference in survival or risk of fibrotic transformation between *CALR*⁻ and *JAK2*-mutated ET [160, 176, 177]. Patients with *JAK2*^V617F- ET do not commonly progress to become *JAK2*^V617F+ [178].

Disease progression and prognosis

Median survival for ET patients is approximately 20 years (32.7 years for patients younger than 60 years) and is higher than in PV (13.5 years) and PMF (5.9 years) [25]. Despite the long survival in patients with ET, their life expectancy is inferior to age- and sex-matched population. The mutational status (*JAK2* versus *CALR* versus *MPL* versus triple negative) does not influence survival in ET patients [25]. A transformation of ET to AML, MDS or myelofibrosis is a relatively rare event and occurs in 1–5% of all patients [161, 179–184]. Diagnostic criteria for post-ET myelofibrosis (post-ET-MF) are presented in Table 21.5. The risk of blastic transformation (BT) is low in the first 10 years (1.4% and 9.1%, respectively) but increased substantially in the second (8.1% and 28.3%, respectively) and third (24.0% and 58.5%, respectively) decades of the disease [179]. Overall, BT is reported in 1.4%–4.1%, and fibrotic transformation 9% to 10% [25].

Differential diagnosis of ET

Differential diagnosis of ET includes

- Reactive thrombocytosis
- PMF
- PV
- CML
- MDS/MPN with ring sideroblasts and thrombocytosis (MDS/MPN-RS-T)
- MDS with 5q deletion (5q⁻ syndrome)

Algorithmic approach to thrombocytosis is presented in Figure 21.2.

Reactive thrombocytosis

Causes for secondary thrombocytosis include acute hemorrhage, inflammatory disorders (rheumatoid arthritis, rheumatoid arthritis, systemic lupus erythematosus (SLE), sarcoidosis, or inflammatory bowel disease), after splenectomy, surgery or other form of trauma, marrow recovery after toxic insult (e.g., treatment, drugs etc.), bleeding, hemolytic anemia, iron deficiency anemia, some malignancies (lymphoma), therapy with steroids, and in paraneoplastic syndromes, especially accompanying hepatocellular

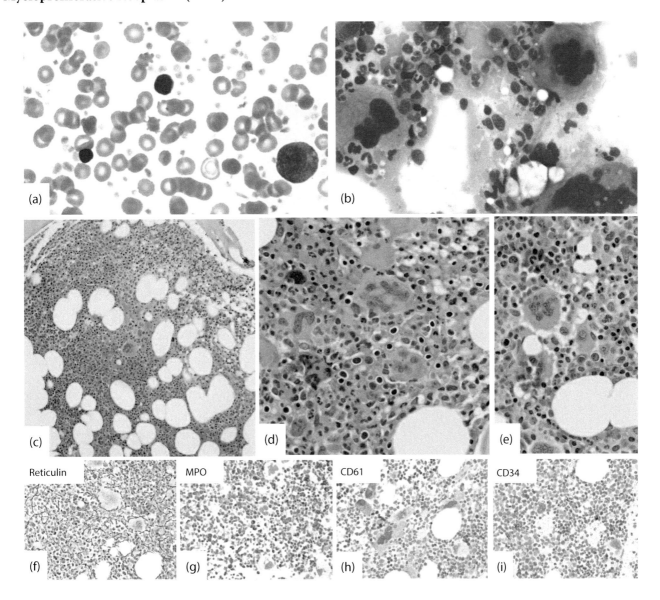

FIGURE 21.21 Essential thrombocythemia (ET). (A) Blood film with thrombocytosis. (b) hypercellular BM aspirate with promi-nent megakaryocytes. (c—e) BM core biopsy showing mildly hypercellular BM with myeloid hyperplasia and megakaryocytic atypia in the form of loose clusters and large megakaryocytes with hyperlobated nuclei. (f) Silver staining depicts mild diffuse increase in reticulin fibers. (g—i) Immunohistochemistry shows predominance of myeloid cells (g), atypical megakaryocytes (CD61 staining; h) and rare blasts (CD34 staining; i).

TABLE 21.5: Diagnostic Criteria for Post-ET Myelofibrosis (WHO)

Required criteria

1. Documentation of a previous diagnosis of WHO-defined ET
2. Bone marrow fibrosis grade 2–3 (on 0–3 scale) or grade 3–4 (on 0–4 scale)

Additional criteria (Two are required)

1. Anemia and >2g/dL decrease from baseline hemoglobin level
2. Leukoerythroblastic peripheral blood picture
3. Increasing splenomegaly
4. Increased lactate dehydrogenase
5. Development of >1 of 3 constitutional symptoms: >10% weight loss in 6 months, night sweats, unexplained fever (>37.5°C)

carcinoma, non-small cell lung cancer or POEMS (polyneuropa-thy, organomegaly, endocrinopathy, M-protein, skin changes). Secondary thrombocythemia is not associated with organomeg-aly in most cases. Evaluation of BM (core biopsy), blood smear and genetic testing (*JAK2, BCR/ABL1,* other*)* helps to confirm or exclude MPN in patients with thrombocytosis.

PMF

The histologic features characteristic of ET includes the presence of large and hypersegmented megakaryocytes with voluminous cytoplasm (including staghorn megakaryocytes), normal overall cellularity, and loose megakaryocyte clustering. In contrast, pre-PMF and PMF are characterized by the presence of prominent often cohesive megakaryocytes clusters (>3 cells), with marked atypia including immature, cloudlike, dysplastic, and hyper-chromatic nuclei, and increased marrow cellularity. The fibrosis in pre-PMF is mild and focal but still is slightly more prominent than in ET, which rarely shows any degree of reticulin fibrosis. Presence of splenomegaly favors the diagnosis of PMF/pre-PMF. Risk of thrombosis or hemorrhage in pre-PMF is similar to those in PV or ET. Without clinical history it is not possible to differentiate between post ET myelofibrosis with PMF. In some cases of MPNs, there may be overlap of features typical for ET with those seen in prefibrotic PMF (e.g. large number of staghorn megakaryocytes in hypercellular marrow or pyknotic loosely clustered megakaryocytes), and therefore it might be difficult to reliably distinguish those two entities [170]. No differences could be discerned between patients labeled as having "prefibrotic myelofibrosis" or "true ET" in clinical and laboratory features at presentation, *JAK2* status, survival, thrombosis, major hemorrhage, or myelofibrotic transformation [170].

MDS/MPN-RS-T

Among disorders with thrombocytosis, ET is much more common than MDS/MPN-RT-T. The BM in ET is usually normocellular to only mildly hypercellular, without prominent reticulin fibrosis and contains typical hyperlobulated (staghorn-like) giant megakaryocytes. CBC data in ET show usually thrombocytosis without significant leukocytosis, whereas MDS/MPN-RS-T may show leukocytosis and anemia (in addition to thrombocytosis). The presence of ring sideroblasts differentiates between ET and MDS/MPN-RS-T. The majority of ET cases have JK2, MPL, or CALR mutation, and the majority of MDS/MPN-RS-T have SF3B1 mutations (60%–90%), often in conjunction with JAK2 mutation (>60%).

PV

There is significant morphologic overlap between ET and PV, especially early phase of PV. Transformation of *JAK2*-mutated ET to PV has been reported, while no transformation to PV was observed in *CALR*-mutated ET patients [160]. The hemoglobin levels ≥16.5g/dL in men and 16.0g/dl in women or a Hct level of 49% in men and 48% in women indicate PV. The BM in ET is usually normocellular or only slightly hypercellular, whereas all PV cases display age-adjusted increased hematopoietic cellularity due to panmyelosis (proliferation of all three lineages) [125]. In ET, megakaryocytes are dispersed individually or rarely in loose small groups, and mostly large (giant) with hyperlobulated (staghorn) nuclei, while PV shows cytologic pleomorphism among megakaryocytes, which vary in size and occasionally may show feature reminiscent of PMF. Reticulin staining is also helpful in differential diagnosis with ET showing no increase in reticulin fibers (<5%) and PV usually showing mild increase in fibrosis (<20%) [125]. *JAK2* mutation is seen in 100% of PV cased and in 64% of ET. The presence of *MPL*, CALR, or lack of *JAK2*, *CALR*, and *MPL* (triple negative status) indicate ET.

CML

All cases with thrombocytosis, regardless of white blood cell count, need to be tested for *BCR-ABL1* to exclude (or confirm) CML.

MDS with 5q deletion

MDS with isolated deletion of 5q is characterized morphologically by small hypolobated megakaryocytes (micromegakaryocytes), which differ significantly from cytologic features of giant megakaryocytes in ET. The presence of MPN-specific mutations (*JAK2, CALR, MPL*) would favor the diagnosis of ET over MDS.

Primary myelofibrosis

Introduction

PMF is an uncommon clonal stem cell disorder characterized by the autonomous proliferation of myeloid and granulocytic elements with panmyelosis, marked and diffuse BM fibrosis (due to cytokine-induced non-neoplastic fibroblast proliferation), leukoerythroblastic blood picture with teardrop poikilocytosis and extramedullary hematopoiesis with progressive hepatosplenomegaly [2, 15, 26, 122, 185]. Patients with history of PV or ET and myelofibrosis are classified as post-PV-MF and post-ET-MF, respectively. Patients with PMF are usually diagnosed late in life (median age is 66 years), and usually present with symptoms of BM failure such as fatigue and dyspnea (due to ineffective erythropoiesis leading to severe anemia), bleeding (associated with thrombocytopenia), night sweats, and fever. Other common clinical manifestations of PMF include prominent hepatosplenomegaly, thrombosis, pruritus, and bone pain. Extramedullary hematopoiesis ("myeloid metaplasia") is the main cause of organomegaly. The BM is hypercellular with panmyelosis, diffuse reticulin fibrosis and clusters of highly atypical (often bizarre and hyperchromatic) megakaryocytes. WHO criteria for PMF are presented in Table 21.6. The discovery of the *JAK2* mutation and the development of *JAK2* inhibitors (such as Ruxolitinib) provide clinicians with a new effective treatment option for patients with PMF. Treatment options include also allogeneic stem cell transplant (ASCT).

Prognostic factors and leukemic transformation

Patient outcome in PMF is significantly influenced by karyotype. Current prognostication in PMF is based on the Dynamic International Prognostic Scoring System (DIPSS)-plus that uses eight parameters, including karyotype, age, hemoglobin level, leukocyte count, platelet count, circulating blasts, constitutional symptoms, and need for transfusion [186]. The prognosis of PMF is poor, with median survival ranging from 3.5 to 5.5 years [187–189]. Most PMF patients will progress and finally die from cause related to the disease, including BM failure, thromboembolic events, portal hypertension, cardiac failure, progressive cachexia,

---

TABLE 21.6: WHO Criteria for Fibrotic Stage of PMF

Major criteria:

1. Megakaryocytic proliferation and atypia with either reticulin and/or collagen fibrosis, grades 2 or 3
2. Not meeting WHO criteria for *BCR-ABL1*⁺ CML, PV, ET, MDS or other myeloid neoplasms
3. Presence of *JAK2, CALR* or *MPL* mutation (or in the absence of these mutations, presence of either another clonal marker or, absence of reactive myelofibrosis)

Minor criteria (presence of at least one of the following in two consecutive determination):

1. Anemia not attributed to a comorbid condition
2. Leukocytosis ≥11x10⁹/L
3. Palpable splenomegaly
4. LDH increased to above upper normal limit
5. Leukoerythroblastosis

Diagnosis of overt PMF requires all three major criteria, and at least one minor criterion

infections, and leukemic progression (BP) [187, 190]. The reported incidence of BP ranges from 5% to 30% (some cases of acute leukemia may be related to prior therapy) [187, 189, 190].

Poor prognostic factors for overall survival at the time of diagnosis include hemoglobin <10 g/dL, leukopenia <4 × 10⁹/L, leukocytosis >30 × 10⁹/L, constitutional symptoms, presence of circulating blasts (≥1%), age older than 65 years and abnormal karyotype. Significant adverse time-dependent prognostic factors for the risk of death were the time to onset of anemia (hemoglobin <10 g/dL), leukocytosis (>30 × 10⁹/L), thrombocytopenia (<150 × 10⁹/L), presence of circulating blasts, and time to splenectomy [187]. The first three factors (especially leukocytosis) and the time to chemotherapy initiation are prognostic factors for the risk of BP. Patients with leukocytosis should be closely monitored. Development of monocytosis in patients with established PMF is associated with rapid disease progression and these patients should be considered as a high-risk group associated with short survival [191, 192].

Mutations involving *EZH2*, *IDH1*, *SRSF2*, and *ASXL1* have been associated with poor survival, but only ASHL1 mutations remained significant in the context of DIPSS [193]. Mutations involving *JAK2*, *MPL*, *TET2*, or *SF3B1* do not influence the prognosis. Mutations in *CALR* are associated with better prognosis, whereas triple-negative cases (*CALR⁻*, *JAK2⁻*, and *MPL⁻*) have worst prognosis [29, 176]. In a study by Tefferi et al., the median survival in *CALR*-mutated PMF was 16 years and in "triple-negative" patients only 2.3 years [25]. In the same study, blast transformation for *CALR*-mutated and triple-negative PMF was 6.5% and 25%, respectively.

Morphology

Fibrotic PMF. Table 21.6 lists WHO criteria for overt PMF. In the fibrotic stage of PMF, the peripheral blood shows leukoerythroblastosis, prominent red blood cell anisocytosis, poikilocytosis, and dacrocytosis (tear-drop erythrocytes). The BM is variably cellular but mostly hypocellular with predominance of fibrotic areas or adipose tissue and focal areas with increased cellularity showing hematopoietic elements with highly atypical megakaryocytes. PMF in fibrotic stage is characterized by osteosclerosis, diffuse reticulin fibrosis, collagen fibrosis, and dilated sinuses which often show intrasinusoidal hematopoiesis (Figure 21.22). The semiquantitative grading system for reticulin fibrosis is presented in Table 21.7. In fibrotic stage of PMF, the BM shows at least grade 2 of reticulin fibrosis (in the pre-fibrotic stage the reticulin fibrosis is either normal or only focally increased; Grade 0 to 1). Megakaryocytes are increased in number with prominent atypia, including bizarre hyperchromatic forms, as well as nuclei with immature features, often described as "cloud-like." Clusters

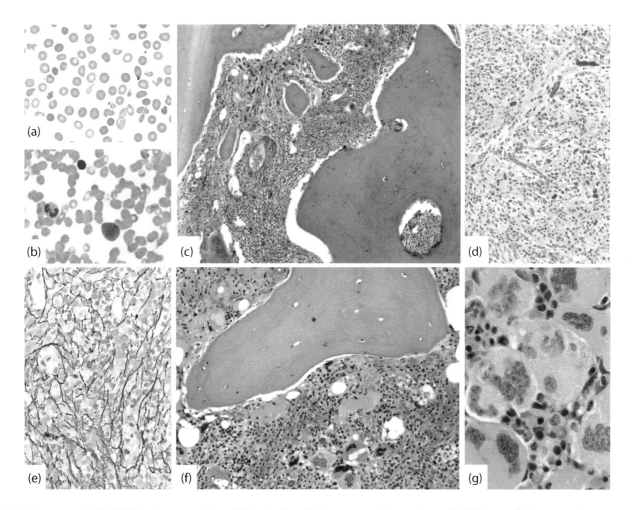

FIGURE 21.22 PMF. (A) blood smear with red blood cell poilkilocytosis and tear-drop cells. (b) hypocellular, aspicular BM aspirate (c) hypercellular marrow with osteosclerosis and megakaryocytosis. (d) the cells appear to "stream", due to fibrosis. (e) increased reticulin fibers (silver staining). (f–g) clusters of atypical megakaryocytes.

TABLE 21.7: WHO Grading for Reticulin Fibrosis in BM

Grade 0 (MF-0)	Scattered linear reticulin with no intersections (crossovers), corresponding to normal BM
Grade 1 (MF-1)	Loose network of reticulin with many intersections, especially in perivascular areas
Grade 2 (MF-2)	Diffuse and dense increase in reticulin with extensive intersections, occasionally with focal bundles of thick fibers mostly consistent with collagen and/or associated with focal osteosclerosis
Grade 3 (MF-3)	Diffuse and dense increase in reticulin with extensive intersections and coarse bundles of thick fibers consistent with collagen, usually associated with osteosclerosis

TABLE 21.8: WHO Criteria for Pre-PMF

Major criteria:

Megakaryocytic proliferation and atypia without reticulin fibrosis >grade 1, accompanied by increased age-adjusted BM cellularity, granulocytic proliferation, and often decreased erythropoiesis

Not meeting WHO criteria for *BCR-ABL1*+ CML, PV, ET, MDS, or other myeloid neoplasms

Presence of *JAK2, CALR,* or *MPL* mutation (or in the absence of these mutations, presence of either another clonal marker, or absence of minor reactive BM reticulin fibrosis)

Minor criteria:

Anemia not attributed to a comorbid condition

Leukocytosis $\geq 11 \times 10^9$/L

Palpable splenomegaly

LDH increased to above upper normal limit.

Diagnosis of pre-PMF requires all three major criteria, and at least one minor criterion

or even sheets of megakaryocytes are easily identifiable. The AP is diagnosed with blasts number between 10% and 19% (blood or BM) and BP with ≥20% blasts.

The prefibrotic PMF (pre-PMF). In 2016, pre-PMF was introduced as a separate variant of PMF [1]. The pre-PMF is characterized by hypercellular marrow with increased myeloid to erythroid ratio and megakaryocytic hyperplasia with prominent atypia. Megakaryocytes display similar morphologic feature to those observed in the fibrotic stage. There is no reticulin fibrosis or only minimal fibrosis (mostly around the blood vessels. Grade 0 or 1). Table 21.8 lists WHO criteria for pre-PMF.

Extramedullary hematopoiesis. Extramedullary hematopoiesis is common in PMF. The most common sites include spleen, liver, and lymph nodes. The spleen shows expansion of the red pulp by myeloid and erythroid precursors and megakaryocytes. The latter often predominate and display marked atypia. Extramedullary sites may show features typical for extramedullary myeloid tumor (EMT; granulocytic sarcoma).

PMF with monocytosis. Monocytosis in PMF patients can be seen at presentation, or appear later, especially during disease progression (often with development of dysplasia) [194]. Comparison of PMF patients with and without monocytosis revealed significant associations between monocytosis and older age, higher leukocyte count, low platelet count, higher circulating blast count, and higher prognostic score [192].

PMF with ring sideroblast (PMF-RS). Dyserythropoiesis is not a typical feature of PMF, but minor subset of cases may display dyserythropoiesis, mostly in the form of ring sideroblasts (PMF-RS). PMF-RS cases often show *SRSF2* and/or *SF3B1* mutations. Ring sideroblasts and/or *SRSF2/SF3B1* mutations may occur either de novo or during disease progression.

PMF in spent phase. As fibrosis progresses, marrow elements may be patchy or markedly decreased with predominance of dense reticulin and collagen fibers, adipose tissue, and/or dilated sinuses.

PMF with accompanying disorders. PMF may be accompanied by storage disorders or metastatic carcinoma. Some metastatic carcinomas (e.g., breast, prostate) may produce significant reactive marrow fibrosis with extramedullary hematopoiesis and splenomegaly, mimicking PMF.

Flow cytometry

In contrast to ET or PV, FC analysis often shows phenotypic abnormalities in patients with PMF (the findings may be similar to post PV-MF and post ET-MF), including presence of circulating blasts, aberrant phenotype of neutrophils (blood) or maturing myeloid precursors (BM), decreased side scatter of myeloid cells, and/or aberrant phenotype of monocytes. It is not unusual to identify higher percentage of blasts in samples from blood when compared to blast enumeration in BM (either due to extramedullary hematopoiesis or abnormal blasts trafficking in fibrotic marrow). BM samples are often suboptimal (due to fibrosis) and mostly represent blood elements. Figure 21.23 shows an example of BM analysis by FC from patient with early (pre-fibrotic) PMF. In the series reported by Feng et al., granulocytes and monocytes from PMF cases exhibited multiple dysplastic features overlapping with those of MDS with accompanying reticulin fibrosis (MDS-f) and included low side scatter, aberrant CD56 expression

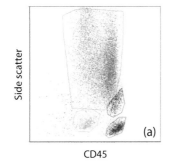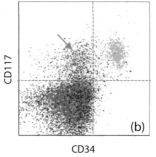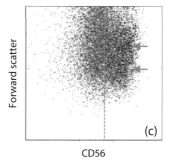

FIGURE 21.23 Early PMF – flow cytometry of BM. Blasts (a–b; green dots) are slightly increased. They are positive for CD34 and CD117 (b). Granulocytes (gray dots; arrows) show aberrant expression of CD117 on minor subset (b) and aberrant expression of CD56 on prominent population (c).

in granulocytes and monocytes, and an abnormal CD13/CD16 maturation pattern [52]. Although the percentage of CD56⁺ granulocytes and monocytes did not correlate with *JAK2*(V617F) or cytogenetic abnormalities, a subset analysis of 36 cases revealed that median fluorescence intensity of CD56 expression correlated positively with the presence of cytogenetic abnormalities [52].

Genetic features

Karyotype. The cytogenetic data on PMF are scanty with few distinct recurrent cytogenetic aberrations being identified, most often partial trisomy 1q, 13q-, 20q-, trisomy 8, and abnormalities of chromosomes 1, 7, and 9. Chromosomal abnormalities are reported in ~30%–56% of patients with PMF [195–199]. Unfavorable karyotype is associated with complex karyotype or sole or two abnormalities that include +8, −7/7q−, i(17q), inv(3), 5/5q−, 12p−, or 11q23 rearrangement. Three characteristic defects, namely, del(13q) (9 cases), del(20q) (eight cases), and partial trisomy 1q (seven cases) are present in ~65% (24 of 37) of patients with clonal abnormalities [195]. Tefferi et al., reported worse prognosis for patients with chromosomal abnormalities (other than interstitial deletions involving the long arm of chromosome 13 or 20) when compared to patients with normal karyotype or interstitial deletions involving chromosome 13 or 20 [197]. Mark et al., reported a case of PMF associated with a reciprocal t(3;9) translocation with the 3q21 and 9p24 breakpoints disrupting the *JAK2* gene [200].

Genetic profile. Mutations reported in PMF include *JAK2*, *CALR*, *SF3B1*, *SRSF2*, *ASXL1*, *EZH2*, *IDH*, *TET2*, *U2AF1*, and *MPL* [7, 13, 26, 41, 174, 193, 201, 202]. The most frequent mutations, *JAK2* and *CALR*, are mutually exclusive. *IDH*, *EZH1*, *ASXL1*, and *SRSF2* mutations are associated with poor prognosis [13, 14, 26, 193, 201, 202]. In contrast to *SRSF2*, mutations in *SF3B1*, another component of RNA splicing machinery, lack prognostic significance (in both MDS and PMF). *SRSF2* mutations are frequent in PMF (17%), may be accompanied by ring sideroblasts, cluster with *IDH* mutations, and are independently predictive of poor prognosis [202]. They are present in hypercellular and prefibrotic stage of PMF. $JAK2^{V617F}$ mutation has been found in ~50%–60% of patients with PMF [32, 129, 203]. Kroger et al., described a new, highly sensitive (≥0.01%) real-time PCR to monitor and quantify $JAK2^{V617F}$−positive cells after dose-reduced allogeneic stem cell transplantation [204]. After 22 allogeneic stem cell transplantation procedures in 21 $JAK2^{V617F+}$ patients with myelofibrosis, 78% became PCR negative with a significant inverse correlation between $JAK2V^{617F}$-positivity and donor-cell chimerism [204]. *CALR* exon 9 insertions/deletions represent the second most common mutation in PMF. Their overall frequency is estimated between 25% and 35% [25, 29, 174, 176, 177], ~70% of patients with PMF without *JAK2* or *MPL* mutations [174]. The mutation of MPL^{W515} occur in 8% and $IDH_{1/2}$ in 4% [203]. None of the mutations are specific for PMF.

Differential diagnosis of PMF

The differential diagnosis of PMF includes

- Reactive processes with marrow fibrosis
- CML (CML, *BCR-ABL1*⁺)
- PV
- ET
- MDS with fibrosis (MDS-f)
- Transient post-treatment megakaryocytic hyperplasia with *JAK2* mutation
- CMML
- SM

- Acute megakaryocytic leukemia
- Acute panmyelosis with myelofibrosis
- Hodgkin lymphoma, classic (cHL) and non-Hodgkin lymphoma with marrow fibrosis
- Hairy cell leukemia (HCL)
- PCM with marrow fibrosis
- MDS/MPN with ring sideroblasts and thrombocytosis (MDS/MPN-RS-T)
- Unclassifiable MDS/MPN with fibrosis (MDS/MPN-U-f)
- Metastatic carcinoma with marrow fibrosis

Numerous reactive and malignant conditions are associated with BM fibrosis, including MPNs, acute megakaryoblastic leukemia, SM, acute panmyelosis with myelofibrosis, infectious disease (granulomas), MDS with fibrosis, HCL, non-Hodgkin lymphoma, cHL, HIV infection, SLE and other autoimmune disorders leading to marrow fibrosis (autoimmune fibrosis), treatment with hematopoietic growth factors, reactive changes following BM damage (necrosis, irradiation, fracture), some metabolic disorders, and metastatic tumors. Most pronounced reticulin fibrosis is seen in PMF. Advanced (fibrotic) stages of ET, PV, and CML may also show marrow fibrosis.

CML, BCR-ABL1⁺

CML is characterized by prominent leukocytosis with basophilia. Thrombocytosis may also be present. In contrast to often large and hyperchromatic megakaryocytes with hyperlobulated or bulbous nuclei, CML reveals characteristic hypolobated micromegakaryocytes (dwarf megakaryocytes). Positive Philadelphia chromosome by metaphase cytogenetic (*BCR/ABL1* fusion by FISH or PCR) confirms the diagnosis of CML.

PV

PV is a disorder which is most difficult to differentiate from PMF based on the histomorphologic features alone (especially between PV and pre-PMF, and post-PV-MF and typical PMF). Similar to PMF, BM is hypercellular with increased megakaryocytes, which display prominent atypia and clustering. Fibrosis is often present. Correlation with clinical and laboratory information, including historical CBC data, may be essential to establish proper diagnosis. Patients who otherwise fulfill the diagnostic criteria for PV, even when there is substantial BM fibrosis, should be diagnosed as PV [26, 168].

ET

Without any history of prior MPN, the presence of significant reticulin fibrosis excludes the diagnosis of ET. Differential diagnosis between post ET myelofibrosis and PMF is based on clinical history. Main morphologic challenge is to differentiate ET from prefibrotic phase of PMF. The median age at diagnosis is similar. Palpable splenomegaly is higher in pre-fibrotic PMF cases, but this parameter alone cannot be used to discriminate the two disorders. ET shows thrombocytosis, which can be also prominent in pre-PMF. Pre-PMF shows more often lower hemoglobin levels and higher white blood cell count than ET. Some PMFs present with prominent leukocytosis, which is rarely seen in ET. Both the lactate dehydrogenase (LDH) level and CD34⁺ cell count are higher in pre-PMF [185]. Increased marrow cellularity with presence of mild reticulin fibrosis (grade MF-1), lymphoid aggregates in the stroma, megakaryocytic clustering (>7 cells), markedly atypical, bulbous or balloon shaped nuclei with maturation defects and hyperchromasia, and variable size of megakaryocytes would favor the diagnosis of pre-PMF. Presence of giant megakaryocytes with hyperlobulated nuclei without maturation defects, complete lack of fibrosis, and normal marrow cellularity would favor the diagnosis of ET. In difficult cases, it is suggested to render the diagnosis of MPN, unclassifiable, and to re-evaluate BM periodically for a more definite subclassification [185].

MDS with fibrosis (MDS-f)

MDS differs from PMF by presence of dyserythropoiesis and dysgranulopoiesis, cytomorphology of megakaryocytes, M:E ratio, findings on blood smear, spleen status and genetic (mutational) profile. In both pre-PMF and overt PMF, megakaryocytes are much more atypical then in MDS or other MPNs, and tend to cluster with >7 cells, often adjacent to either bone trabeculae or sinuses. Megakaryocytes are variably in size, mostly large, with irregularly shaped hyperchromatic nuclei with bulbous, cloud-like or balloon-like appearance. The presence of large hyperlobulated megakaryocytes is typical for PMF and small hypolobulated megakaryocytes for MDS. Intrasinusoidal hematopoiesis is often seen in PMF. In PMF, BM cellularity varies, but generally marrow is less cellular than in typical MDS, with only focal areas of hypercellular marrow elements between fibrous stroma or fat. The myeloid to erythroid ratio (M:E) is usually higher in PMF and low or reversed in MDS-f. Lymphoid aggregates are seen more often in PMF than in MDS-f. In advanced stages of PMF, fibrosis and osteosclerosis replace normal marrow elements. PMF is accompanied by splenomegaly, extramedullary hematopoiesis, and leukoerythroblastosis on blood smear, features not associated with MDS. The presence of thrombocytosis and leukocytosis would also favor PMF over MDS. No genetic change is specific for PMF, but presence of *JAK2*, *CALR*, or *MPL* mutation would highly favor PMF over MDS. Fibrosis in MDS is usually associated with more advanced MDS (such as MDS-EB). In MDS with fibrosis, the degree of marrow fibrosis and megakaryocytic atypia is less pronounced than in MPF. Typical morphologic features of megakaryocytes in MDS include small forms with hypolobated or bilobed nuclei, micromegakaryocytes, or megakaryocytes with multiple well-separated nuclei. The presence of marrow fibrosis and dyserythropoiesis with ring sideroblasts in patient with thrombocytosis should raise the possibility of MDS/MPN-RS-T. On molecular level, presence of driver mutation (*JAK2*, *CALR*, or *MPL*) would favor the diagnosis of PMF. In triple negative PMF (*JAK2−*, *MPL−*, *CALR−*), *TP53* mutations and spliceosome mutations are less common than in MDS-f.

MDS/MPN-SF3B1-T

MDS/MPN-SF3B1-T may show reticulin fibrosis which in conjunction with prominent megakaryocytic atypia raises the possibility of non-CML MPN, including PMF. PMF usually shows increased M:E ratio due to myeloid hyperplasia and lack of significant dyserythropoiesis, although rare cases of PMF may show ring sideroblasts (PMF-RS), which together with thrombocytosis observed in some PMF-RS require differential diagnosis from MDS/MPN-SF3B1-T. Blood smears form PMF show often leukoerythroblastosis, rarely observed in MDS/MPN-SF3B1-T. The most typical histomorphologic features of PMF include megakaryocytic hyperplasia with marked atypia and clustering (>7 cells), often around bone trabeculae or sinuses, and intrasinusoidal hematopoiesis. Those features are rarely observed in MDS/MPN-SF3B1-T. On the molecular level, *JAK2* mutation is common in both neoplasms, whereas the presence of *SF3B1* mutation together with *JAK2*, *CALR,* or *MPL* mutation strongly supports the diagnosis of MDS/MPN-SF3B1-T [2]. *SF3B1* mutation has been reported in PMF (and late fibrotic stages of ET or PV). Splenomegaly is seen in majority of patients with PMF and is only rarely observed in MDS/MPN-SF3B1-T.

CMML

Features overlapping in CMML and PMF are fibrosis, monocytosis, presence of leukocytosis, and splenomegaly (in CMML, splenomegaly is usually associated with infiltration of spleen by leukemic CMML cells). Megakaryocytes in PMF show much more pronounced atypia than those in CMML. Also prominent clustering is a typical feature of PMF. Megakaryocytes in CMML are either normal or show dysplastic features characterized by dwarf megakaryocytes and/or megakaryocytes with hypolobated or abnormally lobated nuclei. The dysplastic variant of CMML usually shows erythroid hyperplasia with dyserythropoiesis, while PMF is most often characterized by erythroid hypoplasia. Genetic (mutational) profile also shows an overlap between PMF and CMML. The presence of MPN-associated "driver" mutations (*JAK2*, *MPL*, or *CALR*) favors the diagnosis of PMF with monocytosis [2]. Those mutations, however, are not specific for PMF, as they may be present in CMML. PMF may also acquire secondary mutations, such as *TET2, DNMT3A, EZH2, ASXL1, SRSF2,* and *U2AF1*, which occur also commonly in CMML. In comparison to PMF with monocytosis, patients with CMML are older, have lower platelet count, higher BM blasts, presence of micromegakaryocytes (or hypolobated forms), and a higher frequency of *TET2* mutations. Prior history of PMF or early PMF (pre-PMF) excludes CMML, but if monocytosis is present at initial diagnosis of PMF, it is difficult to distinguish between those two neoplasms. The neoplasms with overlapping features between PMF with monocytosis and CMML represent either "gray-zone" neoplasm (hybrid between PMF and CMML) or unusual PMF with monocytosis, dysplasia, and CMML-like mutations [2, 176, 192, 194, 203].

HCL

HCL is often associated with pancytopenia and circulating atypical lymphoid cells, which on occasion may be difficult to differentiate from myeloid precursors. FC analysis of peripheral blood and/or immunostaining of the BM provides clues to establish the correct diagnosis. HCL cells are positive for B-cell markers, CD11c, CD25, CD103, CD123, and annexin-A1. Majority of HCL cases have *BRAF* mutation.

"Acute myelofibrosis"

Acute megakaryocytic leukemia and acute panmyelosis with myelofibrosis are characterized by sudden onset of severe constitutional symptoms, pancytopenia, no or only mild splenomegaly and high number of circulating blasts.

Hodgkin lymphoma, classic (cHL) and non-Hodgkin lymphoma with marrow fibrosis

Clinical data and immunohistochemical staining of the BM with CD30, PAX5, B-cell, and T-cell markers help to differentiate between PMF and secondary fibrosis associated with lymphoma.

Systemic mastocytosis (SM)

BM biopsy in SM shows increased mast cells (which can be visualized by staining with mast cell tryptase, CD2, CD25, and CD117) and eosinophilia. SM may be accompanied by other hematopoietic neoplasms (including MDS or MPN).

PCM with marrow fibrosis

Rare cases of PCM may display prominent marrow fibrosis. FC or immunohistochemical analysis of cellular infiltrate with plasma cell makers establishes the diagnosis.

Metastatic carcinoma with marrow fibrosis

Immunostaining with specific solid tumor markers (e.g., cytokeratin, TTF1, estrogen receptor, PSA, S100, pan-melanoma, etc.)

is essential to diagnose metastatic neoplasm with accompanying marrow fibrosis in the BM.

MDS/MPN-U-f

MDS/MPN-U-f is a rare entity characterized by marrow fibrosis and overlapping morphologic features between MDS and MPN. It shows hypercellular marrow with myeloid hyperplasia, reticulin fibrosis, focal megakaryocytic clustering with predominantly small (MDS-like) hypolobulated megakaryocytes. Blood shows anemia, thrombocytopenia, and mild to moderate leukocytosis. Circulating blasts are usually present.

Transient post-treatment megakaryocytic hyperplasia with JAK2 mutation

Rare cases of AML followed by complete remission but post-treatment BM showing typical morphologic features of either PMF or ET with *JAK2* mutation have been reported [205, 206]. It is uncertain whether this represents a case of AML transformed from pre-existing MPN or development of separate hematopoietic clone after treatment of AML.

Chronic neutrophilic leukemia

Introduction

CNL is a rare and distinct *BCR-ABL1*-negative chronic MPN defined by sustained (mature) neutrophilia [15, 88, 207–210]. It affects mostly elderly patients and is characterized by splenomegaly, hepatomegaly, persistent neutrophilic leukocytosis without

significant leftward shift, toxic granulation and Döhle bodies, elevated LAP, and vitamin B12 levels. Diagnostic criteria of CNL include (1) peripheral blood neutrophilic leukocytosis (≥25 × 10^9/L) with segmented neutrophils and bands >80%, myeloblasts <1% and immature granulocytes (promyelocytes, myelocytes, and metamyelocytes) <10%; (2) hypercellular BM with normal maturation pattern, less than 5% myeloblasts and increased M:E ratio; (3) hepatosplenomegaly; (4) no identifiable secondary etiology for neutrophilia; (5) lack of Philadelphia chromosome (*BCR-ABL1* fusion); (6) lack of rearrangement of *PDGFRA*, *PDGFRB,* or *FGFR1*; (7) no evidence of classic chronic MPN (PV, ET, or PMF); and (8) no evidence of MDS (features of dyspoiesis) or monocytosis (monocytes <1 × 10^9/L) [88].

The most common clinical features include splenomegaly, bleeding from mucocutaneous surfaces, pruritus, and hepatomegaly [207, 208, 211–213]. Vitamin B12 and alkaline phosphatase levels are elevated. CNL has heterogeneous clinical course with a definite risk of death from either BT, brain hemorrhage, or progressive neutrophilic leukocytosis, and therefore the prognosis is generally poor [211, 214]. Usually the neutrophilia is slowly progressive followed by anemia and thrombocytopenia, worsening organomegaly, and BT. The median survival is 23.5 months (range, 1–106 months), and median time to AML transformation is 21 months (range, 3–96) [208, 215].

Morphology

Blood smear shows marked neutrophilia with minimal left shift, predominance of segmented forms and bands (≥80%), prominent

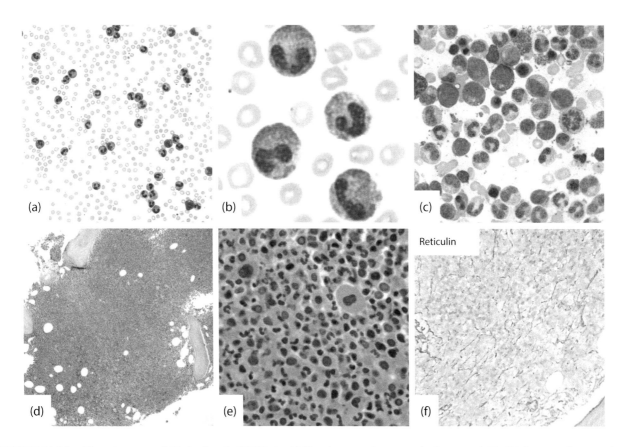

FIGURE 21.24 Chronic neutrophilic leukemia (CNL). (a–b) blood smear shows marked neutrophilia (high magnification shows typical toxic appearance of neutrophils with numerous cytoplasmic granules. (c) BM aspirate smear shows markedly increased m:E ratio due to myeloid hyperplasia. (d–e) core biopsy shows hypercellular marrow with predominance of granulocytic cells without increased number of blasts. There is mild reticulin fibrosis (f).

toxic granules (Figure 21.24), and Döhle bodies. There is no thrombocytosis, prominent basophilia and eosinophilia, monocytosis, circulating myeloblasts, or dyspoietic (Pelgeroid) features of neutrophils. Monocytes may be present but are $<1 \times 10^9$/L The BM is hypercellular with increased M:E ratio due to expansion of neutrophilic granulopoiesis with granulocytic maturation pattern and without excess of myeloblasts or promyelocytes (<5% blasts in BM and <1% in blood). There is no evidence of dysplasia or striking reticulin fibrosis. Megakaryocytes appear normal without overt atypia or clustering. No hypolobated micromegakaryocytes are present.

Genetic features
Some patients with CNL may harbor the *JAK2* mutations [216]. Cytogenetic and molecular studies have demonstrated the clonal nature of the disease in individual cases, although most patients have normal karyotype by conventional cytogenetics at the time of diagnosis [208, 211, 217]. Reported isolated chromosomal abnormalities include +8, +9, del(20q), del(11q14), +21, and complex karyotypes [208, 211–213]. Approximately 80%–90% of patients with CNL harbor mutations in the receptor of colony-stimulating factor 3 (*CSF3R*) [218]. The most common *CSF3R* mutations in both CNL and aCML is the membrane proximal mutation, T6181 [210].

Differential diagnosis of CNL
The exclusion of underlying *BCR-ABL1*-driven oncogenesis is an essential component in the diagnosis of this chronic leukemic process [219]. Apart from CML, the differential diagnosis includes aCML (*BCR-ABL1⁻*) and reactive neutrophilia/leukemoid reaction. The presence of *BCR-ABL1* differentiates CML from CNL. The e19/a2 type *BCR-ABL1* mRNA transcript (p230) may be seen in an unusual "neutrophilic" variant of CML. In both CNL and aCML, trisomy 8 and del(20q) are the most common nonspecific chromosomal changes observed at the time of diagnosis or disease progression. The *CSF3R* mutations occur in up to 40% of aCML. aCML differs from CNL by myeloid left shift, prominent granulocytic dysplasia (including hypogranular and hypolobated neutrophils, and pseudo-Pelger-Hüet cells). Exclusion of the leukemoid reaction, which is defined as a persistent neutrophilic leukocytosis $>50 \times 10^9$/L when the cause is other than leukemia, may be difficult and require careful correlation with clinical history and presentation. The major causes of leukemoid reactions are severe infections, intoxications, malignancies, severe hemorrhage, or acute hemolysis [220]. Severe neutrophilia may be associated with PCM [221–223].

Chronic eosinophilic leukemia

Introduction
CEL is very rare MPN characterized by clonal proliferation of eosinophil precursors leading to persistent eosinophilia in blood, BM and peripheral tissues [2, 15, 224–227]. Diagnosis of CEL requires sustained eosinophil count $≥1.5 \times 10^9$/L in the blood, blasts are <20% (blood or BM), exclusion of specific neoplasms which may be associated with eosinophilia (e.g., AML with inv16, *BCR-ABL⁺* CML, PV, ET, PMF, CNL, CMML, *BCR-ABL1⁻* aCML, MDS, and MPNs with *PDGFRA*, *PDGFRB*, or *FGFR1*.), evidence of clonality by chromosomal or molecular studies and presence of dysplasia in BM [2, 224, 225, 227].

Cases with sustained eosinophilia but without evidence of clonality or dysplasia are classified as HES. Cases fulfilling the criteria for HES but without tissue damage are classified as idiopathic hypereosinophilia. The clinical presentation of HES/CEL is variable with cardiovascular, cutaneous, and/or neurologic systems being most often involved. CEL is a multisystem disorder with eosinophilia and tissue infiltrate by eosinophils leading to organ damage. Some patients have constitutional symptoms such as fever, fatigue, muscle pain, pruritus, angioedema, and diarrhea. Serious complications include endomyocardial fibrosis (leading to restrictive cardiomyopathy), scaring of the heart valves, peripheral neuropathy, and pulmonary dysfunction.

WHO diagnostic criteria of CEL:

- Eosinophilia ($≥1.5 \times 10^9$/L)
- WHO criteria for *BCR-ABL⁺* CML, PV, ET, PMF, CNL, CMML, MDS/MPN-n are not met
- No rearrangement of *PDGFRA*, *PDGFRB*, or *FGFR1* and no *PCM1-JAK2*, *ETV6-JAK2*, or *BCR-JAK2* fusion
- Blasts are <20% in blood and BM
- No evidence of inv(16), t(16;16)(p13.1;q22), t(8;21) (q22;q22.1), t(15;17), or other features diagnostic of AML
- There is a clonal genetic abnormality (cytogenetic or molecular) abnormal BM morphology (dysplasia)

Morphology
Blood. Blood smear shows prominent eosinophilia with predominance of mature forms Occasional cases may also show neutrophilia, monocytosis, or mild basophilia. BM is hypercellular and show prominent eosinophilia and often Charcot-Leyden crystals. There is normal maturation pattern, but some cases may show increased blasts (<20%) or fibrosis.

Bone marrow. BM is hypercellular with eosinophilia, megakaryocytic hyperplasia with cytologic atypia of megakaryocytes, and mild reticulin fibrosis (Figure 21.25). Presence of megakaryocytic or erythroid dysplasia is required for the diagnosis.

Immunophenotype
FC analysis shows very characteristic pattern of eosinophilia (although does not allow to differentiate between malignant and reactive processes). Eosinophils are negative for CD10 and CD16, positive for CD11b, CD13, CD15, CD33, and CD45 (bright), and have low forward scatter and high side scatter (Figure 21.26). They show typically non-specific staining with viability dyes, imitating non-viable elements (Figure 21.27). Eosinophils differ from neutrophils by much lower forward scatter, slightly higher side scatter, and negative expression of CD10 and CD16.

Genetic features
Cytogenetic abnormalities are common and may include trisomy 8, complex karyotype, del(20q), del(3q), monosomy 7, and chromosome 1 abnormalities [224]. CEL may be associated with *ASXL1*, *IDH1*, *TP53*, *SRSF2*, *SH2B3*, *STAT5B*, *KDM6A*, *NF1*, or *JAK2* mutations [36, 224]. In some elderly individuals, low level mutations in *TET2*, *ASXL1*, and *DNMT3A* (and less often other genes) may occur in the absence of any hematological abnormalities (so-called CHIP), and therefore WHO classification recommends to exclude all possible causes of reactive eosinophilia, before diagnosing the patient with CEL [2, 18–21, 227].

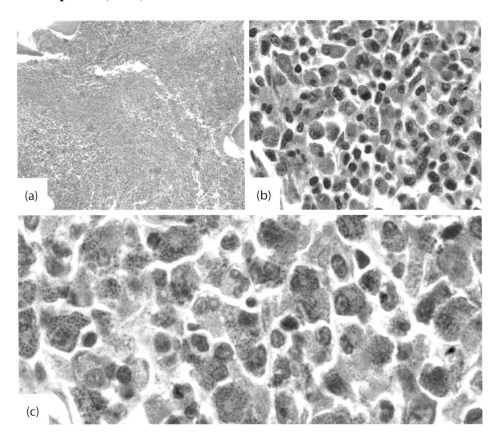

FIGURE 21.25 Chronic eosinophilic leukemia (CEL). Hypercellular BM with predominance of mature-appearing eosinophils (a–b, H&E section at low and high magnification; c, giemsa staining).

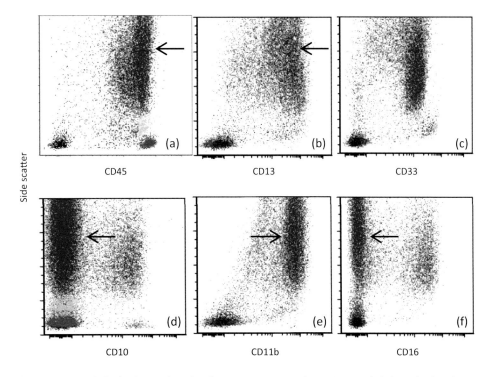

FIGURE 21.26 Chronic eosinophilic leukemia (CEL) – flow cytometry analysis. Eosinophils have high side scatter (a–f), are positive for CD45 (a), CD13 (b), CD33 (c), and CD11b (e). They do not express CD10 (d) and CD16 (f).

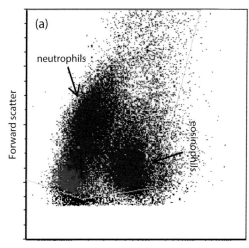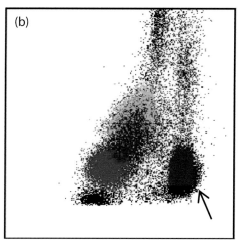

FIGURE 21.27 Comparison of eosinophils (a) with granulocytes and non-viable cells based on forward scatter versus viability staining. Eosinophils (a) have much lower forward scatter and show non-specific staining with viability dye, mimicking non-viable elements (b; negative control shows truly necrotic cells with much brighter expression of the viability dye, aqua V450 (arrow).

Differential diagnosis of CEL

The algorithmic approach to patients with eosinophilia is presented in Figure 21.5. Differential diagnosis includes secondary (reactive) eosinophilia, primary (clonal) eosinophilia, and idiopathic eosinophilia.

Secondary etiology for eosinophilia includes

- Allergic disorders (asthma, atopic dermatitis/eczema, hay fever)
- Dermatologic disorders (non-allergic)
- Drugs (certain antibiotic and anticonvulsants)
- Infectious diseases (parasitic infections and fungal infections, chronic tuberculosis, resolving scarlet fever)
- Gastrointestinal disorders (eosinophilic esophagitis, chronic pancreatitis, inflammatory bowel disease, coeliac disease)
- Rheumatological disorders and vasculitides (SLE, eosinophilic fasciitis, rheumatoid arthritis, polyarteritis nodosa)
- Respiratory disorders (Löffler syndrome, allergic bronchopulmonary aspergillosis, and sarcoidosis)
- Hematological and non-hematological neoplasms with secondary (non-clonal) eosinophilia (solid tumors, ALL, lymphomas, SM with non-clonal eosinophils)
- Lymphocytic variant of HES (L-HES)
- Other miscellaneous causes

The disorders in which eosinophilia is part of the neoplastic clone (primary eosinophilia) include

- Myeloid and lymphoid neoplasms associated with rearrangement of *PDGFRA*, *PDGFRB*, or *FGFR1*
- CEL, not otherwise specified (CEL, NOS)
- Myeloid neoplasms with *ETV6-ABL1*, *ETV6-FLT3*, or *ETV6-ACSL6*
- MDS/MPN-n with eosinophilia
- CMML with eosinophilia (CMML-Eo)
- CML in AP or transformation

- Other MPN in transformation
- AML with eosinophilia, e.g., AML with t(8;21) or inv(16)
- SM (in which eosinophils are clonal)

Secondary (non-clonal) eosinophilia

Secondary (hyper)eosinophilia is associated with reactive expansion of eosinophils due to either parasitic infestation, drugs, allergies, or certain malignant neoplasm (most often cHL, T-cell lymphomas, ALL, and some solid tumors such as renal cell carcinoma, breast cancer, lung cancer, and transitional cell carcinoma).

Primary (clonal) hypereosinophilia

Primary hypereosinophilia includes CEL, MPNs with *PDGFRA*, *PDGFRB*, *FGFR1*, or with *PCM1-JAK2*, HES (Figure 21.28) differs from CEL by lack of evidence of clonality and blasts <2% in blood and <5% in BM. Idiopathic hypereosinophilia (with eosinophils ≥1.5 × 10⁹/L) differs from HES by lack of associated tissue damage. L-HES is associated with presence of clonal T-cell population with aberrant phenotype and reactive eosinophilia. Abnormal T-cell population usually shows the positive (bright) CD2 and CD5, lack of CD3, dim or negative CD7, and positive CD4 expression.

Neoplasms with ETV6-ACSL6 fusion. Myeloid neoplasms with *ETV6-ACSL6* fusion occur predominantly in men and mainly present with myeloproliferative and myelodysplastic disorders with increased eosinophils (and/or basophils) and are characterized by poor prognosis.

Neoplasms with ETV6-ABL1 fusion. Myeloid neoplasms with *ETV6-ABL1* fusion are rare and include B-cell and T-cell ALL (B-ALL, T-ALL), AML, and MPNs [2, 227, 228]. MPNs with *ETV6-ABL1* fusion often mimic CML due to marked leukocytosis with myeloid leftward shift, eosinophilia with basophilia, and presence of hypolobated megakaryocytes. In B-ALL, the morphologic and clinical features resemble Philadelphia chromosome⁺ B-ALL, hence the designation *BCR-ABL1*-like B-ALL in current WHO classification.

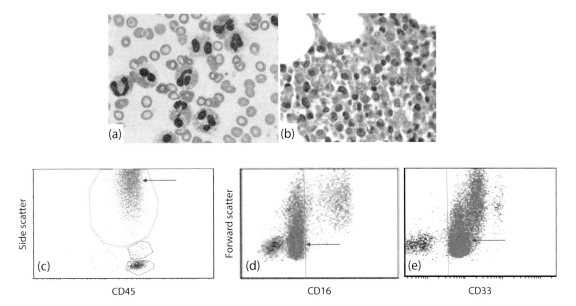

FIGURE 21.28   HES (blood). (A) Blood with prominent eosinophilia (WBC = 104 k/uL). (b) BM biopsy shows hypercellular marrow with eosinophilia and without increased blasts. (c–e) Flow cytometry shows eosinophils (arrow) with increased side scatter (c), negative CD16 (d) and dim CD33 (e). Cytogenetics, FISH (BCR-ABL, PDGFRA/B, FGFR1), and next gene sequencing studies were negative.

References

1. Arber, D.A., et al., *The 2016 revision to the World Health Organization classification of myeloid neoplasms and acute leukemia.* Blood, 2016. **127**(20): p. 2391–405.

2. Swerdlow, S.H., et al., ed. *WHO classification of tumors of haematopoietic and lymphoid tissues.* 2016, IARC: Lyon.

3. Adeyinka, A. and G.W. Dewald, *Cytogenetics of chronic myeloproliferative disorders and related myelodysplastic syndromes.* Hematol Oncol Clin North Am, 2003. **17**(5): p. 1129–49.

4. Mertens, F., et al., *Karyotypic patterns in chronic myeloproliferative disorders: report on 74 cases and review of the literature.* Leukemia, 1991. **5**(3): p. 214–20.

5. Werner, M., et al., *Karyotype findings and molecular analysis of the bcr gene rearrangement supplementing the histologic classification of chronic myeloproliferative disorders.* Lab Invest, 1995. **72**(4): p. 405–10.

6. Skov, V., *Next generation sequencing in MPNs. Lessons from the past and prospects for use as predictors of prognosis and treatment responses.* Cancers (Basel), 2020. **12**(8): p. 2194.

7. Alvarez-Larran, A., et al., *Genomic characterization in triple-negative primary myelofibrosis and other myeloid neoplasms with bone marrow fibrosis.* Ann Hematol, 2019. **98**(10): p. 2319–28.

8. Abdel-Wahab, O., et al., *Genetic characterization of TET1, TET2, and TET3 alterations in myeloid malignancies.* Blood, 2009. **114**(1): p. 144–7.

9. Bench, A.J., et al., *Molecular diagnosis of the myeloproliferative neoplasms: UK guidelines for the detection of JAK2 V617F and other relevant mutations.* Br J Haematol, 2012. **160**(1): p. 25–34.

10. Green, A. and P. Beer, *Somatic mutations of IDH1 and IDH2 in the leukemic transformation of myeloproliferative neoplasms.* N Engl J Med, 2010. **362**(4): p. 369–70.

11. Hobbs, G.S. and R.K. Rampal, *Clinical and molecular genetic characterization of myelofibrosis.* Curr Opin Hematol, 2015. **22**(2): p. 177–83.

12. Taylor, J., W. Xiao and O. Abdel-Wahab, *Diagnosis and classification of hematologic malignancies on the basis of genetics.* Blood, 2017. **130**(4): p. 410–23.

13. Tefferi, A., *Novel mutations and their functional and clinical relevance in myeloproliferative neoplasms: JAK2, MPL, TET2, ASXL1, CBL, IDH and IKZF1.* Leukemia, 2010. **24**(6): p. 1128–38.

14. Tefferi, A., et al., *IDH mutations in primary myelofibrosis predict leukemic transformation and shortened survival: clinical evidence for leukemogenic collaboration with JAK2V617F.* Leukemia, 2012. **26**(3): p. 475–80.

15. Tefferi, A., R. Skoda, and J.W. Vardiman, *Myeloproliferative neoplasms: contemporary diagnosis using histology and genetics.* Nat Rev Clin Oncol, 2009. **6**(11): p. 627–37.

16. Tefferi, A. and W. Vainchenker, *Myeloproliferative neoplasms: molecular pathophysiology, essential clinical understanding, and treatment strategies.* J Clin Oncol, 2011. **29**(5): p. 573–82.

17. Caponetti, G.C. and A. Bagg, *Mutations in myelodysplastic syndromes: core abnormalities and CHIPping away at the edges.* Int J Lab Hematol, 2020. **42**(6): p. 671–84.

18. Valent, P., *ICUS, IDUS, CHIP and CCUS: diagnostic criteria, separation from MDS and clinical implications.* Pathobiology, 2019. **86**(1): p. 30–8.

19. Steensma, D.P., et al., *Clonal hematopoiesis of indeterminate potential and its distinction from myelodysplastic syndromes.* Blood, 2015. **126**(1): p. 9–16.

20. Heuser, M., F. Thol, and A. Ganser, *Clonal hematopoiesis of indeterminate potential.* Dtsch Arztebl Int, 2016. **113**(18): p. 317–22.

21. Link, D.C. and M.J. Walter, *'CHIP'ping away at clonal hematopoiesis.* Leukemia, 2016. **30**(8): p. 1633–5.

22. Hummel, J.M., et al., *Concomitant BCR-ABL1 translocation and JAK2(V617F) mutation in three patients with myeloproliferative neoplasms.* Diagn Mol Pathol, 2012. **21**(3): p. 176–83.

23. Pieri, L., et al., *Concomitant occurrence of BCR-ABL and JAK2V617F mutation.* Blood, 2011. **118**(12): p. 3445–6.

24. Barraco, D., et al., *Molecular correlates of anemia in primary myelofibrosis: a significant and independent association with U2AF1 mutations.* Blood Cancer J, 2016. **6**: p. e416.

25. Tefferi, A., et al., *Long-term survival and blast transformation in molecularly annotated essential thrombocythemia, polycythemia vera, and myelofibrosis.* Blood, 2014. **124**(16): p. 2507–13.

26. Tefferi, A., *Primary myelofibrosis: 2013 update on diagnosis, risk-stratification, and management.* Am J Hematol, 2013. **88**(2): p. 141–50.

27. Bartels, S., et al., *Mutations associated with age-related clonal hematopoiesis in PMF patients with rapid progression to myelofibrosis.* Leukemia, 2020. **34**(5): p. 1364–72.

28. Bartels, S., et al., *Fibrotic progression in polycythemia vera is associated with early concomitant driver-mutations besides JAK2.* Leukemia, 2018. **32**(2): p. 556–8.

29. Klampfl, T., et al., *Somatic mutations of calreticulin in myeloproliferative neoplasms.* N Engl J Med, 2013. **369**(25): p. 2379–90.

30. Lacronique, V., et al., *A TEL-JAK2 fusion protein with constitutive kinase activity in human leukemia.* Science, 1997. **278**(5341): p. 1309–12.

31. Peeters, P., et al., *Fusion of TEL, the ETS-variant gene 6 (ETV6), to the receptor-associated kinase JAK2 as a result of t(9;12) in a lymphoid and t(9;15;12) in a myeloid leukemia.* Blood, 1997. **90**(7): p. 2535–40.

32. Baxter, E.J. and L.M. Scott, *Acquired mutation of the tyrosine kinase JAK2 in human myeloproliferative disorders.* Lancet, 2005. **365**: p. 1054–61.

33. Levine, R.L., et al., *The JAK2V617F activating mutation occurs in chronic myelomonocytic leukemia and acute myeloid leukemia, but not in acute lymphoblastic leukemia or chronic lymphocytic leukemia.* Blood, 2005. **106**(10): p. 3377–9.

34. Kralovics, R., et al., *A gain-of-function mutation of JAK2 in myeloproliferative disorders.* N Engl J Med, 2005. **352**(17): p. 1779–90.

35. James, C., et al., *A unique clonal JAK2 mutation leading to constitutive signalling causes polycythaemia vera.* Nature, 2005. **434**(7037): p. 1144–8.

36. Jones, A.V., et al., *Widespread occurrence of the JAK2 V617F mutation in chronic myeloproliferative disorders.* Blood, 2005. **106**(6): p. 2162–8.

37. Michiels, J.J., et al., *Current diagnostic criteria for the chronic myeloproliferative disorders (MPD) essential thrombocythemia (ET), polycythemia vera (PV) and chronic idiopathic myelofibrosis (CIMF).* Pathol Biol (Paris), 2007. **55**(2): p. 92–104.

38. Michiels, J.J., et al., *The 2001 World Health Organization and updated European clinical and pathological criteria for the diagnosis, classification, and staging of the Philadelphia chromosome-negative chronic myeloproliferative disorders.* Semin Thromb Hemost, 2006. **32**(4 Pt 2): p. 307–40.

39. Scott, L.M., et al., *Prevalance of JAK2 V617F and exon 12 mutations in polycythaemia vera.* Br J Haematol, 2007. **139**(3): p. 511–2.

40. Pietra, D., et al., *Somatic mutations of JAK2 exon 12 in patients with JAK2 (V617F)-negative myeloproliferative disorders.* Blood, 2008. **111**(3): p. 1686–9.

41. Lasho, T.L., et al., *Concurrent MPL515 and JAK2V617F mutations in myelofibrosis: chronology of clonal emergence and changes in mutant allele burden over time.* Br J Haematol, 2006. **135**(5): p. 683–7.

42. Pardanani, A.D., et al., *MPL515 mutations in myeloproliferative and other myeloid disorders: a study of 1182 patients.* Blood, 2006. **108**(10): p. 3472–6.

43. Pikman, Y., et al., *MPLW515L is a novel somatic activating mutation in myelofibrosis with myeloid metaplasia.* PLoS Med, 2006. **3**(7): p. e270.

44. Bennett, M. and D.F. Stroncek, *Recent advances in the bcr-abl negative chronic myeloproliferative diseases.* J Transl Med, 2006. **4**: p. 41.

45. Moliterno, A.R., et al., *Molecular mimicry in the chronic myeloproliferative disorders: reciprocity between quantitative JAK2 V617F and Mpl expression.* Blood, 2006. **108**(12): p. 3913–5.

46. Cools, J., et al., *A tyrosine kinase created by fusion of the PDGFRA and FIP1L1 genes as a therapeutic target of imatinib in idiopathic hypereosinophilic syndrome.* N Engl J Med, 2003. **348**(13): p. 1201–14.

47. Pardanani, A., et al., *FIP1L1-PDGFRA fusion: prevalence and clinicopathologic correlates in 89 consecutive patients with moderate to severe eosinophilia.* Blood, 2004. **104**(10). p. 3038–45.

48. Pardanani, A., et al., *CHIC2 deletion, a surrogate for FIP1L1-PDGFRA fusion, occurs in systemic mastocytosis associated with eosinophilia and predicts response to imatinib mesylate therapy.* Blood, 2003. **102**(9): p. 3093–6.

49. Klion, A.D., et al., *Molecular remission and reversal of myelofibrosis in response to imatinib mesylate treatment in patients with the myeloproliferative variant of hypereosinophilic syndrome.* Blood, 2004. **103**(2): p. 473–8.

50. Arnoulet, C., et al., *Four- and five-color flow cytometry analysis of leukocyte differentiation pathways in normal bone marrow: A reference document based on a systematic approach by the GTLLF and GEIL.* Cytometry B Clin Cytom, 2010. **78**(1): p. 4–10.

51. van Lochem, E.G., et al., *Immunophenotypic differentiation patterns of normal hematopoiesis in human bone marrow: reference patterns for age-related changes and disease-induced shifts.* Cytometry B Clin Cytom, 2004. **60**(1): p. 1–13.

52. Feng, B., et al., *Aberrant myeloid maturation identified by flow cytometry in primary myelofibrosis.* Am J Clin Pathol, 2010. **133**(2): p. 314–20.

53. Bellos, F., et al., *Evaluation of flow cytometric assessment of myeloid nuclear differentiation antigen expression as a diagnostic marker for myelodysplastic syndromes in a series of 269 patients.* Cytometry B Clin Cytom, 2012. **82**(5): p. 295–304.

54. Porwit, A., *Role of flow cytometry in diagnostics of myelodysplastic syndromes–beyond the WHO 2008 classification.* Semin Diagn Pathol, 2011. **28**(4): p. 273–82.

55. Cherian, S., et al., *Flow-cytometric analysis of peripheral blood neutrophils: a simple, objective, independent and potentially clinically useful assay to facilitate the diagnosis of myelodysplastic syndromes.* Am J Hematol, 2005. **79**(3): p. 243–5.

56. Gorczyca, W., et al., *Immunophenotypic pattern of myeloid populations by flow cytometry analysis.* Methods Cell Biol, 2011. **103**: p. 221–66.

57. Han, X., et al., *Immunophenotypic study of basophils by multiparameter flow cytometry.* Arch Pathol Lab Med, 2008. **132**(5): p. 813–9.

58. Kussick, S.J. and B.L. Wood, *Using 4-color flow cytometry to identify abnormal myeloid populations.* Arch Pathol Lab Med, 2003. **127**(9): p. 1140–7.

59. Loken, M.R., et al., *Flow cytometry in myelodysplastic syndromes: report from a working conference.* Leuk Res, 2008. **32**(1): p. 5–17.

60. Lorand-Metze, I., et al., *Detection of hematopoietic maturation abnormalities by flow cytometry in myelodysplastic syndromes and its utility for the differential diagnosis with non-clonal disorders.* Leuk Res, 2007. **31**(2): p. 147–55.

61. Malcovati, L., et al., *Flow cytometry evaluation of erythroid and myeloid dysplasia in patients with myelodysplastic syndrome.* Leukemia, 2005. **19**(5): p. 776–83.

62. Ogata, K., *Diagnostic flow cytometry for low-grade myelodysplastic syndromes.* Hematol Oncol, 2008. **26**(4): p. 193–8.

63. Ogata, K., et al., *Diagnostic utility of flow cytometry in low-grade myelodysplastic syndromes: a prospective validation study.* Haematologica, 2009. **94**(8): p. 1066–74.

64. Stetler-Stevenson, M. and C.M. Yuan, *Myelodysplastic syndromes: the role of flow cytometry in diagnosis and prognosis.* Int J Lab Hematol, 2009. **31**(5): p. 479–83.

65. Wood, B.L., *Myeloid malignancies: myelodysplastic syndromes, myeloproliferative disorders, and acute myeloid leukemia.* Clin Lab Med, 2007. **27**(3): p. 551–75, vii.

66. Ouyang, J., et al., *Flow cytometry immunophenotypic analysis of philadelphia-negative myeloproliferative neoplasms: Correlation with histopathologic features.* Cytometry B Clin Cytom, 2014. **88**(4): p. 236–43.

67. Wood, B., *Multicolor immunophenotyping: human immune system hematopoiesis.* Methods Cell Biol, 2004. **75**: p. 559–76.

68. Quintas-Cardama, A. and J.E. Cortes, *Chronic myeloid leukemia: diagnosis and treatment.* Mayo Clin Proc, 2006. **81**(7): p. 973–88.

69. Sawyers, C.L., *Chronic myeloid leukemia.* N Engl J Med, 1999. **340**(17): p. 1330–40.

70. Druker, B.J., et al., *Efficacy and safety of a specific inhibitor of the BCR-ABL tyrosine kinase in chronic myeloid leukemia.* N Engl J Med, 2001. **344**(14): p. 1031–7.

71. Savage, D.G. and K.H. Antman, *Imatinib mesylate–a new oral targeted therapy.* N Engl J Med, 2002. **346**(9): p. 683–93.

72. Baccarani, M., et al., *Evolving concepts in the management of chronic myeloid leukemia: recommendations from an expert panel on behalf of the European LeukemiaNet.* Blood, 2006. **108**(6): p. 1809–20.

73. Thiele, J., H.M. Kvasnicka, and A. Orazi, *Bone marrow histopathology in myeloproliferative disorders–current diagnostic approach.* Semin Hematol, 2005. **42**(4): p. 184–95.

74. Thiele, J. and H.M. Kvasnicka, *A critical reappraisal of the WHO classification of the chronic myeloproliferative disorders.* Leuk Lymphoma, 2006. **47**(3): p. 381–96.

75. Georgii, A., G. Buesche, and A. Kreft, *The histopathology of chronic myeloproliferative diseases.* Baillieres Clin Haematol, 1998. **11**(4): p. 721–49.

76. Cortes, J., *Natural history and staging of chronic myelogenous leukemia.* Hematol Oncol Clin North Am, 2004. **18**(3): p. 569–84, viii.

77. Cortes, J.E., M. Talpaz, and H. Kantarjian, *Chronic myelogenous leukemia: a review.* Am J Med, 1996. **100**(5): p. 555–70.

78. Handa, H., et al., *Bcl-2 and c-myc expression, cell cycle kinetics and apoptosis during the progression of chronic myelogenous leukemia from diagnosis to blastic phase.* Leuk Res, 1997. **21**(6): p. 479–89.

79. Shet, A.S., B.N. Jahagirdar, and C.M. Verfaillie, *Chronic myelogenous leukemia: mechanisms underlying disease progression.* Leukemia, 2002. **16**(8): p. 1402–11.

80. Hirsch-Ginsberg, C., et al., *RAS mutations are rare events in Philadelphia chromosome-negative/bcr gene rearrangement-negative chronic myelogenous leukemia, but are prevalent in chronic myelomonocytic leukemia.* Blood, 1990. **76**(6): p. 1214–9.

81. Bi, S., F. Lanza and J.M. Goldman, *The involvement of "tumor suppressor" p53 in normal and chronic myelogenous leukemia hemopoiesis.* Cancer Res, 1994. **54**(2): p. 582–6.

82. Griesshammer, M., et al., *Karyotype abnormalities and their clinical significance in blast crisis of chronic myeloid leukemia.* J Mol Med, 1997. **75**(11-12): p. 836–8.

83. Furukawa, Y., et al., *Heterogeneous expression of the product of the retinoblastoma susceptibility gene in primary human leukemia cells.* Oncogene, 1991. **6**(8): p. 1343–6.

84. Bernstein, R., *Cytogenetics of chronic myelogenous leukemia.* Semin Hematol, 1988. **25**(1): p. 20–34.

85. Johansson, B., T. Fioretos, and F. Mitelman, *Cytogenetic and molecular genetic evolution of chronic myeloid leukemia.* Acta Haematol, 2002. **107**(2): p. 76–94.

86. Cortes, J., et al., *Erythropoietin is effective in improving the anemia induced by imatinib mesylate therapy in patients with chronic myeloid leukemia in chronic phase.* Cancer, 2004. **100**(11): p. 2396–402.

87. Druker, B.J., et al., *Five-year follow-up of patients receiving imatinib for chronic myeloid leukemia.* N Engl J Med, 2006. **355**(23): p. 2408–17.

88. Swerdlow, S.H., E. Campo, N.L. Harris, E.S. Jaffe, S.A. Pileri, H. Stein, J. Thiele, and J.W. Vardiman, ed. WHO classification of tumors of haematopoietic and lymphoid tissues. 2008, IARC: Lyon.

89. Faderl, S., et al., *Chronic myelogenous leukemia: biology and therapy.* Ann Intern Med, 1999. **131**(3): p. 207–19.

90. Faderl, S., et al., *The biology of chronic myeloid leukemia.* N Engl J Med, 1999. **341**(3): p. 164–72.

91. Kantarjian, H.M., et al., *Treatment of chronic myelogenous leukemia in accelerated and blastic phases with daunorubicin, high-dose cytarabine, and granulocyte-macrophage colony-stimulating factor.* J Clin Oncol, 1992. **10**(3): p. 398–405.

92. Beard, M.D., et al., *Blast crisis of chronic myeloid leukaemia (CML). I. Presentation simulating acute lymphoid leukaemia (ALL).* Br J Haematol, 1976. **34**(2): p. 167–78.

93. Cervantes, F., et al., *'Lymphoid' blast crisis of chronic myeloid leukaemia is associated with distinct clinicohaematological features.* Br J Haematol, 1998. **100**(1): p. 123–8.

94. O'Brien, S.G., et al., *Imatinib compared with interferon and low-dose cytarabine for newly diagnosed chronic-phase chronic myeloid leukemia.* N Engl J Med, 2003. **348**(11): p. 994–1004.

95. Kantarjian, H., et al., *Hematologic and cytogenetic responses to imatinib mesylate in chronic myelogenous leukemia.* N Engl J Med, 2002. **346**(9): p. 645–52.

96. Kantarjian, H.M., et al., *Long-term survival benefit and improved complete cytogenetic and molecular response rates with imatinib mesylate in Philadelphia chromosome-positive chronic-phase chronic myeloid leukemia after failure of interferon-alpha.* Blood, 2004. **104**(7): p. 1979–88.

97. Baccarani, M., et al., *Chronic myeloid leukemia: an update of concepts and management recommendations of European LeukemiaNet.* J Clin Oncol, 2009. **27**(35): p. 6041–51.

98. Cortes, J. and H. Kantarjian, *How I treat newly diagnosed chronic phase CML.* Blood, 2012. **120**(7): p. 1390–7.

99. Sawyers, C.L., et al., *Imatinib induces hematologic and cytogenetic responses in patients with chronic myelogenous leukemia in myeloid blast crisis: results of a phase II study.* Blood, 2002. **99**(10): p. 3530–9.

100. Talpaz, M., et al., *Imatinib induces durable hematologic and cytogenetic responses in patients with accelerated phase chronic myeloid leukemia: results of a phase 2 study.* Blood, 2002. **99**(6): p. 1928–37.

101. Rosti, G., et al., *Molecular response to imatinib in late chronic-phase chronic myeloid leukemia.* Blood, 2004. **103**(6): p. 2284–90.

102. Alvarez, R.H., H. Kantarjian, and J.E. Cortes, *The biology of chronic myelogenous leukemia: implications for imatinib therapy.* Semin Hematol, 2007. **44**(1 Suppl 1): p. S4–14.

103. Schmid, C., et al., *Comparison of bone marrow histology in early chronic granulocytic leukemia and in leukemoid reaction.* Eur J Haematol, 1990. **44**(3): p. 154–8.

104. Cappetta, M., et al., *Concomitant detection of BCR-ABL translocation and JAK2 V617F mutation in five patients with myeloproliferative neoplasm at diagnosis.* Int J Lab Hematol, 2013. **35**(1): p. e4–5.

105. van de Loosdrecht, A.A., et al., *Standardization of flow cytometry in myelodysplastic syndromes: report from the first European LeukemiaNet working conference on flow cytometry in myelodysplastic syndromes.* Haematologica, 2009. **94**(8): p. 1124–34.

106. Wells, D.A., et al., *Myeloid and monocytic dyspoiesis as determined by flow cytometric scoring in myelodysplastic syndrome correlates with the IPSS and with outcome after hematopoietic stem cell transplantation.* Blood, 2003. **102**(1): p. 394–403.

107. Borowitz, M.J., et al., *U.S.-Canadian Consensus recommendations on the immunophenotypic analysis of hematologic neoplasia by flow cytometry: data analysis and interpretation.* Cytometry, 1997. **30**(5): p. 236–44.

108. Stetler-Stevenson, M., et al., *Diagnostic utility of flow cytometric immunophenotyping in myelodysplastic syndrome.* Blood, 2001. **98**(4): p. 979–87.

109. Gorczyca, W., *Flow cytometry immunophenotypic characteristics of monocytic population in acute monocytic leukemia (AML-M5), acute myelomonocytic leukemia (AML-M4), and chronic myelomonocytic leukemia (CMML).* Methods Cell Biol, 2004. **75**: p. 665–77.

110. Borowitz, M.J., et al., *Guidelines for the diagnosis and monitoring of paroxysmal nocturnal hemoglobinuria and related disorders by flow cytometry.* Cytometry B Clin Cytom, 2010. **78**(4): p. 211–30.

111. Thurau, A.M., et al., *Identification of eosinophils by flow cytometry.* Cytometry, 1996. **23**(2): p. 150–8.

112. Truong, F., et al., *The utility of flow cytometric immunophenotyping in cytopenic patients with a non-diagnostic bone marrow: a prospective study.* Leuk Res, 2009. **33**(8): p. 1039–46.

113. van de Loosdrecht, A.A., T.M. Westers, and G.J. Ossenkoppele, *Flowcytometry in myelodysplastic syndromes: towards a new paradigm in diagnosis and prognostication?* Leuk Res, 2008. **32**(2): p. 205–7.

114. Vikentiou, M., et al., *Distinct neutrophil subpopulations phenotype by flow cytometry in myelodysplastic syndromes.* Leuk Lymphoma, 2009. **50**(3): p. 401–9.

115. Wells, D.A. and K. Ogata, *On flow cytometry in myelodysplastic syndromes, with caveats.* Leuk Res, 2008. **32**(2): p. 209–10.

116. Matsushima, T., et al., *Prevalence and clinical characteristics of myelodysplastic syndrome with bone marrow eosinophilia or basophilia.* Blood, 2003. **101**(9): p. 3386–90.

117. Galton, D.A., *Haematological differences between chronic granulocytic leukaemia, atypical chronic myeloid leukaemia, and chronic myelomonocytic leukaemia.* Leuk Lymphoma, 1992. **7**(5–6): p. 343–50.

118. Lacronique-Gazaille, C., et al., *A simple method for detection of major phenotypic abnormalities in myelodysplastic syndromes: expression of CD56 in CMML.* Haematologica, 2007. **92**(6): p. 859–60.

119. Thomason, R.W., et al., *Identification of unsuspected PNH-type cells in flow cytometric immunophenotypic analysis of peripheral blood and bone marrow.* Am J Clin Pathol, 2004. **122**(1): p. 128–34.

120. Richards, S.J., A.C. Rawstron, and P. Hillmen, *Application of flow cytometry to the diagnosis of paroxysmal nocturnal hemoglobinuria.* Cytometry, 2000. **42**(4): p. 223–33.

121. Dransfield, I., et al., *Neutrophil apoptosis is associated with a reduction in CD16 (fc gamma RIII) expression.* J Immunol, 1994. **153**(3): p. 1254–63.

122. Tefferi, A., J. Thiele, and J.W. Vardiman, *The 2008 world health organization classification system for myeloproliferative neoplasms: order out of chaos.* Cancer, 2009. **115**(17): p. 3842–7.

123. Tefferi, A., *A contemporary approach to the diagnosis and management of polycythemia vera.* Curr Hematol Rep, 2003. **2**(3): p. 237–41.

124. Barbui, T., et al., *Discriminating between essential thrombocythemia and masked polycythemia vera in JAK2 mutated patients.* Am J Hematol, 2014. **89**(6): p. 588–90.

125. Kvasnicka, H.M., et al., *European LeukemiaNet study on the reproducibility of bone marrow features in masked polycythemia vera and differentiation from essential thrombocythemia.* Am J Hematol, 2017. **92**(10): p. 1062–7.

126. McMullin, M.F., et al., *A guideline for the diagnosis and management of polycythaemia vera. A british society for haematology guideline.* Br J Haematol, 2019. **184**(2): p. 176–91.

127. Spivak, J.L., *How I treat polycythemia vera.* Blood, 2019. **134**(4): p. 341–52.

128. Barbui, T., et al., *Masked polycythemia vera (mPV): results of an international study.* Am J Hematol, 2014. **89**(1): p. 52–4.

129. Levine, R.L., et al., *Activating mutation in the tyrosine kinase JAK2 in polycythemia vera, essential thrombocythemia, and myeloid metaplasia with myelofibrosis.* Cancer Cell, 2005. **7**(4): p. 387–97.

130. Scott, L.M., et al., *JAK2 exon 12 mutations in polycythemia vera and idiopathic erythrocytosis.* N Engl J Med, 2007. **356**(5): p. 459–68.

131. Passamonti, F., et al., *Molecular and clinical features of the myeloproliferative neoplasm associated with JAK2 exon 12 mutations.* Blood, 2011. **117**(10): p. 2813–6.

132. Aladag, E., et al., *Unclassifiable non-CML classical myeloproliferative diseases with microcytosis: findings indicating diagnosis of polycythemia vera masked by iron deficiency.* Turk J Med Sci, 2019. **49**(5): p. 1560–3.

133. Kambali, S. and A. Taj, *Polycythemia vera masked due to severe iron deficiency anemia.* Hematol Oncol Stem Cell Ther, 2018. **11**(1): p. 38–40.

134. Georgii, A., et al., *Classification and staging of Ph-negative myeloproliferative disorders by histopathology from bone marrow biopsies.* Leuk Lymphoma, 1996. **22 Suppl 1**: p. 15–29.

135. Georgii, A., et al., *Chronic myeloproliferative disorders in bone marrow biopsies.* Pathol Res Pract, 1990. **186**(1): p. 3–27.

136. Thiele, J., et al., *Clinicopathological impact of the interaction between megakaryocytes and myeloid stroma in chronic myeloproliferative disorders: a concise update.* Leuk Lymphoma, 1997. **24**(5–6): p. 463–81.

137. Thiele, J., H.M. Kvasnicka, and J. Vardiman, *Bone marrow histopathology in the diagnosis of chronic myeloproliferative disorders: a forgotten pearl.* Best Pract Res Clin Haematol, 2006. **19**(3): p. 413–37.

138. Thiele, J., et al., *Polycythemia rubra vera versus secondary polycythemias. A clinicopathological evaluation of distinctive features in 199 patients.* Pathol Res Pract, 2001. **197**(2): p. 77–84.

139. Barosi, G., et al., *Proposed criteria for the diagnosis of post-polycythemia vera and post-essential thrombocythemia myelofibrosis: a consensus statement from the international working group for myelofibrosis research and treatment.* Leukemia, 2008. **22**(2): p. 437–8.

140. Alvarez-Larran, A., et al., *Postpolycythaemic myelofibrosis: frequency and risk factors for this complication in 116 patients.* Br J Haematol, 2009. **146**(5): p. 504–9.

141. Herborg, L.L., et al., *Distinguishing myelofibrosis from polycythemia vera and essential thrombocythemia: the utility of enumerating circulating stem cells with aberrant hMICL expression by flow cytometry.* Int J Lab Hematol, 2018. **40**(3): p. 320–5.

142. Maugeri, N., et al., *Clearance of circulating activated platelets in polycythemia vera and essential thrombocythemia.* Blood, 2011. **118**(12): p. 3359–66.

143. Dewald, G.W. and P.I. Wright, *Chromosome abnormalities in the myeloproliferative disorders.* Semin Oncol, 1995. **22**(4): p. 341–54.

144. Diez-Martin, J.L., et al., *Chromosome studies in 104 patients with polycythemia vera.* Mayo Clin Proc, 1991. **66**(3): p. 287–99.

145. Swolin, B., A. Weinfeld, and J. Westin, *A prospective long-term cytogenetic study in polycythemia vera in relation to treatment and clinical course.* Blood, 1988. **72**(2): p. 386–95.

146. Najfeld, V., et al., *Exploring polycythaemia vera with fluorescence in situ hybridization: additional cryptic 9p is the most frequent abnormality detected.* Br J Haematol, 2002. **119**(2): p. 558–66.

147. Rege-Cambrin, G., et al., *A chromosomal profile of polycythemia vera.* Cancer Genet Cytogenet, 1987. **25**(2): p. 233–45.

148. Bench, A.J., et al., *Myeloproliferative disorders.* Best Pract Res Clin Haematol, 2001. **14**(3): p. 531–51.

149. Zamora, L., et al., *Is fluorescence in situ hybridization a useful method in diagnosis of polycythemia vera patients?* Cancer Genet Cytogenet, 2004. **151**(2): p. 139–45.

150. Berk, P.D., et al., *Increased incidence of acute leukemia in polycythemia vera associated with chlorambucil therapy.* N Engl J Med, 1981. **304**(8): p. 441–7.

151. Najean, Y. and J.D. Rain, *The very long-term evolution of polycythemia vera: an analysis of 318 patients initially treated by phlebotomy or 32P between 1969 and 1981.* Semin Hematol, 1997. **34**(1): p. 6–16.

152. Fruchtman, S.M., et al., *From efficacy to safety: a polycythemia vera study group report on hydroxyurea in patients with polycythemia vera.* Semin Hematol, 1997. **34**(1): p. 17–23.

153. Kiladjian, J.J., et al., *Long-term outcomes of polycythemia vera patients treated with pipobroman as initial therapy.* Hematol J, 2003. **4**(3): p. 198–207.

154. Fruchtman, S.M., et al., *Anagrelide: analysis of long-term efficacy, safety and leukemogenic potential in myeloproliferative disorders.* Leuk Res, 2005. **29**(5): p. 481–91.

155. Finazzi, G., et al., *Acute leukemia in polycythemia vera: an analysis of 1638 patients enrolled in a prospective observational study.* Blood, 2005. **105**(7): p. 2664–70.

156. Passamonti, F., *How I treat polycythemia vera.* Blood, 2012. **120**(2): p. 275–84.

157. Marchioli, R., et al., *Vascular and neoplastic risk in a large cohort of patients with polycythemia vera.* J Clin Oncol, 2005. **23**(10): p. 2224–32.

158. Hernandez-Boluda, J.C., et al., *A polymorphism in the XPD gene predisposes to leukemic transformation and new nonmyeloid malignancies in essential thrombocythemia and polycythemia vera.* Blood, 2012. **119**(22): p. 5221–8.

159. Theocharides, A., et al., *Leukemic blasts in transformed JAK2-V617F-positive myeloproliferative disorders are frequently negative for the JAK2-V617F mutation.* Blood, 2007. **110**(1): p. 375–9.

160. Rumi, E., et al., *JAK2 or CALR mutation status defines subtypes of essential thrombocythemia with substantially different clinical course and outcomes*. Blood, 2014. **123**(10): p. 1544–51.

161. Tefferi, A., *Essential thrombocythemia: scientific advances and current practice*. Curr Opin Hematol, 2006. **13**(2): p. 93–8.

162. Harrison, C.N. and A.R. Green, *Essential thrombocythemia*. Hematol Oncol Clin North Am, 2003. **17**(5): p. 1175–90, vii.

163. Kutti, J. and H. Wadenvik, *Diagnostic and differential criteria of essential thrombocythemia and reactive thrombocytosis*. Leuk Lymphoma, 1996. **22 Suppl 1**: p. 41–5.

164. Murphy, S., et al., *Experience of the polycythemia vera study group with essential thrombocythemia: a final report on diagnostic criteria, survival, and leukemic transition by treatment*. Semin Hematol, 1997. **34**(1): p. 29–39.

165. Sanchez, S. and A. Ewton, *Essential thrombocythemia: a review of diagnostic and pathologic features*. Arch Pathol Lab Med, 2006. **130**(8): p. 1144–50.

166. Thiele, J., et al., *Follow-up examinations including sequential bone marrow biopsies in essential thrombocythemia (ET): a retrospective clinicopathological study of 120 patients*. Am J Hematol, 2002. **70**(4): p. 283–91.

167. Finazzi, G. and C. Harrison, *Essential thrombocythemia*. Semin Hematol, 2005. **42**(4): p. 230–8.

168. Tefferi, A., et al., *Proposals and rationale for revision of the world health organization diagnostic criteria for polycythemia vera, essential thrombocythemia, and primary myelofibrosis: recommendations from an ad hoc international expert panel*. Blood, 2007. **110**(4): p. 1092–7.

169. Campbell, P.J., et al., *Reticulin accumulation in essential thrombocythemia: prognostic significance and relationship to therapy*. J Clin Oncol, 2009. **27**(18): p. 2991–9.

170. Wilkins, B.S., et al., *Bone marrow pathology in essential thrombocythemia: interobserver reliability and utility for identifying disease subtypes*. Blood, 2008. **111**(1): p. 60–70.

171. Michiels, J.J. and J. Thiele, *Clinical and pathological criteria for the diagnosis of essential thrombocythemia, polycythemia vera, and idiopathic myelofibrosis (agnogenic myeloid metaplasia)*. Int J Hematol, 2002. **76**(2): p. 133–45.

172. Gianelli, U., et al., *Essential thrombocythemia or chronic idiopathic myelofibrosis? A single-center study based on hematopoietic bone marrow histology*. Leuk Lymphoma, 2006. **47**(9): p. 1774–81.

173. Wolanskyj, A.P., et al., *JAK2 mutation in essential thrombocythaemia: clinical associations and long-term prognostic relevance*. Br J Haematol, 2005. **131**(2): p. 208–13.

174. Nangalia, J., et al., *Somatic CALR mutations in myeloproliferative neoplasms with nonmutated JAK2*. N Engl J Med, 2013. **369**(25): p. 2391–405.

175. Tefferi, A., et al., *An overview on CALR and CSF3R mutations and a proposal for revision of WHO diagnostic criteria for myeloproliferative neoplasms*. Leukemia, 2014. **28**(7): p. 1407–13.

176. Tefferi, A., et al., *CALR vs JAK2 vs MPL-mutated or triple-negative myelofibrosis: clinical, cytogenetic and molecular comparisons*. Leukemia, 2014. **28**(7): p. 1472–7.

177. Rotunno, G., et al., *Impact of calreticulin mutations on clinical and hematological phenotype and outcome in essential thrombocythemia*. Blood, 2014. **123**(10): p. 1552–5.

178. Campbell, P.J., et al., *Mutation of JAK2 in the myeloproliferative disorders: timing, clonality studies, cytogenetic associations, and role in leukemic transformation*. Blood, 2006. **108**(10): p. 3548–55.

179. Wolanskyj, A.P., et al., *Essential thrombocythemia beyond the first decade: life expectancy, long-term complication rates, and prognostic factors*. Mayo Clin Proc, 2006. **81**(2): p. 159–66.

180. Gangat, N., et al., *Risk stratification for survival and leukemic transformation in essential thrombocythemia: a single institutional study of 605 patients*. Leukemia, 2007. **21**(2): p. 270–6.

181. Cervantes, F., et al., *Acute transformation in nonleukemic chronic myeloproliferative disorders: actuarial probability and main characteristics in a series of 218 patients*. Acta Haematol, 1991. **85**(3): p. 124–7.

182. Chim, C.S., et al., *Long-term outcome of 231 patients with essential thrombocythemia: prognostic factors for thrombosis, bleeding, myelofibrosis, and leukemia*. Arch Intern Med, 2005. **165**(22): p. 2651–8.

183. De Sanctis, V., et al., *Long-term evaluation of 164 patients with essential thrombocythaemia treated with pipobroman: occurrence of leukaemic evolution*. Br J Haematol, 2003. **123**(3): p. 517–21.

184. Passamonti, F., et al., *Blast phase of essential thrombocythemia: a single center study*. Am J Hematol, 2009. **84**(10): p. 641–4.

185. Curto-Garcia, N., J.C. Ianotto, and C.N. Harrison, *What is pre-fibrotic myelofibrosis and how should it be managed in 2018?* Br J Haematol, 2018. **183**(1): p. 23–34.

186. Gangat, N., et al., *DIPSS plus: a refined dynamic international prognostic scoring system for primary myelofibrosis that incorporates prognostic information from karyotype, platelet count, and transfusion status*. J Clin Oncol, 2011. **29**(4): p. 392–7.

187. Morel, P., et al., *Identification during the follow-up of time-dependent prognostic factors for the competing risks of death and blast phase in primary myelofibrosis: a study of 172 patients*. Blood, 2010. **115**(22): p. 4350–5.

188. Tefferi, A., *Myelofibrosis with myeloid metaplasia*. N Engl J Med, 2000. **342**(17): p. 1255–65.

189. Cervantes, F., et al., *New prognostic scoring system for primary myelofibrosis based on a study of the international working group for myelofibrosis research and treatment*. Blood, 2009. **113**(13): p. 2895–901.

190. Dupriez, B., et al., *Prognostic factors in agnogenic myeloid metaplasia: a report on 195 cases with a new scoring system*. Blood, 1996. **88**(3): p. 1013–8.

191. Boiocchi, L., et al., *Development of monocytosis in patients with primary myelofibrosis indicates an accelerated phase of the disease*. Mod Pathol, 2013. **26**(2): p. 204–12.

192. Tefferi, A., et al., *Monocytosis is a powerful and independent predictor of inferior survival in primary myelofibrosis*. Br J Haematol, 2018. **183**(5): p. 835–8.

193. Vannucchi, A.M., et al., *Mutations and prognosis in primary myelofibrosis*. Leukemia, 2013. **27**(9): p. 1861–9.

194. Chapman, J., et al., *Myeloid neoplasms with features intermediate between primary myelofibrosis and chronic myelomonocytic leukemia*. Mod Pathol, 2018. **31**(3): p. 429–41.

195. Reilly, J.T., *Idiopathic myelofibrosis: pathogenesis, natural history and management*. Blood Rev, 1997. **11**(4): p. 233–42.

196. Reilly, J.T., *Cytogenetic and molecular genetic abnormalities in agnogenic myeloid metaplasia*. Semin Oncol, 2005. **32**(4): p. 359–64.

197. Tefferi, A., et al., *Prognostic diversity among cytogenetic abnormalities in myelofibrosis with myeloid metaplasia*. Cancer, 2005. **104**(8): p. 1656–60.

198. Strasser-Weippl, K., et al., *Prognostic relevance of cytogenetics determined by fluorescent in situ hybridization in patients having myelofibrosis with myeloid metaplasia*. Cancer, 2006. **107**(12): p. 2801–6.

199. Djordjevic, V., et al., *Cytogenetics of agnogenic myeloid metaplasia: a study of 61 patients*. Cancer Genet Cytogenet, 2007. **173**(1): p. 57–62.

200. Mark, H.F., et al., *Chronic idiopathic myelofibrosis (CIMF) resulting from a unique 3;9 translocation disrupting the janus kinase 2 (JAK2) gene*. Exp Mol Pathol, 2006. **81**(3): p. 217–23.

201. Guglielmelli, P., et al., *EZH2 mutational status predicts poor survival in myelofibrosis*. Blood, 2011. **118**(19): p. 5227–34.

202. Lasho, T.L., et al., *SRSF2 mutations in primary myelofibrosis: significant clustering with IDH mutations and independent association with inferior overall and leukemia-free survival*. Blood, 2012. **120**(20): p. 4168–71.

203. Tefferi, A., et al., *One thousand patients with primary myelofibrosis: the Mayo Clinic experience*. Mayo Clin Proc, 2012. **87**(1): p. 25–33.

204. Kroger, N., et al., *Monitoring of the JAK2-V617F mutation by highly sensitive quantitative real-time PCR after allogeneic stem cell transplantation in patients with myelofibrosis*. Blood, 2007. **109**(3): p. 1316–21.

205. Wang, S., et al., *Myeloproliferative neoplasm or reactive process? A rare case of acute myeloid leukemia and transient posttreatment megakaryocytic hyperplasia with JAK-2 mutation.* Case Rep Hematol, 2016. 2016: p. 6054017.

206. Ding, W., et al., *Essential thrombocythemia during treatment of acute myeloid leukemia with JAK2 V617F mutation: a case report of a CARE-compliant article.* Medicine (Baltimore), 2018. **97**(27): p. e11331.

207. Elliott, M.A., *Chronic neutrophilic leukemia: a contemporary review.* Curr Hematol Rep, 2004. **3**(3): p. 210–7.

208. Elliott, M.A., *Chronic neutrophilic leukemia and chronic myelomonocytic leukemia: WHO defined.* Best Pract Res Clin Haematol, 2006. **19**(3): p. 571–93.

209. Haferlach, T., et al., *The diagnosis of BCR/ABL-negative chronic myeloproliferative diseases (CMPD): a comprehensive approach based on morphology, cytogenetics, and molecular markers.* Ann Hematol, 2008. **87**(1): p. 1–10.

210. Gotlib, J., et al., *The new genetics of chronic neutrophilic leukemia and atypical CML: implications for diagnosis and treatment.* Blood, 2013. **122**(10): p. 1707–11.

211. Elliott, M.A., et al., *Chronic neutrophilic leukemia (CNL): a clinical, pathologic and cytogenetic study.* Leukemia, 2001. **15**(1): p. 35–40.

212. Froberg, M.K., et al., *Demonstration of clonality in neutrophils using FISH in a case of chronic neutrophilic leukemia.* Leukemia, 1998. **12**(4): p. 623–6.

213. Matano, S., et al., *Deletion of the long arm of chromosome 20 in a patient with chronic neutrophilic leukemia: cytogenetic findings in chronic neutrophilic leukemia.* Am J Hematol, 1997. **54**(1): p. 72–5.

214. Bohm, J. and H.E. Schaefer, *Chronic neutrophilic leukaemia: 14 new cases of an uncommon myeloproliferative disease.* J Clin Pathol, 2002. **55**(11): p. 862–4.

215. Elliott, M.A., et al., *WHO-defined chronic neutrophilic leukemia: a long-term analysis of 12 cases and a critical review of the literature.* Leukemia, 2005. **19**(2): p. 313–7.

216. Kako, S., et al., *Early relapse of JAK2 V617F-positive chronic neutrophilic leukemia with central nervous system infiltration after unrelated bone marrow transplantation.* Am J Hematol, 2007. **82**: p. 386–90.

217. Reilly, J.T., *Chronic neutrophilic leukaemia: a distinct clinical entity?* Br J Haematol, 2002. **116**(1): p. 10–8.

218. Maxson, J.E., et al., *Oncogenic CSF3R mutations in chronic neutrophilic leukemia and atypical CML.* N Engl J Med, 2013. **368**(19): p. 1781–90.

219. Haferlach, T., et al., *The diagnosis of BCR/ABL-negative chronic myeloproliferative diseases (CMPD): a comprehensive approach based on morphology, cytogenetics, and molecular markers.* Ann Hematol, 2008. **87**(1): p. 1–10.

220. Sakka, V., et al., *An update on the etiology and diagnostic evaluation of a leukemoid reaction.* Eur J Intern Med, 2006. **17**(6): p. 394–8.

221. Federici, L., C. Blondet, and E. Andres, *Aggressive form of multiple myeloma presenting with specific pleural effusion, neutrophilia, and eosinophilia.* Eur J Intern Med, 2007. **18**(4): p. 348–9.

222. Fukuno, K., et al., *Chronic neutrophilia preceding overt aggressive light chain multiple myeloma.* Leuk Lymphoma, 2006. **47**(4): p. 762–4.

223. Kohmura, K., et al., *Granulocyte colony stimulating factor-producing multiple myeloma associated with neutrophilia.* Leuk Lymphoma, 2004. **45**(7): p. 1475–9.

224. Morsia, E., et al., *WHO defined chronic eosinophilic leukemia, not otherwise specified (CEL, NOS): a contemporary series from the Mayo clinic.* Am J Hematol, 2020. **95**(7): p. E172–E174.

225. Noel, P., *Eosinophilic myeloid disorders.* Semin Hematol, 2012. **49**(2): p. 120–7.

226. Valent, P., *Pathogenesis, classification, and therapy of eosinophilia and eosinophil disorders.* Blood Rev, 2009. **23**(4): p. 157–65.

227. Wang, S.A., *The diagnostic work-up of hypereosinophilia.* Pathobiology, 2019. **86**(1): p. 39–52.

228. Zaliova, M., et al., *Characterization of leukemias with ETV6-ABL1 fusion.* Haematologica, 2016. **101**(9): p. 1082–93.

22

ACUTE MYELOID LEUKEMIA, DEFINED BY DIFFERENTIATION

Based on World Health Organization (WHO) criteria, ≥20% blasts (or blasts equivalents) are needed for the diagnosis of acute myeloid leukemia (AML) [except for AML with t(15;17), t(16;16/inv(16) and t(8;21) which can be diagnosed with <20% blasts]. AMLs with <20% blasts, which otherwise fulfill WHO criteria for the diagnosis, are sometimes called "oligoblastic" AMLs. Myeloid neoplasms with ≥20% blasts and prominent dyspoiesis (in ≥50% cells) are classified as AML with myelodysplasia-related changes (AML-MRC) and myeloid neoplasms with 5%–20% blasts in the bone marrow (BM) and dyspoiesis are classified as myelodysplastic neoplasms with excess blasts (MDS-EB; see Chapter 19). Figure 5.1 in Chapter 5 presents an algorithm to the diagnosis and subclassification of acute leukemias. The WHO classifies AML based on genetic, immunophenotypic, and clinical characteristics into four major categories:

- AML with defining genetic abnormalities
- Therapy-related myeloid neoplasms and
- AML, defined by differentiation

AMLs with recurrent genetic abnormalities are discussed in Chapter 23. AML, defined by differentiation is subdivided further based on morphologic criteria (similar to prior French–American–British classification; FAB) to:

- AML with minimal differentiation (FAB: AML-M0)
- AML without maturation (FAB: AML-M1)
- AML with maturation (FAB: AML-M2)
- Acute myelomonocytic leukemia (AMML; FAB: AML-M4)
- Acute monoblastic (monocytic) leukemia (FAB: AML-M5)
- Acute erythroid leukemia (AEL) (pure erythroid leukemia; FAB: AML-M6)
- Acute megakaryoblastic leukemia (AMKL) (FAB: AML-M7)
- The identification of myeloblasts by flow cytometry (FC) and their differential diagnosis are presented in Chapter 5.

Acute myeloid leukemia with minimal differentiation

Phenotype of AML with minimal differentiation: s.CD3⁻, c.CD3⁻, CD4⁻, CD7⁺/⁻, CD11b⁻, CD11c⁻, CD13⁺, CD14⁻, CD15⁻, CD19⁻, c.CD22⁻, CD33⁺/⁻, CD34⁺, CD38⁺, CD36⁻, CD56⁻, CD64⁻, CD65⁻, c.CD79a⁻, CD117⁺, HLA-DR⁺, MPO⁻/few blasts⁺, TdT⁺/⁻

AML with minimal differentiation is an acute leukemia with no cytomorphologic or cytochemical evidence of myeloid differentiation [1]. Cytochemical staining for myeloperoxidase (MPO) or Sudan Black B (SBB) are negative (<3% blasts are positive). Myeloid differentiation is confirmed by immunophenotyping and by exclusion of all other acute leukemias as defined by WHO, especially AML without maturation and acute undifferentiated leukemia (AUL).

Morphology
Blasts (≥20%) are poorly differentiated without cytoplasmic granules. The nuclei may be round or indented and show fine (delicate) chromatin and often prominent nucleoli. Irregular blasts with "hand-mirror" appearance or smaller blasts with more condensed chromatin resembling lymphoblasts may be present. BM is most often hypercellular showing total replacement of normal elements by blasts (Figure 22.1).

Immunophenotype
FC immunophenotyping most often reveals predominance of blasts which have low side scatter (SSC) and moderate CD45, although occasional cases have dim or negative CD45 (Figures 22.1 and 22.2). Rare cases may show blasts and residual maturing myeloid cells (granulocytes). Blasts are positive for pan-myeloid antigens (CD13 and/or CD33), blastic markers (CD34, CD117, CD133), HLA-DR, CD38, and often also TdT. Markers associated with myeloid maturation (CD11b, CD10, CD16) or monocytic maturation (CD11b, CD14, CD15, CD64, and CD65) are negative. Cytoplasmic lymphoid markers (c.CD22, c.CD79a, and c.CD3) are negative. Similar to other types of AML, CD7 may be expressed.

Differential diagnosis of AML with minimal differentiation
Differential diagnosis includes:

- AML without maturation
- AML with MRC (AML-MRC)
- B-cell acute lymphoblastic leukemia (B-ALL)
- T-cell acute lymphoblastic leukemia (T-ALL)
- Mixed phenotype acute leukemia (MPAL)
- AEL (pure erythroid leukemia)
- AMKL
- Plasma cell myeloma (PCM)
- Large B- and T-cell lymphomas in leukemic phase or prominent BM involvement
- Blastic plasmacytoid dendritic cell neoplasm (BPDCN)
- AUL

The expanded immunophenotyping, cytomorphology, and clinical history allow to differentiate AML with minimal differentiation from other acute leukemias or hematologic neoplasms with blastoid appearance. Subset of AML with minimal differentiation is negative for CD33 and rare cases may be negative for both CD13 and CD33. In those cases, positive CD117 and lack of lymphoid markers favors the diagnosis of AML with minimal differentiation rather than B-ALL (c.CD22⁺, c.CD79a⁺, CD19⁺, CD10⁺), T-ALL (surface or cytoplasmic CD3⁺) or AUL (CD34⁺, TdT⁺, CD38⁺ and HLA-DR⁺ only). AMLs may display dim (weak) CD19 and often show aberrant expression of CD2, CD5 or CD7, and B- and T-ALLs may be positive for CD13, CD33, and/or CD117 and therefore differential diagnosis often requires extensive immunophenotyping. Since AML with minimal differentiation is MPO⁻, positive staining with CD117 and CD13 and/or CD33 in conjunction with lack of monocytic markers (non-specific esterase [NSE],

DOI: 10.1201/9781003197935-22

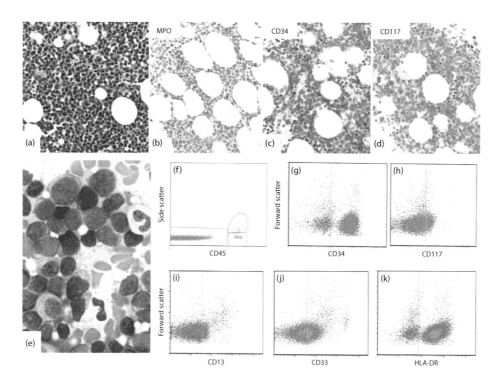

FIGURE 22.1   AML with minimal differentiation. (a–d) BM is totally replaced by blasts (a), which are negative for MPO (b) and positive for CD34 (c) and CD117 (d). (e) Aspirate smear shows small to medium-sized blasts with scanty basophilic cytoplasm and round to occasionally irregular nuclei with fine chromatin pattern. (f–k) Flow cytometry analysis shows blasts (green dots) with SCC, negative CD45 (a), bright CD34 (b), negative to dim CD117 (c), negative CD13 (d), dim CD33 (e), and positive HLA-DR (f).

CD11b, CD11c, CD14, and CD64), surface or cytoplasmic CD3 expression and strong expression of CD19 with positive CD79a, cCD22 and strong CD10 help to diagnose AML with minimal differentiation and exclude acute monoblastic leukemia, T-ALL, B-ALL, and MPAL. Blasts expressing CD4 and CD56 without co-expression of CD13, CD33. and CD117 suggest BPDCN, positive expression of CD41 and CD61 indicates acute megakaryoblastic leukemia and positive GPHA, E-cadherin, CD71, and/or hemoglobin A indicates AEL or high-grade MDS with EBs and erythroid hyperplasia. PCM which often shows aberrant expression of CD56 and/or CD117 (and rarely CD13 or CD33) is distinguished by cytomorphology, bright expression of CD38 and/or CD138, presence of cytoplasmic light chain immunoglobulins (kappa or lambda), negative CD45, and presence of paraprotein in blood. The immunophenotype of AML with minimal differentiation is similar to AML without maturation. The latter more often show lack of CD34 and especially TdT expression, and less often is negative for CD33. The presence of 3% or blasts expressing MPO and/or SBB indicates AML without maturation. AUL expresses HLA-DR, CD34, CD38, and often TdT [1–3]. They are negative for markers

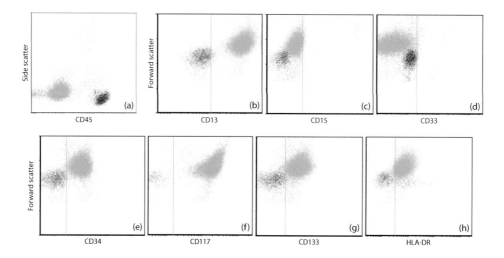

FIGURE 22.2   Minimally differentiated AML. Blasts (green dots) show the following phenotype: dim CD45$^+$ (a), CD13$^+$ (b), CD15$^-$ (c), CD33$^-$ (d), CD34$^+$ (e), CD117$^+$ (f), CD133$^+$ (g) and HLA-DR$^+$ (h).

associated with specific leukemias, mentioned above (e.g., MPO, CD3, CD13, CD33, CD14, cCD22, cCD79a, CD19, CD64, and CD56). MPAL is characterized by expression of MPO (or two of the monocytic markers; CD11c, CD14, CD64, and NSE) and either CD3 or B-cell markers (strong CD19 with strong expression of CD79a, cCD22, or CD10; or weak CD19 with strong expression of two of the following: CD79a, cCD22, and CD10) [1, 3–7].

AML without maturation

Phenotype of AML without maturation: CD2$^{-/rarely+}$, s.CD3$^-$, c.CD3$^-$, CD4$^{-/+}$, CD7$^{+/-}$, CD11b$^{-/rarely+}$, CD13$^+$, CD14$^-$, CD15$^-$, CD19$^{-/rarely+}$, c.CD22$^-$, CD33$^{+/-}$, CD34$^{+/rarely-}$, CD38$^{+/rarely-}$, CD36$^-$, CD64$^-$, CD65$^-$, c.CD79a$^-$, CD117$^+$, CD133$^{+/-}$, HLA-DR$^{+/rarely-}$, MPO$^{rare\ blasts+}$, TdT$^{+/-}$

AML without maturation is defined by ≥90% blasts of non-erythroid lineage (<10% of the marrow cells manifest evidence of maturation to promyelocytes or more mature myeloid cells) with ≥3% blasts being positive for MPO or SBB [1].

Morphology
BM is hypercellular with predominance of blasts (Figure 22.3). Blasts are medium to large with round or irregular nuclei, fine chromatin, and occasional cytoplasmic granules. Some cases may show blasts resembling lymphoblasts.

Immunophenotype
Blasts are positive for MPO, CD13, CD33, and CD117, and usually express CD34 and HLA-DR (Figure 22.4). Majority of cases are negative for markers associated with neutrophilic (CD10, CD15, CD65) or monocytic (CD14, CD64) maturation. CD11c may be dimly expressed, and rare cases show aberrant expression of CD11b (Figure 22.5). Cytoplasmic lymphoid markers (cCD22, cCD79a) and CD3 are negative, but CD2, CD4, CD7, CD19, and/

or CD56 may be occasionally expressed. Occasional cases may show aberrant lack of CD13 or CD33 expression.

Differential diagnosis of AML without maturation
The immunophenotype of AML without maturation is similar to AML with minimal differentiation (see above), and it is difficult to differentiate those two entities based on FC analysis of blasts alone. AML with minimal differentiation has less than 3% of blasts expressing MPO and/or SBB. AML with maturation shows distinct population of maturing myeloid precursors (≥10%). Blasts in AML with maturation are more often negative for TdT and/or CD34, and less often negative for CD33. AMML is distinguished by ≥20% of cells with monocytic differentiation.

AML with maturation

Phenotype of AML with maturation: CD2$^{-/rarely+}$, s.CD3$^-$, c.CD3$^-$, CD4$^{-/+}$, CD7$^{+/-}$, CD11b$^{-/rarely+}$, CD11c$^{-/+}$, CD13$^+$, CD14$^-$, CD15$^{-/rarely+}$, CD19$^{-/rarely+}$, c.CD22$^-$, CD33$^{+/-}$, CD34$^{+/rarely-}$, CD38$^{+/rarely-}$, CD36$^-$, CD56$^{-/rarely+}$, CD64$^-$, CD65$^{-/rarely+}$, c.CD79a$^-$, CD117$^{+/rarely-}$, CD133$^{+/-}$, HLA-DR$^{+/rarely-}$, MPO$^+$, TdT$^{-/+}$

AML with maturation is defined by ≥20% blasts and evidence of myeloid maturation (promyelocytes and subsequent stages) in ≥10% of the BM cells [1].

Morphology
The myeloblasts vary from medium-sized to large. The cytoplasm may be agranular to paucigranular (myeloblast types 1 and 2). Single Auer rods are occasionally seen. BM biopsy shows hypercellular marrow with sheets of immature cells and scattered (rare) maturing myeloid and erythroid precursors (Figure 22.6). In occasional cases of AML with maturation, the BM may be hypocellular.

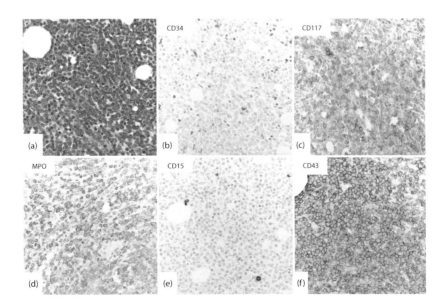

FIGURE 22.3 AML without maturation. The BM section (a) shows sheets of blasts. There is no evidence of maturing marrow elements. Blasts are negative for CD34 (b), positive for CD117 (c), MPO (d), and CD43 (f). CD15 is not expressed (e).

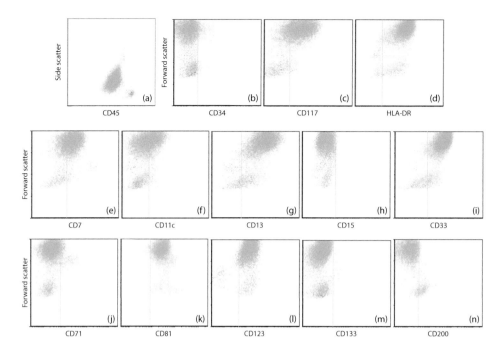

FIGURE 22.4 AML without maturation. Blasts (green dots) are characterized by low side scatter (a) and high forward scatter (b–n) and show the following phenotype: CD45$^+$ (moderate expression, a), CD34$^-$ (b), CD117$^+$ (c), HLA-DR$^+$ (d), CD7$^+$ (e), CD11c$^+$ (dim/partial expression, f), CD13$^+$ (g), CD15$^-$ (h), CD33$^+$ (i), CD71$^+$ (j), CD81$^+$ (k), CD123$^+$ (l), CD133$^-$ (m), and CD200$^-$ (n).

Immunophenotype

Phenotyping by FC reveals blasts with SCC and moderate CD45 and admixture of maturing myeloid precursors and neutrophils (Figure 22.7). Blasts are positive for myeloid markers (CD13, CD33, and MPO), CD34, CD117, and HLA-DR in majority of cases. Occasional cases show aberrant expression of maturation markers, CD11b, CD15, and/or CD65 or aberrant loss of one of the blasts markers, CD34, CD117, or CD133 (Figure 22.8). CD11c may be positive (usually dim), and subset of cases show dim expression of CD64 (bright CD11b, CD11c, and CD64 is typical for acute monoblastic leukemia). There may be aberrant expression of CD7, CD56, and CD4 and less often CD19. Subset of AML with or without maturation may be negative for HLA-DR and CD34. The presence of invaginated nuclear morphology in blasts and lack of HLA-DR, CD34, and CD133 expression is often seen in AML with *FLT3*-ITD (Figure 22.9). Similar phenotype may be associated with *NPM1* mutations, but those leukemias show often monocytic differentiation (see Chapter 23). AML with *FLT3* mutations including internal tandem duplication does not constitute specific AML category in WHO classification, since *FLT3* mutations often coincide with other genetic changes.

Differential diagnosis of AML with maturation

Differential diagnosis includes:

- AML without maturation
- AML with MRC (AML-MRC)
- AMML
- Chronic myelomonocytic leukemia (CMML)
- MDS/MPN with neutrophilia (MDS/MPN-n)
- AML with *NPM1* mutation
- MDS with increased blasts (MDS-IB)
- Myeloproliferative neoplasm (MPN) in accelerated or blast phase
- AML with t(8;21)/*RUNX1-RUNX1T1*

Correlation with genetic studies, cytologic evaluation of dysplasia, blood smear (absolute number of monocytes), prior medical

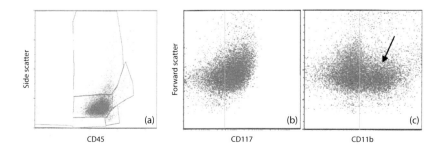

FIGURE 22.5 AML without maturation. Blasts (green dots) show low side scatter and moderate CD45 (a), positive CD117 (b), and aberrant expression of CD11b on subset (c; arrow).

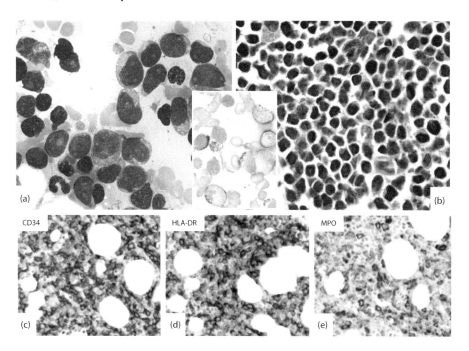

FIGURE 22.6 AML with maturation. (a) BM aspirate shows large blasts with abundant granular cytoplasm, irregular nuclei and several nucleoli (inset: positive staining with MPO). (b) Histology section shows replacement of the marrow by immature mononuclear cells. Blasts are positive for CD34 (c), HLA-DR (d), and MPO (e) by immunohistochemistry.

history and extensive immunophenotyping helps to differentiate AML with maturation from other neoplasms with increased blasts. AMML differs by the presence of ≥20% monocytes and their precursors. MDS with EBs has <20% blasts, and AML-MRC is defined by having ≥20% blasts and ≥50% cells with dysplasia (or prior history of MDS, or MDS-related cytogenetic abnormalities). MPN in accelerated phase has <20% blasts), and MPN in blast phase (≥20% blasts phase) is distinguished by clinical history. AML with t(8;21)/*RUNX1-RUNX1T1* is confirmed by genetic testing (this variant often shows aberrant expression of CD19 and CD56 by blasts). AML cases with history of toxic therapy or radiotherapy are diagnoses as therapy-related myeloid neoplasms. CMML-2 shows <20% blasts (BM or blood) and absolute monocytosis in blood (≥1 × 10^9/L) and MDS/MPN-n differs by having <20% blasts.

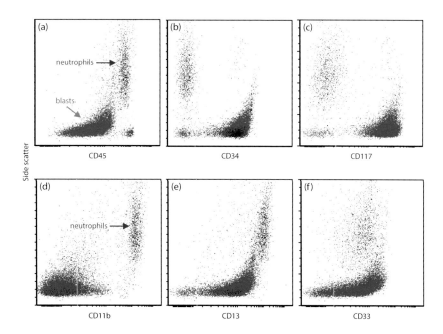

FIGURE 22.7 AML with maturation. Blasts (blue dots) show dim CD45 (a), positive CD34 (b), positive CD117 (c), negative CD11b (d), and positive CD13 (e) and CD33 (f). Granulocytes (purple dots) are strongly positive for CD11b (d) and do not express CD34 or CD117.

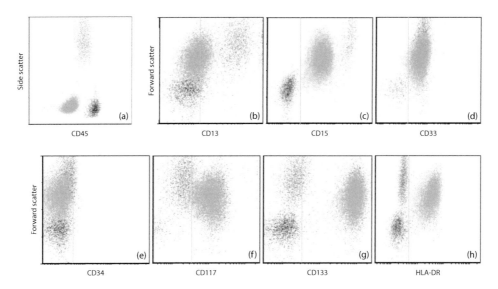

FIGURE 22.8 AML with maturation and aberrant phenotype (CD13$^-$/CD15$^+$/CD34$^-$). Blasts (green dots) show low side scatter and moderate expression of CD45 (a). Neutrophils/maturing myeloid precursors (gray dots, a, arrow) show high side scatter and brighter expression of CD45 when compared to blasts. Blasts show the following phenotype: CD13$^-$ (b), CD15$^+$ (c), CD33$^+$ (d), CD34$^-$ (e), CD117$^+$ (f), CD133$^+$ (g), and HLA-DR$^+$ (h).

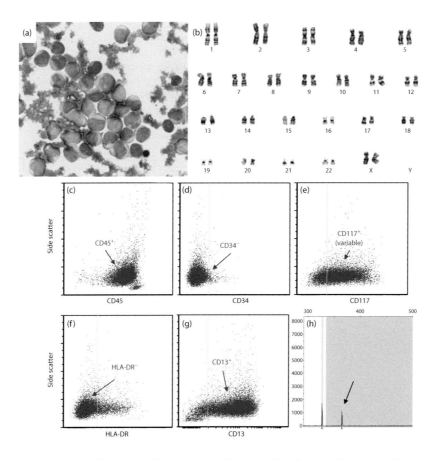

FIGURE 22.9 AML with *FLT3-ITD*. Blasts are rather poorly differentiated with irregular nuclei (a). Metaphase cytogenetics (b) shows normal karyotype (46,XX). Flow cytometry analysis (c–g) shows blasts with the following phenotype: CD45$^+$ (c), CD34$^-$ (d), CD117$^+$ (e), HLA-DR$^-$ (f), and CD13$^+$ (g). PCR analysis was positive for an internal tandem duplication (ITD) between FLT3 exons 14 and 15 (h).

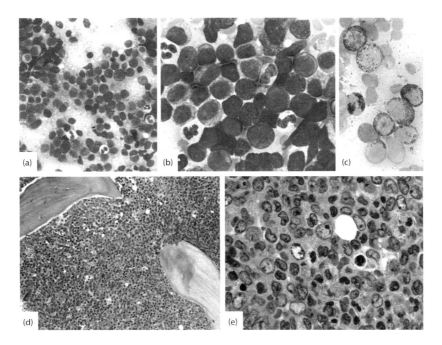

FIGURE 22.10 AMML. (a–b) Cytology shows mixed population of blasts and atypical monocytes. Blasts are MPO⁺ (c). (d–e) Histology section shows hypercellular marrow with predominance of blasts and monocytes.

Acute myelomonocytic leukemia (AMML)

Phenotype of AMML

Myeloblastic component: CD2$^{-/rarely+}$, s.CD3⁻, c.CD3⁻, CD4$^{-/+}$, CD7$^{+/-}$, CD11b$^{-/rarely+}$, CD11c$^{-/+}$, CD13⁺, CD14⁻, CD15$^{-/+}$, CD19$^{-/rarely+}$, c.CD22⁻, CD33$^{+/-}$, CD34$^{+/rarely-}$, CD38$^{+/rarely-}$, CD36⁻, CD56$^{-/rarely+}$, CD64⁻, CD65$^{-/+}$, c.CD79a⁻, CD117$^{+/rarely-}$, CD133$^{+/-}$, HLA-DR$^{+/rarely-}$, MPO⁺, TdT$^{-/+}$

Monocytic component: CD2$^{+/-}$, CD4⁺, CD11b⁺, CD11c⁺, CD14⁺, CD15⁺, CD34⁻, CD36⁺, CD56$^{-/+}$, CD64⁺, CD117⁻, HLA-DR⁺

AMML is characterized by the proliferation of both neutrophil and monocyte precursors with ≥20% blasts (including promonocytes) in the blood or BM, with neutrophils and their precursors and monocytes and their precursors each comprising ≥20% of marrow elements [1]. The number of monocytic cells and their precursors in peripheral blood is usually >5 × 10⁹/L. Myeloid-associated, non-specific cytogenetic abnormalities, for example, +8 are present in most cases. Variant of AMML characterized by increased number of abnormal eosinophils is positive for t(16;16) (p13;q22) or inv(16)(p13q22) and constitute a specific category of AML with *CBFB-MYH11* rearrangement (see Chapter 23).

Morphology

The BM is hypercellular and contains a mixed population of monocytes and their precursors and granulocytes and their precursors (Figure 22.10). The monoblasts are slightly larger than myeloblasts, have abundant cytoplasm, round nuclei with delicate lacy chromatin, and one or more large prominent nucleoli. The promonocytes have a more irregular and delicately convoluted nuclear configuration; the cytoplasm is usually less basophilic and sometimes more obviously granulated with occasional large azurophilic granules and vacuoles (Figure 22.11). The myeloblasts and maturing myeloid precursors show morphologic features similar to AML with maturation. At least 3% blasts are MPO⁺. Monocytic precursors are positive for NSE.

Immunophenotype

FC (Figures 22.12–22.14) reveals two distinct populations: blasts (moderate CD45 and SCC) and monocytic cells (bright CD45 and slightly increased side scatter). The monocytic component is positive for CD11b, CD11c, CD13, CD14, CD33, CD64, and HLA-DR and myeloblasts are positive for CD13, CD33, CD34, CD117, and HLA-DR. A subset of cases shows expression

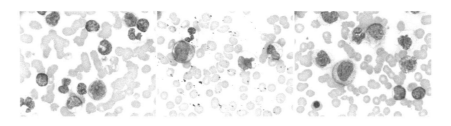

FIGURE 22.11 AMML (cytology). BM aspirate smear show mixed population of blasts and monocytes at different stages of maturation.

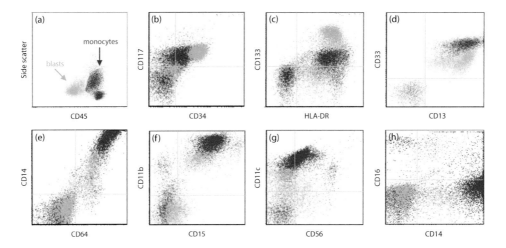

FIGURE 22.12 AMML is characterized by presence of blasts (≥20%) and monocytes (≥20%), Blasts (green dots) have moderate CD45 (a) and low side scatter (a), and monocytes (blue dots) have bright CD45 and minimally increased side scatter (a). Blasts show the following phenotype: CD34+ (b), CD117+ (b), CD133+ (c), HLA-DR+ (c), CD13+/CD33+ (d), CD14−/CD64− (e), CD11b−/CD15− (f), CD11c dimly+ (g), and CD14−/CD16− (h). Monocytes show the following phenotype: CD34-/CD117+/CD133+ (b-c), HLA-DR+ (c), CD13+/CD33+ (d), CD14+/CD64+ (e), CD11b+/CD15+ (f), CD11c bright+ (g), and CD14+/CD16− (h).

of CD2, CD7, CD34, and CD56 by atypical monocytes. The expression of CD56 is less common in neoplastic monocytes from AMML than in monocytes from either CMML or acute monoblastic leukemia (~26% in AMML versus ~70% in CMLL versus ~86% in acute monoblastic leukemia). Monocytic population from AMML usually does not display aberrant lack of CD11b, CD14, and HLA-DR, or positivity for CD16, CD23, and CD117, observed more frequently in acute monoblastic leukemia and CMML [8]. In occasional cases, monocytes may display expression of CD117 and/or CD133. Similar to CMML, monocytes in AMML show usually the phenotype of classical (MO1) monocytes (CD14^{high+}/CD16$^-$) with decreased fraction of "intermediate" monocytes (CD14+/CD16+, MO2) and "non-classical" monocytes (CD14$^{dim+/-}$/CD16+, MO3).

Differential diagnosis of AMML

The differential diagnosis includes:

- AML with inv(16)/t(16;16)
- AML-MRC
- Acute monocytic (monoblastic) leukemia
- CMML
- MPN in accelerated or blasts phase
- MDS/MPN-n
- AML with maturation
- AML with *NPM1* mutation

AML with inv(16)/t(16;16) and AML with NPM1 mutation are excluded by genetic testing, while MPN in blast phase are

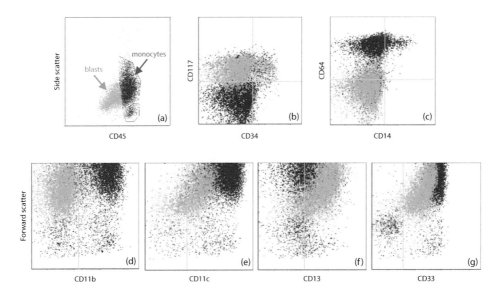

FIGURE 22.13 Acute myelomonocytic leukemia (AMML) – flow cytometry. Blasts (green dots) and monocytes (blue dots) predominate. Blasts show low side scatter and moderate CD45 (a), positive CD117 (b), negative CD34 (b; rare blasts are positive), negative CD14 and CD64 (c), negative CD11b (d), dim CD11c (e), positive CD13 (f), and positive CD33 (g). Monocytes show bright CD45 (a), negative CD34 and CD117 (b), bright CD64 (c), negative CD14 (c), positive CD11b (d), bright CD11c (e), dim CD13 (f), and bright CD33 (g).

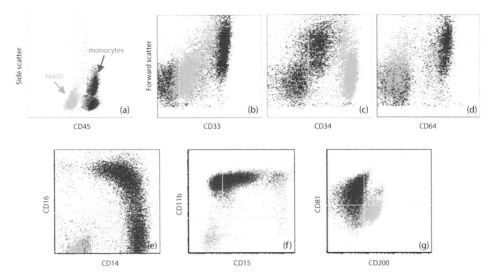

FIGURE 22.14 AMML – flow cytometry. Blasts (green dots) show low side scatter and moderate CD45 (a), dim CD33 (b), bright CD34 (c), negative CD64 (d), negative CD14 and CD16 (e), negative CD11b and CD15 (f) and positive CD200 (g). Monocytes (blue dots) show bright CD45 (a), bright CD33 (b), aberrant expression of CD34 (c), bright CD64 (d), positive CD14 (e), partially positive CD16 (e), bright CD11b (f), and positive CD81 (g). Note presence of classical and non-classical monocytes (e).

excluded by clinical history. Both high-grade MDS (MDS-EB-2) and MPN in accelerated phase have blasts <20%. The most difficult differential diagnosis is between AMML, AML-MRC, and CMML, due to the presence of myeloid and erythroid leftward shift with dyspoiesis in all three lineages and monocytosis with leftward shift. AML-MRC differs from AMML by ≥50% cells with dysplasia, prior history of MDS, or MDS-related cytogenetic abnormalities. Proper identification of myeloblasts, monoblasts, promonocytes, and dysplastic proerythroblasts in good quality BM aspirate smears plays the key role in differential diagnosis of AMML and CMML-2. In contrast to AMML, CMML has <20% myeloblasts, monoblasts, and promonocytes.

Cytologic features of immature cells in AMML and CMML

Myeloblasts. Myeloblasts vary in size but are generally large, round cells with high nuclear-cytoplasmic ratio, round to oval nucleus (occasionally irregular) with fine chromatin, smooth nuclear membrane, and often more than one nucleolus. The cytoplasm is generally moderately basophilic with azurophilic cytoplasmic granules or less often Auer rods.

Monoblasts. Monoblasts are large cells with round or oval nuclei with regular outlines, fine chromatin, and one or more prominent nucleoli. Cytoplasm is pale basophilic, usually without granules, but sometimes with vacuoles and/or pseudopods formation.

Promonocytes. Promonocytes are large (often slightly larger than myeloblasts or monoblasts), have pale cytoplasm, delicate chromatin, and small (indistinct) nucleolus. The main difference between monoblasts and promonocytes is the presence of irregular nuclear outlines in promonocytes (convoluted, folded, or grooved nuclei resembling wrinkled paper). Mature monocytes, which often show cytologic atypia, differ from promonocytes by more hyperchromatic nuclei with clumped chromatin, smaller size, more granular, grayish cytoplasm, and lack of nucleoli.

Proerythroblasts. The proerythroblasts are medium sized to large cells with deep blue, agranular cytoplasm, which may be vacuolated or show perinuclear clear area (hof). The nuclei are round with evenly dispersed chromatin and one or more nucleoli.

Acute monoblastic (monocytic) leukemia

Phenotype of acute monoblastic (monocytic) leukemia: CD2$^{-/+}$, s.CD3$^-$, c.CD3$^-$, CD4$^+$, CD7$^{+/-}$, CD11b$^{+(variable)/rarely-}$, CD11c$^+$, CD13$^+$, CD14$^{-/+(variable)}$, CD15$^+$, CD19$^-$, c.CD22$^-$, CD33$^+$, CD34$^{-/rarely+}$, CD38$^{+/rarely-}$, CD36$^+$, CD56$^{+/rarely-}$, CD64$^+$, CD65$^+$, c.CD79a$^-$, CD117$^{-/rarely+}$, CD133$^-$, HLA-DR$^{+/rarely-}$, MPO$^{-/rarely+}$

Acute monoblastic (monocytic) leukemia is defined as AML in which ≥80% of the leukemic cells are of monocytic lineage (monoblasts, promonocytes, and monocytes) and with ≥20% blasts (including myeloblasts, monoblasts, and promonocytes) [1]. Acute monoblastic leukemia has ≥80% monoblasts, and acute monocytic leukemia shows mostly promonocytes and monocytes (with monoblasts <80%). Acute monoblastic leukemia often involves extramedullary sites, including lymph nodes, skin, gingiva, gonads, and central nervous system (CNS).

Morphology
Leukemic monocytes have abundant cytoplasm that may show irregular borders with pseudopods and cytoplasmic vacuoles (Figure 22.15). The monoblasts have large and usually round nuclei with one or several prominent nucleoli. Promonocytes tend to have irregular folded nuclei, pale, slightly basophilic cytoplasm with occasional azurophilic granules. NSE is positive in most cases, although it may be weak. MPO is negative (some cases may show dim MPO staining). Hemophagocytosis (erythrophagocytosis) may be observed and suggests an associated t(8;11). The BM core biopsy is hypercellular and usually completely replaced by monoblasts and/or promonocytes (Figures 22.16 and 22.17).

Immunophenotype
Immunohistochemistry. Acute monoblastic leukemias are positive for CD45, muramidase (lysozyme), CD68, CD43, and CD11c. CD4 and CD56 are often positive. Less differentiated leukemias may be positive for CD117 and/or CD34. CD123 may also

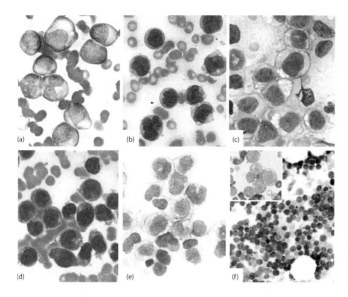

FIGURE 22.15 Acute monoblastic leukemia – cytology and cytochemistry. Examples of acute monoblastic leukemia (a–e). Note abundant cytoplasm, occasional cytoplasmic vacuoles and prominent nuclear irregularities. (f) Cytochemistry shows strong staining with NSE (*inset* negative MPO).

be positive. In contrast to mature monocytes, CD163 is usually negative in monoblastic leukemia or shows only scattered positive cells. MPO, CD71, and CD15 are negative in most cases, but rare cases may show aberrant MPO positivity (Figures 22.16 and 22.17).

Flow cytometry. Based on the CD45 versus orthogonal SSC display, majority of cases (~60%) are characterized by bright CD45 and increased side scatter ("monocytic" gate; Figures 22.17–22.20). Subset of cases (~34%) shows moderate CD45 placing tumor cells in "blast" gate and very few cases may show loss of CD45 or only partial CD45 expression (Figure 22.21). Rare cases (~5%) display high side scatter similar to APL, placing leukemic cells in "granulocytic" gate. CD33 is most often brightly positive. Majority of cases are positive for CD11c (~99%), CD64 (~99%), HLA-DR (~89%), CD4 (~93%), and CD11b (~92%). CD13 is positive in 78% of cases. Other myeloid markers often positive include CD15 and CD65. The expression of CD14 and CD300e depends on the stage of maturation of monocytes, being strong in more mature cells (CMML, acute monocytic leukemia) and absent or partial in immature variant (acute monoblastic leukemia). In contrast to benign monocytes which have bright CD14 expression, leukemic cells in acute monoblastic leukemia are often negative for CD14 (44%). Among CD14+ cases, the expression often is present only on subset (~15%) or has characteristic "smeared" pattern (variable expression; ~15%); only ~20% of cases have moderate and/or bright

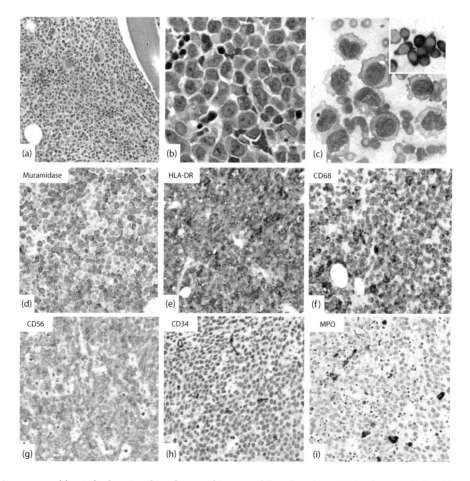

FIGURE 22.16 Acute monoblastic leukemia – histology and immunohistochemistry. BM is hypercellular (a) and on high magnification shows predominance of atypical mononuclear cells replacing normal elements (b). Aspirate smear (c) shows monoblasts with irregular nuclei and nucleoli (*inset*: positive NSE). Immunohistochemistry (d–i) shows positive muramidase (d), HLA-DR (e), CD68 (f) and CD56 (g) and negative CD34 (h) and MPO (i).

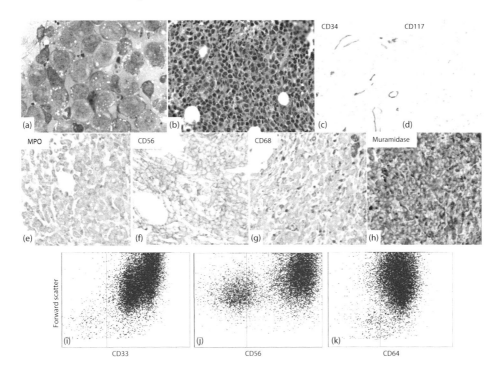

FIGURE 22.17 Acute monoblastic leukemia with prominent phenotypic atypia. (a) Aspirate smear shows highly atypical large monoblasts with nucleoli and cytoplasmic vacuoles. (b) BM core biopsy shows marrow replacement by sheets of monoblasts. (c–h) Immunohistochemistry: monoblasts are negative for CD34 (c) and CD117 (d) and positive for MPO (e), CD56 (f), CD68 (g), and muramidase (h). (i–k) Flow cytometry analysis shows bright CD33 expression (i), bright CD56 expression (j), and positive CD64 (k).

CD14. CD56 is positive in ~68% cases and CD123 in 28%. A subset of cases shows positive expression of CD2, CD7, CD10, and/or CD23. CD34 is positive in ~13% and CD117 in ~23% of cases (only very few cases are positive for both markers). The FC profile of acute monoblastic leukemia differs from acute monocytic leukemia with CD34, CD117, and CD7 being most often positive in acute monoblastic leukemia, while CD14, CD11b, CD15, and CD36 are more often strongly positive in acute monocytic leukemia. Aberrant expression of CD56 and CD123 is comparable in both variants. Acute monoblastic leukemia more often shows diminished expression of CD11b, CD13, CD14, CD33, CD36, and

CD300e when compared to acute monocytic leukemia. Table 22.1 presents the summary of the immunophenotypic profile of acute monoblastic leukemia.

Genetic features

Majority of cases shows non-specific, often complex, myeloid associated cytogenetic abnormalities. There is a strong association with deletions or translocations involving *MLL* gene at chromosome 11q23, which are identified in 12%–31% of patients (Figure 22.22). Trisomy 8 is also frequently found in acute monoblastic leukemia (Figure 22.23). Haferlach et al., analyzed

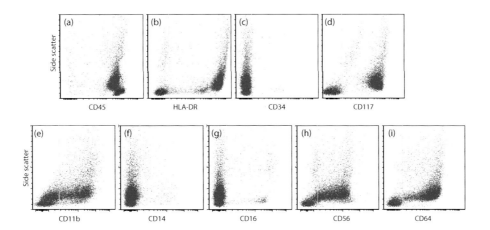

FIGURE 22.18 Acute monoblastic leukemia – flow cytometry. Monoblasts (blue dots) are positive for CD45 (a), HLA-DR (b; bright), CD117 (d), CD11b (e; variable expression), CD56 (h), and CD64 (i). They do not express CD34 (b), CD14 (f), and CD16 (g).

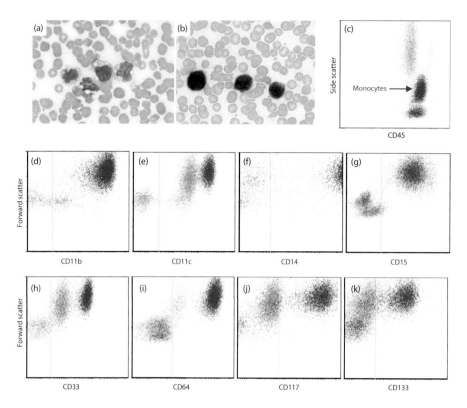

FIGURE 22.19 Acute monocytic leukemia. The smear (a) shows atypical monocytes with irregular nuclei and vacuolated cytoplasm, which are positive for non-specific esterase (NSE; b). Monocytes are positive for CD45 (c), CD11b (d), CD11c (e), CD14 (f), CD15 (g), CD33(h), CD64 (i), CD117 (j), and CD133 (k).

58 patients with *de novo* acute monoblastic leukemia and 66 patients with *de novo* acute monocytic leukemia and found an aberrant karyotype in ~76% and ~29% of cases, respectively [9].

Differential diagnosis of acute monoblastic leukemia

Based on cytomorphology, histomorphology, and immunophenotype, the differential diagnosis of acute monoblastic leukemia includes APL (microgranular variant), AML with minimal differentiation, AML without maturation, CMML, acute megakaryoblastic leukemia, AMML, granulocytic (monoblastic) sarcoma, large cell lymphomas, and non-hematopoietic tumors. Extramedullary myeloid tumors (EMT) with monocytic differentiation (monoblastic sarcoma) may be mistaken with large cell lymphoma, carcinoma, melanoma, or sarcoma. Examples of tumors mimicking acute monoblastic leukemia cytologically are presented in Figure 22.24.

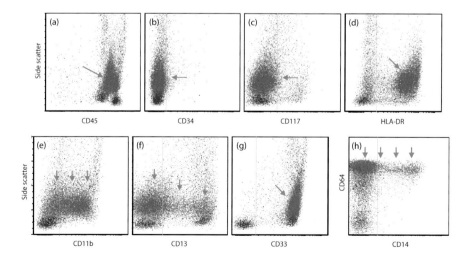

FIGURE 22.20 Acute monoblastic leukemia – flow cytometry. Monoblasts (green dots, arrow) show bright expression of CD45 and slightly increased side scatter (a). CD34 and CD117 are not expressed (b–c). HLA-DR is positive (d) and both CD33 and CD64 are brightly expressed (g–h). There is aberrant expression of CD11b (e: variable with subset negative and dimly positive), CD13 (f: mostly negative, only minor population is positive) and CD14 (h: mostly negative with only minute population showing variable expression).

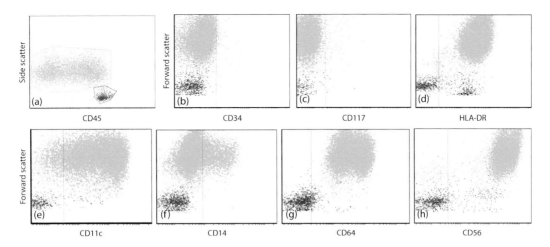

FIGURE 22.21 Acute monocytic leukemia with aberrant (partial) loss of CD45 expression (flow cytometry). Monoblasts (green dots) are negative to partially dimly positive CD45 (a), negative for CD34 (b) and CD117 (c), positive for HLA-DR (d) and CD11c (e), mostly negative for CD14 (f; minor subset is dimly⁺), and positive for CD64 (g) and CD56 (h).

The differential diagnosis of acute monoblastic leukemia based on cytomorphology and flow cytometry includes:

- Acute promyelocytic leukemia, microgranular variant (APL-v)
- AML, especially AML with *NPM1* mutation

TABLE 22.1: Immunophenotypic Profile of Acute Monocytic (Monoblastic) Leukemia (*n* = 94)

Marker	Frequency	Comments
CD2⁺	34%	Usually dim or partial expression
CD4⁺	93%	Usually dim expression
CD7⁺	2%	
CD10⁺	3%	
CD11b⁺	92%	Including bright expression in 29.9%; moderate in 29.9%; dim in 8%, variable in 17.2%, and partial in 6.9%
CD11c⁺	99%	Including bright expression in 64.4%; moderate in 26.4%; dim in 3.4%, variable in 2.3%, and partial in 2.3%,
CD13⁺	78%	Including bright expression in 4.6%; moderate in 24.1%; dim in 14.9%, variable in 16.1%, and partial in 17.2%,
CD14⁺	55%	Including bright expression in 14.9%; moderate in 3.5%; dim in 3.5%, variable in 19.5%, and partial in 12.6%,
CD16⁺	8%	
CD19⁺	0	
CD23⁺	15%	
CD33⁺	100%	Including bright expression in 73.6%, moderate in 24.1%, and variable in 2.3%,
CD34⁺	13%	May be partial expression
CD45⁺	99%	Predominantly bright or moderate expression
CD56⁺	68%	
CD64⁺	99%	Mostly bright expression, rarely moderate or dim
CD117⁺	23%	May be partial expression
CD123⁺	28%	
HLA-DR⁺	89%	

- MDS
- AMML
- CMML
- AEL (pure erythroid leukemia)
- Plasma cell leukemia and poorly differentiated PCM
- Diffuse large B-cell lymphoma in leukemic phase (DLBCL)
- "Double hit lymphoma" (high grade B-cell lymphoma with *MYC* and *BCL2* rearrangement, HGBL-R)
- Burkitt lymphoma (BL)
- Metastatic tumors (rhabdomyosarcoma; poorly differentiated carcinoma, melanoma)
- BPDCN
- "Blastoid" variants of mature B- and T-cell lymphoproliferative disorders, such as T-cell lymphomas, hairy cell leukemia (HCL), or mantle cell lymphoma (MCL)

APL and other non-monocytic AMLs. Myeloblasts and abnormal promyelocytes are strongly MPO⁺, whereas monocytes are either weakly positive or negative. Monoblasts and promonocytes usually are positive for NSE, but a significant subset of acute monoblastic leukemias is NSE⁻. Therefore, the definite diagnosis often requires correlation with CBC data, cytologic features and cytochemistry with additional techniques such as immunophenotyping by FC, cytogenetics/FISH, and molecular tests. Hypogranular APL (APL-v) is distinguished from acute monoblastic leukemia by strong expression of MPO, negative NSE, FC immunophenotypic pattern and positive *PML-RARA* rearrangement by genetic testing. Presence of CD11b, CD11c, CD14, and HLA-DR differentiates acute monoblastic leukemia form APL (APL cases are negative for all these markers). CD64, typical for acute monoblastic leukemia is often positive in other types of AML, including APL; the expression of CD64 in other types of leukemia is usually dim or positive only on subset. Positive CD11b, CD11c, CD14, and CD64 favor acute monoblastic leukemia over AML with or without maturation, especially when expression is strong (myeloblasts may be positive for both CD11c and CD64, but expression is dim). Figure 22.25 compares the FC features of acute monoblastic leukemia and hypogranular variant of APL and Figure 22.26 compares FC features of myeloblasts and monoblasts.

AML with NPM1 mutation. AMLs with *NPM1* mutation often show monocytic differentiation and both phenotypic and

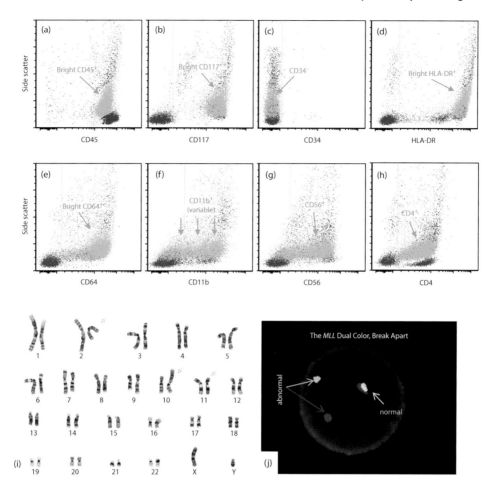

FIGURE 22.22 Acute monoblastic leukemia from a four-year-old boy. Flow cytometry analysis shows immature monocytic cells expressing CD45 (a) and CD117 (b), lack of CD34 (c), positive HLA-DR (d), CD64 (e), CD11b (f), CD56 (g), and CD4 (h). Metaphase cytogenetics (i) shows unusual three-way translocation involving *MLL* gene: 46,XY,t(2;10;11)(q23;p11.2;q23). FISH studies confirmed rearrangement of *MLL* at 11q23 (j). The three-way translocation involving *MLL* gene is rare, the most common being t(9;11). AML with 10p12/11q23 rearrangements are more common in males and mainly found in infants and children.

cytologic features may be indistinguishable from acute monocytic leukemia. Correlation with next generation sequencing for *NPM1* is necessary for final subclassification (see Chapter 23).

CMML. CMML is composed of mostly mature monocytes with rare (if any) monoblasts or promonocytes. FC analysis compliments morphologic diagnosis. When compared to CMML and AMML, acute monoblastic leukemias show predominance

of monocytic population in flow sample. In CMML monocytes are mature without overt cytological atypia. The aberrant immunophenotype of monocytic population is more often seen in acute monoblastic leukemia than in CMML or AMML. Loss of CD14 expression in acute monoblastic leukemia, CMML and AMML is seen in ~45%, ~4%, and 10%, respectively. Aberrant expression of CD56 is seen in majority of acute monoblastic leukemias (~76%),

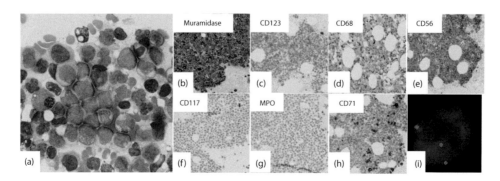

FIGURE 22.23 Acute monoblastic leukemia with trisomy 8. (a) Aspirate smear shows predominance of monoblasts and promonocytes. B-h) Immunohistochemistry performed on clot section shows the following phenotype: muramidase+ (b), CD123+ (c; dim), CD68+ (d; focal), CD56+ (e), CD117− (f), MPO− (g), and CD71− (h). (i) FISH testing showed trisomy 8 (CEP8 red probe).

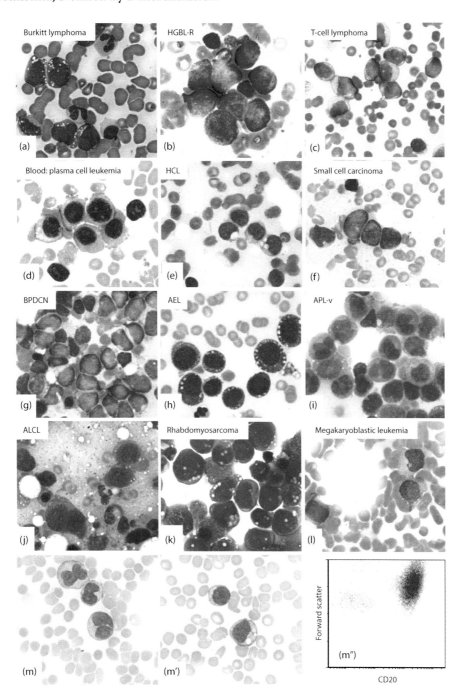

FIGURE 22.24 Cytologic differential diagnosis of acute monoblastic leukemia: (a) Burkitt lymphoma; (b) high grade B-cell lymphoma with *MYC* and *BCL2* rearrangement (HGBL-R, double hit lymphoma); (c) T-cell lymphoma with unusual "blastoid" appearance; (d) plasma cell leukemia with abundant cytoplasm mimicking monoblasts; (e) hairy cell leukemia with unusual "blastoid" cytologic features; (f) small cell carcinoma; (g) blastic plasmacytoid dendritic cell neoplasm (BPDCN); (h) acute erythroid leukemia (AEL); (i) hypogranular APL; anaplastic large cell lymphoma (j); alveolar rhabdomyosarcoma (k); acute megakaryoblastic leukemia (l) and diffuse large B-cell lymphoma with leukemic blood involvement (m-m′, cytology; m″, flow cytometry).

and in ~70% of CMML and only ~26% of AMML. Aberrant expression of CD10, CD16, and CD23 is comparable in all three disorders, but only acute monoblastic leukemia show expression of CD117 (~20% of cases) or CD34 (~8% of cases). Lack of HLA-DR is noted in ~8%, ~19%, and ~14% of acute monoblastic leukemia, CMML, and AMML, respectively. In contrast to acute monoblastic leukemia, AMML show significant population of myeloblasts, in addition to monocytic cells. The number of myeloblasts in CMML varies but by definition is below 20% (≥20% blasts qualified the leukemia to acute group). Promonocytes are considered blasts equivalents.

AMML. AMML differs by distinct populations of myeloblasts (≥20%) and monocytes. AML with inv(16)/t(16;16) shows increased number of atypical and immature eosinophils (see Chapter 23).

BPDCN. BPDCN shares with acute monoblastic leukemia some of the clinical, morphologic and immunophenotypic characteristics (Figure 22.27). BPDCN originates in the skin with

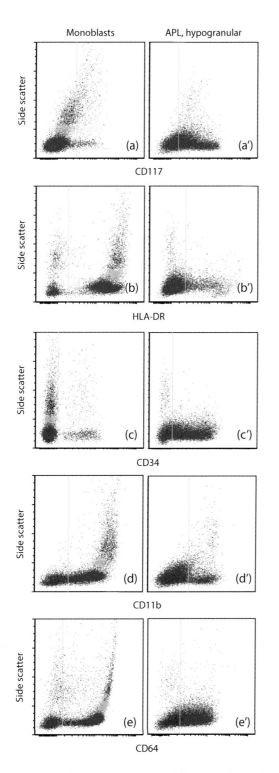

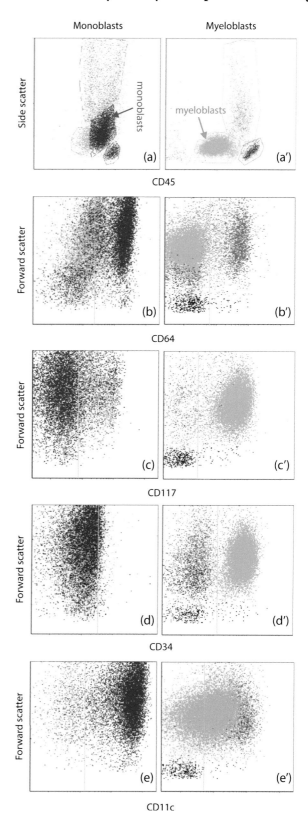

FIGURE 22.25 Comparison of monoblasts (a–e) with hypogranular APL (a′–e′). In contrast to hypogranular promyelocytes in APL, monoblasts are usually CD117 negative (a), HLA-DR positive (b), CD34 negative (c), CD11b positive (d) and CD64 brightly positive (e). Hypogranular APL show positive CD117 (a′), negative HLA-DR (b′), positive CD34 (c)′, negative CD11b (c′; minor subset of cells show non-specific staining), and dim (not bright) CD64 (e′). Since neoplastic promyelocytes in APL tend to display non-specific staining, correlation with isotypic controls and with markers known to be negative in AMLs (such as CD8, CD20, kappa, lambda etc.) is recommended for reliable analysis of phenotypic profile.

FIGURE 22.26 Comparison of monoblasts (a–e; blue dots) and myeloblasts (a′–e′; green dots). Monoblasts differ from myeloblasts by brighter expression of CD45 a–a′), bright expression of CD64 (b), often negative CD117 (c) and CD34 (d), and brighter expression of CD11c (e). Myeloblasts are either CD64 negative (b′) or show dim CD64, are usually positive for CD117 (c′) and CD34 (d′) and show negative or dim expression of CD11c (e′).

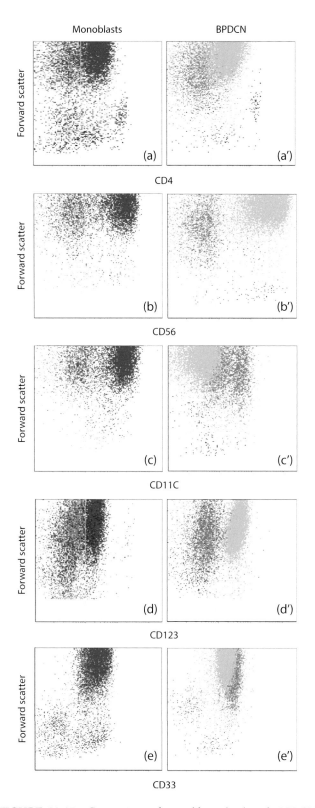

Monoblasts   BPDCN

Forward scatter   (a)   (a')

CD4

Forward scatter   (b)   (b')

CD56

Forward scatter   (c)   (c')

CD11C

Forward scatter   (d)   (d')

CD123

Forward scatter   (e)   (e')

CD33

FIGURE 22.27 Comparison of monoblasts (a–e) with BPDCN (a'–e'). The phenotype of monoblasts (blue dots) and blastic plasmacytoid dendritic cells (green dots) is similar. Monoblasts are often positive for CD4 (a) and CD56 (b), expression of which is the hallmark of BPDCN (a'–b'). In contrast to monoblasts, BPDCNs are negative for CD11c (c–c') and CD11b (not shown). CD123 is typically positive in BPDCN but maybe also expressed in acute monoblastic leukemia (d–d'). Rare BPDCNs may be positive for CD33 (e–e').

frequent involvement of BM and blood. It is positive for CD4, CD56, CD45, and CD123, and may be positive for CD7, and/or CD117. It is negative for NSE and majority of monocytic markers (CD11b, CD11c, CD14, CD36, CD64, lysozyme).

B-cell lymphoproliferations. Diffuse large B-cell lymphoma, BL and high-grade B-cell lymphomas, as well as unusual "blastoid" variants of HCL or MCL may resemble cytologically immature monocytic cells. FC immunophenotyping helps to distinguish between monoblasts and B-cell neoplasms (Figure 22.28).

Poorly differentiated plasma cell myeloma. Rare cases of PCM or plasma cell leukemia may display blastic or monocytoid cytomorphology requiring differential diagnosis with AML. Both plasma cell neoplasms and acute monoblastic leukemia may be CD56+ and/or CD117+. Plasma cell neoplasms differ by usually negative CD45, bright CD38 and CD138, negative HLA-DR and monocytic markers (CD11c, CD14, CD64), and clonal expression of cytoplasmic light chain immunoglobulins. See also Figures 5.32 and 5.33 in Chapter 5.

MDS. Occasionally, granulocytes with phenotypic features of dysmaturation may have similar phenotype to neoplastic monocytes. Lack of CD4 and CD56 and positive expression of CD10 and CD16 on subset favor granulocytes, whereas expression of CD4 and bright CD56 favor monocytes. Final diagnosis of equivocal cases should be based on cytomorphologic features and cytochemical staining for MPO and NSE. Although CD45 expression is most often bright on monocytic population, subset of acute monoblastic leukemias may display moderate CD45 expression, similarly to myeloblasts or dysplastic granulocytes.

Other tumors. Differential diagnosis also includes other hematopoietic (anaplastic large cell lymphoma; Langerhans cell histiocytosis, etc.) and non-hematopoietic tumors (carcinomas, rhabdomyosarcoma) which in rare occasions may mimic cytologically acute monoblastic leukemia on blood film or BM aspirate smear. Correlation with FC, cytochemistry, medical history, and BM morphology help in establishing the correct diagnosis.

Acute erythroid leukemia (AEL)

Phenotype of AEL: CD45$^{-/rarely+}$, CD71$^{+bright}$, GPHA$^{-/+}$, CD117$^{+(often\ dim)/rarely-}$, CD34$^{-/rarely+}$, CD36$^+$, CD56$^{-/rarely+}$, HLA-DR$^{-/rarely+}$, TdT$^-$

AEL (pure erythroid leukemia) is a rare variant of AML defined by >80% erythroid precursors among all nucleated marrow cells with ≥30% proerythroblasts [1]. The prior neoplasms classified as erythroleukemia (erythroid/myeloid type) are now diagnosed as either MDS or AML-MRC. Cases with ≥20% blasts of all marrow cells and the presence of either morphologic evidence of significant multilineage dysplasia, specific MDS-related cytogenetic abnormalities, or a history of MDS (or a myelodysplastic/MPN), irrespective of erythroid hyperplasia are now classified as AML with MRC (AML-MRC). Cases with blasts comprising <20% are diagnosed as MDS.

Morphology

Aspirate smear. The erythroid precursors predominate and comprise at least 30% proerythroblasts, which are large with dense basophilic, agranular and often vacuolated cytoplasm, fine chromatin, and one or more nucleoli (Figure 22.29). Cytoplasmic

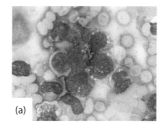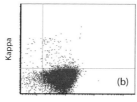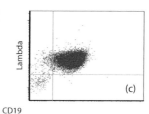

FIGURE 22.28 DLBCL mimicking acute monoblastic leukemia on aspirate smear (a). Flow cytometry (b–c) shows clonal (lambda⁺) B cells.

pseudopods, similar to those of acute megakaryoblastic leukemia, may be present. Nuclei are round or irregular with lobation and multinucleation and prominent megaloblastoid chromatin. The neoplastic cells often show chromatin accentuation at the periphery of the nuclear membrane. Ring sideroblasts are often present (~50%) on iron preparations (Figure 22.30) [10]. The blastoid cells in AEL are negative for MPO and SBB but are positive for PAS (periodic acid Shiff) and acid phosphatase. Some cases may show smaller blasts resembling ALL or AML but showing erythroid differentiation by immunophenotyping (Figure 22.31). Megakaryocytes display dysplastic features in most AEL cases.

BM biopsy. The BM core biopsy is hypercellular with sheets of erythroid precursors replacing medullary space (Figure 22.32). BM may be fibrotic leading to hemodilution of aspirate smears (with <80% of erythroid precursors and <30% proerythroblasts). In those cases, the presence of sheets of immature erythroid cells (with ≥30% proerythroblasts) expressing CD71 and/or E-cadherin confirms the diagnosis of AEL [1]. An intrasinusoidal or intravascular infiltrate pattern is seen in some cases of AEL.

Immunophenotype

Immunohistochemistry. Erythroblasts are strongly positive for CD71, hemoglobin A, e-cadherin, and may express glycophorin A (GPHA; CD235a). GPHA may be weak or negative, as it tends to stain more mature erythroid precursors and red blood cells (in contrast to both CD71 and e-cadherin, which stain early precursors). Erythroid precursors lack MPO, HLA-DR, CD34,

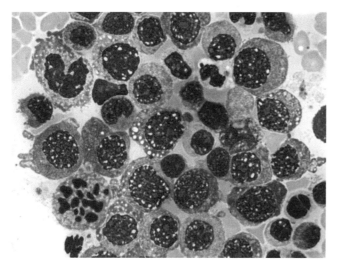

FIGURE 22.29 Pure erythroid leukemia – cytology. Numerous immature erythroid precursors with cytoplasmic vacuoles and occasionally irregular cytoplasmic borders are present.

pan-myeloid antigens, and usually CD45. CD117, CD43, and epithelial membrane antigen (EMA) are often positive (Figures 22.33 and 22.34). The early erythroblasts show coarse granular positivity with PAS. When AEL is poorly differentiated and shows no cytological evidence of erythroid maturation, the diagnosis may be difficult, as blasts are negative for CD34, CD45, and HLA-DR and express only CD71, E-cadherin, and CD117, which are not lineage specific (see differential diagnosis below).

Flow cytometry. FC (Figures 22.33, and 22.35–22.37) shows strong CD71 expression and partial CD117 expression. CD34, CD45, and HLA-DR are usually negative, but less differentiated leukemias may be positive for some or all of these markers. GPHA expression varies from positive to partial to negative, depending on the degree of maturation, as GPHA tends to stain more mature erythroid precursors, whereas both CD71 and CD117 are positive in early precursors. Rare cases may be CD56⁺.

Genetic features

AEL has no specific chromosomal changes but may show numerous unbalanced and balanced abnormalities, the former being more common [11–14]. In a series of 75 cases reported by Lessard et al., hypodiploidy was the most frequent numerical abnormality (48% cases with abnormal karyotype), associated with complex karyotypes (37%) [11]. Chromosomes 5 and 7 are most frequently involved (complete monosomy 5 in 26% and complete monosomy 7 in 38%), followed by chromosomes 8, 16, and 21 [11]. Trisomy 8 is the most frequent complete trisomy in erythroleukemia. In a series of 124 cases reported by Hasserjian et al., the most common specific cytogenetic abnormalities included monosomy 7, deletion 7q, monosomy 5, deletion 5q, trisomy 8, deletion 20q, deletion 9q, and deletion 12p [15]. The karyotypic changes are somewhat similar to those observed in high-grade MDS (refractory anemia with EBs) with the following changes observed only in AEL: der(9)t(1;19)(q11;p13), i(3)(q10), t(3;5)(q25;q35), inv(6)(p23q12), and t(7;11)(q11;p15) [11]. Figure 22.38 presents AEL with deletion of 5q and 7q.

Prognosis

AEL has poor prognosis with median survival of 4 to 6 months. The pathological diagnosis of AEL does not impart by itself a worse outcome, and rather prognosis should rely on classical AML prognostic factors. By univariate analysis, the following factors are associated with worse disease-free survival and overall survival: older age, intermediate risk cytogenetics, poor-risk cytogenetics, lower hemoglobin, lower platelets, poor performance status, history of MDS, and previous radiotherapy or chemotherapy [16]. The number of cytopenias in AEL patients did significantly correlate with survival, as patients with a single cytopenia had a better survival than those with 2 or 3 cytopenias [15].

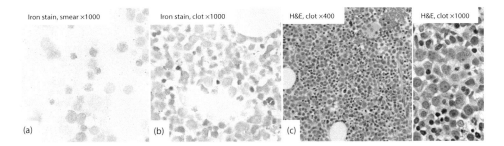

FIGURE 22.30 AEL with ring sideroblasts. The iron staining of the aspirate smear (a) and clot section (b) shows numerous ring sideroblasts. BM is packed with immature erythroid cells (c).

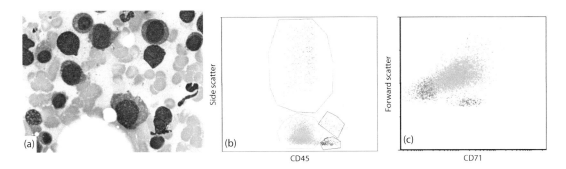

FIGURE 22.31 AEL with erythroid precursors resembling myeloblasts (a). Flow cytometry analysis shows moderate expression of CD45 (b) and positive CD71 (c).

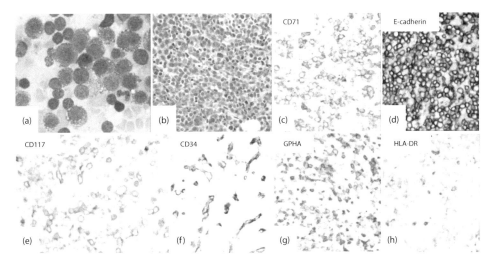

FIGURE 22.32 Acute erythroid leukemia (AEL). Aspirate smear (a) and BM core biopsy (b) shows predominance of proerythroblasts. They are positive for CD71 (c), e-cadherin (d) and focally CD117 (e). They do not express CD34 (f), GPHA (g), and HLA-DR (h).

Differential diagnosis of AEL
Differential diagnosis (Figure 22.39) includes:

- AML with minimal differentiation
- AUL
- AMKL
- AML-MRC
- MDS-EB with erythroid hyperplasia
- Acute panmyelosis with myelofibrosis (APMF)
- MDS with increased blasts and fibrosis (MDS-IB-f)
- Blast phase of MPN

- BPDCN
- Poorly differentiated PCM
- Metastatic tumors (alveolar rhabdomyosarcoma, melanoma, other)
- Benign process with prominent erythroid hyperplasia with leftward shift

MDS
The differential diagnosis includes MDSs, especially MDS-IB with erythroid hyperplasia, MDS-IB with diffuse reticulin fibrosis or MDS evaluated after recent treatment with erythropoietin.

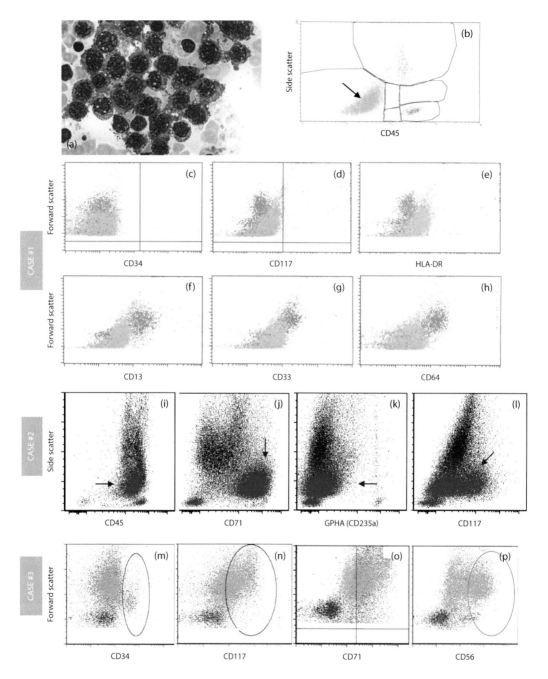

FIGURE 22.35 Pure erythroid leukemia – flow cytometry (three cases). (a–h) Neoplastic erythroid precursors (a, aspirate smear) are negative for CD45 (b, orange dots), CD34 (c), CD117 (d), HLA-DR (e), CD13 (f), CD33 (g), and CD64 (h). (i–l) Some erythroid leukemias may be positive for CD45 (I; blue dots), CD71 (j), and partially CD117 (l). GPHA is negative (k). (m–p) Erythroblasts (green dots) show minute population with CD34 expression (m), positive CD117 (n; dim expression), positive CD71 (o) and aberrant expression of CD56 on majority of blasts (p).

Morphology

Cytomorphologic features vary, depending on the degree of maturation of megakaryoblasts. In the more differentiated cases, megakaryoblasts are medium sized to large with round or slightly irregular nucleus and basophilic, agranular cytoplasm with distinct blebs (pseudopods; Figure 22.40). In poorly differentiated cases, megakaryoblasts resemble myeloblasts or lymphoblasts and their lineage can be revealed by immunophenotyping. The spectrum of morphologic features of acute megakaryoblastic leukemia in BM core biopsy varies from predominance of poorly differentiated blasts to sheets of atypical megakaryocytes with predominance of micromegakaryocytes (Figure 22.41).

Genetic features

AMKL is characterized by higher complexity and incidence of chromosomal abnormalities than in the other subtypes of AML [17–21]. In a series of 281 patients with AML reported by Athale et al., acute megakaryoblastic leukemia was diagnosed in 14.6%

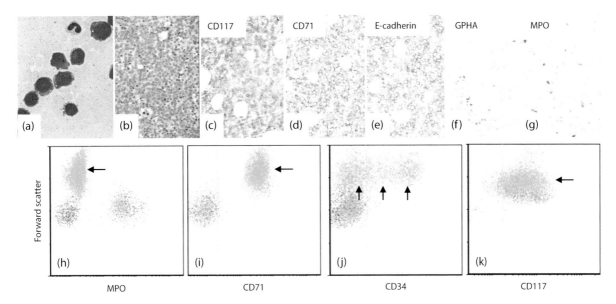

FIGURE 22.36 Acute erythroid leukemia. Aspirate smears shows immature erythroid precursors with vacuolated cytoplasm (a). Histology shows total BM replacement by erythroid precursors (b). Immunohistochemistry (c–g) shows positive expression of CD117 (c), CD71 (d), and E-cadherin (e), and negative GPHA (f), and MPO (g). Flow cytometry (h–k) shows lack of MPO (h), bright CD71 (i), partial CD34 expression of J0 and positive CD117 (k).

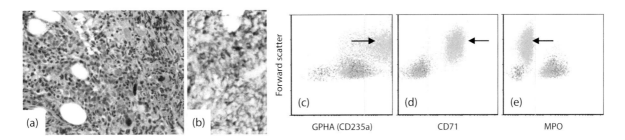

FIGURE 22.37 Acute erythroid leukemia. Histology (a) shows predominance of blasts, which express CD71 (b). Flow cytometry (c–e, arrow) shows bright expression of CD235a (GPHA) and CD71, and negative MPO.

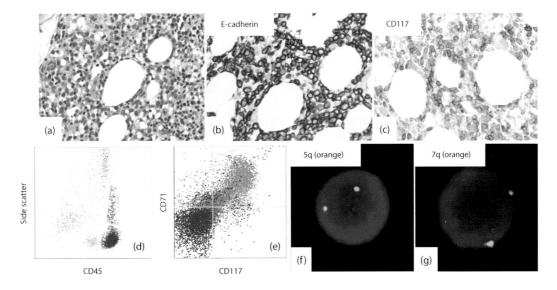

FIGURE 22.38 AEL with deletion of 5q and 7q. (a) Histology shows sheets of immature mononuclear cells replacing normal marrow elements. (b–c) Immunohistochemistry shows strong expression of E-cadherin and CD117. (d–f) Flow cytometry shows blasts (orange dots) with negative CD45 (d), positive CD117 (e) and bright expression of CD71 (e). FISH show deletion of 5q (f) and deletion of 7q (g).

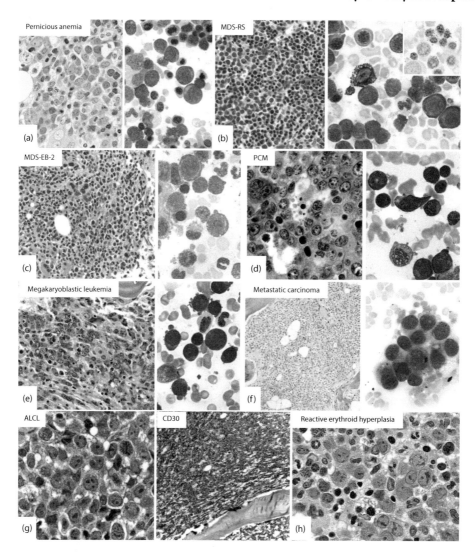

FIGURE 22.39 AEL – differential diagnosis. (a) Erythroid hyperplasia with megaloblastoid features (B12/folate deficiency). (b–c) MDS (b, MDS with ring sideroblasts; c, MDS with excess blasts 2. (d) Plasma cell myeloma (PCM). (e) Acute megakaryoblastic leukemia. (f) Metastatic carcinoma. (g) Anaplastic large cell lymphoma (ALCL). (h) Reactive erythroid hyperplasia (patient with hemolytic anemia).

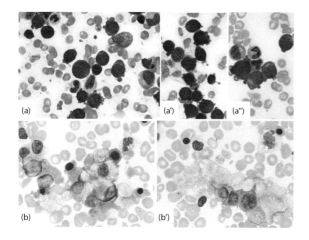

FIGURE 22.40 Acute megakaryoblastic leukemia – cytology (two cases). (a–a″) BM aspirate smear shows numerous blasts with basophilic cytoplasm with distinct blebs or pseudopod formation. (b–b′) Blood smears show leukoerythroblastosis with large blasts, giant platelets, and immature nucleated erythroid cells.

(six patients with Down syndrome, six had secondary leukemia, and 29 represented *de novo* leukemia) [21]. The most frequent chromosomal changes reported in AMKL include ⁻7/del(7q), ⁻5/del(5q), +8, +19 (or +19q), +21, followed by i(12)(p10), t(9;22)(q34;q11), t(10;22)(q26;q11), t(13;20), del(20)(q11), der(7)/t(7;17), t(1;22)(p13;q13), t(6;11)(q24.1;p15.5), t(17;22)(q21;q13), and 11q23 abnormalities [17, 18, 22–27]. Dastugue et al., identified nine cytogenetic groups in patients with AMKL: normal karyotypes (group 1); patients with Down syndrome (group 2); numerical abnormalities only (group 3), t(1;22)(p13;q13) or *OTT/MAL* transcript (group 4); t(9;22)(q34;q11) (group 5); 3q21q26 (group 6); ⁻5/del(5q) or ⁻7/del(7q) or both (group 7); i(12)(p10) (group 8), and other structural changes (group 9) [17]. Groups 1, 2, 3, and 4 were exclusively seen in children (except one adult in group 3), whereas groups 5, 6, 7, and 8 were mainly made up of adults [17]. Based on current WHO classification, AML-MRC, AML with t(1;22), AML with inv(3), AML with t(3;3), or Down syndrome-related leukemias are excluded from acute megakaryoblastic leukemia category. AMKL not associated with Down syndrome harbors a number of driving rearrangements, many of which are unique to this form of AML, including *RBM15-MKL1*, *CBFA2T3-GLIS2*,

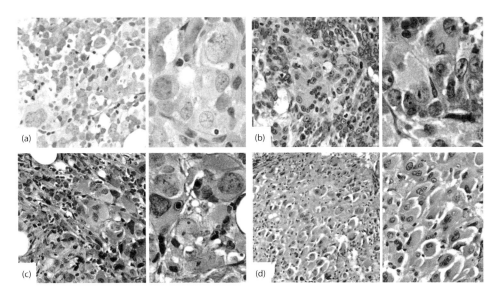

FIGURE 22.41 Acute megakaryoblastic leukemia – histologic features of four different cases. Histologic features in acute mega-karyoblastic leukemia vary from case to case. In some cases, poorly differentiated blasts predominate (a). In other, there is mixed population of highly atypical megakaryocytes, megakaryoblasts, and blasts (b–c). In some leukemias, highly dysplastic (hypolobated) megakaryocytes predominate (d).

and *NUP98-KDM5A* fusions in addition to *KMT2A* rearrangements [28].

Immunophenotype

Majority of AMKLs are positive for CD38, CD71, CD61, and CD117 and often positive for CD34, CD41, and CD45. Subset of blasts shows co-expression of CD34 and megakaryocytic markers. In contrast to bright expression of CD71 in erythroid precursors, the expression of this marker in acute megakaryoblastic leukemia is dimmer. HLA-DR is often negative but may be dim. Some cases show CD56 expression. MPO, CD15, and TdT are most often negative. FC analysis is often quite characteristic and shows blasts with moderate CD34, dim CD117, negative to dim HLA-DR, negative CD13 and MPO, bright CD33, and dim CD64 (Figure 22.42). CD41 and CD61 are expressed (Figure 22.43; expression of CD41 and CD61 has to be interpreted with caution due to potential

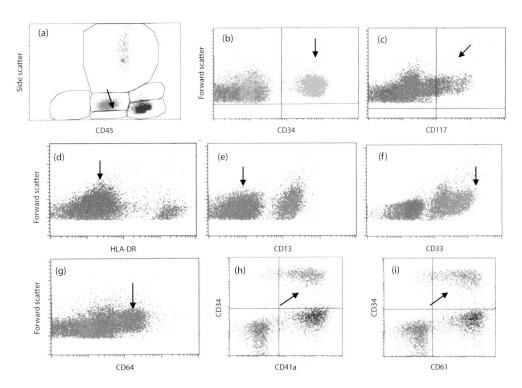

FIGURE 22.42 Acute megakaryoblastic leukemia – flow cytometry. Although the phenotypic pattern may vary, most cases show the following phenotype: low side scatter (a, arrow), CD34+ (moderate expression; b), negative to dim expression of CD117 (c), negative HLA-DR (d), negative CD13 (e), bright expression of CD33 (f), dim expression of CD64 (g), and co-expression of CD41a and CD61 (h–i).

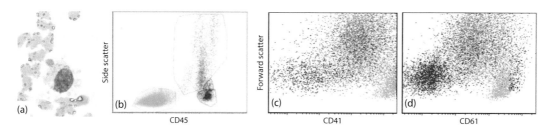

FIGURE 22.43 Acute megakaryoblastic leukemia (flow cytometry). Blasts (green dots) show negative to dim CD45 expression (a), and positive CD41 (b) and CD61 (c).

non-specific adsorption of platelets on other cells). Some poorly differentiated acute megakaryoblastic leukemias may be negative for most of the markers except CD41, CD61, and dim CD34. AMKL associated with Down syndrome is more likely to express CD7, CD11b, CD13, CD33, and CD36 when compared to cases not associated with Down syndrome [29].

Differential diagnosis of acute megakaryoblastic leukemia
The differential diagnosis includes:

- AML with minimal differentiation
- AUL
- AEL
- AML-MRC
- APMF
- MDS with increased blasts and fibrosis (MDS-IB-f)
- Blast phase of MPN and PMF
- B-ALL and T-ALL
- MPAL

AML with minimal differentiation, B-ALL, T-ALL
Poorly differentiated AMKL needs to be differentiated from AML with minimal differentiation, AUL, MPAL, B-ALL, and T-ALL. In AML with minimal differentiation, blasts are positive for pan-myeloid antigens (CD13 and/or CD33), blastic markers (CD34, CD117, CD133), HLA-DR, CD38, and often also TdT. B-ALL expressed CD34 and/or TdT with B-cell lineage markers (CD19, CD22, CD79a) and often CD10. T-ALL is positive for cytoplasmic CD3, CD7, and one or more blastic markers (CD34, TdT, CD1a).

AUL
AUL is diagnosed after exclusion of all other types of acute leukemia after immunophenotypic, cytochemical, and genetic studies. Blasts are often positive only for CD34, HLA-DR, and/or CD38.

Acute erythroid leukemia (AEL)
AEL is defined by >80% erythroid precursors among all nucleated marrow cells with ≥30% proerythroblasts. Erythroblasts are strongly positive for CD71, hemoglobin A, E-cadherin, and may express glycophorin A (GPHA; CD235a). GPHA may be weak or negative, as it tends to stain more mature erythroid precursors and red blood cells. They do not express megakaryocytic markers (CD41, CD61).

APMF
Based on WHO classification, APMF is characterized by fibrotic marrow, multilineage myeloid proliferation (panmyelosis), increased blasts, atypical megakaryocytes, and diffuse reticulin fibrosis. In contrast to APMF which shows variable degrees of expansion of erythroid, myeloid, and megakaryocytic precursors, AMKL usually shows rather monomorphic proliferation of mega-karyoblasts without significant number of other lineages (i.e., no panmyelosis). Megakaryocytes in APMF are predominately of small size showing variable degrees of atypia including the presence of hypolobulated or nonlobulated nuclei [30].

MDS-IB-f and AML-MRC
The presence of grades 2 or 3 reticulin fibrosis classifies the findings as MDS with fibrosis (MDS-f), if other criteria for MDS are fulfilled. Most cases represent MDS with increased blasts (MDS-IB). Differential diagnosis between MDS-IB-f, AML-MRC, PMF, and APMF may be difficult and require careful morphologic and immunophenotypic analysis, clinical correlation (prior diagnoses, exclusion of toxic therapy, infections, autoimmune disorders), and genetic testing (specific chromosomal changes or the presence of certain mutations). As smears are often inadequate in those disorders, morphologic analysis is usually limited to core biopsy. Immunohistochemistry staining with CD34, CD117, MPO, CD61, CD71, and E-cadherin helps to determine number of blasts and their phenotype. Number of blasts <20% indicates MDS-EIB, while number of blasts ≥20% is diagnostic of AML-MRC. In some cases of prominent marrow fibrosis, number of blasts present in BM may be lower than in peripheral blood (as revealed by FC or smear analysis). This phenomenon may be due abnormal "blast trafficking" due to fibrosis, extramedullary hematopoiesis, and/or uneven distribution of blasts in BM. The blasts in acute megakaryoblastic leukemia express one or more of the platelet glycoproteins, CD41, CD61, and CD42b, and are negative for MPO, and usually negative for CD45 and HLA-DR (CD13 and CD33 may be occasionally positive). Megakaryocytes in acute megakaryoblastic leukemia usually have round or slightly irregular nuclei with fine chromatin, while megakaryocytes in MDS typically show hypolobated or bilobed nuclei, multinucleation, and micromegakaryocytes. AML-MRC differs from MDS-IB-f, by having ≥20% blasts. Evaluation of blasts with CD34 in MDS-IB and AML-MRC must be correlated with other markers (e.g., MPO, CD33, CD45, and CD61), as dysplastic megakaryocytes are often CD34+.

PMF and blast phase of MPN
Prior history of MPN helps to identify blasts phase, regardless of morphologic and phenotypic features of leukemia. Primary myelofibrosis (PMF) typically is associated with splenomegaly, usually has blasts <5% and is often positive for either *JAK2*, *MPL*, or *CALR* mutation. PMF is characterized by leukoerythroblastosis, while in acute megakaryoblastic leukemia may show in blood smear circulating micromegakaryoblasts, megakaryoblast fragments,

dysplastic large platelets, and hypogranular neutrophils [1]. Megakaryocytes in PMF are typically large and show prominent cytologic atypia in the form of hyperchromasia, bulbous, cloud-like or balloon-shaped nuclei. Megakaryocytes in AMKL usually have round or slightly irregular nuclei with fine chromatin.

Acute panmyelosis with myelofibrosis

APMF is a rare and not well-defined variant of AML with clinical, morphologic, and immunophenotypic features overlapping with acute megakaryoblastic leukemia, AML with MRC (AML-MRC), MDS with EBs (MDS-EB), and PMF, especially PMF in accelerated phase. Based on WHO classification, APMF is characterized by a multilineage myeloid proliferation with increased blasts, increased atypical megakaryocytes, and diffuse reticulin fibrosis. Patients are present with abrupt onset with pancytopenia and without splenomegaly. The diagnosis is based on clinicopathological features and the exclusion of other myeloid malignancies, in particular AML with myelodysplasia-associated changes. There is no history of MPN or MDS, exposure to radiation or cytotoxic drugs.

Morphology

BM biopsy usually shows hypercellular BM with panmyelosis (i.e., trilineage myeloid proliferation) with dysplastic erythropoiesis, abundant atypical (dysplastic) megakaryocytes, and overt diffuse fibrosis (Figures 22.44 and 22.45). In some cases, marrow may be normocellular or even hypocellular. Megakaryocytes (CD61+) are mostly small and dysplastic (hypolobulated) without highly atypical hyperchromatic, cloud-like, or balloon-shaped nuclei typical for PMF. Megakaryocytes show focal clustering, but not to the extent seen in PMF. Less differentiated (immature) megakaryocytes may be present but are not as prominent as in acute megakaryoblastic leukemia. Erythroid precursors are leftward shifted with megaloblastoid features. The stroma shows an inflammatory reaction (perivascular plasmacytosis, lymphoid nodules, many macrophages, iron deposits) in about 50% of the samples. In contrast to

PMF, there is no intrasinusoidal hematopoiesis. CD34+ blasts are increased (≥20%) and are often arranged in clusters. Peripheral blood shows pancytopenia with dysplastic and leftward-shifted granulocytes and occasional circulating blasts (usually <5%). Red blood cells do not display prominent poikilocytosis (there are no dacrocytes). Leukoerythroblastic features may be present.

Immunophenotype

Blasts are positive for CD34, CD117, HLA-DR, and myeloid antigens (CD13, CD33). Variable proportion of blasts is MPO+.

Differential diagnosis of acute panmyelosis with myelofibrosis

The differential diagnosis of acute panmyelosis includes:

- AMKL
- MDS with increased blasts (MDS-IB)
- MDS with fibrosis
- AEL
- PMF
- MPNs in accelerated or blast phase
- Toxic myelopathy
- AML with MRC (AML-MRC)

Differentiation of APMF from AML-MRC, acute megakaryoblastic leukemia, and MDS-EB and marrow fibrosis may be difficult. Clinical and hematopathologic findings in APMF and acute megakaryoblastic leukemia partially overlap. The number of blasts in acute megakaryoblastic leukemia is higher than in acute panmyelosis, they are less often CD34+, and more often positive for megakaryocytic markers (CD41/CD61, CD42b) [30]. Blasts in APMF are positive for CD34 without expression of megakaryocytic markers[30]. PMF shows in blood smear prominent red blood cell anisocytosis with many dacrocytes, and in BM biopsy marked megakaryocytic atypia and variable size, clustering and presence of intrasinusoidal hematopoiesis. In contrast to PMF,

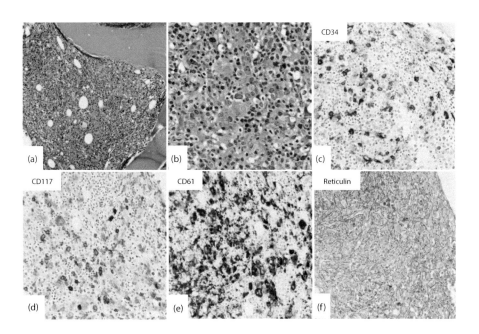

FIGURE 22.44 Acute panmyelosis with myelofibrosis. BM is hypercellular with myeloid and erythroid leftward shift (a–b), increased blasts (c–d), megakaryocytic hyperplasia with atypia (e), and diffuse reticulin fibrosis (f).

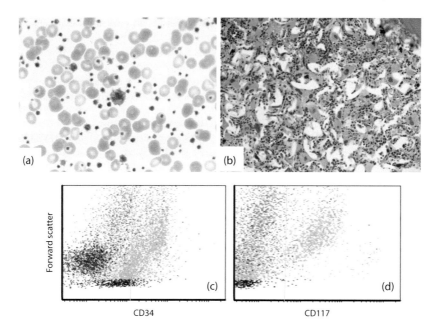

FIGURE 22.45 Acute panmyelosis with myelofibrosis in patient with COVID infection. (a) Blood smear shows thrombocytosis with prominent cytologic atypia of platelets. (b) BM core biopsy shows hypercellular marrow with megakaryocytic hyperplasia and increased blasts. (c–d) Flow cytometry. Blasts (green dots) are increased; they are CD34+ (c) and CD117+ (d).

patients with APMF have minor splenomegaly or no organomegaly at all. Megakaryocytes may look similar in APMF, MDS-EB, and AML-MRC (micromegakaryocytes with hypolobated nuclei). MDS-EB and fibrosis is usually excluded based on abrupt clinical presentation typical for APMF, <20% CD34+ blasts, and the presence of numerous small atypical megakaryocytes with nonlobulated or hypolobulated nuclei). AML-MRC differs by the presence of marked dyspoiesis. The presence of ⁻5/del(5q) and/or ⁻7/del(7q) favors the diagnosis of AML with MDS-associated changes over acute panmyelosis. See also differential diagnosis of acute megakaryoblastic leukemia, above.

Acute basophilic leukemia

Acute basophilic leukemia is very rare form of acute leukemia with predominance of immature basophils (Figure 22.46). It has to be differentiated from CML (especially in accelerated or blast phase; Figure 22.47), chronic basophilic leukemia, other acute leukemias with basophilia, and MDS-EB with basophilia.

Extramedullary myeloid tumor (EMT)

EMT (myeloid sarcoma, granulocytic sarcoma, chloroma) is a tumor mass composed of immature myeloid cells (myeloblasts or monoblasts), which occur outside the BM. It occurs in 2.5% to 9.1% of patients with AML [31, 32]. EMT occurs concomitantly, following or rarely, antedating the onset of systemic AML. EMT may be also associated with MDS or MPN. Myeloid sarcoma may be the first evidence of AML or precede it by months or years. EMT can also develop at relapse (with or without BM involvement); the incidence of patients developing EMT after allogeneic hematopoietic stem cell transplantation has been reported to be 0.2% to 1.3% with poor overall survival [33, 34]. AML with t(8;21) has been associated with a higher frequency of EMT [35]. The most common type of EMT is the granulocytic sarcoma which has the phenotype similar to AML with or without maturation. EMT with the phenotype similar to acute monoblastic leukemia is termed monoblastic sarcoma. EMT involves lymph nodes (Figure 22.48), skin (Figure 22.49), bone, periosteum, paranasal

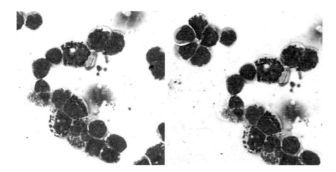

FIGURE 22.46 Acute basophilic leukemia – cytology. Numerous immature cells with basophilic granules are present.

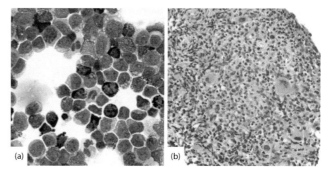

FIGURE 22.47 CML – myeloid blast phase with basophilia (a, cytology; b, histology).

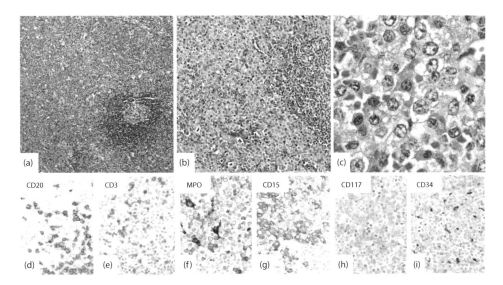

FIGURE 22.48 Extramedullary myeloid tumor (granulocytic sarcoma) – lymph node. (a) Atypical large cell infiltrate in the interfollicular area. (b–c) Higher magnification shows mononuclear cells with blastoid appearance. Neoplastic cells have the following phenotype: CD20$^-$ (d), CD3$^-$ (e), MPO$^+$ (f), CD15$^+$ (g), CD117$^+$ (h; dim), CD34$^+$ (i).

sinuses, testis, GI tract (Figure 22.50), and CNS. Occasional EMT may display features of MPAL (Figures 22.51 and 22.52). EMT with T-lymphoblastic component and AML component (especially when both populations express CD3) needs to be differentiated from bilineal lymphoma/leukemia associated with myeloid and lymphoid neoplasms with *FGFR1* abnormalities (8p11 myeloproliferative syndrome).

In a series of EMT patients reported by Pileri et al., 27% (25 patients) presented as *de novo* myeloid sarcoma, 35% (32 patients) had simultaneous AML, chronic MPN or MDS, and the remaining 38% (35 patients) had a previous history of AML, polycythemia vera (PV), essential thrombocythemia (ET), PMF, CML, mastocytosis, or MDS [36]. Cytogenetic analysis revealed normal karyotype in 13 of 28 patients (46%), whereas 15 of 28 patients (54%) showed chromosomal abnormalities which included add(6)(q24), add(8)(p23), del(9), del(2), inv(16), $^-$16, $^-$18, t(1;12), t(9;11), t(9;22), t(11;11), t(15;17), +8, +10, +21 [36]. FISH analysis showed clonal abnormalities in 25 of 49 cases (54%). Based on the FISH

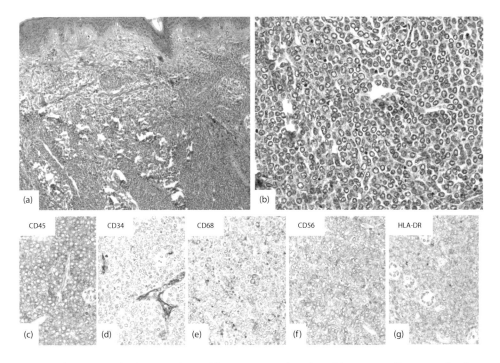

FIGURE 22.49 Extramedullary myeloid tumor (monoblastic sarcoma) – skin. (a) Dense infiltrate in the dermis without epidermotropism. (b) High magnification shows mononuclear cells with irregular nuclei. Tumor cells are positive for CD45 (c), negative for CD34, positive for CD68 (e), CD56 (f), and HLA-DR (g).

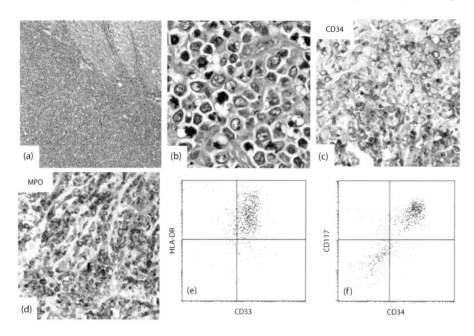

FIGURE 22.50   Extramedullary myeloid tumor (granulocytic sarcoma) involving small intestine. Histology (a–b) shows diffuse large cell infiltrate immunoreactive with CD34 (c) and MPO (d). Flow cytometry (e–f) shows blasts expressing CD33, HLA-DR, CD34, and CD117.

and cytogenetics, monosomy 7(10.8%), trisomy 8(10.4%), and mixed lineage leukemia-splitting (8.5%) were the commonest abnormalities in that series, whereas t(8;21) was rare (2.2%) [36]. However, the t(8;21) translocation was the most common cytogenetic abnormality reported by others [35, 37]. In children, the t(8;21) has been associated with orbital EMT [38, 39]. The inv(16) is another cytogenetic abnormality with a higher incidence of EMT involvement, particularly in abdomen [40].

AML with myelodysplasia-related changes (AML-MRC)

The diagnosis of AML-MRC requires one of the following:

- Previous history of MDS or MDS/MPN (e.g., CMML, MDS/MPN-n)
- ≥50% cells in two or more myeloid lineages with dyspoiesis

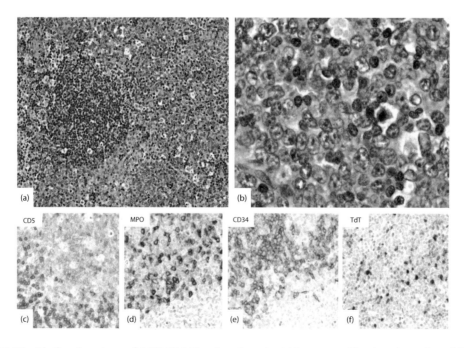

FIGURE 22.51   EMT with the phenotype of AML/T-ALL – lymph node. (a) Low magnification shows interfollicular/paracortical infiltrate. (b) High magnification shows blastic appearance of neoplastic cells. The phenotype of blasts fulfilled the criteria proposed by European Group for the Immunologic Classification of Leukemia for acute biphenotypic leukemia. Immunohistochemistry (c–f) shows positive expression of CD5 (c), MPO (d), CD34 (e), and TdT (f).

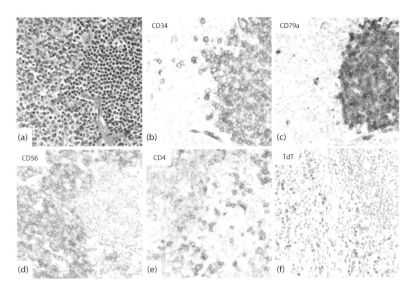

FIGURE 22.52 EMT with features of biphenotypic acute leukemia (B-ALL and AML with monocytic differentiation). (a) Histology with atypical mononuclear infiltrate (mostly large cell type on the left, and small cell type on the right). B-lymphoblastic component is positive for CD34 (b) and CD79a (c), whereas myeloid component expresses CD56 (d), CD4 (e), and TdT (f).

- MDS-related chromosomal abnormality:
  - complex karyotype (three or more chromosomal abnormalities)
  - unbalanced changes: ⁻7 or del(7q); ⁻5 or del(5q); i(17q) or t(17p); ⁻13 or del(13q); del(11q), del(12p) or t(12p); idic(X)(q13)
  - balanced changes: t(11;16)(q23;p13.3); t(3;21)(q26.2; q22.1); t(1;3)(p36.3;q21.1); t(2;11)(p21;q23); t(5;12)(q33; p12); t(5;7)(q33;q11.2); t(5;17)(q33;p13); t(5;10)(q33;q21) t(3;5)(q25;q34)

In addition to cytogenetic changes, recent publication has described molecular alterations in AML patients that are highly suggestive of antecedent MDS or therapy-induced AML even in the absence of overt dysplasia: *SF3B1, SRSF2, U2AF1, ZRSR2, ASXL1, EZH2, BCOR,* and *STAG2* [41]. If the diagnosis of AML-MRC is based on only multilineage dysplasia, then mutational analysis is required to exclude patients with *NPM1* and biallelic *CEBPA* mutations. Outcomes for patients with AML-MRC are poor compared to patients with many other AML subtypes. Figure 22.53 shows an example of AML-MRC. AML-MRC may display phenotype

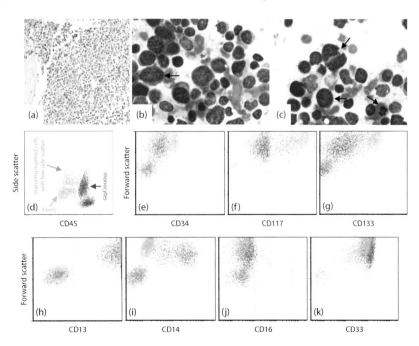

FIGURE 22.53 AML-MRC. Bone marrow (a) is hypercellular with myeloid and erythroid leftward shift. Aspirate smear (b–c) shows increased blasts and prominent dyserythropoiesis (arrows). Flow cytometry (d–k) shows increased blasts (green dots), increased monocytes (dark blue dots) and neutrophils and maturing myeloid precursors (gray dots) with low side scatter. Blasts are positive for CD45 (d), CD34 (e), CD117 (f), CD133 (g), CD13 (h), and CD33 (k). Monocytes are positive for CD13 (h), CD14 (i), and CD33 (k). Neutrophils/maturing myeloid precursors show aberrant down-regulation of CD16 (j).

compatible with AUL or AML, NOS (often AML with minimal differentiation, AML with maturation or AMML).

Therapy-related myeloid neoplasms

Therapy-related myeloid neoplasms include therapy-related acute myeloid leukemia (tAML), therapy-related myelodysplastic syndrome (tMDS), therapy-related myeloproliferative neoplasm (t(MPN)), and tMDS/MPN occurring as late complications of cytotoxic chemotherapy and/or radiation therapy. Excluded from this category is transformation of MPN to AML since it is often not possible to determine if this is a disease evolution or de novo therapy-related neoplasm.

Morphology

Most patients present with tAML/tMDS associated with multi-lineage dysplasia, history of treatment with alkylating agents and/or radiation therapy and cytogenetics revealing abnormalities of chromosome 5 and/or 7, or a complex karyotype [42–47]. Dysplasia may be seen in some patients with balanced translocations. Blood shows anemia, poikilocytosis, and macrocytosis in majority of cases. Neutrophils show hypolobation of nuclei and hypogranular cytoplasm. Basophilia is frequently seen. BM may be hypercellular, normocellular, or hypocellular with occasional reticulin fibrosis. Majority of cases show dysgranulopoiesis, dysmegakaryopoiesis, and/or dyserythropoiesis. Ringed sideroblasts are frequently seen. Number of blasts varies. Subset of patients presents with features of tMDS/MPN, such as CMML. In 20%–30% of cases, the first manifestation of therapy-related myeloid neoplasm is overt acute leukemia without a preceding myelodysplastic phase.

Immunophenotype

FC shows increased blasts and prominent features of dyspoiesis on granulocytes/maturing myeloid precursors (Figures 22.54–22.56).

Blasts may display increased side scatter and often show aberrant phenotype, including expression of CD7, CD11b, CD19, and CD56, lack of CD34 or HLA-DR, and abnormal expression of pan-myeloid markers. Dyspoietic features on granulocytes are similar to those seen in MDS (see Chapter 19).

Genetic features

The leukemic cells show abnormal karyotype in 90% of patients with tAML/tMDS. Approximately 70% of patients have unbalanced chromosomal aberrations, mainly whole or partial loss of chromosome 5 and/or 7, that are often associated with one or more additional abnormalities [e.g., del(13q), del(20q), del(11q), del(3p), 017, ‾18, ‾21, +8]. Balanced translocations include rearrangements of 11q23 [e.g., t(9;11) and t(11;19)], 21q22 [t(8;21); t(3;21)] and other abnormalities, including t(15;17) and inv(16). The balanced translocations are generally associated with a short latency period, most often present as over AML without a preceding myelodysplastic phase and are associated with prior topoisomerase-II inhibitor therapy. The majority of these cases are associated with balanced translocations that frequently involve 11q22 (*MLL*) or 21q22 (*RUNX1*). Some leukemias show cytogenetic abnormalities associated with AML with recurrent chromosomal abnormalities, including t(15;17) [t-APL] or t-AML with t(9;11). Cases of lymphoblastic leukemia also occur in this group, usually associated with a t(4;11).

Prognosis

Therapy-related myeloid neoplasm has poor prognosis comparable to AML with MRC (AML-MRC). However, secondary APL has similar morphologic, immunophenotypic, and cytogenetic findings to those of *de novo* APL (including comparable rates of *FLT3* mutations, recurrent disease, and death), which differentiates it from other therapy-related myeloid neoplasms [43].

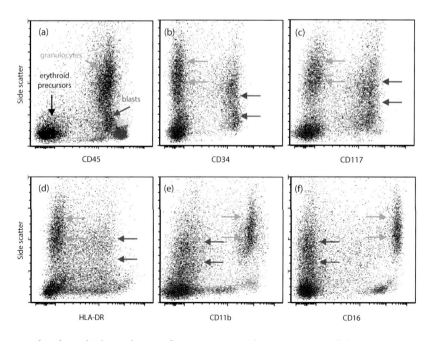

FIGURE 22.54 Therapy-related myeloid neoplasm – flow cytometry. Flow cytometry of the BM aspirate from patient with a history of B-cell lymphoma after cytotoxic therapy shows increased blasts (red arrows), increased CD45-negative erythroid precursors (a; black dots), down-regulation of CD45 on granulocytes (a), increased side scatter of CD34+ (b), CD117+ (c), and HLA-DR+ (d) myeloblasts (positive CD34 and HLA-DR excludes promyelocytes). Granulocytes (green arrows) can be separated from blasts be positive CD11b (e) and CD16 (f), and lack of CD34 (b), CD117 (c), and HLA-DR (d).

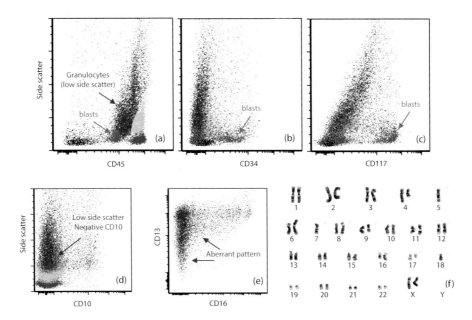

FIGURE 22.55 Therapy-related myeloid neoplasm: flow cytometry and cytogenetics. Bone marrow from patient with history of follicular lymphoma (stage IV) after cytotoxic therapy. Flow cytometry (a–e) shows increased blasts (blue dots; a–c) and phenotypic features of dyspoiesis on granulocytes (purple dots), including decreased side scatter (a), down-regulation of CD10 (d), and aberrant pattern of CD13 versus CD16 expression (e). Metaphase cytogenetics (f) shows complex changes including monosomy 5 and monosomy 7: 42~44,XX,add(4)(q21),⁻5,add(6)(p22),⁻7, t(8;17)(p22;q12), t(9;16)(q22;q22), add(12)(p11.2),⁻18.

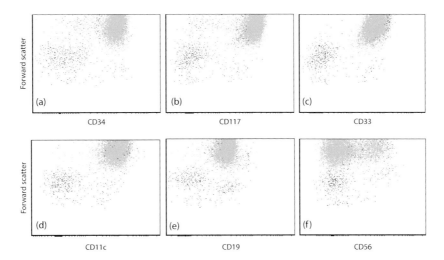

FIGURE 22.56 Therapy-related myeloid neoplasm (AML after therapy for breast carcinoma) – flow cytometry. Blasts (green dots) are positive for CD34 (a), CD117 (b), CD33 (d), CD11c (d), CD19 (e), and partially CD56 (f). Cytogenetic and FISH studies were negative for t(8;21)/*RUNX1-RUNX1T1*.

References

1. Swerdlow, S.H., et al., ed. *WHO classification of tumors of haematopoietic and lymphoid tissues.* 2016, IARC: Lyon.
2. Bernier, M., et al., *Immunological definition of acute minimally differentiated myeloid leukemia (M0) and acute undifferentiated leukemia (AUL).* Leuk Lymphoma, 1995. **18 Suppl 1**: p. 13–7.
3. Porwit, A. and M.C. Bene, *Acute leukemias of ambiguous origin.* Am J Clin Pathol, 2015. **144**(3): p. 361–76.
4. Borowitz, M.J., *Mixed phenotype acute leukemia.* Cytometry B Clin Cytom, 2014. **86**(3): p. 152–3.
5. Fuda, F. and W. Chen, *Lineage determination in mixed phenotype acute leukemia: response to Marcondes et al.* Cytometry B Clin Cytom, 2014. **86**(3): p. 150–1.
6. Porwit, A. and M.C. Bene, *Multiparameter flow cytometry applications in the diagnosis of mixed phenotype acute leukemia.* Cytometry B Clin Cytom, 2019. **96**(3): p. 183–94.
7. Raikar, S.S., et al., *Isolated myeloperoxidase expression in pediatric B/myeloid mixed phenotype acute leukemia is linked with better survival.* Blood, 2018. **131**(5): p. 573–7.
8. Gorczyca, W., *Flow cytometry immunophenotypic characteristics of monocytic population in acute monocytic leukemia (AML-M5), acute*

myelomonocytic leukemia (AML-M4), and chronic myelomonocytic leukemia (CMML). Methods Cell Biol, 2004. **75**: p. 665–77.

9. Haferlach, T., et al., *Distinct genetic patterns can be identified in acute monoblastic and acute monocytic leukaemia (FAB AML M5a and M5b): a study of 124 patients.* Br J Haematol, 2002. **118**(2): p. 426–31.

10. Wang, W., et al., *Pure erythroid leukemia.* Am J Hematol, 2017. **92**(3): p. 292–6.

11. Lessard, M., et al., *Cytogenetic study of 75 erythroleukemias.* Cancer Genet Cytogenet, 2005. **163**(2): p. 113–22.

12. Preiss, B.S., et al., *Cytogenetic findings in adult de novo acute myeloid leukaemia. A population-based study of 303/337 patients.* Br J Haematol, 2003. **123**(2): p. 219–34.

13. Cuneo, A., et al., *Morphologic, immunologic and cytogenetic studies in erythroleukaemia: evidence for multilineage involvement and identification of two distinct cytogenetic-clinicopathological types.* Br J Haematol, 1990. **75**(3): p. 346–54.

14. Olopade, O.I., et al., *Clinical, morphologic, and cytogenetic characteristics of 26 patients with acute erythroblastic leukemia.* Blood, 1992. **80**(11): p. 2873–82.

15. Hasserjian, R.P., et al., *Acute erythroid leukemia: a reassessment using criteria refined in the 2008 WHO classification.* Blood, 2010. **115**(10): p. 1985–92.

16. Santos, F.P., et al., *Adult acute erythroleukemia: an analysis of 91 patients treated at a single institution.* Leukemia, 2009. **23**(12): p. 2275–80.

17. Dastugue, N., et al., *Cytogenetic profile of childhood and adult megakaryoblastic leukemia (M7): a study of the Groupe Francais de Cytogenetique Hematologique (GFCH).* Blood, 2002. **100**(2): p. 618–26.

18. Cuneo, A., et al., *Multipotent stem cell involvement in megakaryoblastic leukemia: cytologic and cytogenetic evidence in 15 patients.* Blood, 1989. **74**(5): p. 1781–90.

19. Tallman, M.S., et al., *Acute megakaryocytic leukemia: the Eastern Cooperative Oncology Group experience.* Blood, 2000. **96**(7): p. 2405–11.

20. Ribeiro, R.C., et al., *Acute megakaryoblastic leukemia in children and adolescents: a retrospective analysis of 24 cases.* Leuk Lymphoma, 1993. **10**(4-5): p. 299–306.

21. Athale, U.H., et al., *Biology and outcome of childhood acute megakaryoblastic leukemia: a single institution's experience.* Blood, 2001. **97**(12): p. 3727–32.

22. Chan, W.C., et al., *Acute megakaryoblastic leukemia in infants with t(1;22)(p13;q13) abnormality.* Am J Clin Pathol, 1992. **98**(2): p. 214–21.

23. Tosi, S., et al., *Characterization of 6q abnormalities in childhood acute myeloid leukemia and identification of a novel t(6;11)(q24.1;p15.5) resulting in a NUP98-C6orf80 fusion in a case of acute megakaryoblastic leukemia.* Genes Chromosomes Cancer, 2005. **44**(3): p. 225–32.

24. Ohyashiki, K., et al., *Cytogenetic findings in adult acute leukemia and myeloproliferative disorders with an involvement of megakaryocyte lineage.* Cancer, 1990. **65**(4): p. 940–8.

25. Kaloutsi, V., et al., *Occurrence of a variant Philadelphia translocation, t(10;22), in de novo acute megakaryoblastic leukemia.* Cancer Genet Cytogenet, 2004. **152**(1): p. 52–5.

26. Alvarez, S., et al., *Frequent gain of chromosome 19 in megakaryoblastic leukemias detected by comparative genomic hybridization.* Genes Chromosomes Cancer, 2001. **32**(3): p. 285–93.

27. Chitlur, M.B., et al., *Acute megakaryoblastic leukemia with t(17;22)(q21;q13) and liver dysfunction.* Cancer Genet Cytogenet, 2004. **154**(2): p. 167–8.

28. de Rooij, J.D., et al., *Pediatric non-Down syndrome acute megakaryoblastic leukemia is characterized by distinct genomic subsets with varying outcomes.* Nat Genet, 2017. **49**(3): p. 451–6.

29. Wang, L., et al., *Acute megakaryoblastic leukemia associated with trisomy 21 demonstrates a distinct immunophenotype.* Cytometry B Clin Cytom, 2015. **88**(4): p. 244–52.

30. Orazi, A., et al., *Acute panmyelosis with myelofibrosis: an entity distinct from acute megakaryoblastic leukemia.* Mod Pathol, 2005. **18**(5): p. 603–14.

31. Neiman, R.S., et al., *Granulocytic sarcoma: a clinicopathologic study of 61 biopsied cases.* Cancer, 1981. **48**(6): p. 1426–37.

32. Wiernik, P.H. and A.A. Serpick, *Granulocytic sarcoma (chloroma).* Blood, 1970. **35**(3): p. 361–9.

33. Szomor, A., et al., *Myeloid leukemia and myelodysplastic syndrome relapsing as granulocytic sarcoma (chloroma) after allogeneic bone marrow transplantation.* Ann Hematol, 1997. **75**(5-6): p. 239–41.

34. Bekassy, A.N., et al., *Granulocytic sarcoma after allogeneic bone marrow transplantation: a retrospective European multicenter survey. Acute and Chronic Leukemia Working Parties of the European Group for Blood and Marrow Transplantation.* Bone Marrow Transplant, 1996. **17**(5): p. 801–8.

35. Tallman, M.S., et al., *Granulocytic sarcoma is associated with the 8;21 translocation in acute myeloid leukemia.* J Clin Oncol, 1993. **11**(4): p. 690–7.

36. Pileri, S.A., et al., *Myeloid sarcoma: clinico-pathologic, phenotypic and cytogenetic analysis of 92 adult patients.* Leukemia, 2007. **21**(2): p. 340–50.

37. Sugimoto, Y., et al., *Acute myeloid leukemia with t(8;21)(q22;q22) manifesting as granulocytic sarcomas in the rhinopharynx and external acoustic meatus at relapse after high-dose cytarabine: case report and review of the literature.* Hematol J, 2004. **5**(1): p. 84–9.

38. Bonig, H., U. Gobel, and W. Nurnberger, *Bilateral exopthalmus due to retro-orbital chloromas in a boy with t(8;21)- positive acute myeloblastic acute leukemia.* Pediatr Hematol Oncol, 2002. **19**(8): p. 597–600.

39. Schwyzer, R., et al., *Granulocytic sarcoma in children with acute myeloblastic leukemia and t(8;21).* Med Pediatr Oncol, 1998. **31**(3): p. 144–9.

40. Zhang, X.H., R. Zhang, and Y. Li, *Granulocytic sarcoma of abdomen in acute myeloid leukemia patient with inv(16) and t(6;17) abnormal chromosome: case report and review of literature.* Leuk Res, 2010. **34**(7): p. 958–61.

41. Lindsley, R.C., et al., *Acute myeloid leukemia ontogeny is defined by distinct somatic mutations.* Blood, 2015. **125**(9): p. 1367–76.

42. Swerdlow, S.H., Campo, E., Harris, N. L., Jaffe, E. S., Pileri, S. A., Stein, H., Thiele, J., Vardiman, J. W., ed. WHO classification of tumors of haematopoietic and lymphoid tissues. 2008, IARC: Lyon.

43. Duffield, A.S., et al., *Clinical and pathologic features of secondary acute promyelocytic leukemia.* Am J Clin Pathol, 2012. **137**(3): p. 395–402.

44. Li, S., et al., *Myelodysplastic Syndrome/Acute Myeloid Leukemia With t(3;21)(q26.2;q22) Is Commonly a Therapy-Related Disease Associated With Poor Outcome.* Am J Clin Pathol, 2012. **138**(1): p. 146–52.

45. Orazi, A., et al., *Therapy-related myelodysplastic syndromes: FAB classification, bone marrow histology, and immunohistology in the prognostic assessment.* Leukemia, 1993. **7**(6): p. 838–47.

46. Schoch, C., et al., *Karyotype is an independent prognostic parameter in therapy-related acute myeloid leukemia (t-AML): an analysis of 93 patients with t-AML in comparison to 1091 patients with de novo AML.* Leukemia, 2004. **18**(1): p. 120–5.

47. Side, L.E., et al., *RAS, FLT3, and TP53 mutations in therapy-related myeloid malignancies with abnormalities of chromosomes 5 and 7.* Genes Chromosomes Cancer, 2004. **39**(3): p. 217–23.

23

ACUTE MYELOID LEUKEMIA WITH DEFINING GENETIC ABNORMALITIES

Acute promyelocytic leukemia (APL)

PHENOTYPE OF APL

APL (hypergranular): CD2$^-$, s.CD3$^-$, c.CD3$^-$, CD4$^{-/+}$, CD7$^{+/-}$, CD11b$^-$, CD11c$^-$, CD13$^+$, CD14$^-$, CD15$^{-/rarely+(dim)}$, CD19$^-$, c.CD22$^-$, CD33$^{+bright}$, CD34$^-$, CD38$^+$, CD36$^-$, CD56$^{-/rarely+}$, CD64$^{-/dim+}$, CD65$^{-/rarely+}$, c.CD79a$^-$, CD117$^{+(may\ be\ dim)}$, CD133$^{-/rarely+}$, HLA-DR$^-$, MPO$^+$

APL-v (hypogranular): CD2$^{+/rarely-}$, s.CD3$^-$, c.CD3$^-$, CD4$^{-/+}$, CD7$^{+/-}$, CD11b$^-$, CD11c$^-$, CD13$^+$, CD14$^-$, CD15$^{-/rarely+(dim)}$, CD19$^-$, c.CD22$^-$, CD33$^{+bright}$, CD34$^{+/rarely-}$, CD38$^+$, CD36$^-$, CD56$^{-/rarely+}$, CD64$^{-/dim+}$, CD65$^{-/rarely+}$, c.CD79a$^-$, CD117$^{+(may\ be\ dim)}$, CD133$^{-/rarely+}$, HLA-DR$^-$, MPO$^+$

Introduction

Acute promyelocytic leukemia (APL) is a distinct subtype of acute myeloid leukemia (AML) with characteristic biologic and clinical features that is now highly curable due to the ability of neoplastic promyelocytes to undergo differentiation and apoptosis with exposure to retinoic acid and arsenic trioxide. It occurs more often in young patients. APL is characterized by maturation arrest at promyelocytic stage, t(15;17)/*PML-RARA* and response to maturation inducing treatment with all trans-retinoic acid (ATRA) [1–4]. APL accounts for ~8%–10% of AML cases. Distinctive features of APL include leukopenia coexisting with a marrow replacement by atypical promyelocytes, disseminated intravascular coagulopathy (DIC), and lack of HLA-DR antigen expression by neoplastic cells. The introduction of ATRA and arsenic trioxide (As$_2$O$_3$), which target the underlying molecular changes, dramatically changed the clinical course of APL, from invariably fatal to one of the most curable type of acute leukemia.

Morphology

Cytology

The peripheral blood smear often shows pancytopenia with rare circulating promyelocytes, which usually have abundant azurophilic granules. Bone marrow (BM) aspirate is hypercellular and usually shows maturation arrest at promyelocytic stage. Promyelocytes usually show irregular, bilobed, or reniform nuclei. Based on the cytomorphologic features, APL can be divided into hypergranular (classical) APL and hypogranular variant (APL-v). The hypergranular variant of APL contains abnormal promyelocytes with numerous azurophilic granules. A subset of promyelocytes may contain one or typically for APL, multiple Auer rods (Figure 23.1). APL-v is characterized by atypical promyelocytes with marked nuclear irregularities, mostly in the form of bilobation, folding, or convolution (Figure 23.2). The cytoplasm is either agranular or hypogranular with finer azurophilic granulation when compared to typical APL. Presence of occasional cells with Auer rods or characteristic cytoplasmic protrusions (Figure 23.3) helps to identify APL-v. Presence of multiple Auer rods and bilobed or reniform nuclei helps to differentiate APL from other acute myeloid leukemias with hypergranular blasts.

Histomorphology

The BM biopsy shows hypercellular marrow completely replaced by promyelocytes with abundant pale or eosinophilic cytoplasm with distinct borders mimicking "fried eggs" or plant cells (Figure 23.4).

Genetic features

The balanced reciprocal translocation between chromosomes 15 and 17 (Figure 23.5) characterizes >95% cases of APL [5]. The t(15;17)(q24;q21) disrupts *PML* gene on chromosome 15q24 (15q22-24) and the gene encoding the retinoic acid receptor α (*RARA*) on chromosome 17q21 (17q12-21). The t(15;17) leads to the formation of two reciprocal fusion genes, *PML-RARA* on chromosome 15 and *RARA-PML* on chromosome 17. Depending on the *PML* gene breakpoint in chromosome 15, the transcript subtypes bcr1, bcr2, and bcr3 may be formed. Approximately 50% of APLs have a PML breakpoint in exon 6 (long form; bcr1), 40%–50% in exon 3 (short form; bcr3), and rare cases (<10%) show breakpoint in exon 6 (variable form; bcr2). The resultant *PML-RARA* fusion protein, which retains the retinoic acid receptor-binding domain, plays a role in leukemogenesis but also mediates the response to retinoids [6]. Fluorescence in situ hybridization (FISH; Figure 23.6) and/or PCR testing provide fast confirmation of the APL diagnosis and are also used in disease monitoring. Especially reverse transcription polymerase chain reaction (RT-PCR) is very sensitive, as it allows detecting one malignant cell with *PML-RARA* fusion out of 1×10^5 benign cells.

Apart from most typical t(15;17)/*PML-RARA*, rare cases of APL show the t(11;17)(q23;q21) involving *RARA* and *ZBTB16* (previously *PZLF* or promyelocytic leukemia zinc finger), t(5;17)(q35;q21) involving *RARA* and *NPM1* gene (nucleophosmin), t(17;17)(q11.2;q21) involving *RARA* and *STAT5B*, t(11;17)(q13;q21) involving *RARA* and *NUMA1* gene or three-way translocation, such as t(5;17;15)(q35;q21;q22). APL with both variants of t(11;17) translocation does not respond to ATRA treatment. APL with translocations other than t(15;17) are diagnosed as AML with variant *RARA* rearrangement.

Additional genetic abnormalities including trisomy 8 and complex karyotypic changes can occur in APL. *FLT3*-ITD and tyrosine kinase mutations occur in 30%–40% and are often associated with high blood cell count and APL-v. Presence of additional chromosomal changes in APL does not change the favorable prognosis associated with t(15;17)/*PML-RARA*. The significance of *FLT3*-ITD in APL is still under investigation. Some studies found no significant differences in disease-free survival between patients with and without *FLT3*-ITD [7–10], whereas others reported a tendency toward shorter overall survival and significantly worse disease-free survival for patients with *FLT3*-ITD [11–14], especially with concurrent *RAS* mutations. *FLT3*-ITD is common in pediatric APL and was reported to be associated with poor prognosis [15].

Immunophenotype

Immunohistochemistry. APL is strongly positive for CD117, CD33, and MPO (Figure 23.7), and is negative for HLA-DR and CD11c. Subset of cases (mostly APL-v) shows CD34 and CD2 expression.

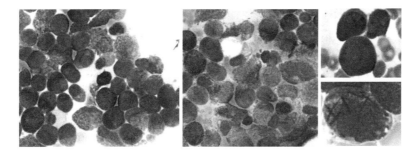

FIGURE 23.1   Acute promyelocytic leukemia (APL) – cytology. Aspirate smear with hypergranular promyelocytes and promyelocytes with numerous Auer rods.

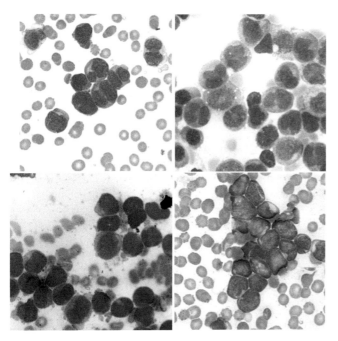

FIGURE 23.2   APL-v – cytology. Hypogranular (microgranular) variant of APL is characterized by agranular cytoplasm and bilobed nuclear shape (four different cases).

Flow cytometry. Because of tendency for disseminated coagulopathy, a life-threatening complication of APL, establishing the correct diagnosis in a timely fashion is critical in the management of patients with APL. The characteristic cytomorphology and flow cytometry (FC) immunophenotype allow for correct identification of cases suggestive of APL, leading to mandatory genetic testing, preferably by both FISH and RT-PCR for definite confirmation of APL diagnosis [3, 5, 16–19]. APLs are positive for CD13, CD33, CD117, CD133, MPO, often dimly positive for CD64 and positive for CD123. The expression of CD13 is variable (heterogeneous) and majority of APL cases show very bright expression of CD33 (much brighter than residual benign neutrophils and/or monocytes, if present in the sample). The APL is negative for HLA-DR, CD11b, CD11c, and often also CD34. Rare APL cases may show very dim or partial CD117 expression by FC despite usually strong CD117 expression by immunohistochemistry in BM core or clot sections. APL with variant translocation(s) may show some aberrant phenotype, which may differ from that seen in typical *PML-RARA*+ APLs. Neoplastic promyelocytes display non-specific background fluorescence with many fluorescent dyes and therefore the expression of any given antigenic marker should be correlated with isotypic negative controls or antigens which are known to be negative in APL (e.g., CD3, CD7, CD10, CD11b, CD14, CD16, CD19, CD20, CD57, kappa, or lambda). Identification of even a few promyelocytes in blood by FC or on blood smear should prompt immediate molecular studies for *PML-RARA* and morphologic BM analysis, as those cases are associated with either BM involvement by APL or imminent development of APL. Figure 23.8 shows an example of minimal blood involvement by APL. Based on flow cytometry findings in blood suggestive of APL, patient underwent immediate BM analysis which confirmed involvement by APL. Figure 23.9 shows an example of rapid progression of APL in blood within a few days. Prompt identification of neoplastic promyelocytes (based on increased side scatter [SSC], positive CD117, and brighter expression of CD33 then in neutrophils), even if their number is low, helps to establish a definite diagnosis by confirmatory molecular testing for *PML-RARA*.

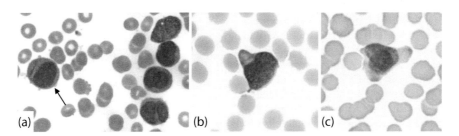

FIGURE 23.3   APL-v – cytology. Even in hypogranular (microgranular) variant of APL occasional promyelocytes with Auer rods can be identified (a, arrow). Another characteristic feature helpful in identification of APL-v is presence of asymmetric cytoplasmic protrusions (which occasionally may contain granules or Auer rods; b–c).

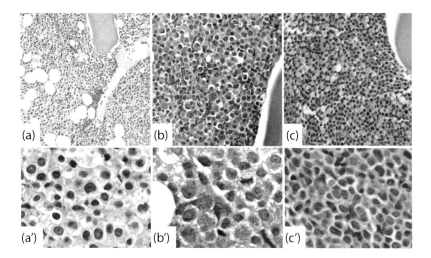

FIGURE 23.4 APL – histomorphology (three different APL cases). BM is replaced by abnormal promyelocytes with abundant pale cytoplasm and conspicuous borders (fried egg or plant-like cells; a), promyelocytes with eosinophilic cytoplasm (b), and APL-v (c).

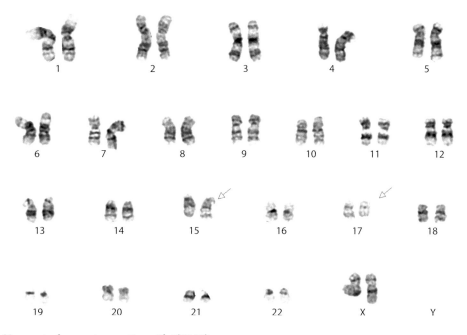

FIGURE 23.5 APL – metaphase cytogenetics with t(15;17).

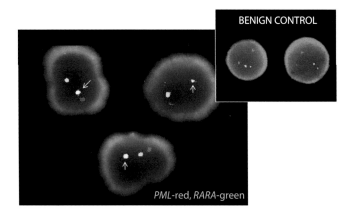

FIGURE 23.6 APL – FISH. FISH analysis shows *PML-RARA* fusion (yellow signal, arrow). Inset shows negative control (note normal pattern with two red and two green signals).

Classic (hypergranular) APL cells have a specific phenotype:

- high SSC
- moderate CD45 expression
- non-specific staining with viability dyes (imitating decreased viability)
- high background (non-specific) fluorescence
- negative HLA-DR expression
- bright CD33 expression (much brighter than in benign neutrophils)
- positive CD117 (may be dim or partial by FC analysis)
- positive CD13
- positive MPO
- dim CD64 (many cases)
- negative CD7, CD10, CD11b, CD11c, CD15 (most cases), CD16, CD19, and CD65

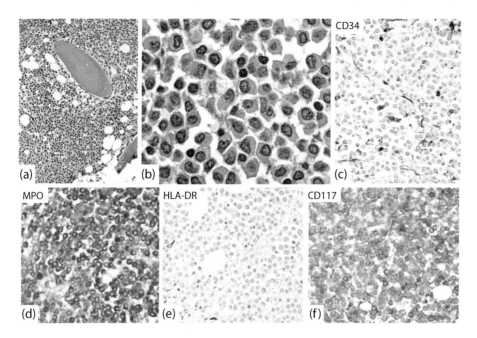

FIGURE 23.7 APL – immunohistochemistry. (a–b) Histologic section shows hypercellular marrow with atypical promyelocytes. Neoplastic cells are negative for CD34 (c) and HLA-DR (e) and are positive for MPO (d) and CD117 (f).

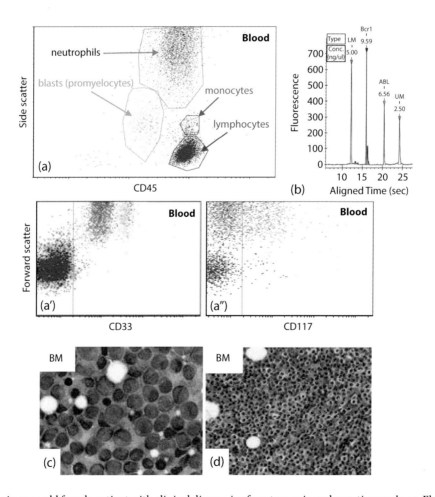

FIGURE 23.8 Sixty-six-year-old female patient with clinical diagnosis of neutropenia and negative work-up. Flow cytometry of blood (a-a″) showed 1.7% blasts with slightly increased SSC (a), bright CD33 (a′) and positive CD117 (a″). Note the typical for APL very bright expression of CD33 (much brighter than in benign neutrophils). Based on flow data, APL was suspected, which was confirmed by PCR for *PML-RARA* (b). Subsequent BM biopsy showed extensive involvement by APL with typical cytologic (c) and histologic (d) findings.

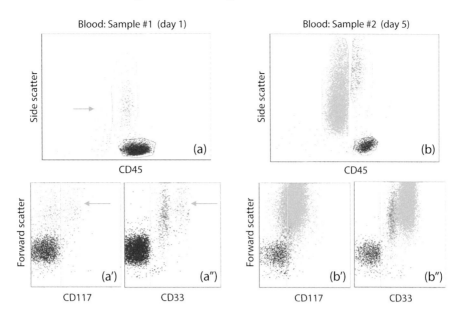

FIGURE 23.9 Rapid progression of APL within 5 days (blood sample). First flow cytometry analysis of blood due to pancytopenia (day 1, a) shows only very few blasts (green dots, arrow) with slightly increased SSC (a), positive CD117 (a′) and bright CD33 (a″). Repeated flow cytometry analysis of blood after few days shows numerous neoplastic promyelocytes (b) with typical high SSC (b), positive CD117 (b′) and bright CD33 (b″). Presence of event very minute population of blasts in blood with positive CD117 and brighter expression of CD33 than in neutrophils (a″) should prompt immediate molecular testing for *PML-RARA* rearrangement.

Based on the immunophenotype and SSC properties, four FC patterns can be recognized in APL [20].

Pattern 1. The majority of cases represent classical (hypergranular) APL (Table 23.1; Figures 23.10 and 23.11). It is characterized by a predominant population of atypical promyelocytes with markedly increased SSC. The first clue to the diagnosis of APL is the pattern on CD45 versus SSC showing population of cells with moderate CD45 (dimmer than in benign neutrophils) and increased SSC placing blasts in "granulocytic gate" (ranging

TABLE 23.1: Immunophenotypic Profile of Hypergranular APL (*n* = 85)

	Frequency (%)	Comments
Side scatter		High ("granulocytic" region on CD45 vs SSC)
CD2+	17	
CD4+	16	Dim expression
CD7+	1.2	
CD11b+	0	
CD11c+	1.2	1 case (1.2%) showed dim expression; additional 5 cases (6%) showed dim expression on minor subset)
CD13+	94	
CD14+	0	
CD16+	0	
CD19+	0	
CD33+	100	Moderate, 15%; bright 85%
CD34+	14	Mostly dim or partial expression
CD45+	100	Moderate expression
CD56+	14	
CD64+	61	Mostly dim expression
CD117+	100	Moderate expression
HLA-DR+	0	

from the area slightly above typical "blast gate" expanding to very high SSC as displayed usually by normal neutrophils). Neoplastic promyelocytes are positive for CD13 (~94%), CD33 (100%), CD64 (~61%; dim expression), CD117 (100%) and are negative for HLA-DR, CD7, CD10, CD11b, CD11c, and CD14. Subset of cases is positive for CD2 (~19%), CD4 (~23%), CD34 (~14%), and CD56 (~14%). It is exceptionally unusual for APL to display CD11c expression (<1% of cases). The expression of CD13 is dim to moderate but may be partial and the expression of CD33 is bright (brighter than in residual benign neutrophils or monocytes). Many cases show dim CD64 expression. The expression of all markers in APL needs to be carefully correlated with isotypic controls, to differentiate between true positive staining from high non-specific background fluorescence (Figure 23.12). Very rare cases may show CD11c expression (6% with dim expression on minor subset and 1.2% cases with dim expression on entire blast population).

Pattern 2. Hypogranular (microgranular) APL (APL-v; Table 23.2; Figures 23.13 and 23.14) is a second most common pattern. It is characterized by low SSC and moderate expression of CD45 (leukemic cells distributed in the "blast" region on CD45 versus SSC dot plot display, similar to blasts in non-APL acute myeloid leukemias). Neoplastic promyelocytes in this variant are positive for CD2 (79%), CD4 (18%), CD13 (94%), CD33 (100%), CD34 (~76%), CD56 (26%), CD64 (79%), and CD117 (100%). HLA-DR, CD10, CD11b, and CD11c are negative. The expression of CD45 is dimmer than in maturing myeloid cells/neutrophils. CD2 and CD34 expression in APL was linked to *FLT3*-ITD and bcr3 isoform [14]. Figure 23.15 shows an example of APL-v with a typical phenotype and high non-specific expression of PerCP-Cy5.5 fluorochrome (conjugated to HLA-DR). Only careful correlation with isotypic controls conjugated with the same fluorochrome allows for correct interpretation of HLA-DR staining as negative.

Pattern 3. The third, much less common FC pattern of APL shows mixture of neoplastic promyelocytes with decreased SSC and positive CD117, and significant proportion of benign

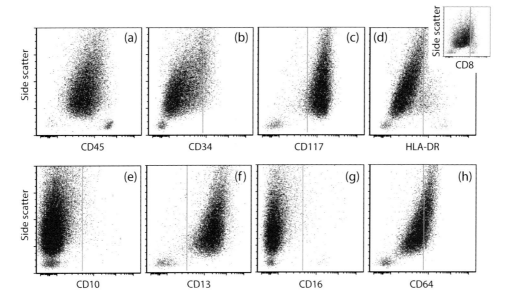

FIGURE 23.10   APL – flow cytometry of hypergranular variant (pattern 1). Neoplastic promyelocytes are characterized by very high SSC and moderate CD45 (a), negative CD34 (b), positive CD117 (c), negative HLA-DR (d; compare with negative staining with the same fluorochrome for CD8, inset), negative CD10 (e), positive CD13 (f), negative CD16 (g), and dim CD64 (h).

(residual) maturing myeloid cells (granulocytes) with typical high SSC, negative CD117, and positive (on most mature elements) CD10, CD11b, and CD16 (Figures 23.16 and 23.17). The immunophenotype of neoplastic cells in pattern 3 is usually similar to that observed in hypogranular APL, but occasional cases show pattern 3 with classic (hypergranular) APL (Figure 23.18).

Pattern 4. The least common immunophenotypic variant of APL (mixed variant; Figure 23.19) shows two neoplastic populations, one with high SSC and the other with low SSC. Both populations are positive for CD13, CD33, and CD117 and negative for HLA-DR and CD11c. The cells with high SSC express CD45 (dim), CD13 (dim), CD33 (bright), and CD64 (dim), and cells with low SSC express CD45 (moderate; brighter than cells with high SSC) and are positive for CD13 (dim), CD33 (moderate to bright), and are exclusively positive for CD34 and CD2.

CD56 expression in APL. CD56 is positive from 11% to 20% of APL (≥20% of leukemic cells) [21, 22]. It is more common in hypogranular variant (Figure 23.15). CD56⁺ APL was reported to be significantly associated with high white blood cell counts; low albumin levels; bcr3 isoform; and the co-expression of CD2, CD34, CD7, HLA-DR, CD15, and CD117 antigens [21]. The expression of CD56 antigen in APL blasts has been associated with short remission duration and extramedullary relapse [21, 23–25]. In a series reported by Montesinos et al., for CD56⁺ APL, the 5-year relapse rate was 22%, compared with a 10% relapse rate for CD56⁻ APL, and CD56⁺ APL also showed a greater risk of extramedullary relapse [21].

Differentiation syndrome (DS). Unusual myelomonocytic population can be found in rare cases of APL after treatment with ATRA (Figures 23.20–23.22). These atypical myelomonocytic cells, while *PML-RARA*⁺ differ from residual APL (neoplastic promyelocytes) by positive CD11b and CD11c expression and lack of CD2, HLA-DR, CD34, and CD117 expression. CD10, CD14, and CD16 are usually negative, but partial expression of CD14 or CD16 may be present. They differ from benign neutrophils by lack of CD10, positive CD64, partial CD14, and negative or only

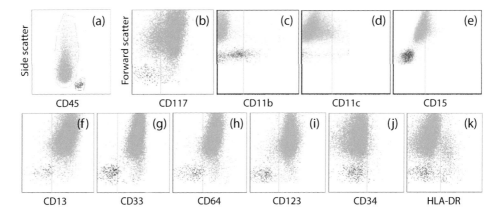

FIGURE 23.11   APL – flow cytometry. Neoplastic promyelocytes (green dots) show increased SSC (a) and moderate expression of CD45 (a). They are positive for CD117 (b), negative for CD11b (c), CD11c (d) and CD15 (e), positive for CD13 (f), CD33 (g), CD64 (h), and CD123 (i) and do negative for CD34 (j) and HLA-DR (k).

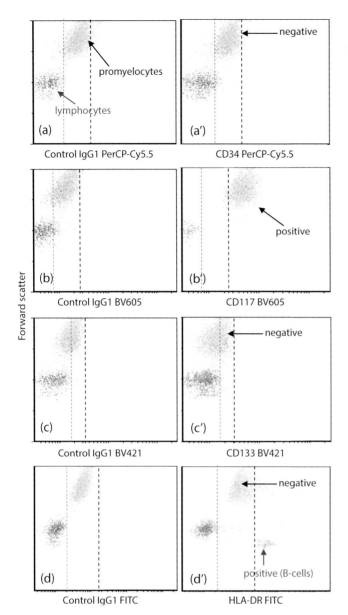

Forward scatter

(a) Control IgG1 PerCP-Cy5.5
(a') CD34 PerCP-Cy5.5 — negative

(b) Control IgG1 BV605
(b') CD117 BV605 — positive

(c) Control IgG1 BV421
(c') CD133 BV421 — negative

(d) Control IgG1 FITC
(d') HLA-DR FITC — negative, positive (B-cells)

promyelocytes
lymphocytes

FIGURE 23.12 Neoplastic promyelocytes in APL are characterized by high (non-specific) background fluorescence (left column; compare the staining of lymphocytes and APL cells). The classification of each marker to negative or positive category needs to be based on careful correlation with isotypic controls. Based on background staining of promyelocytes (gray dots, black dotted line), the expression of CD34 is negative (a-a'), CD117 is positive (b-b'), CD133 is negative (c-c') and HLA-DR is negative (d-d'). If one would evaluate expression of each marker based on controls set up on lymphocytes (red dotted line), CD34 and HLA-DR would be classified mistakenly as positive.

partial CD16 expression. In contrast to benign (mature) monocytes, this population shows occasional CD16 expression and is either negative or only partially positive for CD14. They represent *PML-RARA*+ myelomonocytic cells with atypical maturation patterns ("differentiated" blasts) induced by ATRA (or arsenic) therapy and their presence is often associated with differentiation syndrome (DS; also known as cytokine release syndrome or retinoic acid syndrome) [26, 27].

TABLE 23.2: Immunophenotypic Profile of Hypogranular APL (APL-v; $n = 34$)

	Frequency (%)	Comments
Side scatter		Low ("blastic" region)
CD2+	79	Dim expression
CD4+	18	Dim expression
CD7+	0	
CD11b+	0	
CD11c+	0	
CD13+	94	Dim, 30%; moderate 65%; negative 6%
CD14+	0	
CD16+	0	
CD19+	0	
CD33+	100	Moderate expression, 10%; bright expression,90%
CD34+	76.5	8 cases (23.5%) were completely negative 3 cases showed dim expression on minor subset
CD45+	100	Moderate expression
CD56+	26	
CD64+	79	Mostly dim expression
CD117+	100	
HLA-DR+	0	

DS is a potentially fatal complication of induction chemotherapy in patients with APL. ATRA is thought to lead to a release of a variety of cytokines (IL1, IL6, IL8 TNFα, cathepsin G) by differentiating blast cells and induce a change in adhesive properties of blasts [26]. Another plausible explanation could be increased levels of leptin, insulin, or IGF1 or due to altered ATRA metabolism which have tendency to be stored in fat tissue resulting in a slow release of ATRA over time and continuous blast differentiation [27–29]. Clinically, patients with DS as defined by Frankel et al., have the following symptoms: dyspnea, weight gain (>5kg), unexplained fever (not attributable to infection), respiratory distress (hypoxemia), cardiac involvement, unexplained hypotension, hepatic dysfunction (hyperbilirubinemia), acute renal failure and/or radiological findings suggesting interstitial infiltrates and pleural or pericardial effusions [27, 30]. Morphologically, there is an extensive interstitial and intra-alveolar pulmonary infiltration by maturing myeloid cells, endothelial cell damage, intra-alveolar edema, inter-alveolar hemorrhage, and fibrinous exudates.

Differential diagnosis of APL
Morphologic differential diagnosis of APL
Hypergranular (classic) APL needs to be differentiated with AML composed of blasts with numerous cytoplasmic granules and/or Auer rods. In particular, AML with t(8;16) often resembles cytologically and clinically APL due to the presence of heavily granulated blasts in the BM or blood, and features of DIC [31]. Also, AML with t(8;21) shows occasional Auer rods in the cytoplasm. The major differential diagnosis of APL-v includes acute monoblastic leukemia (Figure 23.23). Cytochemistry (MPO+/NSE−), cytology (presence of rare blasts with granular cytoplasm, Auer rods and cytoplasmic protrusions) and flow cytometry (lack of CD11b, CD11c, HLA-DR, and positive CD117; see below) would favor APL-v over acute monoblastic leukemia. The diagnosis of APL has to be definitively confirmed by FISH and/or molecular studies for *PML/RARA*.

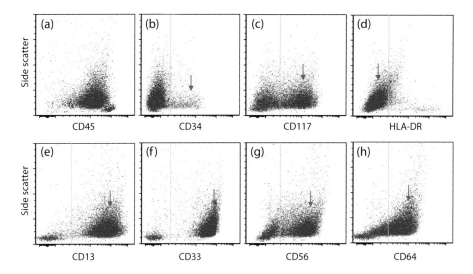

FIGURE 23.13 APL-v (hypogranular variant) – flow cytometry (pattern 2). Neoplastic promyelocytes show slow SSC (a) with the following phenotype: CD34 partially⁺ (b; minor population), CD117⁺ (c), HLA-DR⁻ (d), CD13⁺ (e), CD3⁺ (f), CD56⁺ (g), and CD64⁺ (h).

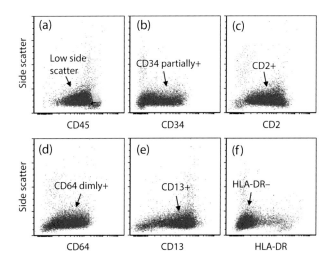

FIGURE 23.14 APL-v (hypogranular variant) – flow cytometry (pattern 2). Neoplastic promyelocytes (blue dots) are characterized by low SSC (a), positive CD45 (a), positive CD34 (b), positive CD2 (c), dimly positive CD64 (d), positive CD13 (e), and lack of HLA-DR (f).

Flow cytometric differential diagnosis of APL
The FC differential diagnosis of APL includes:

- HLA-DR⁻ AML
- Acute monoblastic leukemia
- Maturing myeloid precursors with leftward shift and/or dysgranulopoiesis
- BM with reactive promyelocytic hyperplasia
- Immature plasma cell myeloma
- AML with *NPM1* mutation
- AML with *FLT3* mutation
- "Maturing blasts" and atypical myelomonocytic cells in differentiation syndrome (after treatment with ATRA)

Phenotypic (flow cytometric) differential diagnosis of APL is presented in Table 23.3 and also in Chapter 5.

Classic (hypergranular) APL. Classic APL (pattern 1) has well recognized FC pattern with increased SSC (placing blasts in "granulocytic" gate with dimmer CD45 expression than in benign neutrophils), lack of expression of HLA-DR, CD11a, CD11b, CD18, positive CD117, negative or weakly positive CD15 and CD65, negative CD34, often positive (dim or partial) CD64, variable

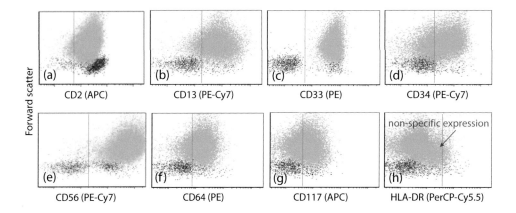

FIGURE 23.15 APL-v with typical phenotype and aberrant expression of CD56: CD2⁺ (a), CD13⁺ (b), CD33⁺ (c), CD34⁺ (d), CD56⁺ (e), CD64⁺ (f), CD117⁺ (g), and HLA-DR⁻ (h).

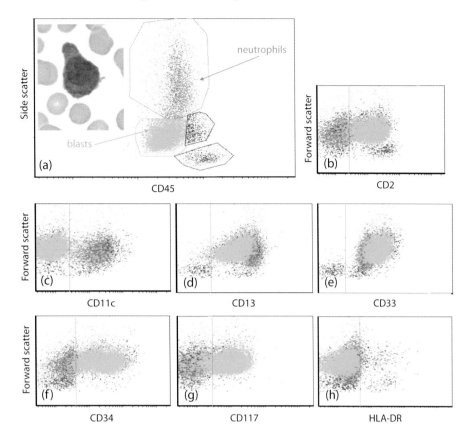

FIGURE 23.16   APL with pattern 3 (partial involvement). Flow cytometry analysis of blood (a) shows mixed population of blasts (green dots), neutrophils (gray dots), monocytes (dark blue dots) and lymphocytes (red dots) [inset show typical hypogranular promyelocyte with bilobed nucleus]. Blasts (promyelocytes) show the phenotype of APL-v: CD2+ (b), CD11c− (c; neutrophils are positive), CD13+ (d), CD33+ (e), CD34+ (f), CD117+ (g), and HLA-DR− (h).

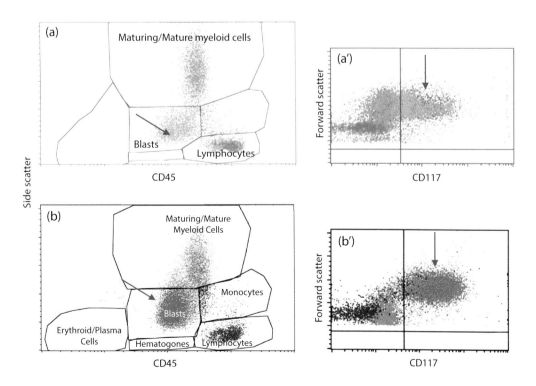

FIGURE 23.17   APL – flow cytometry (pattern 3). Two cases of APL (a and b) showing partial bone marrow involvement. Neoplastic promyelocytes (green dots; arrow) are CD117+ (a′, b′). Neutrophils (gray dots) are CD117−.

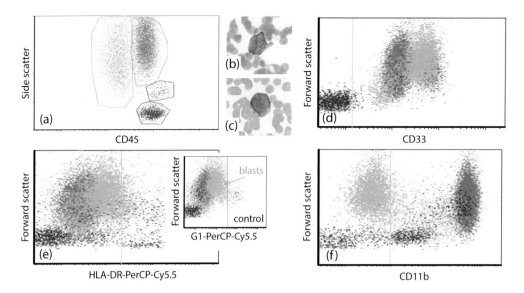

FIGURE 23.18 APL (pattern 3). Flow cytometric analysis of blood (a) shows neoplastic promyelocytes (green dots) with high SSC, mixed with benign blood elements (neutrophils, monocytes, and lymphocytes). Blood smear shows scatter hypergranular promyelocytes (b-c). APL cells shows typical bright CD33 expression (much brighter than in benign neutrophils (d), negative HLA-DR (e, compare with negative isotypic control, inset), positive (dim), and negative CD11b (f).

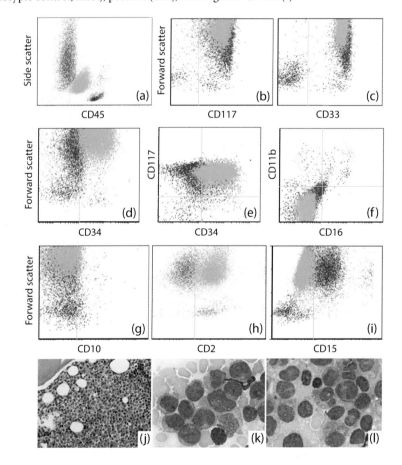

FIGURE 23.19 APL (pattern 4). Unusual variant of APL composed of hypergranular promyelocytes with high SSC (a; magenta dots) and hypogranular promyelocytes with low SSC (a; green dots). Both populations express CD117 (b) and are brightly positive for CD33 (c). CD34 is expressed only by hypogranular subset of neoplastic promyelocytes (d–e; green dots). In contrast to neutrophils and benign myeloid precursors, hypergranular promyelocytes (magenta dots) are negative for CD11b. Apart from CD34 expression, both populations differ in the expression of CD2 (h) and CD15 (i) with hypogranular promyelocytes being positive for CD2 (h, green dots) and hypergranular promyelocytes being positive for CD15 (I; magenta dots). Histology section of the bone marrow core biopsy shows diffuse infiltrate of neoplastic promyelocytes (j). Aspirate smear (k–l) shows two distinct promyelocytes, hypogranular cells with irregular nuclei and basophilic cytoplasm without granules, and hypergranular blasts with numerous cytoplasmic granules and occasional Auer rods.

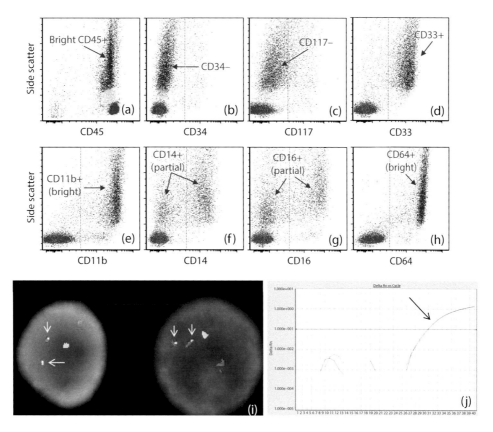

FIGURE 23.20 Atypical myelomonocytic population (CD117⁻/CD11b⁺/CD33⁺/CD64⁺/*PML-RARA*⁺) after treatment with ATRA compatible with "differentiation syndrome" (recent history of APL). Flow cytometry shows very atypical myelomonocytic cells with high SSC, bright CD45 (a), negative CD34 (b) and CD117 (c), bright CD33 (d), bright CD11b (e), partial CD14 (f) and CD16 (g), and bright CD64 (h). FISH studies (i) showed rearrangement of *RARA* at 17q21 (48%). *PML-RARA* rearrangement was also confirmed by PCR (j).

(heterogeneous) CD13 and bright CD33 [20]. Differential diagnosis of hypergranular APL includes normally maturing myeloid cells, BM with myelodysplasia, MPNs with myeloid leftward shift, benign marrow proliferation (e.g., recovering marrow after treatment with promyelocytic hyperplasia), occasional cases of acute monoblastic leukemia with high SSC (Figure 23.24), rare cases of AML with maturation, which have high SSC, positive CD117 and lack of both CD34 and HLA-DR expression (Figure 23.25) and rare cases of B-ALL with unusual high SSC. The phenotypic features which do not favor the diagnosis of APL in those cases include the presence of HLA-DR expression on minor subset of blasts, positive CD11c expression, lack of dim CD64 expression, lack of increased staining with viability dyes, strong CD4 expression, aberrant CD7 expression and/or lack of very bright CD33 expression. Evaluation of *PML-RARA* by FISH and/or PCR testing helps in establishing a definite diagnosis in difficult cases.

Analysis of CD10, CD11b, CD11c, CD16, CD33, CD45, CD117, and HLA-DR helps to distinguish benign processes from APL. Neutrophils and benign maturing myeloid precursors show high scatter, variable expression of CD45 (brighter on neutrophils and dimmer on promyelocytes, myelocytes, and metamyelocytes), and in contrast to APL, partially positive expression of CD10, CD11b, CD11c, and CD16. Typical for APL is a very bright expression of CD33 with much higher fluorescence intensity when compared to residual benign neutrophils and monocytes. Neutrophilic maturation from blasts through promyelocytes, myelocytes, metamyelocytes, bands, and neutrophils is characterized by loss of CD34 and HLA-DR expression at promyelocytic stage and loss

CD117 expression at myelocyte stage, and acquisition of CD11b and CD11c expression at myelocytic stage, and CD10 and CD16 expression by neutrophils. CD64 is expressed by promyelocytes through metamyelocytes. In contrast to APL, granulocytes are positive for CD10, CD11b, CD11c, and CD16 and are negative for CD117. Granulocytes/maturing myeloid precursors with dyspoiesis (e.g., MDS) and/or leftward shift (e.g., CML) may display aberrant down-regulation of CD10, CD11b, and CD16, but in contrast to neoplastic promyelocytes lack CD117 expression and are (at least partially) CD11c⁺. Similar to hypergranular APL, eosinophils have also high SSC, but in contrast to APL, they have characteristic low forward scatter (FSC).

Hypogranular APL (APL-v). Differential diagnosis of hypogranular APL (pattern 2) includes acute myeloid leukemia with or without maturation, acute monoblastic leukemia, AML with *NPM1* mutation, AML with *FLT3* mutation and MDS with prominent dysgranulopoiesis (agranular or hypogranular cytoplasm). Subset of AML with or without maturation may be HLA-DR⁻, but they differ from hypogranular APL by often positive CD11c and/or rarely CD11b, dimmer CD33, and negative CD2. HLA-DR⁻/CD34⁻ phenotype in AML may be associated with *FLT3* mutation (internal tandem duplication; *FLT3*-ITD) [32]. Albano et al., reported an association of CD34 expression with the hypogranular APL variant and higher proportion of CD2⁺ and HLA-DR⁺ cases [33]. In the same study, CD34⁺ APL patients had a significantly higher percentage of peripheral blood leukemic promyelocytes at presentation, were more frequently female and had a higher proportion of bcr3 expression, but there were no

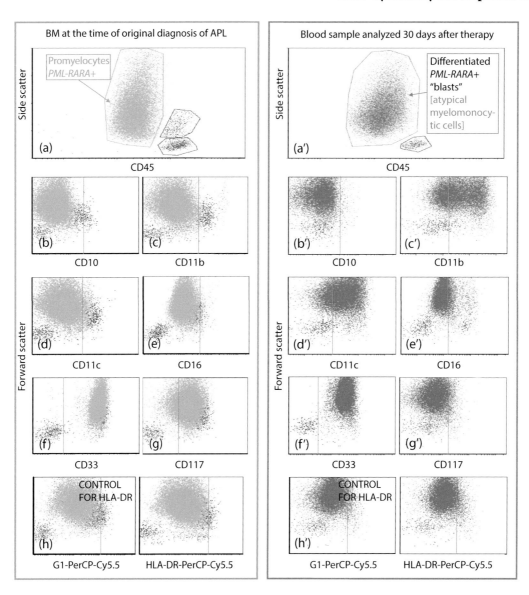

FIGURE 23.21 APL (left column; BM sample at the time of diagnosis) and APL after treatment (right column; blood sample 30 days after therapy). Both samples are positive for *PML-RARA* by FISH analysis. Neoplastic promyelocytes show typical flow cytometric features of APL: high SSC (a), negative CD10 (b), CD11b (c), CD11c (d) and CD16 (e), brightly expressed CD33 (f), positive CD117 (g) and negative HLA-DR (h; compare with isotypic negative control showing high background, non-specific fluorescence). "Differentiation syndrome" shows atypical myelomonocytic cells with high SSC (a'), negative CD10 (b'), positive CD11b (c'), positive CD11c (d'), negative CD16 (e'), positive CD33 (f'), negative CD117 (g'), and negative HLA-DR (h').

differences between the two groups in terms of complete remission, overall survival and disease-free survival [33].

Expression of HLA-DR, CD11b, CD11c, CD14, and CD64 helps to differentiate phenotypically acute monoblastic leukemia (CD2$^{+/-}$, CD4$^+$, HLA-DR$^+$, CD11b$^+$, CD11c$^+$, CD14$^{+(variable)/-}$, CD64$^{+ (bright)}$) from the hypogranular variant of APL (CD2$^{-/+}$, CD4$^-$, HLA-DR$^-$, CD11b$^-$, CD11c$^-$, CD14$^-$, CD64^{+dim}). Monoblasts are often positive for CD11b, have bright CD11c, may show positive (often variable or partial) expression of CD14, and are often positive for CD56, whereas CD56 is only rarely expressed in APL. All APL cases express CD117, whereas CD117 is positive only in subset of less differentiated acute monoblastic leukemias. Majority of acute monoblastic leukemias show moderate to bright HLA-DR and only rare cases are HLA-DR$^-$. Acute monoblastic leukemia is characterized by bright CD64 expression and positive CD11c, whereas CD64

expression in APL is usually dim or negative, and APL cases are CD11c$^-$. In most cases of acute monoblastic leukemia, the expression of CD45 is brighter than in APL. The SSC of monoblastic leukemia is only slightly increased (in contrast to classic APL). Only occasional cases of acute monoblastic leukemia show high SSC. CD2 may be positive in both leukemias, but in contrast to acute monoblastic leukemias, APLs are negative for CD4.

One of the major problems in FC differential diagnosis of hypogranular APL (pattern 2) is differentiating it from a subset of AML with *NPM1* mutation and APL-like FC pattern (Figure 23.26). Some AML with *NPM1* mutation shows CD117 expression, positive CD13 and CD33, and lack of both HLA-DR and CD34. High SSC. Lack of CD11c expression and brighter CD33 expression favor the diagnosis of APL, but correlation with molecular testing is needed for a definite subclassification.

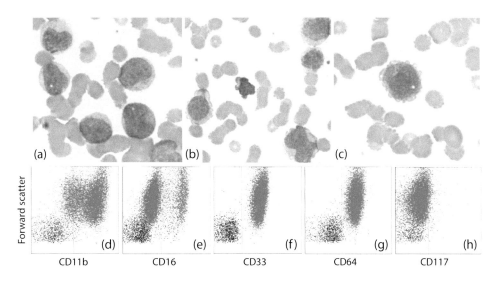

FIGURE 23.22 APL after therapy with atypical myelomonocytic cells compatible with "differentiation syndrome". Aspirate smear shows highly atypical immature cells with monocytic and myelocytic features (a–c). Based on flow cytometry analysis (d–h), the cells show phenotype overlapping between neutrophils and monocytes with partially positive CD11b (d) and CD16 (e), positive CD33 (f) and CD64 (g), and negative CD117 (h). FISH studies were positive for *PML-RARA* rearrangement.

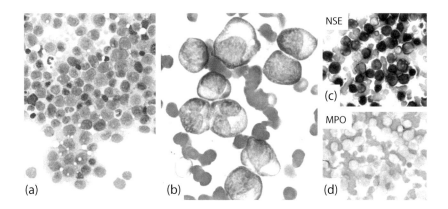

FIGURE 23.23 Acute monoblastic leukemia. Monoblasts (a–b) have irregular nuclei, which look similar to hypogranular promyelo-cytes. In contrast to APL, monocytic cells are NSE⁺ (c) and MPO⁻ (d).

TABLE 23.3: Differential Diagnosis of APL by FC

	Classic APL	Hypogranular APL	Differentiation Syndrome	*NPM1*⁺ AML[a]	Benign Neutrophils	Benign Monocytes
CD2	–	+/(–)	–	–	–	+/–
CD10	–	–	–	–	+bright	–
CD11b	–	–	+	–	+	+bright
CD11c[b]	–	–	+	+	+	+bright
CD13	+	+	+	+	+	+
CD14	–	–	–/+	–	–	+bright
CD16	–	–	–/+	–	+bright	–
CD33	+bright	+bright	+	+	+	+
CD34	–	+/(–)	–	+/–	–	–
CD64	+dim/–	+dim/–	+/–	–	–	+bright
CD117	+	+	–	+	–	–
HLA-DR	–	–	–	–/+	–	+

Abbreviations: APL, acute promyelocytic leukemia, AML, acute myeloid leukemia

Notes: +, positive; (+), rarely positive; –, negative; (–), rarely negative.

[a] Variable phenotype, including cases with monocytic differentiation.

[b] CD11c is positive in APL in very rare cases (~1%).

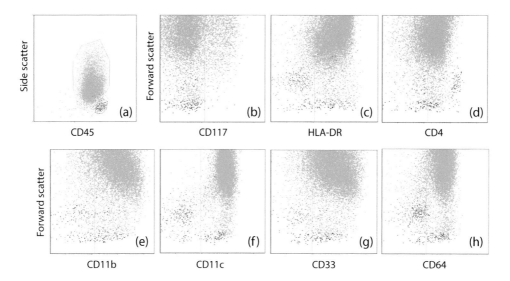

FIGURE 23.24 Acute monocytic (monoblastic) leukemia. Neoplastic monocytes (green dots) show slightly increased SSC and moderate CD45 (a), negative CD117 on majority of cells (b; minor population is positive), positive HLA-DR (c), positive CD4 (d), positive CD11b (e), positive CD11c (f), positive CD33 (g) and positive (bright) CD64 (h). Neoplastic promyelocytes (APL) are positive for CD117, negative for CD4, CD11b, and CD11c, show brighter CD33 and dimmer CD64.

Very rare poorly differentiated plasma cell myelomas with plasmablastic features show expression of CD45, CD33, and CD117, which in conjunction with lack of HLA-DR may mimic hypogranular APL (Figure 23.27). Cytologic features and often bright expression of CD38 and CD56 helps to exclude APL

Differentiation syndrome. "Maturing blasts" in differentiation syndrome (atypical *PML-RARA*+ myelomonocytic cells after treatment with maturation inducing agents) differ from residual APL by lack of CD117 expression, positive CD11b and CD11c expression, which may be partial.

Acute myeloid leukemia with t(8;21) [*RUNX1-RUNX1T1*]

Phenotype of AML with t(8;21): CD2$^{-/rarely+}$, s.CD3$^-$, c.CD3$^-$, CD4$^{-/+}$, CD7$^{+/rarely-}$, CD11b$^{-/rarely+}$, CD11c$^{-/+}$, CD13$^{+/rarely-}$, CD14$^-$, CD15$^{-/rarely+}$, CD19$^{+/rarely-}$, c.CD22$^-$, CD33$^{+/rarely-}$, CD34$^{+/rarely-}$, CD38$^{+/rarely-}$, CD36$^-$, CD56$^{+/rarely-}$, CD64$^-$, CD65$^{-/rarely+}$, CD79a$^{+/rarely-}$, CD117$^{+/rarely-}$, CD133$^{+/-}$, HLA-DR$^{+/rarely-}$, MPO$^+$, TdT$^{-/rarely+}$

Morphology

Acute myeloid leukemia with t(8;21)(q22;q22) [*RUNX1-RUNX1T1*] most often displays the morphology of AML with maturation [1]. Blasts are large with abundant basophilic cytoplasm and variable, often increased number of azurophilic granules and frequent Auer rods. Large granules (pseudo-Chédiak-Higashi granules) are often present. Maturing elements often show dysgranulopoiesis (including pseudo-Pelger-Huët nuclei). The AML with t(8;21) is associated with a higher incidence of myeloid sarcoma (extramedullary myeloid tumor) [34].

Immunophenotype

Phenotypically, AML with t(8;21) is positive for pan-myeloid antigens (CD13, CD33), HLA-DR, blastic markers (CD34, CD117, CD133) and characteristically for B-cell antigens (CD19, PAX5 and/or CD79a) and often also CD56 and/or CD7 (Figures 23.28–23.30). Rare cases may be dimly TdT positive. Occasional cases may show dim CD33, lack of surface pan-myeloid antigens, or aberrant expression of CD15 and/or CD65. The expression of CD34 is often strong.

Genetic features

The t(8;21) (Figure 23.31) is one of the most frequent structural chromosomal abnormalities seen in AML. AML with t(8;21)

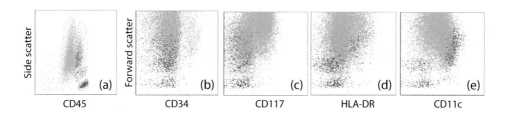

FIGURE 23.25 AML with increased SSC. Occasional cases of AML may "mimic" APL by displaying increased SSC (a; green dots), negative CD34 (b), and positive CD117 (c). In contrast to APL, minor population of blasts in this AML shows dim HLA-DR expression (d) and major population of blasts is CD11c$^+$ (e).

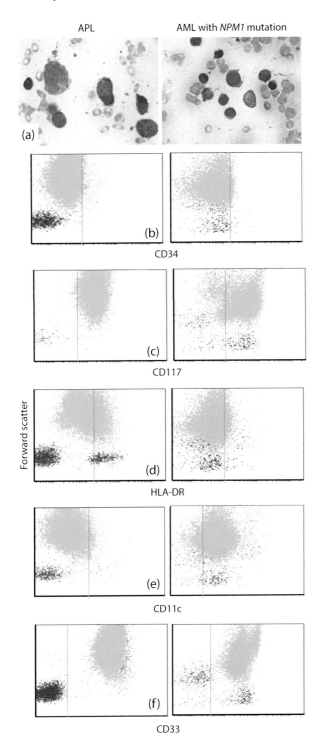

APL   AML with *NPM1* mutation

(a)

(b)

CD34

(c)

CD117

Forward scatter

(d)

HLA-DR

(e)

CD11c

(f)

CD33

FIGURE 23.26 Comparison between APL (left column) and *NPM1*+ AML (right column). APL and subset of *NPM1*+ AML (a; aspirate smear) may show similar phenotype, including lack of CD34 (b), positive CD117 (c) lack of HLA-DR (d), and positive CD33 (f). The subtle flow cytometric differences include the presence of CD11c expression by *NPM1*+ AML (e) and brighter expression of CD33 by APL (f). The threshold for positive versus negative expression is established based on isotypic negative controls, as APL blasts tend to show high non-specific background fluorescence with many of the fluorochromes. Molecular testing for *PML-RARA* and *NPM1* is crucial in establishing the final diagnosis.

represents approximately 5%–12% of de novo AMLs. The t(8;21) results in fusion between *RUNX1* gene (Runt-related gene family; formerly termed *AML1* gene) and *RUNX1T1* gene (also known as *ETO* gene *for* eight twenty-one) [35–37]. AML with t(8;21) belongs to a group of core-binding factor (CBF) leukemias. CBF is also rearranged in AML with t(3;21) and t(16;16)/inv(16). This subtype of AML is associated with favorable prognosis [37–39]. Gustafson et al., studied 13 cases of t-AML/t(8;21) and 38 adult cases of *de novo* AML/t(8;21) [40]. Of 13 t-AML/t(8;21) cases, 11 had previously received chemotherapy with or without radiation for malignant neoplasms and 2 received radiation alone. The median latency to t-AML onset was 37 months (range, 11–126 months). Compared with patients with de novo AML/t(8;21), patients with t-AML/t(8;21) were older and had a lower WBC count, substantial morphologic dysplasia, and comparable CD19/CD56 expression. The *RUNX1-RUNX1T1* fusion was demonstrated in all 10 cases assessed. With a median follow-up of 13 months, 10 patients with t-AML-t(8;21) died; the overall survival was significantly inferior to that of patients with de novo AML/t(8;21) (19 months vs. not reached). These findings suggest that t-AML/t(8;21) shares many features with de novo AML/t(8;21)(q22;q22), but affected patients have a worse outcome [40].

Prognosis

Prognosis of AML with t(8;21) is good. Despite overall good prognosis, ~40% of cases relapse. The white blood cell count at initial diagnosis, additional chromosomal aberrations such as del(9), loss of sex chromosomes and CD56 positivity have been reported as adverse prognostic factors. The presence of *KIT* mutations is associated with worse outcome (intermediate prognosis) [41–43].

AML with *CBFB-MYH11*

PHENOTYPE OF AML WITH *CBFB-MYH11*

Blasts: CD2[-/rarely+], s.CD3[-], c.CD3[-], CD4[-/+], CD7[+/rarely-], CD11b[-/rarely+], CD11c[-/+], CD13[+/rarely-], CD14[-], CD15[-/rarely+], CD19[-], c.CD22[-], CD33[+/rarely-], CD34[+/rarely-], CD38[+/rarely-], CD36[-], CD56[+/-], CD64[-], CD65[-/rarely+], CD79a[-], CD117[+/rarely-], CD133[+/-], HLA-DR[+/rarely-], MPO[+], TdT[-/rarely+]

Monocytes: CD4[+], CD11b[+], CD11c[+], CD13[+], CD14[+], CD33[+], CD45[+], CD56[-/+], CD64[+(bright)]

Eosinophils: FSC[low], SSC[high], CD10[-], CD13[+], CD16[-], CD33[+], CD123[+/rarely-]

Inversion (16)(p13.1q22), t(16;16)(p13.1;q22), and del(16)(q22) [*CBFB-MYH11*] are nonrandom abnormalities associated with acute myelomonocytic leukemia with eosinophilia, and rarely with other subsets of AML. It is more often diagnosed in younger patients.

Morphology

This leukemia has increased blasts and monocytic cells and is characterized by increased atypical (often immature) eosinophils with large basophilic granules intermixed with more typical eosinophilic granules (Figure 23.32). In some cases, blasts are large with irregular nuclei and prominent cytoplasmic granules, and occasional Auer rods (mimicking cytologically APL; Figure 23.33).

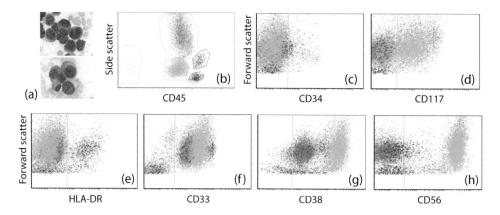

FIGURE 23.27 Plasmablastic plasma cell myeloma (a) with aberrant phenotype mimicking hypogranular APL. Plasma cells (green dots) display the following phenotype: CD45+ (b), CD34− (c), CD117+ (d), HLA-DR− (e), CD33+ (f), CD38+ (g), and CD56+ (h). Lack of HLA-DDR, strong expression of CD33 and positive CD117 may suggest APL based on flow data alone.

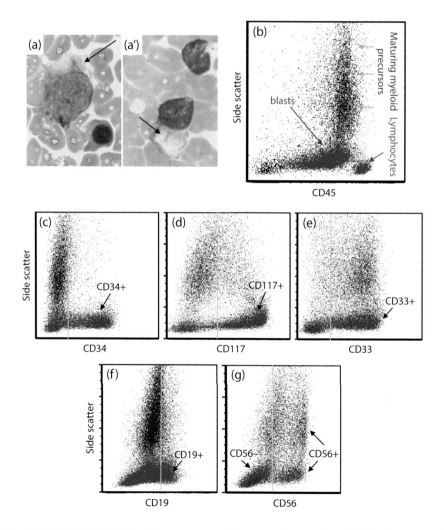

FIGURE 23.28 AML with *RUNX1-RUNX1T1* – flow cytometry. Blasts are large with nucleoli and occasional Auer rods (a; smear from flow sample). Flow cytometry (b-g) reveals phenotypic features of AML with maturation (b; blasts are represented by blue dots and maturing myeloid precursors by purple dots). Blasts are positive for CD45 (b), CD34 (c), CD117 (d), CD33 (e), CD19 (f; partial), and CD56 (g; partial). Granulocytes show aberrant CD56 expression on subset (g).

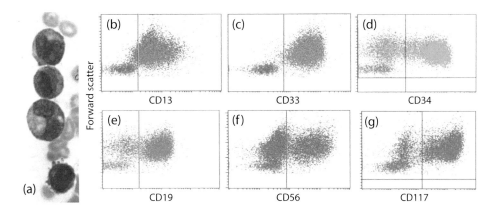

FIGURE 23.29 AML with t(8;21) – flow cytometry. Myeloblasts have granular cytoplasm (a). They are positive for CD13 (b; green dots), CD33 (c), CD34 (d), CD19 (e), CD56 (f), and CD117 (g).

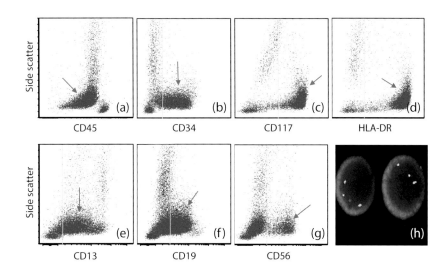

FIGURE 23.30 AML with t(8;21)/*RUNX1-RUNX1T1*. The flow cytometry pattern is often similar to AML with maturation. Blasts (blue dots; arrow) are positive for CD45 (a), CD34 (b), CD117 (c), HLA-DR (d), and CD13 (e). Blasts in AML with t(8;21)/*RUNX1-RUNX1T1* often show aberrant expression of CD19 (f) and CD56 (g; partial positivity). FISH studies (h) revealed fusion between *RUNX1-RUNX1T1* (yellow signal).

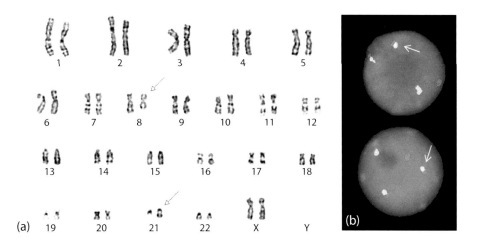

FIGURE 23.31 AML with t(8;21) [*RUNX1-RUNX1T1*] translocation (a, cytogenetics; b, FISH).

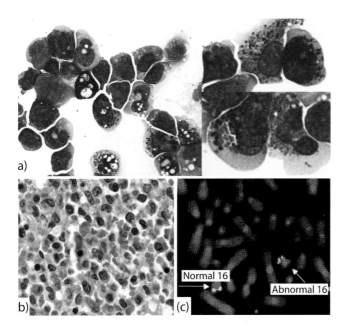

FIGURE 23.32 AML with inv(16)(p13q22. Aspirate smear (a) shows abnormal eosinophils with immature, large basophilic colored granules. Histologic section (b) shows mixed population of blasts, maturing myeloid precursors and eosinophils. FISH studies (c) shows inv(16).

Genetic features
The diagnosis of AML with *CBFB-MYH11* is confirmed by metaphase cytogenetic and/or FISH studies (Figure 23.34).

Immunophenotype
Flow cytometry shows mixed populations of blasts, monocytes, maturing myeloid cells and atypical and immature (CD123+) eosinophils (Figures 23.33 and 23.35). Blasts are positive for

CD13, CD33, CD34 and CD117, and often also HLA-DR and CD2. They may display aberrant expression of CD7, CD15, CD56 and CD65, and/or lack of HLA-DR. Monocytic cells are most often positive for CD11b, CD11c, CD13, CD14, CD64, and HLA-DR. Eosinophils are characterized by high SSC, low FSC, negative CD10 and CD16, and positive CD13, CD33, and often CD123.

Prognosis
Abnormalities of chromosome 16 in AML have been associated with high complete remission and survival rates and favorable prognosis [38, 44]. The t(16;16) or inv(16) results in the fusion of *MYH11* at 16p13 with part of *CBFB* gene at 16q22. Additional karyotypic abnormalities may be present in up to 50% of AML with t(16;16)/inv(16) and most often include trisomies of chromosome 8 (16%), 21, and 22 (22%) [45]. Majority of patients harbor at least one gene mutation, with RAS being affected in 53%, followed by KIT (37%) and FLT3 (17%; FLT3-TKD in 14% and FLT3-ID in 5%) [45]. These additional karyotypic and/or molecular changes do not influence the achievement of complete remission. The overall outcome of patients having additional genetic changes was reported to be similar to patients with sole chromosome 16 aberrations [38, 46], but new data suggest that *KIT* mutation and trisomy 22 influence relapse-free survival and *FLT3* mutation, trisomy 22, trisomy 8, age and therapy-related AML influence overall survival [45]; trisomy 22 is associated with better prognosis, and *FLT3* mutations and trisomy 8 is associated with worse prognosis. The co-existence of t(9;22) and inv(16) in CML appears to correlate with more rapid transformation into blast phase (BP) [47]. Presence of deletion 7q does not change the prognosis (including overall survival) in inv(16)+ AML.

AML with *MLLT3-MLL*

AML with t(9;11) is usually associated with monocytic or myelomonocytic features, is more common in children and patients may present with disseminated intravascular coagulation. Monoblasts

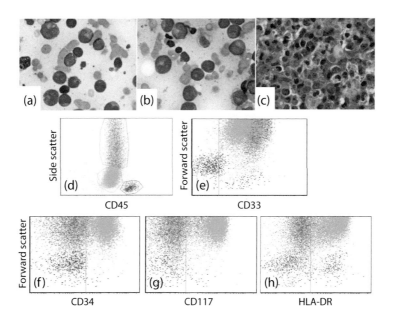

FIGURE 23.33 AML with *CBFB-MYH11*. Aspirate smear (a–b) shows large blasts with irregular nuclei and prominent cytoplasmic granules and occasional Auer rods (mimicking APL). BM core biopsy (c) shows hypercellular marrow with sheets of blasts and increased eosinophils. Flow cytometry analysis (d–h) shows blasts (green dots) with low SSC (d), dim CD33 (e), positive CD34 (f), CD117 (g), and HLA-DR (h).

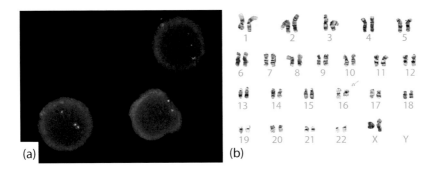

FIGURE 23.34   AML with inv(16) (a, FISH; b, cytogenetic).

and promonocytes typically predominate. Phenotypically they express CD13 (dim), CD33 (strong), CD65, CD4, HLA-DR, and monocytic markers (CD11b, CD11c, CD14 and CD64). CD56 and blastic markers (CD34 and CD117) may be expressed.

AML with *RPN1-EVI1*

AML with inv(3)(q21q26.2) or t(3;3)(q21;q26.2) is recognized as a distinct entity in WHO classification. It is associated with fusion of *EVI1* (ecotropic virus integration-1) with *RPN1* gene. These patients often present with anemia and the platelet count can be normal or increased. The BM often shows increased small hypolobated (or monolobated) megakaryocytes and multilineage dysplasia (Figure 23.36). There are no specific immunophenotypic findings, as blasts may display myeloid, megakaryocytic, or monocytic differentiation. Patients are often refractory to conventional therapy and have short overall survival.

AML with mutated *NPM1*

Phenotype of AML with *NPM1* mutation: CD2$^{-/rarely+}$, s.CD3$^-$, c.CD3$^-$, CD4$^{-/+}$, CD5$^{+/-}$, CD7$^{+/-}$, CD11b$^{-/rarely+}$, CD11c$^+$, CD13$^{+/rarely-}$, CD14$^{-/rarely+}$, CD15$^{-/rarely+}$, CD19$^-$, c.CD22$^-$, CD33$^+$, CD34$^{-/rarely+}$, CD36$^-$, CD38$^+$, CD56$^{+/-}$, CD64$^{-/+}$, CD65$^{-/rarely+}$, CD79a$^-$, CD117$^+$, CD133$^{+/-}$, HLA-DR$^{-/+}$, MPO$^{+/-}$

AML with nucleophosmin 1 (*NPM1*) mutation is associated with good prognosis. The *NPM1* gene is located on chromosome 5q35. Acute myeloid leukemias with *NPM1* mutations often show monocytic differentiation, but sporadically other morphologic variants of AML have been reported. Blasts show monocytic immunophenotype and are typically CD34$^-$. Acute myeloid leukemia with

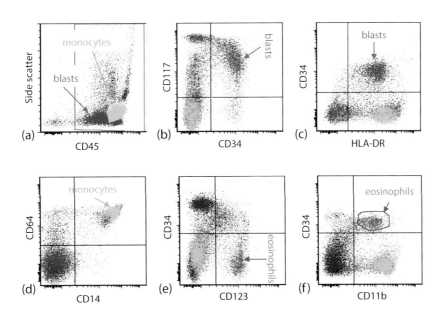

FIGURE 23.35   AML with *CBFB-MYH11* – flow cytometry. Flow cytometry analysis shows increased blasts (blue dots) and monocytes (green dots). In addition, maturing myeloid cells (gray dots) and atypical eosinophils (pink dots) are present. Blasts show dimmer CD45 when compared to monocytes (a); they are positive for CD34 (b), CD117 (b), and HLA-DR (c). Monocytes are negative for CD34 and CD117 (b) and are positive for HLA-DR (c; brighter expression than in blasts), CD14 (d), CD64 (d), and CD11b (f). Atypical (immature) eosinophils are positive for CD123 (e) and CD11b (f; dimmer expression than in monocytes).

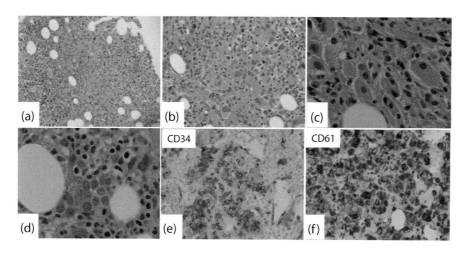

FIGURE 23.36   AML with t(3;3). BM (a–d, at low intermediate and high magnification) shows clusters of blasts (CD34$^+$, e) and prominent megakaryocytic hyperplasia (CD61$^+$, f).

NPM1 mutations is considered low-risk leukemia (in both adults and children). *NPM1* mutations are more common in adults; they have been detected in 5%–8% of children with AML and ~30% of adults AML (~50% of AML with normal karyotype). *NPM1* mutations may be associated with internal tandem duplication of *FLT3* and normal karyotype. Prognosis in children is similar to core binding factor leukemia (overall survival >80%).

Morphology

AML with *NPM1* mutations most often shows morphologic features of acute monocytic leukemia or acute myelomonocytic leukemia, but cases with morphologic features of other types of AML can be also present (including AML without maturation, AML with maturation, or acute erythroid leukemia). The diagnosis of AML with *NPM1* mutation can only be established by molecular testing.

Flow cytometry patterns of *NPM1*$^+$ AML

AML with NPM1 mutations shows variable phenotypic features (based on 141 cases analyzed by the author) and can be subdivided into six categories:

- AML without maturation-like (17 cases; 12.1%)
- AML with maturation-like (47 cases; 33.3%)
- Hypogranular APL-like (35 cases; 24.8%)
- Acute myelomonocytic leukemia-like (17 cases; 12.1%)
- Acute monocytic leukemia-like (15 cases; 10.6%)
- Other (10 cases; 7.1%)

In *NPM1*$^+$ AMLs, the expression of CD34 is identified in 23.4%, CD38 in all 100% and CD117 in 85.1% of cases (Table 23.4). Slightly more than half of the cases (56%) are positive for HLA-DR, CD13 is positive in 73% and the majority of cases expressed CD11c (90.1%), and CD33 (95.7%). CD2, CD5, CD7, CD11b, CD14, CD56, and CD64 are positive in 6.4%, 21.3%, 17%, 12.8%, 5.7%, 22%, and 17.7% of cases, respectively. The SSC is mostly low (97/141) or low to slightly increased (44/141). Flow cytometry detection of *NPM1* exon 12 mutations using high-resolution melting polymerase chain reaction has been recently proposed [48].

***NPM1*$^+$ AML with AML without maturation-like phenotype.** In this category, FC analysis shows predominance of blasts (80.5%; range: 65%–92%). Blasts are positive for CD117 in 16/17 cases,

CD34 in 9/17 cases and HLA-DR in 16/17 cases (the only case negative for CD117, showed positive expression of CD34, negative HLA-DR, positive CD13 and negative CD33). CD13 and CD33 are positive in majority of cases (15/17 and 16/17, respectively) and monocytic markers, CD14 and CD64 are negative except for one case showing dim CD64 expression on subset of blasts. Almost half of the cases (47%) show aberrant expression of CD7 by blasts and none of the cases show CD56 expression.

***NPM1*$^+$ AML with AML with maturation-like phenotype.** In *NPM1*$^+$ cases with AML with maturation-like pattern the number of blasts ranges from 20% to 67% (average, 39%) and granulocytes from 11% to 67% (average, 34.7%). All cases are CD117$^+$, whereas CD34 and HLA-DR are expressed in 14/47 (29.8%) and 36/47 (76.6%), respectively. All cases are CD33+ and only 4/47 cases (8.5%) show aberrant loss of CD13 expression. CD7 is positive in 29.8% and CD56 in 4.3% of cases. The maturing myeloid elements show frequently atypical phenotype suggestive of dysgranulopoiesis and/or leftward shift: CD10 is down-regulated in the majority of cases with the average 78.6% of cells lacking CD10 expression; CD11b is down-regulated in 34/47 cases (72.3%), CD16 is down-regulated in 36/47 cases (76.6%), and CD56 is up-regulated in 4/47 cases (8.5%).

***NPM1*$^+$ AML with hypogranular APL-like phenotype.** *NPM1*$^+$ AML with hypogranular APL-like phenotype shows predominance of blasts. Blasts, granulocytes, and monocytes comprise 70.6%, 12.2%, and 1.5% of all events, respectively (FC analysis). This category is characterized by positive CD117, negative HLA-DR, and often negative CD34 (Figure 23.37). CD34 is positive in 17.1%, CD11c in 82.9%, and CD56 in 34.3% of cases. Rare cases may be positive for CD7 (2.9%) and CD64 (11.4%). The SSC is low (24/35 cases) or low to slightly increased (11/35 cases).

***NPM1+ AML with acute myelomonocytic leukemia-like phenotype.** 17 cases showed the immunophenotype similar to acute myelomonocytic (AMML; Figure 23.38). Number of blasts ranges from 20% to 52% (average: 27.1%); granulocytes from 4% to 55% (average: 26.2%) and monocytes from 10% to 52% (average: 29.2%). In all cases, blasts are positive for CD117 and CD33, and only one case showed negative CD13 expression by blasts. HLA-DR is positive in 13/17 cases (76.5%) and CD34 in only 3/17 cases (23.5%; partial expression). There is no aberrant CD7 or CD56 expression by blasts. Monocytes show prominent phenotypic atypia in the majority of cases, including loss of CD13, CD14, and/or HLA-DR expression, partial or variable expression of CD11b or CD14, and

TABLE 23.4: The Immunophenotype of Blasts in *NPM1*⁺ AMLs

Antigen Expression by Blasts	All Cases n = 141	AML without Maturation-like n = 17	AML with Maturation-like n = 47	Hypogranular APL-like n = 35	AMML-like n = 17	Acute Monocytic Leukemia-like n = 15	Other n = 10
CD2	**6.4%**	0	0	0	0	60%	0
CD4	**21.3%**	35.3%	12.8%	0	11.8%	93.3%	20%
CD7	**17%**	47%	29.8%	2.9%	0	0	10%
CD11b	**12.8%**	5.9%	2.1%	0	0	100%	10%
CD11c	**90.1%**	94.1%	89.4%	82.9%	94.1%	100%	90%
CD13	**73%**	88.2%	91.5%	57.1%	94.1%	26.7%	50%
CD14	**5.7%**	0	0	0	0	53.3%	0
CD33	**95.7%**	94.1%	100%	94.3%	100%	100%	70%
CD34	**23.4%**	52.9%	29.8%	17.1%	23.5%	0	0
CD56	**22%**	0	4.3%	34.3%	0	66.7%	70%
CD64	**17.7%**	5.9%	4.3%	11.4%	5.9%	100%	20%
CD117	**85.1%**	94.1%	100%	100%	100%	6.7%	40%
HLA-DR	**56%**	100%	76.6%	0	76.5%	86.7%	10%

Abbreviations: AML, acute myeloid leukemia; APL, acute promyelocytic leukemia; AMML, acute myelomonocytic leukemia

positive expression of CD56. All cases show bright CD64 and CD11c expression by monocytes. CD11b is either bright (9 cases), moderate (3 cases), or variable (4 cases). CD13 can be bright or moderate but is negative in more than half of the cases (9 cases). CD14 is usually negative (13 cases) but occasional cases may be positive (partial in 2 and variable in 2 cases). HLA-DR is most often positive but rare cases may be negative.

***NPM1*⁺ AML with acute monocytic leukemia-like phenotype.** In 15 out of 141 cases, the FC phenotype may be reminiscent of acute monoblastic (monocytic) leukemia (Figure 23.39). The number of neoplastic monocytes ranges from 41% to 85% (average 64.2%). All cases are negative for CD34, and positive for CD11b, CD11c, CD33, and CD64, and all except one were negative for CD117 (one case showed dim CD117 on a minute subset of monocytes). The majority of cases are positive for HLA-DR (13/17; 86.7%), CD2 (9/19; 60%), CD4 (16/17; 93.3%), and CD56 (10/17; 66.7%). There is no aberrant expression of CD7 by neoplastic monocytes.

"Other" phenotypes. Ten out of one hundred and forty one cases in my collection could not be further subclassified. Four

of those cases showed phenotype vaguely resembling blastic plasmacytoid dendritic cell neoplasm (BPDCN) with positive CD56 expression and negative HLA-DR, CD11b, CD14, CD34, and CD64 (Figure 23.40). One case showed 26% blasts and a predominant population of eosinophils (Figure 23.41), and one cases showed blasts without expression of CD11b, CD13, CD33, CD14, CD33, CD56, CD64, HLA-DR, and CD117. The immunophenotype of the cases in "other" category is presented in Table 23.5.

Genetic features

Among 125 cases with *NPM1* mutation with available cytogenetic data, 19 cases (15.2%) showed abnormal karyotype by metaphase cytogenetics. The abnormalities are often complex and include inv(3)(p13p24)del(3)(q21q22), ins(7;3)(p15;p14p25), t(1;19)(q21;q13.1), t(2;4)(p23;q25), t(2;12)(p21;q13), t(3;5;7)(p14;q33;p13), t(4;6)(q27;p15.1), t(10;12)(q22;p13), t(11;17)(p14;q11.2), del(1)(p13p31),del(5)(q13q31), del(12)(p12) [2 cases], del(13)(q12q22), del(15)(q11.2q22), del(20)(q11.2) [2 cases], der(1)t(1;2;10)(p22;q11.2;p11.2), der(7)t(3;5;7), trisomy 5, 6, 8 [3 cases], 10, 18, and 19.

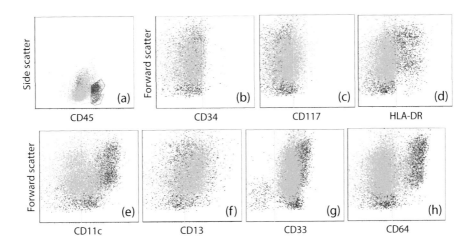

FIGURE 23.37 AML with *NPM1* mutation (hypogranular APL-like flow cytometry pattern). Blasts (green dots) show low SSC (a), negative CD34 (b), dim (partial) CD117 (c), negative HLA-DR (d), dim CD11c (e), dim CD33 (f), positive CD33 (g), and negative CD64 (h).

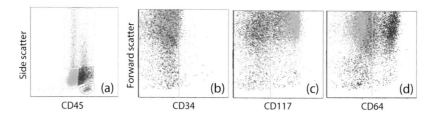

FIGURE 23.38   AML with *NPM1* mutation (AMML-like flow cytometry pattern). Blasts (green dots) show low SSC (a), negative CD34 (b), and positive CD117 (c). Monocytes (blue dots) show bright CD45 (a), negative CD34 (b), negative CD117 (c), and bright CD64 (d).

Differential diagnosis of *NPM1*⁺ AML

Since the phenotype of AML with *NPM1* mutations is very heterogeneous, the differential diagnosis is broad and includes the majority of AML subtypes, especially those with monocytic differentiation (component) and hypogranular APL. When compared to control cases (*NPM1*⁻ AMLs), *NPM1*⁺ AMLs are characterized by less frequent expression of CD34 (23.4% versus 46.8%), CD13 (73% versus 92.8%), CD2 (6.4% versus 23%),

and CD64 (17.7% versus 50.4%), and more frequent expression of CD11c (90.1% versus 37.4%) and CD7 (17% versus 4%).

When compared to *NPM1*⁻ AML without maturation, *NPM1*⁺ AML with AML without maturation-like phenotype showed more frequent expression of CD7 (47% versus 28%), CD11c (94% versus 55.6%), CD33 (94% versus 72.2%), and less frequent expression of CD34 (52.3% versus 77.8%), and CD56 (0 versus 28%). *NPM1*⁺ AML with AML with maturation-like phenotype differed

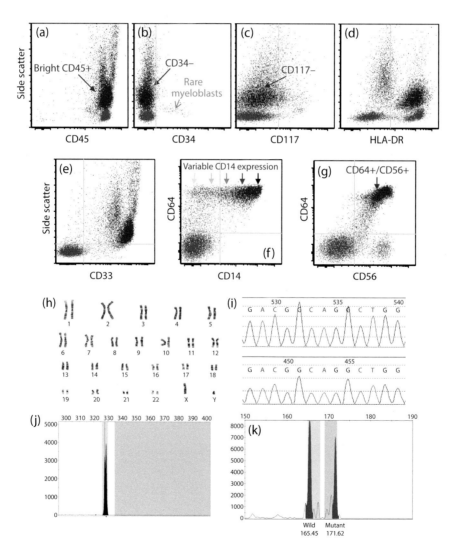

FIGURE 23.39   AML with *NPM1* mutation. Flow cytometry analysis (a–g) shows acute monoblastic leukemia-like pattern. Blasts are positive for CD45 (a), HLA-DR (d), CD33 (e), CD64 (f; bright), CD14 (g; variable expression), and CD56 (g). CD34 and CD117 are negative (b–c). Metaphase cytogenetics shows normal karyotype (e; 46,XY) and molecular results are negative for *CEBPA* (i) and *FLT3*-ITD (j) mutations and positive for *NPM1* mutations (k).

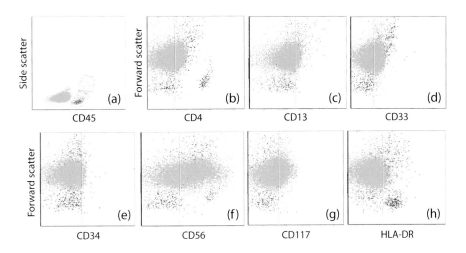

FIGURE 23.40 AML with *NPM1* mutation (BPDCN-like flow cytometry pattern). Blasts (green dots) show low SSC (a), dim CD45 (a), negative to dim CD4 (b), negative CD13 (c), negative to dim CD33 (d), negative CD34 (e), positive CD56 (f), negative to dim CD117 (g), and negative HLA-DR (h).

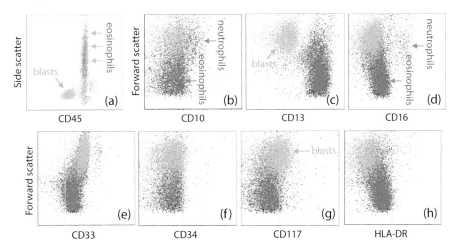

FIGURE 23.41 AML with *NPM1* mutation and eosinophilia. Blasts (green dots) show low SSC (a) and high FSC (b–h). Eosinophils show high SSC (a) and low FSC (b-h) and rare neutrophils show high FSC (b, d). Apart from low FSC, eosinophils are characterized by negative CD10 (b), bright CD13 (c), negative CD16 (d), and positive CD33 (e). Blasts are positive for CD13 (c; dim expression), CD33 (e) and CD117 (g, partial expression), and are negative for CD34 (f) and HLA-DR (h).

TABLE 23.5: The Immunophenotype of *NPM1*+ AML Cases with Unclassifiable Phenotype ("Other" Category; *n* = 10)

Antigen	\multicolumn{10}{c}{Case Number}
	1	2	3	4	5	6	7	8	9	10
CD2	–	–	–	–	–	–	–	–	–	–
CD4	D	–	–	–	–	–	–	–	D	–
CD7	–	–	–	–	–	–	–	–	M	–
CD11b	–	–	–	–	–	–	–	–	S	–
CD11c	S	D	S	D	–	D	D	S	D	D
CD13	M	–	–	D	–	–	–	D	B	M
CD14	–	–	–	–	–	–	–	–	–	–
CD33	M	M	M	–	M	–	–	D	B	M
CD34	–	–	–	–	–	–	–	–	–	–
CD38	M	M	M	D	D	D	M	M	D	M
CD56	B	B	B	V	M	–	–	S	–	M
CD117	–	–	S	–	M	M	–	S	–	–
HLA-DR	–	–	–	–	–	–	–	–	M	–

Notes: –, negative; D, dim; M, moderate; B, bright; V, variable; S, subset.

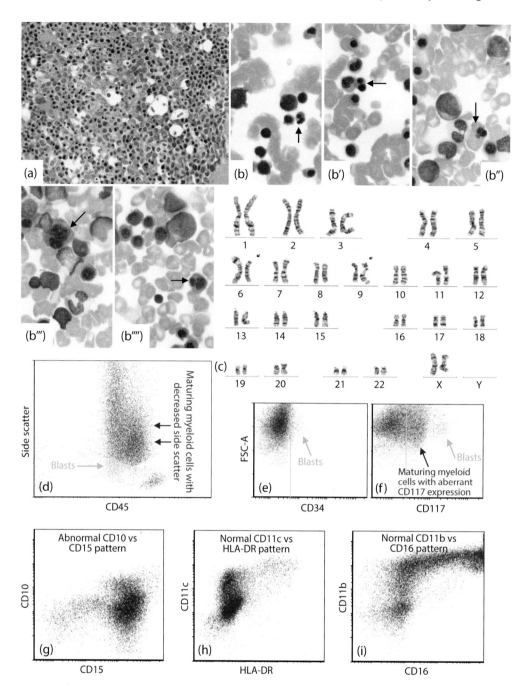

FIGURE 23.42 Myeloid neoplasm with the translocation t(6;9). BM sample from 29-year-old patient with severe anemia (6 months after delivering a baby). BM core biopsy (a) shows hypercellular marrow with myeloid and erythroid leftward shift and decreased M:E ratio due to erythroid hyperplasia. Aspirate smear (b–b''') shows marked dyserythropoiesis (arrows) and leftward shift of both myeloid and erythroid precursors (myeloblasts comprised <5% of marrow elements confirmed with CD34 immunostaining on both core and clot sections, not shown). Metaphase cytogenetic (c) shows the translocation t(6;9), known to be associated with *DEK* (located at 6p22) and *NUP214* (CAN located at 9q34) gene rearrangement. Flow cytometry (d–i) shows rare blasts (green dots, d) positive for CD34 (e) and CD117 (f). Neutrophils and maturing myeloid precursors (brown dots) show decreased SSC (d), partial expression of CD117 (f), and down-regulation of CD10. The expression of CD11b, CD11c, CD15, CD16, and HLA-DR by myeloid cells did not show overt abnormalities.

from *NPM1⁻* AML with maturation by more frequent expression of CD7 (29.8% versus 12%), CD33 (100% versus 88%), and less frequent expression of CD11b (2.1% versus 16%), CD34 (29.8% versus 88%), CD56 (4.3% versus 28%), and CD64 (4.3% versus 24%).

None of *NPM1⁺* AML without HLA-DR expression displayed high orthogonal SSC to revoke the diagnosis of classic

(hypergranular) APL. Thirty-five cases, however, showed positive CD117, low SSC, and negative HLA-DR, reminiscent of hypogranular APL. In contrast to hypogranular variant of *PML-RARA⁺/NPM1⁻* APL, *NPM1⁺* AML with hypogranular APL-like phenotype shows lack of CD2 (0 versus 76.7%) and CD4 (0 versus 20%) expression, less frequent expression of CD13 (57.1% versus

93.3%) and CD64 (11.4% versus 76.7%), frequent expression of CD11c (82.9% versus 0) and more frequent expression of CD56 (34.3% versus 13.3%).

17 *NPM1*⁺ cases showed increased both blasts and monocytes with phenotypic features reminiscent of AMML. They differ from control *NPM1*⁻ AMMLs by higher frequency of CD11c expression (94.1% versus 59.5%), and lower frequency of the expression of CD34 (23.5% versus 85.6%), and slightly less common expression of both CD56 (0 versus 7.1%) and CD64 (5.9% versus 16.7%). *NPM1*⁺ AMLs with monoblastic features differed from *NPM1*⁻ acute monoblastic leukemia by higher frequency of CD2 expression (60% versus 48%), higher frequency of negative CD13 (73.3% versus 16%), and slightly less often expression of CD117 (6.7% versus 24%) and CD34 (0 versus 12%).

AML with mutated *CEBPA*

The prognosis of AML with double mutated *CEBPA* is favorable. The *CEBPA* gene is located on chromosome 19q31.1. *CEBPA* mutations are detected in 10% of AML. Morphologically and phenotypically, AML with *CEBPA* mutation resemble AML with or without maturation.

Immunophenotype
Flow cytometry shows mixed populations of blasts, monocytes, maturing myeloid cells and atypical and immature (CD123⁺) eosinophils. Blasts are positive for CD13, CD33, CD34, and CD117, and often also HLA-DR. They may display aberrant expression of CD2, CD7, CD15, CD56, CD65, and/or lack of HLA-DR [49]. Monocytic cells are most often positive for CD11b, CD11c, CD13, CD14, CD64, and HLA-DR, and often low expression of CD36. In a series published by Mannelli et al., blasts from *CEBPA* AMLs displayed high and homogeneous expression of CD34, CD117, and HLA-DR, with asynchronous maturation (concomitant high expression of CD15, CD65, CD64, and MPO) and aberrant expression of CD7 [50]. CD7 is usually positive on whole population of blasts. The neutrophilic compartment often shows low SSC, lower expression of CD65, and overexpression of CD64. 31% of cases show CD56 expression on blasts.

AML with *DEK-NUP214*

The t(6;9)(p23;q34) [*DEK-NUP214*] abnormality is found in 0.7%–1.8% of patients with acute myeloid leukemia (AML) or myelodysplastic syndromes (MDS). Acute myeloid leukemia with t(6;9)(p23;q34) [*DEK-NUP214*] is a rare variant of AML with or without monocytic features that is often associated with basophilia (>2% basophils) and multilineage dysplasia [1, 51, 52]. It presents with anemia and thrombocytopenia, and often pancytopenia. It occurs in children and younger adults. Morphologically it has most common features of AML with maturation or acute myelomonocytic leukemia, but it may have features of any other leukemia type except for APL and acute megakaryoblastic leukemia. The translocation t(6;9) is usually the only cytogenetic abnormality detected. Molecularly, ~80% of patients with AML/MDS with t(6;9) are characterized by at least one somatic mutation, often FLT3 but also WT1. Although some authors suggested that all myeloid neoplasms with t(6;9)/*DEK-NUP214* may be considered as AML, even when blast count is <20%, in current WHO classification cases with <20% blasts are not classified as AML in current WHO classification. In a series reported by Fang et al., there was no difference in overall survival between MDS and AML patients with t(6;9), but

the survival curves did show a trend toward favorable survival in MDS patients [52]. Figure 23.42 illustrates morphologic, cytogenetics, and FC features of a myeloid neoplasm with the t(6;9).

References

1. Swerdlow, S.H., et al., ed. *WHO classification of tumors of haematopoietic and lymphoid tissues.* 2016, IARC: Lyon.
2. Tallman, M.S., *Acute promyelocytic leukemia as a paradigm for targeted therapy.* Semin Hematol, 2004. **41**(2 Suppl 4): p. 27–32.
3. Lo-Coco, F. and E. Ammatuna, *The biology of acute promyelocytic leukemia and its impact on diagnosis and treatment.* Hematology Am Soc Hematol Educ Program, 2006. **2006**(1): p. 156–61.
4. Tallman, M.S. and J.K. Altman, *How I treat acute promyelocytic leukemia.* Blood, 2009. **114**(25): p. 5126–35.
5. Larson, R.A., et al., *Evidence for a 15;17 translocation in every patient with acute promyelocytic leukemia.* Am J Med, 1984. **76**(5): p. 827–41.
6. Melnick, A. and J.D. Licht, *Deconstructing a disease: RARalpha, its fusion partners, and their roles in the pathogenesis of acute promyelocytic leukemia.* Blood, 1999. **93**(10): p. 3167–215.
7. Shih, L.Y., et al., *Internal tandem duplication of FLT3 in relapsed acute myeloid leukemia: a comparative analysis of bone marrow samples from 108 adult patients at diagnosis and relapse.* Blood, 2002. **100**(7): p. 2387–92.
8. Schnittger, S., et al., *Analysis of FLT3 length mutations in 1003 patients with acute myeloid leukemia: correlation to cytogenetics, FAB subtype, and prognosis in the AMLCG study and usefulness as a marker for the detection of minimal residual disease.* Blood, 2002. **100**(1): p. 59–66.
9. Schnittger, S., et al., *Clinical impact of FLT3 mutation load in acute promyelocytic leukemia with t(15;17)/PML-RARA.* Haematologica, 2011. **96**(12): p. 1799–807.
10. Kiyoi, H., et al., *Internal tandem duplication of FLT3 associated with leukocytosis in acute promyelocytic leukemia. Leukemia Study Group of the Ministry of Health and Welfare (Kohseisho).* Leukemia, 1997. **11**(9): p. 1447–52.
11. Callens, C., et al., *Prognostic implication of FLT3 and Ras gene mutations in patients with acute promyelocytic leukemia (APL): a retrospective study from the European APL Group.* Leukemia, 2005. **19**(7): p. 1153–60.
12. Gale, R.E., et al., *Relationship between FLT3 mutation status, biologic characteristics, and response to targeted therapy in acute promyelocytic leukemia.* Blood, 2005. **106**(12): p. 3768–76.
13. Au, W.Y., et al., *FLT-3 aberrations in acute promyelocytic leukaemia: clinicopathological associations and prognostic impact.* Br J Haematol, 2004. **125**(4): p. 463–9.
14. Takenokuchi, M., et al., *FLT3/ITD associated with an immature immunophenotype in PML-RARalpha leukemia.* Hematol Rep, 2012. **4**(4): p. e22.
15. Kutny, M.A., et al., *FLT3 mutation status is a predictor of early death in pediatric acute promyelocytic leukemia: a report from the Children's Oncology Group.* Pediatr Blood Cancer, 2012. **59**(4): p. 662–7.
16. Fenaux, P., C. Chomienne, and L. Degos, *Acute promyelocytic leukemia: biology and treatment.* Semin Oncol, 1997. **24**(1): p. 92–102.
17. Grimwade, D. and F. Lo Coco, *Acute promyelocytic leukemia: a model for the role of molecular diagnosis and residual disease monitoring in directing treatment approach in acute myeloid leukemia.* Leukemia, 2002. **16**(10): p. 1959–73.
18. Sucic, M., et al., *Acute promyelocytic leukemia M3: cytomorphologic, immunophenotypic, cytogenetic, and molecular variants.* J Hematother Stem Cell Res, 2002. **11**(6): p. 941–50.
19. Dimopoulos, M.A., et al., *Update on treatment recommendations from the Fourth International Workshop on Waldenstrom's Macroglobulinemia.* J Clin Oncol, 2009. **27**(1): p. 120–6.

20. Gorczyca, W., *Acute promyelocytic leukemia: four distinct patterns by flow cytometry immunophenotyping.* Pol J Pathol, 2012. **63**(1): p. 8–17.

21. Montesinos, P., et al., *Clinical significance of CD56 expression in patients with acute promyelocytic leukemia treated with all-trans retinoic acid and anthracycline-based regimens.* Blood, 2011. **117**(6): p. 1799–805.

22. Gorczyca, W., et al., *Immunophenotypic pattern of myeloid populations by flow cytometry analysis.* Methods Cell Biol, 2011. **103**: p. 221–66.

23. Murray, C.K., et al., *CD56 expression in acute promyelocytic leukemia: a possible indicator of poor treatment outcome?* J Clin Oncol, 1999. **17**(1): p. 293–7.

24. Ferrara, F., et al., *CD56 expression is an indicator of poor clinical outcome in patients with acute promyelocytic leukemia treated with simultaneous all-trans-retinoic acid and chemotherapy.* J Clin Oncol, 2000. **18**(6): p. 1295–300.

25. Ito, S., et al., *Clinical and biological significance of CD56 antigen expression in acute promyelocytic leukemia.* Leuk Lymphoma, 2004. **45**(9): p. 1783–9.

26. Stahl, M. and M.S. Tallman, *Differentiation syndrome in acute promyelocytic leukaemia.* Br J Haematol, 2019. **187**(2): p. 157–162.

27. Nauffal, M., et al., *Rate of differentiation syndrome in patients based on timing of initial all-trans retinoic acid administration.* Leuk Res Rep, 2019. **12**: p. 100189.

28. Berry, D.C. and N. Noy, *All-trans-retinoic acid represses obesity and insulin resistance by activating both peroxisome proliferation-activated receptor beta/delta and retinoic acid receptor.* Mol Cell Biol, 2009. **29**(12): p. 3286–96.

29. Tabe, Y., et al., *PML-RARalpha is associated with leptin-receptor induction: the role of mesenchymal stem cell-derived adipocytes in APL cell survival.* Blood, 2004. **103**(5): p. 1815–22.

30. Frankel, S.R., et al., *The "retinoic acid syndrome" in acute promyelocytic leukemia.* Ann Intern Med, 1992. **117**(4): p. 292–6.

31. Diab, A., et al., *Acute myeloid leukemia with translocation t(8;16) presents with features which mimic acute promyelocytic leukemia and is associated with poor prognosis.* Leuk Res, 2013. **37**(1): p. 32–6.

32. Kussick, S.J., et al., *A distinctive nuclear morphology in acute myeloid leukemia is strongly associated with loss of HLA-DR expression and FLT3 internal tandem duplication.* Leukemia, 2004. **18**(10): p. 1591–8.

33. Albano, F., et al., *The biological characteristics of CD34+ CD2+ adult acute promyelocytic leukemia and the CD34 CD2 hypergranular (M3) and microgranular (M3v) phenotypes.* Haematologica, 2006. **91**(3): p. 311–6.

34. Tallman, M.S., et al., *Granulocytic sarcoma is associated with the 8;21 translocation in acute myeloid leukemia.* J Clin Oncol, 1993. **11**(4): p. 690–7.

35. Erickson, P.F., et al., *The ETO portion of acute myeloid leukemia t(8;21) fusion transcript encodes a highly evolutionarily conserved, putative transcription factor.* Cancer Res, 1994. **54**(7): p. 1782–6.

36. Peterson, L.F. and D.E. Zhang, *The 8;21 translocation in leukemogenesis.* Oncogene, 2004. **23**(24): p. 4255–62.

37. Andrieu, V., et al., *Molecular detection of t(8;21)/AML1-ETO in AML M1/M2: correlation with cytogenetics, morphology and immunophenotype.* Br J Haematol, 1996. **92**(4): p. 855–65.

38. Byrd, J.C., et al., *Pretreatment cytogenetic abnormalities are predictive of induction success, cumulative incidence of relapse, and overall survival in adult patients with de novo acute myeloid leukemia: results from Cancer and Leukemia Group B (CALGB 8461).* Blood, 2002. **100**(13): p. 4325–36.

39. Byrd, J.C. and R.B. Weiss, *Recurrent granulocytic sarcoma. An unusual variation of acute myelogenous leukemia associated with 8;21 chromosomal translocation and blast expression of the neural cell adhesion molecule.* Cancer, 1994. **73**(8): p. 2107–12.

40. Gustafson, S.A., et al., *Therapy-related acute myeloid leukemia with t(8;21) (q22;q22) shares many features with de novo acute myeloid leukemia with t(8;21)(q22;q22) but does not have a favorable outcome.* Am J Clin Pathol, 2009. **131**(5): p. 647–55.

41. Wakita, S., et al., *Importance of c-kit mutation detection method sensitivity in prognostic analyses of t(8;21)(q22;q22) acute myeloid leukemia.* Leukemia, 2011. **25**(9): p. 1423–32.

42. Cairoli, R., et al., *Prognostic impact of c-KIT mutations in core binding factor leukemias: an Italian retrospective study.* Blood, 2006. **107**(9): p. 3463–8.

43. Paschka, P., et al., *Adverse prognostic significance of KIT mutations in adult acute myeloid leukemia with inv(16) and t(8;21): a Cancer and Leukemia Group B Study.* J Clin Oncol, 2006. **24**(24): p. 3904–11.

44. Loffler, H., W. Gassmann, and T. Haferlach, *AML M1 and M2 with eosinophilia and AML M4Eo: diagnostic and clinical aspects.* Leuk Lymphoma, 1995. **18 Suppl 1**: p. 61–3.

45. Paschka, P., et al., *Secondary genetic lesions in acute myeloid leukemia with inv(16) or t(16;16): a study of the German-Austrian AML Study Group (AMLSG).* Blood, 2013. **121**(1): p. 170–7.

46. Marlton, P., et al., *Cytogenetic and clinical correlates in AML patients with abnormalities of chromosome 16.* Leukemia, 1995. **9**(6): p. 965–71.

47. Wu, Y., et al., *Coexistence of inversion 16 and the Philadelphia chromosome in acute and chronic myeloid leukemias: report of six cases and review of literature.* Am J Clin Pathol, 2006. **125**(2): p. 260–6.

48. El-Gamal, R.A.E., et al., *Flow cytometry in detection of Nucleophosmin 1 mutation in acute myeloid leukemia patients: A reproducible tertiary hospital experience.* Int J Lab Hematol, 2021. **43**(1): p. 68–75.

49. Lin, L.I., et al., *Characterization of CEBPA mutations in acute myeloid leukemia: most patients with CEBPA mutations have biallelic mutations and show a distinct immunophenotype of the leukemic cells.* Clin Cancer Res, 2005. **11**(4): p. 1372–9.

50. Mannelli, F., et al., *CEBPA-double-mutated acute myeloid leukemia displays a unique phenotypic profile: a reliable screening method and insight into biological features.* Haematologica, 2017. **102**(3): p. 529–40.

51. Visconte, V., et al., *Clinicopathologic and molecular characterization of myeloid neoplasms with isolated t(6;9)(p23;q34).* Int J Lab Hematol, 2017. **39**(4): p. 409–17.

52. Fang, H., et al., *Myelodysplastic syndrome with t(6;9) (p22;q34.1)/DEK-NUP214 better classified as acute myeloid leukemia? A multicenter study of 107 cases.* Mod Pathol, 2021. **34**(6): p. 1143–52.

24

MEASURABLE (MINIMAL) RESIDUAL DISEASE IN AML

Introduction

Measurable residual disease (MRD) represents a critical parameter in prognostic assessment and in post-remission decision-making process in acute myeloid leukemia (AML) patients. Despite improved diagnosis, molecular characterization, prognostication and treatment (including targeted therapy) of AML and high complete remission rates (close to ~80%), more than 50% of adult patients with AML will undergo disease relapse after initial treatment due to the emergence of therapy-resistant clones [1–3]. The detection and exact quantification of MRD below 5% blast threshold of morphological complete remission (mCR) provides powerful independent prognostic information and risk classification [4–23]. A precise estimate of residual disease below the threshold of mCR MRD denotes the presence of leukemic cells down to the levels of 1:10^4 to 1:10^6 white blood cells (WBCs), compared to 1:20 in morphology-based assessment. MRD detection in AML (1) provides an objective methodology to establish deeper remission status, (2) refine outcome prediction and guide postremission treatment, (3) identify impending relapse and enable early intervention, (4) allow more robust posttransplant surveillance, and (5) is used as a surrogate end point to accelerate drug testing and approval [7]. Sensitivity of MRD detection by flow cytometry (FC) can approach 1 leukemic cell per 10^4–10^5 normal cells [8, 13, 24]. Based on the level of MRD (number of residual tumor cells determined by FC), San Miguel et al., suggested 4 risk categories for disease-free and overall survival in AML: very low-risk (<10^{-4}), low risk (10^{-3}–10^{-4}), intermediate risk (10^{-2}–10^{-3}), and high risk (>10^{-2}) [25]. The relapse-free survival rates at 3 years for these risk groups were 100%, 85%, 55%, and 25%, respectively. Levels of MRD, as determined after induction therapy also seem to correlate with the quality of peripheral recovery at the time of morphologic remission. In 178 patients who achieved an CR after intensive induction, the MRD level assessed at days 16–18 after induction was associated with outcome: the 5-year relapse-free survival was 16% for MRD$^+$ patients and 43% for MRD$^-$ patients [26]. In a large cohort of younger patients, low MRD values distinguished patients with relatively favorable outcomes from those with a high relapse rate, short relapse-free and overall survival. Multivariate analysis confirmed that high MRD (>0.1% of WBC) was associated with a greater risk of relapse [6]. MRD analysis before or after hematopoietic stem cell transplantation (HSCT) identifies adults with AML at risk of poor outcomes. Zhou et al., analyzed 279 adults receiving myeloablative allogeneic HSCT in first or second remission who survived at least 35 days and underwent 10-color flow FC analyses of marrow aspirates before and 28 (+/–7 days) after transplantation [27]. The 214 MRD$^-$ patients had excellent outcomes, whereas those with MRD positivity before or after HSCT had a high risk of relapse and poor survival. The occurrence of relapse in a proportion of patients achieving MRD$^-$ status, roughly ranging between 20 and 25%, still represents a major drawback of all MRD studies [17, 28]. Presence of a small subset of cells in a patient with leukemia, termed leukemic stem cells (LSCs), which may be more therapy-resistant than majority of leukemic cells, have been shown to be responsible for the proliferation of disease.

Methods of MRD detection

The presence of MRD in AML patients in mCR can be identified based on abnormal karyotype/gene rearrangement, gene mutations/abnormal gene expression and immunophenotypic atypia of blasts [8–12, 22, 25, 29–39] using:

- Real time quantitative polymerase chain reaction (RT-qPCR)
- Digital droplet PCR (ddPCR)
- Next generation sequencing (NGS)
- Multiparameter FC

Molecular MRD monitoring includes quantification of *PML-RARA, RUNX1-RUNX1T1, CBFB-MYH11*, and mutated *NPM1*. The PCR approach is characterized by high sensitivity and is considered currently a gold standard. However, it is limited to the ~40% of AML patients that harbor 1 or more suitable abnormalities, including commonest fusion transcripts, mutated genes, and overexpressed genes. In APL, molecular assessment of MRD has become standard practice [11, 34, 40]. Patients with t(8;21)(q22;q22), inv(16), t(6;9), t(9;11) and other translocations can be monitored using leukemia-specific and unique fusion transcripts arising from those translocation (e.g., *RUNX1-RUNX1T1, CBFB-MYH11, DEK-NUP214, MLL-MLLT3*) [41–45]. Other markers for molecular MRD assessment include analysis of mutated genes (such as *NPM1, TET2, RUNX1)* or overexpressed genes (e.g., *WT1*). NGS can be potentially applicable to all AML patients, given high rate of mutations identifiable in AML. Presence of some mutations identified after therapy (e.g., *DNMT3A*) does not correlate with risk of relapse during follow-up and therefore cannot be *used for MRD*. Multiparameter FC which has sensitivity between 1 in 10^{-3} to 10^{-5}, offers an advantage over RT-qPCR, as it is less expensive, can be applicable to >90% of AML patients and has faster turnaround time allowing for real-time treatment decision-making [23, 46]. Sensitivity of RT-qPCR is 1 in 10^4–10^6 and sensitivity of NGS varies.

Leukemia-associated immunophenotype (LAIP)

Myeloblasts display variable phenotype, depending on the type of leukemia (see Chapter 5). In majority of AML, blasts are positive for CD34, CD38, CD117, HLA-DR, CD13 and CD33. LSCs are either CD34$^+$/CD38$^+$, CD34$^+$/CD38$^-$, or CD34$^-$ (CD34$^+$/CD38$^-$ being most difficult to eradicate with treatment). In contrast to blasts in normal or regenerating bone marrow (BM), CD123 is expressed by 97% of AML CD34$^+$/CD38$^-$ LSCs [47]. Blasts often display aberrant immunophenotype (LAIP; leukemia-associated immunophenotype) which helps to differentiate MRD from normal marrow precursors. Among antigens most commonly being aberrantly expressed by blasts in AML are CD2, CD7, and CD56, followed by CD5, CD11b, CD11c, CD10, CD15, CD19, CD45, CD65, and HLA-DR. The recognition of LAIP can be used to monitor patients following chemotherapy or BM transplant and to help distinguish recovering BM form residual disease [8, 9, 20, 22, 30,

DOI: 10.1201/9781003197935-24

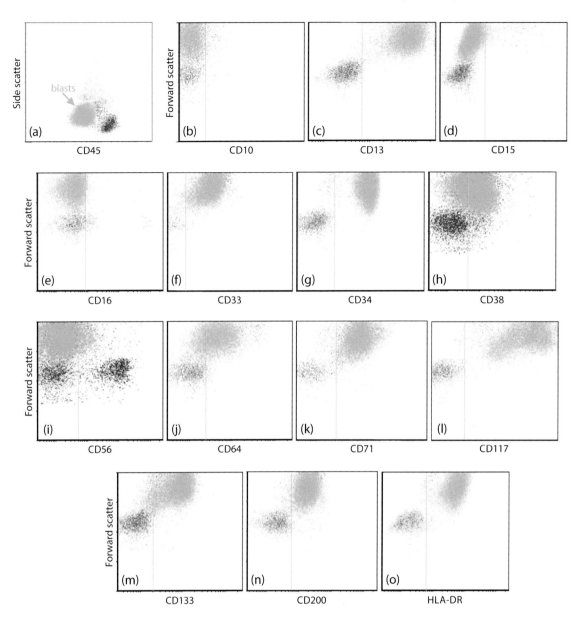

FIGURE 24.1 AML without aberrant phenotype (negative for LAIP). Blasts (green dots) show low side scatter (a), moderate expression of CD45 (a), negative CD10 (b), positive CD13 (c), negative CD15 (d), negative CD16 (e), positive CD33 (f), positive CD34 (g), positive CD38 (h), negative CD56 (i), positive CD64 (j), positive CD71 (k), positive CD117 (l), positive CD133 (m), positive CD200 (n), and positive HLA-DR (o).

48–55]. LAIP (e.g., asynchronous antigen expression, lineage infidelity, antigen overexpression, absence of lineage specific antigen, aberrant light-scatter properties) can be identified in 60%–94% of patients with AML [8, 56, 57]. Figure 24.1 illustrates AML without LAIP and Figure 24.2 AML with positive LAIP (numerous phenotypic abnormalities). In series reported by Al-Mawali et al., the most common LAIPs identified were CD117+/CD15+, CD117+/CD65+, CD34+/CD15+, and CD34+/CD65+ (these were present in 49%, 43%, 39%, and 29% of AML cases, respectively) [8].

LAIP can be divided into the following categories:

- Asynchronous antigen expression
  - Presence of mature myeloid markers such as CD11b, CD15, CD65 on CD34+ and/or CD117+ blasts
  - Asynchronous expression of CD13 and CD33 by myeloblasts
  - Asynchronous expression of CD33 and CD38
  - Asynchronous expression of CD11b, CD11c, CD14, and/or CD64 by monoblasts
  - Aberrant co-expression of myeloid and monocytic antigens by blasts (for example, co-expression of CD11b, CD14, or CD56 antigens is no found in normal CD34+ BM cells)
- Lineage infidelity or cross-lineage expression
  - Expression of T-cell markers (CD2, CD7)
  - Expression of B-cell markers (CD19)
  - Expression of NK-cell markers (CD56)
- Lack of antigen expression
  - Lack of CD45, HLA-DR, CD34, and/or CD33 on myeloblasts
  - Negative HLA-DR, CD11b, CD11c, and/or CD14 on monoblasts

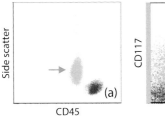 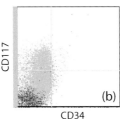 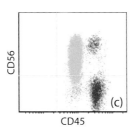 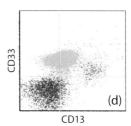 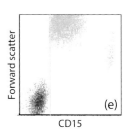

FIGURE 24.2 AML positive for LAIP. Blasts (green dots, arrow) show low side scatter and moderate CD45 (a), partial/dim CD117 (b), negative CD34 (b), positive CD56 (c), dim/partial CD13 (d), and positive CD15 (e).

- Very dim or partial antigen expression (CD13, CD14, CD33, CD38, HLA-DR, CD34, CD117)
- Overexpression of antigen (e.g., very bright expression of CD33, CD34, CD117, and/or CD123)
- Aberrant light-scatter properties (e.g., unusually high side scatter)

LAIP can be identified in 60%–94% of patients with AML [8, 15, 56–58], approaching 90%–95% with newer 8–10 color FC methods. Asynchronous expression is reported in 60%–70%, cross-lineage expression in 30%–40%, overexpression in 20%–30% and lack of expression in 20%–30%. LAIP is usually absent or expressed at low frequency in blasts from normal BM. The most common LAIP includes (in order of frequency) positive CD7 expression, positive CD56 expression, positive CD19 expression, lack of HLA-DR, asynchronous expression of CD13 and CD33 (CD13+/CD33− or CD13−/CD33+), asynchronous expression of CD34 and CD117, positive CD15, and positive CD11b.

Blasts may display immunophenotypic shift during the course of disease. These immunophenotypic changes reflect either reduction/loss or increment/gain of antigen expression. The change in the immunophenotype of blasts in AML between the diagnosis and relapse is associated with either (sub)clonal selection and/or evolution (e.g., an outgrowth of therapy-resistant sub-clones characterized by immunophenotypic aberrancies distinct from the original clone) and has important consequences for MRD detection [59–62]. The antigens most frequently lost are CD11b, CD14, CD15, while those more frequently acquired are CD34 and CD117 [55, 63–65]. At least one LAIP can be identified in 90% AML patients (LAIP is used if present in over 10% blasts). In series reported by Macedo et al., 21 out of 40 AML cases analyzed (73%) showed the existence of at least one aberrant phenotype: in 15 cases the myeloid blast cells co-expressed lymphoid-associated antigens (CD2, CD5, CD7, and/or CD19) lineage infidelity; asynchronous antigen expression was detected in 25 patients (CD34+CD56+, CD34+CD11b+, CD34+CD14+, CD117+CD15+, CD33−CD13+, CD13−CD15+, HLADR+ CD15+, HLA-DR− CD14+CD11b+CD4+); seven cases displayed antigen overexpression (CD13, CD33, CD15, or CD14); and in 13 patients leukemic cells had an abnormal FSC/SSC distribution according to their phenotype [57]. In series reported by Al-Mawali et al., the most common LAIPs identified were CD117+/CD15+, CD117+/CD65+, CD34+/CD15+, and CD34+/CD65+ (these were present in 49%, 43%, 39%, and 29% of AML cases, respectively) [8].

Most frequent LAIPs in AML:

- CD34+/CD117+/CD7+
- CD34+/CD117+/CD7+/CD33−
- CD34+/CD117+/CD13−/dim+
- CD34+/CD117+/CD33−/dim+

- CD34+/CD117+/CD19+
- CD34+/CD117+/CD19+/CD56+
- CD34+/CD117+/CD13bright+
- CD34+/CD117+/CD33bright+
- CD34−/CD117+
- CD34+/CD117−
- CD34+/CD117+/HLA-DR−
- CD34+/CD117+/CD15+
- CD34+/CD117+/CD56+
- CD34−/CD117+/CD56+
- CD34+/CD117+/CD65+
- CD34+/CD117+/CD2+
- CD34+/CD117+/CD38−

In normal (benign) BMs most CD34+ blasts co-express CD38 (96.7% +/− 5.7%), HLA-DR (81.6% +/− 14.0%), CD33 (84.7% +/− 18.3%), CD13 (84.6% +/− 16.2%), and CD71 antigens (65.5% +/− 9.1%) [66]. In addition, almost half of CD34+ blasts are CD117+ (60% +/− 26.8%). Only a small proportion of CD34+ blasts co-express CD4 (15.5% +/− 11.7%), CD36 (31.7% +/− 6.2%), CD61 (16.3% +/− 12.9%), CD41 (6.5% +/− 5.5%) or the lymphoid associated markers CD10 (18.6% +/− 11.8%), and CD19 (12.3% +/− 13.2%). Reactivity for the CD15 antigen is observed in a small population of CD34+/HLA-DR+ blasts (11.6% +/− 11.2%) although its intensity of expression is lower than that of the more mature granulocytic cells. No normal CD34+ blasts express CD14, CD65, CD20, strong CD22, CD3, and CD56 antigens [66].

Flow cytometry analysis of MRD

FC provides a quick and relatively inexpensive method for MRD detection, which in contrast to molecular methodology is applicable to the vast majority of patients with AML. Two separate approaches have been used to identify MRD in AML patients by FC:

1. **Leukemia-associated immunophenotype (LAIP)** approach, which defines LAIP at diagnosis and tracks them in subsequent (post-treatment) samples; and
2. **Different from normal (DfN)** approach based on standardized combination of antibodies, regardless of LAIP, to identify an aberrant differentiation/maturation profiles of blasts outside the maturation patterns of normal BM. DfN approach can be applied if information at diagnosis is not available and in AML cases in which blasts show either disappearance of aberrancies identified at diagnosis or appearance of new aberrancies ("immunophenotype shift").

LAIP and DfN-LAIP can be further categorized as diagnostic, follow-up (based on diagnosis information), follow-up (no diagnosis information) and changed (i.e., new aberrancy compared with diagnostic LAIP) [7]. Although the DfN is often contrasted with the use of LAIP, DfN is really a simplified variant of LAIP approach. Nevertheless, the difference between those two approaches is likely to disappear if an adapted, sufficiently large panel of antibodies (preferable ≥8 colors) is used. The most robust approach to the detection of MRD incorporates DfN both at diagnosis (LAIP) and after therapy, taking into considerations the post-therapeutic changes in immunophenotype (antigenic switch).

With current 8–10 color next generation FC protocols, aberrant phenotype of blasts (LAIP) can be identified in ≥85% of cases. For proper classification and identification LAIP for disease monitoring, FC panel should be broad and include CD2, CD3 (surface CD3; s.CD3), CD4, CD5, CD7, CD10, CD11b, CD11c, CD13, CD14, CD15, CD16, CD19, CD22, CD33, CD34, CD38, CD45, CD56, CD64, CD71, CD117, CD123, CD133, HLA-DR, and TdT. Other markers, such as cytoplasmic CD3 (c.CD3), glycophorin A (GPHA; CD235a), CD41, CD61, CD79a, and myeloperoxidase (MPO) can be used if blasts show only CD34 expression or overlapping phenotype (myeloid/lymphoid). Minimum 8-color FC analysis is recommended for MRD detection in AML. The use of blood at present cannot be recommended [7, 67]. To maximize the assay sensitivity, it is mandatory to avoid hemodilution of BM samples and therefore is recommended to submit the first BM pull for MRD analysis, preferably using the sample volume across time points and patients. The presence of >90% mature neutrophils (high SSC, strong expression of CD10 and CD16) and lack of CD34+ blasts/progenitor cells or CD38+ plasma cells in a BM sample indicates significant hemodilution [67–70]. Most validated methods recommend acquiring from 500,000 to 1 million evens (excluding all CD45- cells and debris). Recent studies showed that after induction and consolidation therapy, the findings in BM and blood were concordant [71, 72]. In the study by Zeijlemaker et al., primitive blast (CD34+/CD117+/CD133+) frequency was significantly lower in blood indicating that blood MRD detection is more specific than BM [72]. Cumulative incidence of relapse 1 year after induction therapy was 29% for blood MRD- and 89% for blood MRD+ patients, and three-year overall survival was 52% for MRD- and 15% for MRD+ patients. Similar differences were found after consolidation therapy [72].

Markers used in analysis of MRD:

- Precursor (blastic) markers include CD34, CD117, CD133, and TdT
- Myeloid markers include cytoplasmic myeloperoxidase (MPO), CD13, and CD33
- Granulocytic differentiation markers include CD10, CD11b, CD15, CD16, and CD65
- Monocytic and dendritic cell-associated antigens include CD11b, CD11c, CD14, CD36, CD64, CD68, CD123, and CD163
- Megakaryocytic markers include CD41, CD61, and CD42
- Erythroid markers include CD235a (glycophorin A), CD71, and hemoglobin A
- Activation and non-specific markers include HLA-DR, CD38, CD71
- B-cell markers include CD10, CD19, and CD22
- T-cell markers include CD2, surface and cytoplasmic CD3, CD4, CD5, and CD7

Potential new phenotypic markers, which are aberrantly expressed in AML but not by normal blasts include ILT3 (CD85k), CD9,

CD18, CD32, CD44, CD47, CD52, CD54, CD59, CD64, CD86, CD93, CD96, CD99, CD123, CD200, CD300a/c, CD366, CD371, and CxCR1 [23, 73].

Recommendation for MRD analysis by flow cytometry

Several different strategies have been used to quantify the MRD burden with the following recommendations [7]:

1. Use the BM samples only (the use of blood at present cannot be recommended [7, 67]). To maximize the assay sensitivity, it is mandatory to avoid hemodilution of BM samples and therefore is recommended to submit the first BM pull for MRD analysis, preferably using the sample volume across time points and patients. The presence of >90% mature neutrophils (high SSC, strong expression of CD10 and CD16) and lack of CD34+ blasts/progenitor cells or CD38+ plasma cells in a BM sample indicates significant hemodilution [67–70]. Presence of hemodilution needs to be mentioned in MRD flow report.

2. Most validated methods recommend acquiring at least 500,000 events (excluding all CD45- cells and debris).

3. Use of 8–10 color FC with large panel of antibodies, which combines LAIP and DfN approaches – it allows to detect any aberrancies in blasts phenotype, regardless of if they have been present *de novo* (original LAIP) or represent new aberrancies (emerging at follow-up studies; DfN-LAIP). In cases in which only subset of blasts shows LAIP, it is allowed to include all blasts (with and without LAIP) provided they form a single clustered population. If the LAIP at the time of diagnosis is available, use diagnostic LAIP and use DfN if any new abnormalities are noted in follow-up sample.

4. Use the best (most specific and/or highest frequency) LAIP for assessing MRD frequency; in case of multiple, non-overlapping LAIPs, frequencies of individual LAIPs should be added. Relate LAIP events to the leukocyte population of CD45+ cells

5. A cutoff of 0.1% was found relevant in most studies and therefore it is recommended using 0.1% as the threshold to distinguish MRD+ from MRD- patients. However, it should be noted that MRD quantified below 0.1% may still be consistent with residual leukemia, and several studies have shown prognostic significance of MRD levels below 0.1% [16, 53, 74, 75]

6. FC gating recommendation: gate the viable CD45+ cells leaving out cells with low FSC (non-viable cells and erythroid cells; Figure 24.3). Use CD34 (and CD117) markers to help ascertain the final position of the blasts in the CD45dim+ region (Figure 24.3). Gate the CD45dim+ cells and back gate the cells in the FSC/SSC plot. Remove the CD34 gate (and CD117 gate) while reporting the percentage of cells in this gate as percent of blasts. Show the blasts in SSC/CD34 (and SSC/CD117) plot and gate the CD34+ cells (and CD117+ cells). Plot CD34+ cells (and CD117+ cells) in new plot with specific markers to identify LAIP (e.g., CD7 versus CD33, CD56 versus CD33, CD19 versus CD33, etc.).

7. Calculation of MRD level: use LAIP based on cross lineage aberrancy, asynchronous differentiation, overexpression of antigen, underexpression of antigens, asynchronous expression of CD34 and CD117 and abnormal side scatter (SSC). Use the best (most specific and/or highest frequency) LAIP for assessing MRD frequency; in case of multiple,

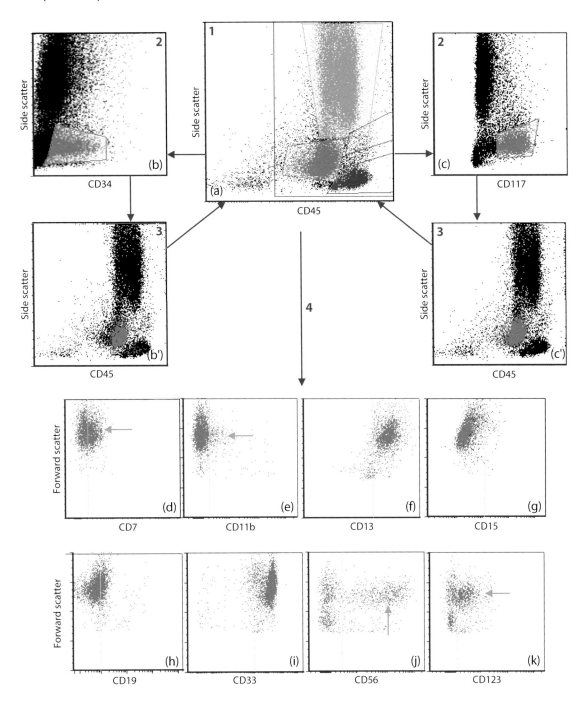

FIGURE 24.3 MRD+ AML after treatment. Simplified illustration of the strategy for analysis of MRD in AML. (a) BM sample is gated on the viable CD45+ cells (without cells with low FSC, non-viable cells, and erythroid cells). The staining with CD34 (b) and CD117 (c) help to identify the final position of the blasts in the CD45dim+ region (b′, c′). The CD45dim+ cells are back gated in the CD45/SCC and FSC/SSC plots. Blasts (green dots) defined by CD45dim+ cells, CD34+ cells and CD117+ cells are analyzed for the expression of different markers to identify aberrant phenotype of blasts. In this case, blasts showed partially dim expression of CD7 (d), minimally positive expression of CD11b (e), normal expression of CD13 (f), CD15 (g), CD19 (h) and CD33 (i), aberrant expression of CD56 (j), and CD123 (k), indicating presence of measurable minimal AML. The threshold for positive and negative expression of an antigens are set up based on staining with isotypic control antibodies on lymphocytes, blasts, and myeloid cells.

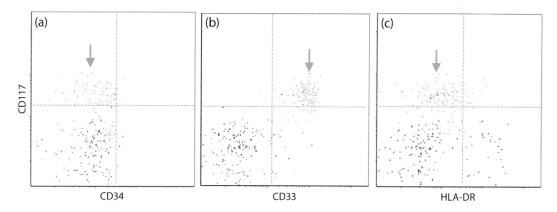

FIGURE 24.4 MRD+ APL after treatment. Neoplastic promyelocytes (green dots; arrow) are positive for CD117 (a–c) and CD33 (b), and do not express CD34 (a) and HLA-DR (c).

non-overlapping LAIPs, frequencies of individual LAIPs should be added. For non-APL and non-monoblastic AMLs use the aberrant expression of the following markers for LAIP reporting: CD2+, CD7+, CD11b+, CD15+, CD19+, CD34bright+, CD56+, HLA-DR–, asynchronous CD13/CD33 expression, asynchronous CD34/CD117 expression. For classic (hypergranular) APL, use gating on CD117+/CD34–/HLA-DR– population with increased SSC (Figure 24.4 shows MRD+ APL). For CD34–/CD117– acute monoblastic leukemia use bright CD64+ cells and report frequencies of individual LAIPs: CD14– CD11b– or dim+, CD11c– or dim+, CD56+, HLA-DR– For CD34+ and/or CD117+ acute monoblastic leukemia, determine the LAIP based number of bright CD64+ monocytes expressing CD34 and/or CD117. Relate LAIP events to the leukocyte population of CD45+ cells.

8. Reporting of MRD by FC: (a) Flow cytometry MRD not possible; (b) Flow cytometry MRD positive (≥0.1%); (c) Flow cytometry MRD negative (no MRD identified) and (d) Flow cytometry MRD detectable and quantifiable but of uncertain significance (<0.1%).

References

1. Burnett, A.K., et al., *Curability of patients with acute myeloid leukemia who did not undergo transplantation in first remission.* J Clin Oncol, 2013. **31**(10): p. 1293–301.

2. Komanduri, K.V. and R.L. Levine, *Diagnosis and therapy of acute myeloid leukemia in the era of molecular risk stratification.* Annu Rev Med, 2016. **67**: p. 59–72.

3. Dohner, H., D.J. Weisdorf, and C.D. Bloomfield, *Acute myeloid leukemia.* N Engl J Med, 2015. **373**(12): p. 1136–52.

4. Tierens, A., et al., *Residual disease detected by flow cytometry is an independent predictor of survival in childhood acute myeloid leukaemia; results of the NOPHO-AML 2004 study.* Br J Haematol, 2016. **174**(4): p. 600–9.

5. Vidriales, M.B., et al., *Minimal residual disease evaluation by flow cytometry is a complementary tool to cytogenetics for treatment decisions in acute myeloid leukaemia.* Leuk Res, 2016. **40**: p. 1–9.

6. Terwijn, M., et al., *High prognostic impact of flow cytometric minimal residual disease detection in acute myeloid leukemia: data from the HOVON/SAKK AML 42A study.* J Clin Oncol, 2013. **31**(31): p. 3889–97.

7. Schuurhuis, G.J., et al., *Minimal/measurable residual disease in AML: a consensus document from the European LeukemiaNet MRD Working Party.* Blood, 2018. **131**(12): p. 1275–1291.

8. Al-Mawali, A., et al., *Incidence, sensitivity, and specificity of leukemia-associated phenotypes in acute myeloid leukemia using specific five-color multiparameter flow cytometry.* Am J Clin Pathol, 2008. **129**(6): p. 934–45.

9. Al-Mawali, A., D. Gillis, and I. Lewis, *The role of multiparameter flow cytometry for detection of minimal residual disease in acute myeloid leukemia.* Am J Clin Pathol, 2009. **131**(1): p. 16–26.

10. Corbacioglu, A., et al., *Prognostic impact of minimal residual disease in CBFB-MYH11-positive acute myeloid leukemia.* J Clin Oncol, 2010. **28**(23): p. 3724–9.

11. Grimwade, D. and S.D. Freeman, *Defining minimal residual disease in acute myeloid leukemia: which platforms are ready for "prime time"?* Blood, 2014. **124**(23): p. 3345–55.

12. Kern, W., et al., *Monitoring of minimal residual disease in acute myeloid leukemia.* Cancer, 2008. **112**(1): p. 4–16.

13. Kern, W. and S. Schnittger, *Monitoring of acute myeloid leukemia by flow cytometry.* Curr Oncol Rep, 2003. **5**(5): p. 405–12.

14. Kern, W., et al., *Monitoring of minimal residual disease in acute myeloid leukemia.* Crit Rev Oncol Hematol, 2005. **56**(2): p. 283–309.

15. Ommen, H.B., *Monitoring minimal residual disease in acute myeloid leukaemia: a review of the current evolving strategies.* Ther Adv Hematol, 2016. **7**(1): p. 3–16.

16. Ossenkoppele, G. and G.J. Schuurhuis, *MRD in AML: does it already guide therapy decision-making?* Hematology Am Soc Hematol Educ Program, 2016. **2016**(1): p. 356–65.

17. Paietta, E., *Should minimal residual disease guide therapy in AML?* Best Pract Res Clin Haematol, 2015. **28**(2-3): p. 98–105.

18. Paietta, E., *Minimal residual disease in AML: Why has it lagged behind pediatric ALL?* Clin Lymphoma Myeloma Leuk, 2015. **15 Suppl**: p. S2–6.

19. Perea, G., et al., *Prognostic value of minimal residual disease (MRD) in acute myeloid leukemia (AML) with favorable cytogenetics [t(8;21) and inv(16)].* Leukemia, 2006. **20**(1): p. 87–94.

20. San-Miguel, J.F., M.B. Vidriales, and A. Orfao, *Immunological evaluation of minimal residual disease (MRD) in acute myeloid leukaemia (AML).* Best Pract Res Clin Haematol, 2002. **15**(1): p. 105–18.

21. Weisser, M., et al., *Risk assessment by monitoring expression levels of partial tandem duplications in the MLL gene in acute myeloid leukemia during therapy.* Haematologica, 2005. **90**(7): p. 881–9.

22. Voso, M.T., et al., *MRD in AML: The Role of New Techniques.* Front Oncol, 2019. **9**: p. 655.

23. Dix, C., et al., *Measurable residual disease in acute myeloid leukemia using flow cytometry: A review of where we are and where we are going.* J Clin Med, 2020. **9**(6): p. 1714.

24. Kern, W., et al., *Detection of minimal residual disease in unselected patients with acute myeloid leukemia using multiparameter flow*

cytometry for definition of leukemia-associated immunopheno-types and determination of their frequencies in normal bone marrow. Haematologica, 2003. **88**(6): p. 646–53.

25. San Miguel, J.F., et al., *Early immunophenotypical evaluation of minimal residual disease in acute myeloid leukemia identifies different patient risk groups and may contribute to postinduction treatment stratification.* Blood, 2001. **98**(6): p. 1746–51.

26. Kohnke, T., et al., *Early assessment of minimal residual disease in AML by flow cytometry during aplasia identifies patients at increased risk of relapse.* Leukemia, 2015. **29**(2): p. 377–86.

27. Zhou, Y., et al., *Pre- and post-transplant quantification of measurable ('minimal') residual disease via multiparameter flow cytometry in adult acute myeloid leukemia.* Leukemia, 2016. **30**(7): p. 1456–64.

28. Paietta, E., *Consensus on MRD in AML?* Blood, 2018. **131**(12): p. 1265–66.

29. Allen, C., et al., *The importance of relative mutant level for evaluating impact on outcome of KIT, FLT3 and CBL mutations in core-binding factor acute myeloid leukemia.* Leukemia, 2013. **27**(9): p. 1891–901.

30. Campana, D. and E. Coustan-Smith, *Minimal residual disease studies by flow cytometry in acute leukemia.* Acta Haematol, 2004. **112**(1-2): p. 8–15.

31. Cilloni, D. and G. Saglio, *WT1 as a universal marker for minimal residual disease detection and quantification in myeloid leukemias and in myelodysplastic syndrome.* Acta Haematol, 2004. **112**(1-2): p. 79–84.

32. Gorello, P., et al., *Quantitative assessment of minimal residual disease in acute myeloid leukemia carrying nucleophosmin (NPM1) gene mutations.* Leukemia, 2006. **20**(6): p. 1103–8.

33. Grimwade, D., et al., *Minimal residual disease detection in acute promyelocytic leukemia by reverse-transcriptase PCR: evaluation of PML-RAR alpha and RAR alpha-PML assessment in patients who ultimately relapse.* Leukemia, 1996. **10**(1): p. 61–6.

34. Grimwade, D., J.V. Jovanovic, and R.K. Hills, *Can we say farewell to monitoring minimal residual disease in acute promyelocytic leukaemia?* Best Pract Res Clin Haematol, 2014. **27**(1): p. 53–61.

35. Schnittger, S., et al., *Analysis of FLT3 length mutations in 1003 patients with acute myeloid leukemia: correlation to cytogenetics, FAB subtype, and prognosis in the AMLCG study and usefulness as a marker for the detection of minimal residual disease.* Blood, 2002. **100**(1): p. 59–66.

36. van der Velden, V.H., et al., *Detection of minimal residual disease in acute leukemia.* J Biol Regul Homeost Agents, 2004. **18**(2): p. 146–54.

37. Venditti, A., et al., *Level of minimal residual disease after consolidation therapy predicts outcome in acute myeloid leukemia.* Blood, 2000. **96**(12): p. 3948–52.

38. Venditti, A., et al., *Multidimensional flow cytometry for detection of minimal residual disease in acute myeloid leukemia.* Leuk Lymphoma, 2003. **44**(3): p. 445–50.

39. Zeleznikova, T. and O. Babusikova, *The value of dot plot patterns and leukemia-associated phenotypes in AML diagnosis by multiparameter flow cytometry.* Neoplasma, 2005. **52**(6): p. 517–22.

40. Grimwade, D. and F. Lo Coco, *Acute promyelocytic leukemia: a model for the role of molecular diagnosis and residual disease monitoring in directing treatment approach in acute myeloid leukemia.* Leukemia, 2002. **16**(10): p. 1959–73.

41. Kayser, S., et al., *Minimal residual disease-directed therapy in acute myeloid leukemia.* Blood, 2015. **125**(15): p. 2331–5.

42. Gabert, J., et al., *Standardization and quality control studies of 'real-time' quantitative reverse transcriptase polymerase chain reaction of fusion gene transcripts for residual disease detection in leukemia - a Europe Against Cancer program.* Leukemia, 2003. **17**(12): p. 2318–57.

43. Ostergaard, M., et al., *WT1 gene expression: an excellent tool for monitoring minimal residual disease in 70% of acute myeloid leukaemia patients - results from a single-centre study.* Br J Haematol, 2004. **125**(5): p. 590–600.

44. Tobal, K. and J.A. Liu Yin, *Diagnosis and monitoring of AML1-MTG8 (ETO)-positive acute myeloid leukemia by qualitative and real-time quantitative RT-PCR.* Methods Mol Med, 2006. **125**: p. 149–61.

45. Tobal, K., L. Frost, and J.A. Liu Yin, *Quantification of DEK-CAN fusion transcript by real-time reverse transcription polymerase reaction in patients with t(6;9) acute myeloid leukemia.* Haematologica, 2004. **89**(10): p. 1267–9.

46. Bueno, C., et al., *CD133-directed CAR T-cells for MLL leukemia: on-target, off-tumor myeloablative toxicity.* Leukemia, 2019. **33**(8): p. 2090–2125.

47. Vega-Garcia, N., et al., *Measurable residual disease assessed by flow-cytometry is a stable prognostic factor for pediatric T-cell acute lymphoblastic leukemia in consecutive SEHOP protocols whereas the impact of oncogenetics depends on treatment.* Front Pediatr, 2020. **8**: p. 614521.

48. Fleming, D.R., et al., *Diagnostic and clinical implications of lineage fidelity in acute leukemia patients undergoing allogeneic stem cell transplantation.* Leuk Lymphoma, 2000. **36**(3-4): p. 309–13.

49. Jennings, C.D. and K.A. Foon, *Flow cytometry: recent advances in diagnosis and monitoring of leukemia.* Cancer Invest, 1997. **15**(4): p. 384–99.

50. Vidriales, M.B., et al., *Minimal residual disease monitoring by flow cytometry.* Best Pract Res Clin Haematol, 2003. **16**(4): p. 599–612.

51. Coustan-Smith, E., et al., *Clinical significance of residual disease during treatment in childhood acute myeloid leukaemia.* Br J Haematol, 2003. **123**(2): p. 243–52.

52. Al-Mawali, A., et al., *The presence of leukaemia-associated phenotypes is an independent predictor of induction failure in acute myeloid leukaemia.* Int J Lab Hematol, 2009. **31**(1): p. 61–8.

53. Olaru, D., et al., *Multiparametric analysis of normal and postchemotherapy bone marrow: Implication for the detection of leukemia-associated immunophenotypes.* Cytometry B Clin Cytom, 2008. **74**(1): p. 17–24.

54. Voskova, D., et al., *Use of five-color staining improves the sensitivity of multiparameter flow cytomeric assessment of minimal residual disease in patients with acute myeloid leukemia.* Leuk Lymphoma, 2007. **48**(1): p. 80–8.

55. Voskova, D., et al., *Stability of leukemia-associated aberrant immunophenotypes in patients with acute myeloid leukemia between diagnosis and relapse: comparison with cytomorphologic, cytogenetic, and molecular genetic findings.* Cytometry B Clin Cytom, 2004. **62**(1): p. 25–38.

56. Reading, C.L., et al., *Expression of unusual immunophenotype combinations in acute myelogenous leukemia.* Blood, 1993. **81**(11): p. 3083–90.

57. Macedo, A., et al., *Characterization of aberrant phenotypes in acute myeloblastic leukemia.* Ann Hematol, 1995. **70**(4): p. 189–94.

58. Lee, D., G. Grigoriadis, and D. Westerman, *The role of multiparametric flow cytometry in the detection of minimal residual disease in acute leukaemia.* Pathology, 2015. **47**(7): p. 609–21.

59. Zeijlemaker, W., J.W. Gratama, and G.J. Schuurhuis, *Tumor heterogeneity makes AML a "moving target" for detection of residual disease.* Cytometry B Clin Cytom, 2014. **86**(1): p. 3–14.

60. Chen, X. and B.L. Wood, *Monitoring minimal residual disease in acute leukemia: Technical challenges and interpretive complexities.* Blood Rev, 2017. **31**(2): p. 63–75.

61. Ho, T.C., et al., *Evolution of acute myelogenous leukemia stem cell properties after treatment and progression.* Blood, 2016. **128**(13): p. 1671–8.

62. Bachas, C., et al., *The role of minor subpopulations within the leukemic blast compartment of AML patients at initial diagnosis in the development of relapse.* Leukemia, 2012. **26**(6): p. 1313–20.

63. Langebrake, C., et al., *Immunophenotypic differences between diagnosis and relapse in childhood AML: Implications for MRD monitoring.* Cytometry B Clin Cytom, 2005. **63**(1): p. 1–9.

64. Baer, M.R., et al., *High frequency of immunophenotype changes in acute myeloid leukemia at relapse: implications for residual disease detection (Cancer and Leukemia Group B Study 8361).* Blood, 2001. **97**(11): p. 3574–80.

65. van der Velden, V.H., et al., *Clinical significance of flowcytometric minimal residual disease detection in pediatric acute myeloid leukemia patients treated according to the DCOG ANLL97/MRC AML12 protocol.* Leukemia, 2010. **24**(9): p. 1599–606.

66. Macedo, A., et al., *Phenotypic analysis of CD34 subpopulations in normal human bone marrow and its application for the detection of minimal residual disease.* Leukemia, 1995. **9**(11): p. 1896–901.

67. Loken, M.R., et al., *Normalization of bone marrow aspirates for hemodilution in flow cytometric analyses.* Cytometry B Clin Cytom, 2009. **76**(1): p. 27–36.

68. Delgado, J.A., et al., *A simple flow-cytometry method to evaluate peripheral blood contamination of bone marrow aspirates.* J Immunol Methods, 2017. **442**: p. 54–8.

69. Brooimans, R.A., et al., *Flow cytometric differential of leukocyte populations in normal bone marrow: influence of peripheral blood contamination.* Cytometry B Clin Cytom, 2009. **76**(1): p. 18–26.

70. Aldawood, A.M., et al., *A Novel Method to Assess Bone Marrow Purity is Useful in Determining Blast Percentage by Flow Cytometry in Acute Myeloid Leukemia and Myelodysplasia.* Ann Hematol Oncol, 2015. **2**(5): p. 1038.

71. Maurillo, L., et al., *Monitoring of minimal residual disease in adult acute myeloid leukemia using peripheral blood as an alternative source to bone marrow.* Haematologica, 2007. **92**(5): p. 605–11.

72. Zeijlemaker, W., et al., *Peripheral blood minimal residual disease may replace bone marrow minimal residual disease as an immunophenotypic biomarker for impending relapse in acute myeloid leukemia.* Leukemia, 2016. **30**(3): p. 708–15.

73. Eveillard, M., et al., *Major impact of an early bone marrow checkpoint (day 21) for minimal residual disease in flow cytometry in childhood acute lymphoblastic leukemia.* Hematol Oncol, 2017. **35**(2): p. 237–43.

74. Freeman, S.D., et al., *Prognostic relevance of treatment response measured by flow cytometric residual disease detection in older patients with acute myeloid leukemia.* J Clin Oncol, 2013. **31**(32): p. 4123–31.

75. Walter, R.B., et al., *Significance of minimal residual disease before myeloablative allogeneic hematopoietic cell transplantation for AML in first and second complete remission.* Blood, 2013. **122**(10): p. 1813–21.

25

ACUTE LEUKEMIAS OF AMBIGUOUS LINEAGE

Acute undifferentiated leukemia (AUL)

Introduction

Majority of cases of acute leukemia belong to the category of either acute myeloid leukemia (AML) or acute lymphoblastic leukemia (ALL). ALL is further subdivided into B-cell acute lymphoblastic leukemia (B-ALL; Chapter 17) and T-cell acute lymphoblastic leukemia (T-ALL; Chapter 18). Since there is often an aberrant antigen expression in acute leukemias (phenotypic overlap between major three lineages, myeloid, B-lymphoblastic, and T-lymphoblastic) such as expression of myeloid antigens (CD13, CD33) in ALL or B- and T-cell antigens (CD7, CD19, and CD56) in AML, often referred to as lineage infidelity, WHO proposed strict criteria for lineage assignment. Myeloid lineage is defined by expression of myeloperoxidase (MPO) or evidence of monocytic differentiation (with positive non-specific esterase, NSE; CD11c, CD14, or CD64). T-lineage is defined by expression of surface or cytoplasmic CD3. B-lineage is defined (1) strong expression of CD19 with ≥1 of the following strongly expressed: CD79a, cytoplasmic CD22 and CD10 or (2) weak CD19 expression with ≥2 of the following strongly expressed: cytoplasmic CD79a, cytoplasmic CD22 and CD10. Only minor subset of acute leukemias show either lack of clear evidence of myeloid or lymphoid differentiation (acute undifferentiated leukemia; AUL) or show blasts with evidence of mixed lineage phenotype (mixed phenotype acute leukemia; MPAL). Both AUL and MPAL belong to the category of acute leukemias of ambiguous lineage in current WHO classification (Table 25.1) [1–10]. Those leukemias represent a heterogeneous group of rare leukemias with adverse prognosis. The diagnosis of AUL is made only if there is no expression of lineage-specific markers and less than two myeloid-associated markers (CD13, CD33, and/or CD117) [1, 10].

Acute leukemias of ambiguous lineage includes:

- Acute undifferentiated leukemia (AUL)
- Mixed phenotype acute leukemia (MPAL)
- MPALs with gene rearrangements
- Acute leukemias of ambiguous lineage, not otherwise specified
- *(Acute myeloid/T-lymphoblastic leukemia, AMTL; proposed category)*

Morphology of AUL

Agranular blasts have non-descript cytology without cytochemical positivity for myeloid or monocytic markers (MPO and non-specific esterase). Some cases may show cytoplasmic vacuolation.

Phenotype of AUL

AUL is a rare variant of acute leukemia, which is positive for CD34 (>90% of cases), TdT (>60% of cases), CD38, and HLA-DR, and does not express markers specific for myeloid or lymphoid lineages (Figure 25.1), except for occasional cases being positive for CD7 or one myeloid marker (CD13, CD33, or CD117). Dim and/or partial expression of CD10 or CD123 may also be seen. In a series reported by Heesch et al. (16 cases), most AULs showed expression of CD34, TdT, and HLA-DR [3]. In a series by Kurosawa et al. (12 cases), expression of CD13 was present in 60% of patients [11].

In series by Weinberg et al. (24 cases), 23/24 cases showed CD34 expression, 6 cases lack myeloid markers (CD117, CD13, CD33), and 15 showed partial or full expression of 1 myeloid marker, and 3 showed expression of 1 myeloid marker plus weak/partial expression of another myeloid marker on the blasts [10]. There was no expression of B-cell markers, with only 5/24 cases showing partial expression of cytoplasmic CD22 or cytoplasmic CD79a. None of the cases showed expression of surface or cytoplasmic CD3, but 11/24 cases were positive for other T-cell antigens (most often CD7). None of AUL in Weinberg series showed expression of two or more monocytic markers, but 2/24 cases were partially positive for CD11b, and 1/24 cases showed partial NSE staining.

Genetic features of AUL

AULs shows overexpression of *BAALC*, *ERG*, *MN1*, *WT1*, and *IGFBP7* genes when compared to T-ALL, B-ALL, and AML [3]. Genetic mutations or gene rearrangements commonly seen in AMLs or ALLs, such as *FLT3*, *WT1*, *KMT2A* (*MLL*), or *BCR-ABL1* are not seen in AUL [1, 3].

Differential diagnosis of AUL

Differential diagnosis of AUL includes:

- AML with minimal differentiation
- AML with myelodysplasia-related changes (AML-MRC)
- Acute megakaryoblastic leukemia
- Acute erythroid leukemia (AEL)
- Acute monoblastic leukemia
- Mixed phenotype acute leukemia (MPAL)
- B-cell acute lymphoblastic leukemia (B-ALL)
- T-cell acute lymphoblastic leukemia (T-ALL)
- Blastic plasmacytoid dendritic cell neoplasm (BPDCN)
- Aggressive NK-cell leukemia
- Large cell lymphoma in leukemic phase
- Poorly differentiated non-hematopoietic tumor

Acute myeloid leukemia with minimal differentiation

Presence of either MPO expression, at least two monocytic markers (NSE, CD11b, CD11c, CD14, and CD64) or two of additional myeloid markers (CD13, CD33, and/or CD117) indicates AML and excludes AUL (Figure 25.2). AML with minimal differentiation may show similar morphology to AUL without cytochemical evidence of myeloid differentiation, i.e., there is no MPO positivity (<3% blasts are MPO⁺). Since AML with minimal differentiation is negative for MPO, this variant of AML is diagnosed when there is an expression of at least two myeloid-associated markers (CD13, CD33, and/or CD117). In the study by Weinberg et al., comparing AUL and AML with minimal differentiation, AULs were characterized by more frequent mutations in *PHF6* and more frequent expression of TdT on blasts, while AML with minimal differentiation cases had more frequent CD123 expression [10].

AML-MRC

AML-MRC is diagnosed based on karyotype (MDS-related clonal changes), AML developing in patients with history of MDS or MDS/MPN (e.g., CMML, aCML) or presence of dysplasia in ≥50%

TABLE 25.1: WHO Classification of Acute Leukemias of Ambiguous Lineage

	B-lineage (CD19)[a]	T-lineage (CD3)	Myeloid Lineage (MPO)[b]
Acute undifferentiated leukemia	−	−	−
MPAL with t(9;22)/*BCR-ABL1*	+	+/−	+
MPAL with t(v;11q23)/*KMT2* (*MLL*)	+	−	+
MPAL (B/myeloid), NOS	+	−	+
MPAL (T/myeloid), NOS	−	+	+
MPAL, NOS (other)	+	+	+

Abbreviations: KMT2 (mixed lineage leukemia gene, MLL); MPAL, mixed phenotype acute leukemia.

[a] B-lineage is determined by (1) strong expression of CD19 with ≥1 of the following strongly expressed: CD79a, cytoplasmic CD22, and CD10; (2) weak CD19 expression with ≥2 of the following strongly expressed: cytoplasmic CD79a, cytoplasmic CD22, and CD10.

[b] MPO positivity in ≥3% of blasts by cytochemistry or ≥10% by flow cytometry (some authors use 13% threshold). Myeloid lineage may be also represented by monocytic differentiation (≥2 of the following: non-specific esterase, CD11c, CD14, CD36, CD64 lysozyme). If MPO is negative myeloid differentiation in AML can be also confirmed by strong expression of at least two myeloid-associated markers (CD13, CD33, and/or CD117).

cells in two or more myeloid lineages. AML-MRC may display phenotype compatible with AUL or AML not otherwise specified (often AML with minimal differentiation).

Acute monoblastic leukemia
Acute monocytic (monoblastic) leukemia is confirmed by positive expression of two or more monocytic markers (NSE, lysozyme, CD11b, CD11c, CD14, CD36, and CD64).

Acute megakaryoblastic leukemia and acute erythroid leukemia (AEL)
Acute megakaryoblastic leukemia is confirmed by positive expression of CD41 and CD61 expression and AEL is confirmed by positive CD71 (bright expression), hemoglobin A, e-cadherin, and GPHA expression.

Mixed phenotype acute leukemia (MPAL)
MPAL is positive for myeloid and lymphoid lineages, as defined by WHO (see section of MPAL, below). Figure 25.3 illustrates poorly differentiated acute leukemia, which is difficult to subclassify based on current criteria (lack of MPO expression does not favor MPAL and lack of CD3 does not favor T-ALL). Positive CD19 and partial cytoplasmic CD79a expression may suggest B-ALL differentiation (component), but there is also CD2 and CD117 expression, which overall raise the possibility of an unusual hybrid between MPAL and AUL.

Acute lymphoblastic leukemia
Negative surface or cytoplasmic CD3 excludes T-ALL and early T-cell precursor acute lymphoblastic leukemia (ETP-ALL). B-ALL is excluded by negative CD19, cytoplasmic CD22, and CD79a expression.

Other tumors
BPDCN is excluded by lack of co-expression of CD4 and CD56. Aggressive NK-cell leukemia is excluded by negative CD2, cytoplasmic CD3, CD16 and CD56 expression. Large B-cell or T-cell lymphomas in leukemic phase are excluded by lack of B- and T-cell markers.

Mixed phenotype acute leukemia

Introduction
Definition. Mixed phenotype acute leukemia (MPAL, biphenotypic acute leukemia) is a very rare disease [1–5, 9, 12, 13]. Two pattern of antigen expression by flow cytometry (FC) analysis are associated with MPAL. Co-expression of antigens classically associated with different lineages on the same cells (biphenotypic leukemia) or co-occurrence in the same sample of two or more blast populations from different lineages (bilineal leukemia). The WHO criteria for bilineal MPAL require that the sum of the two blast populations is at least 20% of nucleated cells [1].

Lineage criteria. In the WHO classification, only markers considered most lineage-specific have been retained for lineage assignment (Table 25.2) [1]. The B-lineage is confirmed by strong expression of CD19 and positive at least one of the following markers: cytoplasmic CD22, cytoplasmic CD79a or CD10. If the expression of CD19 is dim, two those additional markers are needed for B-lineage assignment. T-lineage is confirmed by either surface or cytoplasmic CD3 expression. Myeloid lineage is confirmed by positive MPO staining. If MPO is negative, MPAL can be diagnosed if blasts show strong expression of two of the other myeloid markers, including CD117, CD33, or CD13, or if the blasts display monocytic differentiation by showing expression of non-specific esterase (NSE), CD11c, CD14, CD64, or lysozyme. MPAL co-expresses myeloid (or monocytic) markers with B- or T-cell lineage specific marker. It is often positive for CD34, TdT, and HLA-DR. Although current WHO classification omits threshold for MPO or other markers positivity, in most published series the threshold for MPO positivity is 3% by cytochemistry and 10% or 13% by FC (when using isotype control to define the negative control population) [6, 14, 15]. Guy et al. compared the MPO threshold when isotype negative control with the threshold determined by normal lymphocytes as an internal negative control and found a significantly higher threshold of 28% [13, 15]. This higher threshold may be explained by greater autofluorescence of blasts when compared to mature lymphocytes leading to blasts having higher median fluorescence intensity than a negative lymphocyte population [13]. The most sensitive method for detection of MPO is reverse transcription-polymerase chain reaction, followed by immunohistochemistry, while both FC and cytochemistry are less specific. Based on WHO recommendation, if there is a weak expression of MPO by FC, "the diagnosis of MPAL may not be appropriate for cases that otherwise have typical precursor B-cell lymphoid phenotype with only a single blast population present" [1]. In those cases, correlation with other markers (CD117, CD13, and CD33) or immunohistochemistry staining for MPO on BM core or clot sections is recommended for final subclassification.

Lineage plasticity. MPAL, especially with *KMT2A* (*MLL*) rearrangements show ability to switch lineage between myeloid and lymphoid differentiation [16–22].

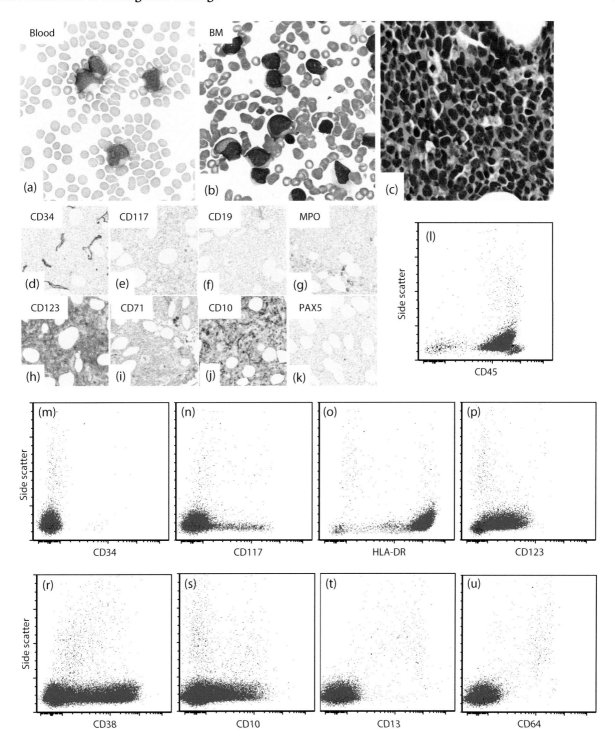

FIGURE 25.1   AUL. Blood (a) and BM aspirate smear (b) shows large blasts with irregular nuclei and prominent nucleoli. BM biopsy (c) shows replacement of the BM by sheets of immature cells. Based on immunohistochemistry (d–k) and flow cytometry (l–u), blasts are positive for CD45 (l), HLA-DR (o), CD123 (h, p), CD38 (r), and partially CD10 (j, s). Few blasts show CD117 expression (n).

Morphology

MPAL cells appear usually as morphologically undifferentiated agranular blasts, blasts with slight granulation, blasts with promonocytic features or rarely display two distinct populations of blasts with different size and morphology suggestive of a bilineal leukemia [5]. In large series of 100 patients with MPAL published by Matutes et al., morphology was consistent with ALL in 43%

and AML in 42% (remaining 15% of patients had inconclusive cytomorphology) [12].

Immunophenotype

In large series reported by Matutes et al., the phenotype was either B/myeloid (59%), T/myeloid (35%), B/T (4%) or B/T/myeloid (trilineage; 2%) [12]. In the same series, TdT was positive in 89%,

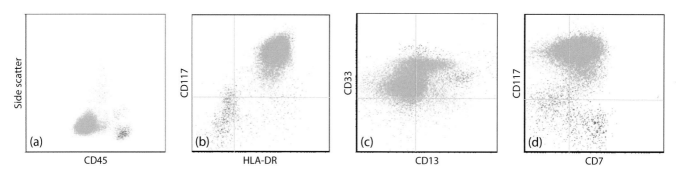

FIGURE 25.2 Minimally differentiated AML with dim CD45 (a, green dots), positive HLA-DR (b), positive CD117 (b), dim CD33 (c), mostly negative CD13 (c) and positive CD7 (d). Both AUL and AML with minimal differentiation are MPO negative but expression of two of myeloid markers (CD13, 33 and/or CD117) support the diagnosis of minimally differentiated AML.

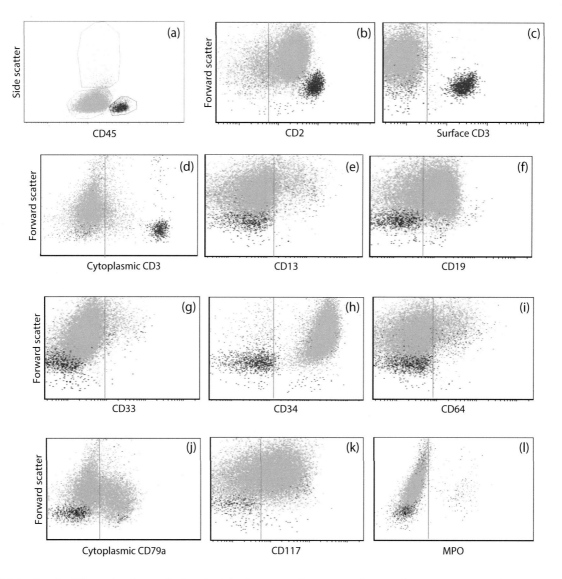

FIGURE 25.3 Poorly differentiated acute leukemia with phenotypic features overlapping between MPAL and AUL. Blasts (green dots) show the following phenotype: CD45+ (a), CD2+ (b), surface and cytoplasmic CD3− (c−d), CD13− (e), CD19+ (f), CD33− (g), CD34+ (h), CD64− (i), cytoplasmic CD79a partially positive (j), CD117+ (k) and MPO− (l). NGS studies showed mutations in *PHF6*, *TP53*, and *NRAS* genes.

TABLE 25.2: Phenotypic Markers to Define Mixed Phenotype Acute Leukemia (MPAL)

Myeloid Lineage[a]	MPO or evidence of monocytic differentiation (at least two of the following: NSE, CD11c, CD14, CD64, lysozyme
B-lineage	1. CD19 (strong) with at least one of the following: cytoplasmic CD79a, cytoplasmic CD22, CD10, or
	2. CD19 (weak) with at least 2 of the following: cytoplasmic CD79a, cytoplasmic CD22, CD10
T-lineage	CD3 (surface or cytoplasmic)

[a] MPO positivity in ≥3% of blasts by cytochemistry or ≥10% by flow cytometry (some authors use 13% threshold). AML with minimal differentiation does not show cytochemical evidence of myeloid differentiation, i.e., there is no MPO positivity (<3% blasts are MPO+). The myeloid differentiation in AML without MPO expression can be also confirmed by strong expression of at least two myeloid-associated markers (CD13, CD33, and/or CD117).

HLA-DR (human leukocyte antigen-D-related) in 92% and CD34 in 74%. Among cases with myeloid differentiation, MPO was expressed in at least 5% of blasts in 98% of cases and in >20% of blasts in 76% of the cases. In B-myeloid cases, CD19 was positive in 93% and was always associated with the expression of CD10, cytoplasmic CD22 and/or cytoplasmic CD79a. In leukemias with *KMT2A* rearrangements monocytic blast population often co-exist with ALL blasts and therefore special attention should be paid to differentiated normal (mature) monocytes from neoplastic monocytes using extended FC panel (CD2, CD11b, CD11c, CD14, CD34, CD56, CD64, CD117, and CD123). Relative frequency of MPAL subtype based on published series is 57% for B-ALL/AML (range 45%–73%), 34% for T-ALL/AML (range 22%–45%), 4% for B-ALL/T-ALL/AML (range 0.7%–3.6%), and 4% for B-ALL/T-ALL (range 0%–12%), as summarized by Porwit and Bene [5]. Figures 25.4–25.7 show examples of biphenotypic leukemia and Figure 25.8 shows an example of bilineal leukemia.

Genetic features

Genetics studies show t(9;22) (20%–30%), 11q23 *KTM2A* rearrangement (8%), *WT1* mutations (18%), complex changes (32%), or normal karyotype (13%) [3, 12].

Differential diagnosis of MPAL

The differential diagnosis between MPAL, AUL, and some other acute leukemias is presented in Table 25.3. Some ALL categories may express myeloid antigens, yet usually with a weaker intensity then in AML. CD13 and CD33 are the myeloid antigens most often expressed on the most immature B-ALL (B-I and B-II according to EGIL) as well as the most immature T-ALL (T-I) and ETP-ALL [23]. B-ALL cases are often homogeneous in their immunophenotypic characteristics. The issue of MPO-only positive B-ALL (cases where the general immunophenotype of blasts is consistent with B-ALL but a fraction of blasts appears to be MPO+) is of uncertain clinical significance [5, 24, 25]. In a study

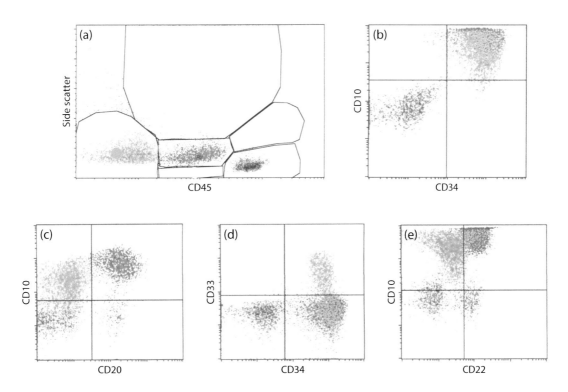

FIGURE 25.4 Bilineal mixed phenotype acute leukemia (MPAL; AML/B-ALL) – BM (flow cytometry). Side scatter versus CD45 (a) shows two populations of blasts: CD45+ blasts (green dots) and CD45- blasts (orange dots). CD45+ blasts have phenotype compatible with B-ALL: CD34+ (b and d), bright CD10+ (b–c), CD20+ (c), CD33− (d), and CD22+ (e). The other population of blasts (CD45−) is CD34+ (b and d), CD33+ (d), and negative for B-cell markers (c, e).

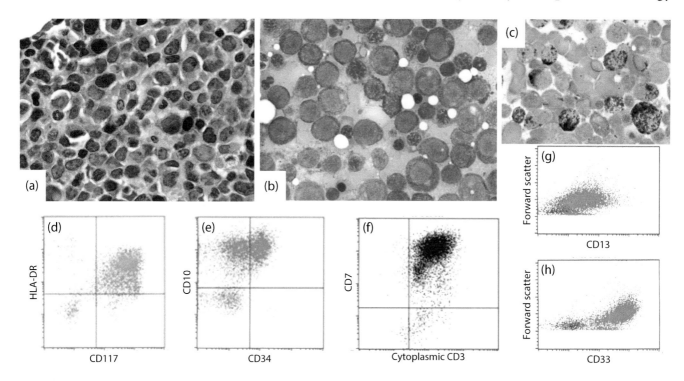

FIGURE 25.5   MPAL (AML/T-ALL) – BM. (a) Hypercellular bone marrow showing complete replacement by large blasts. (b) Aspirate smear showing blasts and rare erythroid precursors. (c) Blasts are positive for MPO. (d-h) Flow cytometry analysis shows the following phenotype of blasts: HLA-DR+ (d), CD117+ (d), CD34+ (e), CD10+ (e), CD7+ (f), cytoplasmic CD3+ (f), CD13+ (g; dim), and CD33+ (h).

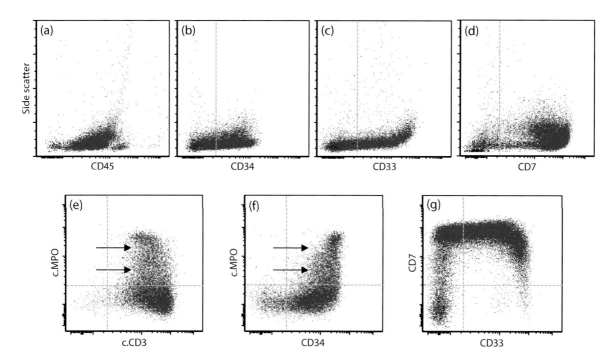

FIGURE 25.6   MPAL (AML/T-ALL) – flow cytometry. Blasts have the following phenotype: CD45+ (a), CD34+ (b), CD33+ (c), CD7+ (d), cytoplasmic CD3+ (e), and cytoplasmic MPO+ (e–f; partial). Note bright expression of CD7 and variable ("smeary") expression of CD33 (g).

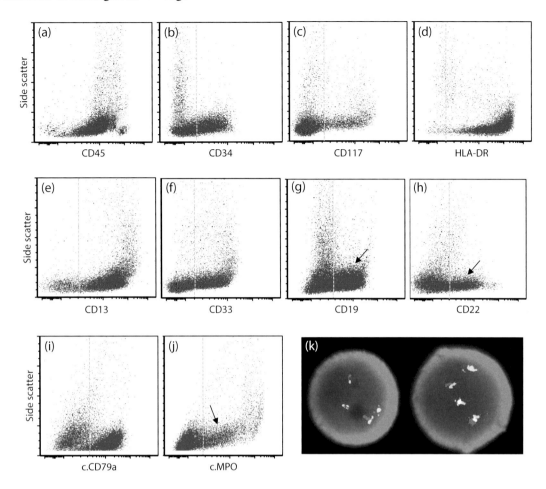

FIGURE 25.7 MPAL (AML/B-ALL; *BCR-ABL1*⁺) – flow cytometry and FISH. Blasts are positive for CD45 (a), CD34 (b), CD117 (c; partial expression), HLA-DR (d), CD13 (e), CD33 (f), CD19 (g), CD22 (h), cytoplasmic CD79a (i), and partially MPO (j). FISH studies showed *BCR-ABL1* fusion (k; aqua, arginosuccinate synthetase 1 gene on 9q34; green, *BCR* gene on chr.22; and red, *ABL1* gene on chromosome 9; yellow signal indicates *BCR-ABL1* fusion).

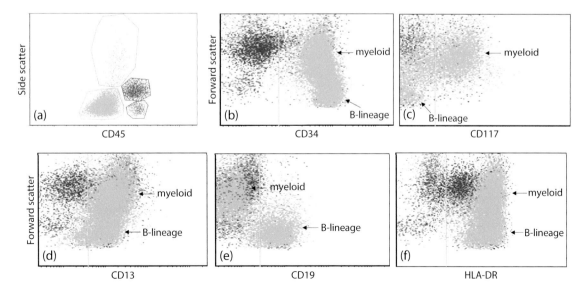

FIGURE 25.8 Bilineal MPAL composed of blasts with AML phenotype and separate population of blasts with B-ALL phenotype. Blasts (green dots) show low side scatter and moderate CD45 (a). They are positive for CD34 (b), with blasts of lineage showing slightly brighter expression. Blasts of myeloid lineage are positive for CD117 (c) and CD13 (d), negative for CD19 (e), and positive for HLA-DR (f). Blasts with B-phenotype are negative for CD117 (c), positive for CD13 (d), positive for CD19 (e), and positive for HLA-DR (f).

TABLE 25.3: Differential Diagnosis of AUL and MPAL

	AUL	AML Minimally Differentiated[a]	ETP-ALL	T-ALL[b]	B-ALL	MPAL (T-ALL/AML)	MPAL (B-ALL/AML)
CD1a+	–	–	–	+/–	–	–	–
CD2+	–	–/(+)	–/(+)	+/–	–	+/–	–
c.CD3+	–	–	+	+	–	+	–
CD4+	–	–/(+)	–	b	–	–/+	–
CD5+	–	–	–/(+)<75%	+/–	–	+/–	–
CD7+	–	–/+	+	+/(–)	–	+/–	–
CD8+	–	–	–	b	–	–	–
CD10+	–	–	–/(+)	–/+	+/(–)	–	+/–
CD11b+	–	–	+/(–)	–	–	–	–
CD13+	–	+	+/–	–/+	–/+	+/(–)	+/–
c.CD22+		–	–	–	+	–	+/–
CD33+	–	+	+/–	–/+	–/+	+/(–)	+/–
CD34+	+	+	+	+/–	+/(–)	+	+
CD56+	–	–/(+)	–	–/(+)	–	–/(+)	–
c.CD79+a	–	–	–	–	+	–	+/–
CD117+	–	+/–	+/(–)	–/(+)	–	+/(-)	+/–
HLA-DR+	+	+/(–)	+/–	–/(+)	+	+/–	+/–
MPO+	–	–	–	–	–	+	+

Abbreviations: AUL, acute undifferentiated leukemia; ETP-ALL, early T-cell precursor acute lymphoblastic leukemia; T-ALL, T-cell acute lymphoblastic leukemia (not including ETP-ALL); MPAL, mixed phenotype acute leukemia; AML, acute myeloid leukemia; MPO, myeloperoxidase.

Notes: +, positive (+), rarely positive; –, negative; (–) rarely negative.

[a] In AML with minimal differentiation MPO is negative (<3% blasts are positive) and myeloid lineage is confirmed by strong expression of two of the following markers: CD13, CD33 and CD117.

[b] Either dual CD4/CD8+ or dual CD4/CD8–.

by Oberley et al., this group had an increased rate of relapse and a worse event-free survival than the patients with B-ALL who did not express MPO [24]. In majority of these cases, MPO cannot be detected by cytochemistry and/or IHC. Most probably, cases with only a single blast population should not be considered MPAL if weak MPO expression by flow cytometry is the only evidence of myeloid differentiation [1, 5]. The proportion of MPO positive cells is controversial, but a 3% cutoff is the level retained in cytochemistry. Identifying the MPO expression by flow cytometry is not completely equal to assessing the enzymatic activity, but the suggested threshold in flow cytometry is 10% [6].

References

1. Swerdlow, S.H., et al., ed. *WHO classification of tumors of haematopoietic and lymphoid tissues*. 2016, IARC: Lyon.
2. Bene, M.C. and A. Porwit, *Acute leukemias of ambiguous lineage*. Semin Diagn Pathol, 2012. **29**(1): p. 12–8.
3. Heesch, S., et al., *Acute leukemias of ambiguous lineage in adults: molecular and clinical characterization*. Ann Hematol, 2013. **92**(6): p. 747–58.
4. Porwit, A. and M.C. Bene, *Acute leukemias of ambiguous origin*. Am J Clin Pathol, 2015. **144**(3): p. 361–76.
5. Porwit, A. and M.C. Bene, *Multiparameter flow cytometry applications in the diagnosis of mixed phenotype acute leukemia*. Cytometry B Clin Cytom, 2019. **96**(3): p. 183–94.
6. van den Ancker, W., et al., *A threshold of 10% for myeloperoxidase by flow cytometry is valid to classify acute leukemia of ambiguous and myeloid origin*. Cytometry B Clin Cytom, 2013. **84**(2): p. 114–8.
7. Gutierrez, A. and A. Kentsis, *Acute myeloid/T-lymphoblastic leukaemia (AMTL): a distinct category of acute leukaemias with common pathogenesis in need of improved therapy*. Br J Haematol, 2018. **180**(6): p. 919–24.
8. Inukai, T., et al., *Clinical significance of early T-cell precursor acute lymphoblastic leukaemia: results of the Tokyo Children's Cancer Study Group Study L99-15*. Br J Haematol, 2012. **156**(3): p. 358–65.
9. Noronha, E.P., et al., *T-lymphoid/myeloid mixed phenotype acute leukemia and early T-cell precursor lymphoblastic leukemia similarities with NOTCH1 mutation as a good prognostic factor*. Cancer Manag Res, 2019. **11**: p. 3933–43.
10. Weinberg, O.K., et al., *Clinical, immunophenotypic, and genomic findings of acute undifferentiated leukemia and comparison to acute myeloid leukemia with minimal differentiation: a study from the bone marrow pathology group*. Mod Pathol, 2019. **32**(9): p. 1373–85.
11. Kurosawa, S., et al., *Outcome of patients with acute undifferentiated leukemia after allogeneic hematopoietic stem cell transplantation*. Leuk Lymphoma, 2018. **59**(12): p. 3006–9.
12. Matutes, E., et al., *Mixed-phenotype acute leukemia: clinical and laboratory features and outcome in 100 patients defined according to the WHO 2008 classification*. Blood, 2011. **117**(11): p. 3163–71.
13. Charles, N.J. and D.F. Boyer, *Mixed-Phenotype Acute Leukemia: Diagnostic Criteria and Pitfalls*. Arch Pathol Lab Med, 2017. **141**(11): p. 1462–8.
14. Bennett, J.M., et al., *Proposals for the classification of the acute leukaemias. French-American-British (FAB) co-operative group*. Br J Haematol, 1976. **33**(4): p. 451–8.
15. Guy, J., et al., *Flow cytometry thresholds of myeloperoxidase detection to discriminate between acute lymphoblastic or myeloblastic leukaemia*. Br J Haematol, 2013. **161**(4): p. 551–5.
16. Sakaki, H., et al., *Early lineage switch in an infant acute lymphoblastic leukemia*. Int J Hematol, 2009. **90**(5): p. 653–5.
17. Hanley, B.P., et al., *Lineage switch from acute myeloid leukemia to T cell/myeloid mixed phenotype acute leukemia: First report of an adult case*. Am J Hematol, 2018. **93**(12): p. E395–7.
18. Marco-Ayala, J., et al., *Lineage switch from B lymphoblastic leukemia with KMT2A-rearranged to mixed-phenotype acute leukemia under daratumumab*. Blood Res, 2020. **55**(2). p. 75.

19. Rossi, J.G., et al., *Lineage switch in childhood acute leukemia: an unusual event with poor outcome.* Am J Hematol, 2012. **87**(9): p. 890–7.

20. Ciolli, S., et al., *Mixed acute leukemia with genotypic lineage switch: a case report.* Leukemia, 1993. **7**(7): p. 1061–5.

21. van den Ancker, W., et al., *Uncommon lineage switch warrants immunophenotyping even in relapsing leukemia.* Leuk Res, 2009. **33**(7): p. e77–80.

22. Nomani, L., J.R. Cook, and H.J. Rogers, *Very rare lineage switch from acute myeloid leukemia to mixed phenotype acute leukemia, B/Myeloid, during chemotherapy with no clonal evolution.* Int J Lab Hematol, 2019. **41**(4): p. e86–8.

23. Bene, M.C., et al., *Proposals for the immunological classification of acute leukemias. European group for the immunological characterization of leukemias (EGIL).* Leukemia, 1995. **9**(10): p. 1783–6.

24. Oberley, M.J., et al., *Clinical significance of isolated myeloperoxidase expression in pediatric B-lymphoblastic leukemia.* Am J Clin Pathol, 2017. **147**(4): p. 374–81.

25. Raikar, S.S., et al., *Isolated myeloperoxidase expression in pediatric B/myeloid mixed phenotype acute leukemia is linked with better survival.* Blood, 2018. **131**(5): p. 573–7.

Blastic plasmacytoid dendritic cell neoplasm (BPDCN)

BPDCN phenotype by flow cytometry: CD2$^{-/rarely+}$, s.CD3$^-$, c.CD3$^-$, CD4$^+$, CD7$^{-/+}$, CD11b$^-$, CD11c$^{-/rarely+}$, CD13$^-$, CD14$^-$, CD16$^-$, CD33$^{-/rarely+}$, CD34$^-$, CD36$^{-/+}$, CD43$^+$, CD45$^+$, CD56$^+$, CD64$^-$, CD117$^{-/rarely+}$, CD123$^{+bright}$, CD303$^{+/-}$, HLA-DR$^+$TdT$^{+/-}$

Introduction
Blastic plasmacytoid dendritic cell neoplasm (BPDCN; synonyms: blastic NK-cell lymphoma/leukemia; DC2 acute leukemia; CD4$^+$/CD56$^+$ hematodermic neoplasm) is a highly aggressive neoplasm derived from the precursors of plasmacytoid dendritic cells (PDC) which involves the skin and often disseminates into other organs with leukemic blood and bone marrow (BM) involvement [1–6]. It occurs at any age but most often affects mainly elderly patients (7th decade) who present with isolated skin lesion that rapidly evolves to multiple sites, including BM, blood, CNS, spleen, liver, lungs and kidneys [7–9]. Due to frequent and extensive BM involvement, most patients have anemia and neutropenia [7, 8]. The ontogenic origin has not been clearly identified, but it has been suggested that it arises from transformed CD56$^+$ "plasmacytoid" monocyte-like dendritic cells (pDC; DC-2) [10–13]. About 10%–20% of cases is associated with or develops into a myelomonocytic leukemia or AML. FISH for 9p21.3 locus is useful in prognostication, since patients with homozygous loss of 9p21.3 have a worse prognosis than those with hemizygous loss [14].

Morphology
Cytomorphology. Tumors are composed of intermediate-sized immature-looking mononuclear cells with blastic morphology, which are pleomorphic and may vary in size from small to intermediate to large (Figure 26.1). The nuclei are round with nucleolus and cytoplasm is abundant and pale basophilic without granules. Myeloperoxidase (MPO), non-specific esterase (NSE), and butyrate esterase cytochemical staining is negative.

Skin. Skin (Figure 26.2) shows diffuse infiltrate by medium-sized cells with blastoid features (fine chromatin pattern and nucleoli).

Lymph nodes. Lymph nodes may be involved (Figure 26.3) and show either diffuse or paracortical pattern of involvement by poorly differentiated blastoid cells.

Bone marrow. Prominent BM involvement (Figure 26.4) is seen in a majority of cases of BPDCN [7, 9, 12].

Immunophenotype
BPDCN show low side scatter and dim to moderate CD45 expression falling into the "blast" gate on CD45 versus SCC display. Typically, BPDCNs express CD4, CD56, CD123, TCL1, HLA-DR, and TCF4 (Figures 26.5–26.8). Blasts of BPDCN can be distinguished from their mature counterparts (benign PDC) by morphology and expression of CD56 and CD33. The expression of

CD4 and/or CD56 may be dim or partial in rare cases. Subset of cases are positive for CD2, CD7, TdT, CD36, CD303, CD33, or CD117. The intensity of expression of CD123 is stronger than in CD123$^+$ cases of AML or ALL. There is no surface or cytoplasmic CD3, B-cell markers, MPO, CD11b, CD11c, plasma cell markers, monocytic markers (CD14, CD64), and TCRαβ or TCRγδ. In reported series, tumor cells expressed CD56, CD43, HLA-DR, and CD4, as well as the following markers: CD45 (dim to moderate expression), CD116, CD123 (IL-3α receptor), CD45RA, BDCA-2 (blood dendritic cell antigen-2; CD303), BDCA-4 (CD304), and ILT-3 (immunoglobulin-like transcript-3) [2, 7, 11, 12, 15–19]. In the series reported by Wang et al., CD303 was positive in 44%, CD7 in 64%, CD2 in 19%, CD33 in 48%, TdT in 25%, CD36 in 57%, and partial CD117 in 9% of cases [20]. Aberrant phenotype of BPDCNs, which is seen in subset of cases, includes positive expression of CD7, CD33, CD34, CD117, CD36, and/or CD79a, decreased or negative CD38, negative CD2, bright HLA-DR, and decreased CD123. Case with lack of CD4 expression has been reported [21]. BPDCNs are negative for CD3, CD13, CD16, CD19, CD20, and MPO. Very rare cases of BPDCN may be CD10$^+$.

Genetic features
Integrated genomic analysis using expression profiling and array-based CGH demonstrated that BPDCN shows distinct gene expression profiles and distinct patterns of chromosomal aberrations when compared to acute myelomonocytic leukemia involving skin; BPDCN was characterized by recurrent deletion of regions on chromosome 4 (4q34), chromosome 9 (9p13-p11 and 9q12-q34), and chromosome 13 (13q12-q31), that contain several tumor suppressor genes with diminished expression (*Rb1*, *LATS2*) [22]. The balanced translocation t(3;5)(q21;q31) appears to be specific for BPDCN [23]. Leroux et al. reported clonal, mostly complex chromosome aberrations in 66% of patients with BPDCN [15]. The recurrent abnormalities involved long arm of chromosome 5 (targeting two regions, 5q21 or 5q34; 72%), 12p (64%), 13q (64%), −6q/del(6q23-qter) (50%), −15q, (43%), and −9 (28%) [15]. In a series reported by Lucioni et al., there was a mean of 7 copy number alterations per case (21 cases analyzed), with prevalence of losses over gains [14]. Most affected were chromosomes 9 (71%), 13 (61%), 12 (57%), 5 (19%), 7 (19%), 14 (19%), and 15 (15%). Deletion of 9p21.3 locus was identified in 14 patients (66.6%), 5 homozygous and 9 hemizygous and containing *CDKN2A*, *CDKN2B*, and *MTAP* [14]. Median overall survival was 11 months for cases with homozygous loss, compared with 26 months for homozygous loss. BPDCN harbors a gene expression profile similar to AML and has mutations in genes commonly altered in myeloid neoplasms, such as *TET2*, *ASXL1*, RNA-splicing factors, and *TP53*.

Differential diagnosis
Differential diagnosis of BPDCN includes:

- Mature plasmacytoid dendritic cell proliferations
- Acute monoblastic (monocytic) leukemia,
- Acute myeloid leukemia (AML)
- Extramedullary myeloid tumor (EMT), especially monoblastic sarcoma,

DOI: 10.1201/9781003197935-26

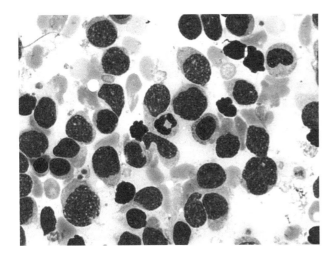

FIGURE 26.1 Blastic plasmacytoid dendritic cell neoplasm – cytology. Bone marrow aspirate with predominance of blasts. Tumor cells have irregular nuclei, inconspicuous nucleoli and pale baso-philic cytoplasm.

- Cutaneous involvement by chronic myelomonocytic leukemia (CMML)
- Large B- and T-cell lymphomas
- Extranodal T/NK-cell lymphoma (nasal type)
- Plasmablastic lymphoma (PBL)
- Poorly differentiated plasma cell myeloma (PCM)
- B-cell and T-cell acute lymphoblastic leukemia/lymphoma (B-ALL, T-ALL)
- Histiocytic sarcoma
- NK/T-cell lymphoma/leukemia
- Non-hematopoietic small "blue cell" tumors

Differential diagnosis of BPDCN based on CD56 expression includes:

- Extranodal T/NK-cell lymphoma, nasal type (ENKTCL)
- Peripheral T-cell lymphoma (PTCL), subset
- T-LGL leukemia
- NK-cell proliferations
- Anaplastic large cell lymphoma (ALCL), subset
- Hepatosplenic T-cell lymphoma (HSTL)

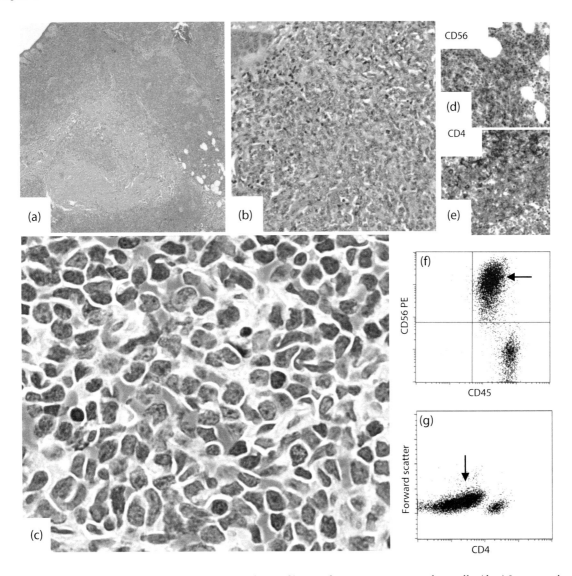

FIGURE 26.2 BPDCN – skin. (a–c) Histology shows diffuse infiltrate of immature mononuclear cells. (d–g) Immunophenotyping (flow cytometry and immunohistochemistry) shows expression of CD56 (d, f) andCD4 (e, g).

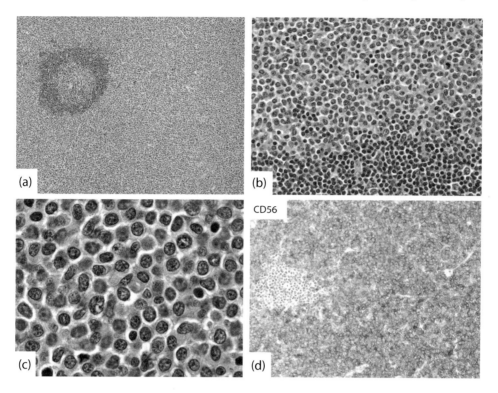

FIGURE 26.3 BPDCN – lymph node. (a) Low magnification shows dense interfollicular infiltrate. (b–c) Higher magnification shows predominance of blasts with round nuclei, prominent nucleoli, and scanty to moderate cytoplasm. (d) Blasts are strongly positive for CD56.

- Monomorphic epitheliotropic intestinal T-cell lymphoma (MEITL)
- Enteropathy-associated T-cell lymphoma (EATL), subset
- Primary cutaneous γδ T-cell lymphoma (PCGD-TCL)
- Plasma cell myeloma (PCM)
- AML, most often AML with t(8;21)
- Acute monoblastic leukemia

Differential diagnosis of BPDCN based on CD123 expression includes:

- AML; subset
- CMML, subset
- B-ALL, T-ALL, subset
- Hairy cell leukemia (HCL)
- NK-cell malignancies

Mature plasmacytoid dendritic cell proliferations

Mature plasmacytoid dendritic cell proliferations are composed of mature PDC, which are CD4+, CD123+, CD68+, CD71+, CD43+, TCL1+ and negative for T-cells antigens (CD2, CD3, CD5, and CD7), B-cell antigens (CD19, CD20), CD30, myeloid antigens (CD13, CD33), CD11b, CD11c, CD14, CD56, and blastic markers (CD34 and CD117) [3, 4, 24–26]. Reactive PDCs can be detected routinely in the BM. They are be associated with myeloid neoplasms, especially CMML and may be increased also in reactive processes (inflammatory processes, non-specific lymphadenopathies or Kikuchi lymphadenitis), post treatment BMs, and in lymphomas (including Hodgkin lymphoma, marginal zone lymphoma, and other) [26]. The concurrent myeloid neoplasm dominates the clinical and morphological features. Scattered PDCs or even small clusters can be seen in normal BM, but larger, well demarcated tumor forming aggregates have been described in association with CMML and other myeloid neoplasms with monocytic differentiation and may occur in lymph nodes, skin, spleen, or BM [24, 26]. In rare cases, the infiltrate of PDCs may be diffuse, effacing the underlying architecture, but in contrast to BPDCN, there is no CD56 and TdT expression. Clusters of CD123+ PDC have been observed in primary cutaneous marginal zone lymphoma and in majority of reactive cutaneous lymphoid hyperplasia but only in a minority of primary cutaneous follicle center lymphoma (13%) and not in primary cutaneous diffuse large B-cell lymphoma, leg type. [27]. Wang et al. reported 10-color flow cytometry panel which allowed for distinction between reactive PDC and BPDCN [20]. In their series, normal (reactive) PDC were positive for CD4, CD38, CD45, CD123, CD303, and HLA-DR, and negative for CD64 [20]. Subset of normal PDC was positive for CD2 (with bimodal pattern ranging from negative to positive cells) and CD7 (median 13%; range 0.3% to 21% of cells positive). CD56 was observed in a subset of normal(reactive) cells (median 4.5%; range 1.3% to 20%), and all CD7+ normal PDC were negative for CD56 [20]. Compared to reactive PDC, BPDCNs show brighter expression of HLA-DR (69%), lower expression of CD123 (78%) and CD38 (78%), and more often negative CD303 (44% in BPDCN, 100% in reactive cells) and CD33 (48% in BPDCN, 100% in reactive) [20]. CD56+ reactive PDC were uniformly positive for CD2, had bright expression of CD38 and negative CD7, while BPDCN cells were often negative for CD2 (81%), positive for CD7 (64%) and showed decreased or negative expression of CD38 (82%) [20].

AML and EMT

BPDCN shares with acute monoblastic leukemia some of the clinical, morphologic and immunophenotypic characteristics. Acute monoblastic leukemia may present with extramedullary location,

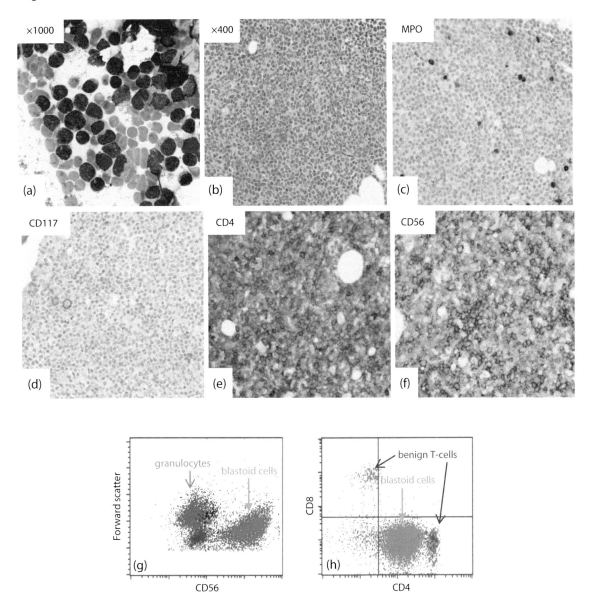

FIGURE 26.4 BPDCN – BM involvement. Poorly differentiated cells resembling myeloblasts and/or monoblasts are present in the BM aspirate smear (a). BM core biopsy shows diffuse replacement of the marrow elements by immature cells (b). Tumor cells are negative for MPO (c) and CD117 (d) and express CD4 (e and g) and CD56 (f) [c–f, immunohistochemistry; g–h, flow cytometry].

including skin (monoblastic sarcoma) and is often positive for CD4 and CD56 (Figure 26.9) and may be positive for both CD123 and CD68. In contrast to acute monoblastic leukemia (monoblastic sarcoma), BPDCN is negative for NSE and majority of monocytic markers (CD11b, CD11c, CD14, CD64, and lysozyme). Although BPDCNs may show aberrant expression of individual myeloid or monocytic markers, in contrast to AMLs they are negative for CD13 and MPO and do not show strong co-expression of both CD33 and CD117. Strong expression of CD123 in conjunction with co-expression of CD4 and CD45, weak expression of CD45 and lack of MPO is typical for BPDCN and helps to exclude AML. Hamadeh et al. described AML cases with plasmacytoid dendritic cell differentiation, with or without monocytic differentiation based on expression of CD34, CD45, CD123, and CD304 [19]. In contrast to BPDCN, all acute leukemia cases with plasmacytoid dendritic cell differentiation lack the expression of CD56. Four of those cases had circulating PDC in blood.

Cutaneous involvement by chronic myelomonocytic leukemia (CMML)

In CMML cases involving skin, Vittae et al., distinguished four clinicopathologic categories of skin involvement [28]:

* Myelomonocytic tumors (MMCT)
* Mature plasmacytoid dendritic cell proliferations
* Blastic plasmacytoid dendritic cell neoplasms (BPDCN)
* Blastic indeterminate dendritic cell tumors

Small clusters of mature PDC are often intermixed with a frequent reactive component consisting of histiomonocytes, lymphocytes, plasma cells and eosinophils. In some cases there is also often an accumulation of scattered or clustered large cells with large, pale, and irregular nucleoli, morphologically similar to large histiocytes or Langerhans cells and corresponding to the definition of indeterminate dendritic cells (IDC) [28]. These

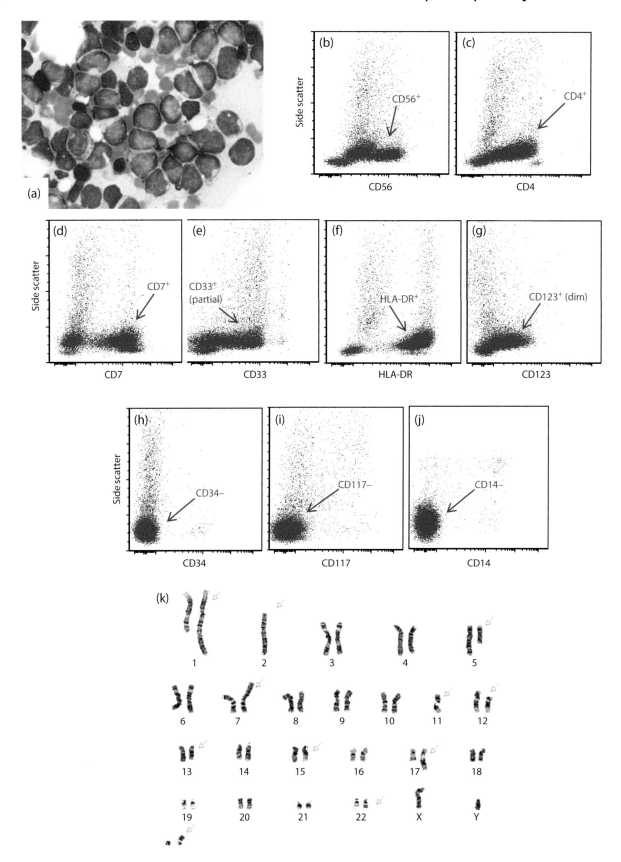

FIGURE 26.5 BPDCN – flow cytometry of the BM aspirate. Neoplastic cells (a; aspirate smear) are positive for CD56 (b), CD4 (c), CD7 (d), CD33 (e; partial), HLA-DR (f), CD123 (g), and do not express CD34 (h), CD117 (i) and CD14 (j). Metaphase cytogenetics (k) shows complex karyotypic abnormalities: 44~46,XY, add(1)(q23),−2, del(5)(q13q33), add(7)(p11.2), −11, del(12)(p11.2p13), del(13)(q12q14), add(15)(q22), add(17)(q21), add(22)(q13),+2mar.

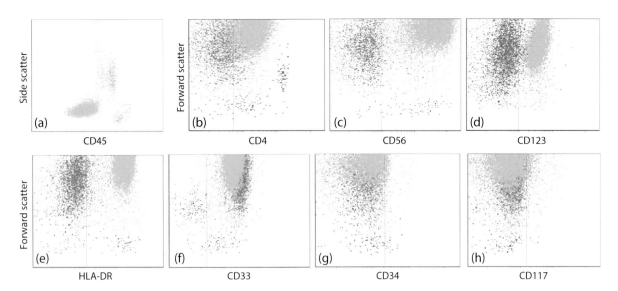

FIGURE 26.6 BPDCN – flow cytometry (BM). Blasts (green dots) show dim to moderate CD45 and low side scatter (a), positive CD4 (b), CD56 (c), CD123 (d), and positive HLA-DR (e), as well as aberrant expression of CD33 (f). CD34 (g) and CD117 (h) are negative.

clusters of IDCs are intermixed or surrounded by PDCs. PDCs display typical phenotype with CD123, CD303, TCL1, and granzyme B expression. IDCs are positive for CD1a.

Large B- and T-cell lymphomas

Expression of some T-cell markers (CD2 and CD7) and B-cell markers (CD79a) can be observed in BPDCN, but lack of CD3 and CD19/CD20 helps to exclude mature T- and B-cell lymphomas. Some variants of large B-cell lymphomas are usually negative for B-cell markers (CD20, CD79a, and PAX5), including ALK+ large B-cell lymphoma (ALK+ LBCL), PBL, and primary effusion lymphoma (PEL). ALK+ LBCL does not express CD4 and CD56 and can be confirmed by ALK staining. PBL most often involves head and neck areas (oral cavity) and is typically positive for plasma cell markers (CD138, MUM1), EBER and in subset of cases CD56. PEL most commonly involves pleural, pericardial and peritoneal cavities and is characterized by expression of HHV8 and EBER.

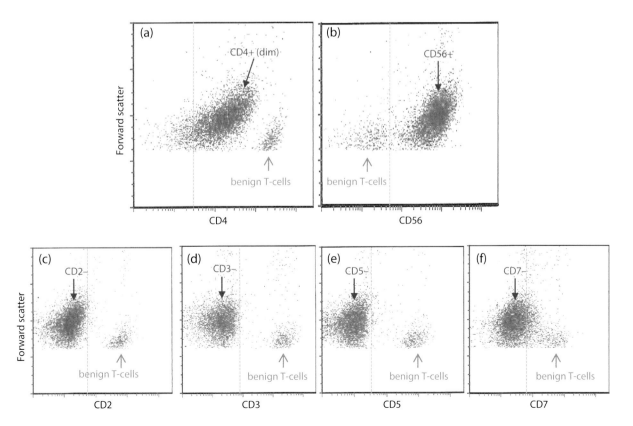

FIGURE 26.7 BPDCN (skin) – flow cytometry. Neoplastic cells are positive for CD4 (a) and CD56 (b). Pan-T-cell markers are negative (c–f).

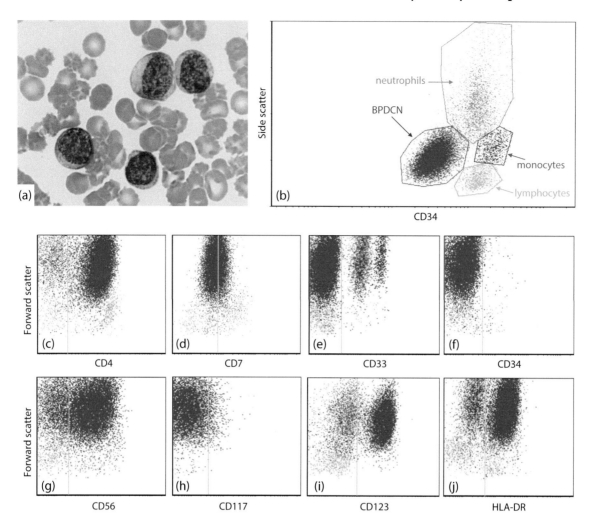

FIGURE 26.8 BPDCN (blood sample from 76-year-old patient with skin lesion and leukocytosis). Blood smear (a) shows numerous blasts. Flow cytometry (b-j) shows the following phenotype of blasts (magenta dots): CD45+ (b), CD4+ (c), CD7−/+ (d), CD33− (e), CD34− (f), CD56+ (g), CD117− (h), CD123+ (j), and HLA-DR+ (k).

Extranodal T/NK-cell lymphoma, nasal type (ENKTL)

ENKTL has always extranodal localization, including typically nasal cavity but also skin, gastrointestinal tract, and soft tissues. Advanced cases show dissemination to lymph nodes, blood and BM. Tumor cells are positive for EBV (EBER), CD2, CD56, and cytoplasmic CD3. CD4 is negative. In contrast to ENKTL, BPDCNs are negative for EBV antigens and EBV-encoded small RNA (EBER).

Poorly differentiated plasma cell myeloma (PCM)

Poorly differentiated PCMs with CD56 expression may mimic cytologically and phenotypically BPDCN. They differ by presence of serum monoclonal protein, positive plasma cell markers (CD138, MUM1), lack of HLA-DR, and most often CD45 and expression of cytoplasmic light and heavy chain immunoglobulins.

B-cell and T-cell acute lymphoblastic leukemia/lymphoma (B-ALL, T-ALL)

B-ALL can be differentiated by immunophenotyping, showing expression of CD19, CD22, CD79a (and occasionally CD20), blastic markers, (CD34 and/or TdT) and in many cases CD10. T-ALL is rarely CD56+ and shows either dual CD4/CD8 positivity or lack of both CD4 and CD8. It is frequently positive for CD7, but in

contrast to BPDCN is usually HLA-DR−, shows cytoplasmic CD3 expression and presence of one or more of immature markers (CD1a, CD34, and/or TdT).

Histiocytic sarcoma

Histiocytic sarcomas (HSs) are often CD4+, but usually do not express CD56. They are positive for one or more of the histiocytic markers (CD68, CD163, and lysozyme), CD45 and HLA-DR.

NK/T-cell lymphoma/leukemia

Aggressive NK-cell tumors, including aggressive NK-cell leukemia or disseminated ENKTL may involve any organs and are characterized by monotonous, diffuse proliferation of medium to large cells with CD56 expression, which can mimic BPDCN. They show NK-cell phenotype (CD2+, cytoplasmic CD3+, CD5−, and CD56+) and co-expression of EBER.

Non-hematopoietic small "blue cell" tumors

Non-hematopoietic tumors with CD56 expression can be differentiated from BPDCN by showing expression of cytokeratins (e.g., small cell carcinoma, Merkel cell carcinoma), S100 and HMB45 (melanoma) and specific sarcoma markers (e.g., desmin in rhabdomyosarcoma).

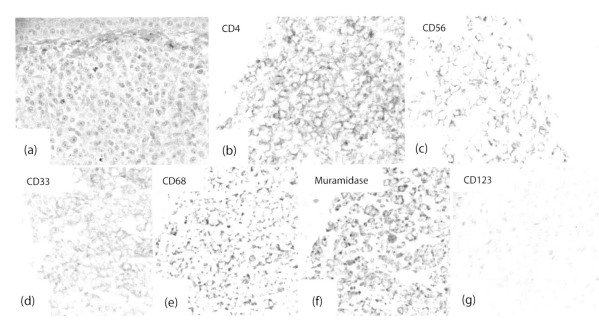

FIGURE 26.9 Skin with monoblastic sarcoma. (a) Histology shows diffuse infiltrate by large blasts. (b–g) Immunohistochemistry. Similar to BPDCN, acute monoblastic leukemia (monoblastic sarcoma) is often positive for CD4 (b) and CD56 (c), but presence of monocytic and myeloid markers, including CD33 (d), CD69 (f), and muramidase (f) and lack of CD123 expression (g) help to exclude BPDCN and confirm monocytic differentiation.

Follicular dendritic cell neoplasms

Follicular dendritic cells are located in the B-cell follicles of secondary lymphoid follicles. Follicular dendritic cell sarcoma is a rare tumor that typically arises within lymph nodes but can also occur in extranodal sites (Figures 26.10–26.12). It is a spindle cell neoplasm showing variety of growth patterns (whorled, storiform, fascicular, and nodular) [29–35]. Both low- and high-grade features may predominate. Tumor cells are positive for CD21, CD23, CXCL13, CD35, clusterin, fascin, desmoplakin, vimentin and epidermal growth factor receptor (EGFR). They usually lack CD45. B- and T-cell markers and CD30 are

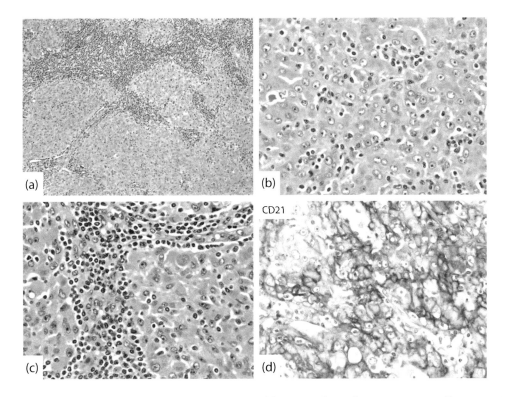

FIGURE 26.10 Follicular dendritic cell sarcoma. (a–c) Histology. (d) Immunohistochemistry: tumor cells are positive for CD21.

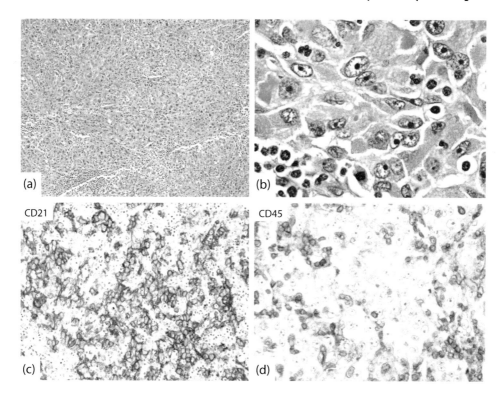

FIGURE 26.11 Follicular dendritic cell sarcoma. (a) Low magnification shows nests of atypical plump cells with abundant eosinophilic cytoplasm. (b) High magnification shows pleomorphic cells with abundant eosinophilic and somewhat granular cytoplasm. Nuclei have prominent nucleoli. (c–d) Immunohistochemistry: tumor cells are positive for CD21 (c) and negative for CD45 (d).

negative. Occasional cases may express S100, EMA, BCL1 (cyclin D1), and CD68. Tumors are negative for CD1a, lysosome, MPO, CD34, CD3, CD79a, and HMB45. Ki-67 ranges from 1% to 25%. It occurs primarily in lymph nodes but extranodal sites have been reported. Lymph nodes contain clusters or sheets of spindle cells with elongated nuclei, eosinophilic cytoplasm and mild to moderate pleomorphism. Nucleoli are present and may

be conspicuous. The tumor cells are mixed with small lymphocytes, with a prominent perivascular cuffing. The uninvolved lymphoid tissue contains small lymphocytes with occasional germinal centers. The behavior of follicular dendritic cell sarcoma is more reminiscent of a low-grade soft tissue sarcoma than a malignant lymphoma and is characterized by local recurrence and occasional metastases.

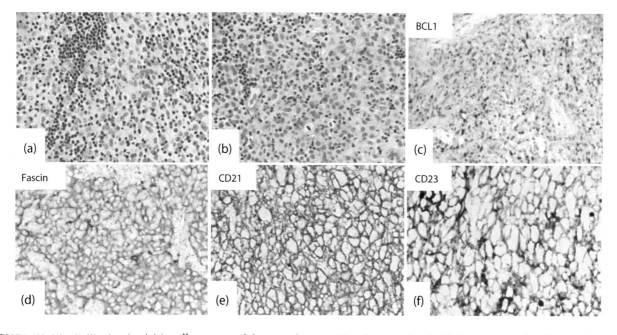

FIGURE 26.12 Follicular dendritic cell sarcoma of the nasopharynx. Histology section (a–b) shows atypical infiltrate of irregular and spindle cells. Expressing BCL1 (cyclin D1, c), fascin (d), CD21 (e), and CD23 (f).

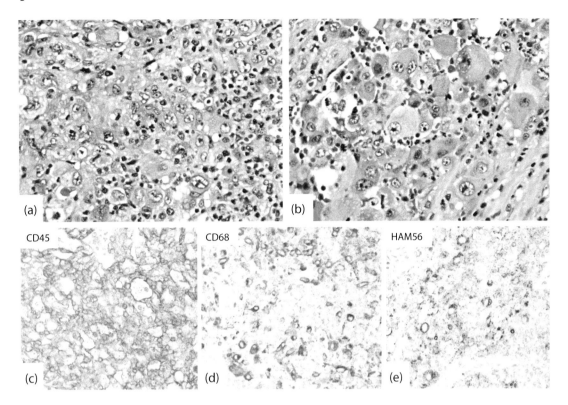

FIGURE 26.13 Histiocytic sarcoma – gallbladder. (a–b) Histologic sections show diffuse infiltrate of large pleomorphic cells with abundant cytoplasm and highly atypical nuclei. (c–e) Immunohistochemistry: tumor cells are positive for CD45 (c) and histiocytic/macrophage markers (CD68 and HAM56; d–e).

Histiocytic sarcoma

HS is a malignant tumor of the macrophage lineage. It occurs in lymph nodes and extranodal locations including skin, abdominal organs (intestinal tract), soft tissue, bone, and spleen. Morphologically HS consists of large cell with diffuse, non-cohesive growth pattern or intrasinusoidal pattern (lymph nodes, spleen, and liver). The cytomorphologic features are highly variable. The neoplastic cells are large and pleomorphic or spindle with abundant eosinophilic or foamy cytoplasm and bizarre nuclei (Figure 26.13). Nucleoli are prominent. Many cells are multinucleated. The overall morphologic features resemble ALCL or malignant melanoma. HSs are positive for CD4, CD11c, CD14, CD43, CD45, CD68, CD163, HAM56, lysozyme, and HLA-DR. Neoplastic cells lack the immunoreactivity with B- and T-cell markers, epithelial markers (EMA, cytokeratin), blastic markers (CD34, TdT, and CD117), HMB-45, CD1a, CD13, CD21, CD23, CD30, CD33, CD35, ALK, langerin (CD207), and MPO. Staining with S100 may be positive (in ~50%) but is usually focal and weak. The diagnosis of HS is largely based on marked cytologic atypia, exclusion of DLBCL, ALCL, melanoma, and carcinoma, and expression of CD45 and histiocytic markers.

Langerhans cell histiocytosis

Classification

The World Health Organization (WHO) classification of histiocytic and dendritic neoplasms recognizes the following tumors [1]:

- Histiocytic sarcomas
- Tumors derived from Langerhans cells (LC)

- Indeterminate dendritic cell tumors
- Interdigitating cell sarcoma
- Follicular dendritic cell sarcoma
- Fibroblastic reticular cell tumor
- Disseminated juvenile xanthogranuloma (JXG)
- Erdheim-Chester disease (ECD)

Rosai-Dorfman disease (RDD) has not been included in WHO classification.

A novel classification of histiocytoses has been recently proposed, defining five subgroups based on clinical and/or phenotypic criteria [24, 36, 37]:

- Langerhans-type histiocytosis
- Cutaneous and mucocutaneous histiocytosis
- Malignant histiocytosis
- Hemophagocytic lymphohistiocytosis (HLH)/macrophage activation syndromes
- Rosai-Dorfman disease (RDD).

Introduction

Langerhans cell histiocytosis (LCH) is an "inflammatory" heterogeneous myeloid neoplasm of CD1a+/CD207+/S100+ dendritic cells (Langerhans cells) involving various organs in both children and adults. Approximately 60% of patients with LCH carry the somatic mutation of *BRAF* V600E [38]. Most of the cases without *BRAF* V600E have other genetic changes, including other *BRAF* mutations, and mutations in other components of RAS-RAF-MEK-ERK cell signaling pathway such as *MAP2K1* mutations. Unifocal tumors, termed eosinophilic granulomas, usually involve bone, lung and less often skin, and lymph nodes. Multifocal

LCH of bone is also known as Hand-Schüller-Christian disease and frequently involves the base of the skull. Disseminated disease, termed Letterer-Siwe disease occurs predominantly in children and involves the bone, liver, spleen, skin, and lymph nodes. Patients with disease that is localized to skin, bone, and lymph node (defined as "nonrisk" organs) generally have a good prognosis and require minimal treatment. However, patients with lesions in "risk" organs (liver, spleen, lung, BM) have a worse overall prognosis regarding mortality and morbidity. Likewise, patients with LCH in the central nervous system (CNS), vertebrae, facial bones or bones of the anterior or middle cranial fossa are at higher risk for morbidity and recurrent disease. LCH in the orbit, mastoid or temporal skull regions are classified as "CNS risk" because of an increased frequency of developing diabetes insipidus and other endocrine abnormalities or parenchymal brain lesions [39]. Currently, stratification is being further advanced by the analysis of *BRAF* V600E mutation in blood of patients with LCH [38, 40].

Morphology

Morphologically, Langerhans cell histiocytosis is recognized by the presence of Langerhans cells (Figure 26.14), which are oval, polygonal or elongated, bean-shaped cells with characteristic nuclear grooves (linear nuclear clefts and indentations) with abundant pale cytoplasm with vacuoles, seen in an inflammatory background of eosinophils, histiocytes, neutrophils, and small lymphocytes. LCH typically presents with multifocal bone and/or BM involvement, with the skull bones being the most frequently affected. Lymph nodes show either an intrasinusoidal distribution or prominent paracortical involvement (Figure 26.15). Figure 26.16 shows BM involvement by LCH.

Immunophenotype

Langerhans cells express CD1a, S100, CD207, vimentin, HLA-DR, Langerin, and CD45. The expression of CD68 is weak and focal.

Differential diagnosis of LCH

Differential diagnosis of Langerhans cell histiocytosis includes other histiocytic lesions, such as Rosai-Dorfman disease, Erdheim-Chester disease, dermatopathic lymphadenitis, metastatic tumors and malignant lymphoma, especially those with a sinusoidal distribution, such as anaplastic large cell lymphoma (ALCL) or malignant lymphoma with erythrophagocytosis.

Langerhans cell sarcoma

Langerhans cell sarcoma is extremely rare and aggressive high-grade hematopoietic neoplasm with a dismal prognosis. It can arise *de novo* or from prior Langerhans cell histiocytosis [41]. The Langerhans cell sarcoma shows pleomorphic cytology, a high mitotic rate and characteristic immunohistochemical staining pattern with positive expression of Langerin, S100 and CD1a (Figures 26.17 and 26.18). Langerhans cell sarcomas are also positive for CD68, CD207, factor VIII, and occasionally CD4 [41].

Metastatic tumors to the bone marrow

The most common tumors metastasizing to the BM include carcinoma of the breast, prostate, lung, followed by kidney, melanoma, adenocarcinoma of gastrointestinal tract and other tumors. Figure 26.19 presents morphologic and immunophenotypic features of metastatic tumors in the BM.

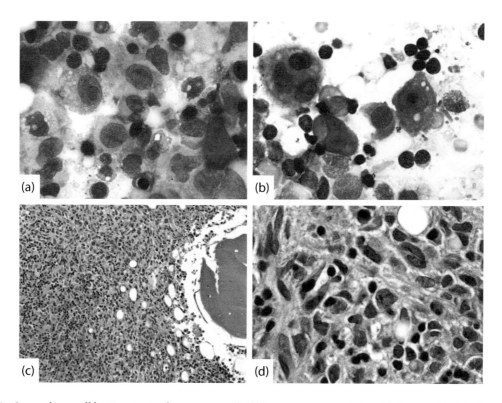

FIGURE 26.14 Langerhans cell histiocytosis – bone marrow. (a–b) Bone marrow aspirate with large cells with abundant cytoplasm, prominent nucleoli, and occasional nuclear irregularities. (c–d) Bone marrow core biopsy. Diffuse large cell infiltrate replacing normal bone marrow elements (c). High magnification shows characteristic nuclear irregularities (d). Scattered eosinophils are present.

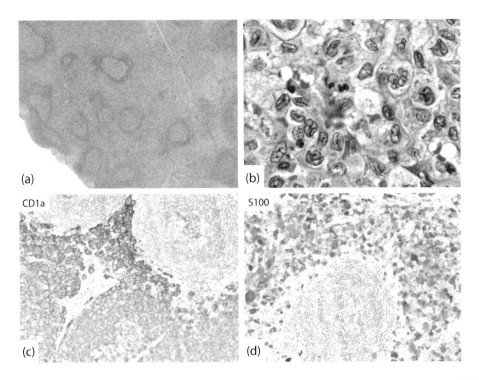

FIGURE 26.15 Langerhans cell histiocytosis – lymph node. (a) Low magnification shows prominent interfollicular/paracortical infiltrate. (b) High magnification displays typical nuclear grooves (folding). (c–d) Immunohistochemistry: tumor cells are positive for CD1a (c) and S100 (d).

Flow cytometry of non-hematopoietic tumors

Routine flow cytometry (FC) can identify non-hematopoietic tumors by showing distinct CD45⁻ population with increased side scatter (Figure 26.20). Flow cytometry is most often positive in poorly differentiated carcinomas with neuroendocrine differentiation, malignant melanoma, and rhabdomyosarcoma [42–44].

Carcinomas with prominent desmoplastic reaction (e.g., breast, prostate) are negative by flow cytometry.

Neuroendocrine carcinoma

Neuroendocrine carcinomas, both small and large cell type are characterized by increased side scatter, negative CD45, positive

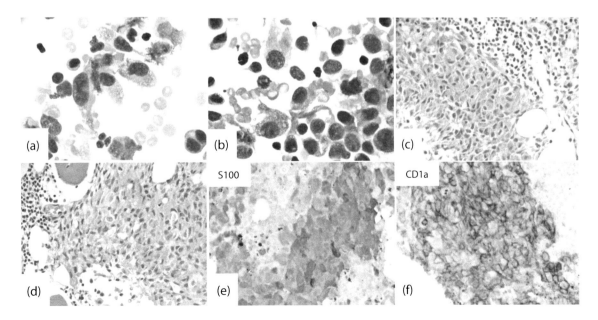

FIGURE 26.16 LCH involving the BM. (a–b) Aspirate smear show numerous atypical Langerhans cells with abundant cytoplasm. (c–d) Histoloy section (BM core biopsy) shows aggregates woth Langerhans cells with irregular, elongated nuclei. Tumor cells are positive for both S100 (e) and CD1a (f).

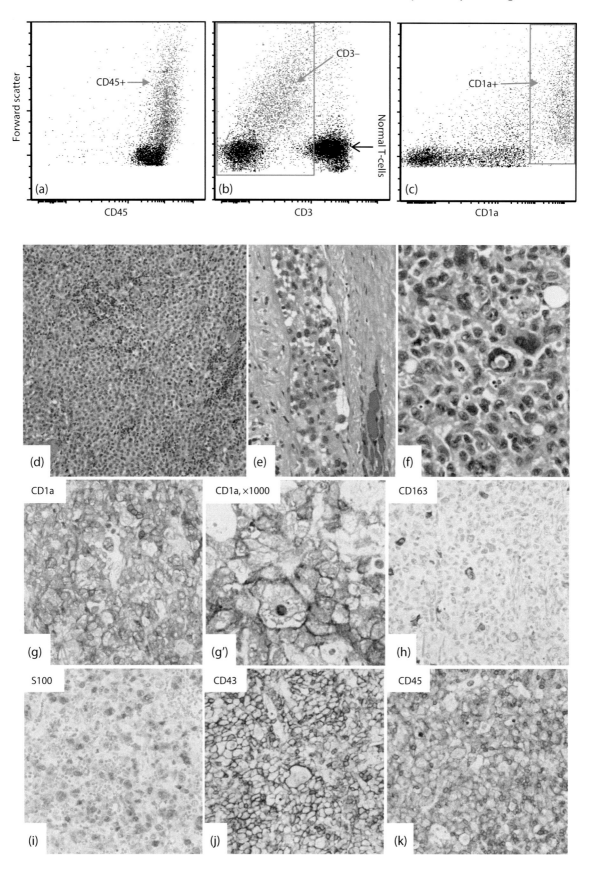

FIGURE 26.17 Langerhans cell sarcoma (axillary lymph node from 88-year-old male patient). (a–c) Flow cytometry analysis shows large CD45+ cells (a), which are negative for CD3 (b) and positive for CD1a (c). Histology sections (d–f) show highly atypical and pleomorphic infiltrate of large cells with focal intrasinusoidal distribution (e). Tumor cells express CD1a (g), S100 (i), CD43 (j), and CD45 (k). CD163 is negative (h).

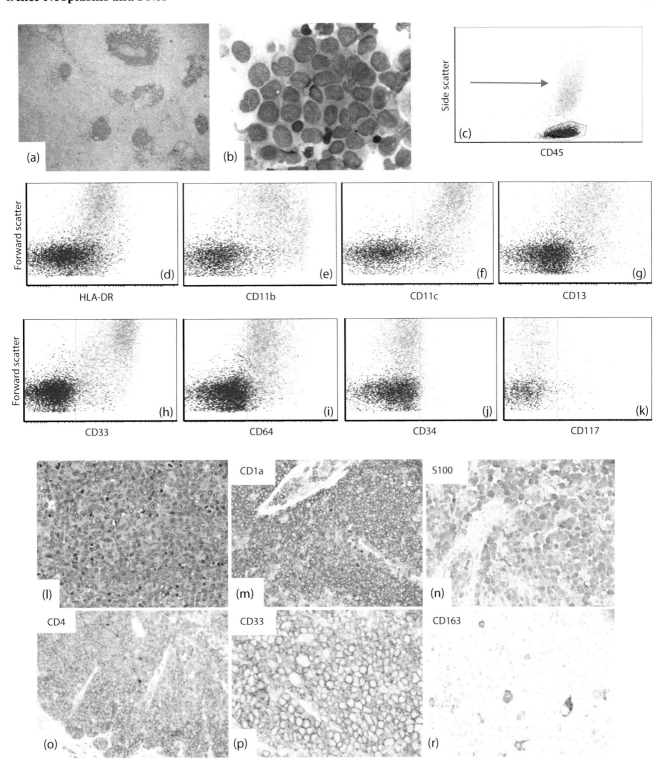

FIGURE 26.18 Lymph node with Langerhans cell sarcoma. (a) Histology (low magnification) shows expansion of paracortical area. (b) Touch smear shows atypical Langerhans cells with irregular nuclei. (c–k) Flow cytometry analysis shows tumor cells (purple dots) with high side scatter (a) and forward scatter (d–k), positive CD45 (c), HLA-DR (d), CD11b (e), CD11c (f), CD13 (g), CD33 (h) and CD64 (i), and negative CD34 (j) and CD117 (k). (l) High magnification of lymph node section shows diffuse infiltrate by atypical oval to spindle to irregular cells with mitotic figures. (m–r) Immunohistochemistry shows tumor cells expressing CD1a (m), S100 (n), CD4 (o), CD33 (p) with negative CD163 expression (r).

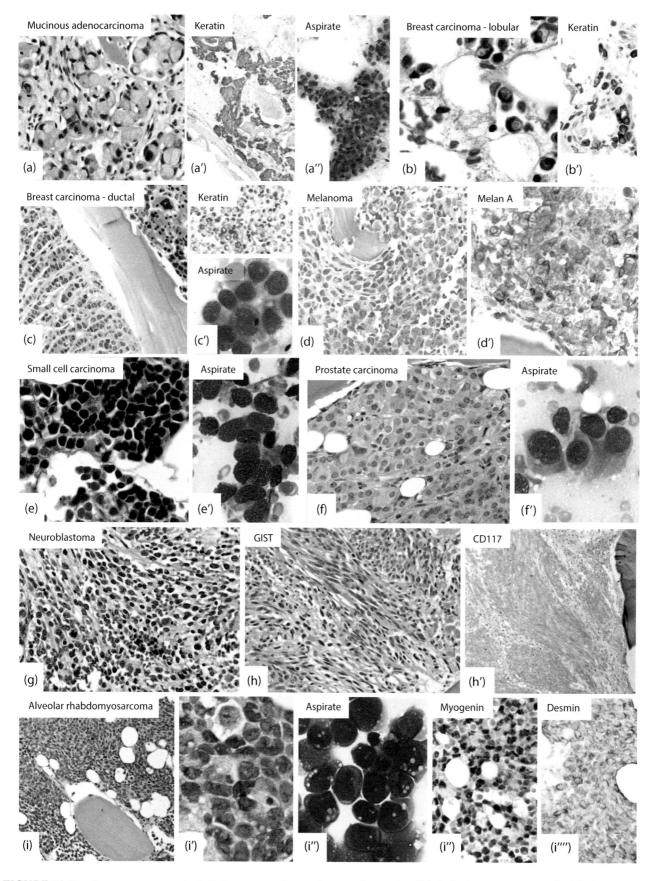

FIGURE 26.19   Bone marrow – metastatic tumors: mucinous adenocarcinoma (a–a″), lobular breast carcinoma (b–b′), ductal breast carcinoma (c–c′), melanoma (d–d′), small cell carcinoma (e–e′), prostate carcinoma (f–f′), neuroblastoma (g), GIST (gastrointestinal stromal tumor; h–h′), alveolar rhabdomyosarcoma (i–i″″).

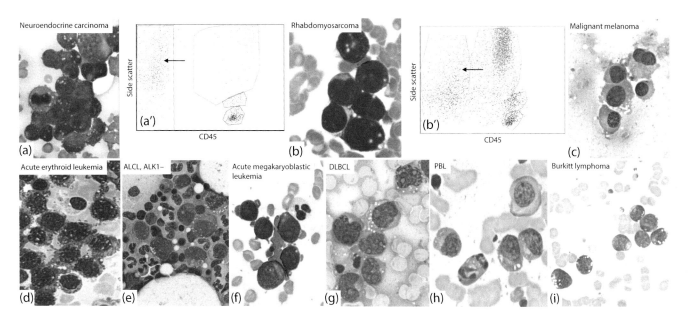

FIGURE 26.20 Metastatic tumors to the bone marrow. Two examples of positive flow cytometry in case of metastatic tumor to BM. (a) Metastatic large cell neuroendocrine carcinoma (a, smear with cohesive clusters of large cells with some cytoplasmic vacuoles, a′ flow cytometry). Flow cytometry shows CD45-negative population (arrow) with increased side scatter. Metastatic carcinomas are often positive for CD56 and may be positive for CD38 (dim) and CD117, mimicking plasma cell neoplasms. (b) Metastatic rhabdomyosarcoma to the bone marrow (b, touch smear; b′, flow cytometry). Rhabdomyosarcoma cells are negative for CD45 (b, arrow) and may be positive for CD56 and CD117. On aspirate smear or touch smear preparation of bone marrow, metastatic tumors need to be differentiated form plasma cell myeloma, melanoma (c), acute erythroid leukemia (d), anaplastic large cell lymphoma (e), acute megakaryoblastic leukemia (f), diffuse large B-cell lymphoma (g), plasmablastic lymphoma (h), and Burkitt lymphoma (i) or other high-grade lymphomas.

CD71 and strong expression of CD56. Subset of tumors may be positive for CD117, CD200, CD38 (dim), and rarely myeloid markers. Cytoplasmic staining with cytokeratin by flow cytometry helps in confirming epithelial origin of a tumor [43]. Positive CD56 and CD117 and lack of CD45 requires differential diagnosis from PCM and positive expression of CD117 and myeloid markers raise the possibility of myeloid neoplasm. Correlation with other markers (e.g., cytoplasmic light chain immunoglobulins, HLA-DR, CD34, CD133, CD11c, and MPO) and morphology helps in differential diagnosis. Acosta et al. evaluated the efficiency of flow cytometry to detect malignant epithelial cells in 238 fresh samples, including effusions, lymph node biopsies, fine needle aspirates, BM aspirates, cerebrospinal fluid, among others tumor to distinguish between monocyte/macrophages (CD45+/CD33+/CD326−), mesothelial cells (CD45±dim/CD33−/CD326−) and epithelial cells (CD45−/CD33−/CD326+) and concluded that the detection of CD326+ cells using FC is strongly indicative of the presence of carcinoma cells [44].

Malignant melanoma

Melanoma cells can be identified by FC by showing CD45− population with high side scatter. Subset of melanomas may be positive for CD10, CD56, CD57, and/or CD117. Using HMB-45 by FC increases the detection rate.

Other tumors

- Rhabdomyosarcomas: CD45−, CD56+, CD90+, CD117+/−, myogenin+
- Neuroblastoma: CD45−, CD56+, CD2+, CD81+
- Primitive neuroectodermal tumors/Ewing sarcoma: CD45−, CD271+, CD99+

- Wilms' tumor: CD45−, CD56+
- Germ cell tumors: CD45−, CD56+, CD10+.

Mastocytosis

Mastocytosis is a heterogeneous group of BM-derived disorders characterized by proliferation of the clonally transformed mast cells, often associated with somatic activating point mutations within *KIT*, and a broad spectrum of clinical and morphologic features ranging from a self-limiting benign disorder (i.e., juvenile cutaneous mastocytosis or urticaria pigmentosa) to highly aggressive neoplasms like mast cell leukemia [1,45–48]. The symptoms observed in mastocytosis are related to the spontaneous or triggered release of mast cell mediators or due to consequences of pathological accumulation of mast cells in tissues. Basically, mastocytosis can be divided into two main subtypes: cutaneous mastocytosis (CM) and systemic mastocytosis (SM), the latter mainly involving the BM. The WHO divides SM into several major subtypes: cutaneous mastocytosis (CM), indolent systemic mastocytosis (ISM), systemic mastocytosis with an associated clonal hematological non-mast-cell disorder (SM-AHN), aggressive systemic mastocytosis (ASM), mast cell leukemia, mast cell sarcoma and extracutaneous mastocytoma [49–53].

Morphology

Majority of patients with mastocytosis have evidence of skin involvement. BM is involved in SM. Other sites of involvement include spleen, lymph nodes, liver, and gastrointestinal tract. Normal mast cells are typically round and mononuclear with prominent metachromatic granules in the cytoplasm. Mast cell progenitors (ungranulated, tryptase-positive blasts, metachromatic, blasts and promastocytes) are rarely seen. In the mastocytosis mast cells may be round to polygonal with prominent cytoplasmic granules, but atypical forms, including spindle cells, multilobed cells and metachromatically granulated blast-like cells may be present. Systemic and more aggressive variants of mast cell disease more often display atypical cytomorphologic features.

SM-AHN. SM may be associated with other (non-mast cell) hematopoietic neoplasms, such as AML, myelodysplastic syndrome (MDS), malignant lymphoma, plasma cell neoplasm, myeloproliferative neoplasms (MPN), and mixed MPD/MPN neoplasms such as CMML and MDS/MPN with ring sideroblasts and thrombocytosis (MDS/MPN-RS-T). Both neoplasms must fulfill diagnostic criteria defined by WHO [1]. In SM-AHN, the hematologic neoplasm can be diagnosed before, after, or concurrently with SM. The reported frequency of this category varies widely from 5% to 40% of all SM cases, with myeloid neoplasms comprising most of the cases (80%–90%).

Immunophenotype
Use of antibodies against tryptase, CD117, and CD25 is recommended in every suspected case. Because most cases of systemic mastocytosis show a very low degree of infiltration of the BM, mast cell tryptase, and anti-CD117 are of major importance for screening and quantification of mast cells, in particular to detect even small compact infiltrates as the only major diagnostic criterion for mastocytosis. Expression of CD25 on mast cells is defined as a minor diagnostic criterion and is usually seen only in mastocytosis and not in reactive states of mast cell hyperplasia. Immunophenotypic studies of neoplastic mast cells reveal expression of CD2, CD25, CD43, CD45, CD68, CD117, and mast cell tryptase. Normal (benign) mast cells lack the expression of CD2 and CD25. CD30 expression by mast cells is usually associated with aggressive systemic mastocytosis or mast cell leukemia, but less may be seen in other variant of SM including indolent forms [45, 54]. By flow cytometry (FC) analysis mast cells appear as brightly CD117+ and CD45+ cells with increased side scatter.

Genetic features
With conventional cytogenetics about 35%–40% of the patients have chromosomally abnormal clones in BM cells including which are similar to those observed in other hematological neoplasms [55, 56]. Following chromosomal abnormalities were described: del(5q), del(7q), del(11q), del(20q), -Y, +8, +14 [55, 56]. Activating codon 816 mutations (*D816V*) in the *KIT* receptor tyrosine kinase gene resulting in deregulation of the c-kit receptor are present in a majority of patients [57–60]. Activating mutations of platelet-derived growth factor receptor-alpha (*PDGFRA*) are identified in a significant number of SM cases that have associated eosinophilia. Detection of codon 816 *KIT* mutation is a minor diagnostic criterion of SM [50].

Simultaneous bi-lineage hematologic malignancies

Composite hematopoietic tumors (simultaneous bi-lineage hematologic malignancies) are rarely seen and the prognosis is worse than single lineage lymphoma or myeloid leukemia. Composite lymphoma is defined as more than one distinct lymphoma variant occurring in the same anatomic site irrespective of clonal relationship between those components. The most frequent type of composite lymphoma is a combination of two different types of B-cell lymphoma. The concurrence of Hodgkin lymphoma and B-cell lymphoma or composite lymphoma composed of T- and

B-cell lymphoma occurs less often. Figures 26.21–26.23 depict the examples of simultaneous bi-lineage hematologic malignancies.

Paroxysmal nocturnal hemoglobinuria (PNH)

PNH is a rare, clonal, acquired hematopoietic stem cell disorder with a partial or absolute deficiency of all glycophosphatidylinositol (GPI)-linked proteins leading to a complement-mediated hemolytic anemia with recurrent crises, predisposition for venous and arterial thrombosis) (often in unusual sites), BM failure (cytopenias), a thrombophilia, or any combination of the above [61–66]. PNH is caused by an acquired mutation in the phosphatidylinositol-N-acetylglucosaminyltransferase-subunit-A (*PIGA*) gene. This mutation leads to the deficiency of cellular anchors for complement inhibitor proteins CD55 and CD59, predisposing red blood cells to hemolysis by the complement system. There is strong correlation between PNH and BM failure syndromes, such as MDS or aplastic anemia (AA) and screening for PNH has become a part of clinical work-up for those conditions. The classical approach to diagnosis of PNH by flow cytometry involves the loss of at least two GPI-linked antigens on red blood cells (RBCs) and neutrophils with a FLAER-based FC assay being considered the gold standard [61–65, 67, 68]. With current treatment using a monoclonal antibody that blocks terminal complement at C5 (eculizumab), survival of patients with PNH is similar to that of aged-matched controls [62]. Subclinical PNH can be present in patients with BM failure like AA and MDS.

Flow cytometry of PNH
PNH flow cytometry evaluates the expression of GPI-anchored proteins on erythrocytes, granulocytes, and monocytes [61, 63–70]. The demonstration of the absence of GPI-linked proteins in a significant fraction (large clone) of peripheral blood erythrocytes, neutrophils and monocytes is diagnostic of PNH [61, 66]. The abnormal red blood cell clones are designated as PNH type III, and PNH type II, while normal clone is named PNH type I (Figure 26.24). Type I red blood cells are normal cells with bright CD59 expression and a lifespan of ~120 days. Type III PNH red blood cell clone have complete lack of GPI protein (negative CD59 expression) while type II PNH clone shows partial CD59 deficiency. The consensus guidelines for PNH analysis by FC were published by Borowitz et al. [61] and more recently by Sutherland et al. [66].

The following, are the recommendations for PNH analysis based on those two articles [61, 66]:

- For the analysis of red blood cells, the forward scatter (FSC) and side scatter (SSC) voltages should be set up in logarithmic mode and voltages adjusted to place red blood cell population just beyond the center of the plot and above any FSC threshold.
- For white blood cells, light scatter voltages should be set in linear mode at such values that all leukocytes subsets scatter above the FSC threshold.
- FLAER is an Alexa488 conjugate and specific compensation setting are required for this conjugate. Setting optimized for FITC must not be used because of the different spillover of Alexa488 and FITC.
- Whole anticoagulated peripheral blood is diluted 1:100 with phosphate buffered saline (PBS). EDTA is preferred but Heparin or ACD anticoagulants are also acceptable.
- Red blood cells are identified by expression of CD235a (glycophorin A; GPHA).

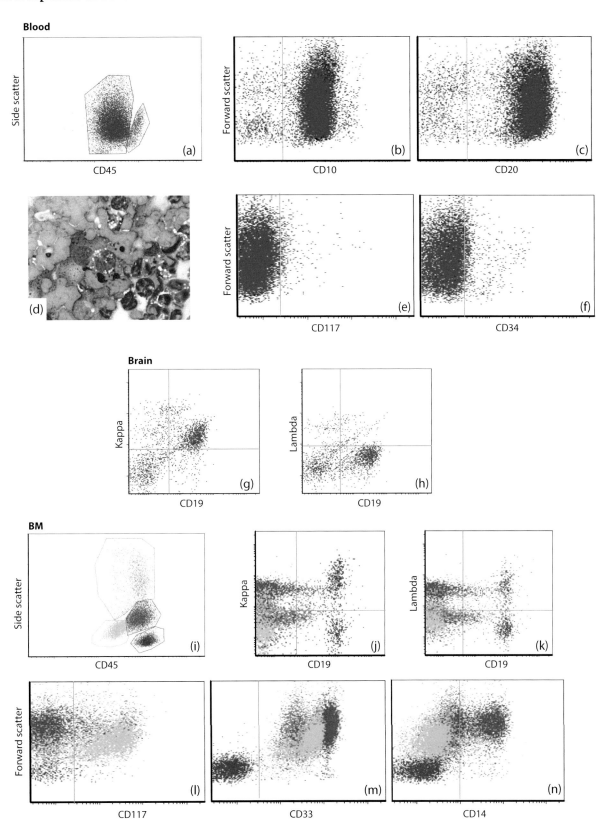

FIGURE 26.21 Composite hematopoietic neoplasm: AML with *NPM1/FLT3* mutations (BM) and high-grade B-cell lymphoma, double-hit (brain + blood). Patient with brain mass and leukocytosis. Flow cytometry analysis of blood showed predominance of large B-cells with moderate expression of CD45 (a, blue dots), positive CD10 (b) and CD20 (c). Smear showed large lymphoid cells with cytoplasmic vacuoles (d). There was no evidence of acute leukemia or circulating CD34+ and/or CD117+ blasts (e–f). Concurrent analysis of brain mass showed clonal B-cells (kappa+, g–h, blue dots), with similar phenotype to that observed in blood sample. BM send subsequently for staging, showed AML with monocytic component (i) positive for *NPM1* and *FLT3* mutations. BM did not reveal involvement by high grade B-cell lymphoma (j–k) and showed CD117+ (l) and CD33+ (m) blasts (green dots) and increased monocytes (CD33+ and CD14+, m–n, pink dots) compatible with AML.

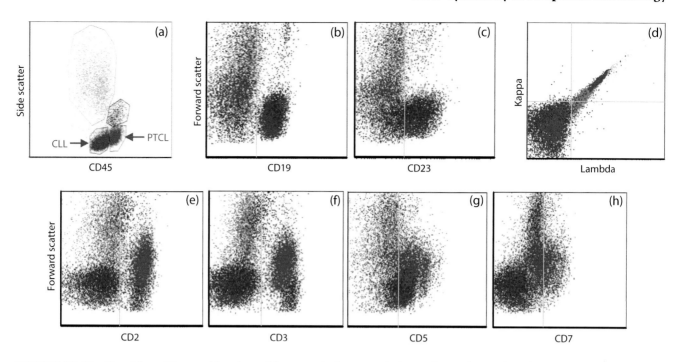

FIGURE 26.22 Blood from 89-year-old patient with composite hematopoietic neoplasm: chronic lymphocytic leukemia (CLL) and peripheral T-cell lymphoma (PTCL). CLL cells (red dots) show dimmer expression of CD45 when compared to PTCL (a), are positive for CD19 (b) and CD23 (c) and lack the expression of surface light chain immunoglobulins (d). PTCL (magenta dots) are positive for all pan T-cell markers (e–h) with dim expression of CD5 (g) and partial expression of CD7. CLL cells are also dim CD5+ (g).

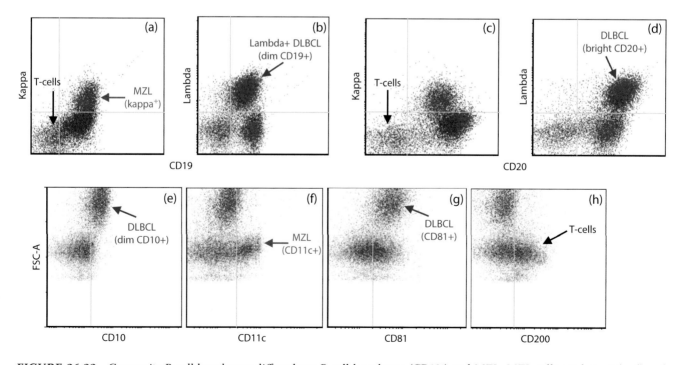

FIGURE 26.23 Composite B-cell lymphoma: diffuse large B-cell lymphoma (CD10+) and MZL. MZL cells are kappa+ (a–d) and DLBCL cells are lambda+ (a–d). The expression of CD19 is brighter in MZL than in DLBCL and the expression of CD20 is brighter in DLBCL than in MZL. Both lymphomas can be easily distinguished based on forward scatter (e–h). DLBCL is dim CD19+ (e) and MZL is dim CD11c+ (f). The expression of CD81 is positive in DLBCL and expression of CD200 is negative in both lymphomas (T cells are dim CD200+, h).

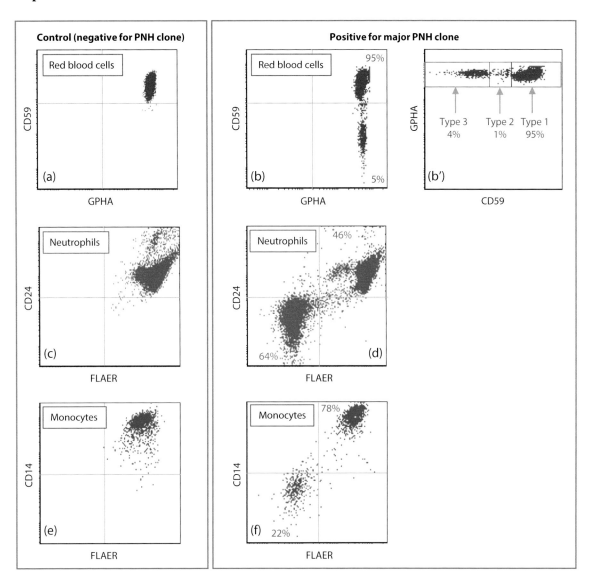

FIGURE 26.24 PNH analysis by flow cytometry. PNH analysis includes evaluation of red blood cells (identified by bright GPHA expression; a–b), neutrophils (identified by positive CD15 expression; c–d) and monocytes (e–f; identified by bright CD64 expression. The results of patient's sample for each lineage are compared with negative controls (presented in a, c, and e panels). Flow cytometry revealed the presence of major PNH clone: 5% of CD59⁻ red blood cells (b), 64% of CD24⁻/FLAER⁻ neutrophils (d), and 22% of CD14⁻/FLAER⁻ monocytes (f).

- CD59 marker provides the best means to delineate and enumerate PNH clones in red blood cells (types I, II, and III). It is recommended to report the percentages of type II versus type III PNH clones.
- Compensation is set by removing fluorescence spillover into the PE channel with a red blood cell sample stained only with CD235a-FITC, and spillover of PE into the FITC channel is removed using a sample stained only with CD59-PE.
- The type III gate is established using a normal (control) sample stained only with CD235a-FITC, and the upper limit of the type II gate is established using a normal sample stained with cocktailed CD235a-FITC and CD59-PE.
- White blood cells are evaluated using FLAER, CD24, CD15, and CD45 (for neutrophils), and FLAER, CD14, CD64, and CD45 (for monocytes).

- CD45 is recommended as part of any gating strategy to identify specific subsets of leukocytes, CD15 is recommended for identifying neutrophils and CD64 for identifying monocytes.
- At least two GPI-linked markers per white blood cell lineage must be analyzed, one of them being FLAER. For neutrophils, combinations of FLAER-Alexa488 with CD24-PE or FLAER-Alexa488 with CD157-PE are recommended. For monocytes, FLAER can be used in combination with CD14-PE or CD157-PE are recommended.
- Recommended terminology of reporting PNH clones:
  - No PNH population identified (negative screening for PNH)
  - PNH clones identified (PNH population >1%)
  - Minor PNH clone identified (PNH population between 0.1% and 1%)
  - Rare cells with GPI-deficiency (PNH population <0.1%)

Identification of a minute PNH clone

A small population of PNH cells called a PNH clone can be present in patients with BM failure who show no clinical or laboratory signs of hemolysis. High-resolution FC protocols can detect small PNH clones at a sensitivity level of ~0.01% in red cells and neutrophils. The International PNH group has defined the presence of this PNH clone in AA and MDS as subclinical PNH [71]. Consensus guidelines recommend that 20 definitive GPI-negative events should be considered the minimum number of events required to report a detectable population of PNH cells by FC [66].

References

1. Swerdlow, S.H., et al., ed. *WHO classification of tumors of haematopoietic and lymphoid tissues.* 2016, IARC: Lyon.
2. Garnache-Ottou, F., et al., *Extended diagnostic criteria for plasmacytoid dendritic cell leukaemia.* Br J Haematol, 2009. **145**(5): p. 624–36.
3. Julia, F., et al., *Blastic plasmacytoid dendritic cell neoplasms: clinico-immunohistochemical correlations in a series of 91 patients.* Am J Surg Pathol, 2014. **38**(5): p. 673–80.
4. Martin-Martin, L., et al., *Classification and clinical behavior of blastic plasmacytoid dendritic cell neoplasms according to their maturation-associated immunophenotypic profile.* Oncotarget, 2015. **6**(22): p. 19204–16.
5. Pagano, L., et al., *Blastic plasmacytoid dendritic cell neoplasm: diagnostic criteria and therapeutical approaches.* Br J Haematol, 2016. **174**(2): p. 188–202.
6. Pagano, L., et al., *Blastic plasmacytoid dendritic cell neoplasm with leukemic presentation: an Italian multicenter study.* Haematologica, 2013. **98**(2): p. 239–46.
7. Jacob, M.C., et al., *CD4+ CD56+ lineage negative malignancies: a new entity developed from malignant early plasmacytoid dendritic cells.* Haematologica, 2003. **88**(8): p. 941–55.
8. Garnache-Ottou, F., J. Feuillard, and P. Saas, *Plasmacytoid dendritic cell leukaemia/lymphoma: towards a well defined entity?* Br J Haematol, 2007. **136**(4): p. 539–48.
9. Willemze, R., et al., *WHO-EORTC classification for cutaneous lymphomas.* Blood, 2005. **105**(10): p. 3768–85.
10. Lucio, P., A. Parreira, and A. Orfao, *CD123hi dendritic cell lymphoma: an unusual case of non-Hodgkin lymphoma.* Ann Intern Med, 1999. **131**(7): p. 549–50.
11. Chaperot, L., et al., *Identification of a leukemic counterpart of the plasmacytoid dendritic cells.* Blood, 2001. **97**(10): p. 3210–7.
12. Feuillard, J., et al., *Clinical and biologic features of CD4(+)CD56(+) malignancies.* Blood, 2002. **99**(5): p. 1556–63.
13. Petrella, T., et al., *'Agranular CD4+ CD56+ hematodermic neoplasm' (blastic NK-cell lymphoma) originates from a population of CD56+ precursor cells related to plasmacytoid monocytes.* Am J Surg Pathol, 2002. **26**(7): p. 852–62.
14. Lucioni, M., et al., *Twenty-one cases of blastic plasmacytoid dendritic cell neoplasm: focus on biallelic locus 9p21.3 deletion.* Blood, 2011. **118**(17): p. 4591–4.
15. Leroux, D., et al., *CD4(+), CD56(+) DC2 acute leukemia is characterized by recurrent clonal chromosomal changes affecting 6 major targets: a study of 21 cases by the Groupe Francais de Cytogenetique Hematologique.* Blood, 2002. **99**(11): p. 4154–9.
16. Chaperot, L., et al., *Leukemic plasmacytoid dendritic cells share phenotypic and functional features with their normal counterparts.* Eur J Immunol, 2004. **34**(2): p. 418–26.
17. Garnache-Ottou, F., et al., *Expression of the myeloid-associated marker CD33 is not an exclusive factor for leukemic plasmacytoid dendritic cells.* Blood, 2005. **105**(3): p. 1256–64.
18. Gopcsa, L., et al., *Extensive flow cytometric characterization of plasmacytoid dendritic cell leukemia cells.* Eur J Haematol, 2005. **75**(4): p. 346–51.
19. Hamadeh, F., et al., *Flow cytometry identifies a spectrum of maturation in myeloid neoplasms having plasmacytoid dendritic cell differentiation.* Cytometry B Clin Cytom, 2020. **98**(1): p. 43–51.
20. Wang, W., et al., *Immunophenotypic characterization of reactive and neoplastic plasmacytoid dendritic cells permits establishment of a 10-color flow cytometric panel for initial workup and residual disease evaluation of blastic plasmacytoid dendritic cell neoplasm.* Haematologica, 2021. **106**(4): p. 1047–55.
21. Ng, A.P., et al., *Primary cutaneous CD4+/CD56+ hematodermic neoplasm (blastic NK-cell lymphoma): a report of five cases.* Haematologica, 2006. **91**(1): p. 143–4.
22. Dijkman, R., et al., *Gene-expression profiling and array-based CGH classify CD4+CD56+ hematodermic neoplasm and cutaneous myelomonocytic leukemia as distinct disease entities.* Blood, 2007. **109**(4): p. 1720–7.
23. Emadali, A., et al., *Haploinsufficiency for NR3C1, the gene encoding the glucocorticoid receptor, in blastic plasmacytoid dendritic cell neoplasms.* Blood, 2016. **127**(24): p. 3040–53.
24. Tzankov, A., et al., *Plasmacytoid dendritic cell proliferations and neoplasms involving the bone marrow: Summary of the workshop cases submitted to the 18th Meeting of the European Association for Haematopathology (EAHP) organized by the European Bone Marrow Working Group, Basel 2016.* Ann Hematol, 2017. **96**(5): p. 765–77.
25. Facchetti, F., et al., *Neoplasms derived from plasmacytoid dendritic cells.* Mod Pathol, 2016. **29**(2): p. 98–111.
26. Jegalian, A.G., F. Facchetti, and E.S. Jaffe, *Plasmacytoid dendritic cells: physiologic roles and pathologic states.* Adv Anat Pathol, 2009. **16**(6): p. 392–404.
27. Kutzner, H., et al., *CD123-positive plasmacytoid dendritic cells in primary cutaneous marginal zone B-cell lymphoma: diagnostic and pathogenetic implications.* Am J Surg Pathol, 2009. **33**(9): p. 1307–13.
28. Vitte, F., et al., *Specific skin lesions in chronic myelomonocytic leukemia: a spectrum of myelomonocytic and dendritic cell proliferations: a study of 42 cases.* Am J Surg Pathol, 2012. **36**(9): p. 1302–16.
29. Chan, J.K., et al., *Follicular dendritic cell sarcoma. Clinicopathologic analysis of 17 cases suggesting a malignant potential higher than currently recognized.* Cancer, 1997. **79**(2): p. 294–313.
30. Chan, J.K., et al., *Follicular dendritic cell tumors of the oral cavity.* Am J Surg Pathol, 1994. **18**(2): p. 148–57.
31. Choi, P.C., et al., *Follicular dendritic cell sarcoma of the neck: report of two cases complicated by pulmonary metastases.* Cancer, 2000. **89**(3): p. 664–72.
32. Hollowood, K., et al., *Extranodal follicular dendritic cell sarcoma of the gastrointestinal tract. Morphologic, immunohistochemical and ultrastructural analysis of two cases.* Am J Clin Pathol, 1995. **103**(1): p. 90–7.
33. Perez-Ordonez, B., R.A. Erlandson, and J. Rosai, *Follicular dendritic cell tumor: report of 13 additional cases of a distinctive entity.* Am J Surg Pathol, 1996. **20**(8): p. 944–55.
34. Perez-Ordonez, B. and J. Rosai, *Follicular dendritic cell tumor: review of the entity.* Semin Diagn Pathol, 1998. **15**(2): p. 144–54.
35. Soriano, A.O., et al., *Follicular dendritic cell sarcoma: a report of 14 cases and a review of the literature.* Am J Hematol, 2007. **82**(8): p. 725–8.
36. Emile, J.F., et al., *Revised classification of histiocytoses and neoplasms of the macrophage-dendritic cell lineages.* Blood, 2016. **127**(22): p. 2672–81.
37. Tzankov, A., et al., *Histiocytic cell neoplasms involving the bone marrow: summary of the workshop cases submitted to the 18th Meeting of the European Association for Haematopathology (EAHP) organized by the European Bone Marrow Working Group, Basel 2016.* Ann Hematol, 2018. **97**(11): p. 2117–28.
38. Badalian-Very, G., et al., *Recurrent BRAF mutations in Langerhans cell histiocytosis.* Blood, 2010. **116**(11): p. 1919–23.
39. Allen, C.E. and K.L. McClain, *Langerhans cell histiocytosis: a review of past, current and future therapies.* Drugs Today (Barc), 2007. **43**(9): p. 627–43.

40. Heritier, S., et al., *New somatic BRAF splicing mutation in Langerhans cell histiocytosis.* Mol Cancer, 2017. **16**(1): p. 115.

41. Nakamine, H., et al., *Langerhans cell histiocytosis and Langerhans cell sarcoma: Current understanding and differential diagnosis.* J Clin Exp Hematop, 2016. **56**(2): p. 109–18.

42. Pillai, V. and D.M. Dorfman, *Flow cytometry of nonhematopoietic neoplasms.* Acta Cytol, 2016. **60**(4): p. 336–43.

43. Cornfield, D., et al., *The potential role of flow cytometry in the diagnosis of small cell carcinoma.* Arch Pathol Lab Med, 2003. **127**(4): p. 461–4.

44. Acosta, M., J. Pereira, and M. Arroz, *Screening of carcinoma metastasis by flow cytometry: A study of 238 cases.* Cytometry B Clin Cytom, 2016. **90**(3): p. 289–94.

45. Chiu, A. and A. Orazi, *Mastocytosis and related disorders.* Semin Diagn Pathol, 2012. **29**(1): p. 19–30.

46. Georgin-Lavialle, S., et al., *Mast cell leukemia.* Blood, 2013. **121**(8): p. 1285–95.

47. Gotlib, J., et al., *International working group-myeloproliferative neoplasms research and treatment (IWG-MRT) & European competence network on mastocytosis (ECNM) consensus response criteria in advanced systemic mastocytosis.* Blood, 2013. **121**(13): p. 2393–401.

48. Horny, H.-P., K. Sotlar, and P. Valent, *Differential diagnoses of systemic mastocytosis in routinely processed bone marrow biopsy specimens: a review.* Pathobiology, 2010. **77**(4): p. 169–80.

49. Valent, P., et al., *Diagnosis and treatment of systemic mastocytosis: state of the art.* Br J Haematol, 2003. **122**(5): p. 695–717.

50. Valent, P., et al., *Diagnostic criteria and classification of mastocytosis: a consensus proposal.* Leuk Res, 2001. **25**(7): p. 603–25.

51. Metcalfe, D.D., *Mast cells and mastocytosis.* Blood, 2008. **112**(4): p. 946–56.

52. Horny, H.-P., *Mastocytosis: an unusual clonal disorder of bone marrow-derived hematopoietic progenitor cells.* Am J Clin Pathol, 2009. **132**(3): p. 438–47.

53. Swerdlow, S.H., et al, ed. WHO classification of tumors of haematopoietic and lymphoid tissues. 2008, IARC: Lyon.

54. Valent, P., K. Sotlar, and H.P. Horny, *Aberrant expression of CD30 in aggressive systemic mastocytosis and mast cell leukemia: a differential diagnosis to consider in aggressive hematopoietic CD30-positive neoplasms.* Leuk Lymphoma, 2011. **52**(5): p. 740–4.

55. Gupta, R., B.J. Bain, and C.L. Knight, *Cytogenetic and molecular genetic abnormalities in systemic mastocytosis.* Acta Haematol, 2002. **107**(2): p. 123–8.

56. Swolin, B., S. Rodjer, and G. Roupe, *Cytogenetic studies in patients with mastocytosis.* Cancer Genet Cytogenet, 2000. **120**(2): p. 131–5.

57. Metcalfe, D.D. and C. Akin, *Mastocytosis: molecular mechanisms and clinical disease heterogeneity.* Leuk Res, 2001. **25**(7): p. 577–82.

58. Barbie, D.A. and D.J. Deangelo, *Systemic mastocytosis: current classification and novel therapeutic options.* Clin Adv Hematol Oncol, 2006. **4**(10): p. 768–75.

59. Nagata, H., et al., *Identification of a point mutation in the catalytic domain of the protooncogene c-kit in peripheral blood mononuclear cells of patients who have mastocytosis with an associated hematologic disorder.* Proc Natl Acad Sci U S A, 1995. **92**(23): p. 10560–4.

60. Valent, P., et al., *Mastocytosis: pathology, genetics, and current options for therapy.* Leuk Lymphoma, 2005. **46**(1): p. 35–48.

61. Borowitz, M.J., et al., *Guidelines for the diagnosis and monitoring of paroxysmal nocturnal hemoglobinuria and related disorders by flow cytometry.* Cytometry B Clin Cytom, 2010. **78**(4): p. 211–30.

62. Brodsky, R.A., *How I treat paroxysmal nocturnal hemoglobinuria.* Blood, 2021. **137**(10): p. 1304–9.

63. Brodsky, R.A., et al., *Improved detection and characterization of paroxysmal nocturnal hemoglobinuria using fluorescent aerolysin.* Am J Clin Pathol, 2000. **114**(3): p. 459–66.

64. Richards, S.J. and D. Barnett, *The role of flow cytometry in the diagnosis of paroxysmal nocturnal hemoglobinuria in the clinical laboratory.* Clin Lab Med, 2007. **27**(3): p. 577–90, vii.

65. Seth, N., et al., *Utility of FLAER and CD157 in a five-color single-tube high sensitivity assay, for diagnosis of Paroxysmal Nocturnal Hemoglobinuria (PNH)-A standalone flow cytometry laboratory experience.* Int J Lab Hematol, 2021. **43**(2): p. 259–65.

66. Sutherland, D.R., et al., *ICCS/ESCCA consensus guidelines to detect GPI-deficient cells in paroxysmal nocturnal hemoglobinuria (PNH) and related disorders part 2 - reagent selection and assay optimization for high-sensitivity testing.* Cytometry B Clin Cytom, 2018. **94**(1): p. 23–48.

67. Richards, S.J., A.C. Rawstron, and P. Hillmen, *Application of flow cytometry to the diagnosis of paroxysmal nocturnal hemoglobinuria.* Cytometry, 2000. **42**(4): p. 223–33.

68. Sutherland, D.R., et al., *Use of a FLAER-based WBC assay in the primary screening of PNH clones.* Am J Clin Pathol, 2009. **132**(4): p. 564–72.

69. Kwong, Y.L., et al., *Flow cytometric measurement of glycosylphosphatidyl-inositol-linked surface proteins on blood cells of patients with paroxysmal nocturnal hemoglobinuria.* Am J Clin Pathol, 1994. **102**(1): p. 30–5.

70. van der Schoot, C.E., et al., *Deficiency of glycosyl-phosphatidylinositol-linked membrane glycoproteins of leukocytes in paroxysmal nocturnal hemoglobinuria, description of a new diagnostic cytofluorometric assay.* Blood, 1990. **76**(9): p. 1853–9.

71. Wang, S.A., et al., *Detection of paroxysmal nocturnal hemoglobinuria clones in patients with myelodysplastic syndromes and related bone marrow diseases, with emphasis on diagnostic pitfalls and caveats.* Haematologica, 2009. **94**(1): p. 29–37.

INDEX

Page numbers in *italics* and **bold** refer to figures and tables, respectively.